Sport and Exercise Psychology

Julia Schüler • Mirko Wegner • Henning Plessner
Robert C. Eklund
Editors

Sport and Exercise Psychology

Theory and Application

Springer

Editors
Julia Schüler
University of Konstanz
Constance, Germany

Mirko Wegner
University of Hamburg
Hamburg, Germany

Henning Plessner
Ruprecht-Karls-University of Heidelberg
Heidelberg, Germany

Robert C. Eklund
Florida State University
Tallahassee, FL, USA

ISBN 978-3-031-03923-2 ISBN 978-3-031-03921-8 (eBook)
https://doi.org/10.1007/978-3-031-03921-8

This Springer imprint is published by the registered company Springer Nature Switzerland AG
The registered company address is: Gewerbestrasse 11, 6330 Cham, Switzerland

Preface

Dear Readers,

Sport and various other related forms of fitness and recreational engagement in physical activity have fascinated people in many ways since time immemorial. These engagements can be a splendid way to express excellence in motoric performance (e.g., at the Olympic Games), to experience or exhibit the sensuousness of bodily movement (e.g., dancing), and/or to interact with other people (e.g., as part of a running club). Regular physical activity is also indispensable for physical and mental health. These engagements can be identity-forming (e.g., being a fan or member of a soccer club) or simply "just" leisure activity.

Sport and Exercise Psychology is a scientific discipline that aims to describe, explain, predict, and ultimately—if it seems reasonable—to change human experience and behavior in the context of physical activity. How can it be, for example, that we can observe people who simply do not want to have any involvement in physical activity at all, let alone on a regular basis, while others seem to be almost addicted to sport or exercise? How can sporting (non)behavior be predicted, and how might interventions be designed to lead to healthy, high-performance sporting activity? In this textbook, many such scientifically as well as socially relevant questions about various phenomena of sport and physical activity more broadly are posed and answered.

Needless to say, as teachers and researchers in the field of Sport and Exercise psychology, we are biased toward believing that it is one of the most interesting, challenging, and promising subjects. We are enthusiastic about sport and exercise psychology so please understand this bias as something that has animated our own interests in the field, as well as our interests as faculty to share our fascination with the subject as broadly as possible.

This textbook has been written for **students** of *Psychology* and *Sports and Exercise Science* as well as for **practitioners** who would like to understand topics in sport and exercise psychology in greater detail and depth. Students can use this book as a comprehensive and optimal preparation for their exam in Sport and Exercise Psychology. Readers might also want to use this book for deepening their understanding in individual research fields. This book is relevant for examination preparation and, at the same time, it is intended to provide valuable impulses for critical thinking and deeper contemplation.

This book is suitable for students and practitioners at different levels of expertise. Differentiating the *learning goals* and the *learning control questions* in the chapters into "*basic*" (undergraduate students, first years of bachelor program, rookies in sports practice), "*advanced*" (undergraduate students, second half of bachelor program, practitioners with little experience), and "*expert*" (graduate students, experienced practitioners) provides a useful framework to help students and their supervisors as well as practitioners to identify what is important for them and enables them to find the right level of learning (**"one-book-for-all principle"**).

Our search for an optimal format for this resource was grounded in the following imperatives: To write a high-quality textbook (**"brain candy"**) covering precisely selected content areas representative of the array of very different topics of interest in sport and exercise psychology that addresses the most important classical and current theories, research findings, and application fields. Questions about which theoretical models would be preferred, and which lines of research, which studies, which methodological novelties, and which current trends would be cited in the subject areas remained daunting. Our answer to these daunting but exemplary questions was to draw on "insiders" (i.e., people with high research and teaching expertise in very specific content areas). This basic idea motivated us to adopt the format of an edited book in which renowned topical experts served as authors for chapters in their content areas. This was already the basis for the first edition of the book in German. In the English-language edition of this book, we have purposefully formed **"tandem partnerships"** for each chapter consisting of authors from different countries or continents to ensure an international perspective on the teaching and research content. We found commonalities to predominate in the observation and scientific investigation of relevant phenomena of interest, but also some differences for which integrative solutions were provided within the chapters. An illustrative example is already evident in the title of this book. In Germany, the term "Sportpsychologie" includes both sport and exercise, but non-European understandings can be more differentiated with more explicit distinctions between sport and exercise being made. In addition, some chapters of the health section of this book deal with the promotion of physical activity in everyday life, which, although related, does not fall cleanly into the categories of sport or exercise. We elaborate upon these terms in the introductory chapter, however, to provide additional clarity. Nonetheless, in order to avoid over complicating matters, we have chosen to use "Sport and Exercise" in the title of our book and leave the authors to make the necessary conceptual distinctions in their chapters according to their own priorities.

The nature of an edited book also means that while each chapter is a necessary element for understanding Sport and Exercise psychology as a whole, it still needs to be self-contained on its own. The book can therefore be read well in its entirety (e.g., in preparation for an exam), and also be suitable for reviewing individual content areas, particularly due to the numerous cross-references within the book. If interested in delving deeper into a single topic, we recommend following the references provided by the authors in the book. Those references lead to related content, and link theory and practice.

In addition to the quality of the content, a textbook should of course also be appealing and invite reading **("eye candy").** The didactic elements such as *Learning Objectives*, *Definitions*, *Key Points*, *Study Boxes*, *Method Boxes*, *Self-Reflection*, *Side Stories*, *For Sports Practice*, *Learning Control Questions,* and other illustrations (*Figures, Tables*) make this textbook attractive but, above all, also support structuring the knowledge and processing it more actively (e.g., making personal references, recognizing application benefit, and promoting theoretical reflection).

Julia Schüler
Constance, Germany

Mirko Wegner
Hamburg, Germany

Henning Plessner
Heidelberg, Germany

Robert C. Eklund
Tallahassee, FL, USA

Acknowledgments

Completing a textbook such as this requires intrinsically motivated hard work done excellently by many people. It is to these people that we would like to express our gratitude. First and foremost, we thank the authors of the book chapters for their willingness to contribute their expertise to our textbook, for their participation in our internal peer review process, and for their constant desire to improve. We also offer many thanks for their always pleasant and courteous cooperation.

We also thank our student assistant, **Svea Gründel**, who took a critical student perspective and provided constructive feedback, and who also is responsible for numerous formal and coordinating tasks throughout the enterprise. **Madison Ehmann** has our thanks for her important contribution in ► Chap. 20.

Finally, we express our sincere gratitude for the continuous, kind, and competent support of our book project by **Sofia Geck**, **Rachel Daniel**, **Clement Wilson Kamalesh**, and **Lavanya Devgun** of Springer Nature Switzerland. Thank you.

We hope you enjoy reading this book and gain many new insights.

The Editors

Julia Schüler, Mirko Wegner, Henning Plessner, and Robert C. Eklund

Contents

Part IV Personality and Development

Part V Social Processes

Part VI Competitive Sport

Part VII Exercise and Health

Contributors

Mitja D. Back University of Münster, Münster, Germany

Adam Beavan TSG ResearchLab gGmbH, Zuzenhausen, Germany

Jürgen Beckmann Technical University of Munich, Munich, Germany

Denise Beckmann-Waldenmayer Peak Performance Academy, Holzkirchen, Germany

Alex Bertrams University of Bern, Bern, Switzerland

Kerstin Brinkmann University of Geneva, Geneva, Switzerland

Rouwen Cañal-Bruland Friedrich-Schiller Universität Jena, Jena, Germany

Flora Colledge University of Basel, Basel, Switzerland

Achim Conzelmann University of Bern, Bern, Switzerland

Joan L. Duda University of Birmingham, Birmingham, UK

David W. Eccles Florida State University, Tallahassee, FL, USA

Felix Ehrlenspiel Technical University of Munich, Munich, Germany

Robert C. Eklund Florida State University, Tallahassee, FL, USA

Anne-Marie Elbe University of Leipzig, Leipzig, Germany

Chris Englert University of Frankfurt, Frankfurt, Germany

Daniel Erlacher University of Bern, Bern, Switzerland

M. Blair Evans Western University Canada, London, ON, Canada

Mark Eys Wilfrid Laurier University, Waterloo, Canada

Philip Feichtinger Eberhard Karls University of Tübingen, Tübingen, Germany

Philip Furley German Sport University Cologne, Köln, Germany

Markus Gerber University of Basel, Basel, Switzerland

Katharina Geukes University of Münster, Münster, Germany

Iris Güldenpenning University of Paderborn, Paderborn, Germany

Kyra Hamilton Griffith University, Brisbane, Australia

Thomas Hannan Medical School Hamburg, Hamburg, Germany

Stephanie J. Hanrahan The University of Queensland, St. Lucia, QLD, Australia

Matthew P. Herring University of Limerick, Limerick, Ireland

Hans-Dieter Hermann Eberhard-Karls University Tübingen, Tübingen, Germany

Oliver Höner Eberhard Karls University of Tübingen, Tübingen, Germany

Ross Julian University of Münster, Muenster, Germany

Stefanie Klatt German Sport University Cologne, Cologne, Germany

Sarah Jakowski Ruhr-Universität Bochum, Bochum, Germany

Martin Kopp University of Innsbruck, Innsbruck, Austria

Daniel Krause University of Paderborn, Paderborn, Germany

Carina Kreitz German Sport University Cologne, Cologne, Germany

Ulrich Kühnen Jacobs University Bremen, Bremen, Germany

Dieter F. Kutz University of Münster, Muenster, Germany

Sylvain Laborde German Sport University Cologne, Cologne, Germany

Andrew Lane University of Wolverhampton, Wolverhampton, UK

Paul Larkin Victoria University, Melbourne, VIC, Australia

Andreas Lau Martin-Luther University Halle-Wittenberg, Halle, Germany

Thorsten Leber Eberhard Karls University of Tübingen, Tübingen, Germany

Jonna Löffler German Sport University Cologne, Cologne, Germany

Clare MacMahon La Trobe University, Melbourne, Australia

David Mann Vrije Universiteit Amsterdam, Amsterdam, The Netherlands

Jan Mayer Coaching Competence Cooperation, Schwetzingen, Germany

Daniel Memmert German Sport University Cologne, Cologne, Germany

Christopher Mesagno Victoria University, Melbourne, VIC, Australia

Edda van Meurs University of Münster, Münster, Germany

Martin Niedermeier University of Innsbruck, Innsbruck, Austria

Claudio R. Nigg University of Bern, Bern, Switzerland

Jeannine Ohlert German Sport University Cologne, Cologne, Germany

Ines Pfeffer Medical School Hamburg, Hamburg, Germany

Henning Plessner Heidelberg University, Heidelberg, Germany

Markus Raab German Sport University Cologne, Cologne, Germany

Ryan E. Rhodes University of Victoria, Victoria, Canada

Claudio Robazza University of Chieti and Pescara, Chieti, Italy

Catherine M. Sabiston University of Toronto, Toronto, ON, Canada

Mirko Schmidt University of Bern, Bern, Switzerland

Julia Schüler University of Konstanz, Constance, Germany

Geoffrey Schweizer Heidelberg University, Heidelberg, Germany

Hamsini Sivaramakrishnan University of Southern Denmark, Odense, Denmark

Kathrin Staufenbiel German Gymnastics Federation, Frankfurt, Germany

Bernd Strauss University of Münster, Münster, Germany

Kelley Strohacker University of Tennessee, Knoxville, TN, USA

Gorden Sudeck Eberhard Karls University Tübingen, Tübingen, Germany

Ian Taylor Loughborough University, Loughborough, UK

Ansgar Thiel Eberhard Karls University Tübingen, Tübingen, Germany

Cecilie Thøgersen-Ntoumani University of Southern Denmark, Odense, Denmark

Claudia Voelcker-Rehage University of Münster, Muenster, Germany

Manfred Wegner University of Kiel, Kiel, Germany

Mirko Wegner University of Hamburg, Hamburg, Germany

Matthias Weigelt University of Paderborn, Paderborn, Germany

Svenja Anna Wolf Florida State University, Tallahassee, FL, USA

Wanja Wolff University of Konstanz, Constance, Germany

Christian Zepp German Sport University Cologne, Cologne, Germany

Introduction: Sport and Exercise Psychology—Theory and Application

Julia Schüler, Mirko Wegner, Henning Plessner and Robert C. Eklund

Contents

J. Schüler et al. (eds.), *Sport and Exercise Psychology*, https://doi.org/10.1007/978-3-031-03921-8_1

Learning Objectives

Basic:
- You are able to define the term sport psychology and reproduce the subject matter in your own words.
- You know about the most important key points of the history of sport psychology.

Advanced:
- You are able to generate examples of sport psychological questions from the different perspectives of psychology (subdisciplines).
- You are able to explain in your own words why theory and practice of sport psychology are intertwined.

Experts:
- You are able to describe the systematization of sport psychology according to its mother disciplines. You understand why one and the same phenomenon can be viewed very differently depending on the scientific perspective taken.
- You know the function of professional societies and other forms of institutionalization of sport psychology.

1.1 World Athletes of the Year?

To get in the mood for this book, please take a look at the homepage of *the International Association of Athletics Federation* (► https://www.worldathletics.org/awards) and its listing of the world athletes of the year. Allow yourself a few minutes to drift a bit through the world of high-performance sports.

- Do you *see* (e.g., in the listing of world records in the long jump) how excellent performance can be translated into numbers and thus only becomes measurable and comparable?
- Do you *feel* inspired by the photos of winning poses and addressed by the usually very strong performance-related words (brilliant, unique, unbelievable, unprecedented, world record, series of successes, top performance)?
- Do you literally *hear* the cheering of the fans on the last meters of the 100 m sprint?
- Do you still *taste* the bitter defeat of your own sporting failure when you see emotional pictures of the losers?
- Or does high-performance sport *smell* too commercial to you and you prefer more recreational and health-oriented sports?

The fact that we can perceive and hopefully mostly enjoy sports with all of our senses, whether as active participants or as spectators, already suggests that sports are about more than the "activity of muscle groups." In this textbook, we aim to show that our involvements with sport implicate all psychological dimensions (cognition, emotion, motivation), our personality traits, the state of our physical development, and with all intertwined with our social environment.

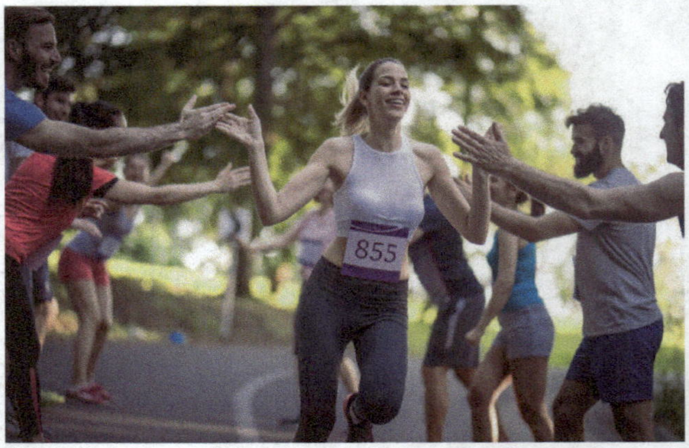

Fig. 1.1 Perceive the sport with all senses. (© skynesher/Getty Images/iStock)

This book is designed to pique your interest in wanting to understand the psychological aspects of sport in more detail. Most likely, you will never become an athlete or sportsperson of the year. Instead, use this book for a goal that is at least as important: use the knowledge gained to describe, explain, and predict sports-related behavior in a "better" way (better = scientifically sound) (Fig. 1.1).

1.2 Sport Psychology: Definition and Subject Area

1.2.1 Describing, Explaining, Predicting, and Changing

The goal of sport psychology is to describe, explain, predict, and ultimately change human experience and behavior in the context of sporting activity.

Describing Describing provides the foundation for everything (i.e., explaining, predicting, and changing). This is true in psychological science just as it is in the building industry. If the foundation is not stable, nothing built upon it will be stable either. To describe phenomena, psychological terms are used that do not necessarily differ greatly from those used in everyday language. For example, a lay person might describe "self-control" (or "team cohesion") more as "willpower" (or "good team chemistry"), although probably be a bit more lenient with what might be included in each instance. Assignment of technical terms, however, requires a thorough analysis and classification of facts in a clear and consistent manner. In the best case, this leads to clear definitions that serve to simplify further scientific processes. For example, team cohesion is more formally defined as the effort of a group to stay united, to stick together to achieve common goals, and to ensure the satisfaction of all group members (Carron et al., 1998, p. 213).

Explaining The next task is to explain the phenomena described. Why, for example, do teams differ in their cohesiveness? Which factors favor cohesion and which undermine cohesiveness? To answer these questions, sport psychology uses theories from which phenomena can be inferred. The logic of research (a book title by the science theorist Karl Popper, 1902–1994) consists of formulating general laws (e.g., about cause-effect relationships) without contradiction, followed by attempts to disprove those formulated laws. This principle of *falsification* leads to holding on to explanations only until a falsification attempt is successful (Popper, 1935).

Predicting Hypotheses such as "Team building activities increase team cohesion" and "High team cohesion leads to better team performance" are, in themselves, predictions. Most of the time, these coincide with explanatory models. Hypotheses need to be tested, and the results are used to infer whether or not the assumptions are true under the very specific circumstances of data collection (e.g., age of study participants, type of sport), with probabilities of error specified.

Changing Knowledge about cause-effect relationships (e.g., that team cohesion and team performance are causally related) allows for the derivation of interventions for change. Complex intervention strategies aimed, for example, at increasing motivation to participate in sports among elementary school children are often based on a combination of several theories (e.g., theories of self-control, group cohesion).

1.2.2 Central Definitions

We have introduced the idea that clear definitions are the most important prerequisite for the scientific process. Unfortunately, the practice of theory building turns out to be more difficult than the simple principle mentioned above. There are numerous definitions of sport psychology, which are shaped by different theoretical perspectives or understandings of science. In the present textbook, we consider the following, relatively broadly accepted definitions, to be appropriate.

Sport Psychology

The American Psychological Association (APA, 2008, ► https://www.apa.org/ed/graduate/specialize/sports) defines sport psychology as follows:

"**Sport psychology** is a proficiency that uses psychological knowledge and skills to address optimal performance and well-being of athletes, developmental and social aspects of sports participation, and systemic issues associated with sports settings and organizations." This is a definition that is perhaps especially linked to sports as competitive rule-governed physical activities (Eklund & Tenenbaum, 2014). A brief characterization of the content and methods of sport psychology can also be found on the pages of the American Psychological Association. (APA, 2008, ► https://www.apa.org/ed/graduate/specialize/sports).

A common European definition of sport psychology, which is more scientifically oriented is the following:

"**Sport psychology** is an empirical science that investigates the conditions, processes, and consequences of the psychological regulation of sporting actions and derives possibilities for influencing them" (Nitsch, 1978, p.6).

These definitions already show that sport psychology is both a basic and application-oriented scientific discipline. It aims to apply its theoretical findings in practice.

Sport psychology is to be distinguished from exercise psychology. Whereas "sport" is competitive and often achievement goal-oriented, "exercise" is planned, structured, often repetitive, and purposefully intended to maintain or improve physical fitness.

Exercise Psychology

"Exercise psychology…tends to be focused on psychological factors implicated in participation in regimented programs of physical activity to improve or maintain health-related physical fitness" (Eklund & Crocker, 2018, p.4).

There are other types of physical activity too (e.g., recreation activity, active transportation, chores, active playing of children) which are not necessarily competitive in orientation nor inherently intended to increase physical fitness. An umbrella term covering human movement is "physical activity."

"Physical activity includes all movements produced by skeletal muscles that result in the expenditure of energy" (USDHHS, 1996).

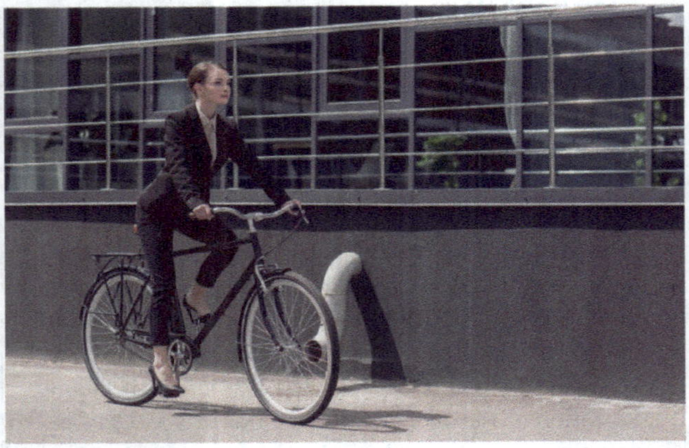

Fig. 1.2 "Physical activity" also includes everyday activities such as riding a bike to work. (© LightFieldStudios/Getty Images/iStock)

Physical activity is an umbrella term including sport and exercise but also other everyday physical activities such as recreational activities, riding a bike to work, taking stairs, gardening, or taking the stairs (Fig. 1.2).

1.3 Subdisciplines of Sport Psychology and Their Research Questions

Probably the roughest division of sport psychology is into its **theoretical foundations**, presented in the first part of this book, and its **fields of application**, elaborated in the second part of this book. However, this necessary systematization is an oversimplification, because it cannot express the close interweaving of theory, empiricism, and practical application. Our recommendation for this textbook is, therefore, to combine theory and practice. Better understanding of the practical application aspects in the second part of the book if they are built upon the corresponding theoretical foundation is provided in the first part of the book. Conversely, a deeper understanding of theories and models often occurs when they become tangible through practice.

1.3.1 Differentiation According to Theoretical Perspectives

Subdisciplines of the parent discipline of psychology serve as the organizing principle of the **theoretical foundations of sport psychology**.

Psychology is divided into subdisciplines. These include:
- Cognitive psychology
- Motivational psychology
- Psychology of emotions
- Psychology of individual differences/personality
- Developmental psychology
- Social psychology

The subdisciplines differ in the perspective from which phenomena in sport are viewed. Cognitive, motivational, emotion, personality, developmental, and social psychologists, for example, already differ in the questions they ask themselves when observing phenomena in sport (see Side Story).

Side Story

Choking Under Pressure: The View from Different Perspectives

Choking under pressure is one phenomenon that can be used to illustrate the differences in the perspectives of the psychological subdisciplines. Choking under pressure is said to occur when people are not able to call up their very good training performance in competition (i.e., precisely when it matters). What questions would the representatives of the various disciplines think of first?

- **Cognitive Psychology**: The focus of cognitive psychology is on information processing processes.

  Is information processed more poorly in the competitive situation? For example, can necessary knowledge content not be retrieved? How is the situation perceived and evaluated?
- **Motivation Psychology**: The focus of motivational psychology is on analyzing the goal-directedness of behavior.

  Does avoidance motivation (just don't fail!) throw a spanner in the works of the real-world championship? Or do unrealistic goals inhibit performance in competition (goals that are too easy or too difficult)?
- **Psychology of Emotions**: The focus of psychology of emotions is on the origin and effect of emotions and emotion regulation.

  Are emotions, for example, competitive anxiety, the cause of the choking under pressure phenomenon?
- **Psychology of Individual Differences/Personality**: The focus of the psychology of individual differences/personality is upon stable characteristics of a person and differences between persons.

  What personality traits characterize chokers, and what distinguishes them from athletes who succeed in delivering their (best) performance in competition?
- **Developmental Psychology**: The focus of developmental psychology is on the observation of developmental and change processes over the life span.

  Are there age groups in which social comparison processes are particularly relevant and identity-forming? Is choking under pressure age-related?
- **Social Psychology**: The focus of social psychology is on the person in his interaction with the social environment.

  Under what circumstances does the presence of other people (competitors/spectators) lead to performance losses and when does it contribute to performance enhancement?

The aforementioned subdisciplines in turn branch out into different, sometimes quite heterogeneous, subject areas. To illustrate these topics, the subchapters in this textbook are briefly listed below.

Cognitive psychology deals with information processing, more specifically with states and processes that are located between the reception of stimuli to experience and behavior. In this textbook, the central cognitive processes of *perception and attention* (▶ Chap. 2), *learning and memory* (▶ Chap. 3), and *judgment and decision-making* (▶ Chap. 5) are detailed. In addition, the chapters on *neurocognition* (interface of neurobiology and cognitive psychology) and *movement* (▶ Chap. 4) and *embodied cognition* (interplay of body and cognition) (▶ Chap. 6) provide space for topics that have developed rapidly in sport psychology research in recent years.

Motivational psychology asks about the motivations for behavior. More specifically, it deals with goal-directed behavior, its direction, intensity, and persistence. The chapters describe *motivation and goals* (▶ Chap. 7) and distinguish between *intrinsic and extrinsic motivation* (▶ Chap. 8). While these content areas are assigned to general psychology, that is, they attempt to explain and predict general regularities, the chapter *Implicit Motives* (▶ Chap. 9) is based on a differential psychological view by focusing on interindividual differences. The chapter *Volition* (▶ Chap. 10) emphasizes that sport often also requires self-control and further volitional processes.

Psychology of emotions is concerned with the description, explanation, and prediction and change of emotions, feelings, affects, and moods. Two chapters deal with the *basics of emotions* (▶ Chap. 11) and the *emotion anxiety* (▶ Chap. 12), which is highly relevant to sport.

The subject *area of personality psychology* focuses on differences between individuals with respect to various psychological functions and abilities. *Developmental psychology* deals with changes in human experience and behavior over the life span. In ▶ Chap. 13, *Person, Situation and Person-Situation-Interaction in Sport*, it is considered that neither persons, with their characteristics and abilities, nor characteristics of the environment determine human behavior and experience on their own but that person and situation are in a complex interrelationship with each other. In ▶ Chap. 14, it is shown that certain personality traits (e.g., self-concept) can be formed or changed in the context of sport. ▶ Chapter 15, *Physical Activity over the Life Span*, concludes this section by explaining whether, how, and why sporting behavior changes from childhood to adulthood.

Under the main heading *Social Processes*, we find theories and models that originate predominantly from social psychology. Their subject area is the analysis of experience and behavior in social contexts. Typical and well-studied contexts include the examination of *group performance* (▶ Chap. 16), *social influences by spectators* (▶ Chap. 17), and *interaction and communication* (▶ Chap. 18). ▶ Chapter 19, *The Self in Sport* captures concepts around "the self," which is never formed in isolation from, but closely interwoven with, the social context. The chapter covers self-esteem, self-concepts, and self-conscious emotions and ends with a cultural perspective on the self.

Our explanations may give the impression that research questions can always be clearly and unambiguously assigned to subdisciplines and subject areas. Of course, just as often the boundaries are fluid, so the questions and phenomena overlap subdisciplines. Questions such as "How can physical activity be promoted in childhood and adolescence?" are cross-cutting questions to which representatives of several subdisciplines can make significant contributions. Researchers therefore consider, at best, explanatory constructs from different disciplines and their interaction, knowing full well that the categorization categories of cognition, motivation, emotion, personality, development, and social processes are also "only" hypothetical constructs. These categories are attempts at systematization with the aim of simplifying complex states and processes.

Side Story

Where Do the Questions of the Subdisciplines of Sport Psychology Actually Come from?

Some of the questions come from research itself. Research provides answers but also generates questions. Expected and unexpected study results are the basic building blocks for optimized future research questions, research methods, hypothesis formulations, and testing.

The advancement of sport psychology research methods offers new opportunities. Questions cannot be addressed until the measurement tools are available to answer them. For example, the theoretical focus expands because of new ways of measuring (e.g., capturing self-control processes through imaging techniques) with the development of a good questionnaire or other types of measures suddenly making the capture of data for a variable very easy, proven study paradigms subsequently spread, while data processing programs become accessible and more user-friendly.

On the other hand, the questions naturally arise from practical problems in the fields of application of sport psychology and often concern higher-level socially relevant issues. Examples include how can we counteract a physically inactive lifestyle and its associated health-damaging consequences? Which psychological performance requirements do our top athletes have to master at the Olympic Games and how do we train them?

1.3.2 Differentiation According to Fields of Application

In addition to differentiating sport psychology according to theoretical perspectives, it is of course also possible to differentiate according to different fields of application of sport psychology. The application of sport psychology, in order not to be arbitrary and amateurish, must be based on empirically tested psychological theories. Thus, good sport psychology practice asks and answers its questions based on research perspectives of the psychological subtheories outlined above (see also self-reflection). Thus, the application fields "sport and performance" and "sport and health" discussed in this book cannot actually be separated from the theoretical foundations. ◘ Table 1.1 is intended to clarify this fact.

In *sport and performance*, we describe how processes of *self-regulation* (▶ Chap. 20) and *cognitive training* (▶ Chap. 21) can look and succeed in competitive sports. *Group dynamics and team building* (▶ Chap. 22) are highly relevant for team sports, for example. *Talent selection and talent development* (▶ Chap. 23), and *Recovery, Sleep, and Performance* (▶ Chap. 24) are further central topics in competitive sports.

In *sport and health*, we look at the interaction of sport and various facets of mental and physical health. ▶ Chapter 25 gives and overview over models that explain health behavior change in the area of sport and physical activity. ▶ Chapter 26 is about *well-being and mental health*, ▶ Chap. 27 addresses *stress and physical health*, and ▶ Chap. 28 explores *sport in the context of illness and injury*.

Most of the chapters in this textbook also allow for strong application to the *school context*. The actions of teachers include, for example, questions about how to motivate students (motivation), how to help them deal with anger, disappointment, and fear in physical education (emotions), or how to create a positive classroom climate (social processes). The authors of this textbook therefore repeatedly draw on examples from physical education classes. In addition, the readers of this textbook with school reference are of course invited to think of their own examples of application in school.

◘ **Table 1.1** Fields of application and theoretical foundations

	Fields of application	
	Sport and performance	**Sport, exercise, and health**
Cognition	How can refereeing decisions be improved? See ▶ Chap. 2 (Perception and Attention), ▶ Chap. 5 (Judgment and Decision-Making)	How can mental training help you participate in a health exercise class on a sustained basis? See ▶ Chap. 20 (Self-regulation, e.g., mental training)
Motivation	Is a strong achievement motive the secret of success? See ▶ Chap. 7 (Motivation and Goals), ▶ Chap. 9 (Implicit Motives)	How can motivation to exercise be facilitated among "couch potatoes"? See ▶ Chap. 8 (Intrinsic Motivation), ▶ Chap. 15 (Physical Activity Across the Life Span), ▶ Chap. 25 (Health Behavior Models)
Emotion	Which emotions are conducive to peak performance and which are a hindrance? See ▶ Chap. 11 (Emotions), ▶ Chap. 12 (Anxiety in Sports)	Do positive emotions contribute to the maintenance of sport participation? Can sport improve positive emotions and well-being? See ▶ Chap. 11 (Emotions), ▶ Chap. 25 (Health Behavior Models), ▶ Chap. 26 (Sport, Well-being, and Mental Health)
Personality	Are top athletes characterized by special personality traits? See ▶ Chap. 13 (Person, Situation, and Person-Situation Interaction), ▶ Chap. 14 (Personality Development Through Sport), ▶ Chap. 23 (Talent Selection and Development)	Does sports improve students' self-concepts? See ▶ Chap. 13 (Person, Situation, and Person-Situation Interaction), ▶ Chap. 14 (Personality Development Through Sport), ▶ Chap. 23 (Talent Selection and Development)
Development	What factors are important for talent selection and development? See ▶ Chap. 23 (Talent Selection and Development)	Are sport and physical activity behaviors in childhood predictive of sport and activity engagement in adulthood? See ▶ Chap. 14 (Personality Development Through Sport), ▶ Chap. 15 (Physical Activity Across the Life Span)
Social Processes	What kind of team climate leads to peak performance? See ▶ Chap. 16 (Group Performance), ▶ Chap. 18 (Interaction and Communication)	Does social support contribute to healthy exercise behavior? See ▶ Chap. 16 (Group Performance), ▶ Chap. 27 (Sport, stress, and Health)

What's the Hype About "Theory"?

You may have really had enough of theory now already and want to finally get into practice!? You may even believe that practical experiences are much more important for the explanation and treatment of problems—after all, it is easy to believe that theory often cannot be put into practice. We, however, would like to convince you of another point of view.

Kurt Lewin (lived from 1890 to 1947), one of the impressive pioneers of psychology, founder of experimental social psychology, and Gestalt psychologist, recognized and emphatically asserted the lack of mutual consideration of theory and practice to be a serious problem. In his 1951 paper *Problems of Research in Social Psychology*, he states "Many psychologists working today in an applied field are keenly aware of the need for close cooperation between theoretical and applied psychology. This can be accomplished in psychology, as it has been accomplished in physics, if the theorist does not look toward applied problems with highbrow aversion or with fear of social problems, and if the applied psychologist realizes that there is nothing so practical as a good theory" (Lewin, 1951, p. 169). From this source comes his famous quote, "Nothing is more practical than a good theory."

Please answer for yourself: Why is professional sport psychological counseling (e.g., of top athletes or personal coaches in the health sector) based on theory and validated empirical findings? Why do we need "theory"? You might come back to these questions after having read some of the book chapters.

Lewin's statement, on the other hand, also reproaches the theorists who, with intellectual arrogance or fear, ignore problems in practice because it is also just as true—rephrasing Lewin's quote—that nothing is more "theoretical" than practice. Many years of experience and observations in practice are condensed empiricism that could be expressed in regularities. Think of best practice examples from industry (i.e., methods or procedures that have proven themselves in practice and have prevailed over others as a kind of "de facto standard"). The "data" are already available, so to speak, only in an unorganized and undocumented form. Formalizing some best practices could lead to profitable hypotheses that, after further empirical support, could lead to theories.

Look for examples of why theory and practice make a good pair. Why one can't do without the other, even if they often argue?

1.4 A Selective History of Sport Psychology

The historic picture on the development of the field of sport psychology provided here is selective. For a more complete picture, the authors ask the interested reader to refer to Gill and Reifsteck (2014), Kornspan (2012), Landers (1995), Seiler and Wylleman (2009), or Wiggins (1984).

The dynamics and speed of development of a young scientific discipline such as sport psychology (beginning around the end of the nineteenth century) is influenced by a highly complex context consisting of, among other things, societal values (e.g., value of sport) and problems (e.g., physical activity as a method to prevent childhood obesity), economic circumstances (e.g., financial support of sport), innovations in related scientific disciplines (e.g., contribution of basic psychological disciplines; neuroscience), and technical developments (e.g., higher reliability of existing measurement instruments and addition of new valid instruments). The interactions are complex, and the individual contributions are unlikely to be resolved neatly.

We, therefore, review the history of sport psychology rather selectively to highlight particular milestones. For those interested in a more detailed history of development, please refer to the more comprehensive descriptions provided by Bäumler (2009) and Kornspan (2009).

As far as is known, the specific **term** "sport psychology" was first used by **Pierre de Coubertin** (lived from 1863 to 1937) at the turn of the last century (de Coubertin, 1900). Coubertin, inspired by the Olympic Games of antiquity, was instrumental in initiating the Olympic Games of modern times as the founder the International Olympic Committee in 1894. He probably recognized that psychological factors play a decisive role in physical performance in the sense of "Citius, altius, fortius" (motto of the Olympic Games; Latin for *faster, higher, stronger*).

The beginning of *European sport psychological research* stemmed from a strong interest in sport psychological topics by students of **Wilhelm Wundt** (lived from 1832 to 1920), who founded the first Experimental Institute of Psychology at the University of Leipzig in 1879. His student **Edward Wheeler Scripture** (lived from 1864 to 1945), for example, published laboratory experimental studies (e.g., Scripture, 1894) on the question of whether fencers differed from other groups of people in their reaction times ("mental quickness") and movement times (speed of execution of movements). **Norman Triplett** (lived from 1861 to 1931) conducted another of the first published experiments from the birth of experimental psychology which dealt with the question whether, and under which circumstances, the presence of others improves athletic performance (see method box).

The Competition Machine

Norman Triplett gained the inspiration for his series of studies from an analysis of official records of ride times in the 1897 cycling season, which he published in his 1898 article "The dynamogenic factors in pacemaking and competition" in the *American Journal of Psychology*. Triplett noticed that ride times were usually better when the race was run with competitors than when the cyclists competed only against the clock. Triplett tested this observation in an experiment: the core results of which were supported in data obtained using his "Competition Machine" which allowed for accurate recording of performance in a laboratory setting when two people were racing against each other or alone (◘ Fig. 1.3).

Triplett explains the function of the Competition Machine as follows:

"The apparatus for this study consisted of two fishing reels whose cranks turned in circles of one and three-fourths inches diameter. These were arranged on a Y shaped frame work clamped to the top of a heavy table, as shown in the cut. The sides of this frame work were spread sufficiently far apart to permit of two persons turning side by side. Bands of twisted silk cord ran over the well lacquered axes of the reels and were supported at C and D, two meters distant, by two small pulleys. The records were taken from the course A D. The other course B C being used merely for pacing or competition purposes. The wheel on the side from which the records were taken communicated the movement made to a recorder, the stylus of which traced a curve on the drum of a kymograph. The direction of this curve corresponded to the rate of turning, as the greater the speed the shorter and straighter the resulting line." (Triplett, 1898, p. 518)

Triplett's study was more complex than outlined here (e.g., he additionally investigated cycling performance with and without pacesetters), but, as a rough core statement, he concluded that the presence of other people increased performance in a motor task. This phenomenon has led to numerous social psychological studies under the term *social facilitation*.

In Germany, Carl Diem, influenced by Wundt especially through his students Hugo Münsterberg and Robert Werner Schulte, established and directed the first sport psychology laboratory at the newly founded German University of Physical Education in Berlin in 1920 where he served as a sport psychology lecturer in psychology and education. This marked the beginning of the institutionalization of sport psychology in Germany.

The founding of the first American research institute for competitive sport (Athletic Research Laboratory, University of Illinois, Chicago Urbana) in 1925 is considered to be one of the first major milestones in *American sport psychological research*. This founding by Coleman R. Griffith (lived from 1893 to 1966) is typically considered to be "the birth" of American sport psychology. Shortly thereafter, Griffith published *Psychology of Coaching* (Griffith, 1926) and *Psychology of Athletics: A General Survey for Athletes and Coaches* (Griffith, 1928), in which he sought to scientifically explain his experiences with professional sport teams and to apply scientific findings to practice. Griffith worked for the Chicago CUBS (Chicago Cubs Baseball Club) beginning in 1938 but met some resistance with his psychological approach to sport performance (see Green, 2003).

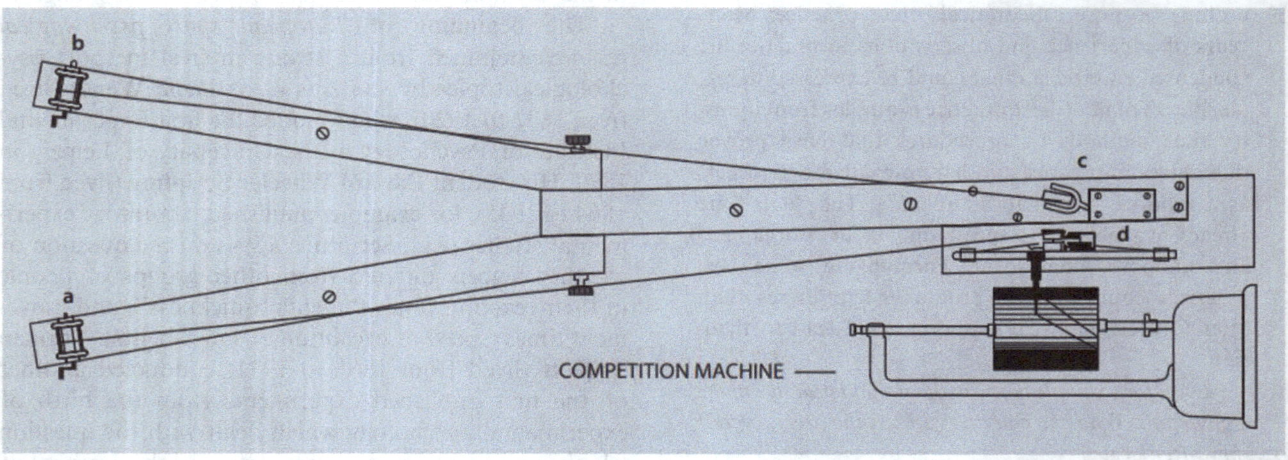

◘ **Fig. 1.3** Triplett's Competition Machine (adapted from Triplett, 1898, p. 519). The meaning of a, b, c, d is explained in the text

The value Griffith placed on psychological processes for peak athletic performance and their social consequences is expressed in the following quote.

> » "The more mind is made use of in athletic competition, the greater will be the skill of our athletes, the finer will be the contest, the higher will be the ideals of sportsmanship displayed, the longer will our games persist in our national life, and the more truly will they lead to those rich personal and social products which we ought to expect of them." (C. R. Griffith, 1925, p.193)

The first World Congress of Sport Psychology took place in Rome, Italy, in 1965. At that time, proximity enabled networking among sport psychologists from different European countries. At the congress, the International Society of Sport Psychology (ISSP) was founded. Three years later, in 1968, the European Federation of Sport Psychology (FEPSAC) was established. In 1970, the first sport psychology journal was published under the name "International Journal of Sport Psychology." "The Journal of Sport Psychology" of the North American Society for Psychology of Sport and Physical Activity (NASPSPA) which later became the influential "Journal of Sport and Exercise Psychology" was the second sport psychology journal first issued in 1979.

In his Senior Lecture at the annual meeting of the German Society of Sport Psychology, Roland Seiler (2018), former FEPSAC President, summarized the development of the number of publications in sport psychology journals since the 1970s (◘ Fig. 1.4a). Seiler also showed that predominantly English-speaking nations have been very active in publishing in sport psychology journals and to a much lesser extent European countries (◘ Fig. 1.4b).

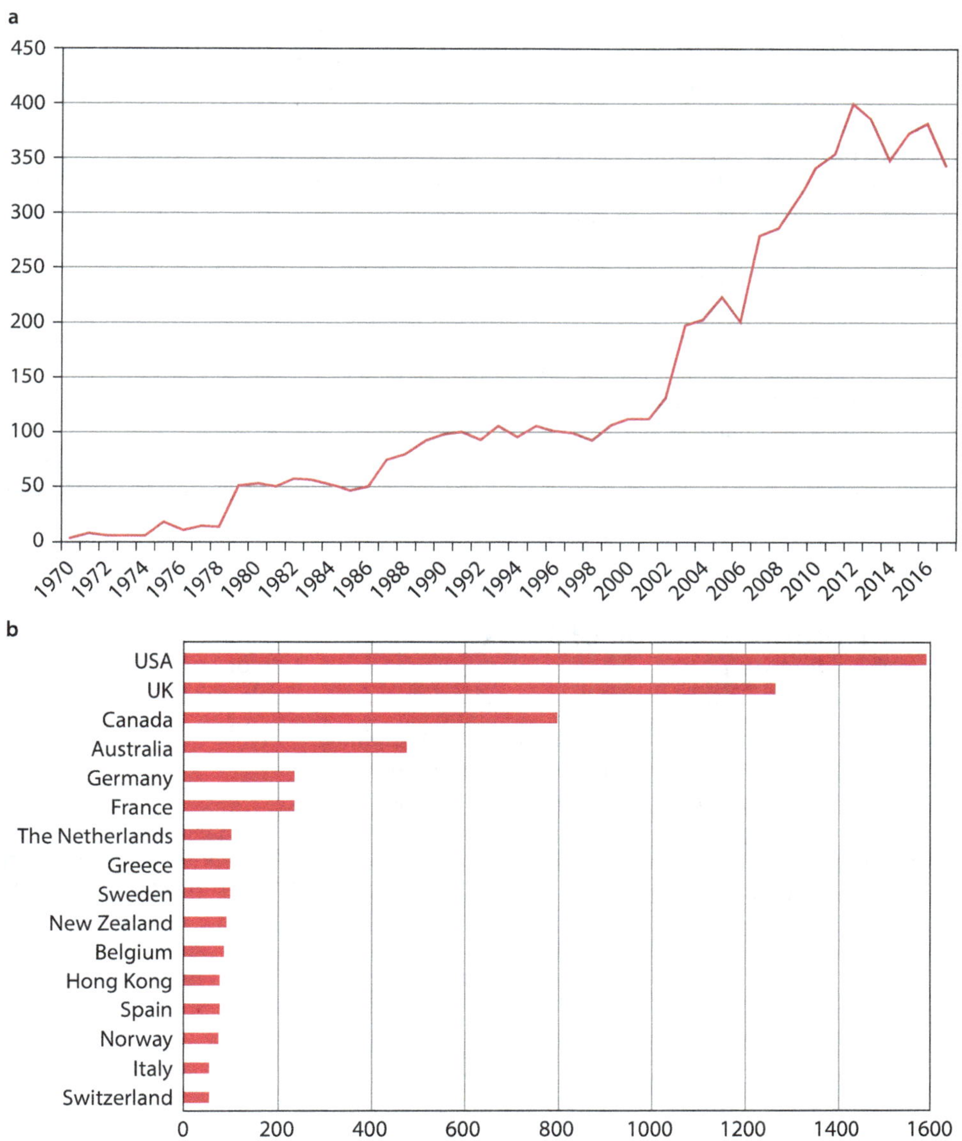

◘ **Fig. 1.4** **a** International development of number of publications in sport psychology journals (data base PsycInfo: Journal word [sport] and [psychology], date of retrieval: May, 4, 2021) and **b** contributions in sport psychology journals from authors from different countries (scrtitle [sport] and [psychology] and doctype [ar], date of retrieval: May, 4, 2021) (Seiler, 2018)

Side Story

Sport Psychology: An international Fascination

Dorothee Alfermann, long-time professor of sport psychology at the University of Leipzig, is considered an experienced international expert and European shaper of the scientific discipline of sport psychology. At the 2016 annual meeting of the *Arbeitsgemeinschaft für Sportpsychologie* (asp, German Society for Sport Psychology) in Münster around the time of her retirement as a university lecturer, Professor Alfermann looked back on the development of sport psychology in an honorary lecture entitled *Fascinating Sport Psychology: On the Identity of a Scientific Discipline in an International Context*. She highlighted the increasingly accelerated internationalization of sport psychology over the two preceding decades with, among others, particular reference to the following four indicators. (The explanations provided are as interpreted by the editors).

1. Common Language of Science

   Explanation: Publishing in a common language (English) enables the exchange and dissemination of research findings and methods which invites critical discussions and further developments across countries.

2. Impact Factor (IF)

   Explanation: Internationalization has been influenced by the great importance that the scientific community attaches to a journal's impact factor. The journal impact factor is an indicator of how often articles published in a journal in a given year are cited, on average, by other scientific articles in the 2 subsequent years. Although strongly criticized, it is often used as an index of research performance. Publishing in one's native language, if not English, can present challenges with the IF metric. Non-English language journals often have low IFs simply because of the limitations imposed by numbers of people who can read the implicated language. This serves as a disincentive to publish in non-English language journals but also as an incentive to publish in English—even sometimes as a necessity for progress in one's academic career.

3. Internationally Composed Working Groups

   Explanation: This trend of mixed research teams is not specific to sport psychology but instead is found across most scientific disciplines. An analysis of 19.9 million journal articles over five decades also showed that teams are more successful at generating knowledge, as measured by the frequency of citations of their papers and journal impact factor, than single authors (Wuchty et al., 2007). This may be due, among other things, to the international composition of the working groups and the resulting higher expertise or networking.

4. English Language International Study Programs

   Explanation: The number of international degree programs in sport psychology and sport science has been increasing. This allows students from other countries to be admitted and promotes heterogeneity of exposure in teaching and research. In addition, international degree programs facilitate later professional establishment in research (e.g., PhD) and practice (diagnostics and interventions in rehabilitation, coaching) even across national borders.

1.5 Institutionalization of Sport Psychology

One indicator of how well established a scientific discipline is can be seen in the extent of its institutionalization. So where does sport psychology find a roof of some kind over its head? One example is the association of those working in sport psychology in umbrella organizations and professional societies that represent their interests in science and application. Their tasks include, for example, the organization of conferences, the quality assurance of training curricula, the formulation of ethical guidelines, the promotion of young professionals, the provision of information portals, and public relations. There are very many organizations around the world with different focuses. ◘ Table 1.2 provides examples of some of the longer-standing influential societies of scientific sport psychology in the Africa, Asia, Australia, Europe, and North America.

Table 1.2 Examples of longer-standing influential societies of scientific sport psychology in Africa, Asia, Australia, Europe, North America, and worldwide

	Association	URL
Africa	South African Society of Sport and Exercise Psychology	► sassep.co.za
Asia	Asian-South Pacific Association of Sport Psychology (ASPASP)	► aspasp.org
Australia	Australian Psychological Society—Board of Sport Psychologist	► psychology.org.au
Europe	European Federation of Sport Psychology (FEPSAC)	► fepsac.com
North America	North American Society of Psychology of Sport and Physical Activity (NASPSPA)	► naspspa.com
World-wide	International Society of Sport Psychology (ISSP)	► issponline.org

Learning Control Questions

Basic:

1. What is the aim of sport psychology?
2. Define "sport psychology" and explain its basic and applied components.
3. Give a definition for the term "physical activity." Can you give examples of its sub-facets?
4. What is the meaning of Kurt Lewin's statement that nothing is more practical than a good theory?

Advanced:

5. What does it mean that sport psychology *describes*, *explains*, *predicts*, and ultimately *changes* human experience and behavior in the context of sport and exercise?
6. Which are the subdisciplines of psychology and from which perspectives do they look at phenomena of sport and exercise?
7. Can you trace the history of sport psychology and important names associated with it?
8. What is meant by the "institutionalization" of a scientific discipline? Please give examples of scientific associations of sport psychology

Experts:

9. What reasons can you think of that the transfer from theory to practice and vice versa can be difficult?
10. When you look at the phenomenon of anxiety in physical education classes. How would different subdisciplines of psychology address the phenomenon?
11. Do some research on the homepages of the professional societies. Where do you see similarities and where differences?

References

Bäumler, G. (2009). The dawn of sport psychology in Europe, 1880–1930. In C. D. Green & L. T. Benjamin (Eds.), *Psychology gets in the game: Sport, mind, and behavior, 1880–1960* (pp. 20–77). University of Nebraska Press.

Carron, A. V., Brawley, L. R., & Widmeyer, W. N. (1998). The measurement of cohesiveness in sport groups. In J. L. Duda (Ed.), *Advances in sport and exercise psychology measurement* (pp. 213–226). Fitness Information Technology.

de Coubertin, P. (1900). Psychologie du sport. *Revue des Deux Mondes, 160*(4), 167–179.

Eklund, R. C., & Crocker, P. R. E. (2018). The nature of sport, exercise and physical activity psychology. In T. S. Horn & A. L. Smith (Eds.), *Advances in sport psychology* (4th ed., pp. 3–16). Human Kinetics.

Eklund, R. C., & Tenenbaum, G. (Eds.). (2014). *Encyclopedia of sport and exercise psychology*. Sage.

Gill, D. L., & Reifsteck, E. J. (2014). History of exercise psychology. In R. C. Eklund & G. Tenenbaum (Eds.), *Encyclopedia of sport and exercise psychology* (pp. 340–345). Sage.

Green, C. D. (2003). Psychology strikes out: Coleman r. Griffith and the chicago cubs. *History of Psychology, 6*(3), 267–283.

Griffith, C. R. (1925). Psychology and its relation to athletic competition. *American Physical Education Review, 30*, 193–199.

Griffith, C. R. (1926). *The psychology of coaching: A study of coaching methods from the point of psychology*. Scribner's.

Griffith, C. R. (1928). *Psychology and athletics: A general survey for athletes and coaches*. Scribner's.

Kornspan, A. S. (2009). *Fundamentals of sport and exercise psychology*. Human Kinetic.

Kornspan, A. S. (2012). History of sport and performance psychology. In S. M. Murphy (Ed.), *The Oxford handbook of sport and performance psychology*. Oxford University Press.

Landers, D. M. (1995). Sport psychology: The formative years, 1950–80. *The Sport Psychologist, 9*, 406–419.

Lewin, K. (1951). Problems of research in social psychology. In D. Cartwright (Ed.), *Field theory in social science: Selected theoretical papers*. Harper & Row.

Nitsch, J. R. (1978). Zur Lage der Sportpsychologie [State of sport psychology]. In J. R. Nitsch & H. Allmer (Hrsg.), *Sportpsychologie—Eine Standortbestimmung* (S. 1–11). Köln: bps.

Popper, K. (1935). *Logik der Forschung: Zur Erkenntnistheorie der modernen Naturwissenschaft [Logic of research: On the epistemology of modern natural science]*. Verlag Julius Springer.

Scripture, E. W. (1894). Tests of mental ability as exhibited in fencing. *Studies from the Yale Psychological Laboratory, 2*, 122–124.

Seiler, R. (2018). *50 Jahre Sportpsychologie: Von Wegen und Umwegen (50 Years of sport psychology: Of paths and detours)*. Senior Lecture at the 50th Annual Meeting of the German Society for Sport Psychology, May 10th, 2018, in Cologne.

Seiler, R., & Wylleman, P. (2009). FEPSAC's role and position in the past and in the future of sport psychology in Europe. *Psychology of Sport and Exercise, 10*, 403–409.

Triplett, N. (1898). The dynamogenic factors in pacemaking and competition. *The American Journal of Psychology, 9*(4), 507–533.

U. S. Department of Health and Human Services (USDHHS). (1996). *Physical activity and health: A report of the surgeon general*. USDHHS.

Wiggins, D. K. (1984). The history of sport psychology in North America. In J. M. Silva & R. S. Weinberg (Eds.), *Psychological foundations of sport* (pp. 9–22). Human Kinetics.

Wuchty, S., Jones, J. F., & Uzzi, B. (2007). The increasing dominance of teams in production of knowledge. *Science, 316*, 1036–1039.

Cognition

Contents

Perception and Attention

Daniel Memmert, Stefanie Klatt, David Mann and Carina Kreitz

Contents

J. Schüler et al. (eds.), *Sport and Exercise Psychology*, https://doi.org/10.1007/978-3-031-03921-8_2

2

Learning Objectives

Basic:

- Being able to clearly describe perception and attention processes
- Understanding and differentiating different theoretical models of perception and attention
- Knowing in what ways perception and attention play a role in sports

Advanced:

- Knowing how to measure perception and attention
- Being able to describe how perception and attention can be systematically trained

Experts:

- Knowing about the "attention window" and selective attention
- Knowing about trainability of perception and attention in sports

2.1 Introduction

Our *perception* allows us to use sensory channels (visual, auditory, haptic, olfactory, gustatory) to gather and process information from our environment and body. This sensory information can then be used to adequately adapt our behavior to the perceived circumstances. Since our processing capacity is limited (Cohen et al., 2015; Mack & Rock, 1998), we cannot process and consciously represent all of the countless pieces of information that we are faced with every second, let alone every hour or even day. Chabris and Simons (2010, p. 38/39) illustrate this by writing:

> The structure of the human body does not allow us to fly, just as the structure of our mind does not allow us to consciously perceive everything around us.

Although it may seem to us as if we perceived the world around us in its entirety and in full detail, this is not actually the case (Eitam et al., 2015; Rensink, 2015).

Limitation of Perception

Our processing capacity is limited. Although it seems to us as if we perceive our environment in its entirety and detail, this is not the case.

We are therefore forced to choose the information relevant to us to perceive it selectively. This selection of perceptual contents is performed by our *attention*. The main task of attention is to select and amplify behaviorally relevant stimuli (see Eriksen & Hoffman, 1974; Schweizer et al., 2000). We sometimes intentionally control attention, for example, when we are purposefully looking for a friend in a cinema auditorium. At other times, particular stimuli are so salient that they attract our attention automatically, for example, when hearing loud noises or someone mentioning our name (Koivisto & Revonsuo, 2007; Theeuwes, 2010; Treisman & Gelade, 1980). The selection of perceptual contents implies that we suppress/attenuate some (internal/external) stimuli to work more effectively with other (internal/external) stimuli.

Perception

Perception is the subjective impression of our environment or body created by the processing of stimuli acquired through different sensory modalities. A distinction can be made between conscious and unconscious perception. However, the term usually refers to conscious verbalizable perception (unless specified otherwise).

Attention

Attention refers to the allocation of processing resources to and the amplification of the perception of particular places, objects, or points in time.

As illustrated by the definitions, perception and attention are, on the one hand, clearly separable processes. However, on the other hand, the two processes are also very closely linked. The deliberate or automatic allocation of attention leads to the targeted intensification of information collected by our sensory organs from our environment. This means that the neuronal processing of this sensory representation is *amplified* (Awh et al., 2006; Kiefer et al., 2011; Nobre, 2001; Posner & Driver, 1992). The processing of other information is *weakened* by deliberately averting attention away from information collected by our sensory organs from our environment (inhibition). Our perception is therefore the product of a combination of objective sensory input received through our sensory organs and our distribution of attention. This implies that perception always has a subjective component and that it is unlikely that two people perceive exactly the same thing, even if the sensory input is identical.

Subjective Perception

Subjective perception is a combination of objective input received by our sensory organs and the distribution of our attention.

Due to their central role for our experience, our behavior and our performance perception and attention have long been central objects of basic psychological investigation (e.g., Fechner, 1860; Posner, 1980; Styles, 2008). Perceptual and attentional performance also plays a major role in sports (Williams et al., 1999; Memmert, 2009), a domain in which a lively research culture has developed over the past 30 years (Abernethy et al., 2007; Gray, 2011; Memmert, 2009; Moran, 2003; Nougier & Rossi, 1999; Williams et al., 1999; Wulf, 2007). The importance of visual-perceptual and attentional performance becomes obvious in team sports. Due to the complexity and multitude of stimuli available (teammates, opponents, field markings, goal or net, ball, etc.), team sports demand complex skills in distributing and dividing attention as well as in perceiving patterns of play (both for players and referees). Good referees, for example, need to monitor the movements of 22 soccer players and the ball in real time. They must integrate this information with the percept of their environment (e.g., field markings) and consequently decide, in a matter of seconds, whether any rule violations have occurred (for various explanations of incorrect offside decisions, see ▶ Chap. 5). It is known that experts tend to store and recognize overall patterns common in their sport, while novices tend to process the many individual components (individual playing positions etc.) separately rather than as a whole (Abernethy et al., 2005; Williams & Davids, 1995). This difference in perception leads to experts showing superior pattern perception for game scenarios (Abernethy et al., 1994; Allard & Burnett, 1985; Borgeaud & Abernethy, 1987). The remaining free attentional resources can then be used by experts to, for example, detect unmarked teammates (Furley & Memmert, 2010). However, also in closed-skill sports with closed requirements, perception and attention play a decisive role. In track and field, for example, outstanding coaches are able to recognize, even at far distances, which feature(s) of a complex technique need to be adjusted to increase an athlete's performance.

Perception and Attention in Sports

- The demands on perception and attention are particularly high in complex team sports.
- Experts are better able to cognitively process sport-specific information than novices.

2.2 Perception

Perception is defined as the *subjective impression* of our environment or body shaped by the sensory processing of stimuli by different sensory modalities. Put simply, perception describes the process of receiving and processing different stimuli and forms the basis of human recognition, experience, and action (Marr, 1982). Individual experiences are based on the information a person receives via the senses and then processes and stores in subcortical and cortical recognition structures of the different perceptual systems (Bruce et al., 1996). Human perception works via one or more senses and helps to *identify and classify* the environment. Visual perception plays a particularly important role in many everyday situations as well as in sports. It includes the reception and transmission of various stimuli via the eyes—or in other words, the sense of vision. From a physiological point of view, *visual perception* involves the reception of photons by photoreceptors in the eyes and the conversion of these stimuli into electrical signals. The electrical signals are registered, processed, and interpreted first in the occipital region of the brain and then in many other brain regions. On a psychological level, visual perception refers to the recognition of in particular color, shape/form, and movement. These components constitute one of the most important, if not the most important, way to perceive the environment for humans, since different situations are usually interpreted and decisions are made based on visual perception.

Visual Perception

The eye is the sensory organ that enables visual perception of the environment. Light waves reflected or emitted from objects enter the eye, where they are focused and converted by receptors into electrical signals that can be processed by the brain.

The visual field is divided into central (foveal) vision and peripheral vision. The *fovea centralis* is the area of the retina that produces the sharpest vision but covers only about 2° of the visual field. The rest of the retina covers the area of *peripheral vision*, which allows for the identification of shapes and movements but not for detailed vision. Both areas of perception constitute visual systems operating in parallel and jointly; in conjunction they determine the visual perception of our environment. The interaction of both systems begins with the intake of visual environmental stimuli via the peripheral visual field. The stimuli are selected, and a decision is made as to which area receives the most attention, that is, which area is fixated with central vision. The decision about the next fixation point is based, among other things, on previous experience with the same or similar situations. Moreover, blinking or moving objects tend to attract attention.

2

Foveal and Peripheral Perceptual Area
A distinction is made between the foveal and peripheral areas of visual perception. The foveal perceptual region covers about 2° of the visual field and provides the part of the environment that the eye can perceive most sharply. Outside this area, peripheral vision is used, which is particularly sensitive to movements and changes in our environment and directs eye movements to those areas, if necessary.

In most cases, perception is not an isolated process of passive information reception. Rather, the information intake often serves to *react to the environment* directly or indirectly. Especially in sports, perception often involves an evaluation of the perceived information in relation to one's own body or even one's own movement. When I see a defender of the opposing team running toward me (at a certain speed and from a certain direction), I need to react in a certain way (e.g., adjusting my own speed, my direction, my ball control) and potentially even to adjust this reaction while the information is being acquired. This ability to successfully integrate and coordinate one's own perception and movements is also vital when catching. Results from experimental research show that our ability to assess a ball flying toward us decreases significantly if we lack visual information about the throwing action (Panchuk et al., 2013) or if we are not allowed to move freely during our assessment (Oudejans et al., 1996). In addition, subjects showed better catching performance when they observed the ball for a longer time while in the air (Whiting et al., 1970), when more environmental information was available (Rosengren et al., 1988), when they were allowed to pick up information with both eyes instead of only one (von Hofsten et al., 1992), and when the ball's acceleration was included in their assessment (Michaels & Oudejans, 1992).

In summary, visual perception refers to the process of the intake and processing of stimuli via the photoreceptors of the eye. This process is of enormous importance in many, if not all, areas of life. Visual perception enables a person to form a picture of his or her environment and to adjust his or her reactions to that environment. In almost all everyday situations, visual perception plays a decisive role. The interaction of central and peripheral perception ensures that the human brain does not become overloaded and that people can make "good" decisions quickly. Also, in the context of sports, both foveal and peripheral vision are important for extracting the necessary, constantly changing, relevant pieces of information from the environment (▶ Side Story: Visual Field Versus Field of Vision).

Side Story

Visual Field Versus Field of Vision
When describing a person's range of visual perception, a distinction is made between the person's visual field and their field of vision. The visual field comprises the extent of the environment that can be visually perceived while the head and the eyes are at rest. In contrast, the field of vision represents the area of the environment that can be perceived visually by moving the eyes keeping the head still; thus, it is larger than the visual field.

2.2.1 Peripheral Perception

The process of visual perception is extremely important, also in sports. The perception of both stationary and dynamic elements of our environment can make the difference between victory and defeat, especially in complex team sports. Both where we look and the speed at which the information can be acquired will influence the outcome of the situation, that is, the decision leading to a particular motor action and its success. Therefore, it already becomes obvious that eye fixations on particular targets are a crucial tool for athletes, since stimuli that are fixated centrally are processed most effectively.

But what about peripheral perception? Central and peripheral visual perceptions are two complementary components of a system that facilitates the selective pickup of information from the environment. Nevertheless, focus is almost always on visual fixations and therefore central vision, and as a result the importance of peripheral perception is often neglected. However, especially in complex team sports, players are constantly required to simultaneously perceive a range of stimuli and objects. The perception of a centrally fixated stimulus alone is therefore often insufficient for many decision-making tasks. Since fixation toward several spatially separated stimuli is not possible simultaneously using central vision, peripheral perception is of great importance. Thus, peripheral vision enables not only the *selection of the most appropriate next fixation point* but also the *perception of the game situation as a whole*. This includes stationary objects (e.g., markings of the playing field or targets such as goals and baskets) as well as moving people and objects (e.g., teammates, opponents, the game equipment).

Peripheral Perception

Peripheral perception continuously scans the environment for movements and change. When movements and salient contrasts are detected in the visual field, eye movements redirect the eyes toward those objects to be able to perceive them in detail via foveal vision.

Sport Practice

An easy-to-understand example, which highlights the importance of the different perceptual processes, can be found in a sport rather unknown to Europeans: American Football. The quarterback, who controls the ball at the beginning of a play, looks for the player he/she can throw the ball to in order to gain as much territory as possible. He has to perceive as much of the playing field in front of him as possible to decide which of his teammates is free and ready to receive a pass, but he must also simultaneously observe his immediate surroundings to avoid opposing players trying to tackle him or knock the ball out of his hands. In this case, however, it is sufficient to observe opponents via the peripheral vision, so that, in case of any unusual movements, the visual focus can be altered toward those approaching opponents. This sport-specific example illustrates that both foveal and peripheral perceptions are extremely important in sports, since the simultaneous perception of teammates, opponents, and the ball optimizes a players' decision-making behavior and improves their odds of winning.

This example from American Football can be applied to many sport games (e.g., basketball, football, handball, volleyball) and also to other sports (e.g., automobile sports, synchronized swimming) in which athletes are required to observe several objects or stimuli simultaneously (e.g., other players, objects, markings). The better the athlete is at combining and making use of their foveal and peripheral perception in a meaningful way, the easier it becomes to perform (provided they have the necessary technical and tactical skills), for example, to defend a ball, score a goal, or adapt to the movements of their teammates.

What Influences Peripheral Perception?

- An object or movement suddenly appearing in the periphery attracts attention.
- In stressful situations people's peripheral perception can become restricted (Williams & Andersen, 1997).
- Because of the light sensitivity in the periphery (due to the light-dark sensitive rods of the retinal periphery), peripheral perception is particularly advantageous in poor lighting conditions.

Peripheral perception describes an important process of information pickup in sport and should, therefore, be trained and improved to increase athletes' overall performance (Williams & Davids, 1998). Peripheral perception can be enhanced, for instance, by enhancing primary skills so that the athlete has the necessary attentional capacity to attend to peripheral information (see Dunton et al., 2019), or it can be achieved perhaps surprisingly by initially removing or blurring peripheral vision to first enhance central information pickup (see Ryu et al., 2016).

Sport Practice

Training Peripheral Perception

Particularly in competitive sports, a new scientific approach to improving performance at the top level has been sought in recent years via methods that train visual perception. Indeed, various perceptual skills (such as visual acuity, motion perception, and also peripheral vision) seem to improve via specific training programs in the laboratory. It is still unclear, though, whether such improvements in perceptual skills have a direct influence on actual sports performance, or rather whether sport-specific visual training leads to greater benefits (for an overview see Schapschröer et al., 2011). Nevertheless, many coaches and athletes make use of different exercises in their daily training routines that are meant to improve peripheral vision or the interplay of peripheral and foveal vision, as it is undisputed that the combination of foveal and peripheral perception is of great importance, especially in sport games. This becomes obvious when looking, for instance, at the task description of a setter in volleyball.

The task of a setter in volleyball is to pass the ball to one of their teammates as precisely as possible ready for them to score a direct point. In order to play the ball precisely, it is beneficial to fixate the ball immediately before and at the moment touching/playing it. At the same time, the setter needs to be able to perceive his or her teammates to check if they are ready to receive the ball, as well as the opposing blocking players. Based on the positioning of the opposing blockers, it becomes clear(er) which attacker has the best chance of scoring a point. Thus, while the setter fixates the ball, he or she perceives the positions and movements of the others using peripheral vision. This also gives him or her the opportunity to detect gaps behind the opponent's blockers, so that he or she does not necessarily have to pass the ball to the attackers but can also score a point him- or herself.

2

2.2.2 Failures of Conscious Perception

Our processing capacity is highly limited. This limitation means that the *selection of perceptual content* by attention is essential. Through a combination of deliberate distribution of attention (top-down) and automatic prioritization of certain representations (bottom-up), we are usually able to use our limited capacity efficiently to achieve our behavioral goals. This means that we consciously perceive relevant items and block out irrelevant ones. Sometimes, however, this selective prioritization of perceptual content makes us block out items that we might have wanted to attend to or should have perceived consciously. When made aware of what we missed, we often experience astonishment, particularly when missing very salient (e.g., large or loud) stimuli. Imagine you are watching a short video of two teams of three players each, one team wearing black shirts and one wearing white shirts. The three players of each team are passing a basketball back and forth. Your task is to count how often the three players in white pass the ball back and forth. After a short time, a person in a gorilla costume appears in the video and walks right through the scene. What would you think are the chances of you not noticing the gorilla? Surprisingly, the chance is about 50%; it is as likely that you notice the gorilla as it is that you do not perceive the gorilla consciously at all (Simons & Chabris, 1999; ► Study Box: Overlooking Relevant Events). Attention toward the passing behavior causes many of us to block out what would usually be a highly salient piece of information.

Failures of Awareness
Because our cognitive processing capacity is highly limited, we select perceptual content. This sometimes holds us from consciously perceiving even salient and behaviorally relevant stimuli.

Reflection

Failures of conscious perception are often a consequence of our cognitive structure and occur frequently in everyday life. Most of the time we do not realize how much we miss; after all, we did not consciously perceive it. But do you perhaps know some failures of awareness from your own experience?

- You are looking for a friend in a crowd. You think he is wearing a red jacket. You look and look again, but you cannot find him. When he finally approaches you, he says that he even waved his arms wildly and that you looked directly in his direction several times. That may be true, but he had taken off his red jacket.
- You are completely immersed in a book. Someone is trying to talk to you. It is only when she touches your arm that you realize you have been spoken to.
- There are many mistakes in movies: Sometimes a crew member sneaks into the picture unnoticed, objects change their position as if by an invisible hand, or the actor's hairstyle is not exactly the same in the next scene. But how often do we actually notice these mistakes if nobody explicitly draws our attention to them? Exactly, we almost never notice these changes.

Study Box

Overlooking Relevant Events

In 1995, Boston police officer Kenny Conley was convicted of perjury and obstruction of justice. He had been chasing a suspect during an operation, while two of his colleagues confused another police officer with a suspect and assaulted him. Although Conley walked directly past the attack, he later testified that he had not noticed any of it. However, since the assault happened right in front of him, no one believed his repeated claim not to have witnessed the assault (Lehr, 2009).

Some attention researchers became fascinated by this case. Based on their research on failures of awareness, they were convinced that missing even salient stimuli could indeed occur under certain circumstances and that the question of police officer Conley's guilt could therefore not be automatically inferred.

Chabris et al. (2011) designed a study that was based as closely as possible on the situation described above. Participants were asked to follow another person around the campus at a fixed distance while counting how often this person touched their head. Right next to the path, in direct view of the participants for at least 15 s, a fight was simulated between three men involving much shouting and noise. The results of the study showed that a large proportion of participants were deaf and blind to the fight. The probability of noticing the fight depended both on the difficulty of the task (counting head touches separately for the left and right hand, 42% noticed the fight; counting head touches regardless of the hand, 56% noticed the fight; not having to count head touches at all, 72% noticed the fight) and on the lighting conditions (moderately difficult task in bright day light, 56% noticed the fight; moderately difficult task in the dark, 35% noticed the fight).

Conley was acquitted on appeal. However, the research findings on failures of awareness did not contribute to his acquittal (Lehr, 2009). Of course, research cannot directly prove or disprove a person's innocence. However, the research results do indicate that it is conceivable that Conley could have been telling the truth. Even more so as Hüttermann and Memmert (2012) demonstrated that physical stress (Conley pursued the suspect over a long time) further reduces the probability that an unexpected object or event is noticed.

Several different types of failures of awareness can be identified. On the one hand, there is information that we are not aware of because we *deliberately inhibit* it and, thus, effectively filter it out. This is intentional and, therefore, not a failure. On the other hand, there is information that has such a *low level of sensory energy* (e.g., too small for our eyes or too quiet for our ears) that we cannot consciously perceive it even when we devote our attention to it; these stimuli are subliminal (Dehaene et al., 2006) and are discussed in ► Sect. 2.2.3. Of particular interest are failures of awareness involving stimuli that are consciously perceived or remain unconscious depending on the way attention is distributed. Thus, these stimuli have enough inherent sensory energy to be perceived but do not always reach this threshold—namely, when their representation is not sufficiently amplified by attention. The phenomenon of *change blindness* (Rensink et al., 1997; Simons & Levin, 1997) describes situations in which participants look for the difference in two versions of an image presented in rapid change with a very short black image in between (i.e., the two versions of the image flicker back and forth). As long as the attentional focus does not coincide with the part of the image in which the change occurs, participants have no conscious representation of the change. Thus, change blindness originates from the spatial absence of attention. In contrast, the phenomenon of the *attentional blink* (Raymond et al., 1992; Shapiro et al., 1997) arises from a temporal absence of attention: a target stimulus is not consciously perceived when another target is presented 100–500 ms beforehand. This is not a reaction conflict but appears to be a 100–500 ms long "hole" in the allocation of attention which results in an associated blindness for other target stimuli. Both lines of research (change blindness and attentional blink) have contributed to the advancement of basic scientific theories on attention and perception. However, both phenomena occur primarily in experimental tasks with specific constraints including timing and material and might, therefore, not be easily transferred to everyday life. In contrast, *inattentional blindness* occurs regularly in everyday tasks. By definition, this is a failure of awareness that occurs when a stimulus unexpectedly appears in our visual field while our attention is focused on another task or stimulus (Mack & Rock, 1998; Simons & Chabris, 1999). These conditions are often present in our everyday life as well as in the context of sports. In major sport games, for example, there is often a primary task that demands attention (e.g., controlling the ball or concentrating on a predetermined tactical sequence), which can lead to an unexpectedly free player not being noticed. The transferability to everyday life and sport is additionally increased by studies showing that inattentional blindness occurs with very divergent situational conditions (e.g., with different laboratory tasks, driving simulators, and in naturalistic settings), that it occurs with a wide variety of unexpected objects (from a small black square to a unicycling clown; Hyman et al., 2010; Mack & Rock, 1998), and that it is also robust when the unexpected object is shown for relatively long presentation times (e.g., demonstrations of 200 ms to more than 15 s).

The Most Important Failures of Awareness

- Change blindness
- Inattentional Blindness
- Attentional Blink

Inattentional Blindness

Inattentional blindness refers to the phenomenon that we sometimes miss objects that appear unexpectedly in our view. The more our attention is drawn to another task, the higher the probability that the unexpected object is not consciously perceived.

To date, several studies have specifically addressed the topic of *inattention in sports*. From these studies, some interesting insights can be derived. For example, Memmert (2006) and Furley et al. (2010) were able to show that basketball experts are less prone to inattentional blindness in basketball situations than novices; experts were more likely to notice both a stimulus completely unfitting to the situation (e.g., a gorilla; see Simons & Chabris, 1999) as well a stimulus fitting to the situation (a free player). A study by Memmert et al. (2009) suggests that this increased perceptual capacity is specific to expertise in a particular sport and does not generalize beyond it: their results showed that team athletes, individual athletes, and nonathletes did not differ in their probability to discover an unexpected object in a neutral (i.e., not sports-related) task ► Study Box: Overlooking Unexpectedly Unmarked Teammates).

2

Study Box

Overlooking Unexpectedly Unmarked Teammates

Memmert and Furley (2007) transferred the classic inattentional blindness paradigms (Mack & Rock, 1998; Simons & Chabris, 1999; Most et al., 2001) to the context of sports. To stick as closely as possible to the complex reality of sport games, they developed a study design that incorporated video recordings of handball situations. Participants were asked to put themselves in the position of a specific player in the video and to perform two tasks: (1) to observe their direct opponent and evaluate whether he adopted an offensive or defensive position (primary task requiring attention) and (2) to state what they would have done in this situation to maximize their chance of scoring a goal. After two non-critical videos (i.e., without any unexpected stimulus), participants watched a video in which an unmarked player stood on the court unexpectedly but very obviously. Although this player clearly represented the best solution in this situation and was positioned in the center of the video scene, right next to the opponent that had to be observed, 50% of the participants did not notice him.

In two further experiments, Memmert and Furley (2007) discovered interesting factors influencing the probability of failures of awareness in their sport-specific inattentional blindness task. First, they found that significantly more participants noticed the unmarked player when no additional instructions were given, as opposed to when such instructions were provided (e.g., "If it makes sense, you should take two rules into account. First, if your opponent steps out, try to trick him with a feint. Second, if your opponent remains defensive, try to score a goal with a jump shot."). Potentially, this effect arises from differences in the breadth of the attentional focus: when additional instructions are given, the attentional focus is constricted. Second, they found that the unmarked player was almost always noticed when he was made more salient, by waving his arm. These findings in the specific context of handball have now been replicated in another sport, namely, basketball (Furley et al., 2010; Fig. 2.1).

Which Factors Influencing the Detection of Unexpected Objects Have Been Identified in the Sport Context So Far?

- *Experts* in a specific sport are more likely to detect unexpected objects in the context of their respective sport (Furley et al., 2010; Memmert, 2006).
- *More salient objects* (e.g., a waving teammate) are detected with a higher probability (Memmert & Furley, 2007).
- Specific *tactical instructions* increase the probability that an unexpectedly unmarked teammate is missed (Memmert & Furley, 2007). Conversely, it can be inferred that fewer explicit instructions increase the probability that an unmarked player is detected.
- Memmert (2006, 2014a, 2014b) was able to show that children up to 10 years of *age* are particularly susceptible to missing unexpected objects. Therefore, this topic is of particular relevance for this age group.
- Extremely high or extremely low *physical arousal* leads to more failures of awareness for unexpected objects (Hüttermann & Memmert, 2012).

In order to remain as unpredictable to opponents as possible, it is advantageous for players to have as many *convergent and divergent decision-making solutions* as possible, including those that are unusual and surprising to the opponent. The repertoire of possible tactical solutions for any given situation will increase in alignment

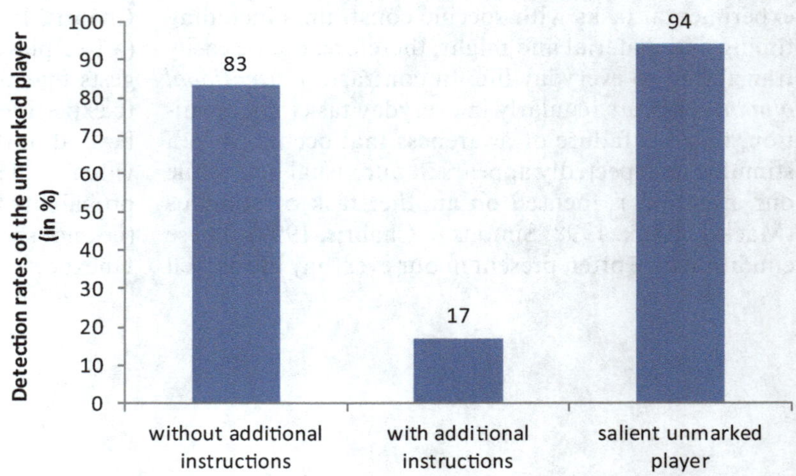

Fig. 2.1 Results of the study by Memmert and Furley (2007). Detection rates of the unexpectedly unmarked player are given as percentages

with the number of players and game patterns that can be simultaneously attended to. A *broad focus of attention* is therefore required of team athletes for them to be able to make tactical decisions and to integrate original solutions into their cognitive decision-making process (Memmert, 2010). For this purpose, it is also necessary that unexpectedly unmarked players are noticed and that the decision-making process is modified adequately based on such additional information. Perceiving and passing the ball to unmarked players often constitutes the best solution in complex game situations.

Coaches' instructions (e.g., tactical routes, well-trained moves)—which are designed to assist the players—can sometimes negatively impact tactical decision-making by narrowing the players' focus of attention and, thus, reducing their flexibility.

Increasing the Number of Action Alternatives

The number of convergent and divergent decision-making solutions in any given situation and, thus, the unpredictability for the opponent will likely increase commensurate with the number of game elements an athlete is able to simultaneously attend to.

Sport Practice

How can the detection of unexpected opportunities be fostered?

General psychological as well as sports-related research on inattentional blindness shows that various situational factors clearly influence whether an unexpected object is noticed or not. The different actors in a sport game can do different things to increase the probability that unexpected opportunities are detected.

As unmarked teammate:

Unmarked teammates need to be aware that they can easily be overlooked, especially when they are free unexpectedly. Even if the passer looks directly at them, this does not automatically mean that he or she will consciously perceive them (Beanland & Pammer, 2010; Memmert, 2006). Salient gestures that draw the attention of the passing player (e.g., hand waving) are recommended.

As coach:

Clear instructions for action as well as tactical instructions from outside the playing field narrow the attentional focus of the player and increase the probability that unexpected chances go unnoticed (Memmert & Furley, 2007). Coaches who wish for their players to find creative solutions and to notice unexpected chances should give as few tactical instructions as possible. Since children under the age of 10 have an even higher susceptibility to inattentional blindness, external instructions should be kept to a minimum in this age group particularly. Otherwise their attentional focus may be fundamentally restricted, rendering original solutions highly unlikely (see Memmert & Furley, 2007).

As player:

Basic research on inattentional blindness has shown that neither personality traits nor individual cognitive abilities can reliably predict whether or not unexpected objects are noticed across different situations (Bredemeier & Simons, 2012; Kreitz et al., 2015a, 2015b). Thus, in this context, it is useless to train one's basic cognitive abilities in a targeted manner. However, it has been shown that expectations have a strong influence on the detection of additional objects (Downing et al., 2004; Kreitz et al., 2015a, 2015b). If objects, persons, or situations are expected, then inattentional blindness hardly occurs. Players should therefore always be aware that unexpected constellations and opportunities can occur in addition to frequently occurring and often practiced situations during a game. This broadening of attention might help to raise the awareness of unexpected chances.

2.2.3 Unconscious Perception

Due to the limitation of our cognitive capacity, we perceive only a small fraction of our environment consciously. Nevertheless, a lot of the information that remains unconscious is processed and can even influence our behavior (Dehaene et al., 1998; Schnuerch et al., 2016). For example, *reaction times* can be shortened if a similar stimulus is previously presented subliminally (Dell'Acqua & Grainger, 1999; Kouider & Dehaene, 2009), the *identification and naming* of very briefly presented stimuli can be promoted if the same stimulus has already been presented before (Bar & Biederman, 1998), and even *decisions* can be systematically influenced: 60% of penalty takers' kicks are directed to the side of the goal with more space when the goalkeeper is slightly displaced form the middle of the goal even though this displacement is not consciously perceived by the penalty takers (Noël et al., 2015; ► Study Box: The Unconscious Shot into the Free Corner).

Influence of Unconscious Perception

- Reaction times can be influenced.
- The identification and naming of weak stimuli can be facilitated.
- Arbitrary decisions can be influenced.

2

Subliminal

The term "subliminal" describes the presentation of stimuli below the threshold of conscious perception. Subliminally presented stimuli are, therefore, processed unconsciously (if at all). Examples of subliminal stimuli are those with very weak contrast, a very short presentation duration, or masked stimuli.

Current research shows that the conscious and unconscious processing of stimuli share several commonalities (Kiefer et al., 2011): for sensory input, many processing steps take place even if we do not consciously perceive the input (Dehaene & Naccache, 2001). We do not even need a conscious representation of the stimulus for semantic (i.e., related to the meaning of a stimulus) processing (Dehaene et al., 1998). Furthermore, we can even process the emotional content of stimuli without perceiving it consciously (Gainotti, 2012; Kiss & Eimer, 2008; Naccache et al., 2005).

? Which Types of Processing Depend on Conscious Perception of a Stimulus?

There seem to be only four types of processing that depend on a conscious representation of a stimulus (Dehaene & Naccache, 2001):

- For information to remain stable over time
- For explicit (e.g., verbal) expression of the information
- For innovative and creative solutions to complex or new issues
- For intentional behavior

A clear influence of subliminal perception on behavior also becomes evident in the context of sports. For example, more than 60% of penalty takers aim at the more open side of the goal, even when they do not consciously perceive that the goalkeeper is standing slightly to one side of the middle of the goal (*off-center effect*).

Off-Center Effect

The off-center effect refers to a slight offset of the goalkeeper from the center of the goal. It increases the probability that the penalty taker will aim at the side with more space, even though the offset is so small that the shooter does not consciously perceive it.

The off-center effect appears to be very robust and has already been demonstrated with schematic computer animations (Masters et al., 2007), with photorealistic goalkeepers (Weigelt & Memmert, 2012; Weigelt et al., 2012), and in field tests with real goalkeepers in real goals (Noël et al., 2015). Although there is no conscious, verbalizable perception of the goalkeeper being off-center, the shooters' behavior changes. This demonstrates a clear dissociation between our conscious perception and our cognition or behavior (▶ Study Box: The Unconscious Shot into the Free Corner).

Study Box

The Unconscious Shot into the Free Corner

In a study by Noël et al. (2015), the off-center effect was examined in a realistic, game-like setting. Participants (soccer players with at least 8 years of experience) were asked to position a goalkeeper precisely in the middle of the goal. They then took 20 penalty kicks. Of course, due to the inherent limitations of human perception, the goalkeeper was never placed exactly in the middle of the goal but usually a few centimeters to the left or right of the actual center. Results showed that over 60% of the shots were kicked to the side with more space, even though the shooters thought the goalkeeper was standing precisely in the middle. The offset of the goalkeeper to one side was so small that it was not consciously perceptible to the shooters. Nevertheless, subliminal processing of the offset apparently took place and influenced the behavior of the shooters (◘ Fig. 2.2).

In addition, the authors examined the influence of common strategies used by penalty takers and goalkeepers on the off-center effect. Half of the participants were instructed to adopt a goalkeeper-independent approach for their penalty kicks (kicking in a predetermined direction irrespective of the movements of the goalkeeper); the other half were asked to use a goalkeeper-dependent strategy (trying to anticipate whether the goalkeeper will jump to the left or right and kicking in the opposite direction). In half of the cases, the goalkeeper was instructed to jump toward one of the corners of the goal early, and in the other half, he was asked to jump late. So, in total, there were four different conditions:

i. shooter has goalkeeper-dependent strategy + goalkeeper jumps early.
ii. shooter has goalkeeper-independent strategy + goalkeeper jumps early.
iii. shooter has goalkeeper-dependent strategy + goalkeeper jumps late.
iv. shooter has goalkeeper-independent strategy + goalkeeper jumps late.

Results showed that the off-center effect occurred independent of the goalkeeper's behavior when the

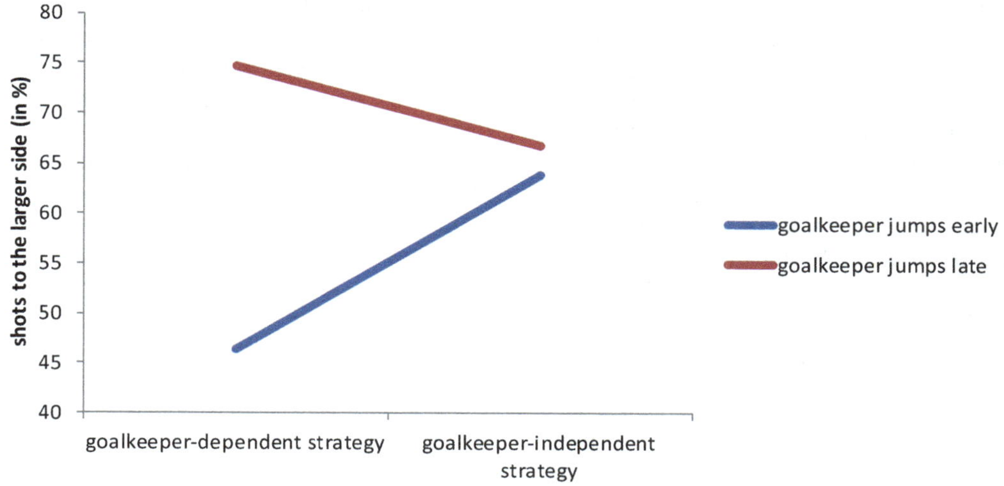

Fig. 2.2 Results of the study by Noël et al. (2015). The shots to the larger side are given as percentages depending on the condition. With a goalkeeper-independent shooting strategy, it makes no difference whether the goalkeeper jumps early or late. With a goalkeeper-dependent strategy, the off-center effect is particularly pronounced if the goalkeeper jumps late

shooter adopted a goalkeeper-independent strategy. However, when the shooter adopted a goalkeeper-dependent strategy, the off-center effect only occurred when the goalkeeper jumped late. Apparently, when a shooter adopts a goalkeeper-dependent strategy, an early-jumping goalkeeper "overwrites" the starting point of the goalkeeper. This makes sense: if you can already see where the goalkeeper is jumping, you do not have to base your decision on whether the goalkeeper has a slight offset in the goal; you have much more relevant information on which to base your decision.

The off-center effect is all-the-more astonishing given that there are many other factors that influence the direction in which penalty takers aim their shot: the kicker's previous success toward the different corners, the personal kicking preferences toward the left or right side, and previous experiences with the respective goalkeeper. It speaks to the strength and robustness of the effect that a significant influence of subliminal perception can nevertheless be consistently found.

Sport Practice

How Can Knowledge About Subliminal Perception Be Applied in a Game Situation?

As a goalkeeper, you could take advantage of the effect by deliberately standing slightly offset but being prepared to jump to the more spacious corner. This could give you some advantage. However, in practice, this can be somewhat tricky, as the offset from the center must be large enough to be perceived subliminally. If the difference is below the threshold of subliminal perception, it is not processed at all and, thus, has no behavioral effect whatsoever. However, if the difference is so big that the shooter consciously perceives it, the shooter can process this information consciously and make tactical decisions accordingly. The area in which subliminal but not conscious perception takes place ranges within a few centimeters (Noël et al., 2015).

In sports, subliminal perception does not only impact penalty situations but forms the basis of a wide range of motor responses (Kibele, 2006): the adaptation of movement sequences during the execution of a movement is mostly based on *unconscious processing* of internal and external cues (Pélisson et al., 1986). *Automated motion sequences* require significantly less processing capacities and predominantly occur outside our conscious perception. That is the reason why experts, whose motor responses have already been automated over the course of many years of training, have additional capacity left to detect new and unexpected stimuli (Memmert, 2006; Memmert & Furley, 2007). Additionally, experts can use tiny hints in the movement of their opponents to rapidly adapt their movement sequences.

Afterward, athletes often report they reacted automatically without having made any conscious decision about the movement in advance. Kibele (2006) assumes that quick motor responses are pre-activated by unconsciously represented movement features embedded in the movement sequence of the opponents or teammates. Relevant visual cues are linked to corresponding quick motor responses over the course of *long-term exercise processes* and can thereafter be activated unconsciously. The benefit of such an unconscious, automated connection of cues with quick movement adaptations is that it works very fast and that hardly any cognitive resources are needed.

Automated Motion Sequences Under Time Pressure

Automated motion sequences are primarily initiated and controlled unconsciously, particularly under time pressure. This means that in some situations athletes react without having made any conscious decision beforehand.

2.2.4 Perceptual Deceptions and Distortions

With increasing performance levels, athletes usually try to optimize their technical skills in such a way that information which might be indicative of their action intentions is minimized. Or they even try to gain performance advantages over opponents by using *deception* or *feints*. In these cases, opponents are deliberately presented with false indications of the intended action (Renshaw & Fairweather, 2000), to entice them to react differently to the actor than they usually would. In the case of successful deception, players obtain a time advantage and thus possibly a performance advantage over their observers/opponents (Schmidt & Lee, 2005; Schmidt & Wrisberg, 2008).

Perceptual Deception

Perceptual deception refers to a player gaining a temporal advantage over his or her opponent by deliberately providing false indications of their intended action.

Two types of possible deception and feint are distinguished: body feints and head fakes. Whereas *body feints* involve the movement of the whole body to deceive the opponent, in many situations the use of misleading glances is sufficient to deceive the opponent. *Such head fakes* increase the reaction time of the opponent and thus delay his or her reactions to the intended action (Alhaj Ahmad Alaboud et al., 2012; Henry et al., 2012).

Deception in Sport Games

In sport games, a distinction is made between two types of deception:

1. Body feint: An action is commenced to mislead the opponent which is then aborted and followed by the truly intended action.
2. Head fake: A player directs his or her gaze in a direction different to that of their intended movement direction.

Perceptual deception is relevant in almost all sports where the aim is to control a ball (e.g., in basketball or football), to target (e.g., in fencing), or to fight (e.g., in boxing). Since the athletes' task can continuously switch from an attacking to a defensive position in the course of a game or competition, not only is the *use* of deceptive movements essential but so too is the *recognition* of possible feints by the opponent. In basketball, for example, pretending to dribble to the left can open space and time to pass to a teammate standing on the right. The opponent on the other hand can negate that advantage by recognizing the movement as a feint and continuing to block the right option.

Scientific studies have found that higher and lower level athletes deal with deception differently. Among other things, it has been shown that *experts* in the sport of rugby are more likely to see through misleading information than less experienced players. They are also more likely to correctly anticipate the movement directions of the opponents, enabling them to make their tackling movement (holding the ball carrier and bringing him/her to the ground) more effectively (Brault et al., 2012; Jackson et al., 2006). Such an advantage of expertise is also found in basketball and handball: experts are more likely to correctly identify body feints than novices (Cañal-Bruland & Schmidt, 2009; Cañal-Bruland et al., 2010). Interestingly, the experience of experts, which leads to a faster and more frequently correct identification of deception and feints, seems to not only affect the expert's own sport but appears to span *across sport types*: experienced soccer players are less influenced by a deceptive movement in basketball than inexperienced soccer players are (Weigelt et al., 2017).

So-called perceptual illusions can be distinguished from perceptual deception; perceptual illusions (which are mostly optical) are not caused by another person's movements of the body or the gaze but by the visual system.

Perceptual Illusion

We sometimes perceive size, distance, or color of stimuli not objectively but distorted by the context they are presented in. Such optical illusions originate from processing in our neuronal system.

Examples of optical illusions are situations in which two identical objects suddenly appear different in size, straight lines appear crooked, the same colors appear lighter or darker, or an observers sees nonexistent items. Among the most well-known visual illusions are the so-called "Ebbinghaus illusion" and the "Müller-Lyer illusion."

Ebbinghaus Illusion

The Ebbinghaus illusion refers to the visual illusion that occurs when two circles of equal size appear to be of different size because one of the circles is surrounded by several larger circles and the other by several smaller circles. The circle surrounded by the larger circles is perceived to be smaller than the circle surrounded by smaller circles.

Müller-Lyer-Illusion

The Müller-Lyer illusion is an optical illusion occurring when two lines of equal length are presented while arrowheads at either end of one line are directed inward and arrowheads at the end of the other line are directed outward. The line with the arrowheads pointing inward is perceived to be longer by the observer.

Various research groups have investigated the effectiveness of using optical illusions in sport training. In their article published in 2016, Cañal-Bruland, van der Meer, and Moerman describe that a training in which the target appears smaller due to an optical illusion (Ebbinghaus illusion) can improve performance in a target task in sport. In contrast, Witt et al. (2011) point out that individuals' self-confidence can be strengthened and consequently that their performance can be improved, by using a target that appears to be larger due to the Ebbinghaus illusion. Indeed, a performance increase has been observed in golf for holes that appear larger (Chauvel et al., 2015). However, with regard to this study, it should be mentioned that the participants had little or no previous experience in the sport of golf. It would, therefore, be interesting to examine the extent to which visual illusions influence the performance of experienced players. Moreover, it is still uncertain whether visual illusions only affect the planning of action regardless of its control (Glover, 2002) or whether they affect both movement planning and control (Mendoza et al., 2005; ▶ Side Story: The Perception-Action Model by Goodale and Milner).

Side Story

The Perception-Action Model by Goodale and Milner

The scientists Melvyn Goodale and David Milner have worked on the concept of conscious and unconscious visual perception since the 1990s. Their *perception-action model* is based on neuroscientific as well as psychological evidence. Milner and Goodale propose that there is not one but two visual systems: one for the conscious perception of our environment on which we base our thought processes and the other with which we unconsciously pick up visual information from the environment to control actions in an online manner.

After brightness and movement stimuli are recorded by the retina, the visual information is transmitted via the visual cortex in the occipital lobe to various areas in the brain primarily through one of two visual streams. These streams run spatially separately and use similar information in different ways (Goodale & Milner, 1992). The so-called ventral stream is responsible for conscious recognition and identification of objects, while the *dorsal stream* unconsciously controls movements. Although both streams process visual information in parallel, it is important to note that people are capable of visually guided actions even without conscious visual perception.

The perception-action model outlines a theory that is particularly interesting in the context of sports. In most sports, visual information is the primary source of information and is therefore crucial for athletes' movement planning. Since the model assumes that visual action control is largely controlled by unconscious perception and, thus, independent of conscious visual perception, illusions or errors that only affect conscious perception should not play a significant role in movement control. Thus, the interesting question arises to what extent it is possible to intervene in unconsciously controlled actions at all.

2

2.3 Attention

Attentional mechanisms can be interpreted as a supporting function of human perception, whose task is to select relevant aspects from a variety of sensory impressions in order to efficiently control actions and thought processes (Posner, 1980). Visual attention, in contrast to basic visual processes, is a *higher cognitive skill*. This classification is supported by the fact that different attentional processes are influenced, for example, by stress, strain on working memory, or competition-oriented selection (Knudsen, 2007; Schweizer et al., 2000). On top of that, performance on attention-demanding tasks appears to be closely related to measures of intelligence, presumably because "higher" mental processes are involved in both domains (Bates & Stough, 1997).

By now, research in sport sciences has provided numerous findings demonstrating superior attentional performance of professional athletes when compared with relatively less experienced athletes (Abernethy & Russell, 1987; Castiello & Umiltà, 1992a, 1992b; Memmert, 2006; Pesce Anzeneder & Bösel, 1998).

Attention theories and models help to describe, explain, and predict sport psychological phenomena. They are important for our (sport-)scientific thinking and our goal-oriented approach to sport practice. Or, as Lewin expressed in 1951 already "There is nothing so practical as a good theory" (▶ Chap. 1). Unsurprisingly, a great number of theories, models, and paradigms exist regarding attention that is discussed both in sport psychology and the wider psychological literature.

In general, *four sub-processes of attention* can be distinguished based on neuroscientific and psychological findings: selective attention, orienting of attention divided attention, and sustained attention (e.g., Coull, 1998; Knudsen, 2007; Mirsky et al., 1991; Van Zomeren & Brouwer, 1994).

Four Sub-processes of Attention

The following sub-processes of attention are often the basis of sport psychological research:

- Selective attention
- Orienting of attention
- Divided attention
- Sustained attention

2.3.1 Selective Attention

Selective attention is responsible for directing our limited processing capacity toward certain locations or events at particular points in time (or within certain time windows), while at the same time suppressing other events (cf. Coull, 1998; Posner & Boies, 1971).

Selective Attention

Selective attention chooses between competing stimuli, locations, and points in time. Thus, specific objects, locations, or points in time are processed preferentially while others are inhibited.

Next to the orienting of attention, selective attention has undoubtedly been the most researched of the subprocesses of attention in sport sciences to date (Memmert, 2009, 2014a, 2014b). This is because (a) the ability to *selectively process certain perceptual contents* and suppress other stimuli is essential in many sport tasks and (b) there is a variety of methodological approaches to investigate selective attention.

On the one hand, studies investigated the gaze behavior of experts during competition (how exactly do they "scan" their surroundings?) to understand how the athletes are able to react as quickly and correctly as possible. *Information-rich areas* (Magill, 1998) contain visual features that can be used particularly well to anticipate movements. In tennis, for example, it is helpful to focus attention not only on regions distant from the body (e.g., the opponent's racket or the ball's trajectory) but also on the opponent's arm and upper body in order to detect important information for the prediction of the ball's trajectory (Rowe & McKenna, 2001).

On the other hand, selective attention was systematically manipulated in video-based laboratory training programs (e.g., Tayler et al., 1994; Abernethy et al., 1999; Williams et al., 2003) and real-world interventions (Hagemann & Memmert, 2006). Here, attention was drawn to information-rich areas by visual or verbal cues (for an overview see Jackson & Farrow, 2005). Conscious, unconscious, and self-discovery strategies support the learning process (Farrow & Abernethy, 2002; Smeeton et al., 2004; Williams et al., 2002, 2003).

Sport Practice

To circumvent the limited information-processing capacity of athletes, exercises can be developed that direct the attention of athletes toward those game features considered especially important by the coach. This way, specific *expectations* can be developed that focus attention toward information-rich areas.

However, specific instructions by the coach (e.g., tactical routes, studied moves) which are supposed to support the athletes' control of their selective attention can also have adverse and unintended effects on tactical decision-making by reducing the attentional *flexibility* of the athlete. Consequently, important features (e.g., unmarked teammates) are more likely to be overlooked (Memmert & Furley, 2007), and solutions become less creative (Memmert, 2007).

2.3.2 Orienting of Attention

Orienting of attention means that attention is directed to salient stimuli or important parts of a stimulus. This allows the attentional focus to quickly shift to different locations and objects. Attention is "logged in" and "logged out" (Tennenbaum & Bar-Eli, 1995). Information that attention has "logged in" on is amplified, while the processing of data outside the attentional focus is impeded (Posner, 1980).

A *processing advantage* can be demonstrated for stimuli that appear in a location to which attention has been drawn previously by a cue stimulus. Reaction times for such stimuli are shorter than for stimuli that appear at other locations in the display (for an overview see Cañal-Bruland, 2007).

Orienting of attention is closely related to selective attention (► Sect. 2.3.1), as both are processes that direct and guide attentional resources. However, the two attentional sub-processes activate different areas of the brain (Posner & Peterson, 1990): selective attention favors certain stimuli over others (i.e., when there is a multitude of stimuli competing for attentional selection), whereas the orienting of attention refers to a single stimulus.

Orienting of Attention

Orienting of attention directs attention to behaviorally relevant stimuli. Such orienting is often accompanied by eye movements (overt orienting of attention) but can also take place in peripheral vision (covert orienting of attention).

Professional athletes from open-skills sports such as boxing (Nougier et al., 1989), hockey (Enns & Richards, 1997), soccer (Lum et al., 2002), or volleyball (Castiello & Umiltà, 1992a, 1992b) show significantly higher flexibility when orienting their attention than novices do (cf. Memmert, 2014a, 2014b). This enables the experienced athletes to pay less attention to probable events in their surroundings and in turn devote more of their attentional resources to unlikely events. Further study results suggest this is not the case for athletes from closed-skills sports (e.g., swimming; Nougier et al., 1996). Furthermore, experts are also better able to modify their attentional resources according to the specific task requirements during competition (e.g., Nougier et al., 1989; Castiello & Umiltà, 1992a, 1992b).

Sport Practice

A processing advantage (i.e., shorter reaction times) can be shown when an athlete's attention is directed to a specific location where a relevant event will take place (e.g., extremity that will hit the ball, point on the field where the ball will land). For everyday training, this means that coaches' instructions and tips, which direct an athlete's attention, should be appropriate for the respective situation and need to be reinforced in the learning process. To convince athletes of the advantages of certain actions in certain situations, coaches should always make their intentions behind the instructions clear.

2.3.3 Divided Attention

In sports, it is often necessary to perform several tasks simultaneously, between which the limited attentional resources must be divided. *Divided attention* enables people to focus on *two or more sources of information* simultaneously (cf. Coull, 1998). This type of attentional skill can be captured by dual-task paradigms (Castaneda & Gray, 2007). Numerous practical requirements in sports presuppose the ability to divide attention and also require a sufficiently broad breadth of attention (► Sect. 2.3.3.1; Memmert, 2014a, 2014b).

Divided Attention

Divided attention refers to the simultaneous distribution of attention to different stimuli.

2.3.3.1 Breadth of Attention

Over the previous decades, several different methods and paradigms have been developed to investigate the distribution of visual attention or determine the spatial breadth of the visual focus of attention. One of the best known and most influential test methods is the so-called useful field of view (UFoV; Ball & Owsley, 1993). When performing this test, participants are required to focus on a centrally presented stimulus while at the same time identifying and locating a stimulus presented in the periphery. The UFoV is mainly used in the context of investigations of attention in driving. It enables the collection of data on the detection, identification, and localization of stimuli in the central and peripheral visual field. However, other everyday situations are not considered, for example, situations in which two peripheral stimuli need to be observed simultaneously. Such situations do not only occur in road traffic, for example, when other road users or events need to be observed to the right and the left of one's own vehicle simultaneously, but also in sports, when teammates, opponents, and the ball have to be simultaneously observed. To be able to assess and measure attention performance during such situations, Hüttermann et al. (2013) developed a new testing, the so-called attention window task. By means of this method, the maximum distance between two peripheral stimuli (i.e., the maximum attention breadth) can be measured. Stimuli are presented along one horizontal, one vertical, and two diagonal axes. The maximum breadth of attention measured along each axis allows the determination of an individual's maximum visual attention window, within which stimuli can be consciously perceived with one look. During the test, two stimuli are presented along one axis, always at the same distance from the center. The limit of the attention window is determined by the maximum attention breadth on each axis, that is, the point up to which both stimuli can still be simultaneously identified correctly with at least 75% response accuracy. Each stimulus consists of four different objects. Combinations of shapes and colors are used to ensure that attention processes are needed in the process. Light and dark grey circles and triangles are presented, and the participants' task is to identify the number (0–4) of light-grey triangles for each of the two stimuli. During the task, participants focus their gaze centrally between the two stimuli and perceive the stimuli peripherally. To prevent jumps of gaze between the two stimuli (and, thus, ensure divided attention), the stimuli are presented for only 300 ms.

Attention Window

Attention window refers to the spatial area of the visual field in which several peripheral stimuli can be consciously perceived simultaneously (▸ Methods: Attention Window Task).

Methods: Attention Window Task

One trial consists of six different display sequences (◘ Fig. 2.3). At the beginning of each trial, a fixation cross is presented at the center of the presentation area for 1000 ms. Subsequently, in the second display sequence, two cue stimuli are shown for 200 ms at precisely the same locations the target stimuli will later appear. In each trial, the stimuli are presented on a selected axis, on opposite sides of and at the same distance from the center of the projection. The separation of the two stimuli varies between trials with viewing angles of 5°–45°. The time interval between the presentation of the peripheral cue stimuli and the target stimuli is 200 ms. The two target stimuli, each consisting of a random combination of four light or dark grey circles or triangles, are presented simultaneously at the locations previously indicated by the cue stimuli. In the fifth and sixth display sequence, participants indicate how many light-grey triangles they perceived in each of the two different object formations.

The stimuli in the attention window task are presented at equal distances from the center of the projection along four axes (one horizontal, one vertical, and two diagonal axes) with eight orientations (0°, 45°, 90°, 135°, 180°, 225°, 270°, and 315°). ◘ Figure 2.4 shows the stimuli on one of the two diagonal axes at a total viewing angle of 30°. (The participants cannot see the individual axes in the real test condition. Only the stimuli on the white screen are visible for them.)

Fig. 2.3 Display sequences of the attention window task

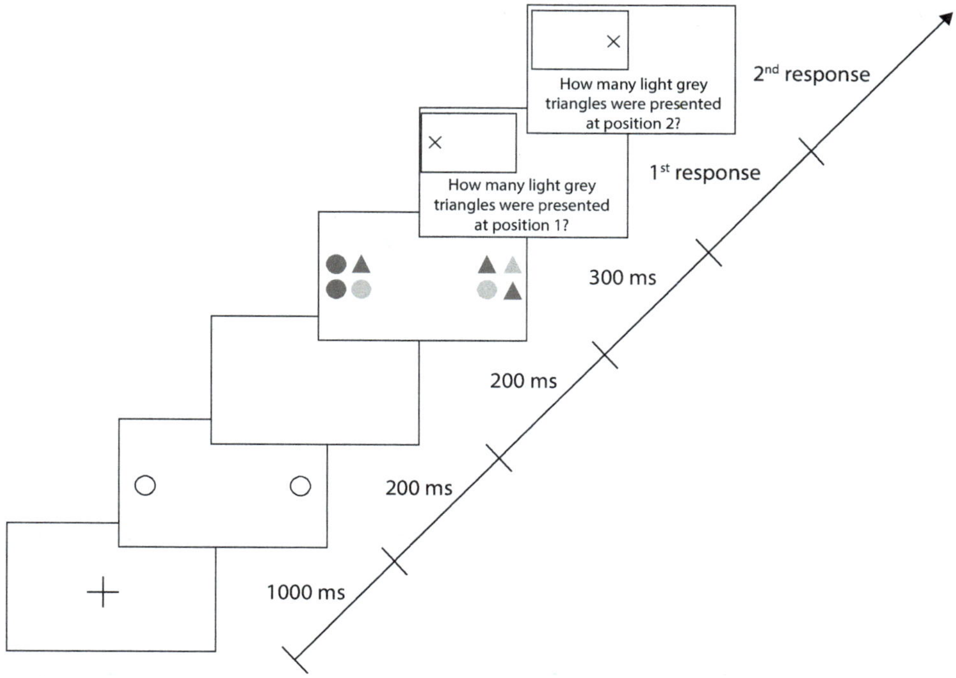

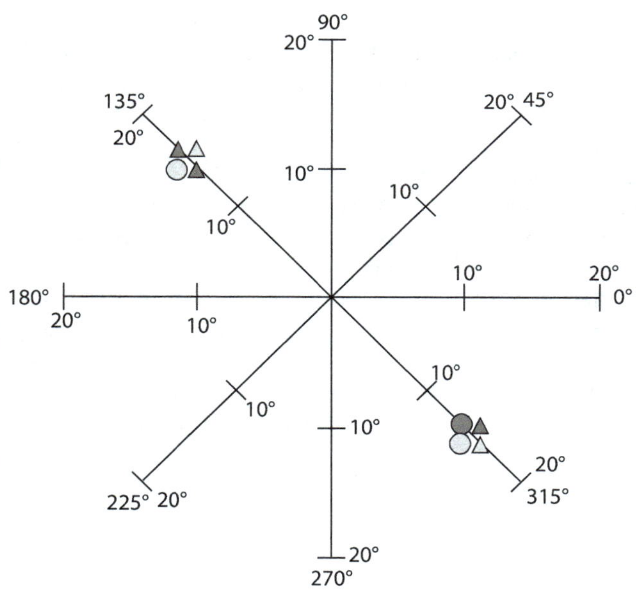

Fig. 2.4 Schematic representation of the axes of the attention window task

Breadth of Attention

Especially in team sports, it is often necessary to perceive several stimuli simultaneously (e.g., teammates and opponents). Difficulties in dealing with such situations indicate that especially large distances between relevant objects exceed our maximum attentional focus. To determine the individual maximum possible breadth of attention when processing two stimuli, Hüttermann et al. (2013) developed the attention window task (► Study Box).

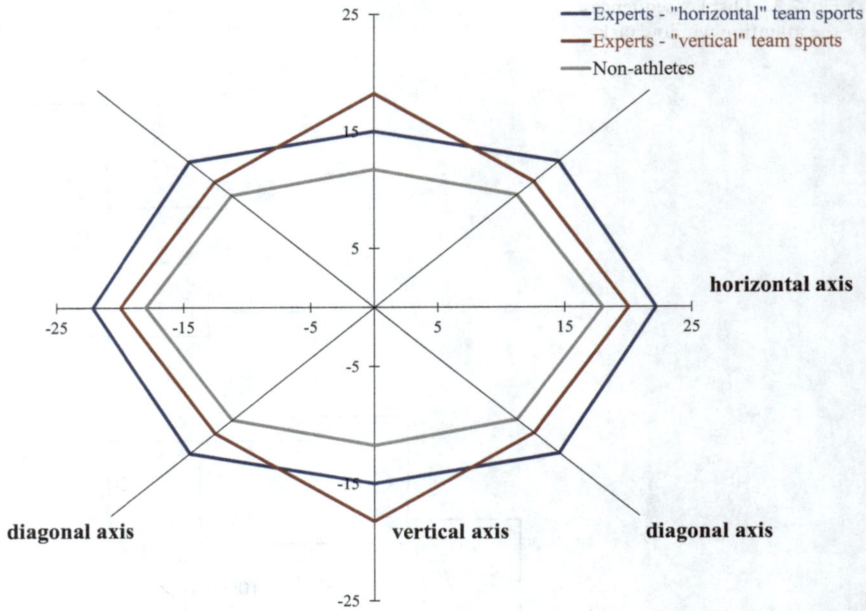

Fig. 2.5 Attention windows of athletes and nonathletes

Study Box

The Breadth of the Attentional Focus of Experts in Different Sports

Various studies indicate that athletes show more efficient performance and more flexible orientation patterns, adapt the size of the attentional focus more quickly, and are able to maintain attention over longer periods of time compared to nonathletes (Pesce Anzeneder & Bösel, 1998; Turatto et al., 1999). By means of the attention window task, Hüttermann et al. (2014) were able to further differentiate the differences in visual attention between experts and novices often mentioned in the literature (e.g., Helsen & Pauwels, 1993; Williams et al., 1994; Ryu et al., 2015; Ryu et al., 2013; Ryu et al., 2016); Williams & Davids, 1998). Their results indicate that athletes have a 25% larger attention window compared to nonathletes (Fig. 2.5). Moreover, there are also differences in the attention window between experts in different sports: experts from sports in which a primarily horizontal distribution of attention seems to be required (e.g., soccer) showed a distribution of visual attention that was 8% wider along the horizontal axis, compared to athletes who mostly need a vertical orientation of attention for a good performance in their sport (e.g., volleyball). In contrast, volleyball players and basketball players showed a 15% greater vertical distribution of attention than soccer players and other athletes who require a primarily horizontal focus in their sport. This finding indicates a systematic relationship between the shape of the attention window found in laboratory tasks and the real-world visual requirements of different expert groups.

Sport Practice

In sports, the necessary orienting of visual attention is dependent on the requirements of the tasks athletes face. *Flexible orienting* of the size of the visual attentional focus can be decisive for performance, especially in the fast-paced team and racket sports. Depending on the game situation, players have to alternate between a *broad focus of attention* (e.g., attending to a wide area on the pitch to discover free teammates) and a *narrow focus* (e.g., fixating the ball during a penalty kick). A narrow focus of attention is essential for perception and recognition of details in situations such as penalty shootouts, for example, to be able to detect potential information about the shooting direction of the penalty taker by observing the position of his or her hips. On the other hand, a broad focus of attention is essential to, for example, be able to integrate the positioning of as many teammates and opponents as possible into the decision-making processes, i.e., to generate tactical decisions and to be able to incorporate the best possible solutions into this cognitive decision-making process (Memmert, 2010).

Athletes in team sports, in which the simultaneous observation of several objects and situations is an ongoing requirement, should in training frequently be confronted with exercises and tasks in which they have to focus their attention on multiple areas simultaneously. The following tips can be carried out in different variations:

1. Implementation of game forms in which team athletes require a broad focus of attention to generate various tactical decisions that allow the players to act creatively.
2. Development of game forms in which unexpected solutions arise for the players (e.g., an additional neutral player); this way, the players can learn to modify their decision-making process based on new, additional information.
3. Increasing the number of elements/objects to be perceived (e.g., teammates, opponents, balls).

Furley and Memmert (2005) describe sample exercises and give further tips for the systematic training of the visual attentional focus of athletes. The suggested exercises are constructed in a way that trains a broader focus of attention.

Training the Breadth of Visual Attention in Sports

Based on the attention window task, in which two peripheral stimuli have to be identified simultaneously, different rules/principles can be established by which an athlete's focus of attention can be trained (narrowed and broadened):

- The more elements of a game a player can consciously perceive simultaneously across a large spatial area, the greater is his/her repertoire of possible tactical solutions for a given situation.
- Too many instructions (e.g., by the coach) can negatively affect the tactical decision-making of players and limit their flexibility in orienting their visual attention.

Which Factors Influence the Breadth of Visual Attention?

- Personal characteristics/developments:
  - Age: Young people have a bigger attention window than older people.
  - Sport expertise: Team sport athletes have a bigger attention window than athletes from individual sports and nonathletes.
- Tasks:
  - Gaze behavior: The attention window is bigger when foveal gaze is directed between two peripheral stimuli, compared to when one of the stimuli is fixated and the other is perceived in the far periphery.
- Situation:
  - Physical stress: During moderate physical stress, people's attention window is bigger than it is during periods of low or high stress.
  - Mood: Positive mood increases the size of the attention window, while negative mood decreases it.

2.3.3.2 Internal/External Focus of Attention

Wulf and Prinz (2001) distinguished between an internal and an external focus of attention while individuals perform sport movements and other motor actions (e.g., Beilock et al., 2004; Rowe & McKenna, 2001). When focusing internally, learners direct their attention to the movement itself (e.g., on the nodal points of the motion sequence when driving in golf). When focusing externally, attention is directed on the effects of the movement, that is, on the target itself (e.g., on the ball or hole when putting in golf). In general, an external focus of attention appears to be superior to an internal, that is, movement-related, focus across different movement skills, skill levels, and target groups (Gray, 2011; Wulf et al., 2001; Wulf, 2007). Accordingly, an external focus of attention leads to better acquisition and learning performance (Wulf et al., 2002; see Gray, 2004, for a more differentiated position). Expert athletes are even more likely to be hindered by an internal focus of attention when performing highly automated motor skills (Beilock et al., 2002).

Internal Focus of Attention

With an internal focus of attention, individuals direct their attention directly toward the movement execution itself (e.g., the movement pattern during the golf swing).

External Focus of Attention

With an external focus of attention, attention is directed to the effect that is supposed to be achieved by the movement or on the movement target (e.g., on the ball or hole when putting in golf).

2.3.4 Sustained Attention

Sustained attention is the sub-process of attention that *maintains* the focus on relevant information, a stimulus, or a location for a sustained period of time (cf. Coull, 1998). The terms "concentration" and "vigilance" are often used synonymously. Vigilance, however, refers to long-lasting attention processes ranging from minutes to hours, while concentration tends to refer to processes lasting from seconds to minutes. An example of concentration in the sport context would be the fixation of the trajectory of a ball during a 60-m pass in soccer to "pluck the ball from the sky." In contrast to selective attention, which operates rather spatially, concentration seems to be a *temporal process* (Fernandez-Duque & Posner, 1997). Although concentration plays a significant role in a large number of sports, surprisingly, there is little established empirical evidence on this subprocess of attention (Memmert, 2014a, 2014b). Moran (1996, 2003, 2004) puts forward some suggestions as to how athletes can improve their ability to concentrate (Tip).

Concentration

Sustained attention which ensures that attention is maintained on a specific stimulus over a certain period of time (seconds to minutes).

Sport Practice

Athletes could train their sustained attention by performing tasks in which attention has to be maintained over a certain period of time (cf. Moran, 2003, 2009, 2011). For example, during serve training in racket sports, it can be instructed that different zones must be hit consistently. On the opposite side of the court, zones (the size depends on the player's level of expertise) are marked in the service courts. These zones must now be hit by performing a precise serve. For each zone that is hit, one point is awarded. The player has to concentrate on the particular target (the specific area on court) over an extended period of time.

2.4 Trainability of Perception and Attention in Sports

Experts in a particular sport are clearly superior to novices in their perceptual and attentional performances in that given sport (Cañal-Bruland et al., 2006; Ericsson & Hagemann, 2007). For example, experts recognize patterns in individual elements of a game situation, a cognitive ability that allows them to process and store more information simultaneously (Abernethy et al., 1994, 2005; Allard & Burnett, 1985; Williams & Davids, 1995). Moreover, experts orient their attention differently compared to novices: they focus their attention less on expected and predictable stimuli and patterns and focus more on unlikely events (Memmert, 2009). In contrast, a large number of studies demonstrate that experts from different sports do *not* differ from novices regarding their general, sport-independent perceptual abilities. General laboratory-based tests of perception typically do not reveal any differences (e.g., Blundell, 1985; Hughes et al., 1993; West & Bressan, 1996). Thus, experts, for example, notice unexpected objects more frequently in sport-specific situations (Memmert, 2006), but not in nonspecific situations (Memmert et al., 2009).

Cognitive Differences Between Experts and Novices

Experts appear to be superior to novices in their sport-specific perceptual and attentional performance. However, they do not appear to be superior in their non-sport-specific cognitive abilities.

Sport Practice

Since the research results described above show that athletes in all probability do not possess better general cognitive abilities, it can conversely be concluded that training general cognitive abilities does presumably not lead to performance advantages in a specific sport. Consequently, the recommendation that can be derived is that perceptual and attentional skills should not be trained in general but rather in a sport-specific way in direct relation to the relevant sport.

How can perceptual abilities be trained in a sport-specific way? An interesting line of research shows that experts are superior to novices in the *anticipation* of actions (Abernethy, 1990; Ripoll, 1991; Rowe et al., 2009; Smeeton & Williams, 2012). Thus, experts are better able to anticipate action outcomes based on the perception of little information. This creates a performance advantage as the athlete can initiate his or her counterreaction more quickly. Anticipatory decision-making can be trained, for example, by means of the occlusion technique (Cañal-Bruland et al., 2005, 2006, 2007). Since both spatial and temporal factors often play an important role in sports, it is possible to work equivalently with both *spatial and temporal occlusion techniques* (▶ Methods: Temporal and Spatial Occlusion Technique).

Methods: Temporal and Spatial Occlusion Techniques

Two methods widely used to determine performance differences between experts and novices in sport psychology are the *temporal* and *spatial* occlusion techniques.

The *temporal occlusion technique* involves the manipulation of the amount of movement information available to the observer. For example, participants are presented with a video clip showing a tennis player performing a serve. The movement/action is interrupted at different points in time (Farrow et al., 2005) or during critical phases of the movement (Müller et al., 2006). The participants' task is to make statements about the likely outcome of the shown action, for example, about the direction of the stroke performed by the tennis player or about the direction of a penalty kick in soccer.

When applying the *spatial occlusion technique*, selected regions (e.g., the torso) are not visible to the observer so that information contained in the respective areas is not available to predict action effects (Müller et al., 2006). The technique is used to better understand the information on which experts base their anticipatory judgments.

In different sports, it was shown that experienced athletes can more frequently predict the correct outcome of an observed action based on early movement information than inexperienced athletes (e.g., Hagemann & Strauß, 2006) and that they can also extract information from different regions more efficiently (e.g., Williams et al., 2009).

Another line of research reliably finds differences in visual attentional performance between experts and novices using the *dual-task paradigm*, that is, when several tasks have to be performed simultaneously (e.g., Castiello & Umiltà, 1992a, 1992b; Helsen & Pauwels, 1993; Hüttermann et al., 2014; McAuliffe, 2004; Williams & Davids, 1998; Williams et al., 1994). Studies using the attention window task (► Sect. 2.3.3.1) not only confirm the performance differences between experts and novices, but they can also quantify those differences.

In sport psychology and in general cognitive research, there has been a controversial discussion for many years about whether the commonly found differences between experts and novices in visual attentional tasks constitute a preexisting characteristic or whether the differences can be explained as consequence of learning and training processes. Some studies assume that preexisting differences in visual attention are responsible for superior athletic performance, that is, the athletes that become successful have had superior attentional abilities from birth (e.g., Maxeiner, 1988). Most researchers though suggest that individual attention ability can be improved over time through experience (e.g., Konzag, 1981) and that experts have optimized the orientation of their visual attention through years of training (Ericsson & Hagemann, 2007). They have developed better "software" (Starkes, 1987, p. 147), meaning more efficient information processing and more extensive knowledge representations, which, among other things, enable them to discover and identify objects or information relevant to decision-making more quickly than novices (Cañal-Bruland et al., 2006; Ericsson et al., 1993).

What Came First?

There are two different explanatory models for the finding that experts show better perceptual and attention performance in their respective sports than novices:

(a) People innately differ with regard to their cognitive abilities and subsequently benefit in their respective sports.
(b) People train and develop their cognitive abilities through sport-specific training.

Most research suggests that (b) is the dominant causal direction.

Assuming that differences in perceptual and attentional performance are preexisting and rather constitute a *selection criterion* in the sport context, the *trainability* of these cognitive abilities must be questioned. However, based on the more widespread assumption that the differences between experts and novices in perception and attention are (at least in part) caused by the years of training, such training should be implemented in a goal- and performance-oriented manner.

Learning Control Questions

Basic:

1. Briefly describe the difference between perception and attention in your own words and substantiate the distinction using examples from the field of sports.
2. What are the characteristics of foveal and peripheral perception? What distinguishes them?

2

3. Use various examples to describe perceptual deception and its importance in sports.
4. What are perceptual illusions? What role do they play in the context of sport?
5. Name the sub-processes of attention. Describe their significance in the context of sport using practical examples.
6. Briefly name and describe some failures of awareness.
7. What is inattentional blindness? Name some influencing factors. To what extent is this phenomenon important in the context of sport?

Advanced:

8. To what extent is unconscious perception relevant in sport?
9. What is an "attention window"? How does the attention window differ in size for sports with different requirements?
10. What is the difference between an internal and external focus of attention? What are advantages and disadvantages of each?

Experts:

11. What is orienting of attention and how is this subprocess of attention relevant in the context of sport?
12. What is selective attention?
13. What is sustained attention? How can it be trained in the context of sport? Give different examples.
14. Describe the occlusion technique. Which conclusions can be drawn from this method?
15. Which perceptual and attentional skills differ between experts and novices in sports and which probably do not?

References

Abernethy, B. (1990). Antisipation in squash: differences in advance cue utilization between expert and novice players. *Journal of Sport Sciences, 8*, 17–34.

Abernethy, B., Baker, J., & Côté, J. (2005). Transfer of pattern recall skills may contribute to the development of sport expertise. *Applied Cognitive Psychology, 19*(6), 705–718.

Abernethy, B., Maxwell, J. P., Masters, R. S. W., van der Kamp, J., & Jackson, R. C. (2007). Attentional processes in skill learning and expert performance. In G. Tenenbaum & R. C. Eklund (Eds.), *Handbook of sport psychology* (3rd ed.). Wiley & Sons.

Abernethy, B., Neal, R. J., & Koning, P. (1994). Visual–perceptual and cognitive differences between expert, intermediate, and novice snooker players. *Applied Cognitive Psychology, 8*, 185–211.

Abernethy, B., & Russell, D. G. (1987). Expert-novice differences in an applied selective attention task. *Journal of Sport Psychology, 9*, 326–345.

Abernethy, B., Wood, J. M., & Parks, S. (1999). Can the anticipatory skills of experts be learned by novices? *Research Quarterly for Exercise and Sport, 70*, 313–318.

Alhaj Ahmad Alaboud, M., Steggemann-Weinrich, Y., Klein-Soetebier, T., Kunde, W., & Weigelt, M. (2012). Täuschungshandlungen im Sport. Eine experimentelle Untersuchung zur Wirkung der Häufigkeitsverteilung auf die Blicktäuschung im Basketball. *Zeitschrift für Sportpsychologie, 19*, 110–121.

Allard, F., & Burnett, N. (1985). Skill in sport. *Canadian Journal of Psychology/Revue canadienne de psychologie, 39*(2), 294.

Awh, E., Vogel, E. K., & Oh, S.-H. (2006). Interactions between attention and working memory. *Neuroscience, 139*, 201–208.

Ball, K. K., & Owsley, C. (1993). The useful field of view test: A new technique for evaluating age-related declines in visual function. *Journal of the American Optometric Association, 63*, 71–79.

Bar, M., & Biederman, I. (1998). Subliminal visual priming. *Psychological Science, 9*, 464–469.

Bates, T., & Stough, C. (1997). Processing speed, attention, and intelligence: effects of spatial attention on decision time in high and low IQ subjects. *Personality and Individual Differences, 23*(5), 861–868.

Beanland, V., & Pammer, K. (2010). Looking without seeing or seeing without looking? Eye movement in sustained inattentional blindness. *Vision Research, 50*, 977–988.

Beilock, S. L., Berenthal, B. I., McCoy, A. M., & Carr, T. H. (2004). Haste does not always make waste: Expertise, direction of attention, and speed versus accuracy in performing sensorimotor skills. *Psychonomic Bulletin & Review, 11*, 373–379.

Beilock, S. L., Carr, T. H., MacMahon, C., & Starkes, J. L. (2002). When paying attention becomes counterproductive: Impact of divided versus skill-focused attention of novice and experienced performance of sensorimotor skills. *Journal of Experimental Psychology: Applied, 8*, 6–16.

Blundell, N. L. (1985). The contribution of vision to the learning and performance of sports skills: Part 1: The role of selected visual parameters. *The Australian Journal of Science and Medicine in Sport, 17*, 3–11.

Borgeaud, P., & Abernethy, B. (1987). Skilled perception in volleyball defense. *Journal of Sport Psychology, 9*, 400–406.

Brault, S., Bideau, B., Kulpa, R., & Craig, C. M. (2012). Detecting deception in movement: the case of the side-step in rugby. *PLoS One, 7*, e37494.

Bredemeier, K., & Simons, D. J. (2012). Working memory and inattentional blindness. *Psychonomic Bulletin & Review, 19*, 239–244.

Bruce, V., Green, P. R., & Georgeson, M. A. (1996). *Visual perception: Physiology, psychology, and ecology* (3rd ed.). Psychology Press.

Cañal-Bruland, R. (2007). Das Hinweisreizparadigma—sportpsychologische Anwendungen im Überblick. *Zeitschrift für Sportpsychologie, 14*, 53–66.

Cañal-Bruland, R., Hagemann, N., & Strauß, B. (2005). Aufmerksamkeitsbasiertes Wahrnehmungstraining zur taktischen Entscheidungsschulung im Fußball. *Zeitschrift für Sportpsychologie, 12*, 39–47.

Cañal-Bruland, R., Hagemann, N., & Strauß, B. (2006). Wahrnehmungstraining im Sport. In M. Tietjens & B. Strauß (Hrsg.), *Handbuch Sportpsychologie* (S. 262–268). Schorndorf: Hofmann.

Cañal-Bruland, R., Hagemann, N., & Strauß, B. (2007). Videobasierte Wahrnehmungstrainings—praktischer Nutzen für Sportler und Schiedsrichter. *Spectrum der Sportwissenschaften, 19*, 51–64.

Cañal-Bruland, R., & Schmidt, M. (2009). Response bias in judging deceptive movements. *Acta Psychologica, 130*, 235–240.

Cañal-Bruland, R., van der Kamp, J., & van Kesteren, J. (2010). An examination of motor and perceptual contributions to the rec-

ognition of deception from others' actions. *Human Movement Science, 29*(1), 94–102.
Castaneda, B., & Gray, R. (2007). Effects of focus of attention on baseball batting performance in players of differing skill levels. *Journal of Sport and Exercise Psychology*, *29*(1), 60–77.
Castiello, U., & Umiltà, C. (1992a). Orienting of attention in volley-ball players. *International Journal of Sport Psychology, 23*, 301–310.
Castiello, U., & Umiltà, C. (1992b). Splitting focal attention. *Journal of Experimental Psychology: Human Perception and Performance, 18*, 837–848.
Chabris, C., & Simons, D. (2010). *The invisible gorilla: And other ways our intuitions deceive us*. Crown Publishing Group.
Chabris, C., Weinberger, A., Fontaine, M., & Simons, D. (2011). You do not talk about Fight Club if you do not notice Fight Club: Inattentional blindness for a simulated real-world assault. *i-Perception, 2*, 150–153.
Chauvel, G., Wulf, G., & Maquestiaux, F. (2015). Visual illusions can facilitate sport skill learning. *Psychological Bulletin & Review, 22*, 717–721.
Cohen, M. A., Nakayama, K., Konkle, T., Stantic, M., & Alvarez, G. A. (2015). Visual aware- ness is limited by the representational architecture of the visual system. *Journal of Cognitive Neuroscience, 27*, 2240–2252.
Coull, J. T. (1998). Neural correlates of attention and arousal: insights from electrophysiology, functional neuroimaging and psychopharmacology. *Progress in Neurobiology, 55*, 343–361.
Dehaene, S., Changeux, J.-P., Naccache, L., Sackur, J., & Sergent, C. (2006). Conscious, pre-conscious, and subliminal processing: A testable taxonomy. *Trends in Cognitive Sciences, 10*, 204–211.
Dehaene, S., & Naccache, L. (2001). Towards a cognitive neuroscience of consciousness: Basic evidence and a workspace framework. *Cognition, 79*, 1–37.
Dehaene, S., Naccache, L., Le Clec'H, G., Koechlin, E., Mueller, M., Dehaene-Lambertz, G., et al. (1998). Imaging unconscious semantic priming. *Nature, 395*, 597–600.
Dell'Acqua, R., & Grainger, J. (1999). Unconscious semantic priming from pictures. *Cognition, 73*, B1–B15.
Downing, P. E., Bray, D., Rogers, J., & Childs, C. (2004). Bodies capture attention when nothing is expected. *Cognition, 93*, B27–B38.
Dunton, A., O'Neill, C., Jermyn, S., Dawson, D., & Coughlan, E. (2019). The Impact of Spatial Occlusion Goggles on the Basketball Crossover Dribble. *European Journal of Sports & Exercise Science, 7*(1), 20–30.
Eitam, B., Shoval, R., & Yeshurun, Y. (2015). Seeing without knowing: task relevance dissociates between visual awareness and recognition. *Annals of the New York Academy of Sciences, 1339*, 125–137.
Enns, J., & Richards, J. (1997). Visual attentional orienting in developing hockey players. *Journal of Experimental Child Psychology, 64*, 255–275.
Ericsson, K. A., & Hagemann, N. (2007). Der "Expert-Performance-Approach" zur Erklärung von sportlichen Höchstleistungen: Auf der Suche nach deliberate practice zur Steigerung der sportlichen Leistung. In N. Hagemann, M. Tietjens, & B. Strauß (Eds.), *Psychologie der sportlichen Höchstleistung. Grundlagen und Anwendungen der Expertiseforschung im Sport* (pp. 17–39). Hogrefe.
Ericsson, K. A., Krampe, R. T., & Tesch-Römer, C. (1993). The role of deliberate practice in the acquisition of expert performance. *Psychological Review, 100*, 363–406.
Eriksen, C. W., & Hoffman, J. E. (1974). Selective attention: Noise suppression or signal enhancement? *Bulletin of the Psychonomic Society, 4*(6), 587–589.
Farrow, D., & Abernethy, B. (2002). Can anticipatory skills be learned through implicit video-based perceptual training? *Journal of Sports Sciences, 20*, 471–485.
Farrow, D., Abernethy, B., & Jackson, R. C. (2005). Probing expert anticipation with the temporal occlusion paradigm: Experimental investigations of some methodological issues. *Motor Control, 9*(3), 332–351.
Fechner, G. T. (1860). *Über einige Verhältnisse des binocularen Sehens* (Vol. 3). S. Hirzel.
Fernandez-Duque, D., & Posner, M. I. (1997). Relating the mechanisms of orienting and alerting. *Neuropsychologica, 35*(4), 477–486.
Furley, P., & Memmert, D. (2005). Provozieren vor instruieren! Zur Aufmerksamkeitsfokussierung im Sportspiel. *Sportpraxis, 6*, 22–24.
Furley, P., & Memmert, D. (2010). The role of working memory in sports. *International Review of Sport and Exercise Psychology, 3*, 171–194.
Gainotti, G. (2012). Unconscious processing of emotions and the right hemisphere. *Neuropsychologia, 50*(2), 205–218.
Glover, S. R. (2002). Visual illusions affect planning but not control. *Trends in Cognitive Sciences, 6*, 288–292.
Goodale, M. A., & Milner, A. D. (1992). Separate visual pathways for perception and action. *Trends in Neurosciences, 15*, 20–25.
Gray, R. (2004). Attending to the execution of a complex sensorimotor skill: Expertise differences, choking, and slumps. *Journal of Experimental Psychology: Applied, 10*, 42–54.
Gray, R. (2011). Links between attention, performance pressure, and movement in skilled motor action. *Current Directions in Psychological Science, 20*, 301–306.
Hagemann, N., & Memmert, D. (2006). Coaching anticipatory skill in badminton: laboratory-versus field-based perceptual training? *Journal of Human Movements Studies, 50*, 381–398.
Hagemann, N., & Strauß, B. (2006). Perzeptive Expertise von Badmintonspielern. *Zeitschrift für Psychologie, 214*, 37–47.
Helsen, W. F., & Pauwels, J. M. (1993). The relationship between expertise and visual information processing in sport. In J. L. Starkes & F. Allard (Eds.), *Cognitive issues in motor expertise* (pp. 109–134). North-Holland.
Henry, G., Dawson, B., Lay, B., & Young, W. (2012). Effects of a feint on reactive agility performance. *Journal of Sports Sciences, 30*, 787–795.
Hughes, P. K., Blundell, N. L., & Walters, J. M. (1993). Visual and psychomotor performance of elite, intermediate and novice table tennis competitors. *Clinical and Experimental Optometry, 76*, 51–60.
Hüttermann, S., & Memmert, D. (2012). Moderate movement, more vision: Effects of physical exercise on inattentional blindness. *Perception, 41*, 963–975.
Hüttermann, S., Memmert, D., & Simons, D. J. (2014). The size and shape of the attentional "spotlight" varies with differences in sports expertise. *Journal of Experimental Psychology: Applied, 20*, 147–157.
Hüttermann, S., Memmert, D., Simons, D. J., & Bock, O. (2013). Fixation strategy influences the ability to focus attention on two spatially separate objects. *PLoS One, 8*, e65673.
Hyman, I. E., Boss, S. M., Wise, B. M., McKenzie, K. E., & Caggiano, J. M. (2010). Did you see the unicycling clown? Inattentional blindness while walking and talking on a cell phone. *Applied Cognitive Psychology, 24*, 597–607.
Jackson, R. C., & Farrow, D. (2005). Implicit perceptual training: How, when and why? *Human Movement Science, 24*, 308–325.
Jackson, R. C., Warren, S., & Abernethy, B. (2006). Anticipation skill and susceptibility to deceptive movement. *Acta Psychologica, 3*, 355–371.
Kibele, A. (2006). Non-consciously controlled decision making for fast motor reactions in sports—A priming approach for motor responses to non-consciously perceived movement features. *Psychology of Sport and Exercise, 7*(6), 591–610.
Kiefer, M., Ansorge, U., Haynes, J.-D., Hamker, F., Mattler, U., Verleger, R., & Niedeggen, M. (2011). Neuro-cognitive mecha-

nisms of conscious and unconscious visual perception: From a plethora of phenomena to general principles. *Advances in Cognitive Psychology, 7*, 55–67.

Kiss, M., & Eimer, M. (2008). ERPs reveal subliminal processing of fearful faces. *Psychophysiology, 45*(2), 318–326.

Knudsen, E. (2007). Fundamental components of attention. *Annual Review of Neuroscience, 30*, 57–78.

Koivisto, M., & Revonsuo, A. (2007). How meaning shapes seeing. *Psychological Science, 18*, 845–849.

Konzag, G. (1981). Zur Bedeutung und Diagnostik der Distribution und Konzentration der Aufmerksamkeit von Sportspielen. In H. Schellenberger (Ed.), *Psychologie im Sportspiel* (pp. 36–59). Sportverlag.

Kouider, S., & Dehaene, S. (2009). Subliminal number priming within and across the visual and auditory modalities. *Experimental Psychology, 56*, 418–433.

Kreitz, C., Furley, P., Memmert, D., & Simons, D. J. (2015a). Inattentional blindness and individual differences in cognitive abilities. *PLoS One, 10*, e0134675.

Kreitz, C., Schnuerch, R., Gibbons, H., & Memmert, D. (2015b). Some see it, some don't: Exploring the relation between inattentional blindness and personality factors. *PLoS One, 10*, e0128158.

Lehr, D. (2009). *The fence: A police cover-up along Boston's racial divide*. Harper-Collins.

Lum, J., Enns, J. T., & Pratt, J. (2002). Visual orienting in the college athletes: Explorations of athlete type and gender. *Research Quarterly for Exercise and Sport, 73*, 156–167.

Mack, A., & Rock, I. (1998). *Inattentional blindness*. MIT Press.

Magill, R. A. (1998). Knowledge is more than we can talk about: Implicit learning in motor skill acquisition. *Research Quarterly for Exercise and Sport, 69*, 104–110.

Marr, D. (1982). *Vision. A computational investigation into the human representation and processing of visual information*. W.H. Freeman.

Masters, R. S. W., van der Kamp, J., & Jackson, R. C. (2007). Imperceptibly off-centre goalkeepers influence penalty-kick direction in soccer. *Psychological Science, 18*, 222–223.

Maxeiner, J. (1988). *Aufmerksamkeit und Sport. Sportpsychologie, 4*, 16–19.

McAuliffe, J. E. (2004). Differences in attentional set between athletes and non-athletes. *Journal of General Psychology, 131*, 426–437.

Memmert, D. (2006). The effects of eye movements, age, and expertise on inattentional blindness. *Consciousness and Cognition, 15*, 620–627.

Memmert, D. (2007). Can creativity be improved by an attention-broadening training program?—An exploratory study focusing on team sports. *Creativity Research Journal, 19*, 281–292.

Memmert, D. (2009). Pay attention! A review of attentional expertise in sport. *International Review of Sport & Exercise Psychology, 2*, 119–138.

Memmert, D. (2010). Creativity, expertise, and attention: Exploring their development and their relationships. *Journal of Sport Science, 29*, 93–104.

Memmert, D. (2014a). Inattentional blindness to unexpected events in 8-15-year-olds. *Cognitive Development, 32*, 103–109.

Memmert, D. (2014b). Training der Aufmerksamkeitsausrichtung und -lenkung im Sportspiel. In K. Zentgraf & J. Munzert (Eds.), *Kognitives Training im Sport* (pp. 117–136). Hogrefe Verlag.

Memmert, D., & Furley, P. (2007). "I spy with my little eye!"—Breadth of attention, inattentional blindness, and tactical decision making in team sports. *Journal of Sport & Exercise Psychology, 29*, 365–347.

Memmert, D., Simons, D. J., & Grimme, T. (2009). The relationship between visual attention and expertise in sports. *Psychology of Sport & Exercise, 10*, 146–151.

Mendoza, J., Hansen, S., Glazebrook, C. M., Keetch, K. M., & Elliott, D. (2005). Visual illusions affect both movement planning and on-line control: a multiple cue position on bias and goal-directed action. *Human Movement Science, 24*, 760–773.

Michaels, C. F., & Oudejans, R. R. (1992). The optics and actions of catching fly balls: Zeroing out optical acceleration. *Ecological Psychology, 4*(4), 199–222.

Mirsky, A. F., Anthony, B. J., Duncan, C. C., Ahearn, M. B., & Kellam, S. G. (1991). Analysis of the elements of attention: A neuropsychological approach. *Neuropsychological Review, 2*, 109–145.

Moran, A. (2004). Attention and concentration training in sport. In C. Spielberger (Ed.), *Encyclopaedia of applied psychology* (pp. 209–215). Academic Press.

Moran, A. P. (1996). *The psychology of concentration in sport performers: a cognitive analysis*. Psychology Press.

Moran, A. P. (2003). *The state of concentration skills training in applied sport psychology*. In Greenlees & A. P. Moran (Eds.), *Concentration skills training in sport* (pp. 7–19). British Psychological Society.

Moran, A. P. (2009). Attention, concentration, and thought management. In B. Brewer (Ed.), *The olympic handbook of sports medicine and science: sport psychology* (pp. 18–29). Wiley-Blackwell.

Moran, A. P. (2011). Concentration. In T. Morris & P. Terry (Eds.), *The new sport and exercise psychology companion* (pp. 309–326). Fitness Information Technology.

Most, S. B., Simons, D. J., Scholl, B. J., Jimenez, R., Clifford, E., & Chabris, C. F. (2001). How not to be seen: The contribution of similarity and selective ignoring to sustained inattentional blindness. *Psychological Science, 12*, 9–17.

Müller, S., Abernethy, B., & Farrow, D. (2006). How do world-class cricket batsmen anticipate a bowler's intention? *Quarterly Journal of Experimental Psychology, 59*, 2162–2186.

Naccache, L., Gaillard, R., Adam, C., Hasboun, D., Clemenceau, S., Baulac, M., et al. (2005). A direct intracranial record of emotions evoked by subliminal words. *Proceedings of the National Academy of Sciences, 102*, 7713–7717.

Nobre, A. C. (2001). Orienting of attention to instants in time. *Neuropsychologia, 29*, 1317–1328.

Noël, B., van der Kamp, J., & Memmert, D. (2015). Implicit goalkeeper influences on goal side selection in representative penalty kicking tasks. *PLoS One, 10*(8), e0135423.

Nougier, V., Ripoll, H., & Stein, J. F. (1989). Orienting of attention with highly skilled athletes. *International Journal of Sport Psychology, 20*, 205–223.

Nougier, V., & Rossi, B. (1999). The development of expertise in the orienting of attention. *International Journal of Sport Psychology, 30*, 246–260.

Nougier, V., Rossi, B., Alain, C., & Taddei, F. (1996). Evidence for strategic effects in the modulation of the orienting of attention. *Ergonomics, 39*, 1119–1133.

Oudejans, R. R. D., Michaels, C. F., Bakker, F. C., & Dolné, M. A. (1996). The relevance of action in perceiving affordances: Perception of catchableness of fly balls. *Journal of Experimental Psychology: Human Perception and Performance, 22*(4), 879–891.

Panchuk, D., Davids, K., Sakadjian, A., MacMahon, C., & Parrington, L. (2013). Did you see that? Dissociating advanced visual information and ball flight constrains perception and action processes during one-handed catching. *Acta psychologica, 142*(3), 394–401.

Pélisson, D., Prablanc, C., Goodale, M. A., & Jeannerod, M. (1986). Visual control of reaching movements without vision of the limb. *Experimental Brain Research, 62*(2), 303–311.

Pesce Anzeneder, C., & Bösel, R. (1998). Modulation of the spatial extent of the attentional focus in high-level volleyball players. *The European Journal of Cognitive Psychology, 10*, 247–267.
Posner, M. I. (1980). Orienting of attention. *Quarterly Journal of Experimental Psychology, 32*, 3–25.
Posner, M. I., & Boies, S. J. (1971). Components of attention. *Psychological Review, 78*, 391–408.
Posner, M. I., & Driver, J. (1992). The neurobiology of selective attention. *Current Opinion in Neurobiology, 2*, 165–169.
Posner, M. I., & Peterson, S. E. (1990). The attention system of the human brain. *Annual Review of Neuroscience, 13*, 25–42.
Raymond, J. E., Shapiro, K. L., & Arnell, K. M. (1992). Temporary suppression of visual pro- cessing in an RSVP task: an attentional blink? *Journal of Experimental Psychology: Human Perception and Performance, 18*, 849–860.
Renshaw, I., & Fairweather, M. M. (2000). Cricket bowling deliveries and the discrimination ability of professional and amateur batters. *Journal of Sports Sciences, 18*, 951–957.
Rensink, R. A. (2015). A function-centered taxonomy of visual attention. In P. Coates & S. Coleman (Eds.), *Phenomenal qualities: Sense, perception, & consciousness*. University Press.
Rensink, R. A., O'Regan, J. K., & Clark, J. J. (1997). To see or not to see: The need for attention to perceive changes in scenes. *Psychological Science, 8*, 368–373.
Ripoll, H. (1991). The understanding-acting process in sport: The relationship between the semantic and the sensorimotor visual function. *International Journal of Sport Psychology, 22*, 221–250.
Rosengren, K. S., Pick, H. L., & von Hofsten, C. (1988). Role of visual information in ball catching. *Journal of Motor Behavior, 20*(2), 150–164.
Rowe, R., Horswill, M. S., Kronvall-Parkinson, M., Poulter, D. R., & McKenna, F. P. (2009). The effect of disguise on novice and expert tennis players' anticipation ability. *Journal of Applied Sport Psychology, 21*, 178–185.
Rowe, R. M., & McKenna, F. P. (2001). Skilled anticipation in real-world tasks: measurement of attentional demands in the domain of tennis. *Journal of Experimental Psychology. Applied, 7*, 60–67.
Ryu, D., Abernethy, B., Mann, D. L., & Poolton, J. M. (2015). The contributions of central and peripheral vision to expertise in basketball: how blur helps to provide a clearer picture. *Journal of Experimental Psychology: Human Perception and Performance, 41*(1), 167–185.
Ryu, D., Abernethy, B., Mann, D. L., Poolton, J. M., & Gorman, A. D. (2013). The role of central and peripheral vision in expert decision making. *Perception, 42*, 591–607.
Ryu, D., Mann, D. L., Abernethy, B., & Poolton, J. M. (2016). Gaze-contingent training enhances perceptual skill acquisition. *Journal of Vision, 21*(2), 1–21.
Schapschröer, M., Holzhey, C., Bund, A., & Sickenberger, W. (2011). Trainierbarkeit der visuellen Wahrnehmung im Sport. *DOZ Optometrie, 1*, 92–96.
Schmidt, R., & Lee, T. (2005). *Motor control and learning: A behavioural emphasis* (4th ed.). Human Kinetics.
Schmidt, R., & Wrisberg, C. (2008). *Motor learning and performance* (4th ed.). Human Kinetics.
Schnuerch, R., Kreitz, C., Gibbons, H., & Memmert, D. (2016). Not quite so blind: Semantic processing despite inattentional blindness. *Journal of Experimental Psychology: Human Perception and Performance, 42*, 459–463.
Schweizer, K., Zimmermann, P., & Koch, W. (2000). Sustained attention, intelligence, and the crucial role of perceptual processes. *Learning and Individual Differences, 12*, 271–286.
Shapiro, K. L., Arnell, K. M., & Raymond, J. E. (1997). The attentional blink. *Trends in Cognitive Sciences, 1*, 291–296.
Simons, D. J., & Chabris, C. F. (1999). Gorillas in our midst: Sustained inattentional blindness for dynamic events. *Perception, 28*, 1059–1074.
Simons, D. J., & Levin, D. T. (1997). Change blindness. *Trends in Cognitive Sciences, 1*, 261–267.
Smeeton, N. J., & Williams, A. M. (2012). The role of movement exaggeration in the anticipation of deceptive soccer penalty kicks. *British Journal of Psychology, 103*, 539–555.
Smeeton, N. J., Williams, A. M., Hodges, N. J., & North, J. (2004). Developing perceptual skill in tennis through explicit, guided-discovery, and discovery methods. *Journal of Sport & Exercise Psychology, 24*(Suppl), 175.
Starkes, J. L. (1987). Skill in field hockey: The nature of the cognitive advantage. *Journal of Sport Psychology, 9*, 146–160.
Styles, E. A. (2008). *The Psychology of Attention*. Psychology Press.
Tayler, M. A., Burwitz, L., & Davids, K. (1994). Coaching perceptual strategy in badminton. *Journal of Sports Sciences, 12*, 213.
Tennenbaum, G., & Bar-Eli, M. (1995). Contemporary issues in exercise and sport psychology research. In S. J. H. Biddle (Ed.), *European perspectives on sport and exercise psychology* (pp. 292–323). Human Kinetics.
Theeuwes, J. (2010). Top-down and bottom-up control of visual selection. *Acta Psychologica, 135*, 77–99.
Treisman, A., & Gelade, G. (1980). A feature-integration theory of attention. *Cognitive Psychology, 12*, 97–136.
Turatto, M., Benso, F., & Umiltà, C. (1999). Focusing of attention in professional women skiers. *International Journal of Sport Psychology, 30*, 339–349.
Van Zomeren, A. H., & Brouwer, W. H. (1994). *Clinical neuropsychology of attention*. Oxford University Press.
von Hofsten, C., Rosengren, K., Pick, H. L., & Neely, G. (1992). The role of binocular information in ball catching. *Journal of Motor Behavior, 24*(4), 329–338.
Weigelt, M., Güldenpenning, I., Steggemann-Weinrich, Y., Alhaj Ahmad Alaboud, M., & Kunde, W. (2017). Control over the processing of the opponent's gaze direction in basketball experts. *Psychonomic Bulletin & Review, 24*(3), 828–834.
Weigelt, M., & Memmert, D. (2012). Goal-side selection in soccer penalty kicking when viewing natural scenes. *Frontiers in Psychology, 3*, 312.
Weigelt, M., Memmert, D., & Schack, T. (2012). Kick it like Ballack: the effects of goalkeeping gestures on goal-side selection in experienced soccer players and soccer novices. *Journal of Cognitive Psychology, 24*, 942–956.
West, K. L., & Bressan, E. S. (1996). The effects of a general versus specific visual skills training program on accuracy in judging length-of-ball in cricket. *International Journal of Sports Vision, 3*, 41–45.
Whiting, H. T. A., Gill, E. B., & Stephenson, J. M. (1970). Critical time intervals for taking in flight information in a ball-catching task. *Ergonomics, 13*(2), 265–272.
Williams, A. M., & Davids, K. (1998). Visual search strategy, selective attention and expertise in soccer. *Research Quarterly for Exercise and Sport, 69*, 111–128.
Williams, A. M., Davids, K., Burwitz, L., & Williams, J. G. (1994). Visual search strategies in experienced and inexperienced soccer players. *Research Quarterly for Exercise and Sport, 65*, 127–135.
Williams, A. M., Davids, K., & Williams, J. G. P. (1999). *Visual perception and action in sport*. Taylor & Francis.
Williams, A. M., Huys, R., Canal-Bruland, R., & Hagemann, N. (2009). The dynamical information underpinning anticipation skill. *Human Movement Science, 28*, 362–370.
Williams, A. M., Ward, P., & Chapman, C. (2003). Training perceptual skill in field hockey: Is there transfer from the laboratory to the field? *Research Quarterly for Exercise and Sport, 74*, 98–103.

Williams, A. M., Ward, P., Knowles, J. M., & Smeeton, N. J. (2002). Anticipation skill in a real-world task: Measurement, training, and transfer in tennis. *Journal of Experimental Psychology: Applied, 8*, 259–270.
Williams, J. M., & Andersen, M. B. (1997). Psychosocial influences on central and peripheral vision and reaction time during demaning tasks. *Behavioral Medicine, 22*, 160–167.
Williams, M., & Davids, K. (1995). Declarative knowledge in sport: A by-product of experience or a characteristic of expertise? *Journal of Sport and Exercise Psychology, 17*, 259–259.
Witt, J. K., Linkenauger, S. A., & Proffitt, D. R. (2011). Get me out of this slump! Visual illusions improve sports performance. *Psychological Science, 23*, 397–399.
Wulf, G. (2007). *Attention and motor skill learning*. Human Kinetics.
Wulf, G., McConnel, N., Gärtner, M., & Schwarz, A. (2002). Feedback and attentional focus: Enhancing the learning of sport skills through external-focus feedback. *Journal of Motor Behavior, 34*, 171–182.
Wulf, G., & Prinz, W. (2001). Directing attention to movement effects enhances learning: A review. *Psychonomic Bulletin & Review, 8*, 648–660.
Wulf, G., Shea, C. H., & Park, J.-H. (2001). Attention in motor learning: Preferences for and advantages of an external focus. *Research Quarterly for Exercise and Sport, 72*, 335–344.

Learning and Memory in Sports

Matthias Weigelt, Daniel Krause and Iris Güldenpenning

Contents

J. Schüler et al. (eds.), *Sport and Exercise Psychology*, https://doi.org/10.1007/978-3-031-03921-8_3

Learning Objectives

Basic:

- To understand the psychological foundations of learning and memory

Advanced:

- To differentiate and describe learning mechanisms and memory processes
- To evaluate practice variables and their effects on learning outcomes in sports

Experts:

- To understand how sport skills are stored and represented in memory

3

3.1 Introduction

Learning and memory are prerequisites for the acquisition, storage, and recall of sport skills. The chapter deals with the psychological foundations of learning and memory. It introduces the central concepts of the psychology of learning and memory and presents the basic theories and models. Furthermore, the most important aspects of the design of teaching and learning processes in sport are discussed, and the representation of complex sport skills is presented. The aim of the chapter is to provide a basic introduction to the topics of learning and memory in sport.

3.2 Fundamentals of the Psychology of Learning

Learning is mirrored in the permanent changes of people's behavior. Such changes are the result of experiences made through simple repetition, systematic training or observation (cf. Squire, 1992). Through experience, people can continuously adapt to changes in their natural and social environment ("learning as adaptation"). According to this common assumption, one can observe from the behavior of other people whether they have learned (or not learned). However, this presupposes the application of the learnt in the execution of behavior. This is referred to as **performance**. Learning can, however, also already be initiated with those changes in the behavioral potential that result from the acquisition of knowledge ("learning as knowledge acquisition"). This also includes learning about regularities, for example, which events are caused by one's own or other's actions in the environment. In this sense, this is referred to as **acquisition**. Whether a behavior is carried out after the acquisition (and thus observable) depends further on external incentives and the varying motivation of a person (Selg & Schermer, 2015; Chaps. 7 and 8).

Learning

Learning refers to a relatively permanent change in a person's behavior or behavioral potential, based on experience and knowledge acquisition.

Learning as Change

Often, learning is perceived primarily as an improvement of knowledge (e.g., language, spelling, and mathematical formulae) and skills (e.g., sewing, cycling, and baking bread), which are associated with an increase in performance in a particular area of life. However, the term should be used broader. For example, learning also means the loss of knowledge or the decrease in the performance of a skill. The latter is not only important in a sport or academic context but also in everyday life. That is, whenever previously learned material is not repeated over a certain period of time, then performance deteriorates again. This means that experience-related changes also occur when experience in a particular field is lacking.

3.2.1 Learning by Association

An essential learning mechanism is based on building links between events (Squire & Kandel, 1999). These connections are called **associations** in learning psychology. Associations can be formed between two events in the environment (e.g., lightning followed by thunder) or between one's own behavior and the resulting effects in the environment (e.g., an inside kick in soccer and a flat trajectory of the ball) (*law of effect*). This elementary learning mechanism enables us, for example, to predict thunder and to protect ourselves after lightning by rushing into a house entrance or to anticipate the lower left corner of the goal for a penalty kick and to shoot the soccer ball with an inside kick (▶ Sect. 3.2.1.3). The strength of association between two events is determined by how reliably they occur together. If two events regularly occur together or in quick succession, then a strong association between these events is formed. In addition to the temporal and spatial proximity of two events (**contiguity**), associations can also be based on their **similarity** or their **contrast**. The formation of associations plays an important role in a number of theories of learning psychology, such as classical conditioning, instrumental learning, observational learning, or implicit learning.

Associations

An association is the elementary connection between two events, based on the laws of contiguity, similarity, and contrast.

Law of Effect

The law of effect goes back to the work of Edward L. Thorndike (1911). According to this law, in certain situations (S), those reactions (R) are strengthened, which repeatedly lead to positive consequences (C). In contrast, those reactions that are not accompanied by positive consequences will be less frequently selected or suppressed in the same situation in the future. This is based on the acquisition of S-R compounds, with a higher associative strength for successful reactions than for unsuccessful reactions.

3.2.1.1 Classical Conditioning

Classical conditioning, as a behavioristic approach to learning, goes back to the observations of Iwan P. Pawlow (1953), who examined salivation in dogs in a series of animal experiments (◘ Fig. 3.1). It starts with innate **reflexes**, which always produce the same reactions to a particular stimulus. Reflexes are therefore elementary S-R connections, which, as **unconditioned stimuli** (US) and **unconditioned responses** (UR), form the basis of human (and animal) behavior. In the case of Pavlov's experiments, the presentation of food (a US) regularly led to a salivation response (an UR). Stimulus and reaction are called unconditioned here, because the presentation of food, as an event in the environment, leads to a physical reaction (i.e., salivation response) in the dog without prior learning. The sound of a bell as a neutral stimulus (NS) initially triggers an orientation reflex in the dog (e.g., putting up the ears). Learning in the sense of classical conditioning occurs when the sound is presented as an additional stimulus together with the food. After some time, this stimulus is associated with the food and can, after a sufficient amount of repetition, also trigger the salivation response alone, which was originally only bound to the US. The sound then acts as a so-called conditioned stimulus (CS), which causes salivary flow as a so-called conditioned response (CR). The basic mechanism of learning by classical conditioning is depicted in ◘ Fig. 3.1.

Important aspects, which influence learning in terms of classical conditioning, are contiguity, stimulus generalization, stimulus discrimination, and extinction. For

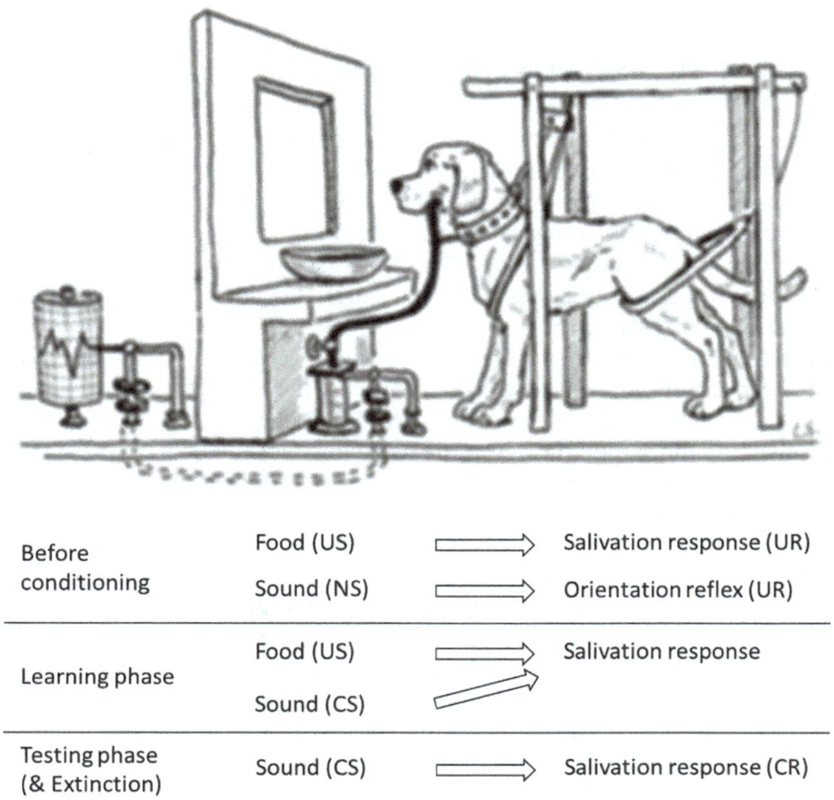

◘ **Fig. 3.1** Apparatus of the animal experiments conducted by Pavlov (taken from Hoffmann & Engelkamp, 2017) and a schematic depiction of the learning process through classical conditioning. In the testing phase, the sound (CS) triggers a salivation response (CR), which was initially only associated with food (US) before conditioning, after the sound (CS) has been associated with food (US) in the learning phase as long as the CS reliably predicts the US, the CR is generated with the same strength (**contiguity**). **Stimulus generalization** takes place, when the CR is activated by a stimulus, which is similar to the previous CS, at the beginning of the learning process. However, as practice continues, the learner learns to differentiate more and more between the stimuli, up to the point, where only the CS is effective as an imperative, triggering stimulus (**stimulus discrimination**). Finally, **extinction** refers to the decrease of the CR, when the CS is no longer paired with the US. In this case, the learner learns that when presenting the CS, the US will not occur, which leads to the extinction of the CR.

Reflex

A reflex is an innate S-R connection, that is, a certain stimulus is always followed by the same physical reaction.

Classical Conditioning

Classical conditioning is a learning process, which is based on the association of a previously neutral stimulus (NS) with an existing connection between an unconditioned stimulus (US) and an unconditioned response (UR), after which the NS, as a conditioned stimulus (CS), leads to a conditioned response (CR).

3.2.1.2 Instrumental Learning (Operant Conditioning)

Instrumental learning (also known as operant conditioning) is also based on Thorndike's (1911) associative learning approach. According to the "law of effect", S-R connections are strengthened when they are accompanied by positive consequences. This was first shown in animal studies on the behavior of cats. Thorndike observed that cats learned to pull on a rope and then push a pedal to free themselves from a cage, according to the **principle of trial and error**. For this, they were rewarded with food outside the cage. When the cats received no more food, however, the behavior weakened again, followed by the extinction of the S-R connections. Thorndike (1911) assumed that the respective reward (food) only strengthened the S-R connections but was not tied to the associations.

Burrhus F. Skinner (1938) changed this paradigm by associating certain behavioral patterns of animals (rats or pigeons) with either a **reward** (positive stimulus) or a **punishment** (negative stimulus) in his so-called Skinner box (◘ Fig. 3.2). The animals thus learned new S-R connections, which increased or decreased in strength depending on the consequences associated with the behavior. **Positive reinforcement** can be observed when a certain behavior (e.g., lever presses) occurs more often, because it is rewarded with a positive stimulus (e.g., food). If a certain behavior is followed by **punishment** (e.g., electric current), however, then the probability for this behavior to occur in the future is reduced. In a similar way, the withdrawal of a positive stimulus (e.g., taking away food) also acts as a kind of punishment and reduces the corresponding behavior. If, however, a negative stimulus can be removed by a certain behavior (e.g., by switching off the electric current), then the probability of this behavior increases. This is called **negative reinforcement**. Learning is **instrumental** in the sense that the learner acquires knowledge about which operant behavior leads to desired or undesired consequences in the environment.

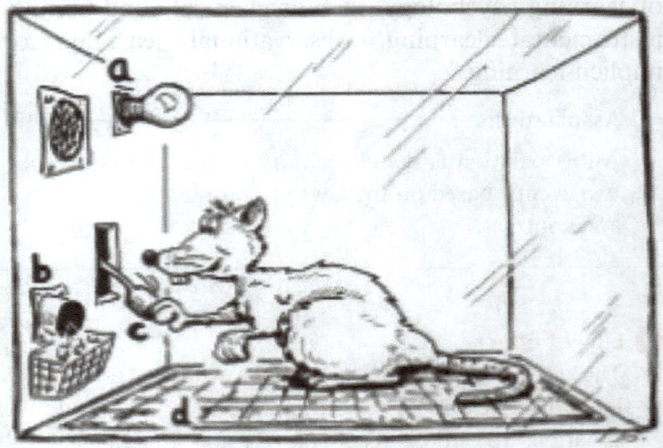

◘ **Fig. 3.2** Depiction of a typical Skinner box, which features **a** a signal light, **b** a food dispenser, **c** a lever, and **d** an electric grid (taken from Hoffmann & Engelkamp, 2017)

Instrumental Learning

During instrumental learning, new behavior is learned through the consequences of behavior, that is, depending on whether a particular association of stimulus and response is reliably rewarded or punished.

3.2.1.3 Learning of Action-Effect Relations

Expanding on the assumptions of Thorndike (1911) and Skinner (1938) on associative learning and instrumental learning, respectively, Joachim Hoffmann (Hoffmann, 1993; Hoffmann et al., 2007) postulated in his "anticipatory behavioral control (ABC)" framework that learning rather depends on the acquisition of complex **situation-**

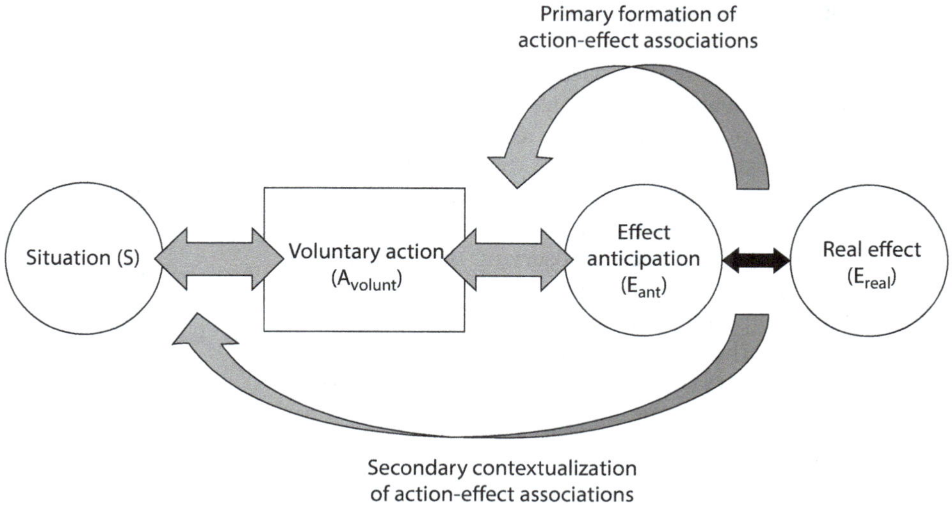

Fig. 3.3 Illustration of the basic framework of action-effect learning that is based on two learning mechanisms, the primary formation of action-effect association and the secondary contextualization of action-effect associations, respectively (adapted from Hoffmann & Engelkamp, 2017)

action effect (SAE) triples. For these SAE triples, the strength of association between **voluntary actions** (A_{volunt}) and **anticipated effects** (E_{ant}) is decisive for the selection of a particular behavior in a given **situation** (S), in order to produce the intended events in the environment (as **real effects** (E_{real})). To this end, those A-E connections are strengthened in the primary learning process, which reliably lead to the desired effect (**primary formation of action-effect associations**). In the secondary learning process, these A-E connections are linked to those situational conditions under which the actions run successfully (**secondary contextualization of action-effect associations**; Fig. 3.3). Based on these learning processes, the counterattack in team handball (as a voluntary action), for example, can be initiated quickly and reliably after a successful goalkeeper parade (situational condition as a triggering stimulus) to score a goal (anticipated effect), for as long as this behavioral routine has been practiced (i.e., learned) in training before. The acquisition of such action-effect relations forms the core of ideomotor approaches to explain human behavior, according to which complex actions are selected depending on intended goal states (Hommel & Nattkemper, 2011; ► Side Story: Anticipative Behavioral Control and flow experience (Hoffmann, 1993)).

Action-Effect Learning

Action-effect relations are established when under certain situational conditions a voluntary behavior reliably leads to the desired event in the environment.

Side Story

Anticipatory Behavioral Control and Flow Experience (Hoffmann, 1993)

In his book entitled *Prediction and Knowledge* (German title *Vorhersage und Erkenntnis*), Joachim Hoffmann (1993) connects the occurrence of predicted behavioral consequences with the so-called flow experience (Csikszentmihalyi, 1985). Such "flow experiences" can happen in sports when a certain action seems to run smoothly and effortlessly and, thus, results in a feeling of deep physical satisfaction. In these situations, athletes are in complete harmony with the environment, and their actions reliably lead to the intended consequences, which is continuously accompanied by positive feedback on one's own actions. The action "is therefore part of a rational system of cause and effect, within which, what it does, has realistic and predictable consequences" (Csikszentmihalyi, 1985, p. 58). One's own physical activity is "in the flow" with the situational conditions that define the frame for behavior as environmental incentives (► Chap. 8).

3

3.2.2 Observational Learning

The development of associations also plays a major role in **observational learning**. However, these are not acquired through one's own activity, as in classical conditioning or in instrumental learning, but by observing other people who perform these actions (as models). Learning is therefore based on those representative experiences, which are made by observing the behavior of others. Because the observation of different models, whose behavioral patterns are imitated, is central to this kind of learning, the term **social cognitive learning** (or social cognitive theory) is often used, which goes back to the work of Albert Bandura (1977).

Social Cognitive Learning

Social cognitive learning is based on the observation of other people, who serve as models and whose behavioral patterns are imitated.

An important prerequisite for social cognitive learning is the ability to **imitate** (Fig. 3.4). For example, it is not difficult for us to try out simple dance steps that we observe in a TV show. This ability to spontaneously imitate an observed behavior is innate. Like the different reflexes, it is part of the basic setup of human (and animal) behavior. For example, newborns already imitate the facial gestures of an adult model person (Meltzoff & Moore, 1977), and preschool children can imitate complex movements (Bekkering et al., 2000) or reproduce action effects, which have been previously generated by an adult model (Gergely et al., 2002).

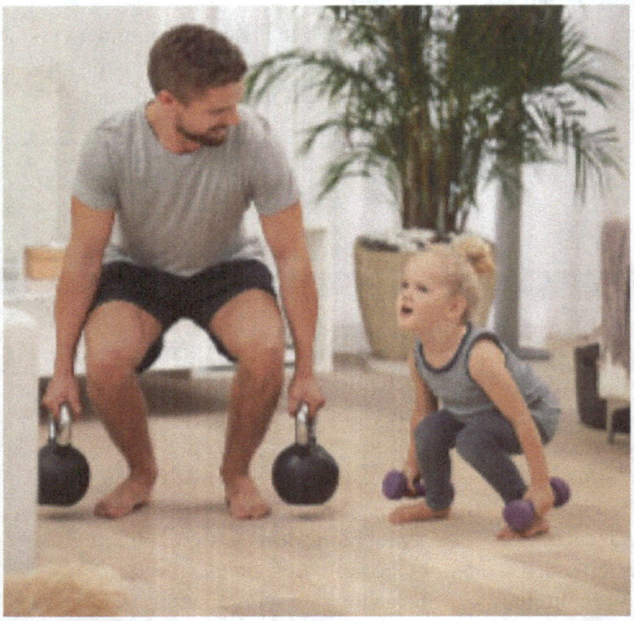

Fig. 3.4 The spontaneous imitation of unfamiliar behavior as a basic learning principle. (© PeopleImages/Getty Images/iStock)

Imitation

Imitation is the spontaneous imitation of an unfamiliar behavior, which is expressed in the reproduction of an observed movement or action effect.

Observational learning goes insofar beyond mere imitation as an instinctive behavior, in that the social consequences of desired or undesired behavior are also taken into account. People copy previously observed behavior of other model persons (e.g., a famous soccer player dives in the penalty area and is awarded a penalty kick), if they hope for a reward and/or recognition in a certain situation (e.g., in case of a slight physical contact in the penalty area, they will also dive to receive a penalty kick). People suppress the same behavior, however, if they fear punishment and/or rejection (e.g., in the same situation, they do not fall, because they had already received a yellow card and want to avoid a second yellow card for diving, which would lead to dismissal).

In Bandura's "social cognitive theory (SCT)" (Bandura, 1977), the imitation of foreign behavior falls into one of three classes of reactions: (1) as a **model effect**, when a new behavior occurs after it has been observed in a model; (2) as an **inhibition or disinhibition effect**, when an undesirable behavior is omitted or a previously inhibited undesirable behavior is displayed after a model has been punished or rewarded; and (3) as a **triggering effect**, when the observation of a model stimulates already acquired behavior in the observer.

According to Bandura (1977), a total of four sub-processes are necessary for social cognitive learning to take place through the observation of a model: the person must perceive the behavior of the model (**attention processes**) and store it (**retention processes**). He or she must also be able to carry out the behavior himself or herself (**reproduction processes**) and be motivated to do so (**motivation processes**). The first two sub-processes control the acquisition; the last two sub-processes are responsible for the performance of the behavioral patterns, which is modeled (Study Box: Bobo Doll Study on Imitating Aggression in Children (Bandura, 1965)).

Case Study

Bobo Doll Study on Imitating Aggression in Children (Bandura, 1965)

The classic finding on observational learning comes from a series of studies from Albert Bandura's laboratory on aggression in preschool children (Bobo doll study; Bandura, 1965). In the Bobo doll study, 4- and 5-year-old children were shown films of a male adult, who behaved verbally or physically aggressive toward a clown doll. The children saw the adult model calling the doll names, hitting, kicking, or lifting the doll up and throwing it onto the floor. After some time, either (A) a second person came into the room, praised the adult for his behavior and gave him sweets; (B) a second person entered the room, blamed the adult for his behavior and punished him with beatings and threats; or (C) the behavior remained uncommented. When the children were then confronted with the plastic doll themselves, they imitated the behavior just observed by the model. Those children, who behaved particularly aggressive, were the ones who had just observed the adult model, which was praised and rewarded. Later, when the experimenter offered children a reward in the form of sweets for their aggressive behavior, all the children showed an increased level of aggression toward the clown doll. This shows that reward and punishment via the mechanisms of operant conditioning also influence social cognitive learning, but the processes of acquisition and performance are affected differently.

3.2.3 Implicit Learning

Implicit learning occurs when learners acquire knowledge without realizing how the acquisition process works. Acquisition is incidental and not influenced by intention. The crucial difference to explicit knowledge acquisition is the absence of awareness. Learning is implicit when people are not aware of the fact that they are learning (Frensch, 2006). A frequently used example is language acquisition. Children learn language and complex grammars long before they acquire explicit knowledge about grammar rules later at school. The same is true for children who learn soccer "on the street" without being specifically instructed about the execution of shooting techniques and the use of offensive and defensive tactics within a training session. Implicit learning has been empirically investigated in experiments on the construction of artificial grammar (Reber, 1989), on learning hidden covariations (Lewicki et al., 1992) or on motor sequence learning (Nissen & Bullemer, 1987). Currently, research on implicit learning is contributing to highlight the role of consciousness in human behavioral control (▶ Side Story: Implicit Learning of Action Sequences).

Side Story

Implicit Learning of Action Sequences

The acquisition of complex sequences of action is often implicit. This is tested in experiments with the so-called serial-reaction-time (SRT) task (Nissen & Bullemer, 1987). For this purpose, participants are presented with stimuli in the form of asterisks at different spatial positions on a screen, one after the other, upon which they must respond with a spatially corresponding reaction (typically with a keystroke). With increasing practice, participants form associations between several elements of the sequence (so-called chunking) and, thus, learn the structural properties of the stimulus-response sequence without being aware of it. This is reflected in shorter SRTs, that is, the individual keystrokes are executed faster for the entire sequence of actions. If the acquired sequence is then replaced by a new sequence in a transfer phase, the SRT rises again. The latter shows that not the mere stimulus-response coupling, but the (whole) action sequence was learned.

3

Implicit Learning

Implicit learning is based on the ability to acquire knowledge without realizing how this knowledge was acquired.

3.3 Designing Teaching and Learning Processes in Sports

Learning processes in sports occur in a variety of fields. These concern not only the acquisition of motor skills but also the acquisition of general knowledge about rules, as well as game and competition tactics. The following sections focus on the field of motor learning. For this, those learning processes will be addressed, which underly the acquisition of motor skills.

3.3.1 Learning Phases and Learning Processes

Motor learning processes represent the changes in memory, relevant for motor control. Corresponding representations change not only in terms of the resulting behavioral competence but also in terms of their **coding** (Hikosaka et al., 1999), the corresponding **neural substrates** (Keele et al., 2003), and the **mode of control** when these representations are recalled for behavioral control (Chein & Schneider, 2012; ◘ Fig. 3.5). There are numerous, mostly two- or three-stage models that differentiate **between early and late learning phases** (e.g., Fitts & Posner, 1967; Chein & Schneider, 2012). According to these models, early phases are dominated by cognitive processes that highly rely on limited information processing resources (e.g., working memory resources). For example, spatially coded representations are postulated, which are recalled at the beginning of a learning process, **depending on working memory** and are gradually transformed into motor commands. In parallel, **working memory independent** representations are also developed (e.g., motor programs; Schmidt, 1976), which usually control motor skills in later phases of learning (Hikosaka et al., 1999). Correspondingly, a **structural shift** in the neuronal substrates (Lohse et al., 2014) and a change in the mode of control, which is less dependent on capacity-limited working memory resources (**non-attentional/automatic control**), can be detected. At the same time, so-called dual-task costs are reduced as learning progresses (Abernethy, 2001; ▶ Methods: Measuring Automatization by Means of Dual-Task Paradigms (Abernethy, 2001).

Methods: Measuring Automatization Using the Dual-Task Paradigm (Abernethy, 2001)

The dual-task paradigm is often used to measure automatization. Here, the motor primary task and a cognitive secondary task (e.g., counting backward in steps of three, tone counting tasks) are tested in single- and dual-task conditions. So-called dual-task costs are determined as the difference in performance between single- and dual-task conditions. High dual-task costs are attributed to a high demand for cognitive control processes, and low dual-task costs are attributed to a high degree of automaticity.

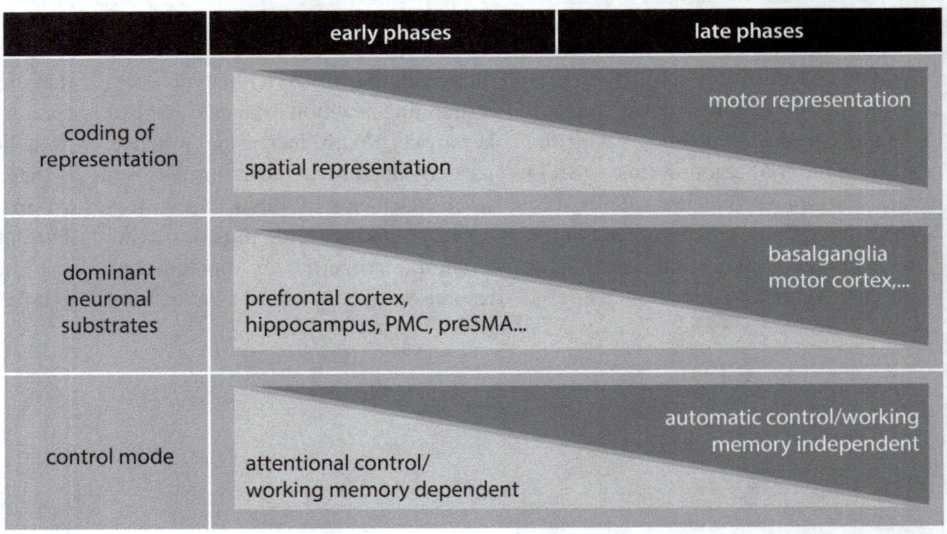

◘ **Fig. 3.5** Changes of the representation of motor skills in early and late phases of learning (mod. Olivier et al., 2013; with permission of Hofmann Publishing)

3.3.2 Instruction and Feedback

Information provided to learners by **extrinsic sources of information** can support or supplement the processing of information perceived by the learners (**intrinsic feedback** based on sensory feedback). A distinction is made here between the future-oriented form of instruction and the past-oriented form of feedback on the movement outcome (**knowledge of results**) or on the movement itself (**knowledge of performance**) (Schmidt et al., 2019). In addition to external persons, such as the coach, external information can be transmitted through various media (e.g., screens, speakers), in various forms of **coding** (e.g., verbal, spatial), and through various **sensory modalities** (e.g., visual, acoustic, kinesthetic, tactile). In the following, selected aspects for providing external information are discussed.

Intrinsic Feedback

Intrinsic feedback refers to sensory impressions that result directly from the execution of the movement.

External Information

External information refers to instructional information and augmented feedback information from external sources (e.g., trainers, videos, diagrams, etc.).

3.3.2.1 Instruction: Variables of Observational Learning

Observational learning is most often based on demonstrations of successful movement executions (e.g., using various forms of video presentation or demonstrations by the instructor). In the case of dynamic-visual demonstrations, it is also referred to as **modeling** (when this practice procedure is deliberately used) or **imitation** (when reenactment occurs rather spontaneously). The observations are processed in two different ways. On the one hand, the observation of the model can result in **visually and spatially coded representations,** which **depend on working memory** and are transformed into motor commands (Rumiati & Tessari, 2002). Thereby, attentional processing requires the learner to select information (i.e., selective attention), because of limited attentional resources. Therefore, attention should be directed to the most relevant elements of the movement. In the case of using screen displays, for example, slow motion, still images, as well as textual and graphical attentional cues can be used to take the limitations of the visual information processing into account. The resulting performance of this **visuomotor transformation process** can thus be significantly increased (Blischke et al., 1999). On the other hand, as well as in addition to this working-memory-dependent route of processing, **ideomotor processes** can also support the imitation of movements. The **mirror neuron system** is regarded as the neuronal substrate for the transformation of visual perceptions into executive motor representations (Fabbri-Destro & Rizzolatti, 2008). Accordingly, action observations evoke corresponding motor representations without the need to immediately execute these movements. The visual perspective of observation modulates these ideomotor effects to a large extent (on the influence of the observation perspective. ◘ Figure 3.6; ► Study Box: Observation Perspective: Neuronal Activation and Imitation Performance).

Case Study

Perspective: Neuronal Activation and Imitation Performance

The observation of hand movements from an egocentric perspective leads to a strong neural resonance of motor representations, where brain areas related to these movements are more activated as compared to when one observes a model person sitting opposite (Jackson et al., 2006). Both, the spatial-temporal imitation of arm movement sequences presented by a video model (Krause & Kobow, 2013) and the comprehension of visual tactical instructions (Koopmann et al., 2017; Krause & Weigelt, 2020) are more effective with low model-observer disparity (◘ Fig. 3.6). Besides the stronger activation of corresponding motor representations in the brain, it can be assumed that an increased model-observer disparity requires mental rotation processes to transform the observation into the own egocentric reference system. Such mental rotation processes seem to interfere with motor planning and execution processes (Wohlschläger, 2001).

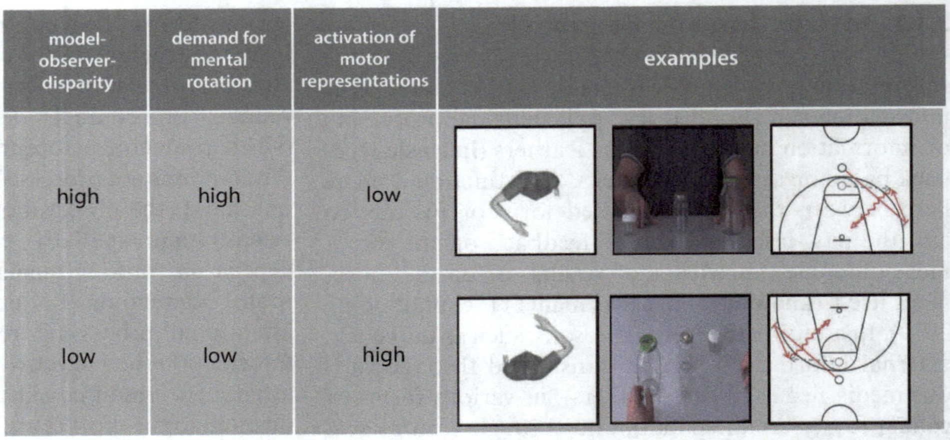

Fig. 3.6 Observational perspectives with varied model-observer-disparity (left, Krause & Kobow, 2013, copyright with permission from Elsevier; middle, Physiofun, 2010, copyright Kaase health GmbH; right, Krause & Weigelt, 2020, copyright with permission from Springer)

In addition to **visual forms of instruction**, which are particularly suitable for conveying corresponding **spatial structures** (Daugs et al., 1989), **acoustic forms of instruction** can also be used, which are particularly suitable for conveying **temporal structures**, since the auditory sense has a very high temporal resolution (Effenberg, 2005). For acoustic instructions, for example, dynamometric or kinematic series of measurements of model movements can be converted to music (so-called sonification). Multimodal models (e.g., audiovisual multimodal models) appear to be particularly effective as compared to unimodal models (e.g., purely visual models) (Effenberg, 2005).

3.3.2.2 Instruction: Focus of Attention

Instructions can be used to direct the **focus of attention** on the body (internal) or on the effects in the environment (external). According to the "constrained action hypothesis" (Wulf et al., 2001), it is assumed that an internal focus of attention tends to induce **attentional, cognitive-dominated control processes** that suppress (constrain) the recall of established automatisms, while an external attention focus leads to more **automatic control**. The latter goes along with a more **efficient execution of movements**, which can have a positive effect on endurance performance, for example in swimming (Freudenheim et al., 2010) or running (Schücker et al., 2009).

> **Internal Focus of Attention**
>
> An internal focus of attention addresses particular aspects of the movement itself (e.g., the arm swing of the tennis serve).

> **External Focus of Attention**
>
> An external focus of attention addresses the action effects, which result from a movement in the environment (e.g., bat-ball contact in baseball).

The impact of the focus of attention on skill acquisition was first shown in the studies of Gabriele Wulf (for a review, see Wulf, 2009). According to these studies, an external focus of attention is generally superior to an internal focus. This can be seen both in the short-term improvement of movement performance (**motor performance**) and in the long-term changes of behavior (**motor learning**). These findings are supported by studies with children, adults, and elderly, as well as patients with various diseases (e.g., Parkinson's disease, stroke, speech disorders). The improved performance due to an external focus of attention is accompanied—among other things—by **more efficient neuromuscular activity and/or coordination**. An external focus of attention benefits novices and experts across a large variety of skills.

3.3.2.3 Instruction: Movement Rules and Analogies

Verbal instructions in the form of **explicit movement rules** can be related to single elements of an action, where the corresponding information details usually require a similar amount of **cognitive effort** to be processed and transformed into a representation. Alternatively, **analogies** can be used as **metaphorical instructions** (e.g., "bend like a bow" at the end of the backswing of a tennis serve). These make it possible to induce a holistic idea of the movement, without all details necessarily becoming conscious and requiring a similar amount of attentional resources during learning and later on, during recall. Instruction by analogies benefits **implicit learning processes** and a rather automatic mode of control (Lam et al., 2009; ▶ Study Box: Analogy Instructions: Robustness in Pressure Situations (e.g., Lam et al., 2009)).

Case Study

Analogy Instructions: Robustness in Pressure Situations (e.g., Lam et al., 2009)

Analogy instructions, like "Shoot as if you are trying to put cookies into a cookie jar on a high shelf!" (set shot in basketball; Lam et al., 2009) and "Move the bat as if it is traveling up the side of a mountain!" (forehand topspin in table tennis; Poolton et al., 2006), induce implicit learning. This is the reason why learners (with comparable acquisition performance) show superior performance in more challenging situations, such as when concurrently solving additional cognitive tasks (i.e., in dual-task scenarios) or when performing under pressure. Learners, on the contrary, who have been trained with explicit movement rules (e.g., "Extend the elbow fully at ball release! Follow-through by snapping wrist forward, so that the palm of shooting hand is facing downward! Release the ball with your fingertips!", Lam et al., 2009) can explicitly describe single movement elements, but due to these explicit attention-demanding memory contents, their performance suffers in dual-task scenarios and under pressure.

3.3.2.4 Feedback: Timing and Frequency

Especially in initial stages of learning, learners are very imprecise when it comes to interpret **intrinsic feedback** (internal information, e.g., kinesthetic, vestibular, or tactile sensory feedback). **Extrinsic feedback** (external information, e.g., feedback from the coach or a technical medium) can reduce information deficits (Schmidt et al., 2019) and supports learners in successfully solving the movement task ("guidance hypothesis"; Salmoni et al., 1984). However, the "**guidance hypothesis**" also states that a high availability of extrinsic feedback may lead to a situation in which the learner becomes dependent on the guidance by extrinsic feedback, while the processing of intrinsic information is neglected. This prevents the development of **error detection mechanisms** and results in a reduced performance whenever the guiding extrinsic information is not available (▶ Study Box: Feedback: "Less Is More!"). The demand for an effective **feedback delay** of about 5–30 s can be argued in a similar way (e.g., Swinnen et al., 1990). Immediate feedback without any delay might prevent the processing of intrinsic feedback, while longer delays (e.g., more than 30 s) are accompanied by the "fading" of intrinsic feedback in short-term memory, so that it can no longer be compared to the extrinsic information (◘ Fig. 3.7). However, the comparison is important to enable the development of error detection mechanisms.

3.3.2.5 Feedback: Positive and Negative Valence

Extrinsic feedback can be perceived by learners with **positive or negative valence**. The valence (i.e., the value of the feedback) can be determined both by the subjective level of aspiration and by the type of feedback. Thus, target areas can be defined for the feedback, within which qualitative-positive feedback can be provided (**bandwidth feedback**, e.g., Sherwood, 1988) or normative reference values can be added (**normative**

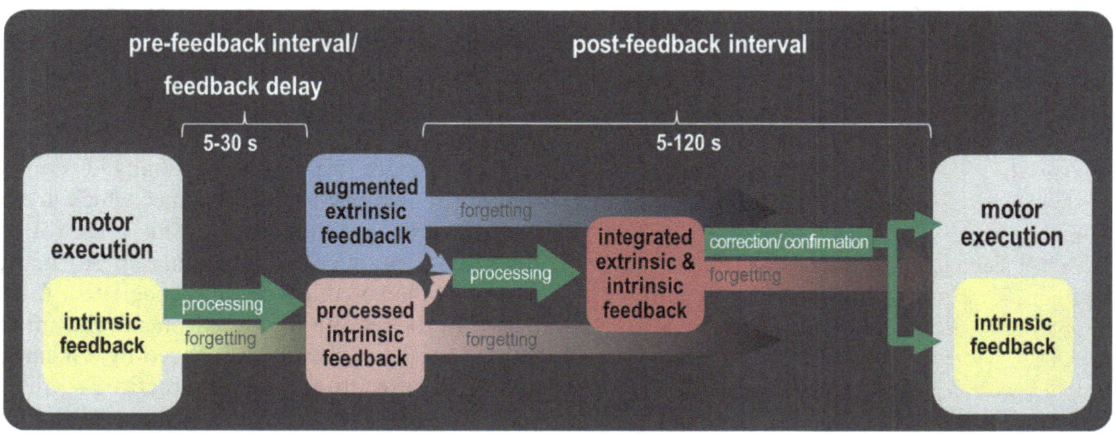

◘ **Fig. 3.7** Processing of extrinsic and intrinsic feedback in motor learning (mod. Krause et al., 2019; with friendly permission of Thieme Publishing)

feedback/social-comparative feedback, e.g., Wulf & Lewthwaite, 2016). Based on the "reward-prediction-error-hypothesis" (Glimcher, 2011), it can be expected that **feedback with (rather unexpected) positive valence** is of higher significance for learning (i.e., reinforcement learning), because it is associated with an increase in the firing rate of dopaminergic neurons in the midbrain, which in turn causes a **dopamine-dependent long-term potentiation** of the neuronal activation patterns correlated with the feedback event. To state it metaphorically: the neuronal activation patterns that led to the successful execution of the action are post-activated somewhat beyond the end of the execution and are "bathed" in the dopamine release (Glimcher, 2011).

For **feedback with (rather unexpected) negative valence**, however, it can be assumed, that it induces an **increase in attention-dependent processes**, in order to reduce sources of error through cognitive strategies, triggered by a decrease in the firing rate of dopaminergic neurons. The cognitive involvement can have a short-term positive influence on practice performance but particularly limit motor automatization—as a partial aspect of long-term learning (▶ Study Box: Feedback Valence and Motor Automatization).

Case Study

Feedback: "Less Is More!"

Numerous experimental studies have shown that acquisition performance is positively influenced by a high availability of extrinsic feedback, but retention performance, which is usually tested without extrinsic feedback, tends to benefit from a reduced frequency (e.g., after 30–60% of the trials). This reversal effect can be observed after larger amounts of practice (more than 90 trials of practice) and for tasks that can be characterized by motor program learning (overview: Marschall et al., 2007). The consequence for teachers is that they should not provide feedback as frequently as possible but should rather deliberately use feedback less frequently, to promote the development of error detection mechanisms. Recent findings also show that more frequent error feedback can limit motor automatization processes (Krause et al., 2018).

Effective Use and Effective Design of Instructions

- Modeling, a procedure to enable observational learning, generates spatial representations of the movement and activates motor representations.
- The spatial disparity between the model and the observer should be as low as possible during modeling.
- Analogies and instructions addressing an external focus of attention induce implicit processes and promote a more automatic control of movements.

Effective Use and Effective Design of Augmented Feedback

- Augmented (extrinsic) feedback directs the learner into the direction of the learning objective by pointing to the discrepancies between the desired state and the actual state of performance and helps by the interpretation of the intrinsic feedback.
- A reduced feedback frequency promotes the development of error detection mechanisms and improves performance without augmented feedback.
- Feedback with negative valence hinders, whereas feedback with positive valence promotes motor automatization.

3.3.3 Practice Schedules

3.3.3.1 Distributed and Massed Practice

Concerning the temporal distribution of practice, a distinction is made **between massed practice,** as practice without interruption, and **distributed practice**, where practice is interrupted by resting periods. In general, distributed practice schedules show better learning effects than massed practice schedules (e.g., Shea et al., 2000). This applies both to the intervals between repeated practice trials within a practice session and to the interruption of practice by longer time intervals, for example, by day- or night-sleep intervals. Several complementary approaches can be used to explain this so-called spacing effect. In case of longer interruptions, **consolidation processes** enable the learner to perform further practice trials by using changed (consolidated) long-term memory representations, which are based on the previous practice before the retention interval. Restarting practice at a higher performance level describes the so-called reminiscence effect (Shea et al., 2000). In the retention intervals, task-relevant representations can be positively influenced by a **mental simulation** of the execution (Mental practice; ▶ Chap. 20). A stagnating performance can be observed when practice is scheduled without interruptions, which is signified by

reactive impedance due to changes in the availability of physical and psychological resources or an accumulation of inhibition potentials (especially in the case of non-reward and high physical demands), so that the learner is no longer able to reach the previous acquired level of performance.

Case Study

Feedback Valence and Motor Automatization

In addition to the learning advantages for movement accuracy and consistency (e.g., Sherwood, 1988), Agethen and Krause (2016) were able to show that the use of feedback with positive valence (in form of bandwidth feedback) leads to increased motor automatization. For this purpose, a dual-task paradigm (see Method Box in ► Sect. 3.3.1) was used in the pretest-posttest design to measure automatization effects. One group of participants, who had received positive qualitative feedback in most of the practice trials and quantitative error feedback in only comparatively few practice trials (approx. 14 %), were able to almost eliminate their dual-task costs completely from pretest to retention test. Another group of participants with a comparable reduced error feedback frequency, but without additional positive qualitative feedback, was able to reduce the dual-task costs by about one half. Yet another group of participants, who received quantitative error feedback after each practice trial, displayed a similar level of dual-task costs in the pretest and the retention test. Accordingly, both, the reduction of the frequency of feedback with negative valence and the addition of feedback with positive valence seem to promote motor automatization.

3.3.3.2 Part Practice and Whole Practice

A strategy to simplify the learning situation is to break down the learning task into single subtasks relative to either the simultaneously (**fractionalization**) or successively (**segmentation**) arranged elements, where the single elements are practiced in **isolation**. This approach is called **part practice**, as opposed to **whole practice**. Like these part practice methods, other simplification strategies can also be differentiated (e.g., using other objects, attentional cues, or rhythmic cues, as well as reducing performance speed). For example, as a simplification strategy, the whole task can be executed, but the learner's attention can be directed to a single aspect or subtask in the sense of a **variable priority training** (Wickens et al., 2013). Part practice seems necessary when the task is very challenging, because of high **task complexity** (relative to the number of sub-elements). Naylor and Briggs (1963) also recommended to take the degree of **organization** (relative to the interdependence of the single sub-elements) into account. An isolated practice of single elements that are highly interdependent (i.e., high degree of organization) can lead to limited transfer when trying to coordinate the individual elements appropriately in the combined execution. For example, problems may arise in case of high biomechanical dependence, especially when the strategies of fractionalization and segmentation are applied. In general, tasks with high complexity and relatively low degree of organization should benefit from part practice strategies (Study Box: Meta-analyses on the Effectiveness of the Part Practice Method (Fontana et al., 2009; Wickens et al., 2013)).

Case Study

Meta-analyses on the Effectiveness of the Part Practice Method (Fontana et al., 2009; Wickens et al., 2013)

Fontana et al. (2009) have analyzed 20 studies and revealed a high degree of heterogeneity in the findings, which, however, fit well with the considerations of Naylor and Briggs (1963). According to this meta-analysis, the effectiveness of the part practice method may be more effective or more ineffective than the whole-practice method, depending on the setting, which is determined by the task characteristics and skill level. For tasks with high complexity and a low degree of organization (e.g., dance sequences), the part practice method appears to be best. For tasks with a high degree of organization (e.g., juggling), the whole-practice approach should be taken instead. The meta-analysis by Wickens et al. (2013) comes to a similar conclusion based on these considerations and demonstrates that part practice often leads to reduced learning effects. More specifically, fractionalization (the practice of task elements) shows on average 29% lower learning effects, as compared to the whole-practice method. Segmentation (the isolated practice of successive task elements) appears to be more effective when the task complexity is low and the skill level requires a part practice method to avoid an informational overload. The variable-priority-training method, focusing on the prioritization of single task elements, has been shown to be the most effective method in this meta-analysis, with on average 27% higher learning effects than the whole-practice method without prioritization of single task elements. Based on both meta-analyses, it can be concluded that the part practice method should only be used in selected settings. Under certain circumstances, alternative simplification strategies may offer a more effective way of practice.

3.3.3.3 Practice Variability

Practice variability can be defined for different aspects of practice. The "schema theory" (Schmidt, 1975) proposes that higher **parameter variability** (e.g., a variation of the force parameter) during practice results in a better development of the motor schema, i.e., the goal-adequate use of the movement parameters, than monotonous practice. According to the "contextual interference hypothesis" (Shea & Morgan, 1979), practice schedules should integrate more frequent changes between different motor programs or parameters to optimize learning effects. Changing tasks in a serial or randomized order significantly affects learning when **motor parameter** (e.g., throwing over different target distances) and/or **motor programs** are varied (e.g., golf putt and golf tee). In addition, the level of contextual interference should be adapted to the expertise to set the optimal level of practice demands (optimal-challenge-point theory; Guadagnoli & Lee, 2004).

The **contextual interference effect** is explained by both, motivational and cognitive mechanisms. According to the "motivational hypothesis", frequent switching between tasks after every trial or a block of a few trials leads to less monotony. With regards to the "elaboration hypothesis", a deeper and more elaborative information processing can be expected because the single tasks can be better related to each other (communalities and distinctions). The "reconstruction hypothesis" assumes, that the repeated reconstruction of the action plan before each execution should lead to better recall and formation of the underlying representations in long-term memory (Schmidt et al., 2019; ► Side Story: The Reversal Effect in Motor Learning with Varying Variability).

Side Story

The Reversal Effect in Motor Learning with Varying Variability

In general, an increase of practice variability leads to poorer initial performance but to better long-term learning (Brady, 2008). For simple movement tasks (e.g., arm movement sequences; Shea & Morgan, 1979) and for complex sport skills (Brady, 2008), blocked practice leads to better acquisition in the beginning. However, when considering performance improvements after a longer retention interval, this effect is reversed in favor of conditions with higher variability during practice (reversal effect).

Another form of practice variability results from **changing the side of the body** for skill execution during acquisition and training **(bilateral practice)**. In many sports, the bilateral use of skills is crucial for success during competition (e.g., dribbling with the left and right hand in basketball). Recent studies reveal that bilateral practice, as compared to unilateral practice, also proves to be advantageous when only the dominant side is used in competition (e.g., for long jump; Focke et al., 2016). If there is a frequent change of the lateral side in bilateral training, the contextual interference effects described above could also be taken to account for these bilateral practice effects. The advantages of bilateral practice can further be explained with the **functional asymmetry of the two brain hemispheres** ("dynamic dominance hypothesis"; Sainburg, 2002). Accordingly, bilateral practice should address the specialized cerebral hemisphere (left hemisphere = temporal-sequencing of the action and dynamic aspects of motor control; right hemisphere = spatial orientation and target coordination), respectively. **Sequential effects**, which can be observed after changing from one side of the body to the other side, can also be viewed in the context of hemispheric specialization. In this regard, it is better to involve that side of the body during early skill acquisition, which activates the brain hemisphere, which is specialized for the processing of the dominant control aspects of the task. ("specialized processing and information transfer model"; Stöckel & Weigelt, 2012; Study Box: Training of One Hand Does Not Automatically Lead to Better Skill Acquisition (Senff & Weigelt, 2011)).

Case Study

Training of One Hand Does Not Automatically Lead to Better Skill Acquisition (Senff & Weigelt, 2011)

In the study conducted by Senff and Weigelt (2011), 10- to 12-year-old schoolchildren were asked to slide coins across a table into a target (aiming task). Two groups of the children were only allowed to use their left or their right index finger for practice, respectively, while another two groups of the children used either their left or their right hand during the first part of practice and then switched to the other hand for the second part, respectively. According to the results, those children learned the motor task best, who first started with the left hand and then switched to the right hand. Practicing with only one hand (or first with the right hand and then with the left hand) did not lead to any long-term learning effects. The authors explained these findings with the early activation of the specialized (right) cerebral hemisphere for processing the spatial information in the aiming task by initial practice with the left hand.

Differential learning goes far beyond the limits of the approaches mentioned so far regarding practice variability (Schöllhorn et al., 2014). According to the differential learning approach, the fluctuations in execution that occur from trial to trial should be increased during practice. Therefore, individual practice trials show high **differences relative to numerous execution variables** (e.g., variation of the initial and final state of a movement, variation of amplitudes, variation of the external and internal rhythm of a movement). The strengthening of the fluctuation is usually induced by instructions for movement variation. The entire range of variation and combination of the execution variables defines the solution space. The **solution space** should be "scanned" at its edges by the differential executions, and in this way, "the system" should be able to interpolate individual optimal solutions for the movement task based upon self-organization processes. The approach of differential learning has been also critically discussed (Künzell & Hossner, 2012; Schöllhorn et al., 2013).

Considerations for the Effective Design of Practice Schedules

- The systematic distribution of practice and practice interruptions (distributed practice) has a positive influence on the learning process.
- Practicing single parts of a task (part practice) can reduce the informational overload during the practice of complex sport skills and positively influence skill learning, for as long as the single elements practiced in isolation do encompass a low degree of organization.
- The variable practice of different execution parameters (schema theory), the frequent change of the movement task (contextual interference, but also differential learning), and the change of the side of the body (bilateral practice) can be used to benefit long-term learning.

Tip

The practice info box provides different examples and additional notes for the practice of the jump shot in basketball with different approaches of variable practice.

Approaches of practice variability	Examples for the practice of jump shots in basketball	Additional important notes
Schema theory	Variation of the distance to the basket: e.g., 2.5 m, 3.0 m, 3.5 m, 4.0 m, 4.5 m	– The schema theory makes no prediction whether the frequency of parameter changes is of any significance for learning (cf. contextual interference).
Contextual interference	Variation with more or less frequent changes between a number of tasks (common number of tasks: $n = 3$) *Example A:* Serial or random trial-to-trial changes between throwing distances (i.e., parameter variation cf. schema theory) *Example B:* serial or random trial-to-trial changes between different techniques, like a jump shot, a chest pass, and a dribbling sequence (i.e., program variation)	– Moderate contextual interference (e.g., shooting mini blocks of three consecutive throws, before the distance is changed) seems to be preferable for learners with low expertise. – For high intra-task variability (two consecutive jump shots show different movement- or outcome-related kinematics), the level of contextual-interference should be kept low. – It is efficient for learning to increase the level of contextual interference from blocked to serial or random practice (e.g., 12 shots from each of three distances in a blocked schedule, followed by a change of distance after mini blocks of three consecutive throws, followed by a distance change after each of the 36 shots).

3

Approaches of practice variability	Examples for the practice of jump shots in basketball	Additional important notes
Bilateral practice	Variation of the throwing arm for the jump shot *Example A:* 40 trials with the left arm, then 40 trials with the right arm *Example B:* Alternate the throwing arm after each of 80 trials	– Frequent changes between the left and right throwing arm (cf. example B) can also be considered as an increased level of contextual interference. – If a blocked schedule is used in bilateral practice, the choice of the side for the first phase of practice affects learning. Accordingly, jump shot practice should start with the left throwing arm, because of the high requirements on spatial precision.
Differential learning	Variation of several kinematic variables with the aim to practice without any repetition of the same movement *Variation A:* Stand with your feet close together/at shoulder width/wider than shoulder width *Example B:* Shoot with full/half extension of your throwing arm *Example C:* Shoot with a steep/normal/flat release angle *Example D:* Combine and interchange the features of Examples A–C	– For some sport skills, the transfer of what has been practiced to what is required during competition might be limited.

3.3.4 Transfer of Learning

Every change in behavior influences past experiences and takes effect upon future learning processes. **Generalization** is assumed to take place when a skill is transferred from the practice condition to a new context, e.g., in rowing when switching from the rowing ergometer to the rowing boat. **Transference** is the transfer of previous learning experiences in task A to the current learning of task B. Hence, **motor learning transfer** refers to the influence of one learning process upon another learning process. Regarding the **kind of transfer performance**, a distinction is made between the transfer of single movement elements, the transfer of actions rules or structures, and effector transfer. Basically, three possibilities of learning transfer can be assumed: (1) **positive transfer** of learning occurs when current learning is facilitated by earlier experiences (e.g., from ice skating to inline skating), (2) **negative transfer** of learning occurs when learning of an earlier task hinders the acquisition of the new task (e.g., two-handed backhand to one-handed backhand in tennis), and (3) for **null transfer**, there is no influence of an earlier task on current learning (e.g., if both tasks are too different, such as the volleyball serve and unicycling). Sometimes it is also necessary to **relearn** an already acquired movement, for example, when the development in a particular sport domain requires a new sporting technique (e.g., from the parallel jump style to the V-style in ski jumping) or when new materials or sport equipment enter the market (e.g., ice speed skating shoes with clap blades). The phenomenon that one learning process can interfere with, inhibit, or cancel another learning process is called **interference** (Sperl & Cañal-Bruland, 2020). There are two kinds of interference: (1) **retroactive interference** means that task A is negatively affected by the following task B. (2) In the case of **proactive interference**, however, task A makes it more difficult to acquire or relearn task B. Transfer and interference effects are often explained by the **similarity of the tasks**. According to the so-called "identical elements theory" (Thorndike & Woodworth, 1901), the greater the number of identical elements between two skills is, the greater should be the transfer from one task to the other task. Here, the identical elements refer to the **motor**, **perceptual**, and **strategic-tactical requirements** of a task.

3.4 Fundamentals of Memory Psychology

The modern psychology of memory is based on the early work of Hermann Ebbinghaus (1885). Among other things, he investigated how long it takes to memorize long lists of meaningless syllables and over which periods of time they are remembered (▶ Study Box: Forgetting Curve (Ebbinghaus, 1885)). As it turned out, some of the syllables are **forgotten** after a short time. This phenomenon is known from many everyday situations, when people forget important information or cannot **remember** certain things, despite intensive reflection. This is not only a matter of **storing** and **recalling** verbal information but also of **recognizing** people, places, and other things, as well as **reproducing** motor skills (Hoffmann & Engelkamp, 2017). Memory is thus crucial for the performance of perception and action, without which mastering the tasks of everyday life would not be possible.

Memory

"Memory refers to processes and systems that are responsible for the storage, retention, retrieval and application of information, as soon as the original source of the information is no longer available" (Gruber, 2018, p. 2 [own translation]).

Study Box

Forgetting Curve (Ebbinghaus, 1885)

In a series of experiments, Hermann Ebbinghaus (1885) himself learned lists of meaningless syllables of three letters. Therefore, he repeated each list until he could reproduce it without mistakes. After a certain time interval (after 20 min, 1 h, 9 h, 1 day, 2 days, 6 days, 31 days), Ebbinghaus then repeated the whole procedure, which then took him less time than the first time to reproduce all the syllables of a list without errors. Accordingly, repeating the exercise after a certain time interval saved (some) time to learn these lists. People therefore refer to this method as to the **saving method** in this context. How big this saving was depended in the experiments of Ebbinghaus (and thereafter in many other studies) on the length of the time interval between both learning sessions. The following relationship emerged: the greater the time interval was, the fewer syllables Ebbinghaus was able to reproduce. From this he derived the so-called forgetting curve, for which the negatively accelerated curve suggests that the loss of memory is greatest in the first hours of memorization.

3.4.1 Representation of Knowledge

Knowledge is represented in human memory in the form of **names** or **concepts** that are assigned to different **category systems**, which include a vertical and a horizontal dimension. The vertical dimension relates to the inclusiveness of an object to a certain category, whereas the horizontal dimension separates different categories from each other at the same level of inclusiveness. The assignment of an exemplar to a category is made by means of common attributes or characteristics, by which a class of objects can be defined. There are two approaches to this assignment: the "prototype theory" and the "exemplar theory".

The "**prototype theory**" put forward by Rosch (1978) assumes that a category system is represented by a set of objects that share some common attributes or characteristics. The averaging of all objects within a category results in the **prototype**. Each new exemplar object is then compared with the prototype and, if there is sufficient **similarity**, is included into the category. Thereby, the prototype is updated again. Thus, in each category system, there are objects, which are more similar to the prototype than others. One can imagine different balls (e.g., a soccer ball, volleyball, basketball, handball, table tennis ball, football, and rugby ball), for example. This results in a specific **family resemblance** of all objects within a category system with more or less typical exemplars.

The "**exemplar theory**" of Medin et al. (1982), instead, assumes that each new exemplar object is compared with all other exemplars in a category, to which the object fits best. Hence, individual object characteristics are compared but without relying on a prototype. The "exemplar theory" thus places higher demands on memory capacity than the "prototype theory."

By assigning objects to category systems, complex taxonomies (i.e., *knowledge representations*) are created, whose exemplars are hierarchically represented on different levels. An example can be found in ◘ Fig. 3.8. On the **basic level**, concepts (i.e., *basic level objects*) are represented with certain characteristics that make them dis-

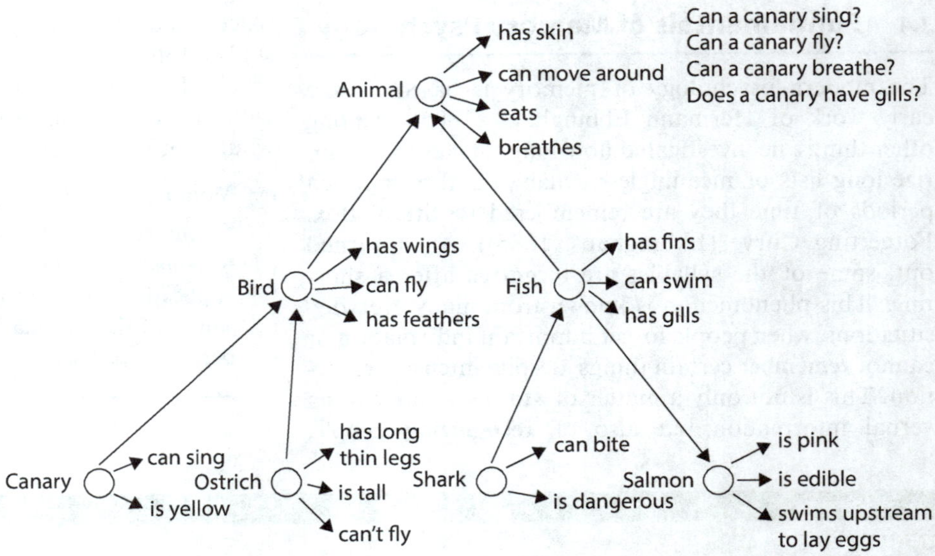

Fig. 3.8 Example of a hierarchical network of representational structures, including different exemplars of two basic level objects (bird and fish), which are organized on different levels (taken from Collins & Quillian, 1969, with permission from Elsevier)

3

tinguishable from other concepts (Rosch, 1978), such as fish or bird. Basic level objects combine a set of exemplars that share these characteristics and are represented on a **subordinate level**. For example, sharks and salmon are fish, because they share a number of common attributes of the concept of "fish" (both have fins and gills, and they are able to swim), although they differ naturally in many other characteristics. Birds and fish also share common characteristics (both breathe, eat, and move). Therefore, they can be assigned to the concept of "animals" at a **superordinate level**.

In memory, entire **networks** of hierarchically organized representational structures are formed in this way (Collins & Quillian, 1969). Within these networks, concepts on the basic level play a special role, as they are acquired earlier and can be recalled more quickly in memory than concepts on other levels of representation. In addition, they are functionally related to our behavior or behavioral potential. Let us consider the concept of "balls" again. A ball can be thrown, rolled, bounced, juggled, caught, etc. Therefore, a ball is always considered as an object with regard to its behavioral potential for the interaction with the environment and can (pre-) activate specific motor actions (▶ Sect. 3.5.2 Structures in Movement Representations). Through action, basic level objects are also integrated into events (i.e., as *action representations*).

Knowledge Representations

Knowledge is represented in human memory in the form of names or concepts within single categories according to common attributes or characteristics and is connected via the vertical organizational structure hierarchically over various levels to other categories.

Knowledge Acquisition from a Developmental Perspective

Put yourself into the mental shoes of a young child, and imagine how he or she acquires knowledge representations about different **animal categories**. When the child begins to speak his or her first words, parents will (most likely) start teaching them about animals by using pointing gestures and referring to different exemplars in a book by naming the animals on the **basic level** of the category systems, like "this is a dog," "this is a cat," "this is a bird," and so on. They will sing the child tune *Old MacDonald had a Farm*, and the child associates specific characteristics to different animal exemplars (e.g., for a cow, the song text goes "With a moo moo here and a moo moo there, …"). Imagine, that during a journey on the weekend, the parents will then take the child to a farm nearby and say, "look, there is a cow," "look, there is a pig," "look, there is a duck," and so on. The child may pet the different animals, feed them, and run after them. Through these interactions, he or she will find out more about the characteristics of these animals, such as the difference between fur and feathers, what the animals eat, and how fast they are while escaping. Back in kindergarten, the child has fun to imitate animals during play, such as when walking like a horse, barking like a dog, or hopping like a rabbit. With more experiences, the number of animal exemplars increases, and the child will form more and more distinct categories, based on **similarity** and **family resemblance**. Soon, he or she will be able to distinguish animals from a particular basic level concept (e.g., birds) on a **subordinate level** (e.g., a duck, from a chicken and a pigeon), according to specific characteristics (e.g., a duck lives near a pond and can swim). Hence, through perceptual and motor interactions as well as language development, the child will form hierarchically organized **knowledge representations** in long-term memory about different animals and other concepts in the world.

3.4.2 Memory Systems

According to the structural approach, memory is divided into several separate systems, which are considered in so-called multistore models of memory. The classical multistore (or modal) model of memory by Atkinson and Shiffrin (1968) distinguishes a sensory memory, a short-term, and a long-term memory system. Today, however, one rather assumes a sensory memory, a working memory, and a long-term memory system. These different memory systems are explained in more detail below.

3.4.2.1 Sensory Memory (or Sensory Register)

The **sensory memory** collects information from the environment or one's own body via the receptors of the different senses (i.e., initially modality-specific) and transforms it into perceptual representations. This results in transient memory traces about the physical properties of the stimuli, which are based on perceptual experience and which are temporarily maintained in different sensory storages, until they either decay or are further processed (via other memory systems) and finally are transformed into permanent representations. The sensory memory is therefore a transient memory system.

Sensory Memory

In sensory memory, information from the environment or one's own body is briefly maintained in different sensory storages as transient memory traces, before either decaying or being transformed into permanent representations in forthcoming processes.

In principle, different sensory memories can be assumed for each of the different senses. However, most of the research work addresses the **visual sensory memory** and the **auditory sensory memory**. From the early experiments of Georg Sperling (1960) on the visual sensory memory, it is known that a 3×4 matrix of letters, which is only being presented for 50 ms, is almost completely represented in the sensory (short-term) storage. However, this iconic image (suggestive of an iconic memory) of the matrix decays within about 1 s. Similar findings were also found for the auditory sensory memory (Darwin et al., 1972). Here, the participants were able to report three auditory lists of three numbers and letters almost completely (suggestive of an echoic memory). The auditory information decays within about 4 s. Overall, the (perceptual) capacity of the sensory memory seems to be relatively large, but the stored information decays rapidly.

3.4.2.2 Working Memory (Short-Term Memory)

Because the information in the sensory memory decays after a short time, it must be transferred to another memory system. The classical multistore model of memory by Atkinson and Shiffrin (1968) assumes a **short-term memory**, which can be characterized as follows: it has a storage capacity of 7 plus/minus 2 items (Miller, 1956), the information can be retained for about 20 s (Murdock, 1961), items from the beginning and end of a list are remembered best (so-called serial position effect; Murdock, 1962), and the search processes in short-term memory are serial and exhaustive (Sternberg, 1966).

For a long time, short-term memory was only regarded as a kind of "buffer" between sensory memory and long-term memory, in which information can be stored by **maintenance rehearsal**, until it is either forgotten or transferred to long-term memory. Newer approaches, however, see the short-term memory rather as a **working memory**, in which the information is not only temporarily stored but can also be transformed, integrated multimodally, structured, and manipulated through **elaborate rehearsal**. This is accompanied by a deeper processing of the information, which is under the influence of long-term memory and enables the processing of complex tasks.

Working Memory

Working memory is a storage system of limited capacity that draws on knowledge representations from long-term memory and, thus, enables information to be available for the processing of complex tasks over a short period of time.

Currently, there are two influential models addressing the structure of working memory: the "three-component model of working memory" and the "embedded processes model".

The "**three-component model of working memory**" was developed by Baddeley and Hitch in 1974 and in its current version (Baddeley, 2003) adopts three systems for the short-term storage of information: the **phonological loop** for storing and transforming auditory verbal information, the **visuospatial sketchpad** for storing visual and spatial information, and the **episodic buffer** as a multimodal storage system for the short-term storage of coherent episodes. For example, basketball players can briefly memorize the next game play (episodic buffer) during a time-out, which the coach verbalizes for them (phonological loop) and draws on the tactic board (visuospatial sketchpad). According to Baddeley (2003), the **central executive** serves as a superordinate structure, which flexibly coordinates the three systems as a kind of control center.

The "**embedded processes model**" by Nelson Cowan (1997) postulates that working memory is an activated part of long-term memory. Individual elements or entire information nodes are activated and thus made available for the working memory. Elements in the focus of attention are consciously perceived (explicit memory), whereas elements outside of attentional focus can become unconsciously effective (implicit memory). Cowan (1997) also assumes a central executive, which primarily controls those cognitive processes that are subject to voluntary control. Both models assume a transient memory system for the working memory.

3.4.2.3 Long-Term Memory

Long-term memory is assumed to store information permanently and (most likely) without capacity limits. According to van der Meer (2006), the content of long-term memory is based either on (1) one's own experiences or observations, (2) on facts and rules conveyed by language (or images), or (3) on one's own insights into facts, based on cognitive operations.

The basic function of long-term memory is to provide information for the organization of one's own behavior or the behavior of groups. This concerns the retrieval of information for decision making, as well as for behavioral control and subsequent evaluation. Basically, long-term memory is divided into a **declarative** and a **non-declarative memory** (Squire & Kandel, 1999; ◘ Fig. 3.9).

Long-Term Memory

The long-term memory is the storage system that stores information permanently and without capacity limitation, whereby a fundamental distinction is made between declarative and non-declarative memory contents.

Declarative memory (explicit memory): The knowledge stored in the **declarative memory** can be accessed consciously, that is, it can be verbalized or visualized and be used flexibly (especially in new situations). With reference to the recall process, declarative memory is also often referred to as **explicit memory**. According to Endel Tulving (1985), a distinction is made within declarative memory between **episodic memory** and **semantic memory**. The episodic memory contains context-specific knowledge about one's own experiences in the past, for example, the memory of the first visit to the indoor climbing hall, the belt examination in martial arts, or the last victory in the ongoing season. The place and time of the event are also stored in an episode. If the memory refers to one's own biography, then it is often referred to as **autobiographic memory**.

If one remembers that he/she wanted to carry out a certain action in the future (e.g., riding a bicycle around a lake the next day for a training session), it is called **prospective memory**, because the episodic content refers to a future event. Our general knowledge of the world is stored in the **semantic memory**. The most important informations stored are names of persons or objects, languages, mathematical formulas, and knowledge about physical laws. As discussed in ► Sect. 3.4.1, Knowledge Representations, this is a form of **conceptual knowledge**, which, on the one hand, is acquired through explicit instruction and with an intention to learn (**intentional learning**) but, on the other hand, also often incidentally and without any instructed intention to learn (**incidental learning**). It is important to note that both episodic and semantic

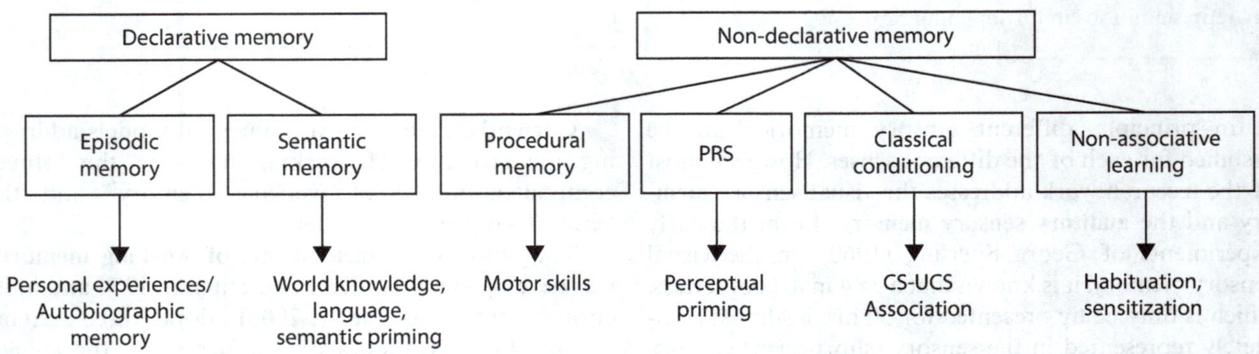

◘ **Fig. 3.9** The illustration shows the organization of long-term memory into different subsystems of storage. (Adapted from Gruber, 2018)

contents can be deliberately retrieved from long-term memory, regardless of how this knowledge was acquired previously.

Non-declarative memory (implicit memory): In contrast to the declarative memory, the **non-declarative memory** is independent from the conscious access of information. To this end, it builds on previous experiences that we cannot verbalize or visualize and controls our behavior unconsciously and involuntarily. It is therefore also called **implicit memory**. An example are the behavioral changes through **habituation** and **sensitization**. Due to regular training, the water's temperature in the lake will not feel as cold after some time for an open-water swimmer, that is, he or she will get used to the temperature (habituation). A non-regular visitor, instead, will tend to perceive the temperature of this lake as being colder, that is, he or she will react more strongly when jumping into the lake (sensitization). Besides of these two nonassociative forms of learning, non-declarative knowledge can also be acquired through classical conditioning (i.e., by associative learning processes).

Two further subsystems are particularly important for coping with everyday life and performing in sports: the **perceptual representation system (PRS)** and the **procedural memory**. The PRS represents the perceptual parts of the non-declarative memory. Information from the environment is being processed on a pre-semantic level, without access to declarative memory, which can be observed when a person initiates a particular behavior, without being aware of it (so-called unconscious priming). Thereby, it is very likely that multiple domain-specific PRSs exist, that is, priming can influence our behavior via almost all sensory modalities. For the visual PRS, for example, it has been shown that even the slightest displacement of a goalkeeper on the goal line influences the choice of goal side during penalty kicks in soccer (Masters et al., 2007). Automated skills, behavioral routines, and habits are stored in the procedural memory. In the broadest sense, this is about the representation of actions and their execution, based on perceptual-motor codes. Examples are cycling, snowboarding, or sailing. Also, such routines as the fast break after a turnover in basketball or returning to the line of scrimmage in American football are actions that are stored in the procedural memory. At this point, it is important to note that many of these actions are first acquired through deliberate practice (being a form of explicit knowledge acquisition), before they are transferred into the procedural memory. Hence, the single subsystems of the long-term memory do not exist separately but interact with each other through different processes.

3.4.3 Memory Processes

In addition to the structural approach, in which memory is divided into several separate systems (Atkinson & Shiffrin, 1968), memory performance can also be viewed from a procedural approach. This approach focuses on the individual processes that take place in the different systems. The following phases are distinguished: (1) **encoding**, (2) **retention**, (3) **consolidation**, (4) **recall**, and (5) **forgetting**. Three aspects are important for the processing of information across the individual phases (Zimmer & Kaernbach, 2006): First, information is processed hierarchically (i.e., it is abstracted from sensory stimulus properties to symbolic-conceptual representations). Second, since the information is received by individual sensory systems, the initial processing is modality-specific, before it is integrated and represented multimodally. Third, the entire processing of information is cascaded (i.e., the output of one process serves as an input for the next process).

3.4.3.1 Encoding

The first phase of information uptake is called **encoding**, where the new information (stimulus) is received and stored by different sensory modalities. Through this, the information enters working memory. This happens, for example, when one watches the presentation of the starting five in basketball on TV. The sensory storage of this information into working memory is disrupted, when the (visual or auditory) presentation of the players finishes. Therefore, the encoding phase only lasts for as long as the stimulus is being presented. How and if information is processed afterward depends upon whether or not the stimulus has been perceived and given attention.

3.4.3.2 Retention

The second phase is about **retention**. After the presentation of the information is finished, it must be retained in working memory, so that it does not immediately vanish again. Therefore, the information can be repeated in the working memory, for example, by internal (subvocal) or loud speech in the phonological loop. In this way, the team's lineup can be recited aloud to oneself again and again. The active maintenance of information is susceptible to interference and requires attention and concentration. At the same time, the next process is initiated, the consolidation (of at least parts) of the information.

3.4.3.3 Consolidation

Maintaining information in the retention phase also leaves traces in long-term memory. The process of transferring information into long-term memory is called **consolidation**, where new information is integrated into existing knowledge. For example, the team lineup of the current match day is compared with that of the previous week. Consolidation processes often take hours, several days, or even several weeks. This process is also prone to disruption.

3.4.3.4 Retrieval

In the fourth phase, the information must be made available or potentially be made available. This is done by the **retrieval** of the information from long-term memory. For this purpose, the information is transferred into working memory, where the information can be used further. For example, one can use it to inform another person, who came too late to watch the beginning of the basketball game, about the team's starting five and possibly point out changes to the last game.

3.4.3.5 Forgetting

Finally, it can happen that certain information is no longer remembered. In this case, **forgetting** means that previously learned content is no longer available. For example, it is very likely, that in a while, one will not remember the starting five of the basketball team from the TV broadcast anymore. On the one hand, this may be due to the decay of memory traces over longer periods of time and, on the other hand, to interference effects that occur when "old" memory content is overwritten by "new" information. However, forgetting can also mean that certain information cannot be accessed temporarily. This often occurs when emotional events suppress certain memories (which illustrates the close connection between emotion and memory) and thus prevent their recall.

3.5 Representation of Motor Skills

As already introduced in ► Sect. 3.4.1, there are very elaborate models for the representation of object and event concepts in long-term memory. These have been advanced for a long time, and therefore today, much is known about how these long-term representation structures are used for cognitive processes (e.g., speaking, thinking). Much less is known, however, about how those representations are structured, which represent the cognitive building blocks of behavioral control for actions of varying complexity, ranging from everyday actions (such as grasping an object) to the control of complex athletic skills (such as multiple twists and somersaults in springboard diving).

Movement Representations

Movement representations are those cognitive units stored in long-term memory that are the building blocks for the control of movement skills.

Knowledge about **movement representations** enables us to look at problems during skill execution in sport practice from a cognitive, inner perspective and not only from a movement-related, outer perspective. For example, there may be a point in time during the acquisition and optimization of the Fosbury Flop in high jump (► Sect. 3.3), at which an athlete cannot perform the movement sequence at the optimal skill level. Repeatedly failing to be successful signals that the goal of the movement (i.e., to clear the bar) has not been achieved. However, the reason for the performance failure may not be always visible from outside. With the application of experimental methods for **measuring cognitive representations of complex sport skills** (Methods: Measurement of Movement Representations), the cognitive causes of movement problems can be uncovered and analyzed. These cognitive representations of complex sport skills also play an important role in **mental training** procedures (also known as imagery training; ► Chap. 21 Excurse: Mental Training).

Mental Training

Mental training is the deliberate, repeated, planned, and conscious imagining of a skilled action, without its simultaneous execution (Eberspächer, 2007, p. 70; own translation).

Side Story

Mental Training

The theoretical assumption, which is central for the effectiveness of mental training, is that both, the execution and the imagination of a movement are based on the same cognitive representation structure. During mental training, those cognitive structures are therefore activated that form the basis for the execution of the action ("theory of mental simulation"; Jeannerod, 2001). As a result, multimodal mental training can improve motor learning and performance (Driskell et al., 1994). An area of application is motor rehabilitation, where neurological patients suffering from movement impairments (e.g., stroke patients) can be supported by mental training of everyday activities (e.g., drinking from a cup) (Braun et al., 2006).

3.5.1 Building Blocks of Complex Skills

When considering the representation of actions, the question of how complex skills are stored in long-term memory to enable the voluntary control of the motor system with its many effectors, muscles, and joints, is of most interest. The following section therefore explains how such cognitive structures are designed to store aspects of both, **action representation** (action knowledge) and **action execution** (control of movement execution).

3.5.1.1 Goal Representations and Effect Representations

The main goal of voluntary actions is to achieve a **distal effect** (i.e., a distal perceptual event) in the environment (e.g., basketball passing through the rim). Such an effect is usually accompanied by **proximal effects** (i.e., a proximal perceptual event) arising from the movement of one's own body (e.g., tactile and kinesthetic sensations of the fingers while throwing the ball). Both, distal effects in the environment and proximal effects of physical sensations are associated with the movement that reliably produces these sensory effects (e.g., a particular basketball free-throw technique). At this point, it is important to understand that this **association** between a particular action and its sensory effects is **bidirectional**. This means that the execution of a certain movement leads to the activation of the corresponding effect representation and, at the same time, that the anticipation of a particular effect representation is sufficient to activate the corresponding action. This idea is fundamental for goal-directed behavior and has been known since the middle of the nineteenth century as the "ideomotor hypothesis" (for a historical overview, see Stock & Stock, 2004; ▶ Methods: Response-Effect Compatibility (Kunde et al., 2004)).

Methods: Response-Effect Compatibility (Kunde et al., 2004)

Many experimental studies, which investigated the so-called response-effect compatibility-effect between motor responses and associated effects, demonstrated the influence of **effect anticipations** on the choice of actions across different tasks. Kunde et al. (2004), for example, showed that pressing a response key softly or powerfully for a green or red stimulus was faster when the key press generated a compatible effect as opposed to an incompatible effect. That is, participants performed the key presses faster if a soft or powerful keystroke was followed by a quiet or loud tone, respectively. The authors argued that response-effect compatibility affected response selection because participants anticipated the sensory effect in advance (i.e., the loudness of the sound). This seems to be the only way to explain how a preceding response is influenced by a subsequent effect. Therefore, the study by Kunde et al. (2004) lends direct support for the "ideomotor hypothesis."

Ideomotor Hypothesis

According to the "ideomotor hypothesis", actions are represented in terms of their sensory effects and are bidirectionally connected to them. The simple imagination or anticipation of these effects can activate the corresponding action (James, 1890).

3.5.1.2 Representation of Biomechanical Parameters

The assumption that actions are represented in terms of their sensory effects includes that these effects are specific to the movement system of the actor (e.g., body size, length of the effectors). For example, children will not produce the same sensory effects as adults do when performing a tennis serve, because the trajectories of the racket's motion differ greatly, due to the different lengths of the limbs. The representations of complex skills must therefore also include the biomechanical parameters of the acting person, representing the boundary conditions of behavioral control.

Another important assumption in this context is based on the work of Wolfgang Prinz (1997) and posits that the perception of actions is mediated by shared representations, which also represent these actions ("common coding theory", Prinz, 1997). This assumption can be tested empirically: Predicting of one's own action effects should be easier than predicting the action effects of other people because the representation of the biomechanical parameters of one's own movement system should convey the perception of one's own movement system more precisely. This assumption was confirmed by Knoblich and Flach (2001) (▶ Study Box: Representation of Biomechanical Parameters (Knoblich & Flach, 2001)).

Common Coding of Perception and Action
Perception and action are coded as perceived and produced perceptual events within shared representations, which provide a direct link between perception and action ("common coding theory"; Prinz, 1997). The "theory of event coding" (TEC; Hommel et al., 2001) assumes that the representation of events conveys the codes of their features, which refer to the distal perceptual events (i.e., sensory action effects).

3

Study Box

Representation of Biomechanical Parameters (Knoblich & Flach, 2001)

Knoblich and Flach (2001) conducted an experimental study to test the hypothesis that predicting one's own actions is more precise than predicting the actions of others. For this purpose, participants observed video sequences in which they threw darts on a dartboard or in which other people threw darts on the board. The throws could hit either the upper, middle, or lower third of the dartboard. Participants only saw the throwing movement (i.e., biomechanical parameters), but not the trajectory or the landing position of the dart. When asked to predict the landing position of the darts (bottom, middle, top), participants were more accurate in predicting own throws compared to the throws of other people. This result suggests that the representation of the biomechanical parameters of one's own movement is used for the prediction of self-observation. However, since the representation does not fit the movement system of another person, the prediction for throws of other people is less accurate.

3.5.1.3 Basic Action Concepts (BACs)

The previous two sections focused on the movement informations, that must be represented in long-term memory, in order to plan, to execute, and to predict actions, and to anticipate their outcomes. The cognitive units that tie this information together in the context of complex actions were called **basic action concepts (BACs)** by Thomas Schack (2004, 2010). BACs represent the **nodes of a certain action** (e.g., Fosbury Flop; ◘ Fig. 3.10), which are central to solve the task. They are (within limits) conscious and explicable, and are often communicated in training processes (e.g., "lift your hips" for the Fosbury Flop). The sensory perceptual effects that a sub-movement causes are stored in and recalled from long-term memory based on these BACs. Thereby, the representation structure of complex actions is defined by the functional relation of the BACs within the execution of the movement.

Basic Action Concepts
Basic action concepts (BACs) are the cognitive building blocks of movement representations and combine the following features of an action: (1) proximal sensory effects, (2) distal sensory effects, and (3) biomechanical parameters of one's own movement system.

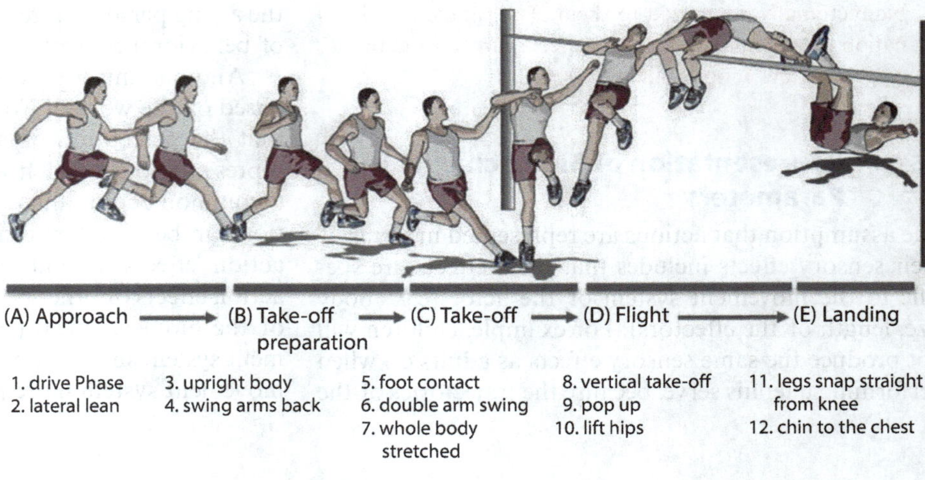

◘ **Fig. 3.10** Functional phases of the Fosbury Flop (A–E) from a biomechanical perspective. Pictures are taken from Göhner (2002) (grey-scaled print, Fig. 17. S. 76, with friendly permission from Ulrich Göhner). The basic action concepts (BACs) of the different movement phases are given in terms of verbal labels (1–12)

3.5.2 Structures in Movement Representations

The **representation of action knowledge in long-term memory** is, like the representation of semantic knowledge (▶ Sect. 3.4.1), the result of learning processes. The information available in motor learning processes, for example, feedback from the trainer (extrinsic feedback) or self-perception (intrinsic feedback), is stored, integrated, and organized in long-term memory. This results in a specific arrangement of the BACs for the execution of the action, namely, a **functional representation structure**, reflecting all phases of movement execution.

For an example of a functional representation structure, consider the biomechanical structure of the high-jump movement (Göhner, 1983, 1996): The main goal in high jump is to clear the bar after a one-legged **takeoff** without tossing it down. Different preparatory phases, namely, the **approach** and the **takeoff preparation**, must be carried out in a way to ensure that the bar is cleared in the **main phase** (flight). During **landing** in the final phase of the movement, the actual task has already been solved.

Each of these movement phases has a function, which serves the main goal. For example, the curve of the run-up serves to lower the body's center of mass to extend the vertical acceleration path. The main goal of the takeoff is to achieve the highest possible takeoff speed. During landing, the primary aim is to transfer the action from a dynamic into a static state (i.e., from dynamic to static balance) and to avoid injuries (Göhner, 2017; ◘ Fig. 3.10).

All cognitive units represented as BACs, which serve the same function (e.g., horizontal acceleration), are represented in long-term memory within so-called clusters. Within a cluster, BACs are linked with each other, if they are functionally related (e.g., "pop up" is the precondition for "lift hips") and if they share similar characteristics (e.g., only by popping up can the hips be lifted and the associated kinesthetic sensations be achieved). Such a representation structure is comparable to other categorical representations of knowledge (▶ Sect. 3.4.1).

Functional Representation Structure

A functional representation structure reflects the biomechanical structure of the movement execution and ensures the achievement of the main goal of the action.

3.5.3 Measurement and Variability of Movement Representations

In the context of motor learning (▶ Sect. 3.3), the question arises of how movement representations change with increasing motor performance. One approach to investigate this question is to conduct learning studies, while the other approach is to use comparative studies with novices, intermediate athletes, and expert athletes. Both approaches require the measurement of cognitive movement representations. For this purpose, Schack (2004) applied the "structural dimensional analysis" **(SDA)**, which is a method of cognitive psychology to measure conceptual structures in long-term memory (Lander & Lange, 1992). For the analysis of movements, the method was called "structural dimensional analysis-motoric" **(SDA-M)** (Schack, 2004).

Studies investigating the movement representations of complex skills have shown (1) that these representation structures develop over the learning process (Frank et al., 2013), (2) that they differ between novices and expert athletes (Schack & Mechsner, 2006) and approach the optimal functional structure relative to the biomechanics of movement execution with increasing expertise (Bläsing et al., 2009), (3) that the SDA-M method is suitable for individual skill diagnostics in high-performance sports (Weigelt et al., 2011), (4) that the representation of team tactics differs between experienced and less experienced athletes (Lex et al., 2015), and (5) that the representation structures can be changed through mental training (Frank et al., 2014).

As can be seen in ◘ Fig. 3.11, dendrograms can be used to visualize different cluster solutions between experts and novices. These dendrograms were obtained for the Fosbury Flop (high jump) using SDA-M (▶ Methods: Measurement of Movement Representations). Each cluster solution is determined by the so-called critical Euclidean distance (horizontal dotted line, d_{crit}). All connections between BACs below d_{crit} are considered as associated concepts. Connections above the critical value are considered as nonassociated concepts. Accordingly, the expert displays a representation structure, which corresponds well with the biomechanical and functional structure of the Fosbury Flop. Hence, in the expert structure, every movement phase of the high-jump movement is represented (◘ Fig. 3.10). Only BAC 8 (vertical takeoff), which marks the beginning of the flight phase, was assigned to the takeoff phase by the expert. In contrast, there are three clusters in the novice structure, which have no plausible correlation to the biomechanical and functional structure of the complex skill.

Methods: Measurement of Movement Representations

Structural Dimensional Analysis—Motoric (SDA-M; Schack, 2010, 2012)

The procedure to analyze a particular action representation within a multistage sorting process using the SDA-M can either be conducted with the SPLIT-software online or offline on a computer. The participants are being presented with a BAC (e.g., "upright body"; ◘ Fig. 3.10) of the movement (either as a picture or verbal label) in the so-called anchor position and must decide whether this BAC is associated with another BAC (e.g., swing arms back), which is displayed in the "reference position." For the comparison, the BAC in the reference position must be "assigned" or "put away" from the BAC in the anchor position. This decision is repeated for every other BAC, after which a new BAC is placed in the anchor position and the assignment procedure starts again for all remaining BACs. After every BAC had been placed in the anchor position and was compared to every other BAC, the sorting process is finished. For movements with 12 BACs, 12 × 11 = 132, decisions must therefore be made by the participants.

To establish the relationships between the BACs, several statistical methods (e.g., hierarchical cluster analysis, factor analysis) are applied to examine the **cluster formation** (structuring) of the BACs. To this end, the SDA-M reveals, which BACs are assigned to the same cluster due to their functional interdependence (functional phases; cf. ▶ Sect. 3.5.2). The cluster solutions are visualized in so-called dendrograms (◘ Fig. 3.11). The cluster solutions and dendrograms can be used to compare participants of different skill level (e.g., to examine the differences between novices and expert athletes) or to evaluate changes in the representation structure using repeated measurements (e.g., to evaluate the effects of intervention and training on the representation structure).

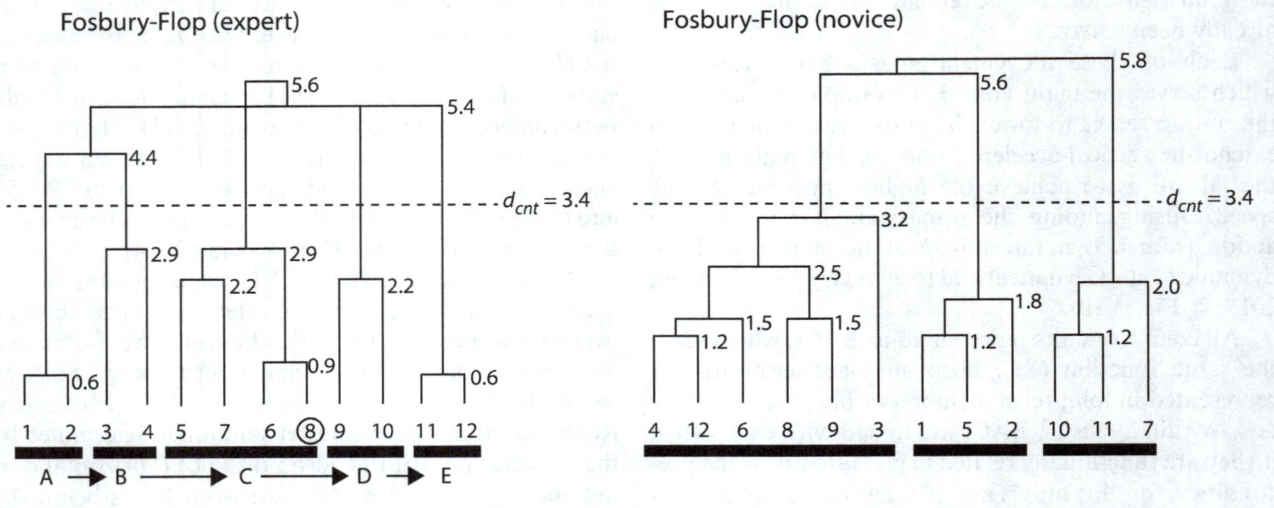

◘ **Fig. 3.11** Dendrogram of an expert (left side) and of a novice (right side). Numbers from 1 to 12 depict the basic action concepts of the Fosbury Flop (1 = drive Phase; 2 = lateral lean; 3 = upright body; 4 = swing arms back; 5 = foot contact; 6 = double arm swing; 7 = whole body stretched; 8 = vertical takeoff; 9 = pop up; 10 = lift hips; 11 = legs snap straight from knee; 12 = chin to the chest). Letters from A to E indicate the biomechanical phases of the high-jump movement (A = approach; B = takeoff preparation; C = takeoff; D = flight; E = landing)

Learning Control Questions

Basic:

1. What are the similarities and differences between the various theoretical approaches for the basic learning mechanisms?
2. Which roles do conscious and unconscious cognitive processes play during the different phases of motor learning? What is motor automatization?
3. How are knowledge representations structured in long-term memory?
4. Which memory systems are distinguished in so-called multistore models of memory?
5. Which memory processes become effective when processing information?

Advanced:

6. Which roles do conscious and unconscious cognitive processes play during the different phases of motor learning? What is motor automatization?
7. Which categories of motor transfer effects can be differentiated, and on which aspects depend the amount and direction of the transfer?
8. How are the cognitive representations of complex sport skills stored in long-term memory?
9. What role do sensory effects play in the control of complex movements according to the ideomotor hypothesis?

Experts:

10. How should the use of external information (instructions and feedback) be designed to effectively promote motor learning processes?
11. What are the differences between the learning mechanisms that effect classical conditioning and the learning of action-effect relations?
12. How does the structure of skill representation differ depending on athletic expertise?

References

Abernethy, B. (2001). Attention. In R. N. Singer, H. A. Hausenblas, & C. M. Janelle (Eds.), *Handbook of Sport Psychology* (2nd ed., pp. 53–85). Wiley.

Agethen, M., & Krause, D. (2016). Effects of bandwidth feedback on the automatization of an arm movement sequence. *Human Movement Science, 45*, 71–83.

Atkinson, R. C., & Shiffrin, R. M. (1968). Human memory: A proposed system and its control processes. In K. W. Spence & J. T. Spence (Eds.), *The Psychology of Learning and Motivation: Advances in Research and Theory* (Vol. 2). Academic Press.

Baddeley, A. (2003). Working memory: Looking back and looking forward. *Nature Review Neuroscience, 4*, 829–839.

Bandura, A. (1965). Influence of models reinforcement contingencies on the acquisition of imitative response. *Journal of Personality and Social Psychology, 1*, 589–595.

Bandura, A. (1977). *Social Learning Theory*. General Learning Press.

Bekkering, H., Wohlschläger, A., & Gattis, M. (2000). Imitation of gestures in children is goal-directed. *Quarterly Journal of Experimental Psychology, 53A*, 153–164.

Bläsing, B., Tenenbaum, G., & Schack, T. (2009). The cognitive structure of movements in classical dance. *Psychology of Sport and Exercise, 10*, 350–360.

Blischke, K., Marschall, F., Muller, H., & Daugs, R. (1999). Augmented information in motor skill acquisition. In Y. Vanden Auweele, F. Bakker, S. Biddle, M. Durand, & R. Seiler (Eds.), *Psychology for Physical Educators* (pp. 257–287). Human Kinetics.

Brady, F. (2008). The contextual interference effect and sport skills. *Perceptual and Motor Skills, 106*, 461–472.

Braun, S. M., Beurskens, A. J., Borm, P. J., Schack, T., & Wade, D. T. (2006). The effects of mental practice in stroke rehabilitation: A systematic review. *Archives of Physical Medicine and Rehabilitation, 87*, 842–852.

Chein, J. M., & Schneider, W. (2012). The brain's learning and control architecture. *Current Directions in Psychological Science, 21*, 78–84.

Collins, A. M., & Quillian, M. R. (1969). Retrieval time from semantic memory. *Journal of Verbal Learning and Verbal Behavior, 8*, 240–247.

Cowan, N. (1997). *Attention and Memory: An Integrated Framework*. Oxford University Press.

Csikszentmihalyi, M. (1985). *Das Flow-Erlebnis—Jenseits von Angst und Langeweile: im Tun aufgehen*. Klett-Cotta.

Darwin, C. J., Turvey, M. T., & Crowder, R. G. (1972). The auditory analogue of the Sperling partial report procedure: Evidence for brief auditory storage. *Cognitive Psychology, 3*, 255–267.

Daugs, R., Blischke, K., Olivier, N., & Marshall. (1989). *Beiträge zum visuomotorischen Lernen im Sport*. Hofmann.

Driskell, J., Copper, C., & Moran, A. (1994). Does mental practice enhance performance? *Journal of Applied Psychology*, 79, 481–492. https://doi.org/10.1037//0021-9010.79.4.481

Ebbinghaus, H. (1885). *Über das Gedächtnis (Untersuchungen zur experimentellen Psychologie)*. Duncker & Humblot.

Eberspächer, H. (2007). *Mentales Training. Das Handbuch für Trainer und Sportler* (p. 7). Copress. Auflage.

Effenberg, A. O. (2005). Movement sonification: Effects on perception and action. *IEEE Multimedia, 12*, 53–59.

Fabbri-Destro, M., & Rizzolatti, G. (2008). Mirror neurons and mirror systems in monkeys and humans. *Physiology, 23*, 171–179.

Fitts, P. M., & Posner, M. I. (1967). *Human Performance*. Brooks/Cole.

Focke, A., Spancken, S., Stockinger, C., Thürer, B., & Stein, T. (2016). Bilateral practice improves dominant leg performance in long jump. *European Journal of Sport Science, 16*, 787–793.

Fontana, F. E., Furtado, O., Jr., Mazzardo, O., & Gallagher, J. D. (2009). Whole and part practice: a meta-analysis. *Perceptual and Motor Skills, 109*, 517–530.

Frank, C., Land, W. M., Popp, C., & Schack, T. (2014). Mental representation and mental practice: experimental investigation on the functional links between motor memory and motor imagery. *PloS One, 9*, e95175.

Frank, C., Land, W. M., & Schack, T. (2013). Mental representation and learning: the influence of practice on the development of mental representation structure in complex action. *Psychology of Sport and Exercise, 14*, 353–361.

3

Frensch, P. A. (2006). Implizites Lernen. In J. Funke & P. A. French (Eds.), *Handbuch der Allgemeinen Psychologie—Kognition* (pp. 229–238). Hogrefe Verlag.

Freudenheim, A. M., Wulf, G., Madureira, F., Pasetto, S. C., & Corrêa, U. C. (2010). An external focus of attention results in greater swimming speed. *International Journal of Sport Science & Coaching, 5*, 533–542.

Gergely, G., Bekkering, H., & Király, I. (2002). Rational imitation in preverbal infants. *Nature, 415*, 755.

Glimcher, P. W. (2011). Understanding dopamine and reinforcement learning: The dopamine reward prediction error hypothesis. *Proceedings of the National Academy of Sciences, 108*, 15,647–15,654.

Göhner, U. (1983). Wie sich sportliche Bewagged analysieren und strukturieren lassen. In: H. Digel (Hrsg.), *Lehren im Sport* (S. 139 ff.). Hamburg: Reinbek.

Göhner, U. (1996). *Bewegungslehre und Biomechnik des Sports*. Tübingen.

Göhner, U. (2017). Springen, Werfen und Laufen aus bewegungstheoretischer und biomechanischer Perspektive. Tübingen.

Göhner, U. (2002). Bewegungslehre und Biomechanik des Sport. Fundamentum mit Hoch- und Weitsprung. Tübingen: U. Göhner.

Gruber, T. (2018). *Gedächtnis (2. Auflage)*. Springer-Verlag.

Guadagnoli, M. A., & Lee, T. D. (2004). Challenge point: A framework for conceptualizing the effects of various practice conditions in motor learning. *Journal of Motor Behavior, 36*, 212–224.

Hikosaka, O., Nakahara, H., Rand, M. K., Katsuyuki, S., Lu, X., Nakamura, K., Miyachi, S., & Doya, K. (1999). Parallel neural networks for learning sequential procedures. *Trends in Neuroscience, 22*, 464–471.

Hoffmann, J. (1993). *Vorhersage und Erkenntnis: Die Funktion von Antizipationen in der menschlichen Verhaltenssteuerung und Wahrnehmung*. Hogrefe.

Hoffmann, J., Berner, M., Butz, M. V., Herbort, O., Kiesel, A., Kunde, W., & Lenhard, A. (2007). Explorations of Anticipatory Behavioral Control (ABC): A report from the Cognitive Psychology Unit of the University of Würzburg. *Cognitive Processing, 8*, 133–142.

Hoffmann, J., & Engelkamp. (2017). *Lern- und Gedächtnispsychologie (2. Auflage)*. Springer-Verlag.

Hommel, B., Müsseler, J., Aschersleben, G., & Prinz, W. (2001). The theory of event coding (TEC). A framework for perception and action. *Behavioral & Brain Sciences, 24*, 849–937.

Hommel, B., & Nattkemper, D. (2011). *Handlungspsychologie: Planung und Kontrolle intentionalen Handelns*. Springer-Verlag.

Jackson, P. L., Meltzoff, A. N., & Decety, J. (2006). Neural circuits involved in imitation and perspective-taking. *Neuroimage, 31*, 429–439.

James, W. (1890). *The Principles of Psychology*. Dover Publications.

Jeannerod, M. (2001). Neural simulation of action: A unifying mechanism for motor cognition. *NeuroImage, 14*, 103–109.

Keele, S. W., Mayr, U., Ivry, R., Hazeltine, E., & Heuer, H. (2003). The cognitive and neural architecture of sequence representation. *Psychological Review, 110*, 316–339.

Knoblich, G., & Flach, R. (2001). Predicting the effects of actions: Interactions of perception and action. *Psychological Science, 12*, 467–472.

Koopmann, T., Steggemann-Weinrich, Y., Baumeister, J., & Krause, D. (2017). Mental rotation of tactical instruction displays affects information processing demand and execution accuracy in basketball. *Research Quarterly for Exercise and Sport, 88*, 365–370.

Krause, D., Agethen, M., & Zobe, C. (2018). Error feedback frequency affects automaticity but not accuracy and consistency after extensive motor skill practice. *Journal of Motor Behavior, 50*, 144–154. https://doi.org/10.1080/00222895.2017.1327406

Krause, D., & Kobow, S. (2013). Effects of model orientation on the visuomotor imitation of arm movements: the role of mental rotation. *Human Movement Science, 32*, 314–327.

Krause, D., Ramme, K., & Weigelt, M. (2019). Erwerb motorischer und sensorischer Kompetenzen. In B. Klemme, U. Weyland, & J. Harms (Eds.), *Praktische Ausbildung in der Physiotherapie* (pp. 59–69). Thieme Verlag.

Krause, D., & Weigelt, M. (2020). The mental rotation of tactic boards in basketball under self-controlled and externally controlled time constraints. *German Journal of Exercise and Sport Research, 50*, 354–365.

Kunde, W., Koch, I., & Hoffmann, J. (2004). Anticipated action effects affect the selection, initiation, and execution of actions. *The Quarterly Journal of Experimental Psychology Section A: Human Experimental Psychology, 57*, 87–106.

Künzell, S., & Hossner, E. J. (2012). Differenzielles Lehren und Lernen: eine Kritik. *Sportwissenschaft, 42*, 83–95.

Lam, W. K., Maxwell, J. P., & Masters, R. (2009). Analogy learning and the performance of motor skills under pressure. *Journal of Sport and Exercise Psychology, 31*, 337–357.

Lander, H.-J., & Lange, K. (1992). Eine differentialpsychologische Analyse begrifflich-strukturierten Wissens. *Zeitschrift für Psychologie, 200*, 181–197.

Lewicki, P., Hill, T., & Czyzewska, M. (1992). Nonconscious acquisition of information. *American Psychologist, 47*, 796–801.

Lex, H., Essig, K., Knoblauch, A., & Schack, T. (2015). Cognitive representations and cognitive processing of team-specific tactics in soccer. *PLoS One, 10*, e0118219.

Lohse, K. R., Wadden, K., Boyd, L. A., & Hodges, N. J. (2014). Motor skill acquisition across short and long time scales: a meta-analysis of neuroimaging data. *Neuropsychologia, 59*, 130–141.

Marschall, F., Bund, A., & Wiemeyer, J. (2007). Does frequent augmented feedback really degrade learning? A meta-analysis. *E-Journal Bewegung und Training, 1*, 74–85.

Masters, R. S. W., van der Kamp, J., & Jackson, R. C. (2007). Imperceptibly off-centre goalkeepers influence penalty-kick direction in soccer. *Psychological Science, 18*, 222–223.

Medin, D. L., Altom, M. W., Edelson, S. M., & Freko, D. (1982). Correlated symptoms of simulated medical classification. *Journal of Experimental Psychology: Learning, Memory, and Cognition, 8*, 37–50.

Meltzoff, A. N., & Moore, M. K. (1977). Imitation of facial and manual gestures by human neonates. *Science, 198*, 75–78.

Miller, G. A. (1956). The magical number seven, plus or minus two: Some limits on our capacity for processing information. *The Psychological Review, 63*, 81–97.

Murdock, B. B. (1961). The retention of individual items. *Journal of Experimental Psychology, 62*, 618–625.

Murdock, J. (1962). The serial position effect of free recall. *Journal of Experimental Psychology, 64*, 482–488.

Naylor, J. C., & Briggs, G. E. (1963). Effects of task complexity and task organization on the relative efficiency of part and whole training methods. *Journal of Experimental Psychology, 65*, 217–224.

Nissen, M. J., & Bullemer, P. (1987). Attentional requirements of learning: Evidence from performance measures. *Cognitive Psychology, 19*, 1–32.

Olivier, N., Rockmann, U. & Krause, D. (2013). *Grundlagen der Bewegungswissenschaft und -lehre* (2., überarb. und erw. Aufl.). Schorndorf: Hofmann.

Pawlow, I. P. (1953). *Ausgewählte Werke*. Akademie-Verlag.

Physiofun. (2010). *Physiofun Senso Move [DVD]*. Kaasa health GmbH.
Poolton, J. M., Masters, R. S., & Maxwell, J. P. (2006). The influence of analogy learning on decision-making in table tennis: Evidence from behavioural data. *Psychology of Sport and Exercise, 7, 677–688.*
Prinz, W. (1997). Perception and action planning. European *Journal of Cognitive Psychology, 9*, 129–154.
Reber, A. S. (1989). Implicit learning and tacit knowledge. *Journal of Experimental Psychology: General, 118*, 219–235.
Rosch, E. (1978). Principles of categorization. In E. Rosch & B. B. Lloyd (Eds.), *Cognition and Categorization* (pp. 27–48). Erlbaum.
Rumiati, R., & Tessari, A. (2002). Imitation of novel and well-known actions. *Experimental Brain Research, 142*, 425–433.
Sainburg, R. L. (2002). Evidence for a dynamic-dominance hypothesis of handedness. *Experimental Brain Research, 142*, 241–258.
Salmoni, A. W., Schmidt, R. A., & Walter, S. B. (1984). Knowledge of results and motor learning: A review and critical reappraisal. *Psychological Bulletin & Review, 95*, 355–386.
Schack, T. (2004). The cognitive architecture of complex movement. *International Journal of Sport and Exercise Psychology, 2*, 403–438.
Schack, T. (2010). *Die Kognitive Architektur menschlicher Bewegung*. Meyer & Meyer Verlag.
Schack, T. (2012). Measuring mental representations. In R. C. E. G. Tenenbaum & A. Kamata (Eds.), *Measurement in Sport and Exercise Psychology* (pp. 203–214). Human Kinetics.
Schack, T., & Mechsner, F. (2006). Representation of motor skills in human long-term memory. *Neuroscience Letters, 391*, 77–81.
Schmidt, R. A. (1975). A schema theory of discrete motor skill learning. *Psychological Review, 82*, 225–260.
Schmidt, R. A. (1976). Control processes in motor skills. *Exercise and Sport Sciences Reviews, 4*, 22.
Schmidt, R. A., Lee, T. D., Winstein, C. J., Wulf, G., & Zelaznik, H. N. (2019). *Motor control and learning: A behavioral emphasis* (6th ed.). Human Kinetics.
Schöllhorn, W. I., Beckmann, H., Eekhoff, A., & Hegen, P. (2013). Differenzielles Lehren und Lernen: (k) eine Kritik–eine Bestätigung. *Sportwissenschaft, 43*, 56–57.
Schöllhorn, W. I., Hegen, P., & Eekhoff, A. (2014). Differenzielles Lernen und andere motorische Lerntheorien. *Spectrum der Sportwissenschaft, 2*, 35–55.
Schücker, L., Hagemann, N., Strauss, B., & Völker, K. (2009). The effect of attentional focus on running economy. *Journal of Sports Sciences, 27*, 1241–1248.
Selg, H. & Schermer, F. J. (2015). Lernpsychologie. In: A. Schütz, M. Brand, H. Selg, & S. Lautenbacher (Hrsg.), *Psychologie—Eine Einführung in ihre Grundlagen und Anwendungsfächer* (5. Auflage, S. 101–116). Stuttgart: Verlag W. Kohlhammer.
Senff, O., & Weigelt, M. (2011). Sequential effects after practice with the dominant and non-dominant hand on the acquisition of a sliding task in schoolchildren. *Laterality, 16*, 227–239.
Shea, C. H., Lai, Q., Black, C., & Park, J. H. (2000). Spacing practice sessions across days benefits the learning of motor skills. *Human Movement Science, 19*, 737–760.
Shea, J. B., & Morgan, R. L. (1979). Contextual interference effects on the acquisition, retention, and transfer of a motor skill. *Journal of Experimental Psychology, 5*, 179–187.
Sherwood, D. E. (1988). Effect of bandwidth knowledge of results on movement consistency. *Perceptual and Motor Skills, 66*, 535–542.
Skinner, B. F. (1938). *The Behavior of Organisms: An Experimental Analysis*. Appleton-Century-Crofts.
Sperl, L., & Cañal-Bruland, R. (2020). Reducing proactive interference in motor tasks. *Journal of Motor Behavior, 52*, 372–381.
Sperling, G. (1960). The information available in brief visual presentations. *Psychological Monographs, 74*, 1–29.
Squire, L. R. (Ed.). (1992). *Encyclopedia of Learning and Memory*. Macmillan.
Squire, L. R., & Kandel, E. R. (1999). *Gedächtnis. Die Natur des Erinnerns*. Spektrum Verlag.
Sternberg, S. (1966). High-speed scanning in human memory. *Science, 153*, 652–654.
Stock, A., & Stock, C. (2004). A short history of ideo-motor action. Psychological Research, 68, 176–188. https://doi.org/10.1007/s00426-003-0154-5
Stöckel, T., & Weigelt, M. (2012). Brain lateralisation and motor learning: Selective effects of dominant and non-dominant hand practice on the early acquisition of throwing skills. *Laterality: Asymmetries of Body, Brain and Cognition, 17*, 18–37.
Swinnen, S. P., Schmidt, R. A., Nicholson, D. E., & Shapiro, D. C. (1990). Information feedback for skill acquisition: Instantaneous knowledge of results degrades learning. *Journal of Experimental Psychology: Learning, Memory, and Cognition, 16*, 706−716.
Thorndike, E. L. (1911). *Animal Intelligence: Experimental Studies*. Macmillan.
Thorndike, E. L., & Woodworth, R. S. (1901). The influence of improvement in one mental function upon the efficiency of other functions. II. The estimation of magnitudes. *Psychological Review, 8*, 384–395.
Tulving, E. (1985). How many memory systems are there? *American Psychologist, 40*, 385–398.
van der Meer, E. (2006). Langzeitgedächtnis. In: J. Funke & P.A. French (Hrsg.), *Handbuch der Allgemeinen Psychologie—Kognition* (S. 346-355). Göttingen: Hogrefe Verlag.
Weigelt, M., Ahlmeyer, T., Lex, H., & Schack, T. (2011). The cognitive representation of a throwing technique in judo experts–Technological ways for individual skill diagnostics in high-performance sports. *Psychology of Sport and Exercise, 12*, 231–235.
Wickens, C. D., Hutchins, S., Carolan, T., & Cumming, J. (2013). Effectiveness of part-task training and increasing-difficulty training strategies: a meta-analysis approach. *Human Factors, 55*, 461–470.
Wohlschläger, A. (2001). Mental object rotation and the planning of hand movements. *Perception & Psychophysics, 63*, 709–718.
Wulf, G. (2009). *Aufmerksamkeit und motorisches Lernen*. Urban & Fischer/Elsevier.
Wulf, G., & Lewthwaite, R. (2016). Optimizing performance through intrinsic motivation and attention for learning: The OPTIMAL theory of motor learning. *Psychonomic Bulletin & Review, 23*, 1382–1414.
Wulf, G., McNevin, N., & Shea, C. H. (2001). The automaticity of complex motor skill learning as a function of attentional focus. *Quarterly Journal of Experimental Psychology A, 54*, 1143–1154.
Zimmer, H.D. & Kaernbach, C. (2006). Ikonischer und auditiver Speicher. In: J. Funke & P.A. French (Hrsg.), *Handbuch der Allgemeinen Psychologie—Kognition* (S. 334–339). Göttingen: Horace Verlag.

Neurocognition and Movement

Claudia Voelcker-Rehage, Dieter F. Kutz and Ross Julian

Contents

J. Schüler et al. (eds.), *Sport and Exercise Psychology*, https://doi.org/10.1007/978-3-031-03921-8_4

Learning Objectives

Basic:

- Knowing the definition of neurocognition
- Be able to reproduce the basic structure of the brain
- Understanding the (neuro-)biological principles of movement control

Advanced:

- Knowing how neurocognition changes over the lifespan
- Knowledge of the importance of physical activity for cognitive processes and the brain

Experts:

- Understanding the concept of neuroplasticity
- Understanding neurophysiological processes
- Knowing about components of executive skills

4.1 Introduction

This chapter focuses on the neurophysiological consideration of motor skills and motor learning. In addition to internal motor control processes themselves, the emphasis is on changes in these processes. The aim is to merge observed behaviour with neuroscientific findings. This is particularly important when permanent changes in coordination competence, i.e. processes of motor learning and motor development, are considered. In this chapter learning is understood as physiological changes of brain functions which are expressed in behaviour, e.g. changed transmission behaviour at synapses, the formation of new synapses or a change of myelinisation of axons. For example, the brain of small children differs noticeably from that of adults, and this difference can certainly be connected with changed prerequisites for complex enhanced coordination and learning performance. Before dealing with single topics of neurocognition and movement, a short overview of relevant neurobiological basics is provided.

Neurocognition

Neurocognition concerns the cognitive performance (e.g. learning, thinking, planning, understanding, etc.) as the result of neuronal processes that are realised in the brain, or rather in the nervous system.

4.2 Movement Control

Our entire behavioural repertoire is made up of movements controlled by motor systems in the brain (see ▶ Side Story: The Brain) and spinal cord. Motor systems should be understood as all areas of the brain that are involved in the planning, execution, and control of a movement or in the success and/or error feedback of a movement.

Motor systems use nerve impulses to generate contraction force in muscles and thus induce movement. These motor systems enable us to maintain posture and balance; to move the body, limbs and eyes; and to communicate through speech, gestures and facial expressions. Even to perform simple movements, such as extending the hand, different joints are moved and the body's centre of gravity shifts. Therefore, stretching the hand forward requires contraction of the leg muscles to compensate for the shift in the centre of gravity. The mechanical properties of the muscles, bones and joints must also be considered (see Ghez & Gordon, 1996).

Motor systems transmit precisely timed commands to many muscle groups. To accomplish these tasks, they continuously receive sensory information about the position and alignment of the body and limbs as well as the degree of muscle contraction. The sensory information from the muscles and joints, the skin and the other sensory organs is transmitted to the brain via the afferent (leading) pathways (sensory feedback). Based on this information, the brain initiates a movement. This motor command is transmitted via the efferent (pathways) to the spinal cord, which is then used for muscle innervation. This is summarised under item of sensory motor feedback.

Side Story

The Brain

The brain is divided into five areas; cerebrum, cerebellum, diencephalon, midbrain and posterior brain. The cerebrum is the largest and most advanced area of the brain. It is made up of one thick strand of nerve fibre (corpus callosum or bar) and is divided in the middle into two hemispheres which are interconnected. The cerebrum consists of the cerebral cortex, a 2- to 4-mm-thick layer of nerve cell bodies (grey matter) and the nerve fibres and tracts (white matter), which processes impulses in a forward trajectory (for further neuroscientific basics, see Bear et al., 2007).The structures and functions of the brain are subject to constant change over the entire lifespan (neuroplasticity). Different stimuli can have an influence on brain plasticity such as stress and non-use. Motor control is particularly related to five areas of the brain: cerebrum, cerebellum, basal ganglia, brain stem and spinal cord.

4.2.1 Hierarchically Organised Motor Control Instances

The motor systems are divided into five control instances: the cerebral cortex, the cerebellum (Crbl), the basal ganglia (BG), the brain stem and the spinal cord (◘ Tab. 4.1), which initiate and control movements in an orderly, cooperative and autonomous manner. For example, at the spinal cord level, without the involvement of the higher centres, reflexes can be generated. On the other hand, in the case of a purposeful arm movement (specific motor activity), for example, the maintenance of balance is controlled via different pathways than the lifting of the arm (◘ Table 4.1).

◘ **Table 4.1** Structure and main functions of movement control in the brain

Structure	Function
Cerebral cortex (cortex)	Decision (if, what), design (how), execution
Cerebellum (Crbl)	Monitoring, fine-tuning
Basal Ganglia (BG)	Evaluation, fine-tuning, forecasting
Brainstem and spinal cord	Execution, reflexes

The example of a ball throw in handball is used to demonstrate how motor systems interact. The planning of the throw is cooperatively carried out by the cortex, the Crbl and the BG, whilst the complex execution is undertaken by the brain stem and spinal cord. The decision whether to throw the ball is made recursively (in feedback loops) in the motivational and limbic parts of the cortex and the BG, which leads to the formation of possible movement patterns. From these preselected movement patterns (e.g. jump throw), a first draft of how the planned movement should be performed is created in the association fields (see Definition in ► Sect. 4.2.2) of the cortex. This draft action is synchronously transmitted to the BG and Crbl, and a final pattern of action is developed. In doing so, the BGs optimise the draft of the throw with regard to a positive prediction error (e.g. the throw arrives exactly at the player; ◘ Fig. 4.1: Basal ganglia/reward learning), and the Crbl refines the spatio-temporal structure of the design based on previous experience of errors (e.g. the throw was too low or too high to be caught by the other player; ◘ Fig. 4.1: cerebellum/supervised learning). Both results are combined in the motor cortex and form the final pattern that is executed by the brainstem and spinal cord.

The feedback signals from Crbl and BG support cortical learning during the execution of movements and also in the subsequent movements (◘ Fig. 4.1: cortex/Hebb's learning). Knowledge gained in subcortical

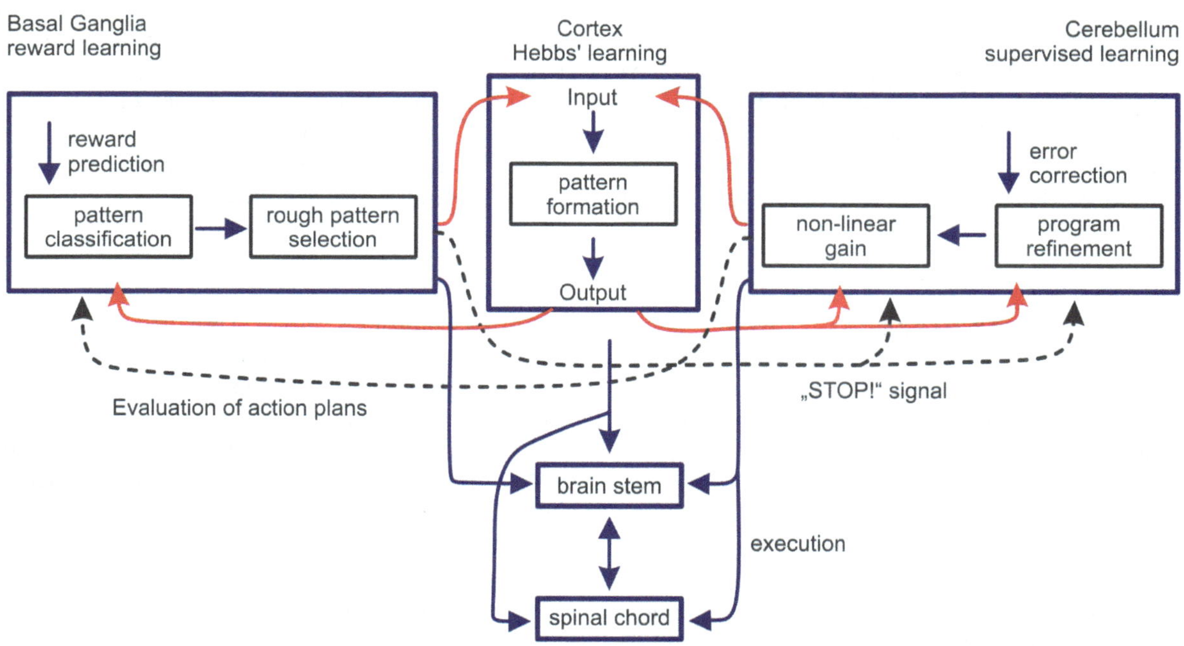

◘ **Fig. 4.1** Schematic representation of the hierarchical organisation of the motor control instances. Blue arrows, projections between and within the control instances; red arrows, cortico-striatal and cortico-cerebellar feedback loop; black dashed arrows, reciprocal connections between BG and Crbl structures is progressively transferred to the cortex by the BG and Crbl. The execution of the throw through the brainstem and spinal cord is also monitored by the BG and Crbl. Furthermore, bidirectional connections between the BG and Crbl have been anatomically proven (◘ Fig. 4.1: dashed lines), whose tasks have not yet been fully clarified. The projection from the Crbl to the BG serves the model-based evaluation of possible actions during reward learning. The path from the BGs to the Crbl provides the Crbl with an internal "Stop!" signal to activate programmes that inhibit current movements, e.g. when an opponent crosses on the planned path of the throw. A strict separation of learning and control is not possible from a physiological perspective.

As the description above shows, every movement control includes a "relearning" of the movement itself. Motor learning in the neurophysiological sense would then be a recurring interlocking of the motor systems, which change the neural processes depending on feedback (internal/external) (see ▶ Side Story: Neurophysiological Forms of Learning).

Side Story

Neurophysiological Forms of Learning

Hebbian learning is assumed to be the learning mechanism for the cortex. Here, if a neuron A excites a neuron B in such a way that neuron B forms action potentials, the synapse from A to B is strengthened. This means that if neuron A is subsequently excited, it becomes more likely that B will also be excited ("What fires together, wires together"). Special forms of this learning can be found in the cerebellum as supervised learning and in the basal ganglia as reward learning.

Supervised learning presupposes that there is a basic pattern of movement with which the planned or to be performed movement is compared. The current model assumes that the cerebellar hemispheres and the deep cerebellar nuclei create a forward model that predicts the outcome of an action (Wolpert et al., 1998). Spatial and temporal deviations are calculated between the model and the real movement. The resulting corrections become visible as an adjustment or adaptation of the current movement. Due to the association of sensory and motor skills, anticipation of movements can also be learned in this way.

Reward learning is found in the mesolimbic system. The neurophysiological basis for today's understanding of reward learning and its pathological malfunction in the form of addiction dates back to the work of Wolfram Schultz and colleagues (Schultz et al., 1997). Dopaminergic neurons of the ventral tegmental area in the midbrain and the substantia nigra compacta (▶ Sect. 4.2.4.1) project to areas of the brain that are relevant for motivation or goal-directed action, such as the striatum of the basal ganglia, the nucleus accumbens and the frontal cortex. These neurons are continuously active, which results in a continuous release of dopamine. The neural activity increases if a reward is given (e.g. something tasty to eat/drink, also catching a ball toss). When there are sensory stimuli that precede the reward, the reward is associated with those stimuli. When the stimulus is given in the future (e.g. seeing that a ball is about to be thrown), the reward is expected, and the neural activity increases already at the time of the stimuli (positive prediction error, e.g. I will catch the ball). If the expected reward is missing (e.g. failure to catch the ball), there is a sharp drop in neural activity (negative prediction error) at the time of the expected reward. Repeated occurrence of this sensorimotor pairing leads to a firm coupling between perception, action and expected success.

4.2.2 Motor Cortex Areas

The neocortex is the most highly organised part of the cerebral cortex and encompasses approximately 90% of the cerebral cortex. In addition to its vertical division into six layers of neurons, it is divided horizontally (two-dimensional) into so-called cortex regions. The division into cortex regions follows the cytoarchitectural work of Korbinian Brodmann (BA for Brodmann areas), who originally divided the cerebral cortex into 52 regions (Brodmann, 1909). In this nomenclature, for example, the primary motor cortex (M1) is called BA 4, whilst the primary visual cortex (V1) is called BA 17. If recent anatomical or functional findings make an additional or different division necessary, specific designation are used (Matelli & Luppino, 1992; Matelli and Luppino 2004; Zilles et al., 1996). The neocortex is involved in higher-order brain functions and is in humans pronounced developed in gyri (brain convolutions) and sulci (furrows).

Sensory information (e.g. visual, acoustic, somatosensory) directly reaches the respective sensory fields (primary visual, auditory or somatosensory cortex) in the cortex. They serve the direct processing of sensory information. Associative fields link different information of the sensory fields with each other and/or with information of the motor fields. In addition to the primary motor cortex (M1), the premotor area (PMA) and the supplementary motor area (SMA), the motor fields include the frontal eye field (frontal eye field, FEF) and the posterior parietal cortex, which is important for sensorimotor integration.

The primary motor cortex (M1), the premotor area (PMA) and the supplementary motor area (SMA) have the same characteristics of a somatotopic structure. This means that all parts of the body are distributed on the M1, SMA and PMA like a map (homunculus). All motor areas together with the primary somatosensory area (S1) form the descending tract (distribution approx. 40% PMA/SMA, 30% M1, 30% S1).

One method used to try to assign properties to cortex areas is transcranial magnetic stimulation (TMS; see ► Study Box: Motor Evoked Potentials (MEPs) by TMS). For example, magnetic stimulation of the hand region, i.e. both via M1 and PMA, can lead to a contraction of the finger muscles on the contralateral side. Electrical stimulation of both areas by microelectrodes in primates, depending on the intensity of the stimulation, not only leads to simple movements (e.g. finger twitches) but also to complex movement patterns (e.g. defensive movement of hand and arm; Graziano, 2016).

Motor Evoked Potentials (MEPs) by TMS

Transcranial magnetic stimulation (TMS) over the hand region of the motor cortex triggers contractions in the associated muscles, which can be measured as motor evoked potentials (MEPs) (◻ Fig. 4.2: upper line of the normal control, NC). In this manner, the integrity of the efferent pathway from the cortex to the hand muscles can be investigated. Conversely, electrical stimulation of the median nerve can be used to measure evoked potentials in the somatosensory cortex using an EEG. These evoked potentials are a measure of the integrity of the afferent pathway. If both methods are combined in such a way that the electrical stimulation is given 20 ms before the TMS pulse, the MEP amplitude is reduced to approx. 41% in normal controls compared to the control condition (◻ Fig. 4.2: lower line of NC). This effect is called short-afferent inhibition and is a consequence of cholinergic (inhibitory) projections from the primary somatosensory cortex to the motor cortex. If the same stimulation protocol is used in Alzheimer's patients, the MEP amplitude is only reduced to approx. 86% of the control condition. This is an indication that the inhibitory cholinergic projections in the neocortex are disturbed in Alzheimer's patients.

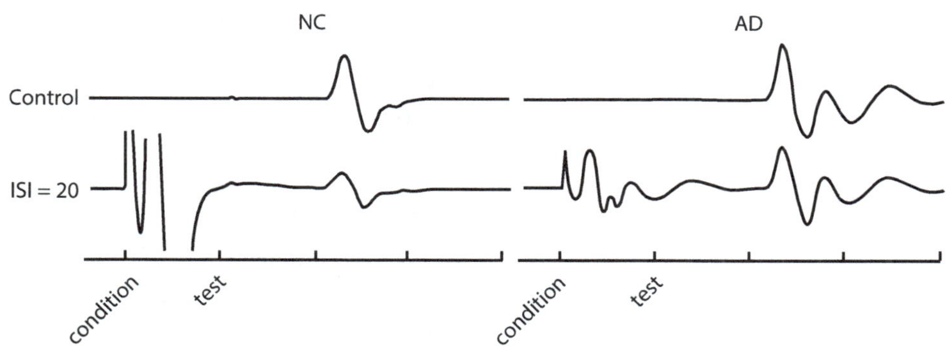

◻ **Fig. 4.2** Original recordings of MEPs of the first M. interosseus in a normal control (NC) and an Alzheimer's patient (AD). Top line ("control"): MEPs during the administration of a single TMS impulse ("test"). The peak-to-peak amplitude is about the same for both subjects. Lower line (ISI = 20): combined stimulation of the median nerve ("condition") and a TMS pulse delayed by 20 ms ("test"). In healthy volunteers, the MEP amplitude is significantly more reduced with combined stimulation than in Alzheimer's patients (Figure from Sakuma et al., 2007; all rights reserved). Sakuma et al., Clinical Neurophysiology 118:1460–1463 (2007)

The PMA is characterised by the fact that it encodes both the target location and the hand to be executed, simultaneously during pointing movements, which is why it is integral in neural movement planning (Beurze et al., 2007). The basis for this is the special neuronal equipment with cells that first encode the location of a target and then the movement to be performed (Crammond & Kalaska, 1994; Gail et al., 2009; Weinrich & Wise, 1982). Planned movements that are to be carried out with a delay are also coded by neurons of the PMA (set-neurons; Bauswein & Fromm, 1992).

One of the special characteristics of SMA is that it is important in the imagination of movements and in the bimanual coordination of movements (Swinnen, 2002). For example, studies on primates demonstrate that following damage to the SMA, they were no longer able to perform two different movements with their hands in a coordinated manner. The SMA is also important for the ability to abort a planned movement due to an external "stop" signal (Logan et al., 2015; Scangos et al., 2013; Stuphorn, 2015).

In such a varied system, several actions can be conducted at the same time. Also, the decision for one of the possible actions seems to be located in the same sensomotoric circuits that perform planning and execution—and not, as often assumed, in the prefrontal cortex (for references see Cisek & Kalaska, 2010). For example, bimanual response-choice tasks in monkeys demonstrated neural activity in the premotor areas of both hemispheres until the hand to be used becomes specified (Hoshi et al., 2000; Hoshi & Tanji, 2006). Similarly, investigations with electroencephalography (EEG) in humans show the simultaneous activation of the premotor and motor areas of both hemispheres until the moment when the subject has decided which hand to use (Henz et al., 2015).

Motor Cortex Areas Are Closely Intertwined

Motor cortex areas are closely interlocked: the individual cortex regions are strongly interlinked with each other, and individual functions can be attributed to them less distinctively than has long been assumed.

4.2.3 Cerebellum

The cerebellum (Crbl) corresponds to about 10% of the cerebral mass and approximately 50–75% of the surface of the cerebral cortex. The functional significance of the Crbl is determined by the number of neurons. It contains about 50% of all neurons of the entire central nervous system. Luigi Rolando (1809) was the first to point out the motor significance of the Crbl. It controls and supports motor functions, especially balance, and coordinates the support of motor function for the target motor function. The cerebellum is also responsible for detecting and correcting errors. Thus, it is active in motor adaptations and in the association of motor tasks and sensors. The calculated correction of performances is projected to the cortex, brain stem and spinal cord. In contrast, there is almost no activity if a learned task is performed correctly.

Functional knowledge of the Purkinje cells is essential for understanding the performance of the cerebellum (Fig. 4.3: blue cells). These cells receive input from the entire sensory system, informing them about planned movements or movements in progress. From this information, the respective adjustment can be calculated.

For a long time, motor tasks were regarded as the only tasks of the Crbl. Only with the work of the American neurologist Schmahmann (1997) a new view of the Crbl began as an important instance for the neurocognition of movement. He hypothesises that the Crbl is critical for the modulation of sensorimotor, cognitive and limbic functions. Damage to the Crbl leads to functional disorders of thinking and the affect (dysmetria of thought) with restricted modulation of intellect and emotion (cerebellar cognitive active syndrome, CCAS). However, people with pure cerebellar lesions do not necessarily show severe cognitive deficits (Timmann-Braun & Maschke, 2003).

4.2.3.1 Anatomy and Function of the Cerebellum

The cerebellum can be macroscopically divided into the cerebellar cortex and the deep cerebellar nuclei (DCN). The cerebellar cortex is divided functionally into three sections to which one or two cerebellar nuclei are assigned (Timmann-Braun & Maschke, 2003). The Crbl has several types of characteristic neurons (Fig. 4.3: Purkinje cell, granule cell, Golgi cell, star cell, basket cell). To understand how it functions, it is important to know that both the Purkinje cells in the cerebellar cortex and the DCN receive the same information from the periphery. The inferior olive uses climbing fibres directly to the Purkinje cells, whereas, nuclei of the pons project to granule cells in the cerebellar cortex. In turn, the granule cells transmit the signal excitatory via parallel fibres (Fig. 4.3: red signal pathways). The Purkinje cells (Fig. 4.3: blue neurons) inhibit the DCN, which are also simultaneously stimulated. In addition, there are interneurons (Fig. 4.3: black neurons) that have an inhibitory effect between the Purkinje cells. The Crbl

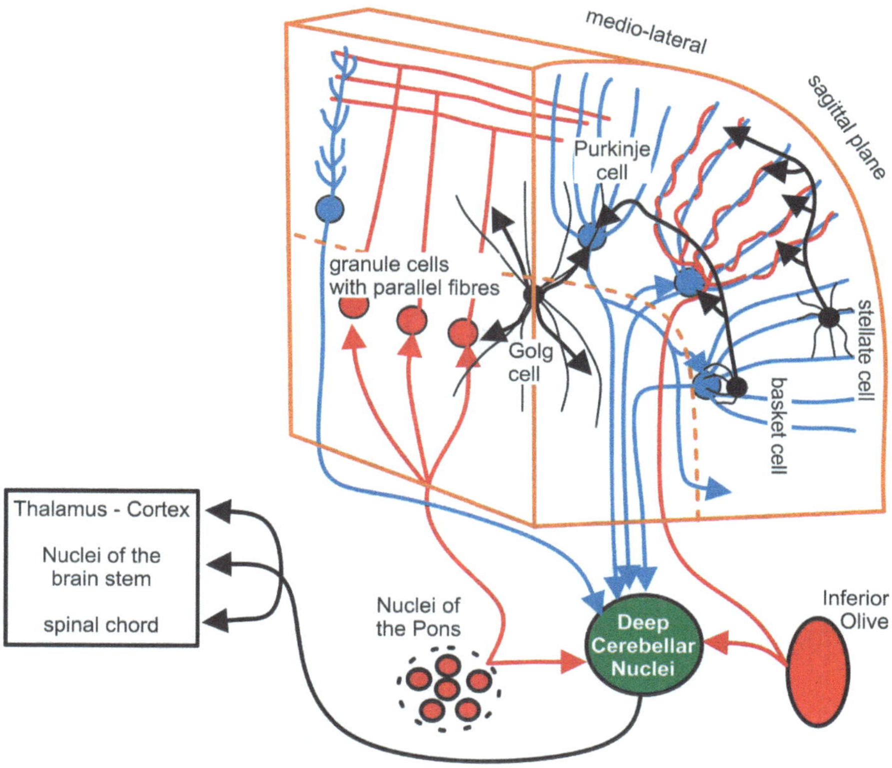

Fig. 4.3 Simplified scheme of the cerebellum. Schematic block cut of the cerebellar hemispheres. Red, entrances from the inferior olive and brain stem nuclei via the granule cells; blue, Purkinje cells; black, inhibitory interneurons of the cerebellar hemisphere

forms a complex feedforward inhibition network that adapts the programmes to be executed to the sensory situation and associates sensory and motor functions together.

Figuratively speaking, the task of the Crbl can be compared to that of a stonemason. Just like a stonemason cuts a figure out of a rough stone, the cerebellum cuts a feasible course of action out of a provisional plan.

4.2.4 Basal Ganglia

The basal ganglia are important in the planning and evaluation of motor tasks. They are responsible for the programmed sequence of slow movements, for which they deliver precisely, spatially and temporally adapted excitation patterns to the performing motor cerebral cortex. This is done via three projection paths in the basal ganglia. The direct pathway (Fig. 4.4: red arrows) promotes movement, whilst the indirect pathway (Fig. 4.4: blue arrows) dampens movement. Dopamine from the substantia nigra compacta (SNc) creates a balance between these two pathways (Fig. 4.4: purple arrows). In addition, there is the hyperdirect pathway (Fig. 4.4: green arrows) from the cortex to the subthalamic nucleus (STN). It is assumed that the function of this path is the choice of action.

The evaluation of movements performed by the basal ganglia does not only question whether the tasks were performed correctly but also assesses whether "I like this movement sequence," "That's the way I want to move" and also "A figure like this gets a better rating." This form of evaluating motor skills is also important when choosing the target of a possible action. The evaluation and planning performances are carried out in a feedback loop with the cortex.

4.2.4.1 Anatomy of the Basal Ganglia

The basal ganglia are a network of functionally interconnected nuclei of the cerebrum, thalamus and brain stem (Fig. 4.4). The entry structure is the striatum, which consists of the caudate nucleus and the putamen and receives entry from the entire cortex (Fig. 4.4). The exit structures are the globus pallidus internus (GPi) and the substantia nigra reticularis (SNr). The basal ganglia also include the globus pallidus externus (GPe), the nucleus subthalamicus (STN) and the substantia nigra compacta (SNc). This network acts as an open-loop as well as a closed-loop network inhibitory or dis-inhibitory on cortical areas and/or brainstem

4

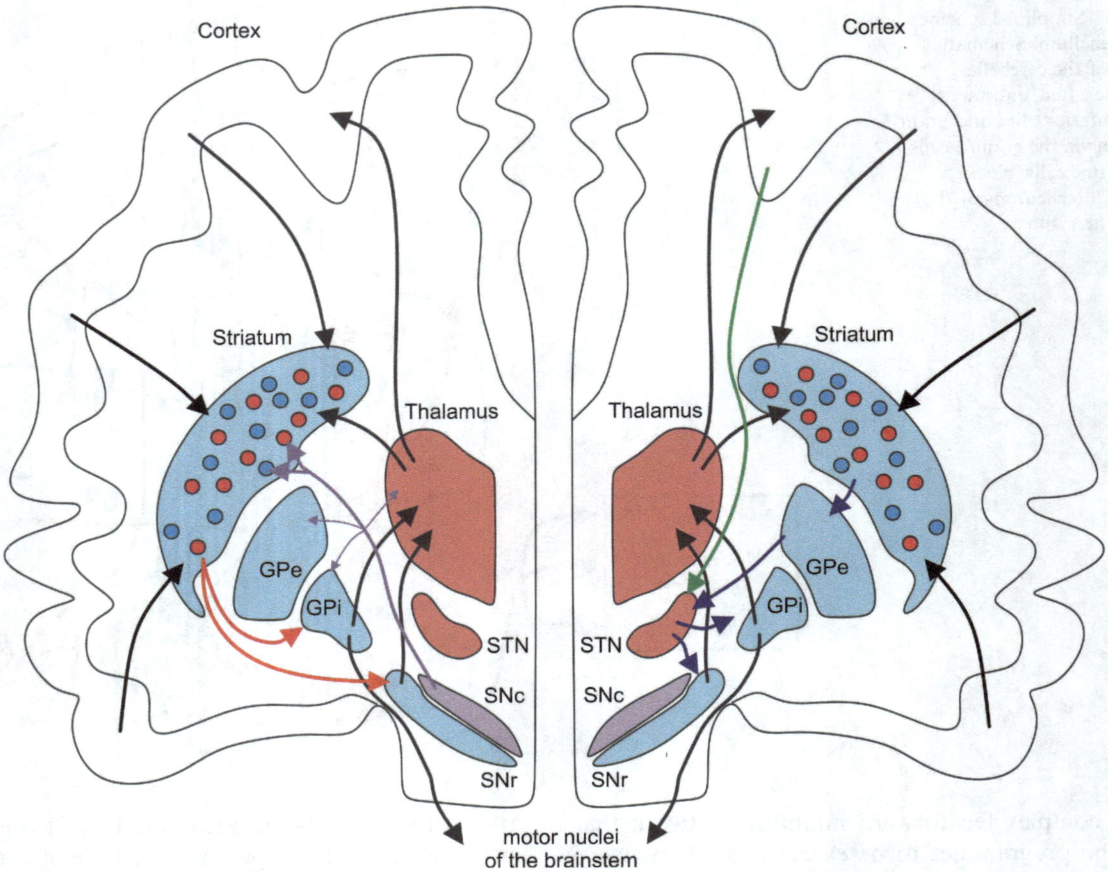

Fig. 4.4 Simplified diagram of the basal ganglia. GPe/GPi, globus pallidus externus/internus; STN, nucleus subthalamicus; SNc/SNr, substantia nigra compacta/reticularis. Core areas that have an excitatory effect on subsequent areas are shown in red; those that have an inhibitory effect are shown in blue. Red circles/arrows, neurons/projections of the direct path; blue circles/arrows, neurons/projections of the indirect pathway; green arrow, hyperdirect pathway; purple arrows, dopaminergic projections from the substantia nigra compacta (SNc); black arrows, input projections and projections belonging to more than one pathway

nuclei to promote or suppress specific actions (Nelson & Kreitzer, 2014). The relationships can be summarised in two functional groups: the direct pathway and the indirect pathway. The direct pathway (Fig. 4.4: red arrows) has a movement-enhancing effect. The starting point is the specific projection neurons of the striatum (Fig. 4.4: red circles), which have an inhibitory effect on the GPi and SNr. The inhibitory effect of GPi and SNr on the thalamus is damped, and its projections to the cortex are promoted. The indirect pathway (Fig. 4.4: blue arrows) has a motion-dampening effect. The starting point here is a second class of specific projection neurons of the striatum (Fig. 4.4: blue circles), which have an inhibitory effect on the GPe. Its inhibitory effect is attenuated upon the STN. The STN has an excitatory effect on GPi and SNr. The reduced inhibition by GPe increases the excitation of the STN, and thus GPi and SNr are more strongly aroused. Their inhibitory effect on the thalamus is thus strengthened, and its projections to the cortex are diminished. The dopaminergic projections of SNc (Fig. 4.4: violet arrows) have a mediating effect between the two pathways. Dopamine has a stimulating effect on striatum neurons of the direct pathway (via D1-receptors) and an inhibiting effect on striatum neurons of the indirect pathway (via D2-receptors). Overall, there is a movement-enhancing effect in the case of dopamine release and a movement-dampening effect in the case of dopamine deficiency (e.g. Parkinson's disease). Additionally, there is a direct projection from the cortex onto the STN which is called a hyperdirect pathway (Fig. 4.4: green arrows). Excitation of the STN excites the GPi and SNr with ultimate inhibition of the thalamus (see above). Hence, the function of gating, i.e. the selection of an action, is attributed to this hyperdirect pathway.

4.2.5 Brainstem and Spinal Cord

The brain stem controls the motor system of posture through its reflex (e.g. vestibulospinal reflex, tonic labyrinthine reflex, righting reflex) and enables targeted movements. It receives information from various centres about muscle length and tension, joint angle position and skin contact, information from the vestibular organ and visual impressions. This enables the body to be raised to an upright position and the gaze (head and eyes) to be held parallel to the horizon. Consequently, the brain stem offers a basic repertoire of movements which can be combined to complex tasks. Furthermore, it is involved in visceromotor tasks such as respiratory and cardiovascular control, which have to be adapted to motor performance.

The spinal cord forms the lowest level of skeletal motor control. By means of reflex arcs, it adjusts given limb positions and muscle contractions and keeps them constant against external perturbations. Furthermore, these reflex arcs enable the spinal cord to perform stimulus-induced complex movement patterns. For example, kicking an object with the foot causes a stiffening of the leg on the opposite side and then leads to lifting of the foot on the irritated side (flexor reflex). This stimulus-response sequence is considered the basic pattern of locomotion.

4.3 Brain Anatomy and Brain Functions in Different Age Ranges

The brain reaches its maximum weight of about 1400 g at the age of about 20 years. Between the 25th and 80th year of life, the weight is then reduced by approximately 20%, whereby weight loss accelerates after the age of 60 (Haug, 1986). The development and change of the brain takes place over the entire lifespan up to old age. Depending on stimuli, new nerve cell networks are constantly being created, converted and degraded. This neuronal plasticity leads to the fact that people can learn over the entire lifespan.

4.3.1 Brain Development in Childhood and Adolescence

Brain development plays a particularly important role in childhood and puberty. By the age of about 6 months, the positioning of the neurons in the motor cortex is completed. At the same time, during the first 2 years of life, there is massive new formation of synapses between cells in many areas of the brain.

By the age of ten months, the number of synapses has more than doubled. Subsequently, the density of synapses in the brain decreases by about two-thirds until puberty, albeit with great regional differences. This happens due to experience-based activation or non-activation. Those synapses that are needed have the best chance of being retained, according to the motto “use it or lose it” (Hebb’s learning). At the same time, a higher conduction speed due to the myelination of the axons leads to increased cognitive and motor capacities. The improvement of cognitive abilities during school age leads, for example, to children and adolescents being able to direct their attention more precisely, better remember instructions and plan their working steps more effectively. Brain physiological maturation also leads to changes in the motor system, such as improved muscle control and faster stimulus perception and processing (see ▶ Study Box: Differentiation-Dedifferentiation Hypothesis).

Differentiation-Dedifferentiation Hypothesis

According to the differentiation-dedifferentiation hypothesis, differentiation processes occur during childhood and adolescence and dedifferentiation processes in old age. These (de-)differentiation processes are described on different levels and for different dimensions. For example, the correlation between different intellectual achievements decreases during childhood and increases again in later adulthood. Eyre et al. (2001) were able to show by means of transcranial magnetic stimulation (TMS) that ipsilateral corticomotor pathways are present in newborns, which regress in the course of early childhood in normal children. In older adults, motor and sensory performances are more prominently associated with intellectual performance than in younger adults (Li & Lindenberger, 2002). For example, brain imaging data show that children and younger adults show very specific activations in the ventral visual cortex for faces, places and words, whereas older people show less specific activations (Park et al., 2004).

4.3.2 Brain Development in Old Age

The development and change of the brain are not limited to childhood but continues over the entire lifespan, up until old age. New nerve cell networks are constantly being created, converted and degraded. In old age, changes occur in anatomy as well as in the functioning of the brain. However, as age increases, individual regions of the brain are affected differently (see ► Side Story: Brain Functions and Connectivity).

4

Side Story

Brain Functions and Connectivity

Functional activations are those activations in the brain that are observed in certain brain structures when solving or performing a certain task or are observed in a certain processing state. Changes in the functional activation of brain regions can be seen, for example, in changes in activation strength, as measured using functional magnetic resonance imaging (fMRI) or functional near-infrared spectroscopy (fNIRS), or in changes in the electrophysiological signals in the EEG (► Methods: Methods of Brain Research). These measurement methods are also used to examine the functional integration or networking of the brain (connectivity analyses). In this context, the anatomical connectivity describes constant connections between brain regions, whilst the functional connectivity describes a statistical connection, and the effective connectivity describes a causal dependence of the neurons in the neural network. The functional and effective connectivity is by no means fixed but is flexibly modulated depending on the situation and is based on sensorimotor and cognitive performance (Stephan et al., 2009).

Brain degenerations are particularly pronounced in areas of the cerebral cortex responsible for vision, hearing and sensorimotor functions, in the Crbl, in the hippocampus (functions in learning, memory and the processing of emotions), in the BG and in the spinal cord. The consequences of these age-related changes are, for example, slower or ineffective information processing, reduced performance in cognitive and motor tasks and a reduced ability to regenerate. The ageing brain is also characterised by changes which may represent attempts to compensate for neurophysiological losses. Accordingly, the brain of older people can compensate for age-related deficits by involving other areas that were not needed for these tasks in younger years. Older people show, for example, an additional prefrontal activation in the execution of motor tasks, which is interpreted as a higher proportion of cognitive control, which, makes the execution of tasks less automated. This is particularly evident in complex tasks.

Side Story

How the Brain and Behaviour Can Be Related

An important question is how neural activation patterns can be related to cognitive, motor and sensory functions. Since there is no linear relationship between neurophysiological and cognitive changes, cognitive changes (gains or deficits) only become visible when a certain threshold of structural and functional changes has been exceeded (Cabeza, 2002). Concurrently, the same cognitive performance in older and younger people can be associated with very different activation patterns. Age research shows that the processes in the brain are not directly and causally related to the observed behaviour of a person. The question remains of how exactly the activation patterns are related to sensory and motor skill.

These phenomena are often investigated with the help of so-called dual-task paradigms (see ► Sect. 4.6), in which a test person is expected to perform a motor and cognitive task simultaneously. Young adult participants often show comparable performance in these dual tasks, as in single tasks. Whereas, in older adults there are greater costs during these dual tasks. This is attributed to the lack of brain resources of the older test persons, i.e. older persons need (more) cognitive resources to perform a motor task, which are then no longer available for the cognitive tasks under dual-task conditions and vice versa (see ► Methods: Brain Research Methods).

Structural Imaging

Structural magnetic resonance imaging (sMRI) provides non-invasive, high-resolution three-dimensional anatomical images of the brain. Based on the magnetic properties of the protons (hydrogen nuclei) and their specific density in the tissue, different structures of the brain (grey matter, white matter, ventricles, air-filled cavities, etc.) can be differentiated and made visible. With suitable measurement sequences and analytical methods, the thickness and volume of the corresponding structures in the entire brain or in individual areas can be determined.

Functional Imaging

Functional MRI (fMRI) is a variant of MRI that can be used to display the activation of areas of the brain during certain tasks or processing procedures. Oxygen bound to haemoglobin changes the magnetic properties of the blood, thus leading to a weakening of the MRI signal in regions with an increased supply of oxygen-saturated blood. The temporal resolution of this so-called BOLD signal (blood oxygenation level dependent; depending on the blood oxygen content) is rather low. Complex statistical procedures and analytical methods nevertheless make it possible to define functional and even causal connectivity patterns between activated brain regions.

A method related to fMRI is functional near-infrared spectroscopy (fNIRS). In contrast to fMRI, fNIRS reveals differences in the light absorption of oxygen-free and oxygen-saturated haemoglobin. For this purpose, near-infrared light is radiated into the skull. This light penetrates 1–2 cm into the brain and is partially absorbed by the haemoglobin. The proportion of light absorbed corresponds to the neuronal activation in the tissue. The disadvantage of this method is the low penetration depth of the light into the brain. As a result, the method is only suitable for making neural activity in the outer layers of the brain visible. One of the advantages is that the method can now be used under very realistic conditions and even in motion.

Neurophysiological Procedures

Electroencephalography (EEG) can be used to record the electrical activity of nerve cells in the brain. The EEG uses electrodes placed on the skull to measure the electrical field that is created by the activity of the nerve cells within the brain. This method has a very high temporal resolution and measures both endogenously generated electrical oscillations in different frequency bands (e.g. alpha 8–13 Hz, beta 14–30 Hz) and task or stimulus-dependent changes (event-related potentials [ERP]) in amplitudes and latencies. The spatial resolution of the EEG depends on the number of electrodes or sensors used. Thirty-two to 128 channels are commonly used in todays practice. EEG systems have now been developed that enable wireless measurements in the field and in motion.

Methods for Influencing Brain Activity

In transcranial magnetic stimulation (TMS), a strong magnetic coil is used to induce an electromagnetic field that can be used to influence the neural activity in its area. This makes it possible, among other things, to record the motor stimulus threshold using so-called motor evoked potentials (MEPs). If the stimulation is repetitive (rTMS), depending on the level of the stimulation frequency, an excitatory (>5 Hz) or inhibitory (<1 Hz) influence can be exerted on the activity of brain areas, such as the primary motor cortex (M1). For example, TMS can be used to disrupt processing in certain areas of the brain (virtual lesion). With behavioural experiments carried out in parallel, it is possible to examine whether the areas concerned are involved in a certain task or function or are even necessary.

In addition to TMS, transcranial direct current stimulation (tDCS) is increasingly being used to a certain extent, to modulate neuronal activity. In this method, a weak direct electrical current is applied to the cortex through electrodes attached to the skull. Depending on the polarity and current strength, the induced electric field can increase or decrease the activity at the synapses in the brain. In contrast to TMS, the electric fields in tDCS are usually too weak to directly induce nerve impulses. Rather, the probability of occurrence of the nerve impulses (action potentials) is increased or decreased. That is why tDCS is also known as a method of neuromodulation.

4

4.4 Neuronal Plasticity

In neurobiology, the term "plasticity" refers to the ability of synapses, nerve cells or entire brain areas to change their characteristics depending on their use. In developmental psychology, plasticity generally describes the changeability (intra-individual variability) within a person.

Neurobiology distinguishes between two forms of learning: non-associative learning and associative learning. Non-associative learning includes habituation (adaptation through repeated identical stimuli), sensitisation (increase in response to a standard stimulus as a result of an intermediate disturbance stimulus) and dishabituation (increase in response to a standard stimulus as a result of an unknown stimulus or because a behavioural response was previously reduced or completely absent through habituation). Associative learning includes classical conditioning, operant conditioning and learning through observation and information.

Plasticity

In neurobiology, the term "plasticity" describes the properties of synapses, nerve cells or entire brain areas that change in their characteristics depending on their use.

In developmental psychology, plasticity generally describes the changeability (intra-individual variability) within a person.

Non-Associative Learning

"Non-associative learning is the behavioural change that occurs over time in response to a single stimulus" (Bear et al., 2007, p. 867). Non-associative learning includes habituation (adaptation through repeated identical stimuli), sensitisation (increase in the response to a standard stimulus as a result of an intervening disturbance stimulus) and dishabituation or weaning (increase in response to a standard stimulus as a result of an unknown stimulus or because a behavioural response was previously reduced or completely absent due to habituation (lack of behavioural reaction).

Associative Learning

"In associative learning, you create connections between events" (Bear et al., 2007, p. 868). Associative learning includes classic conditioning, operant conditioning and observational learning.

All learning processes involve neuroplastic processes. In the case of "so-called" synaptic plasticity, the structure of synapses can change in addition to the number. Therefore, the efficiency of the neuronal circuitry changes. In addition, new contacts between nerve cells can develop or existing contacts can be broken down.

The synaptic changes often result in altered activation patterns, which can be detected in humans using non-invasive methods (e.g. EEG or fMRI). Changes at the molecular level are visible in human studies as functional changes (altered activation patterns) but also as structural changes, such as volume changes of the grey and white matter of the brain. The formation of new nerve cells (neurogenesis) has so far only been demonstrated in individual regions (hippocampus, striatum) of the human brain and at a very low rate (turn-over <3%/year; Ernst et al., 2014; Spalding et al., 2013). The enormous plasticity of our brain is also shown by the fact that, for example, after brain damage (accidents, stroke), the functions of the damaged brain regions can be taken over/compensated by other regions.

Memory content is not stored in specific regions and learning does not take place in certain regions but in a network of those areas which are also involved in recording and processing the information (► Sect. 4.2.2). Learning can change both the size of the representative areas and the supply structures and networks. In the learning process different stages of cognitive processing are distinguished. In the first phase of acquisition, a high cognitive demand is assumed, i.e. the learner has to consciously process and control the movements to be learned (◻ Fig. 4.5). In later learning phases, when a movement is mastered, it is processed automatically (consolidation, automation; Luft & Buitrago, 2005; see ► Sect. 4.3.2).

These differences in the processing or control of motor movements and in the motor learning process can be visualised with brain imaging techniques such as fMRI. Therefore, motor tasks basically display functional activity in the motor areas of the brain described previously (Doyon et al., 2002; Gobel et al., 2011; Hamzei et al., 2012; Kwon et al., 2012; Xiong et al., 2009). Additionally, the acquisition phase of a movement is associated with activation in prefrontal (Doyon et al., 2002; Floyer-Lea & Matthews, 2004; Gobel et al., 2011; Kwon et al., 2012) and parietal areas (Doyon et al., 2002; Floyer-Lea & Matthews, 2004; Gobel et al., 2011; Hamzei et al., 2012; Kwon et al., 2012). This frontal and parietal activation gives an indication of the cognitive contribution in the acquisition phase (Doyon & Benali, 2005). The brain activation then changes with repeated execution of a newly learned movement. The activity in frontal areas is reduced, and the activity in the Crbl remains stable (e.g. Floyer-Lea & Matthews, 2004).

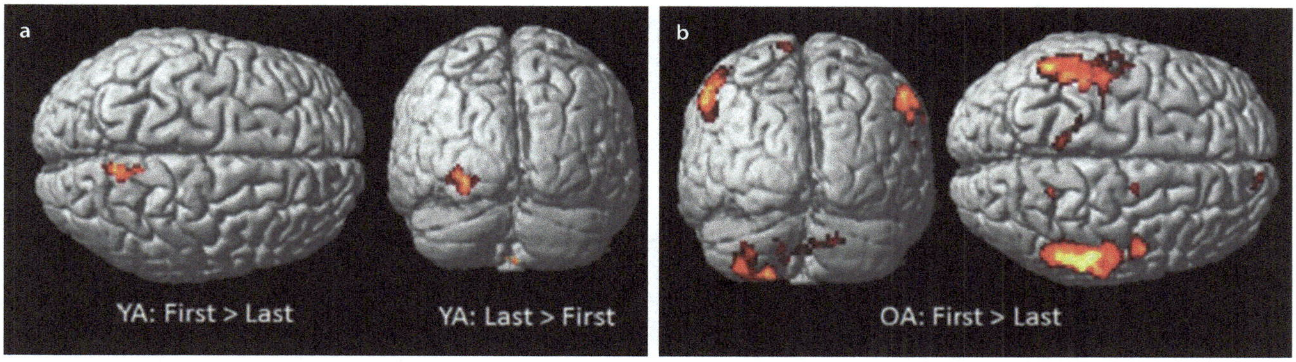

Fig. 4.5 Motor learning of a fine motor precision grip task dependent of age. Age differences in brain activation at the beginning and end of the learning phase of a fine motor power modulation task in precision grip: contrast of the first > last trials. Older adults (OA) show significantly stronger activation in frontal and parietal areas and in the cerebellum at the beginning of the learning task **b**, whereas younger adults (YA) show stronger activation only in the posterior parietal cortex **a** (Godde et al., 2018)

The overall activity is less distributed and more focused, which is interpreted as an indication of efficient movement processing. Such changes in activation patterns demonstrate that learned movements are processed more automatically and require fewer cognitive resources (Doyon et al., 2002; Floyer-Lea & Matthews, 2004; Gobel et al., 2011; Toni et al., 2002). On the behavioural level, the changed activity patterns are accompanied by an improvement in motor performance.

Greater motor performance after training is also associated with improved functional connectivity (▶ Sect. 4.3.2; ▶ Digression: Brain Functions and Connectivity) in motor regions (Coynel et al., 2010; Hamzei et al., 2012; Ma et al., 2010; Vahdat et al., 2011). For example, improved functional connectivity was observed within the "so-called" default mode network (DMN), a functional network that exhibits activity under resting conditions (also resting state network, measured by resting state fMRI or EEG). Ma et al., 2011, demonstrated changes in functional connectivity in central and parietal regions following 4 weeks of daily practicing of a finger sequence task (Ma et al. (2011)). Taubert et al. (2011), observed a change in the fronto-parietal network after only 1 week of two short training sessions for learning a whole-body balance task (Taubert et al., 2011), which was further manifested after 6 weeks. Interestingly, even a one 11-min learning unit (visuomotor joystick tracking task) showed changes in fronto-parietal areas of the DMN (Albert et al., 2009).

In addition to functional adjustments, structural (anatomic) alterations also occur in the brain. For example, after 40 h of golf practice, beginners demonstrated volume increases in the grey matter in cortex regions of the sensorimotor network, such as the central sulcus and the premotor and parietal cortex (Bezzola et al., 2011). Juggling studies have demonstrated changes in the volume of the grey matter in the frontal cortex (Boyke et al., 2008; Driemeyer et al., 2008), temporal cortex (Draganski et al., 2004; Driemeyer et al., 2008) including the hippocampus (Boyke et al., 2008), parietal cortex (Draganski et al., 2004; Driemeyer et al., 2008; Scholz et al., 2009), occipital cortex (Scholz et al., 2009) and nucleus accumbens (Boyke et al., 2008; > Excursus: Motor Learning Depending on Age).

Side Story

Motor Learning Depending on Age

Physical and neurophysiological requirements influence learning and training effects. This includes the experience of previously learned tasks, the personal requirements and the level of development. In childhood, the necessary cognitive, motor and sensory prerequisites must first be developed in order to learn complex movements. Thus, as long as certain prerequisites are not developed, little can be achieved through practice. Therefore, the ability to learn increases with age. It can often be observed that older children have an advantage over younger children/toddlers when it comes to movement learning. This can be illustrated using the example of swimming. Whereby, 5-year-old children learn to perform a swimming movement such as the front crawl, in fewer hours of practice than 2- to 4-year-old children (Blanksby et al., 1995; Parker & Blanksby, 1997). In the case of more complex movements, such as juggling and lacrosse, it was shown that only 9-year-old children achieved clearly visible improvements in performance, following a learning intervention (Voelcker-Rehage, 2008). Of course, younger children also showed performance gains but to a much lesser extent. This also provides hints and recommendations for a sports-specific specialisation. However, simple sequences of movements that do not require any special prior experience or physical fitness are learned in childhood, sometimes even faster than in adolescence and adulthood.

4

4.5 Physical Activity to Promote Cognition

Physical activity is positively related to cognition and brain functions. A distinction must be made between immediate (acute) and long-term (chronic) effects of physical activity. Immediate effects are changes in cognitive performance during or immediately after physical activity. Persistent effects describe the relationship between physical fitness and cognitive performance or the effect of targeted intervention programmes over a period of several weeks or months.

4.5.1 Acute Effects of Physical Activity on Cognition

Acute effects from exercise on cognition were treated with different forms of intervention (endurance activity, coordination training, etc.), different characteristics of the intervention in terms of cognitive measures, different points in time of measurement and different duration and intensity as well as on the basis of different samples (e.g. McMorris et al., 2011).

Immediately after exertion (regardless of the type of exertion), cognitive performance is improved on average, whereas during exertion, depending on duration and intensity, negative effects on cognition tended to be observed (Lambourne & Tomporowski, 2010). These effects appear to be independent of cognitive measures (e.g. executive functions, memory, crystalline intelligence) (Chang et al., 2012).

In addition to the time of measurement, two other important factors contribute to different results regarding acute exercise on cognition. These are the intensity and duration of exercise. A meta-analysis by McMorris and Hale (2012) supports the assumption of an inverse U-shaped relationship between excitation and performance, according to the Yerkes-Dodson law (Yerkes & Dodson, 1908). As such, the best and most robust results of acute exercise on cognition (especially on executive control) are achieved at submaximal moderate intensities, with a duration between 20 and 60 min (Chang et al., 2012; McMorris et al., 2011; Tomporowski, 2003). In contrast, high-intensity exercise seems to be effective in athletes or very active persons, but not in less active individuals (Alves et al., 2014; Budde et al., 2012). These findings suggest that regular physical activity can lead to neurobiological adaptations that enable effects of high-intensity exercise on cognitive processes. The duration of exercise also seems to have an effect. According to this, positive effects on cognition are recorded from the 20th minute up to exertion (Chang et al., 2012).

In addition, training effects differ in terms of the time of cognitive testing after exposure. The effects of acute activity are evident immediately after training and last up to 30–40 min after recovery (Pontifex et al., 2009) but seem to have vanished after 2 h (Hopkins et al., 2012). However, the exercise load also seems to play a role here: in the case of low- to moderate-intensity exercise, the effects are usually only present directly after the exercise, whereas after more intensive exercise (>75% of the maximum heart rate), positive effects are also present after a time delay (Chang et al., 2012).

? Moderating Factors of Acute Effects of Exercise on Cognition

- Time of measurement (during/after exercise)
- Exercise duration
- Exercise intensity
- Cardiovascular fitness status, physical activity behaviour
- Temporal arrangement of cognitive testing after exercise
- Cognitive dimension (e.g. executive functioning, working memory, attention and processing speed)

Studies on the acute effects of exercise have so far mainly been carried out in young adults, but comparable results appear to be achievable in children. In 9- to 10-year-olds, for example, after 20 min of moderate walking on a treadmill, better cognitive performance was measured than under resting conditions (Hillman et al., 2008). Even after a 10-min coordination training session, 13- to 15-year-old schoolchildren were able to demonstrate improved concentration than after a rest condition (Budde et al. 2008). Some studies have also shown positive effects of moderate endurance exercise on information processing speed (Stroop test; Barella et al., 2010) or working memory performance (n-back test; Hogan et al., 2013) in older adults.

Reflection

The Mandatory Sports Lesson

The information that short-, moderate-intensity exercise sessions can improve cognitive function has important implications for various target groups, e.g. for the school context, in the context of active breaks or active lessons. This is especially true for cognitively weaker adolescents (Budde et al., 2010). For example, according to the Folkeskole Act, passed by the Danish Parliament in 1993 and updated in 2014, it is mandatory for Danish primary and lower secondary schools to offer an average of 45 min of physical activity per school day. In addition, a supplementary PE lesson per week was introduced in class 1 and a final exam in class 9. Day care facilities are required to develop an educational curriculum that describes the day care centre's local goals in six thematic areas, one of which is "body and movement."

One aspect that is currently lacking investigation are the sex effects of (physical or cognitive) training on cognition. Previous literature has identified that there are areas of cognitive performance that differ between males and females (Miller & Halpern, 2014). For example, females have been suggested to perform greater during tasks involving perceptual speed, visual memory, verbal fluency and fine motor control, whilst males excel in spatial tasks such as the mental rotations test (Hamson et al., 2016). One explanation could be sex hormones which fluctuate and change in males and females throughout prenatal development, childhood, adolescents and at an older age. This has been an area of consideration since the 1980s. It was hypothesised that cognitive sex differences can be explained by how much of the brain's left or right hemisphere is dominant when performing a specific cognitive task. Prenatal androgens (such as testosterone) were suggested to affect the development of the left hemisphere, meaning that males are possibly dominant than females in their activation of the right hemisphere (slowing down the development). These lateralisation sex differences could be a factor in the differences of cognition between sexes, due to the fact that verbal tasks often rely more on the left hemisphere and spatial tasks more on the right hemisphere (Halpern, 2013). Therefore, it could be assumed that males and females respond differently to (physical or cognitive) training and have subsequent differing changes in cognition. Although this research has not been often directly conducted, a pair of recent meta-analyses on the effects of exercise on cognition have compared research containing high and low numbers of female participants, with equivocal findings. Barha and colleagues (Barha et al., 2017) determined that females respond greater than males in the development of executive functions, regardless of training type (aerobic, resistance and multimodal training), whereas, Ludyga et al. (2020) suggested that a greater effect of a progressive exercise intervention on cognitive functions occurs in samples containing a lower percentage of female participants. These findings in training response alongside the brain development (potentially due to hormones) differences across sexes suggest that sex is an integral element of the training prescription and should be considered greatly.

Side Story

Sex Hormones

The three key hormones that work synergistically throughout prenatal development **up until old** age are progesterone, oestrogen and testosterone. Progesterone is the precursor of both sex-specific hormones. In males there are greater levels of testosterone, whilst females have a greater concentration of oestrogen. These sex hormones act throughout the entire brain of both sexes via hormone-specific receptors and through many cellular and molecular processes. These functions have been identified to alter the structure and function of neural systems and influence behaviour, as well as providing neuroprotection (McEwen & Milner, 2017). Moreover, effect-driven research has indicated that hormones relate to certain cognitive tasks (Colzato & Hommel, 2014). Interestingly, fraternal twins (male and female), whereby the female is exposed to greater androgens, have similar scores as males in tasks such as mental rotation (Heil et al., 2011). In terms of a sporting context, females may be influenced due to the fluctuating concentrations of hormones throughout the menstrual cycle. Previous research has suggested that female footballers may be limited aerobically during the luteal phase (when both oestrogen and progesterone are elevated) (Julian et al., 2017). This has been related to potential thermoregulatory effects of progesterone, which have been noted to raise core body temperature and thus increases cardiovascular strain at same work intensity. These key sex hormones have been identified to affect several physiological, metabolic, thermoregulatory and cognitive functions which in turn could alter physical and athletic functioning (Constantini et al., 2005; Frankovich & Lebrun, 2000; Lebrun et al., 2013).

In several studies, to better understand the underlying brain processes, neurophysiological methods, mainly EEG, were used during or after an acute exercise session. It was repeatedly shown that acute exercise modulates the evoked potentials. Thus, an acute session of moderate intensity is accompanied by an increased P3 amplitude (positive excursion 300–500 ms after stimulus onset) and shorter latencies during a subsequent cognitive task (Drollette et al., 2014; Kamijo et al., 2007; Magnie et al., 2000; Nakamura et al., 1999; Scudder et al., 2012). The increase of the P3 amplitude is interpreted as an increased use of resources (attention control) (for an overview: Kamijo, 2009). Studies that analyse EEG frequency bands (especially alpha frequency) (► Methods: Brain Research Methods) also indicate an increase in neural resources.

4.5.2 Chronic Effects of Physical Activity on Cognition

For school-aged children and adults, there is a positive correlation between physical activity and cognitive performance. The correlation is stronger for children of primary school age than for older children (Sibley & Etnier, 2003). A meta-analysis showed for older adults aged 55 years and older—irrespective of the intervention type, the length of the programme, the amount of training and the cognitive abilities investigated – that physical training increases cognitive performance (Colcombe et al., 2003). Performance improvements can be observed, especially in tasks that require executive control (e.g. response inhibition, updating, task switching; see ► Side Story: Dual/Multitasking Models).

In childhood and adolescence, physical activity also shows a positive correlation with the development of intellectual abilities and school performance (Fig. 4.6). For example, cardiovascular fitness correlates positively with standardised school tests to assess mathematical skills and reading comprehension. One explanation is that good cardiovascular fitness is associated with improved function of the fronto-parietal brain network, which is also used for mathematical skills and reading comprehension (summarised: Hillman et al., 2008).

Not only the functioning of the brain shows a positive correlation with regular physical activity but also its anatomical structure: children with high cardiovascular fitness showed a larger hippocampal volume associated with better memory performance (Chaddock et al., 2010a) and a larger volume of the basal ganglia associated with better attention performance (Chaddock et al., 2010b; Chaddock et al., 2012; see ► Study Box: Physical Frailty and Dementia).

Physical Frailty and Dementia

There are correlations between physical frailty (a measure of muscle strength, walking speed, body composition and fatigue), the risk of Alzheimer's dementia and cognitive decline. Boyle et al. (2010) followed 900 elderly people who were free from dementia at the start of the study for 12 years. Older people with a better overall physical constitution showed a smaller decline in cognitive functions and fewer cognitive impairments and less often suffered from Alzheimer's dementia than people with a higher degree of frailty. The protective effect of a good physical condition remained significant even when various possible influencing factors, such as body mass index, physical activity, lung function, vascular risk factors, vascular diseases and apolipoprotein (E4) levels, were monitored.

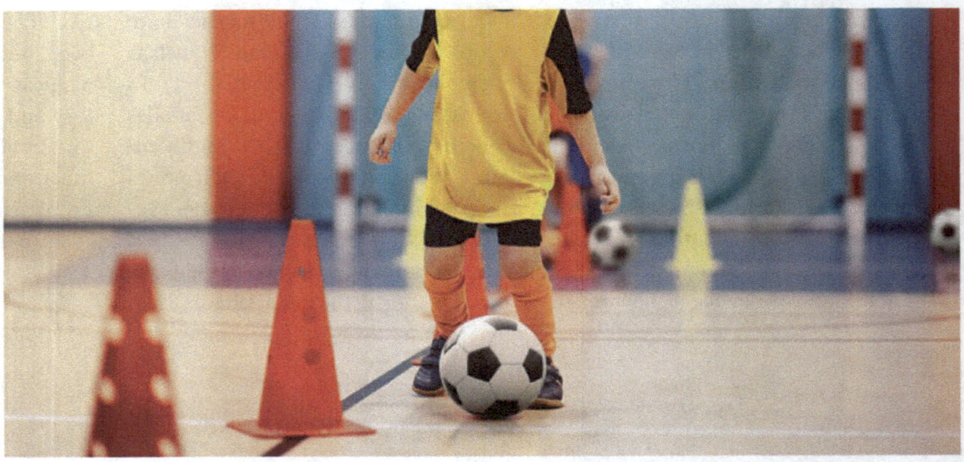

Fig. 4.6 The functioning of the brain in children and adolescents demonstrates a positive correlation with regular physical activity. ((C) matimix/ Getty Images/iStock)

The starting point for studies with older adults are the limitations in cognitive performance observed with age, such as a reduced speed of information processing or a reduced capacity of the working memory. Endurance-trained older people show better cognitive performance, e.g. in tasks concerning selective attention or episodic memory. On a neurophysiological level, functional changes can be observed which indicate faster and more effective information processing. Communication between different areas of the brain also appears to be improved by regular physical training, as connectivity analyses or network analyses show. It is remarkable that regular physical activity/exercise can improve cognitive performance even in previously inactive seniors. Meanwhile, there are indications that not only endurance training but also other forms of training, such as coordination training, can have a positive effect on cognitive functions (Voelcker-Rehage et al., 2011). Regarding the structure of the brain, older subjects with good cardiovascular fitness show significantly lower losses of grey and white matter of the brain than subjects with poor fitness. This is especially apparent in the frontal, parietal and temporal areas and in the hippocampus (Voelcker-Rehage & Niemann, 2013; see ► Self-Reflection: Can I improve my cognitive performance by physical activity?; see ► Side Story: Dose-Effect Relationships Between Physical Activity and Cognitive Control).

Reflection

Can I improve my cognitive performance by physical activity? The cause-and-effect relationships between physical activity and cognitive performance are complex. The biological mechanisms that underlie the effects of physical activity on cognition have so far been primarily investigated in animal experiments. These indicate that endurance training leads to a multitude of physiological changes within the brain, which in turn, may be the basis for the changes in cognitive performance. For example, regular endurance training promotes the formation of new nerve cells (neurogenesis) and their connections in the hippocampus and dental gyrus (synaptogenesis). Further causes are an increasing production of nerve growth factors (neurotrophins), an improvement in capillarisation (angiogenesis) in the hippocampus, Crbl and in the motor cortex, as well as lower cortical losses. One of the tasks of the newly formed capillaries is to transport sufficient nutrients to the existing and newly formed neurons (see for a summary: Voelcker-Rehage & Niemann, 2013).

Physical activity can presumably also have an effect on cognitive performance via other channels, for example, by reducing the risk of illness and increasing emotional well-being. An improvement in motor skills and abilities can also lead to the fact that cognitive resources, which were previously required for the execution of movements, are available for the execution of cognitive tasks.

Changes due to acute exercise are attributed to short-term changes in the activity of the neural networks involved in the cognitive task. It is assumed that physical activity changes the neuronal state of excitation, which means that mental processes run faster and memory processes are facilitated. Changed hormonal conditions, such as an exercise-induced increased release of cortisol and testosterone, can also be responsible for improved cognitive performance. Studies show an inverted U-shaped relationship between cortisol and testosterone levels and cognitive performance.

It can be assumed that an interplay of various factors moderates the influence of physical activity on cognitive functions.

How would you answer the question posed at the beginning? What arguments could you put forward to motivate a person who is not keen on sports to become more physically active? Think of a friend, a neighbour or a member of our family, and prepare your arguments in such a way that they are comprehensible and convincing.

Side Story

Dose–Response Relationship Between Physical Activity and Cognitive Management

So far, little is known about the optimal amount, required intensity and duration of physical activity to promote cognition. Moderate physical activity, two to three times a week, for at least 30 min has been shown to have a positive effect, with positive effects already noticeable after a few weeks. Older people show an almost linear change in their brain activation patterns over 12 months of training. Therefore, it can be assumed that longer-term training leads to further positive effects (Voelcker-Rehage et al., 2011).

4.6 Multitasking

4

In everyday life and sports, one is constantly confronted with double or multiple tasks (dual or multitasking), e.g. when driving a car, making a phone call or crossing a street during a conversation. In sports situations, this becomes apparent when, for example, a throw has to be executed and, at the same time, other players and opponents have to be kept in view. Such multiple tasks are a great challenge for the brain. This is because even a (highly) automated movement, such as walking, requires neural resources. This is particularly observed in older people, since in this population, motor tasks are often less automated in comparison to younger people.

Dual-Task Paradigms in Neuroscientific Research
Dual-tasking paradigms and their neurophysiological correlates are increasingly being studied with the help of brain imaging techniques. Methodologically, it is difficult in an MRI to separate the specific activation under dual-task condition from the activation during a single task. In a dual-task situation under MRI, the performance (brain activation) of both single tasks cannot be considered separately as it is the case in behaviour. In behavioural studies, for example, gait performance and cognitive performance are recorded separately, regardless of whether they were performed under single or dual-task conditions. Szameitat et al. (2011) discuss different approaches to the identifying of DT-specific activation in MRT studies. Therefore, the best approach is to compare the activation under dual-task condition with the sum of the activation under single-task condition.

Motor functions, such as walking and standing, require progressively more cognitive control, attentional resources and executive functions with increasing age (Woollacott & Shumway-Cook, 2002; Yogev-Seligmann et al., 2008). At the same time, older people have fewer cognitive resources available, which can lead to poor performance or problems if two or more tasks have to be completed at the same time, and the available resources have to be distributed between both tasks. Current studies use the "so-called" dual-task paradigm to investigate interactions between motor skills and cognition. The main research areas in gerontology are driving performance, fine motor skills and fall prevention. For example, a motor task (e.g. balance tasks) is combined with other motor tasks (e.g. carrying a tablet) or cognitive tasks (e.g. counting backward) with varying degrees of complexity. In the context of sports, dual-task paradigms are primarily used to investigate the extent to which a movement is automated (► Sect. 4.4; Digression: Dual/Multitasking Models).

Side Story

Dual/Multitasking Models

Several theoretical models describe the mechanisms of motor-cognitive interactions. The common crux is that the various tasks compete for cognitive attentional resources or that the cognitive processing takes place serially and not in parallel. The "theory of the central bottleneck" is based on serial central processing. It states that the information processing of the various task requirements is reaching its limits (bottleneck), since not all information can be processed at the same time. This results in longer processing times, due to the inability of the second task to be processed until the first has been completed (Pashler et al., 2001). The "attentional resource theory" explains the motor-cognitive interferences, by the competition of the subtasks for limited attentional resources (Kahneman, 1973). These unspecific resource theories have been replaced by concepts, such as the four-dimensional "multiple resource model" by Wickens (2002). This model demonstrates that the dual-task interference increases when the tasks have the same or overlapping modalities in the area of information acquisition and processing and/or behaviour production.

Another assumption hypothesises that a superordinate management system distributes the available resources, depending on task requirements and task prioritisation. This superordinate resource management mechanism, called the supervisory attentional system (Norman & Shallice, 1986) or the central executive (Baddeley, 1986), was later divided into distinct components. Undoubtedly the most popular taxonomy differentiates between the components of task switching, updating and response inhibition (Baddeley, 1996; Miyake et al., 2000; Strobach et al., 2014). Some authors have increased the number of executive components. They argue that multitasking is based on a separate executive function (executive function "dual tasking") rather than a mixture of the other three (Enriquez-Geppert et al., 2013; Strobach et al., 2014).

The need for a central executive to monitor the distribution of resources depending on the tasks according to higher-order strategies was recently challenged by the threaded cognition perspective (Salvucci & Taatgen, 2008). It hypothesises that several tasks are processed by the brain according to simple rules: each task requests the required resources and releases them as soon as they are no longer needed. Each resource fulfils the requests in turn, and if there are conflicts, the longest waiting one is processed first. According to this concept, multitasking is the emergent property of a simple algorithmic process and does not need overriding objective setting and decision-making. This process leaves little room for individual differences in multitasking performance. Proponents of the threaded cognition perspective therefore justify inter-individual variability in multitasking performance, with a varying size of resource pools, and not with differences in multitasking ability (Dale & Arnell, 2010; Taatgen et al., 2009). When this is the case, multitasking performance in one condition should not correlate with performance in another condition—a claim for which experimental evidence has varied (Brookings & Damos, 1991). Advocates of the threaded cognition perspective further assume that the neuronal activation under multitasking conditions should not exceed the sum of the activations under the individual tasks (Klingberg, 1998)—another claim for which heterogeneous experimental results are available (Erickson et al., 2005; Szameitat et al., 2002; van Impe et al., 2011).

Learning Control Questions

Basic:

1. Which structures in the CNS are involved in the performance of a movement?
2. What are the respective tasks of the structures that are involved in the performance of a movement?
3. Which neurophysiological mechanisms underlie (motor) learning?
4. What are the Brodmann areas and what is their importance?

Advanced:

5. What are similarities and differences in brain development in childhood and adolescence compared to brain development in old age?
6. What are the differences in motor learning between young and older people?
7. What is the relationship between arousal and performance in the Yerkes-Dodson Law?
8. With which methods can neurophysiological processes be made "visible"?

Experts:

9. What is neuroplasticity? (How) can it be assessed?
10. What is the assumption that the effects of acute physical activity on cognition are based on? Describe the key message of this relationship. What research is needed to advance this field of research?
11. What are the central components of executive skills?

References

Albert, N. B., Robertson, E. M., & Miall, R. C. (2009). The resting human brain and motor learning. *Current Biology, 19*(12), 1023–1027.

Alves, C. R., Tessaro, V. H., Teixeira, L. A., Murakava, K., Roschel, H., Gualano, B., & Takito, M. Y. (2014). Influence of acute high-intensity aerobic interval exercise bout on selective attention and short-term memory tasks. *Perceptual and Motor Skills, 118*(1), 63–72.

Baddeley, A. D. (1986). *Working memory*. Oxford Clarendon Press.

Baddeley, A. D. (1996). The concept of working memory. In S. Gathercole (Ed.), *Models of short-term memory* (pp. 1–28). Hove Lawrence Erlbaum Associates.

Barella, L. A., Etnier, J. L., & Chang, Y. K. (2010). The immediate and delayed effects of an acute bout of exercise on cognitive performance of healthy older adults. *Journal of Aging and Physical Activity, 18*(1), 87–98.

Barha, C. K., Davis, J. C., Falck, R. S., Nagamatsu, L. S., & Liu-Ambrose, T. (2017). Sex differences in exercise efficacy to improve cognition: A systematic review and meta-analysis of randomized controlled trials in older humans. *Frontiers in Neuroendocrinology, 46*, 71–85.

Bauswein, E., & Fromm, C. (1992). Activity in the precentral motor areas after presentation of targets for delayed reaching movements varies with the initial arm position. *The European Journal of Neuroscience, 4*(12), 1407–1410.

Bear, M. F., Connors, B. W., & Paradiso, M. A. (2007). Neurowissenschaften. Berlin: Springer.

Beurze, S. M., de Lange, F. P., Toni, I., & Medendorp, W. P. (2007). Integration of target and effector information in the human brain during reach planning. *Journal of Neurophysiology, 97*(1), 188–199.

Bezzola, L., Merillat, S., Gaser, C., & Jancke, L. (2011). Training-induced neural plasticity in golf novices. *The Journal of Neuroscience, 31*(35), 12,444–12,448.

Blanksby, B. A., Parker, H. E., Bradley, S., & Ong, V. (1995). Children's readiness for learning front crawl swimming. *Australian Journal of Science and Medicine in Sport, 27*(2), 34–37.

Boyke, J., Driemeyer, J., Gaser, C., Buchel, C., & May, A. (2008). Training-induced brain structure changes in the elderly. *The Journal of Neuroscience, 28*(28), 7031–7035.

Boyle, P. A., Buchman, A. S., Barnes, L. L., & Bennett, D. A. (2010). Effect of a purpose in life on risk of incident Alzheimer disease and mild cognitive impairment in community-dwelling older persons. *Archives of General Psychiatry, 67*(3), 304–310.

Brodmann, K. (1909). *Vergleichende Lokalisationslehre der Grosshirnrinde in Ihren Prinzipien Dargestellt auf Grund des Zellenbaues*. Barth.

Brookings, J., & Damos, D. (1991). Individual differences in multiple task performance. In D. Damos (Ed.), *Multiple task performance* (pp. 363–385). Wiley.

Budde, H., et al. (2008). "Acute coordinative exercise improves attentional performance in adolescents." Neuroscience Letters 441, 219–223.

Budde, H., Brunelli, A., Machado, S., Velasques, B., Ribeiro, P., Arias-Carrion, O., & Voelcker-Rehage, C. (2012). Intermittent maximal exercise improves attentional performance only in physically active students. *Archives of Medical Research, 43*(2), 125–131.

Budde, H., Windisch, C., Kudielka, B. M., & Voelcker-Rehage, C. (2010). Saliva cortisol in school children after acute physical exercise. *Neuroscience Letters, 483*(1), 16–19.

Cabeza, R. (2002). Hemispheric asymmetry reduction in older adults: the HAROLD model. *Psychology and Aging, 17*(1), 85–100.

Chaddock, L., Erickson, K. I., Prakash, R. S., Kim, J. S., Voss, M. W., Vanpatter, M., et al. (2010a). A neuroimaging investigation of the association between aerobic fitness, hippocampal volume, and memory performance in preadolescent children. *Brain Research, 1358*, 172–183.

Chaddock, L., Erickson, K. I., Prakash, R. S., VanPatter, M., Voss, M. W., Pontifex, M. B., et al. (2010b). Basal ganglia volume is associated with aerobic fitness in preadolescent children. *Developmental Neuroscience, 32*(3), 249–256.

Chaddock, L., Hillman, C. H., Pontifex, M. B., Johnson, C. R., Raine, L. B., & Kramer, A. F. (2012). Childhood aerobic fitness predicts cognitive performance one year later. *Journal of Sports Sciences, 30*(5), 421–430.

Chang, Y. K., Labban, J. D., Gapin, J. I., & Etnier, J. L. (2012). The effects of acute exercise on cognitive performance: a meta-analysis. *Brain Research, 1453*, 87–101.

Cisek, P., & Kalaska, J. F. (2010). Neural mechanisms for interacting with a world full of action choices. *Annual Review of Neuroscience, 33*, 269–298.

Colcombe, S. J., Erickson, K. I., Raz, N., Webb, A. G., Cohen, N. J., McAuley, E., & Kramer, A. F. (2003). Aerobic fitness reduces brain tissue loss in aging humans. *The Journals of Gerontology. Series A, Biological Sciences and Medical Sciences, 58*(2), 176–180.

Colzato, L. S., & Hommel, B. (2014). Effects of estrogen on higher-order cognitive functions in unstressed human females may depend on individual variation in dopamine baseline levels. *Frontiers in Neuroscience*, 8.

Constantini, N. W., Dubnov, G., & Lebrun, C. M. (2005). The menstrual cycle and sport performance. *Clinics in Sports Medicine, 24*(2), e51–e82, xiii–xiv.

Coynel, D., Marrelec, G., Perlbarg, V., Pelegrini-Issac, M., Van de Moortele, P. F., Ugurbil, K., et al. (2010). Dynamics of motor-related functional integration during motor sequence learning. *NeuroImage, 49*(1), 759–766.

Crammond, D. J., & Kalaska, J. F. (1994). Modulation of preparatory neuronal activity in dorsal premotor cortex due to stimulus-response compatibility. *Journal of Neurophysiology, 71*(3), 1281–1284.

Dale, G., & Arnell, K. M. (2010). Individual differences in dispositional focus of attention predict attentional blink magnitude. *Attention, Perception, & Psychophysics, 72*(3), 602–606.

Doyon, J., & Benali, H. (2005). Reorganization and plasticity in the adult brain during learning of motor skills. *Current Opinion in Neurobiology, 15*(2), 161–167.

Doyon, J., Song, A. W., Karni, A., Lalonde, F., Adams, M. M., & Ungerleider, L. G. (2002). Experience-dependent changes in cerebellar contributions to motor sequence learning. *PNAS, 99*(2), 1017–1022.

Draganski, B., Gaser, C., Busch, V., Schuierer, G., Bogdahn, U., & May, A. (2004). Neuroplasticity: changes in grey matter induced by training. *Nature, 427*(6972), 311–312.

Driemeyer, J., Boyke, J., Gaser, C., Buchel, C., & May, A. (2008). Changes in gray matter induced by learning—Revisited. *PLoS One, 3*(7), e2669.

Drollette, E. S., Scudder, M. R., Raine, L. B., Moore, R. D., Saliba, B. J., Pontifex, M. B., & Hillman, C. H. (2014). Acute exercise facilitates brain function and cognition in children who need it most: an ERP study of individual differences in inhibitory control capacity. *Developmental Cognitive Neuroscience, 7*, 53–64.

Enriquez-Geppert, S., Huster, R. J., & Herrmann, C. S. (2013). Boosting brain functions: Improving executive functions with behavioral training, neurostimulation, and neurofeedback. *International Journal of Psychophysiology, 88*(1), 1–16.

Erickson, K. I., Colcombe, S. J., Wadhwa, R., Bherer, L., Peterson, M. S., Scalf, P. E., & Kramer, A. F. (2005). Neural correlates of dual-task performance after minimizing task-preparation. *NeuroImage, 28*(4), 967–979.

Ernst, A., Alkass, K., Bernard, S., Salehpour, M., Perl, S., Tisdale, J., et al. (2014). Neurogenesis in the striatum of the adult human brain. *Cell, 156*(5), 1072–1083.

Eyre, J. A., Taylor, J. P., Villagra, F., Smith, M., & Miller, S. (2001). Evidence of activity-dependent withdrawal of corticospinal projections during human development. *Neurology, 57*(9), 1543–1554.

Floyer-Lea, A., & Matthews, P. M. (2004). Changing brain networks for visuomotor control with increased movement automaticity. *Journal of Neurophysiology, 92*(4), 2405–2412.

Frankovich, R. J., & Lebrun, C. M. (2000). Menstrual cycle, contraception, and performance. *Clinics in Sports Medicine, 19*(2), 251–271.

Gail, A., Klaes, C., & Westendorff, S. (2009). Implementation of spatial transformation rules for goal-directed reaching via gain modulation in monkey parietal and premotor cortex. *The Journal of Neuroscience, 29*(30), 9490–9499.

Ghez, C., & Gordon, J. (1996). Einführung in die Motorik. In E. Kandel, J. Schwartz, & T. Jessel (Eds.), *Neurowissenschaften* (pp. 499–511). Spektrum.

Gobel, E. W., Parrish, T. B., & Reber, P. J. (2011). Neural correlates of skill acquisition: decreased cortical activity during a serial interception sequence learning task. *NeuroImage, 58*(4), 1150–1157.

Godde, B., Trautmann, M., Erhard, P., & Voelcker-Rehage, C. (2018). Motor practice in a force modulation task in young and middle-aged adults. *Journal of Electromyography and Kinesiology, 38*, 224–231.

Graziano, M. S. A. (2016). Ethological action maps: a paradigm shift for the motor cortex. *Trends in Cognitive Sciences, 20*(2), 121–132.

Halpern, D. F. (2013). *Sex differences in cognitive abilities*. Psychology Press.

Hamson, D. K., Roes, M. M., & Galea, L. A. M. (2016). Sex hormones and cognition: neuroendocrine influences on memory and learning. *Comprehensive Physiology, 6*(3), 1295–1337.

Hamzei, F., Glauche, V., Schwarzwald, R., & May, A. (2012). Dynamic gray matter changes within cortex and striatum after short motor skill training are associated with their increased functional interaction. *NeuroImage, 59*(4), 3364–3372.

Haug, H. (1986). History of neuromorphometry. *Journal of Neuroscience Methods, 18*(1-2), 1–17.

Heil, M., Kavsek, M., Rolke, B., Beste, C., & Jansen, P. (2011). Mental rotation in female fraternal twins: Evidence for intra-uterine hormone transfer? *Biological Psychology, 86*(1), 90–93.

Henz, S., Kutz, D. F., Werner, J., Hurster, W., Kolb, F. P., & Nida-Ruemelin, J. (2015). Stimulus-dependent deliberation process leading to a specific motor action demonstrated via a multi-channel EEG analysis. *Frontiers in Human Neuroscience, 9*, 355.

Hillman, C. H., Erickson, K. I., & Kramer, A. F. (2008). Be smart, exercise your heart: exercise effects on brain and cognition. *Nature Reviews Neuroscience, 9*, 58.

Hogan, C. L., Mata, J., & Carstensen, L. L. (2013). Exercise holds immediate benefits for affect and cognition in younger and older adults. *Psychology and Aging, 28*(2), 587–594.

Hopkins, M. E., Davis, F. C., Vantieghem, M. R., Whalen, P. J., & Bucci, D. J. (2012). Differential effects of acute and regular physical exercise on cognition and affect. *Neuroscience, 215*, 59–68.

Hoshi, E., Shima, K., & Tanji, J. (2000). Neuronal activity in the primate prefrontal cortex in the process of motor selection based on two behavioral rules. *Journal of Neurophysiology, 83*(4), 2355–2373.

Hoshi, E., & Tanji, J. (2006). Differential involvement of neurons in the dorsal and ventral premotor cortex during processing of visual signals for action planning. *Journal of Neurophysiology, 95*(6), 3596–3616.

Julian, R., Hecksteden, A., Fullagar, H. H. K., & Meyer, T. (2017). The effects of menstrual cycle phase on physical performance in female soccer players. *PLoS One, 12*(3).

Kahneman, D. (1973). *Attention and effort*. Prentice-Hall.

Kamijo, K. (2009). Effects of acute exercise on event-related brain potentials. In *Enhancing cognitive functioning and brain plasticity* (pp. 111–132). Champaign, IL.

Kamijo, K., Nishihira, Y., Higashiura, T., & Kuroiwa, K. (2007). The interactive effect of exercise intensity and task difficulty on human cognitive processing. *International Journal of Psychophysiology, 65*(2), 114–121.

Klingberg, T. (1998). Concurrent performance of two working memory tasks: potential mechanisms of interference. *Cerebral Cortex, 8*(7), 593–601.

Kwon, Y. H., Nam, K. S., & Park, J. W. (2012). Identification of cortical activation and white matter architecture according to short-term motor learning in the human brain: functional MRI and diffusion tensor tractography study. *Neuroscience Letters, 520*(1), 11–15.

Lambourne, K., & Tomporowski, P. (2010). The effect of exercise-induced arousal on cognitive task performance: a meta-regression analysis. *Brain Research, 1341*, 12–24.

Lebrun, C., Joyce, S. M., & Constantini, N. (2013). Effects of female reproductive hormones on sports performance. In N. Constantini & A. C. Hackney (Eds.), *Endocrinology of physical activity and sport* (pp. 281–322). Springer.

Li, K. Z., & Lindenberger, U. (2002). Relations between aging sensory/sensorimotor and cognitive functions. *Neuroscience and Biobehavioral Reviews, 26*(7), 777–783.

Logan, G. D., Yamaguchi, M., Schall, J. D., & Palmeri, T. J. (2015). Inhibitory control in mind and brain 2.0: blocked-input models of saccadic countermanding. *Psychological Review, 122*(2), 115–147.

Ludyga, S., Gerber, M., Puhse, U., Looser, V. N., & Kamijo, K. (2020). Systematic review and meta-analysis investigating moderators of long-term effects of exercise on cognition in healthy individuals. *Nature Human Behaviour, 4*(6), 603–612.

Luft, A. R., & Buitrago, M. M. (2005). Stages of motor skill learning. *Molecular Neurobiology, 32*(3), 205–216.

Ma, L., Narayana, S., Robin, D. A., Fox, P. T., & Xiong, J. (2011). Changes occur in resting state network of motor system during 4 weeks of motor skill learning. *NeuroImage, 58*(1), 226–233.

Ma, L., Wang, B., Narayana, S., Hazeltine, E., Chen, X., Robin, D. A., et al. (2010). Changes in regional activity are accompanied with changes in inter-regional connectivity during 4 weeks motor learning. *Brain Research, 1318*, 64–76.

Magnie, M. N., Bermon, S., Martin, F., Madany-Lounis, M., Suisse, G., Muhammad, W., & Dolisi, C. (2000). P300, N400, aerobic fitness, and maximal aerobic exercise. *Psychophysiology, 37*(3), 369–377.

Matelli, M., & Luppino, G. (1992). Anatomo-functional parcellation of the agranular frontal cortex. In R. Caminiti, P. B. Johnson, & Y. Burnod (Eds.), *Control of arm movement in space: neurophysiological and computational approaches* (pp. 85–101). Berlin Springer-Verlag.

Matelli, M., & Luppino, G. (2004). Architectonics of the primates cortex: usefulness and limits. *Cortex, 40*(1), 209–210.

McEwen, B. S., & Milner, T. A. (2017). Understanding the broad influence of sex hormones and sex differences in the brain. *Journal of Neuroscience Research, 95*(1-2), 24–39.

McMorris, T., & Hale, B. J. (2012). Differential effects of differing intensities of acute exercise on speed and accuracy of cognition: a meta-analytical investigation. *Brain and Cognition, 80*(3), 338–351.

McMorris, T., Sproule, J., Turner, A., & Hale, B. J. (2011). Acute, intermediate intensity exercise, and speed and accuracy in working memory tasks: a meta-analytical comparison of effects. *Physiology & Behavior, 102*(3-4), 421–428.

Miller, D. I., & Halpern, D. F. (2014). The new science of cognitive sex differences. *Trends in Cognitive Sciences, 18*(1), 37–45.

Miyake, A., Friedman, N. P., Emerson, M. J., Witzki, A. H., Howerter, A., & Wager, T. D. (2000). The unity and diversity of executive functions and their contributions to complex "Frontal Lobe" tasks: a latent variable analysis. *Cognitive Psychology, 41*(1), 49–100.

Nakamura, Y., Nishimoto, K., Akamatu, M., Takahashi, M., & Maruyama, A. (1999). The effect of jogging on P300 event related potentials. *Electromyography and Clinical Neurophysiology, 39*(2), 71–74.

Nelson, A. B., & Kreitzer, A. C. (2014). Reassessing models of basal ganglia function and dysfunction. *Annual Review of Neuroscience, 37*, 117–135.

Norman, D., & Shallice, T. (1986). Attention to action: willed and automatic control of behavior. In R. Davidson, R. Schwartz, & D. Shapiro (Eds.), *Consciousness and Self-Regulation: Advances in Research and Theory IV*. Plenum Press.

Park, D. C., Polk, T. A., Park, R., Minear, M., Savage, A., & Smith, M. R. (2004). Aging reduces neural specialization in ventral visual cortex. *PNAS, 101*(35), 13091–13095.

Parker, H. E., & Blanksby, B. A. (1997). Starting age and aquatic skill learning in young children: mastery of prerequisite water confidence and basic aquatic locomotion skills. *Australian Journal of Science and Medicine in Sport, 29*(3), 83–87.

Pashler, H., Johnston, J. C., & Ruthruff, E. (2001). Attention and performance. *Annual Review of Psychology, 52*, 629–651. https://doi.org/10.1146/annurev.psych.52.1.629

Pontifex, M. B., Hillman, C. H., & Polich, J. (2009). Age, physical fitness, and attention: P3a and P3b. *Psychophysiology, 46*(2), 379–387.

Rolando, L. (1809). *Saggio sopra la vera struttura del cervello dell'uomo e degli animali e sopra le funzioni del sistema nervoso* (Seconda Edizione, 1828 ed.). Torino.

Sakuma, K., Murakami, T., & Nakashima, K. (2007). Short latency afferent inhibition is not impaired in mild cognitive impairment. *Clinical Neurophysiology, 118*, 1460–1463.

Salvucci, D. D., & Taatgen, N. A. (2008). Threaded cognition: an integrated theory of concurrent multitasking. *Psychological Review, 115*(1), 101–130.

Scangos, K. W., Aronberg, R., & Stuphorn, V. (2013). Performance monitoring by presupplementary and supplementary motor area during an arm movement countermanding task. *Journal of Neurophysiology, 109*, 1928–1939.

Schmahmann, J. D. (1997). *The Cerebellum and Cognition*. Academeic Press.

Scholz, J., Klein, M. C., Behrens, T. E., & Johansen-Berg, H. (2009). Training induces changes in white-matter architecture. *Nature Neuroscience, 12*(11), 1370–1371.
Schultz, W., Dayan, P., & Montague, P. R. (1997). A Neural Substrate of Prediction and Reward. *Science, 275*, 1593–1599.
Scudder, M. R., Drollette, E. S., Pontifex, M. B., & Hillman, C. H. (2012). Neuroelectric indices of goal maintenance following a single bout of physical activity. *Biological Psychology, 89*(2), 528–531.
Sibley, B. A., & Etnier, J. L. (2003). The relationship between physical activity and cognition in children: A meta-analysis. *Pediatric Exercise Science, 15*(3), 243–256.
Spalding, K. L., Bergmann, O., Alkass, K., Bernard, S., Salehpour, M., Huttner, H. B., . . . Frisen, J. (2013). Dynamics of hippocampal neurogenesis in adult humans. Cell, 153(6), 1219–1227.
Stephan, K. E., Friston, K. J. (2009). Functional connectivity. In Squire, L R. (Hrsg.), Encyclopedia of Neuroscience (S. 391–397). New York: Elsevier.
Strobach, T., Salminen, T., Karbach, J., & Schubert, T. (2014). Practice-related optimization and transfer of executive functions: a general review and a specific realization of their mechanisms in dual tasks. *Psychological Research, 78*(6), 836–851.
Stuphorn, V. (2015). The role of supplementary eye field in goal-directed behavior. *Journal of Physiology, 109*(1), 118–128.
Swinnen, S. P. (2002). Intermanual coordination: From behavioural principles to neural-network interactions. *Nature Reviews Neuroscience, 3*, 348.
Szameitat, A. J., Schubert, T., Muller, K., & Von Cramon, D. Y. (2002). Localization of executive functions in dual-task performance with fMRI. *Journal of Cognitive Neuroscience, 14*(8), 1184–1199.
Taatgen, N. A., Juvina, I., Schipper, M., Borst, J. P., & Martens, S. (2009). Too much control can hurt: a threaded cognition model of the attentional blink. *Cognitive Psychology, 59*(1), 1–29.
Taubert, M., Lohmann, G., Margulies, D. S., Villringer, A., & Ragert, P. (2011). Long-term effects of motor training on resting-state networks and underlying brain structure. *NeuroImage, 57*(4), 1492–1498.
Timmann-Braun, D., & Maschke, M. (2003). Das Kleinhirn ganz groß: Über den wichtigsten Zuarbeiter des Großhirns. *Essener Unikate, 22*, 18–29.
Tomporowski, P. D. (2003). Effects of acute bouts of exercise on cognition. *Acta Psychologica, 112*(3), 297–324.
Toni, I., Rowe, J., Stephan, K. E., & Passingham, R. E. (2002). Changes of cortico-striatal effective connectivity during visuomotor learning. *Cerebral Cortex, 12*(10), 1040–1047.
Vahdat, S., Darainy, M., Milner, T. E., & Ostry, D. J. (2011). Functionally specific changes in resting-state sensorimotor networks after motor learning. *The Journal of Neuroscience, 31*(47), 16907–16915.
van Impe, A., Coxon, J. P., Goble, D. J., Wenderoth, N., & Swinnen, S. P. (2011). Age-related changes in brain activation underlying single- and dual-task performance: visuomanual drawing and mental arithmetic. *Neuropsychologia, 49*(9), 2400–2409.
Voelcker-Rehage, C. (2008). Motor-skill learning in older adults - a review of studies on age-related differences. *European Review of Aging and Physical Activity, 5*(1), 5–16.
Voelcker-Rehage, C., Godde, B., & Staudinger, U. M. (2011). Cardiovascular and coordination training differentially improve cognitive performance and neural processing in older adults. *Frontiers in Human Neuroscience, 5*, 26.
Voelcker-Rehage, C., & Niemann, C. (2013). Structural and functional brain changes related to different types of physical activity across the life span. *Neuroscience and Biobehavioral Reviews, 37*(9 Pt B), 2268–2295.
Weinrich, M., & Wise, S. P. (1982). The premotor cortex of the monkey. *The Journal of Neuroscience, 2*(9), 1329–1345.
Wickens, C. D. (2002). Multiple resources and performance prediction. *Theoretical Issues in Ergonomics Science, 3*(2), 159–177.
Wolpert, D. M., Miall, R. C., & Kawato, M. (1998). Internal models in the cerebellum. *Trends in Cognitive Sciences, 2*(9), 338–347.
Woollacott, M., & Shumway-Cook, A. (2002). Attention and the control of posture and gait: a review of an emerging area of research. *Gait & Posture, 16*(1), 1–14.
Xiong, J., Ma, L., Wang, B., Narayana, S., Duff, E. P., Egan, G. F., & Fox, P. T. (2009). Long-term motor training induced changes in regional cerebral blood flow in both task and resting states. *NeuroImage, 45*(1), 75–82.
Yerkes, R. M., & Dodson, J. D. (1908). The relation of strength of stimulus to rapidity of habit-formation. *Journal of Comparative Neurology and Psychology, 18*(5), 459–482.
Yogev-Seligmann, G., Hausdorff, J. M., & Giladi, N. (2008). The role of executive function and attention in gait. *Movement Disorders, 23*(3), 329–342; quiz 472.
Zilles, K., Schlaug, G., Geyer, S., Luppino, G., Matelli, M., Qü, M., et al. (1996). Anatomy and transmitter receptors of the supplementary motor areas in the human and nonhuman primate brain. *Advances in Neurology, 70*, 29–43.

Judgment and Decision-Making

Geoffrey Schweizer, Henning Plessner and Clare MacMahon

Contents

J. Schüler et al. (eds.), *Sport and Exercise Psychology*, https://doi.org/10.1007/978-3-031-03921-8_5

Learning Objectives

Basic:

- Describe theories and models of judgment and decision-making.
- Describe and explain undesirable influences on judgments and decisions in sport.

Advanced:

- Discuss the consequences of errors of judgment and decision-making in sport.
- Describe studies on judgments and decisions in sport and explain their study design.

Experts:

- Make suggestions for improving judgments and decisions in specific sports situations.

5.1 Introduction

When you think of sports psychology, the first thing you probably think of is using imagery, goal-setting, motivation, or team cohesion. Judging and deciding is not an obvious topic that comes to mind in sports psychology. However, sporting activities of all kinds are directly or indirectly influenced by judgments and decisions. Teachers have to assess sporting performance and give marks. Performance in gymnastics is evaluated by a panel of judges. Soccer players must decide whether to pass the ball or to try to score a goal themselves. Goalkeepers choose whether to plant their feet or jump. Referees choose whether or not to call a penalty or to give a yellow or red card. Coaches and managers assess the performance of players and decide whether to recruit them and then if they should select them for an upcoming game. Theories of judgment and decision-making can help explain and understand these judgments and decisions (► Sect. 5.2). They attempt to determine universal mechanisms of judgment and decision-making. At the same time, there are numerous studies that examine more specific situations of judgment and decision-making (► Sect. 5.3). Often these studies identify certain judgment biases. This means that there are factors that influence judgments and decisions when they should not. For example, there is evidence that referees are influenced by the noise of the crowd when they award yellow cards. On the one hand, these studies help to better understand judgments and decisions, and on the other hand, they offer concrete starting points for practical interventions with the aim of improving judgments and decisions (► Sect. 5.4).

Judgments and Decisions

Judgments and decisions are omnipresent in sport and can have a great influence on sporting success and performance in physical education. However, they are susceptible to systematic errors.

5.2 Theoretical Background

5.2.1 Judgments

Judging can be defined as the assignment of judgment objects to values on a judgment dimension (Betsch et al., 2011). A distinction is made between the explicit judgment ("The game was exciting") and the psychological process of assigning the value itself. This is called the judgment process. Both objects of judgment and judgment dimensions can be of a very diverse nature. People, objects, performances, the truth value of statements, the weather, ideas, or future developments can become objects of judgment, to name just a few examples. Judgment dimensions can be evaluative or nonevaluative. In the case of evaluative judgments, the underlying dimension says something about the evaluation of a judgment object. In nonevaluative judgments, the underlying dimension does not initially say anything about the judgment object's rating. However, depending on the context, the same nonevaluative judgment may be good or bad. For example, an athlete's height is initially neither good nor bad. However, depending on whether I am looking for a jockey or a basketball player, the same height may have a different value on an evaluative dimension: tall is good for basketball players, but not good for jockeys. If the underlying dimension describes probabilities, we speak of probability judgments. If the probability of future events is assessed, for example, the outcome of a football game, judgments become predictions. In this case we also speak of predictive judgments.

Judgment

Judgment refers to the psychological process that underlies when people assign a value on a judgment dimension to an object of judgment and explicitly express the resulting judgment (Betsch et al., 2011).

In psychological research on judgments, it is assumed that people are aware of their judgment. However, they do not necessarily have insight into the judgment process, i.e., they do not need to know *how* they made a particular judgment. In research on judgments there are different theories that deal with exactly this question: How do people make judgments? When looking closely, this single question turns into several different ones: What information do people use to make judgments? How do they select this information? Is the information weighted, and if so, how? How is different information translated into values on the judgment scale? Are there undesirable influences on the judging process? In the following chapter, we will focus on those theories and models and the key questions they highlight that give us the most insight into judgment in sports psychology.

Judgments

There are different types of judgments: evaluative judgments contain ratings of judgment objects; non-evaluative judgments do not contain ratings. Predictive judgments refer to the future.

5.2.1.1 Brunswik's Lens Model

A particularly influential model for understanding human judgment is Brunswik's lens model (1952; Doherty & Kurz, 1996). It is suitable for structuring a judgment or decision-making environment and allows conclusions to be drawn about the circumstances under which good judgments result. The basic assumption of the lens model is that people who want to make a judgment usually do not have direct access to the variable to be judged (distal variable or criterion), but must access it—as if looking through a lens—via visible features of the same (proximal variables or cues) (Fig. 5.1). At the same time, the lens model assumes that there is a true state of the criterion that people want to assess as accurately as possible. The agreement between judgment and criterion is called achievement. The lens model is therefore particularly suitable for understanding judgments which actually involve assessing the true state of an object of judgment (i.e., the criterion) as accurately as possible (e.g., medical judgments). Typical examples come primarily from the field of medical diagnostics, where the lens model has had a particular influence (Wigton, 1996). For example, a doctor cannot see directly which disease a patient is suffering from but must derive it from various visible symptoms.

The most important assumption of the lens model is that cues and criteria are not deterministically but probabilistically related (Doherty & Kurz, 1996; Goldstein, 2004). This means that cues and criterion correlate with each other, but these correlations are not perfect. Correlations between cues and criterion are called ecological validities and indicate how well the criterion can be developed based on the cues. Correlations between cues and judgment indicate the extent to which judges use these cues for their judgment (cue usage coefficients). In the lens model, the quality of a judgment is understood as the accuracy with which this judgment maps the respective criterion. This accuracy is called achievement. It is important to note that both sides of the lens play a role in the expression of accuracy, both the ecological validity and the cue use. The higher the cue-criterion correlations are and the more precisely the cue use is oriented toward them, the more likely it is that a judgment will agree with the criterion (be correct). Conversely, it follows that judgments can be imprecise for two reasons: on the one hand, the cue usage of a judge can be incorrect even if there are actually valid cues (i.e., high cue-criterion correlations). On the other hand, if the cue validity is low, this results in an upper limit to the accuracy of the judgment, which judges cannot further improve through their cue use (Cooksey, 1996). This consideration of both the structure of the environment and the cognitive structuring of a judgment is an essential feature of the lens model. It offers a fruitful start-

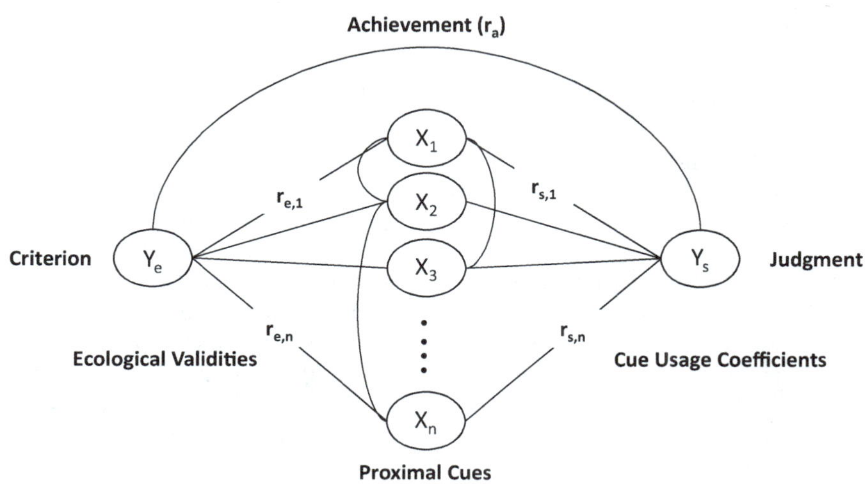

Fig. 5.1 Lens Model by Brunswik

ing point for the analysis of real judgment situations (Hammond, Stewart, Brehmer, & Steinmann, 1975). Consequently, the lens model has also been used to understand judgment situations in sport (e.g., Plessner et al., 2009; Unkelbach & Memmert, 2010; ▶ Side Story: Application of the Lens Model in Sport).

Side Story

Applying the Lens Models to Sports

The lens model can be applied to the activities of referees in the following way (Plessner, Schweizer, Brand & O'Hare, 2009): referees must assess a distal criterion (foul or no foul) by using visible cues. For example, a football referee's decision to call foul may be based on the following observations: player one slips into player two (cue 1), player two falls (cue 2), and the ball had already been played at that moment (cue 3). These cues are probabilistically related to the criterion (it is not a foul every time a player falls). They are also intercorrelated (after a contact between two players, it is more likely than not that one of them will fall). The higher the correlation of the three cues with the criterion (ecological validity), the more confident the referees can be in making their decision if they use the three cues correctly (cue use). Based on the lens model, deeper insights into the decision situation can be gained. For example, analyses can be used to indicate which and how many cues the referee used. Furthermore, attempts can be made to determine the causes of misjudgments (e.g., cue 3 was not used) but also to improve decisions (e.g., training the use of cue 3).

The Lens Model

The lens model assumes that people usually do not have direct access to a variable (criterion) to be judged but that its condition can be deduced from its observable characteristics (cues). The higher the correlations between cues and criterion, the better the judgments that can be made. Judgments are always understood as probabilistic.

5.2.2 Decision-Making

Deciding is the process of choosing between at least two options with the aim of achieving desired consequences and avoiding undesired consequences (Betsch et al., 2011). Options in this case refer to action alternatives between which we have a choice. A decision is made when one of the options has been chosen. Every day we make numerous decisions. The consequences associated with each option can be short-term or long-term, significant or insignificant. In some situations, we are aware that we are making an important decision and we think long and hard about the best option. If the decision seems particularly important, we may try to obtain additional information about the options available. In other situations, we settle for an option that promises sufficiently positive consequences without necessarily trying to find the best one. In many other situations, however, we choose between different options without giving much thought to the options and their consequences and sometimes even without realizing that we have just made a choice. Sometimes the consequences of a single decision are insignificant, but cumulatively (i.e., across many individual decisions), the consequences are severe (▶ Side Story: Judging or Deciding).

Side Story

Judging or Deciding

Despite their different definitions, it is sometimes not clear whether a particular phenomenon is a judgment or a decision. The main difference between judgments and decisions, in terms of definition, is that a decision always involves a choice between at least two options. So, if there is no choice between options in a situation, there can be no decision. Conversely, however, the existence of a choice does not mean that no judgment processes are involved. Thus, there are phenomena which are clearly judgments (e.g., "I like the movie Free Solo a lot") or clearly decisions (e.g., "Do I get up for an early run or do I stay in bed and continue to sleep").

The distinction between judgments and decisions can become complicated when a decision seems to be based on a judgment. For example, a yellow card is given in football for serious foul play. On the one hand, referees must therefore judge the severity of the foul. On the other hand, they have to choose or decide between the options of no card, yellow card, and red card. Whether scientists interpret these phenomena as judgments or decisions depends on which of the two components they consider to be more relevant. If I assume in a refereeing decision that the judging process is decisive for the behavior of the referee because a decision on the severity of the foul necessarily leads to a certain decision, I will try to understand the judging process. However, if I assume that the verdict on the severity of the foul is only one of several pieces of information that the referee must take into account in order to weigh the consequences of the decision options, then I will try to understand the process of weighing the options and thus the decision.

Decision-Making
Deciding is the process of choosing between at least two options with the aim of achieving desired consequences and avoiding undesired consequences. In the best case, the process leads to a decision (choice). An option is selected and the intention to implement it is formed, e.g., to perform an action (Betsch et al., 2011).

5.2.2.1 Expected Utility Theory

Classical decision theories state that for an optimal decision, the option with the highest expected value or utility should be chosen (Betsch et al., 2011). To calculate this, all possible consequences of all options must be assigned a value or a utility. In addition, each possible consequence must be weighted by the probability of its occurrence. The weighted consequences of each option are then added together. The option with the higher expected value or utility is chosen. Therefore, these theories are called "expected value theory" or "expected utility theory." Expected utility or expected value theories are not originally descriptive but normative. They do not imply that people actually calculate the expected value or utility of all options but that optimal decisions choose the option with the highest expected value or utility. Nevertheless, from this perspective, decision behavior presents itself as a conscious and controlled process of complex information integration that serves to maximize the objective value or subjective utility (Baron, 2000; Dawes, 1998; Edwards, 1954; Kahneman & Tversky, 1979).

Let us imagine the following example: Ralf has the choice between two different lottery tickets. With ticket A, he has the chance to win 10,000 Euro, but only one of 100 tickets is a winner. Ticket A therefore has the expected value of 100 Euro. Ticket B only promises the prize of 5000 Euro, but 10 out of 100 tickets are winning tickets. Ticket B therefore has the expected value of 500 Euro. According to the expected value theory, Ralf should choose ticket B. If people actually consciously make or are influenced in making decisions in the way the theories of expected value or expected utility describe, there are some necessary preconditions: first of all, people must be aware of the different consequences of the options and be able to convert them into a uniform scale of value or utility, so to speak. In addition, decision-makers need to know about the probability of the various options occurring. This latter requirement is especially unlikely to be met in reality for many decisions. From the perspective of these theories, good decisions depend on decision-makers being aware of all the possible consequences of the options, on correctly determining their value or utility, on knowing the probabilities of the options occurring, and finally on correctly calculating their value or utility. However, even if people make decisions that are consistent with the predictions of the theories of expected value or utility, this does not necessarily mean that they have actually *consciously* calculated the expected value or benefit of all options (► Side Story: Darwin's Wedding; ► Side Story: Difference Between Value and Utility).

Expected Value and Expected Utility Theories
Theories of expected value state that optimal decisions result if the consequences of all options are assessed and weighted with the probability of their occurrence. Then the evaluated and weighted consequences are added up for each option and the option with the highest value is chosen. Theories of expected utility do not refer to an objective value of an option but to its subjective utility for the decision-maker.

Side Story

Darwin's Wedding

Charles Darwin, the founder of the theory of evolution, proved to be an early follower of the expected utility theories in his private life—perhaps without being aware of it: when Darwin was faced with the choice of whether to marry, he made a list of pros and cons (C. R. Darwin, 1838). This list has been preserved for posterity and is currently in the Cambridge University Library (Cambridge, GB; ► http://darwin-online.org.uk/content/frameset?viewtype=side&itemID=CUL-DAR210.8.2&pageseq=1). Among the arguments for marriage, Darwin lists that a wife could give him children ("children—if it please god") and take care of the house ("home, & someone to take care of home"). Among the arguments against marriage, Darwin argues that a bachelor can go where he wants ("freedom to go where one liked") and is not forced to visit relatives of the wife ("not forced to visit relatives").

Interestingly, both the weighting of the individual arguments and their perceived certainty can be deduced from Darwin's notes. Thus, the main advantage of marriage in his eyes seems to be that it could save him from loneliness, especially in old age. This argument appears several times and is thereby emphasized. The main disadvantage of marriage seems to him to be that marriages take time, because he has underlined "loss of time" several times. It is also interesting that Darwin distinguishes between safe and uncertain consequences, because he has marked the consequence of having children as an uncertain one ("if it please god"). In the end he decided to marry and wrote "Marry—Marry—Marry Q.E.D." on his note. His consideration had almost the status of a mathematical proof for him, as the Q.E.D. (quod erat demonstrandum = what was to be proven) indicates. The marriage with his wife Emma, as far as his biographers know, was a happy one, by the way. His last words to Emma were: "I am not the least afraid of death—Remember what a good wife you have been to me—Tell all my children to remember how good they have been to me" (E. Darwin, 1882). Darwin's hopes, which he had put on paper 44 years earlier as arguments for marriage, seem to have been fulfilled.

5

What Kinds of Decisions Can We Distinguish?

1. Decisions under ignorance: decision-makers do not know all possible consequences.
2. Decisions under certainty: consequences are certain to occur.
3. Decisions under risk: consequences occur with a known probability.
4. Decisions under uncertainty: consequences occur with an unknown probability.

Side Story

The Difference Between Value and Utility

The expected value theory refers to the objective value of the various options (Betsch et al., 2011). Bernoulli further developed this approach by making subjective utility the decisive criterion for a good decision instead of the objective value. The theory of expected value became the theory of expected utility. The difference can be illustrated with the following example: the value of a potential profit of 1000 Euro is always the same and should therefore be included in all decision-makers' calculations in the same way. However, the utility of 1000 Euro depends on how much money I already have. For rich decision-makers, 1000 Euros should therefore have a different utility than for poor decision-makers and should therefore be included differently in a corresponding decision.

5.2.2.2 Heuristics

Within the framework of the bounded rationality approach (Gigerenzer & Selten, 2001; Simon, 1982), the ideas of the theories of expected value or utility were rejected as unrealistic. It has been argued that in most real-life situations, people lack the cognitive capacity to perform such complex computational operations, especially when decision time is limited. Instead of describing how people can make optimal decisions in theory, the focus of psychological theory and empirical research evolved in to understanding how people actually make successful decisions in everyday situations (Gigerenzer & Goldstein, 1996).

Under the influence of bounded rationality, a number of heuristic approaches to human decision-making behavior have emerged (Gigerenzer & Goldstein, 1996; Gigerenzer & Selten, 2001; Gigerenzer, Todd and the ABC Research Group, 1999; Tversky & Kahneman, 1974; Kahneman et al., 1982). These approaches assume that people use simplifying rules, so-called heuristics, to make decisions.

Two of the best known and best-studied of these approaches are the classical heuristics and biases program by Kahneman and Tversky (Tversky & Kahneman, 1974; Kahneman et al., 1982) and the adaptive toolbox (Gigerenzer & Selten, 2001; Gigerenzer, Todd and the ABC Research Group, 1999). The adaptive toolbox emphasizes the functionality of heuristics. The basic idea of the adaptive toolbox is that people have a set of heuristics, each of which is particularly suitable for certain decision situations. From the perspective of this approach, good decisions depend on decision-makers using the most appropriate heuristics for a given situation. When people make decisions based on heuristics, they do not compute all cues in a decision situation according to their respective validities but rely on a single or a reduced number of cues. The available cues are searched according to a certain rule (search rule), and this search is also stopped according to a certain rule (stopping rule). A decision is then made using a decision rule. Such a procedure does not always lead to a perfect decision, but it allows for sufficiently good decisions, especially in situations where people have to make decisions under suboptimal conditions (e.g., time pressure, stress, incomplete information). The heuristics and biases program of

Kahneman and Tversky, on the other hand, emphasizes more strongly that heuristics make people susceptible to systematic errors of judgment and decision, so-called biases (Tversky & Kahneman, 1974; ► Side Story: The Take-The-Best-Heuristics; ► Side Story: Random and Systematic Errors).

Numerous heuristics have also been proposed for decisions in sports (for an overview see Bennis & Pachur, 2006). Some of them represent applications of already existing heuristics to sports settings, while other heuristics have been proposed specifically for sports applications. The first group includes, for example, the application of take-the-first heuristics to the generation and selection of options by athletes (Johnson & Raab, 2003). According to this approach, an expert playmaker would be best off by choosing the first option that comes to his mind in a given game situation while searching for the most valid option on the field.

Heuristic

A heuristic is a rule that simplifies a complex judgment or decision situation by reducing the amount of information that is considered (Gigerenzer, Todd and the ABC Research Group, 1999). Heuristics have rules on how the available information is searched (search rule), how this search is stopped (stopping rule), and which option is selected on the basis of the information searched (decision rule).

Heuristics

People can make good decisions by using heuristics, even if they lack time or other resources. Some research programs emphasize the functionality of heuristics (e.g., the adaptive toolbox), while other research programs emphasize their error-proneness (e.g., the heuristics and biases program).

Side Story

The Take-The-Best-Heuristic

A well-known heuristic is the take-the-best-heuristic (Gigerenzer & Goldstein, 1999). It is often demonstrated using the so-called city size paradigm. Participants are presented with the names of two cities and a range of information on each of these cities. Their task is to decide which of the two cities is the larger. If participants use the take-the-best heuristic, they proceed as follows: they search the information in order of validity (search rule). They stop this search at the first information that distinguishes between the two options (stopping rule). Then they choose the option that has a higher value on this information (decision rule). All other information is ignored. In concrete terms, this means that they rank all information according to its significance for the size of a city and search through it until they find information that distinguishes between the two cities. For example, the participants could first look to see if both cities have an airport. If only one city has an airport, the participants stop searching here, ignore any further information, and choose the city that has an airport as the larger one. If both cities have an airport, they continue searching in the order of perceived significance of the information until they find information that distinguishes between the two cities (e.g., city A has a football stadium, city B does not). The city with the "better value" for this information is taken; all other information is ignored.

The take-the-best-heuristic is therefore non-compensatory. This means that much information pointing to option B as the larger city cannot compensate for the fact that the most valid information points to option A.

Side Story

Random and Systematic Error

In judgment and decision research, two types of errors are distinguished: random errors and systematic errors. While the former type is sometimes labelled as noise (Kahneman et al., 2021), the latter errors are also called biases and represent systematic distortions of judgments and decisions. There are different perspectives on what exactly a bias is. Kahneman and Tversky understand biases as deviations from a theoretically optimal judgment or decision strategy or as the result of applying a heuristic in a situation where it leads to erroneous results (Tversky & Kahneman, 1974). Numerous individual biases have been identified in the psychological literature. For example, the hindsight bias describes the human tendency to overestimate in retrospect how well we have predicted a particular event. For example, many people believe after a football match that it was clear beforehand who would win it. But if they had been asked beforehand, they would not have been as certain.

From the perspective of the lens model, a bias arises when judges use a cue for their judgments that in reality is not correlated with the criterion, or when judges include a cue in their judgments more than is justified by the correlation of that cue with the criterion. A bias would thus be, for example, if a lecturer gave better grades to more attractive students, or if larger football players were considered more aggressive than smaller ones. From this perspective, the distinction between bias and meaningful cue use depends on whether or not cue and criterion correlate in the real world: if taller players are actually more aggressive than smaller ones, the apparent bias becomes meaningful cue use.

5

5.2.2.3 Fast and Slow Decisions

There is a story about Mark Zuckerberg, the founder of Facebook, that he only owns one pair of pants, a t-shirt and a sweater. Mind you—not one copy of each, but one model. This way he doesn't have to think about what to wear in the morning and saves valuable time and resources for the important decisions of the day. There are similar stories about Steve Jobs (founder of Apple) and his black turtleneck sweater or Barack Obama and his ties. These anecdotes may be wrong, but they point to an important point: making decisions can be exhausting. But this is not true for all decisions. Indeed, an important distinction between different types of decisions is how much resource they require (Evans, 2010; Evans & Stanovich, 2013; Furley et al., 2015).

Some decisions are quick, and we simply make them without a conscious process of weighing different options and their consequences. For example, without thinking, we choose our toothbrush instead of our roommates', we step on the brake instead of accelerating at a red light, and we play the ball to a well-positioned teammate in the shortest possible time instead of trying to score a goal ourselves. In some of these situations, we may not even notice that we have just chosen one of several options. Other decisions take time, and we experience them as the result of a conscious process of weighing up the pros and cons. For example, we compare different homes, we weigh up whether or not to get married, and we think long and hard about which players would fit well into our team.

Fast, seemingly effortless decisions are made possible by Type 1 processing (Evans, 2010; Evans & Stanovich, 2013). Type 1 processing is characterized by the fact that it does not require working memory capacity. It is triggered by contextual features and comes to a result without the need for intention or conscious control. Type 1 processing can be modeled as a spreading activity in a network, which is able to process large amounts of information in a very short period of time. In order for Type 1 processing to produce a result in a given situation, learning processes over a longer period of time must have resulted in essential parts of the task being represented in long-term memory. For example, a perception of the cue "red traffic light" leads to the option "brake" being activated and the option "accelerate" being inhibited. This is only possible if both cues and options have become part of the network in long-term memory.

If cues and options are not represented in the network (e.g., a decision with which we have no experience) or if it is not clear which option should be selected in the network (e.g., because of ambiguous learning experiences in the past), Type 2 processing is additionally activated. Type 2 processing is based on working memory capacity. Because working memory capacity is limited, Type 2 processing takes time and can only process a limited amount of information at once. The more information that needs to be considered and the more complicated the available information is to weigh up, the longer Type 2 processing takes, and the more likely it is to produce a suboptimal result. Suboptimal means, in the case of a decision, that the option chosen is not the one that provides the maximum expected benefit. For example, most people have little experience in deciding whether or not to get married. Therefore, they cannot use Type 1 processing to solve this decision. Decisions that rely only to a small extent on Type 2 processing are sometimes referred to as intuitive decisions or routines. Decisions that rely on Type 2 processing in addition to Type 1 processing are sometimes called deliberative decisions (Evans, 2010).

It cannot be said in general terms that one processing mode is superior to the other. Both have their strengths and weaknesses. However, one can deduce the conditions in which each mode is more suitable and should lead to optimal results. The main advantage of Type 1 processing is that it can process large amounts of information in a very short period of time. Decisions based on Type 1 processing are therefore useful in situations where quick decisions have to be made, such as pass decisions or tactical decisions in sports (Furley et al., 2015). However, Type 1 processing only leads to good results if decision-makers have had ample opportunity to learn, i.e., if they have expertise in a particular field. To make good decisions using Type 1 processing, decision-makers must have made many such decisions and received feedback on them.

Type 2 processing leads to good results if decision-makers have the necessary resources to weigh up the advantages and disadvantages of the various options.

These resources are time and working memory capacity. Type 2 processing can also act as a kind of control mechanism for Type 1 processing.

Both processing mechanisms are vulnerable to certain errors. Decisions made using Type 1 processing reflect the circumstances in the situations in which they were learned. In a concrete decision situation they are therefore only meaningful to the extent that the decision situation is similar to the situations in the learning phase. For example, a defender may have learned that an opponent in a certain game situation typically tries to pass to the right. This enables them to react very quickly. If the opponent suddenly passes to the left, the defender will react incorrectly. Decisions made using Type 2 processing are suboptimal if there are not enough resources available.

The distinction between Type 1 and Type 2 processing has a long history in psychology but is new in this form. Therefore, many older decision theories do not say anything about the type of processing they assume. Expected utility theories, for example, only describe when optimal decisions result. However, they do not say anything about how people actually process the underlying information (Betsch et al., 2011). Thus, it can be shown that Type 2 processing is not a prerequisite for the results of decisions to be consistent with the predictions of expected utility theories (Glöckner & Betsch, 2008). Heuristics, on the other hand, are understood by some researchers to be based on Type 1 processing and by others to be based on Type 2 processing (e.g., Betsch, 2008). However, the definition of a heuristic as described above does not really make any statement about the underlying processing mode.

Type 1 Processing

Type 1 processing does not require working memory capacity. It is triggered by context characteristics and comes to a result without the need for intention or conscious control. Multiple pieces of information are processed in parallel, that is, simultaneously. Type 1 processing is fast and based on experience. Decisions based primarily on Type 1 processing are also called intuitive decisions.

Type 2 Processing

Type 2 processing requires working memory capacity. Information is processed serially, that is, one after the other. Decisions that rely heavily on Type 2 processing in addition to Type 1 processing therefore take longer and may resemble a deliberate weighing of the advantages and disadvantages of various options.

5.2.3 Conclusion

It cannot be said in general terms that people always decide on the basis of heuristics or always take all relevant information into account. Similarly, a decision is not necessarily bad because it does not perfectly follow the predictions of the expected utility theory. People probably use different judgment and decision strategies in different situations. For example, people can only rely on intuitions and routines if they have gained extensive experience in a particular area. Conversely, it follows that decision-makers must have extensive experience if they are to make intuitive decisions in a particular area. It can also be useful to make heuristic decisions in some situations. In this case, however, care must be taken that heuristic decisions are not systematically distorted and do not become biases.

Judgment and decision research thus offers us numerous theoretical and model-based ideas. We can use them to understand judgments and decisions and to improve them if necessary. The problem is that the theories of judgment and decision research are often difficult to apply to problems in practice, as will become clear in the following sections. Conversely, research on judgments and decisions in a particular area, such as sport, is often more phenomena-oriented (cf. Raab et al., 2019). This means that one does not try to systematically test the validity of a theory in a field but rather observes an interesting phenomenon and then tries to understand it. In doing so, one can fall back on existing theories of judgment and decision-making or formulate new ones.

5.3 From Athletes to Officials: Who Makes Judgments and Decisions in Sports?

In the second part of this chapter, we present concrete examples of sports psychological research on judgments and decisions and discuss their implications. Although many of the phenomena described have mainly been studied in relation to a specific group of people, they also play a role for other actors in sport. Nevertheless, the organization of the following chapters reflects the focus of the underlying research, which concentrates on the role of the judge or decision-maker: athletes, coaches, and trainers or officials.

5.3.1 Athletes and Coaches

Athletes and coaches make a variety of judgments and decisions, which of course vary greatly depending on the sport. For example, coaches decide on the composition of the team or squad, on the team lineup, on substitutions, and on which tactics are played.

Athletes, for example, assess match situations and decide whether to pass or shoot on goal themselves. They evaluate teammates and opponents and decide on the basis of this for one or the other move. And they can decide to foul or play fair. Although coaches and athletes undoubtedly make serious judgments and decisions, there are comparatively few studies on their decisions.

On the one hand, this may be due to the fact that the decisions mentioned seem to ideally follow the theoretical models of utility maximization presented in the first part of this chapter. Coaches should choose the team, tactic, or formation from which they expect to derive the maximum benefit, i.e., usually the highest probability of winning. Athletes should also choose the most promising pass option.

On the other hand, it may be because athletes' decisions are often examined from a different theoretical perspective than that of decision research. There are numerous studies on the role of perception and attention for tactical decisions (Furley & Memmert, 2012, 2015; ► Chap. 2). Tactical decisions are also examined from the perspectives of creativity and game intelligence (Memmert & Roca, 2019). In this context, creativity refers to the ability to find tactical solutions that are surprising and thus unexpected for the opponents. Game intelligence generally refers to the ability to find the best possible solutions for tactical situations. If one replaces "best possible" with "utility-maximizing," the proximity to classical decision theory is noticeable here as well. Nevertheless, all the areas mentioned (perception, attention, creativity, game intelligence) represent separate fields of research with their own theory formation and methodological approaches.

In the following, we will concentrate on phenomena that are mainly investigated from the theoretical and methodological perspectives of judgment and decision research. A supplementary current collection can be found, for example, in a special issue on judgment and decision-making in sports by the Journal of Economic Psychology (Balafoutas et al., 2019).

5.3.1.1 Sophomore Slump and Regression to the Mean

When assessing sporting performance, especially over longer periods of time, it is important to bear in mind that the performance observed at any given time is always made up of (at least) two factors. This consideration results from the assumptions of classical test theory (e.g., Lord & Novick, 1968; for applications to sports psychology, see, for example, Schweizer et al., 2020; Vaughn et al., 2012). One factor represents the "actual performance" we are interested in when making the assessment. Changes in performance at the expense of this factor are also called systematic changes. At the same time, however, random influences always have an impact on performance: sometimes you have a good day, sometimes a bad one. We humans tend to regard random performance fluctuations as systematic. We commit this error of judgment especially when random influences do not alternate but occur serially. We can easily attribute a single bad game to chance. However, when football players or a football club play a few bad games in a row, experts look for the cause of this "performance deterioration" and possibly even change the training or nutrition of the player. Television analysts begin to call for structural changes in the club. In doing so, they underestimate the proportion of random fluctuation in performance, and they underestimate that positive and negative random influences do not necessarily alternate but can occur in series.

An example of the confusion of random and systematic influences in performance assessment is the so-called sophomore slump. A sophomore slump refers to when a performance in the second year (or second season) is worse than in the first. For example, students might notice a drop in performance in the second year of college, or a Bundesliga club might play worse in the second year in the first division than in the first. Specifically, sophomore slump refers to the observation that college athletes who performed particularly well in their first year (the rookie or freshman year) often perform worse in their second year (the sophomore year). On the one hand, this decline can be understood as a systematic one, and, accordingly, one can start to search for the causes: Is the athlete suffering from homesickness? Do they party too much? Do they have difficulty adapting to the changed life in college? These causes would lead to the demand for appropriate interventions. For example, athletes could be offered psychosocial support, their families might be invited for a visit, or the athletes might be forbidden to party. Before taking such measures, however, it is worth taking a look at the statistics. When doing so, the sophomore slump can be explained as a special case of regression to the mean (Campell & Kenny, 1999). If systematic and random factors always contribute to a specific performance and its respective measurement, then absolute peak performance can only occur if both the systematic and as many of the random factors as possible exert a positive influence. Since the random influencing factors are random, however, they are not correlated across several performances—they will therefore exert a negative influence again at some point after the peak performance has been achieved.

These considerations give rise to a statistical necessity: if a performance was particularly good at a certain point in time, it must deteriorate in the following period (at least if the systematic component does not improve). The same applies, incidentally, to particularly poor performances and can thus explain why football players who change clubs after a particularly bad season virtually flourish with the new club in the following season. These considerations only apply to particularly bad and particularly good performances—but it is precisely these that are often of interest when assessing sporting performance. Moreover, these considerations only apply if the performance or measurement of performance contains a random element.

What do these considerations mean in practice? Individual fluctuations in performance per se should not be overrated. Instead, it is worth looking at the trend, i.e., the average performance development over a period of time. The more single athletic performances are included in the assessment, the more the random fluctuations are averaged out (◘ Fig. 5.2) and the systematic part becomes visible. Under no circumstances should one overreact after a single poor performance and establish extensive changes in training. Otherwise you will end up like the Israeli Air Force, which stopped rewarding its pilots for particularly good flight performances—because it assumed that these rewards were bad for the subsequent efforts of the pilots and thus responsible for the drop in performance in the following flights (see Kahneman, 2011, for this example of overlooked regression to the mean).

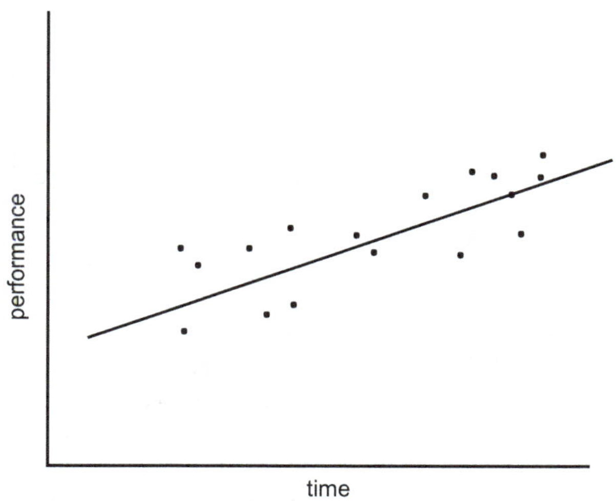

◘ **Fig. 5.2** Random performance fluctuations. This figure shows the development of the true value of an athlete's performance over time (diagonal line). The points represent the performances measured at a given moment. Deviations of the points from the straight line are random variations

Systematic and Random Fluctuations in Performance
People tend to perceive random fluctuations in performance as systematic. This becomes problematic if either changes are made as a result of fluctuations and their interpretation or if the fluctuations themselves are understood as a consequence of measures taken.

Sophomore Slump

Sophomore slump refers to the observation that athletes who have had a particularly good year or season seem to perform worse the following year. This deterioration need not have a systematic cause but can be a random fluctuation.

5.3.1.2 Passing Decisions and the Hot Hand

Basketball players often have to decide which of their teammates they want to pass the ball to. Their goal is to make the decision that will most likely lead to a basket. What information can players use to make the best decision? First of all, they could of course take into account which player is in a favorable throwing position and where the opponents are. They could also take into account that some of their teammates are generally better shooters than others. Finally, they could take into account which of their teammates is the most likely to score at that moment.

In basketball, players and coaches believe that a player has a better chance of scoring a basket if his or her previous attempts were successful than if the previous attempts were not successful. A player who is on a winning streak is "hot." In research, this phenomenon is called the hot hand (Gilovich et al., 1985). Studies suggest that the majority of all athletes and coaches in various sports believe in the hot hand. In addition, coaches as well as athletes use the hot hand for pass decisions: when a player is "hot," he or she is more likely to score a basket, so it makes sense to pass the ball to that player. From the point of view of sports psychology, the hot hand also seems plausible (Bar-Eli et al., 2006): a success should increase the expectation of self-efficacy, and an increased expectation of self-efficacy should in turn increase the probability of success (Bandura, 1997).

Although almost all athletes believe in the hot hand, and although it is consistent with accepted psychological theories, it is surprisingly difficult to find empirical evidence for it. Indeed, the first article on the hot hand concluded that it is a myth (Gilovich et al., 1985): data from several studies showed no evidence of the hot hand, i.e., in these studies the probability of success of an attempt was independent of the success of previous attempts. Therefore, the authors concluded that relying on the hot hand for pass decisions is a potentially harmful error. If the hot hand does not exist, but players make pass decisions based on their belief in the hot hand, they do not use the information that is important (e.g., the general probability of success of a player) for these decisions. In the following decades, numerous studies on the hot hand were conducted in various sports. Almost half of these studies found evidence for the hot hand; the other half did not (Bar-Eli et al., 2006). In spite of these findings, there is still agreement that almost all coaches and athletes believe in the hot hand.

5

But why do so many people believe in the hot hand when in reality it does not exist? One answer to this question is that people are very good at recognizing patterns but very bad at distinguishing systematic from random variation (par. 5.3.1.1). Another answer is that belief in the hot hand could be functional even if the hot hand does not exist (Raab et al., 2012). Even if the hot hand does not exist, athletes with a higher basic probability of success should also have more and longer sequences of successful attempts. In this case, passing the ball to the player who is apparently "hot" would result in passing the ball to the player who is more successful overall. We haven't heard the last word on the hot hand yet, and thus it remains a fascinating research topic at the interface between decision research and sports psychology (▶ Side Story: How to Find Empirical Evidence for the Hot Hand?; ▶ Methods: Hot Hand).

Hot Hand

A person (a player) has the hot hand ("is hot") if their probability of scoring a basket is higher because they have scored in their last *x* (usually three) attempts than if they have not scored in their last x (usually three) attempts (see Gilovich et al., 1985).

In general: A person (a player) has the hot hand ("is hot") if their probability to perform a successful action is higher when their last *x* actions were successful than when their last *x* actions were not successful (cf. Gilovich et al., 1985).

Hot Hand

In many sports, athletes and trainers believe in the hot hand: if an athlete has just had a "run," the probability of further successful actions increases. Therefore, it seems to make sense to pass the ball to the "hot" player. However, the empirical evidence for the hot hand is mixed: some studies find evidence for the hot hand, others do not.

Side Story

How Do You Find Empirical Evidence for the Hot Hand?

The research literature discusses how the hot hand should be defined and assessed. The classical definition of Gilovich et al. (1985) defines the hot hand as a conditional probability. It states that the conditional probability of scoring a basket after three hits ("hits") is higher than the conditional probability of scoring a basket after three misses. Formally this can be expressed as

$$p(\text{Basket} \mid \text{all previous three attempts were hits}) > p(\text{Basket} \mid \text{all previous three attempts were no hits})$$

To search for evidence of the hot hand according to this definition, look at all attempts by a player during a game, and search for all episodes of three hits and three misses. Then, in the next step, you can count whether the player in question has a better ratio of hits to misses after three hits than after three misses (▶ Methods: Hot Hand). So after each sequence of three hits and three misses, both hits and misses are considered.

This method seems intuitively useful, but it is not as trivial to use as one might think, as it involves some subtle mathematical problems that were only described after decades of research (Miller & Sanjurjo, 2015, 2016, for a controversial discussion). Some authors argue that after correcting for these mathematical problems, results that have been interpreted as evidence against the hot hand so far actually represent evidence for the hot hand (Miller & Sanjurjo, 2015, 2016).

There are two further methods to define and thus operationalize the hot hand (Bar-Eli et al., 2006; Gilovich et al., 1985). First, the hot hand can be understood as a correlation between successive attempts ("autocorrelation"). Accordingly, one would look for evidence for the hot hand by correlating successive attempts. Second, the hot hand can be understood as the occurrence of more sequences of consecutive identical events than would be predicted from a player's base rate. Accordingly, one would look for evidence of the hot hand by comparing the number of sequences that actually occur to the number predicted by the baseline.

Methods: Hot Hand

We define the hot hand as follows: a player has the hot hand if his or her probability of having another hit after three misses is higher than his or her probability of having a hit after three misses:

$$p(\mathrm{H}|\mathrm{HHH}) > p(\mathrm{H}|\mathrm{MMM})$$

In ◘ Fig. 5.3, players A and B have a base rate of 0.5, i.e., a total of 50% of their attempts are hits, and 50% are misses. Players C and D have a base rate of 0.65, meaning that a total of 65% of their attempts are hits and 35% are misses.

Players A and C show signs of hot hand (their success rate after hits is higher than their success rate after misses). Players B and D show no signs of the hot hand (their success rate after hits is equal to their success rate after misses).

A sequence may partially overlap with itself. For example, the sequence HHHHM contains two sequences of three hits, the first of which is followed by another hit (HHH – H), the second by a Miss (HHH – M).

5.3.2 Officials

5.3.2.1 Influence of Prior Knowledge

Numerous studies from different areas of human judgment and decision-making suggest that people are influenced by prior knowledge when making judgments and decisions (Betsch et al., 2011). First of all, this is not a bad thing; on the contrary, it is virtually essential for survival: imagine that you had to cope with every situation anew without being able to use your previous experiences! On the positive side, one could say that people fortunately have the ability to incorporate their previous knowledge into current judgments and decisions and to make use of this ability. This useful feature of human judgment and decision-making becomes problematic if either the prior knowledge used is systematically biased or if, in a certain context, rules apply which prohibit the use of prior knowledge. The latter is often the case with judgments and decisions made by officials.

It is important to stress that studies on the influence of prior knowledge on officials do not necessarily show that the use of prior knowledge makes judgments and decisions worse. In fact, the studies in question do not usually investigate this at all. They only show that peo-

◘ **Fig. 5.3** In search of the hot hand: H (Hit) = successful attempt (e.g., basket); M (Miss) = non-successful attempt (e.g., missing the basket); green = all hits and misses following three hits; red = all hits and misses following three misses

Attempt	Player A p(H) = .5	Player B p(H) = .5	Player C p(H) = .65	Player C p(H) = .65
1	H	H	H	H
2	H	M	H	H
3	H	H	H	H
4	H	H	H	M
5	H	H	H	H
6	H	H	M	H
7	M	M	M	H
8	M	H	H	H
9	H	M	H	H
10	M	M	H	M
11	M	M	H	M
12	M	M	M	M
13	M	H	H	M
14	H	H	H	H
15	M	M	M	H
16	M	M	M	M
17	M	H	M	H
18	M	M	M	H
19	H	M	H	M
20	H	H	H	H

ple (e.g., officials) use prior knowledge, and this use is considered problematic because it is considered prohibited in the context studied.

For example, studies suggest that referees consider the reputation of players in their decisions (Jones et al., 2002): if players have a reputation for committing many fouls because they have committed many fouls in the past, referees are more likely to call an ambiguous call that could go either way a foul. On the one hand, this seems to make sense: by using prior knowledge, more correct decisions could be made over many decision situations than without using it. On the other hand, the use of prior knowledge in this case can lead to unfair individual decisions. After all, the player with a bad reputation is always at a disadvantage. Furthermore, the use of prior knowledge leads to a seemingly paradoxical effect: the same incident could be called as a foul in one situation (if a player with a bad reputation was the potential offender) and not in another (if a player with a good reputation was the potential offender). This is probably contrary to the idea of fairness of many fans and would not be in accordance with the rules.

Similarly, studies suggest that judges in gymnastics consider the order of athletes in their judgments (Plessner, 1999). Judges know that coaches usually send the best athlete to the apparatus last. Therefore, they have lower expectations of the first gymnast than of the last. The result is that the same exercise is rated better if it is performed last than if it is performed first. In the literature this is also called sequence or expectation effect. However, the basis of the expectation is the judges' prior knowledge of which athletes will compete when.

Prior knowledge can have a special influence when several judgments have to be made in a sequence. In this case one also speaks of sequential judgments. Examples are referees in football who make up to 200 judgments and decisions per game (Helsen & Bultynck, 2004), judges in gymnastics who evaluate one athlete after another (Plessner, 1999), and also sports teachers who grade all the students in the class one after the other. In the case of sequential judgments, judges have prior knowledge not only of the qualities and characteristics of the athletes to be judged and their performances but also of the judgments they have already made.

Prior Knowledge

Prior knowledge often affects judgments and decisions. This is seen as problematic when prior knowledge is either systematically biased or undesirable. However, prior knowledge does not per se make judgments and decisions better or worse.

Sequential Judgments

Sequential judgment occurs when several judgments are made one after the other or when several objects are judged one after the other.

5.3.2.2 Compensation Decisions

An example of prior knowledge effects in sports is the compensation penalty in football, which every football fan knows. In fact, Plessner and Betsch (2001) were able to show that football referees are more likely to decide on a penalty kick against one team if they have already called a penalty kick against the other team. Conversely, referees are less likely to decide to call a penalty against a team if they have already called a penalty against that team (a kind of "compensation non-penalty"). This pattern has not only been shown in an experiment but has also been confirmed by data from the Bundesliga (Schwarz, 2011).

But why do referees tend to call a compensation penalty and its counterpart, the compensation non-penalty? Plessner and Betsch assume that referees are consciously or unconsciously motivated to influence a football match as little as possible by their decisions (▶ Study Box: An Experiment on Compensation Penalties (Plessner & Betsch, 2001)). Considering that most football matches end with a maximum of one goal difference, a penalty kick represents an intervention in the game that can be decisive in many cases. Referees may then be inclined either to try to compensate for a first significant intervention in the game (the classic compensation penalty) or, after a first significant intervention, try not to influence the game even more in the same direction (the compensation non-penalty). They try, so to speak, to compensate for their own intervention in the course of the game. In basketball, too, referees show a tendency to compensate for their own decisions made in the course of the game so far (Anderson & Pierce, 2009; ▶ Side Story: Are Football Referees Artists or Craftsmen?; ▶ Side Story: Do Compensation Decisions Make the Sport More Aggressive?)

Concession/Compensation Decisions

Referees are expected to influence the course of the game as little as possible. Referees therefore tend to compensate for their own decisions. For example, in football they are more likely to call a penalty kick against one team if they have already called a penalty kick against the other.

Study Box

An Experiment on the Compensation Penalty (Plessner & Betsch, 2001)

Plessner and Betsch (2001) showed a group of football referees videos of contact situations in the penalty area. These videos were selected in such a way that it could not be clearly determined whether the contact shown was a foul or not. When there was a foul in the penalty area, the referees should have awarded a penalty kick. The participating referees were divided into different conditions. All referees had to make decisions on two potential fouls one after the other. In one condition, the first foul was committed by one team and the second foul by the other team (the "compensation penalty kick condition"). In the other condition, both potential fouls were committed by players of the same team (the "compensation non-penalty kick condition"). The decisive factor was how the referees assessed the first potential foul: depending on whether or not they awarded a penalty kick, the decisions on the second potential foul differed drastically.

Side Story

Is Soccer Refereeing a Craft or an Art?

Plessner and Betsch (2001) interpret the compensation penalty as a classic judgment distortion due to prior knowledge and thus as a mistake, since the rules require referees to make independent decisions on penalty offences. Mascarenhas et al. (2002) argue that the effect might not be a misjudgment, but on the contrary the result of a philosophy of adequate game management (refereeing as art). This means that referees must not only make correct decisions but also decisions that are appropriate to the context and that these decisions may deviate from the rules. For example, referees may adapt their decisions to the rigors of the match and at the same time try not to influence the course of the game too much. In a laboratory study such as the study by Plessner and Betsch (2001), this decision-making behavior is then found to be incorrect. Plessner and Betsch (2002), on the other hand, point out that penalty kicks in football, even from the perspective of adequate decisions, are hardly among the situations in which referees have room for interpretation (refereeing as craft). Irrespective of which side one is inclined to agree with in the discussion described above—current thinking on this topic even goes in the direction of assuming that referees systematically change their decision-making style depending on the situation (Raab et al., 2020): it makes it clear that there are sometimes different opinions as to which decision is right and whether the right decision should always be taken.

Side Story

Do Compensation Decisions Lead to More Aggression in Sports?

Anderson and Pierce (2009) discuss the possible consequences of compensation decisions. The purpose of a foul call (or of penalty kicks, free throws, or time penalties) is to punish the respective team for its foul play. However, this punishment will be mitigated if, as a result of a punishment against one team, referees are subsequently more likely to punish the other team. When referees compensate, they increase the incentive for players to commit fouls: the advantage of fouls remains the same, but the disadvantages are reduced. In the medium term, Anderson and Pierce argue that compensation tendencies should therefore lead to more fouls being committed. At least in the American college basketball league NCAA, this trend has been observed. Whether the increasing aggressiveness in the NCAA is actually due to compensation decisions cannot be said with certainty. Nevertheless, the example of Anderson and Pierce shows that it is worth remembering that decisions are not only made with reference to past events but always create incentives for future behavior.

5.3.2.3 Crowd Noise Effects

Studies suggest that in football, referees are influenced by the noise of the spectators. This effect is also called the crowd noise effect. If a foul is accompanied by loud screams from the spectators, the referees are more likely to award a yellow card. This is especially true for fouls committed by the away team. Originally, this effect was explained by motivational forces (Nevill et al., 1999): if spectators react loudly to a foul, they put pressure on the referees to punish the foul. The referees yield to this pressure because they are motivated to avoid negative reactions from spectators and therefore give a yellow card. The referees want to keep the crowd happy, so to speak.

Another view explains the crowd noise effect using the lens model (Unkelbach & Memmert, 2010): the crowd noise correlates with the severity of a foul. This means that the more severe a foul was, the louder the screaming of the spectators. In the course of their career, referees learn this correlation and, conversely, use the crowd noise as an indication of the severity of the foul. Normally this behavior is undesirable, because referees use information that they should not use. Nevertheless, the use of the information "crowd noise" alone should not lead to worse decisions. On the contrary, it could even be that referees who use the cue noise make more correct decisions overall than referees who do not use it. This could be the case if the correlation between crowd noise and the severity of the foul is high and there are otherwise few valid cues. However, the use of the cue "crowd noise" is problematic and becomes a judgment bias because this particular cue is systematically biased at football matches, because there are usually more supporters of the home team than of the away team in the stadium. Football fans, on the other hand, shout louder when fouls are committed against players of their team than when fouls are committed against players of the other team. Referees who use crowd noise as a cue would thus systematically prefer the home team (Unkelbach & Memmert, 2010). Some authors even speculate that the crowd noise effect could contribute to home advantage (Unkelbach & Memmert, 2010). This speculation is supported by the fact that the crowd density in a stadium and the difference in the frequency of yellow cards for the home vs. away team correlate. This means that the more spectators there are in a stadium (relative to the maximum capacity of the stadium), the more yellow cards the away team receives compared to the home team.

5

The crowd noise effect is an excellent example of the importance of basic research for the development of practical interventions. Depending on which theoretical explanation is applicable, very different interventions result to protect referees against the crowd noise effect: if the crowd noise effect occurs because referees yield to the pressure of spectators, the result is the development of a program that makes referees resistant to crowd noise. If the crowd noise effect occurs because the referees have learned a correlation between the crowd noise and severity of the foul, then this results in a different intervention. In this case one could, for example, try to make the referees "unlearn" the learned connection (► Study Box: An Experiment on the Crowd Noise Effect (Unkelbach & Memmert, 2010))

Crowd Noise Effect

Referees use the noise and volume of the spectators in the case of a foul as information about whether they should award a yellow card. The louder the spectators are, the more likely referees are to award a yellow card. Since there are usually more fans of the home team than of the away team in a stadium, this behavior favors the home team.

Study Box

An Experiment on the Crowd Noise Effect (Unkelbach & Memmert, 2010)

Unkelbach and Memmert (2010) investigated the question of whether referees are influenced by crowd noise by means of an experiment. They used videos of 56 fouls from 56 different matches. By doing so, they tried to prevent the later results of the study from being dependent on the particularities of a single match. Half of the incidents used had resulted in a yellow card during the match; the other half had not. In addition, Unkelbach and Memmert used four different audio files, which originally did not belong to one of the 56 fouls. All four audio files contained crowd noise, and all four were used in a quiet and a loud version. The quiet version was 50 decibels quieter than the loud version. Twenty referees of the German Football Association participated in the experiment. They were divided into two equally sized groups. The first group saw all 56 scenes in random order. A computer program randomly assigned a sound to each scene in either the quiet or the loud version. The participating referees were supposed to think that the sound belonged to the respective scene. For each scene, each referee indicated whether he would award a yellow card. The experiment was exactly the same in the second group—with one crucial difference: if a scene in the first group was coupled with high volume (loud) noise, it was coupled with low volume (quiet) noise in the second group and vice versa. This procedure is called yoking in experimental psychology. If under these conditions there was a difference between the quiet and the loud version of the scenes, it could only be due to the volume.

This was exactly what happened: on average, the participating referees were more willing to award a yellow card when a scene was coupled with a loud spectator noise than when it was coupled with a quiet spectator noise. The referees were also more willing to award a yellow card when the incident had actually resulted in a yellow card. However, this effect was independent of the effect of the volume.

5.3.2.4 Assimilation and Contrast

Reflection

Before you read this section, please think about the following problem for a second. Imagine you have an oral exam or a practical sports exam. You can choose whether you want to be examined before or after a particular fellow student. You consider the fellow student to be very good, but you consider yourself to be rather mediocre. Do you want to be tested before or after your fellow student? Most people spontaneously wish to be tested before their very good fellow student. However, this section deals with the best way of answering this question.

In the psychology of perception, two opposite tendencies can be distinguished, namely, assimilation and contrast. Assimilation means that two (or more) objects are perceived to be more similar to each other than they actually are. Contrast means that two (or more) objects are perceived to be more dissimilar than they actually are. The Selective Accessibility Model (SAM) explains how assimilation and contrast can influence judgments and what influence when either assimilation or contrast occurs (Mussweiler, 2003).

The Selective Accessibility Model initially assumes that in a judgment situation, we do not consider all information equally but that some information is systematically more accessible than other information (selective accessibility). If we focus on similarities and neglect differences, assimilation results. If we focus on differences and neglect similarities, contrast results. The "standard mode" that most people use seems to be assimilation. This means that if there is no reason to contrast, we overestimate the similarity between several objects of judgment. In order to contrast, there must be some additional information that leads us to switch from assimilation to contrast.

Assimilation and contrast can also occur in the sequential assessment of athletic or school performance (Damisch et al., 2006). In the simplest case, a judge must assess two athletic performances in succession. When a judge assimilates, he assesses the second performance as more similar to the first performance than it actually is. In the case of a good first performance, the second performance would be judged better than it actually is. In the case of a bad first performance, the second performance would be judged worse than it actually is. If a judge contrasts, then she judges the second performance as less similar to the first performance than it actually is. So in the case of a good first performance, the second performance would be judged worse than it actually is. In the case of a bad first performance, the second performance would be judged better than it actually is.

As an example, imagine an oral examination in sports science. Most candidates will probably not give only right or wrong answers but a mixture of right and wrong answers. If the first candidate was very good and the professor assimilates, then he or she will focus more on the right answers than on the wrong answers in the second candidate. Conversely, if the first candidate was very bad, then the professor will focus more on the second candidate's wrong answers than on the right ones. As a result, the two successive candidates are evaluated more similarly than they would have been in the case of theoretical objective performance recording.

Studies suggest that assimilation and contrast also play a role in the sequential assessment of athletic performance (Damisch et al., 2006). The degree of assimilation or contrast depends on the degree of perceived similarity or difference between successive athletes. If two athletes of the same nationality compete in succession, assimilation is more likely to occur. If, on the other hand, two athletes of different nationalities compete in succession, contrast is triggered. In sports where judges evaluate sporting performance, assimilation and contrast effects can be strong enough to influence who will win a medal. Although these effects are likely to be small, the distances between competitors are also small.

To get back to the initial question: As a tendency, you should therefore enter the exam as second if your fellow student is likely to be very good, because people generally tend to assimilate rather than contrast. You can still support this tendency: dress similarly to your fellow student and emphasize to the professor that you have studied together. The exact opposite is true if you assume that your fellow student is worse than you!

Assimilation and Contrast

In sequential judgments, people can either focus on similarities between the objects of judgment (assimilation) or on differences (contrast). Which one of these is triggered depends on whether successive objects are perceived to be more similar or dissimilar than they actually are.

5.3.2.5 Calibration

Reflection

Again, before you read this section, please think about the following problem for a second. Imagine once again that you have an oral or a practical sports examination. This time you can choose whether you want to have the first examination slot on the day or a later one. Which slot do you choose? Sports psychology research suggests that your choice should depend on whether you hope for an A or even fear failing. You can find out the reason for this in this section.

5

At the beginning of a sequence of judgments, judges shy away from giving extreme judgments. This phenomenon is explained in the literature as calibration (Unkelbach & Memmert, 2014; Unkelbach et al., 2012). When people make judgments, they must first establish ("calibrate") their internal scale of judgment. This means they have to find out which attribute (e.g., which sporting performance) gets which value on the judgment scale (e.g., which grade). In doing so, they strive for consistency. Consistency means that all performances that are worse than others should also receive a worse grade (and vice versa). At the same time, performance assessments should differentiate between different performances. There is therefore often a norm not to award extreme assessments exclusively. The interplay of these two factors results in a tendency for judges not to award extreme judgments at the beginning of a series of judgments in order to keep more options open for later judgments. Once the judgment scale is calibrated, i.e., once the judge has assessed a certain number of performances, extreme judgments become more likely again. The following example illustrates these relationships well: if a professor gives the first student an A, and all subsequent students are at least as good as the first one, then the professor must give all students an A on that day. The same applies if the professor fails the first student. If all subsequent candidates are at least as bad as the first, then the professor must fail all candidates on that day.

The avoidance of extreme judgments at the beginning of judgment sequences has been empirically proven in various areas. Not only judges but also trainers and even referees in football avoid extreme judgments at the beginning of a series of judgments (Fasold et al., 2015; Unkelbach & Memmert, 2008). It has been empirically shown that the avoidance of extreme judgments is actually related to the fact that judges want to keep options open for later judgments: if judges assume that they only have to make a single judgment, they do not show any avoidance of extreme judgments. Only when they anticipate further judgments do they shy away from extreme judgments at the beginning of the sequence. This means that the same (extremely good or extremely bad) performance is judged differently, depending on whether the judges expect to judge further performances or not. At the same time, the same (extremely good or extremely bad) performance is judged differently depending on whether it occurs at the beginning or in the middle of a sequence.

To return to the question from the beginning of this section: If you think that your performance is worthy of an A, then you should try to get a later exam time slot. However, if you are afraid of failing, try to get the first exam slot!

Calibration

Judges strive for consistent and differentiating judgments. They therefore shy away from giving extreme judgments at the beginning of a judgment sequence. This means that the same sporting performance can be judged differently depending on whether it occurs at the beginning or at a later point in the sequence.

5.3.2.6 Offside

Referees in football have to make a very special decision, which also occurs in a similar form in other game sports: the offside decision. It is estimated that approximately 26% of all offside decisions are wrong (Helsen et al., 2006) and wrong offside decisions can have serious consequences for the football match in question. Offside decisions are divided into two different types of error, the flag error (FE) and the non-flag error (NFE). These terms are used because assistants raise their flag to indicate offside. In the case of a flag error, the assistant will display offside even though there is no offside. In the event of a non-flag error, the assistant does not display an offside even though there is an offside.

Offside decisions are very interesting from a psychological point of view, as there are different approaches to explaining how mistakes are made when offside positions are detected. The two most prominent approaches are less related to the theoretical approaches presented in this section: correctly recognizing offside positions is essentially a perceptual task, and thus the corresponding theoretical approaches are of a perceptual psychological nature (▶ Chap. 2).

One approach to understanding offside decisions is based on the so-called flash lag effect (Baldo et al., 2002). The flash lag effect describes the following phenomenon: when people are asked to indicate where a moving object (e.g., a fast-moving clock hand) is at a certain point in time, usually indicated by a short flash, they tend to perceive this object further ahead in its direction of movement than it actually is (▶ http://

www.michaelbach.de/ot/mot-flashLag/index.html). Translated to the offside situation, this means that the moving object is the player running toward the opponent's goal and whose position is to be decided as offside or not offside. The certain point in time is the moment when the ball is played. If the player in question is actually standing on or near the offside line, the flash lag effect would cause the assistant referees to perceive him or her as standing offside, when in fact he or she is not. The flash lag effect is therefore particularly suitable for explaining how flag errors occur.

Another approach to understanding offside decisions is the optical error hypothesis (Oudejans et al., 2000). The starting point of the optical error hypothesis is the observation that offside positions can only be correctly detected if the assistant referee is exactly on the offside line. This is an optical necessity. Depending on whether the assistant referee is in front of or behind the offside line, and depending on whether the attacking player or defender is first in his or her line of vision, different errors occur systematically (Fig. 5.4). The optical error hypothesis thus allows precise predictions to be made as to which error should occur under which circumstances.

There is empirical support for both explanatory approaches. Presumably, both the flash lag effect and the optical error contribute to wrong offside decisions.

Again, basic research has a great influence on the development of interventions for practice. The optical error hypothesis and flash-lag effect lead to completely different training programs: either referee assistants have to work on their positional play, or they have to learn how to correct the flash lag effect with a computer-supported training program. Both interventions exist and are used in practice.

Offside

Both the flash lag effect and the optical error hypothesis can explain how errors occur in offside decisions. Both explanatory approaches have been incorporated into training programs.

Offside

Players are in an offside position if:
- Any part of the head, body, or feet are in the opposing team's half (excluding the halfway line).
- Any part of the head, body, or feet are nearer to the opposing team's goal line than both the ball and the second last opponent.

The hands and arms of all players are not considered.

Players are not in an offside position if level with the:
- Second last opponent
- Last two opponents

Offside is defined in Law 11 of the Laws of the Game (IFAB, 2020).

Flag Error (FE)

The assistant referee indicates offside, although there is no offside.

Non-Flag Error (NFE)

The assistant referee does not indicate offside, although there is offside.

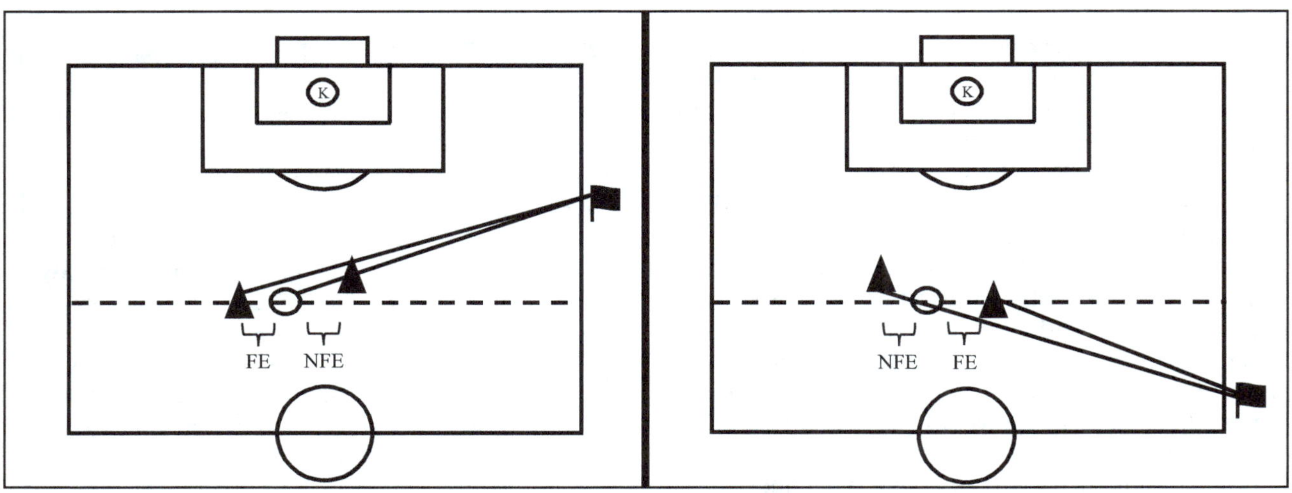

Fig. 5.4 Optical error hypothesis

5

To ◘ Fig. 5.4:

If the assistant is in front of the offside line, then in the example he or she will ◘ Fig. 5.4 (left):

- Make a non-flag error if the attacking player is in front of the defender in his or her line of sight.
- Make a flag error when the attacking player is behind the defender in his or her line of sight.

If the assistant is behind the offside line, then in the example he or she will be in ◘ Fig. 5.4 (right):

- Make a non-flag error if the attacking player is behind the defender in his or her line of sight.
- Make a flag error when the attacking player is in front of the defender in his or her line of sight.

5.3.2.7 Conformity in Group Judgments

So far, we have mainly looked at the judgments and decisions of individuals. However, some judgments and decisions are not made by individuals but by groups. These include, for example, panels of judges in gymnastics. Whenever judgments are made in groups, conformity can occur. Conformity means that individual judges adapt their judgments to those of others in the group.

In the literature a distinction is made between informational and normative conformity (Deutsch & Gerard, 1955). Informational conformity exists when people adapt their judgments to those of the other judges because they are unsure and think the others might know better. Normative conformity exists when people adapt their judgments to those of the others because a norm (i.e., a statement regulating behavior) calls for uniform judgment.

Such a norm can be explicit or implicit. If a norm is explicit, it is openly communicated, and deviations from the norm are officially sanctioned. For example, some sports federations evaluate the performance of their judges based on their deviations from the other judges. In turn, further assignments as judges and the level at which they take place may depend on these evaluations. Implicit standards are not openly communicated but are known to the group members. Violations of implicit standards therefore cannot be officially sanctioned, but they can have far-reaching consequences.

Studies from the fields of gymnastics, synchronized swimming, and skipping suggest that even experienced judges in panels tend to make conforming judgments (Boen et al., 2008; Boen et al., 2006; Vanden Auweele et al., 2004). These studies usually compare a series of scores where the judges learn how the other judges have scored with a series of scores where the judges have no information about the scores of the other judges. The following result is often reported: over several scores, the scores in the group with information about the other scores will increasingly converge, i.e., the variance between the scores will decrease. No such effect occurs in the group without information. Such a pattern is interpreted as evidence of conformity in panels of judges.

While it seems relatively easy to answer the question of whether there are conformity effects in panel judgments, it is much more complicated to decide what consequences should come from these findings. In the literature, it is sometimes suggested that judges should not be given information about their colleagues' evaluations. Apart from the fact that implementing this proposal (if it is possible at all) would entail major changes in the rules of the sports concerned, the question arises as to whether the complete avoidance of conformity effects is actually desirable.

Conformity

When judgments are made in groups (e.g., panels of judges in gymnastics), individual judges adjust their judgments to those of the other group members. In some sports, this effect is reinforced by the fact that uniform judgments are explicitly desired.

Normative Conformity

People adapt their judgments to the judgments of others because they perceive an accepted practice or need to judge as uniformly as possible.

Informational Conformity

People adapt their judgments to the judgments of others because they are uncertain and think that the others might be able to make better judgments.

Reflection

Choose a sport in which conformity effects can be expected. Basically, these are all sports in which several judges give scores and in which they learn how their colleagues have judged. Find out how exactly the scoring system works in the chosen sport. Then make a concrete plan on how to prevent conformity effects in this sport. Please reflect: What advantages would the "new" scoring system have? What disadvantages, costs, or "side effects" do you fear? Please weigh them up: considering the advantages and disadvantages, would you suggest that the sport in question change its scoring system?

5.4 Optimization of Judgments and Decisions

Reflection

On the previous pages, you have learned that numerous factors, which should not, influence your judgments: the order of the objects of judgment (e.g., candidates), the position of the objects of judgment in a sequence, your previous knowledge, and more. At the same time, many readers of this section will probably find themselves in situations in their professional lives where they have to make judgments, e.g., when giving marks at school or evaluating sporting performance in a sports club. What can you practically do to make your judgments as resistant as possible to the above factors? Please think of a situation in which you will have to make judgments later in your professional life. Please make yourself a concrete and practical plan on how you can later make the best possible judgments. This plan should be based on the above-mentioned factors. Do you see possibilities to eliminate previous knowledge? How can you prevent sequence and calibration effects? Can you make your judgments generally more reliable?

In order to improve judgments and decisions, it seems essential to understand the underlying processes and mechanisms. As explained in ▶ Sect. 5.3.2.6, a different training intervention results from the flash lag effect than from the optical error hypothesis. Similarly, referees would need to be trained differently depending on whether the crowd noise effect has motivational causes or is based on a learned correlation between crowd noise and severity of the foul. It is therefore problematic to formulate general rules to improve judgments and decisions. As an overall principle, the specific judgment errors or biases described above can only have an influence if judgments or decisions are made under uncertainty. Instead of trying to "unlearn" a specific error, one can also strive to make a judgment or decision situation fundamentally more secure. An example of this is the so-called calibration effect, in which judges are "calibrated" to a specific line of judgment with the help of videos (Unkelbach & Memmert, 2008). Similar approaches also exist for referees in football and basketball (e.g., Schweizer et al., 2013). An overview of different approaches to optimize decisions by athletes can be found, for example, in Williams and Jackson (2019).

Before deciding to introduce a specific intervention, all potential consequences of the intervention should always be considered—both positive and negative. Thus, whether the advantages of improving a judgment or decision outweigh the disadvantages must be considered. To do this, it is helpful to know the advantages and disadvantages of different psychological processes but also the specifics of different sporting contexts. For example, it could be that a particular intervention makes decisions better but slower. This may be an acceptable price for a video referee in football, but probably not for the referee on the pitch who has to make decisions in a fraction of a second. Moreover, interventions to improve judgments and decisions should be continuously evaluated—as should all other interventions (a fascinating overview of interventions that have achieved exactly the opposite of what they were supposed to achieve is provided by McCord, 2003).

The combination of detailed knowledge of the underlying psychological processes as well as of the specific judgment or decision environment thus promises a basis on which specific judgments or decisions can be improved. It should always be borne in mind that, although science can make statements about the presumed effects of an intervention, only the actors themselves can decide after careful consideration of all advantages and disadvantages whether or not it should ultimately be introduced.

Learning Control Questions

Basics:

1. Define judgments and decisions. What different judgments and decisions are there? What is the difference between judgments and decisions?
2. Describe Brunswik's lens model. Develop an application to a judgment situation in sports.
3. What are heuristics? Why do some scientists assume that people make decisions based on heuristics?
4. What is a bias?
5. What is the difference between Type 1 and Type 2 processing? In which situations are more intuitive decisions beneficial? In which situations are more deliberative decisions beneficial?

Advanced:

6. Name at least two components that each measured sports performance consists of. What are the possible explanations for the sophomore slump?
7. Why or when is the influence of prior knowledge on judgments and decisions problematic?
8. What is meant by compensation decisions? Why could they lead to increased aggressiveness?
9. What is meant by the crowd noise effect? Name at least one explanation of the crowd noise effect.
10. Describe the experiment by Unkelbach and Memmert (2010) on the crowd noise effect.

Experts:

11. Explain the Selective Accessibility Model and its significance for the assessment of sporting performance.
12. What are calibration effects, and how can they be explained theoretically?
13. What different explanations for incorrect offside decisions do you know? Describe why and how the different explanations lead to different interventions.
14. Name the different sources of conformity effects. What are the arguments for and against "eliminating" conformity effects?
15. Describe some concrete ways to optimize judgments and decisions.

5

References

Anderson, K. J., & Pierce, D. A. (2009). Officiating bias: The effect of foul differential on foul calls in NCAA basketball. *Journal of Sports Sciences, 27*, 686–694.

Balafoutas, L., Chowdhury, S. M., & Plessner, H. (2019). Applications of sports data to study decision making [Special Issue]. *Journal of Economic Psychology, 75*(Part B).

Baldo, M. V. C., Ranvaud, R. D., & Morya, E. (2002). Flag errors in soccer games: The flash-lag effect brought to real life. *Perception, 31*, 1205–1210.

Bandura, A. (1997). *Self-efficacy: The exercise of control*. Freeman.

Bar-Eli, M., Avugos, S., & Raab, M. (2006). Twenty years of "hot hand" research. The hot hand phenomenon: Review and critique. *Psychology of Sport and Exercise, 7*, 525–553.

Baron, J. (2000). *Thinking and deciding* (3rd ed.). Cambridge University Press.

Bennis, W. M., & Pachur, T. (2006). Fast and frugal heuristic in sports. *Psychology of Sport and Exercise, 7*, 611–629.

Betsch, T. (2008). The nature of intuition and its neglect in research on judgment and decision making. In H. Plessner, C. Betsch, & T. Betsch (Eds.), *Intuition in judgment and decision making* (pp. 3–22). Lawrence Erlbaum Associates.

Betsch, T., Funke, J., & Plessner, H. (2011). *Denken—Urteilen, Entscheiden, Problemlösen [Thinking—Judging, decision-making, problem-solving]*. Springer.

Boen, F., Van Hoye, K., Vanden Auweele, Y., Feys, J., & Smits, T. (2008). Open feedback in gymnastic judging causes conformity bias based on informational influencing. *Journal of Sports Sciences, 26*, 621–628.

Boen, F., Vanden Auweele, Y., Claes, E., Feys, J., & De Cuyper, B. (2006). The impact of open feedback on conformity among judges in rope skipping. *Psychology of Sport and Exercise, 7*, 577–590.

Campell, D., & Kenny, D. (1999). *A primer on regression artifacts*. Guilford.

Cooksey, R. W. (1996). The methodology of social judgment theory. *Thinking and Reasoning*, 2, 141–173.

Damisch, L., Mussweiler, T., & Plessner, H. (2006). Olympic medals as fruits of comparison? Assimilation and contrast in sequential performance judgments. *Journal of Experimental Psychology: Applied, 12*, 166–178.

Darwin, C. R. (1838). *This is the Question Marry Not Marry* [Memorandum on marriage]. (7.1838) CUL-DAR210.8.2 (Darwin Online, http://darwin-online.org.uk/content/frameset?viewtype=side&itemID=CUL-DAR210.8.2&pageseq=1)

Darwin, E. (1882). *Reminiscences of Charles Darwin's last years*. CUL-DAR210.9 (Darwin Online, http://darwin-online.org.uk/content/frameset?viewtype=side&itemID=CUL-DAR210.9&pageseq=16

Dawes, R. M. (1998). Behavioral decision making and judgment. In D. T. Gilbert, S. T. Fiske, & G. Lindzey (Eds.), *The handbook of social psychology* (4th ed., pp. 497–548). McGraw-Hill.

Deutsch, M., & Gerard, H. B. (1955). A study of normative and informational influence upon individual judgment. *Journal of Abnormal and Social Psychology, 51*, 629–636.

Doherty, M. E., & Kurz, E. M. (1996). Social judgment theory. *Thinking and Reasoning*, 2, 109–140.

Edwards, W. (1954). The theory of decision making. *Psychological Bulletin, 51*, 380–417.

Evans, J. S. B. T. (2010). Intuition and reasoning: A dual-process perspective. *Psychological Inquiry, 21*, 313–326.

Evans, J. S. B. T., & Stanovich, K. E. (2013). Dual-process theories of higher cognition: Advancing the debate. *Perspectives on Psychological Science, 8*, 223–241.

Fasold, F., Memmert, D., & Unkelbach, C. (2015). A theory-based intervention to prevent calibration effects in serial sport performance evaluations. *Psychology of Sport and Exercise, 18*, 47–52.

Furley, P., & Memmert, D. (2012). Working memory capacity as controlled attention in tactical decision making. *Journal of Sport and Exercise Psychology, 34*, 322–344.

Furley, P., & Memmert, D. (2015). Creativity and working memory capacity in sports: working memory capacity is not a limiting factor in creative decision making amongst skilled performers. *Frontiers in Psychology, 6*, 115.

Furley, P., Schweizer, G., & Bertrams, A. (2015). The two modes of an athlete: Dual-process theories in the field of sport. *International Review of Sport and Exercise Psychology, 8*, 106–124.

Gigerenzer, G., & Goldstein, D. G. (1996). Reasoning the fast and frugal way: Models of bounded rationality. *Psychological Review, 103*, 650–669.

Gigerenzer, G., & Goldstein, D. G. (1999). Betting on one good reason. The take the best heuristic. In G. Gigerenzer, P. M. Todd, & The ABC Research Group (Eds.), *Simple heuristics that make us smart* (pp. 75–95). Oxford University Press.

Gigerenzer, G., & Selten, R. (Eds.). (2001). *Bounded rationality: The adaptive toolbox*. MIT Press.

Gigerenzer, G., Todd, P. M., & The ABC Research Group. (1999). *Simple heuristics that make us smart*. Oxford University Press.

Gilovich, T., Vallone, R., & Tversky, A. (1985). The hot hand in basketball: On the misperception of random sequences. *Cognitive Psychology, 17*, 295–314.

Glöckner, A., & Betsch, T. (2008). Multiple-reason decision making based on automatic processing. *Journal of Experimental Psychology: Learning, Memory, and Cognition, 34*(5), 1055–1075.

Goldstein, W. M. (2004). Social judgment theory: Applying and extending Brunswik's probabilistic functionalism. In D. Koehler & N. Harvey (Eds.), *Blackwell handbook of judgment and decision making* (pp. 37–61). Malden, MA: Blackwell Publishing.

Helsen, W., & Bultynck, J. B. (2004). Physical and perceptual-cognitive demands of top-class refereeing in association football. *Journal of Sports Sciences, 22*, 179–189.

Helsen, W., Gilis, B., & Weston, M. (2006). Errors in judging "offside" in football: Test of the optical error versus the perceptual flash-lag hypothesis. *Journal of Sports Sciences, 24*, 512–528.

Hammond, K. R., Stewart, T. R., Brehmer, B., & Steinmann, D. (1975). Social judgment theory. In M. F. Kaplan & S. Schwartz (Eds.), *Human judgment and decision processes* (pp. 271-312). New York: Academic Press.

The International Football Association Board (IFAB). (2020). *The laws of the game 2020/21*. IFAB.

Johnson, J. G., & Raab, M. (2003). Take the first: Option-generation and resulting choices. *Organizational Behavior and Human Decision Processes, 91*, 215–229.

Jones, M. V., Paul, G. C., & Erskine, J. (2002). The impact of a team's reputation on the decisions of association football referees. *Journal of Sports Sciences, 20*, 991–1000.

Kahneman, D. (2011). *Thinking, fast and slow*. Farrar, Straus and Giroux.

Kahneman, D., Sibony, O., & Sunstein, C. R. (2021). *Noise—A flaw in human judgment*. Little, Brown Spark.

Kahneman, D., Slovic, P., & Tversky, A. (Eds.). (1982). *Judgment under uncertainty: Heuristics and biases*. Cambridge University Press.

Kahneman, D., & Tversky, A. (1979). Prospect theory: An analysis of decision under risk. Econometrica, 47, 263–291.

Lord, F. M., & Novick, M. R. (1968). *Statistical theories of mental test scores*. Addison-Weasley.

Mascarenhas, D. R. D., Collins, D., & Mortimer, P. W. (2002). The art of reason versus the exactness of science in elite refereeing: comments on Plessner and Betsch (2001). *Journal of Sport and Exercise Psychology, 24*, 328–333.

McCord, J. (2003). Cures that harm: unanticipated outcomes of crime prevention programs. *Annals of the American Academy of Political and Social Sciences, 587*, 7–30.

Memmert, D., & Roca, A. (2019). Tactical creativity and decision making in sport. In A. M. Williams & R. C. Jackson (Eds.), *Anticipation and decision making in sport* (pp. 203–214). Routledge.

Miller, J. B. & Sanjurjo, A. (2015, July 7). *A cold shower for the hot hand fallacy*. IGIER Working Paper No. 518.

Miller, J. B., & Sanjurjo, A. (2016, November 16). *Surprised by the gambler's and hot hand fallacies? A truth in the law of small numbers*. IGIER Working Paper No. 552.

Mussweiler, T. (2003). Comparison processes in social judgment: Mechanisms and consequences. *Psychological Review, 110*, 472–489.

Nevill, A. M., Balmer, N. J., & Williams, A. M. (1999). Crowd influence on decisions in association football. *Lancet, 353*, 1416–1416.

Oudejans, R. R. D., Verheijen, R., Bakker, F. C., Gerrits, J. C., Steinbrücken, M., & Beek, P. J. (2000). Errors in judging "offside" in football. *Nature, 404*, 33.

Plessner, H. (1999). Expectation biases in gymnastics judging. *Journal of Sport and Exercise Psychology, 21*, 131–144.

Plessner, H., & Betsch, T. (2001). Sequential effects in important referee decisions: The case of penalties in soccer. *Journal of Sport & Exercise Psychology, 23*, 254–259.

Plessner, H., & Betsch, T. (2002). Refereeing in sports is supposed to be a craft, not an art. Response to Mascarenhas, Collins, and Mortimer (2002). *Journal of Sport & Exercise Psychology, 24*, 334–337.

Plessner, H., Schweizer, G., Brand, R., & O'Hare, D. (2009). A multiple-cue learning approach as the basis for understanding and improving soccer referees' decision making. In M. Raab, J. Johnson, & H. Heekeren (Eds.), *Progress in brain research: Mind and motion: The bidirectional link between thought and action* (pp. 151–158). Elsevier Press.

Raab, M., Bar-Eli, M., Plessner, H., & Araújo, D. (2019). The past, present and future of research on judgment and decision making in sport. *Psychology of Sport & Exercise, 42*, 25–32.

Raab, M., Gula, B., & Gigerenzer, G. (2012). The hot hand exists in Volleyball and is used for allocation decisions. *Journal of Experimental Psychology: Applied, 18*, 81–94.

Raab, M., MacMahon, C., Avugos, S., & Bar-Eli, M. (2020). The referee's challenge: A threshold process model for decision making in sport games. *International Review of Sport and Exercise Psychology, 14*(1), 208–228.

Schwarz, W. (2011). Compensating tendencies in penalty kick decisions of referees in professional football: Evidence from the German Bundesliga 1963-2006. *Journal of Sports Sciences, 29*, 441–447.

Schweizer, G., Furley, P., Rost, N., & Barth, K. (2020). Reliable measurement in sport psychology: The case of performance outcome measures. *Psychology of Sport and Exercise, 48*, 101663.

Schweizer, G., Plessner, H., & Brand, R. (2013). Establishing standards for basketball elite referees' decisions. *Journal of Applied Sport Psychology, 25*, 370–375.

Simon, H. A. (1982). *Models of bounded rationality*. MIT Press.

Tversky, A., & Kahneman, D. (1974). Judgment under uncertainty: Heuristics and biases. *Science, 185*, 1124–1131.

Unkelbach, C., & Memmert, D. (2008). Game management, context effects, and calibration: The case of yellow cards in soccer. *Journal of Sport & Exercise Psychology, 30*, 95–109.

Unkelbach, C., & Memmert, D. (2010). Crowd noise as a cue in referee decisions contributes to the home advantage. *Journal of Sport & Exercise Psychology, 32*, 483–498.

Unkelbach, C., & Memmert, D. (2014). Serial position effects in evaluative judgments. *Current Directions in Psychology Science, 23*, 195–200.

Unkelbach, C., Ostheimer, V., Fasold, F., & Memmert, D. (2012). A calibration explanation of serial position effects in evaluative judgments. *Organizational Behavior and Human Decisions, 119*, 103–113.

Vanden Auweele, Y., Boen, F., De Geest, A., & Feys, F. (2004). Judging bias in synchronized swimming: Open feedback leads to non-performance-based conformity. *Journal of Sport and Exercise Psychology, 26*, 561–571.

Vaughn, B. K., Lee, H.-Y., & Kamata, A. (2012). Reliability. In R. C. Eklund, G. Tenenbaum, & A. Kamata (Eds.), *Measurement in sport and exercise psychology*. Human Kinetics.

Wigton, R. S. (1996). Social judgement theory and medical judgment. Thinking and Reasoning, 2, 175–190.

Williams, A. M., & Jackson, R. J. (Eds.). (2019). *Anticipation and decision making in sport*. Routledge.

Embodied Cognition

Markus Raab, Jonna Löffler and Rouwen Cañal-Bruland

Contents

Reprinted from Judgment, Decision Making and Embodied Choices, Raab, Chapter 3 Embodied cognition—How our bodies and movements shape our thinking, Page Nos. 13–28, Copyright (2021), with permission from Elsevier.

J. Schüler et al. (eds.), *Sport and Exercise Psychology*, https://doi.org/10.1007/978-3-031-03921-8_6

Learning Objectives

After having read this chapter, our readers…

Basic:

- Should be able to define embodied cognition and describe its relevance for sports
- Can reflect how movements influence cognition and vice versa
- Know about the differences between classic cognition theories and embodied cognition approaches
- Can describe the theoretical frameworks of embodied cognition and summarize their main characteristics

Advanced:

- Should be able to compare different embodied cognition approaches
- Have acquired knowledge about study designs and methods that can be used to determine the influence of movement on cognition as well as of cognition on movement
- Should be familiar with empirical findings on the interactions of movement, cognition, and perception in sports

Experts:

- Have acquired knowledge about study designs and methods that can be used to determine the influence of movement on cognition as well as of cognition on movement
- Be able to formulate how and why an embodied cognition perspective could change sport psychology research
- Are able to find research gaps and build their own experiments for an added value in this area

6.1 Introduction

> "To say that cognition is embodied means that it arises from bodily interactions with the world. From this point of view, cognition depends on the kinds of experiences that come from having a body with particular perceptual and motor capabilities that are inseparably linked and that together form the matrix within which reasoning, memory, emotion, language, and all other aspects of mental life are meshed." (Thelen et al., 2001, p. 1)

As this quote by Esther Thelen vividly puts it, the term embodied cognition describes a perspective on the human being that assumes substantial interactions between cognition, perception, and movement. A logical consequence of this interaction is that these three cannot be considered independently of each other. In contrast to classic, amodal[1] cognition theories, which consider the brain to be the central governor of mental representations and cognition, embodied cognition approaches postulate that thought processes are not independent of perception and movement processes but are embodied in a multimodal manner. From this assumption it follows that thought processes do not exist exclusively as internal processes in the head but consist of interactions between the body of an individual (and its abilities and skills) and the environment (cf. Rowlands, 2010). By definition, what the environment affords is highly interrelated with the level of the individual's abilities and skills (see also Cañal-Bruland & van der Kamp, 2012). Consequently, from an embodied cognition perspective, the brain is only one part of a broader action system that generates solutions for tasks from all three elements combined: cognition, perception, and movement. A clear example, relevant to sport psychology, is found in baseball: How does an outfielder catch a fly ball? How does the player know where in the field to be and when to be there in order to catch the ball? Amodal cognitive theories would say that the outfielder visually perceives the fly ball and its speed, size, direction, and so on, and the brain uses this information to create an internal model that predicts where the ball will land. The brain then sends instructions to the body to move to that location. According to this solution, the optimal movement toward the ball would be a straight line (because people prefer the shortest distance between two things).

Embodied cognition approaches would seek the solution to the outfielder task by first asking the following question: What resources does the outfielder have to solve the task most efficiently? Yes, the outfielder could build an internal model, but this is a time-consuming and difficult endeavor. The player could likewise use their cognitive, perceptual, and movement capacities in combination, for example, by moving (movement skills) and observing the ball (perceptual skills) with the overall goal (cognitive capacity) of catching it. As soon as the player begins to move, they no longer see the ball first rise and then fall in a parabolic curve. Instead, they sense their own movement and the movement of the flying ball. The player now has several options for adapting their movement to that of the ball and thus getting to the place where the ball will land: One way is to

1 Amodal describes that the neural representation of sensory input such as vision will be transduced to a representation that is not modality specific and therefore amodal such as a semantic network.

match their running trajectory to the trajectory of the ball so that the trajectories zero each other out and the ball looks as if it is flying in a straight line from the outfielder's point of view. Another possibility would be that instead of adjusting their running trajectory, they adjust their running speed to that of the ball: If the outfielder first runs faster and then slows down as soon as the ball loses speed, then from their perspective the ball looks as if it is moving at a constant speed. Both solutions result in the outfielder being in the right place at exactly the right time to catch the ball. If we compare the solutions of the amodal approach and the embodied cognition approach (see ◘ Fig. 6.1), it quickly becomes clear that the solutions of the embodied cognition approach are the ones that reflect reality much better (fielders rarely walk in a straight line at constant speed). Which of the two strategies proposed by embodied cognition approaches (adjusting the movement curve or adjusting the speed of movement) is used depends, among other things, on contextual factors (for a virtual reality study, see Fink et al., 2009; for a seminal paper on catching fly balls, see McBeath et al., 1995; for a study of strategies used by dogs to catch flying objects, see Shaffer et al., 2004). Either way, an embodied cognition perspective can help explain human behavior in a holistic and efficient way.

"Embodied cognition is the theory that many features of cognition, whether human or otherwise, are shaped by aspects of the entire body of the organism" (see ▶ https://en.wikipedia.org/wiki/Embodied_cognition.). The current debate in multiple disciplines indicates that a more specific definition depends on the theoretical perspective and discipline (Newen et al., 2018). We use the term "embodied" based on the seminal definition of Varela et al. (1992, pp. 172–173): "By using the term embodied we mean to highlight two points: first that cognition depends upon the kinds of experience that come from having a body with various sensorimotor capacities, and second, that these individual sensorimotor capacities are themselves embedded in a more encompassing biological, psychological and cultural context."

In the following section, we give an overview of the (philosophical) origins of the embodied cognition perspective and present various newer embodied cognition approaches with their respective relations to sport psychology (▶ Sect. 6.2). This forms the foundation for a discussion of empirical embodied cognition studies that investigate the interactions between movement and cognition (▶ Sect. 6.3) and between movement and perception (▶ Sect. 6.4). At the end of the chapter (▶ Sect. 6.5) we outline how embodied cognition effects can be specified and quantified. Furthermore, the limits of embodied cognition research are discussed and (cautious) predictions about the future of embodied cognition research in the context of sport psychology are proposed.

6.2 Embodied Cognition Approaches: Theoretical Framework

The idea of a holistic understanding of cognition that encapsulates perception and movement is by no means new. Philosophers, especially representatives of phenomenology, laid the foundation for today's embodied cognition approaches. Phenomenologists (e.g., Merleau-Ponty, 1945) placed the *experience of the environment* in the foreground. The central question was determining the meaning of objects, events, the self, or others and how this meaning is created through a person's experience of and interaction with the environment.

What today's embodied cognition approaches have in common is that they agree in their central assumption: Cognition, perception, and movement processes cannot be considered independently of each other but rather influence and condition each other. Today's embodied cognition approaches differ mainly in terms of the role ascribed to the body.

The central assumption of embodied cognition approaches is that cognition, perception, and movement processes are closely interconnected and influence each other.

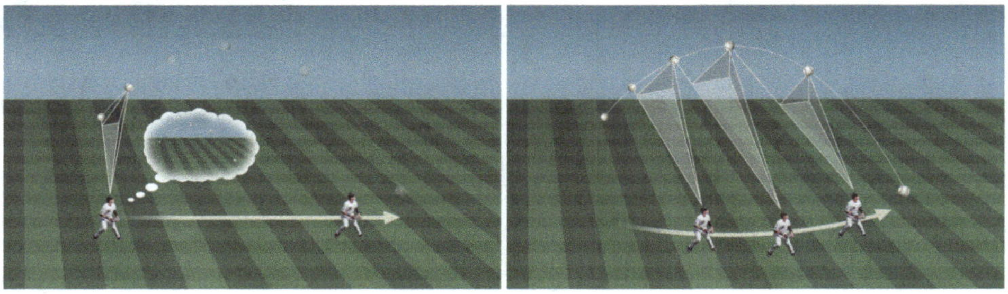

◘ **Fig. 6.1** The outfielder problem: "amodal" solution versus "embodied" solution (adapted from Wang et al., 2015)

Side Story

Maurice Merleau-Ponty

The work of Merleau-Ponty (1908–1961), a French philosopher and one of the most important voices in phenomenology, has had a particular influence on today's embodied cognition approaches. Merleau-Ponty further developed Husserl and Heidegger's basic phenomenological ideas by focusing on the body and its perception ("corporeality") and calling for the abolition of the classic dichotomous division of the body on the one hand and the soul on the other.

> "True reflection presents me to myself not as idle and inaccessible subjectivity, but as identical with my presence in the world and to others, as I am now realizing it: I am all that I see, I am an intersubjective field, not despite my body and historical situation, but, on the contrary, by being this body and this situation, and through them, all the rest." (Merleau-Ponty, 2002, p. 525)

6

Shapiro (2011) distinguished three different perspectives on embodied cognition:
- Conceptualization
- Replacement
- Constitution

In the following we present examples and influential literature for each of the three perspectives.

The conceptualization perspective argues, in general terms, that the way we understand the world depends on the shape of our bodies. Conceptualization predicts that differences between different bodies create different conceptualizations of the world. In other words, different bodies perceive different worlds or lead to different worlds.

An illustrative example is the perception of color. Which colors we perceive and how we perceive them depend on neurophysiological conditions that differ from person to person (Varela et al., 1992; see Arguments for why colors are not in the world but are created by the individual).

Arguments for Why Colors Are Not in the World but Are Created by the Individual (Varela et al., 1992)

1. Color perception is determined by our visual system and does not represent one-to-one the characteristics of the external world.
2. Since our color perception does not correspond to the characteristics of the outer world, but rather colors are created by our individually different visual systems, there are no colors in the world.

What do you think: Is the argument for why colors are not in the world but are created by the individual derived from Varela et al. (1992) logical? (Fig. 6.2)

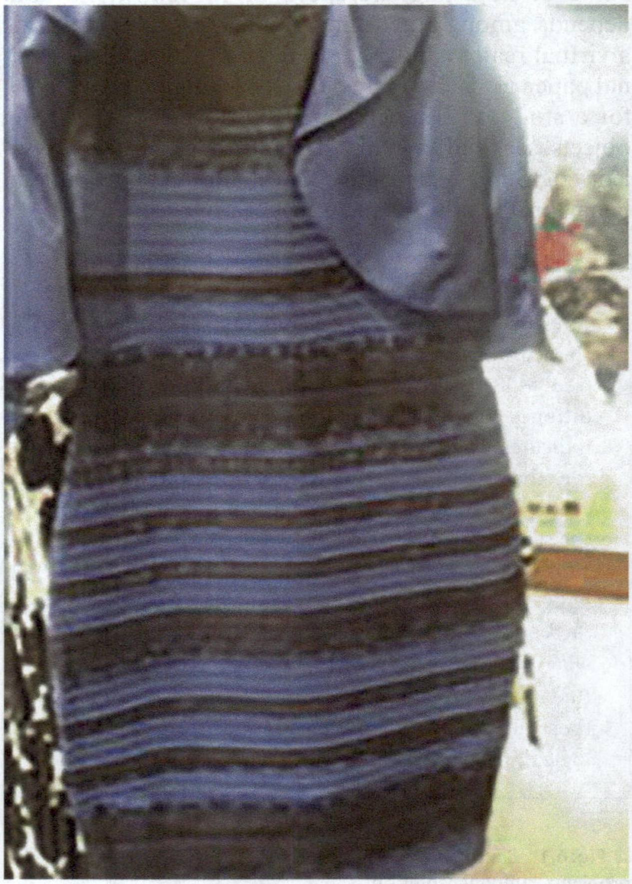

Fig. 6.2 The original photo that caused confusion on social networks. What do you see: a black-and-blue or a white-and-gold striped dress?

The Many Colors of "The Dress"

In 2015, an image of a two-colored dress confused users of social networks worldwide: #TheDress (see ◘ Fig. 6.2). Some saw a black-and-blue striped dress in the photo, others a white-and-gold striped dress. How is it possible that the perception of color differs so drastically between different people?

Karl Gegenfurtner and colleagues examined this phenomenon empirically under controlled light conditions. They found that all participants in their experiment saw similar shades of color that differed only in their brightness. The perceived colors ranged from a very bright light blue to a bright medium blue on one side and from a gold to a dark brown on the other. Both colors of the dress are located in the color circle on the so-called daylight axis: depending on the time of day (or the position of the sun) daylight tends to be bluish (midday) or yellowish (morning and evening). Normally people unconsciously filter out the influence of this bluish or yellowish light and thus correct for the influence of daylight—but for this they need colors as comparison points that lie outside the daylight axis (such as greenish or reddish shades). These are completely missing in #TheDress, and therefore any information about the lighting conditions is missing. The interpretation of the colors depends on the environment in which the dress is situated—it could be a blue dress exposed to warm yellowish light, but it could just as well be a white dress exposed to cool bluish light.

The popular image of the two-colored dress that preoccupied the social networks thus showed in an impressive way that we do not just perceive the pure physical properties through our senses. Rather, we have assumptions about the world that influence our interpretation of sensory stimuli—and these assumptions can be very different across individuals.

A second proposition of the conceptualization perspective is that our ability to form and understand concepts is based on the fact that we move in the world by using our bodies: The concepts of "front" and "back," for example, only make sense to beings who themselves have a front and a back. "If all beings on this planet were uniform stationary spheres floating in some medium and perceiving equally in all directions, they would have no concepts of front and back" (Lakoff & Johnson, 1999, p. 34). Our body with its specific characteristics therefore determines the emergence of concepts (Lakoff & Johnson, 1999). If we take this thought a step further, the question arises whether this also applies to abstract concepts that have no direct relation to our bodies or sensorimotor experiences made through our bodies (such as our concept of time). According to Lakoff and Johnson, the answer is yes, because abstract concepts are grounded in concrete concepts that can be perceived with our sensorimotor system. It is assumed, for example, that the abstract concept of time is based on the concrete concept of space: This is reflected, among other things, in our language: "The evening lies before me" is a sentence with temporal information that is expressed with a spatial expression ("before"). Because in a sport psychological context the connection between movement, time, and space plays an important role, the sport psychological arena is particularly well suited to testing predictions from an embodied cognition perspective. This topic will be further explored in ▶ Sects. 6.3.1 and 6.3.2 of this chapter (see ◘ Fig. 6.3).

A third proposition of the conceptualization perspective (Shapiro, 2011) is an "embodied" response to the "symbol grounding problem" (e.g., Barsalou, 1999; Glenberg, 1997; Glenberg et al., 2005; Glenberg & Kaschak, 2002; Glenberg & Robertson, 2000; Zwaan & Madden, 2005). The symbol grounding problem is about how language acquires meaning for us. A well-known thought experiment is the Chinese room illustrated in ◘ Fig. 6.4. From an embodied cognition perspective, the answer is that language acquires meaning as soon as we move in the world as embodied agents and interact with it. Without interaction we can learn language, but it remains meaningless.

The next perspective explained in Shapiro (2011) is the replacement perspective. The replacement perspective says, in general terms, that the classic understanding of cognition should be replaced with a definition in which the brain has an important function but is downgraded "from a star to a co-star, an equal partner in the creation of cognition alongside body and world" (Shapiro, 2011, p. 137). Proponents of the replacement perspective emphasize the situatedness of cognition. Situatedness of cognition means that the properties of the world (e.g., sunlight) determine what possibilities a person has relative to their body. The properties of the environment thus also determine what information and possibilities the individual has. The term "sunlight" can be used as an example to explain this. The sunlight in the world allows us to see, influences our sleep–wake rhythm, and much more. If the properties of sunlight change, we

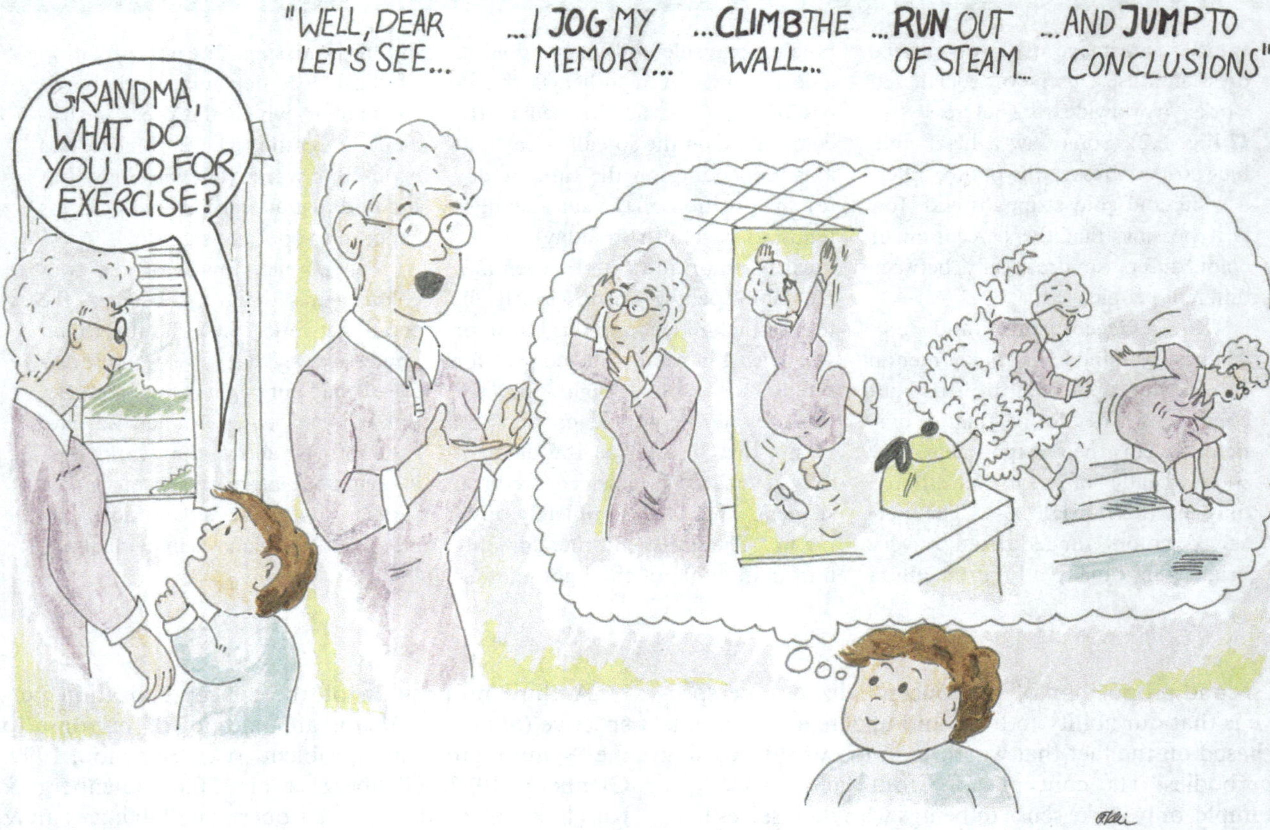
"WELL, DEAR LET'S SEE...
...I JOG MY MEMORY...
...CLIMB THE WALL...
...RUN OUT OF STEAM...
...AND JUMP TO CONCLUSIONS"
GRANDMA, WHAT DO YOU DO FOR EXERCISE?

Fig. 6.3 Movement and metaphors (drawn by Farina Klein, adapted from "The Family Circus")

change too—our bodies, our perceptions, and our cognitive processes.

Brooks (1991) was one of the first to apply the replacement perspective to robotics. The trigger was the robot "Shakey," developed and based on the "sense–model–plan–act" structure: Shakey had a camera in front as a sensor ("sense"). A computer used the input from the camera to construct a symbolic model, which in turn was used by a program ("STRIPS") to give the robot a command to move in a certain direction ("plan") based on the description of the environment, which the robot then executed ("act"). Shakey's task was, among other things, to navigate through a simple space and avoid objects standing around. Shakey was very slow and very bad at this task, because creating a new model was very time-consuming and inefficient. Shakey shows how a robot is built from a classic cognitive theory perspective: The most important steps, the steps that determine the robot's behavior, take place in a computer outside the actual robot body. The "brain" of the robot is thus literally disembodied.

In his attempt to improve the robots existing at the time, Brooks (1991) was inspired by the embodied cognition idea of situatedness. He then constructed the robot "Allen," which was based on a completely different system from Shakey's. Instead of building on the classic sense–model–plan–act structure, he linked perception directly to the robot's action. This new robot was much faster and more efficiently able to perform its task (walking through a room without hitting anything).

The embodied cognition perspective fueled a groundbreaking first step toward increasingly independent moving robots. This can be seen, for example, at the annual Robot Soccer World Cup (RoboCup). There, two robot teams play against each other for the title. The officially formulated goal of the RoboCup is that by 2050 at the latest, the winning team of the RoboCup will win against the best human, professional soccer team at that time (Kitano & Asada, 1998). Even if this ambitious goal is considered unlikely from a sport psychological perspective (see Raab, 2017), the soccer skills of robots are improving at a rapid pace. In fact, the

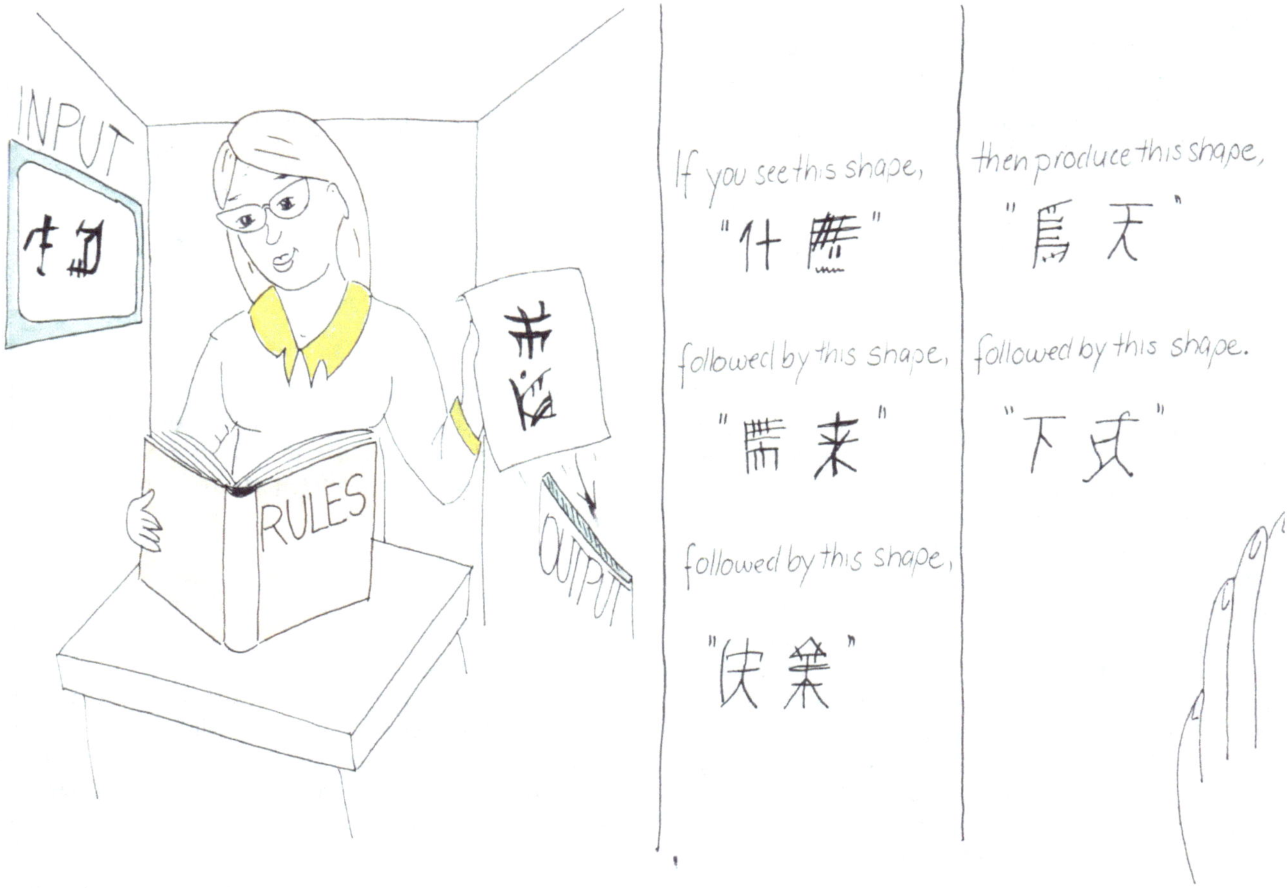

Fig. 6.4 The Chinese Room is a thought experiment demonstrating that human intelligence cannot be simulated by a computer program. It goes like this: Imagine that a person who does not know Chinese is in a room and is slipped a piece of paper through a gap in the wall to the outside with stories and questions about these stories in Chinese. The person in the room has a handbook (in a language that the person understands) with instructions on what to say based on the story and the questions. Using the handbook, the person in the room now answers by returning the responses through the gap to the outside. In doing so, the person gives the correct answers but does not understand the answers they are giving. To someone standing outside the room, however, it seems as if the person inside the room is fluent in Chinese. Transferring this argumentation to the Turing test, the conclusion is that a program that passes the Turing test is not necessarily intelligent; it just appears intelligent. To really develop intelligence, it would have to interact actively with its environment and move within it (drawn by Farina Klein)

RoboCup 2016 was the first time that a robot team won a soccer match against a human soccer team—even if not against a professional one (see ► https://www.youtube.com/watch?v=9CNuTSxVwt4).

The last perspective explained in Shapiro (2011) is the constitution perspective. This perspective claims, in general terms, that cognition basically includes the body (and the environment), rather than cognition being influenced by one's own body and environment. In other words, the body, its movement, and its environment are cognition. Consequently, supporters of the constitution perspective often argue that the term cognition needs to be replaced with a broader definition that includes the body, its movements, and the environment.

Influential proponents of the constitution hypothesis include Clark (2008), O'Regan and Noë (2001), and Wilson (2004). ◘ Figure 6.5 illustrates how cognition is defined according to the classic, amodal perspective versus how it is defined by embodied cognition and the constitution perspective.

A theory particularly relevant to sport psychology is the sensorimotor theory of perceptual experience (O'Regan & Noë, 2001). This theory is based on the view that we perceive the world as we do because we learn sensorimotor contingencies between our movements and the resulting perceived changes in the environment. According to the theory, a ball looks like a ball because it looks like this as soon as we move our eyes.

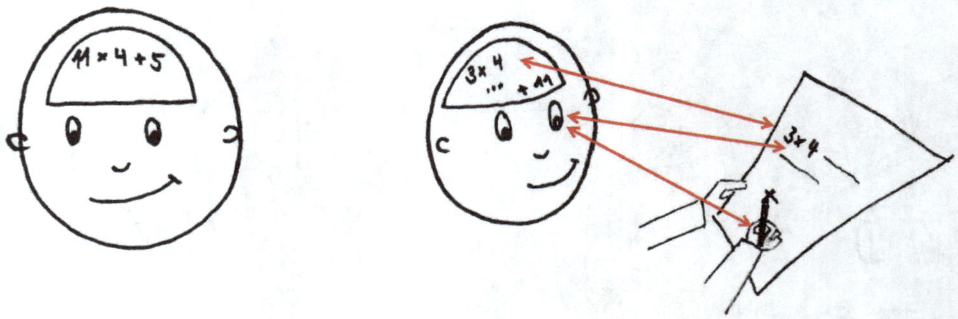

Fig. 6.5 Representation of cognition from two different perspectives. In the left view, all the systems that solve the arithmetic problem are located within the brain, whereas in the right view, the eyes and the environment (i.e., the sheet of paper on which the arithmetic steps are written) contribute to the solution of the problem (Figure: Hannah Haunhorst)

All three embodied cognition approaches presented here (Shapiro, 2011) make it clear that the body, its movements, and its environment should be included in the study of mental processes in order to get to valid conclusions. This applies bidirectionally: When investigating the body and its movements, mental processes and environmental conditions should be considered. The growing importance of embodied cognition is demonstrated by the growing number of discussions about the specification of embodied cognition mechanisms (e.g., Gentsch et al., 2016; Körner et al., 2015; Löffler et al., 2016) and its inclusion in standard textbooks of general psychology (e.g., Müsseler & Rieger, 2016). In the following, we focus on the bidirectional influence of movement and cognition (▶ Sect. 6.3) and the bidirectional influence of movement and perception (▶ Sect. 6.4).

6.3 Movement and Cognition

6.3.1 Influence of Movement on Cognition

General influences of movement on cognition have been known for a long time. Consider, for instance, the well-known phrase, "Mens sana in corpore sano" (a healthy mind in a healthy body). Recent meta-analyses (e.g., Johnson et al., 2016; Kennedy et al., 2017) have shown that this saying of the Roman poet Juvenal, meant to be ironic almost 2,000 years ago, contains at least a bit of truth. Developmental psychology studies have shown that especially children (Bornstein et al., 2013) and older people (Scherder et al., 2014) benefit from regular exercise. These general, long-term influences of movement on cognition do not directly speak to embodied cognition research.

> Embodied cognition research is mainly concerned with very specific, rather short-term effects of exercise on cognition.

Therefore, in the following we report studies that investigated whether certain movements influence cognitive processes and, if so, how. This is particularly important in the context of sport psychology: Does an upright (as in horse show jumping) or bent (as in hockey) posture change my memory processes? Is there any benefit in taking a so-called power pose before a competition to begin the competition with confidence?

Reflection

What do you think of when you see someone walking upright? Probably such concepts as good mood, pride, joy, and self-confidence come to mind. On the other hand, what do you think of when you see someone walking bent over? Probably concepts such as bad mood, humility, sadness, and low self-esteem are more likely. So it seems that certain concepts are automatically associated with certain gait patterns.

Study Box

In a study by Michalak et al. (2015), it was experimentally examined whether positive (or negative) concepts are activated by an upright (or bent) gait. The starting point was the fact that several studies have shown a close connection between a flexed gait and depression (Bader et al., 1999; Lemke et al., 2000; Paleacu et al., 2007; Sloman et al., 1982; Sloman et al., 1987). In a preliminary study, the researchers compared the movements of a group of depression patients in a depressive phase with a group of healthy people. They found that the depressed people walked more slowly, swung their arms less, moved their upper extremities vertically to a lesser extent, swayed more to the left and right with their bodies, and took a more bent and forward-leaning position than healthy people (Michalak et al., 2009; for a demonstration of happy and depressed walking styles, see ▸ https://www.biomotionlab.ca/html5-bml-walker/). Michalak et al. (2015) then manipulated people's gait by letting them walk on a treadmill and giving them online feedback on their gait patterns. A display mounted in front of the participants was programmed so that the bar on the display deflected to the right for one half of the participants when they walked upright and to the right for the other half when they walked bent. The participants were instructed to walk in such a way that the bar in front of them moved to the right. The authors hypothesized that a bent and depressed gait would activate more negatively associated words and an upright and happy gait would activate more positively associated words. This was measured with a memory task: The participants were given 20 words (10 positive, 10 negative) to read before the movement manipulation. After the movement manipulation they were asked to name as many words as possible. Indeed, the participants who walked bent during the movement manipulation remembered more negative words ($M = 6$, $SD = 2.36$) than positive words ($M = 3.8$, $SD = 1.67$) compared to the participants who walked upright (negative words: $M = 5.47$, $SD = 2.23$; positive words: $M = 5.63$, $SD = 2.89$).

Activation of a concept by performing movements associated with this concept is not limited to positive and negative words. Mussweiler (2006) showed that a sluggish gait activates the concept "overweight" and a very slow gait activates the concept "elderly" (but see a current debate on the difficulty of replication of priming studies; Doyen et al., 2012).

What are the mechanisms by which the activation of certain concepts is realized during execution of movement patterns? One possible process is neurophysiological reenactment (Barsalou, 1999). This means that information (e.g., the concept "depression") consists of neuronal activation patterns that include, among other things, certain movements or perceptions. This information is stored by neurons in adjacent associative fields (Damasio & Damasio, 1994). If a certain movement is now carried out, this results in a partial reactivation of the entire concept (e.g., the concept "depression").

> An upright (or bent) gait can activate concepts (e.g., positive, negative, overweight, elderly, depression). The assumed mechanism is neurophysiological reenactment (concepts consists of neuronal activation patterns that also include certain movement. The movement can trigger the whole concept).

Under what circumstances does the mechanism described have an influence on our behavior? Do we perform better if we adopt a so-called power pose before a competition in order to activate the concept of "self-confidence" and accordingly enter the competition with confidence? For some time now, the media (including *The New York Times*; Hochman, 2014) have been propagating the idea that power poses have an influence on various behavioral and hormonal parameters. A high-power pose is a pose that takes up a lot of space, is directed upward, and radiates overall strength and self-confidence. In contrast, a low-power pose is a pose that takes up little space, is directed downward, and overall tends to radiate weakness and low self-confidence (see ▫ Fig. 6.6).

The evidence regarding the effect of power posing is mixed: On the one hand, studies have reported that a high-power pose produces an increased self-reported feeling of strength compared to a low-power pose (Carney et al., 2010), leads to a lower cortisol level and an increased testosterone level (Carney et al., 2010), improves self-esteem and motivation (Fischer et al., 2011; Riskind & Gotay, 1982; Schubert & Koole, 2009), leads to a better performance in a job interview (Cuddy et al., 2015), and increases risk behavior (Huang et al., 2011; Yap et al., 2013) and cognitive bias (e.g., the tendency to remember negative rather than positive words) in depressed people (Michalak et al., 2014). On the other hand, studies have reported that high-power poses do not increase risk behavior compared to low-power poses (Garrison et al., 2016), do not lead to higher testosterone levels (Ronay et al., 2016), and do not produce an increased self-reported feeling of strength (Garrison et al., 2016; Ronay et al., 2016). Differences in the study results show that the activation of a particular concept by a particular movement does not happen at any time and under any circumstances but rather is probably modulated by many factors, such as social (Ranehill et al., 2015) or developmental (Löffler et al., 2016) factors. Accordingly, a challenge for embodied cognition research is to identify these modulating factors and to test them in ecologically valid settings, such as sport settings.

Fig. 6.6 High-power versus low-power pose. High-power poses radiate strength and self-confidence, while low-power poses radiate weakness and low self-confidence

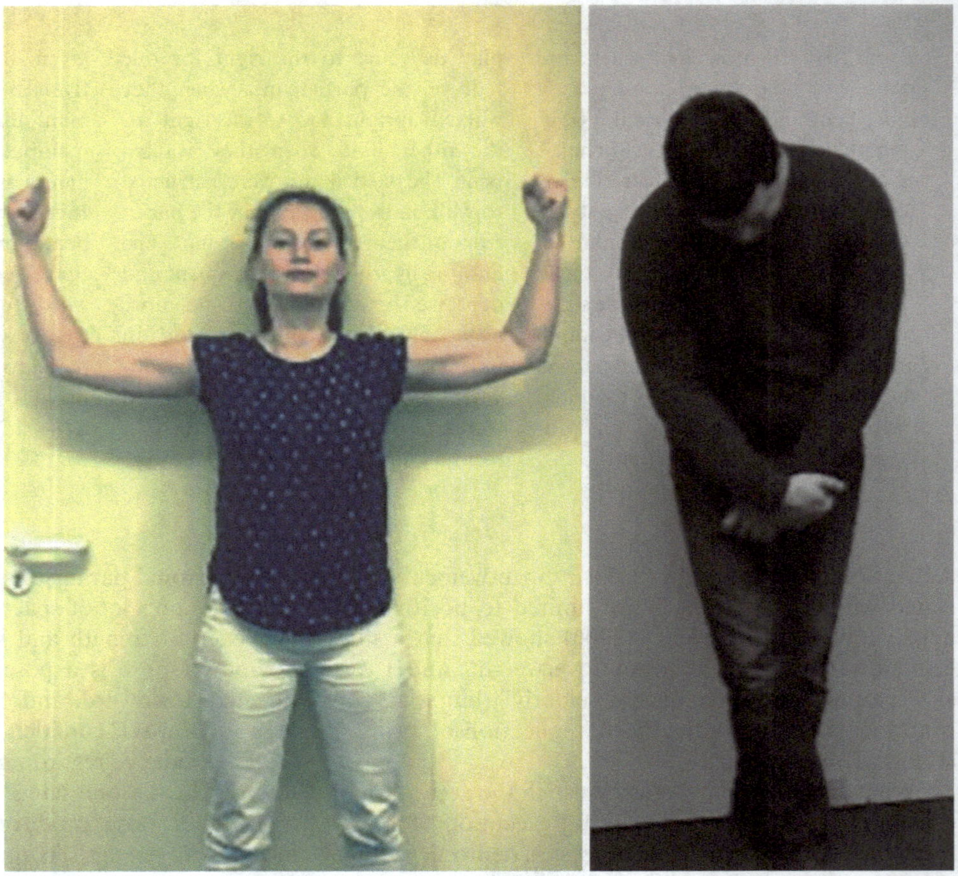

6

> » "I'm an interpreter of space. Every good, successful player, especially an attacking player, has a well-developed sense of space and time. It's not a phenomenon you only find in two or three people on earth. Every great striker knows it's all about the timing between the person who plays the pass and the person making a run into the right zone" (Thomas Müller, former German National Team player and Bayern Munich player, quoted in Hesse, 2016).

This quote by Thomas Müller impressively shows the importance of temporal and spatial concepts in sport. As explained in the section on the theoretical framework of embodied cognition approaches (para. 6.2), one of the assumptions of the embodied cognition perspective is that our ability to form and understand concepts is based on the fact that (and how) we move with our body in the world. Thus, concepts are created by combining bits of information from perception, movement, and mental states and connecting them in a meaningful way. Take the spatial concept "in front," for example: We can *perceive*, say, where a dog has its front. We can *move* forward. And we can *imagine* a ball being shot forward. All this information is combined to form the overall concept "in front." If we now take the temporal concept "future," things become more complicated: We cannot *perceive* the future. We cannot *move* into the future (except with a time machine, of course). But we can still *imagine* the future. So, time has no direct relation to the body, but we still have a concept of time. Are abstract concepts (such as time), which are not directly perceptible through sensorimotor experience, a contradiction to the embodied cognition assumption that concepts are multimodal, created by the sensorimotor experiences of our body? Not necessarily: Lakoff and Johnson (1980) explained that abstract concepts build on more concrete concepts. For time and space, this means that abstract, temporal concepts are built on concrete, spatial concepts. As briefly explained in this chapter's Introduction, this is reflected in the fact that temporal relationships are often represented by spatial expressions. "My 20th birthday is approaching" or "We are moving toward summer" are examples. In both sentences a spatial expression ("something is approaching," "moving toward something") is used to represent a temporal relationship. Looking at the content of these two sentences, it is noticeable that time

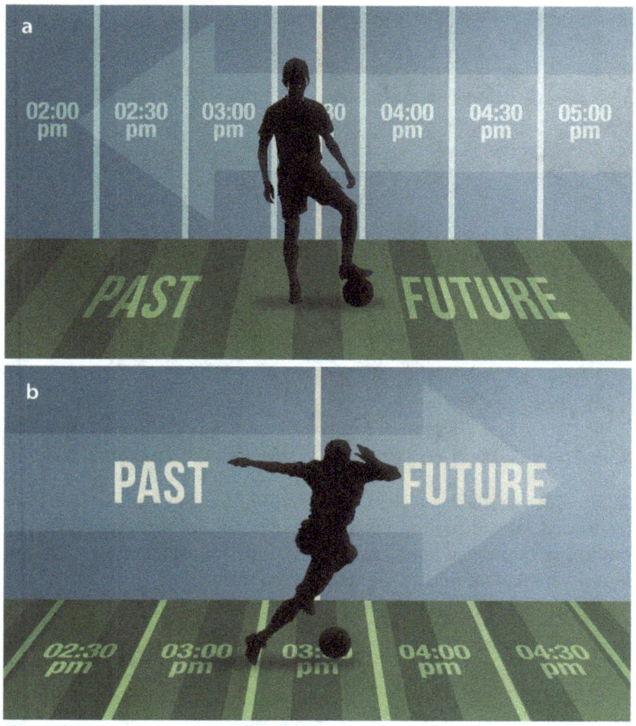

Fig. 6.7 **a, b** How would you spontaneously answer the following question: "The soccer training is usually every day at 3:30 pm. Tomorrow's training has been moved forward 1 h. What time is the training now that it has been rescheduled?" If your answer is "2:30 pm," you are among the 50% of people who answer in a time-moving frame of reference. If your answer is "4:30 pm," you are among the 50% of people who answer in an ego-moving frame of reference (Figure: Max Roebel)

is represented by two different frames of reference (see Boroditsky, 2000). In the first sentence, the person is stationary, and time approaches (time-moving reference frame), while in the second sentence people are actively moving through time (ego-moving reference frame). Through ambiguous, temporal questions, it is now possible to find out what kind of time-moving reference frame someone has (see Fig. 6.7).

> Concepts are created by information from perception, movement, and mental states which are put together to meaningful entities.

Similarly, one can find out what spatial frame of reference someone has by asking ambiguous, spatial questions (see Fig. 6.8). When Boroditsky (2000) asked participants such questions, the answer distribution in English-speaking samples was usually 50/50.

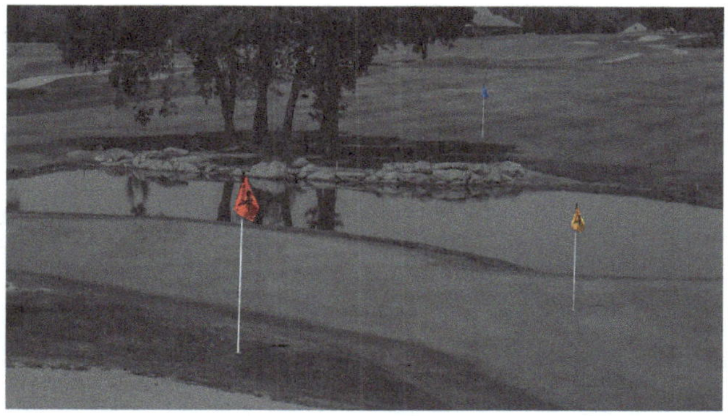

Fig. 6.8 How would you spontaneously answer the following question: "The golf instructor asks Max to putt into the front hole. What color is the hole that Max is supposed to putt into?" If your answer is "red," you are among the 50% of people who answer in a time-moving frame of reference. If your answer is "blue," you are among the 50% of people who answer in an ego-moving frame of reference (picture: Max Roebel)

Whether and under what conditions one or the other frame of reference is preferred depends, among other things, on cultural norms and language (Boroditsky, 2001). Several studies have shown that the spatial frame of reference influences the temporal frame but that the temporal frame of reference does not influence the spatial frame to the same extent (e.g., Casasanto & Boroditsky, 2008; Casasanto et al., 2010). This observation supports Lakoff and Johnson's (1980) assumption that more abstract temporal concepts are based on more concrete spatial concepts and suggests a fundamental space–time asymmetry. Is this asymmetry really a fundamental phenomenon, or does it arise from pieces of information of varying degrees of precision that are represented? One way to find out is to represent the temporal dimension more clearly and distinctly than the spatial dimension. For example, Cai and Connell (2015) asked participants to touch physical sticks while listening to an auditory note and then reproduce either the length of the stick or the duration of the note. In three experiments either participants could only feel the physical stick or they could feel as well as see the stick. Results indicate that when spatial information relies on touch, the effect of time on space is substantially stronger than the effect of space on time. This effect was not found when participants could also see the stick. This indicates that the space–time asymmetry is not a fundamental phenomenon but rather depends on the mode of representation and the associated information content (Löffler et al., 2018).

Reflection

The following two tasks are about estimating space (i.e., size of an object) and time (i.e., length of a sound).

1. Find a playing partner.
2. Close your eyes and ask your partner to put an object into your hands. Then, without looking at the object, estimate its size by holding your fingers apart in the estimated size of the object. Ask your partner to measure the distance between your fingers.
3. Now open your eyes.
4. Repeat Step 2 with another object, but keep your eyes open at all times.
5. Close your eyes and ask your partner to play a sound for a certain time. Then estimate how long the tone was by producing a tone of the same length yourself.
6. Now compare your performance in the spatial and temporal task. How far did both estimates deviate from the actual size of the object or the length of the sound? Did the method of representation have an influence on your performance?

The connection between movement and the associated access to temporal and spatial information is particularly important in the context of sports, when temporal information is transformed into spatial information, as in dance, for example. Music carries mainly temporal information (e.g., rhythm), which is translated into spatial information by the dancer (Ribbat, 2011). A new technological development also makes the other direction possible: Body movements are translated into music in real time (software "Nagual Dance"). Thus, no temporal (acoustic) information is transformed into spatial information, but spatial information is transformed into temporal (acoustic) information (see ◘ Fig. 6.9). This opens new movement horizons and changes the existing transformation flow.

In summary, the interactions between movement, time, and space play an important role in the sport psychology context—be it in instructions ("Please stand in front of the bars"), in the physiological and psychological effects of upright or bent postures, or in dance, where temporal information is translated into spatial information (or vice versa) through movement.

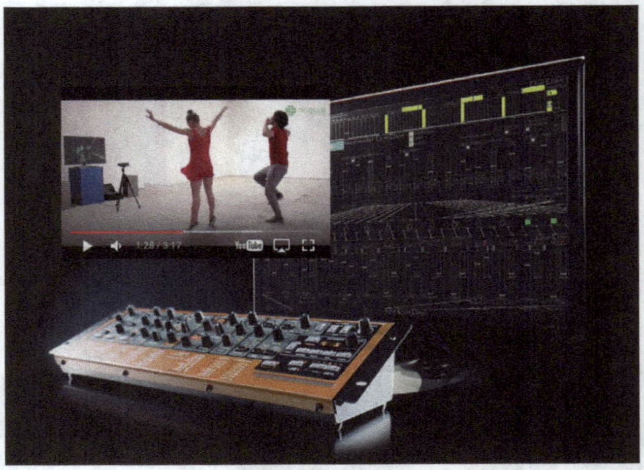

◘ **Fig. 6.9** With the software Nagual Dance, body movements are translated into music in real time, that is, spatial (movement) information is converted into temporal (acoustic) information (Figure: ▸ www.nagualsounds.de, rights of use obtained)

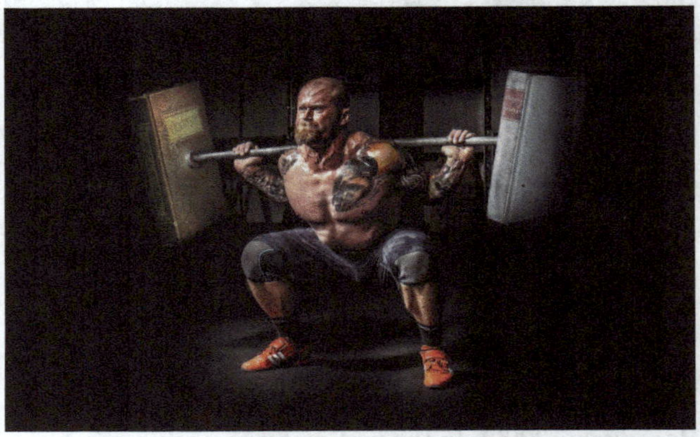

◘ **Fig. 6.10** Illustration of the metaphor learned in Slepian and Ambady (2014), "the past weighs heavily," and the transfer to the assessment of the weight of old books (Figure: Max Roebel)

6.3.2 Influence of Cognition on Movement

In this section, we report on studies that examine whether and how cognitive processes influence movement from an embodied cognition perspective. This is especially important in the context of sport psychology: To what extent do cognitive processes influence our movement patterns? Can we learn movements through mental simulation? When lifting weights, is a weight considered lighter depending on the metaphorical expressions used to describe it?

A methodological difficulty in experimentally answering the second question is that certain multimodal associations are already linked to a metaphor, so previous experience with the metaphor cannot be controlled. Slepian and Ambady (2014) circumvented this problem by having participants learn a new metaphor (see ◘ Fig. 6.10). One half of the participants read a text in which the past was described as very difficult and the present as easy. The other half of the participants read a text in which the past was described as easy and the present as difficult. Afterward they were asked to estimate the weight of an old or new book while either (a) holding the book in their hands or (b) looking at the book (visual presentation). The results showed the presumed interaction between metaphor, book, and representation: Participants who had learned the metaphor that "the past weighs heavily" assessed the old book as heavier than the new book when they interacted with it. If they were asked to evaluate the book only by visual representation, this effect disappeared.

The influence of metaphorical expressions on the estimation of weight has been shown for things other than books (for a failed replication on related research, see Pecher et al., 2015). For example, hard disks with very important information (e.g., of personal importance) were considered heavier than hard disks with unimportant information (Schneider et al., 2014). In practical sport psychology, this means that weightlifters, for example, could use various metaphorical expressions to perceive the lifted weight as lighter or heavier. Further questions include whether the perceived weight also changes performance and what metaphorical expressions have the greatest effect on the perceived weight. The function of metaphorical instructions has been applied and analyzed in martial arts, for example, in judo when learning harai goshi. Harai goshi ("floating hip throw") is a well-known and often used method in judo to overcome an opponent (see ◘ Fig. 6.11). In harai goshi the judoka and their opponent embody a scale: The judoka uses their torso as a lever, which makes the opponent float in a horizontal position. At the point where both together form a kind of scale, the judoka rotates and throws the opponent to the ground. An effective strategy for making this method accessible to a learning judoka is to give metaphorical change information, such as "add weight to throw the scale off balance" (Abrahamson, 2016; Sánchez García & González Álvarez, 2014).

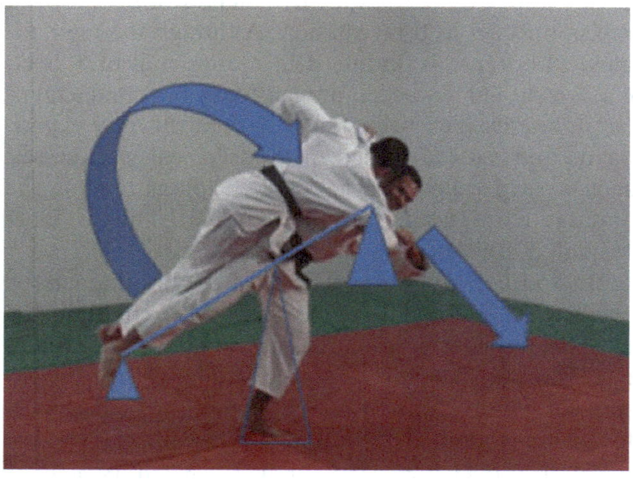

◘ **Fig. 6.11** Metaphorical instruction in judo for harai goshi (Picture: Sánchez García & González Álvarez, 2014, rights of use obtained)

Can thinking about the future or the past unconsciously influence our movements? Does it affect our movements that we associate the future with the space in front of us and the past with the space behind us? In the following, we present preliminary answers to these and other questions and explore this association in the context of sport psychology.

As already discussed in the section on the influence of movement on cognition using the example of movement, space, and time (► Sect. 6.3.1), a unique characteristic of humans is that we can imagine the future in our thoughts. This ability enables us to adapt our behavior in daily life to meet daily challenges (Schacter et al., 2007; Tulving, 2002), such as preparing for future competition through mental simulation (e.g., Guillot & Collet, 2008). According to embodied cognition approaches, notions of abstract things (such as temporal concepts) are based on concrete experiences (such as spatial concepts). That imagining the future has an influence on our movements, as predicted by embodied cognition approaches, has been investigated by Miles et al. (2010), among others. Miles et al. examined whether imagining the future (unconsciously) triggers forward movements and vice versa, whether imagining the past triggers backward movements. For this purpose, participants were asked to stand up in a natural way. Two different instructions followed: They were told to bring to mind what their daily life looked like 4 years ago and to imagine a typical day then or to think about what their daily life will look like in 4 years and to imagine a typical day in the future. While they were imagining the future or the past, a motion sensor above the knee recorded whether the participants leaned forward or backward. The results showed that the participants tended to lean forward when thinking about the future and backward when thinking about the past.

Stins et al. (2016) took up these initial results and expanded the design in various ways. For example, they compared different time intervals (4 days vs. 4 years in the future or past) and measured weight shifts forward or backward with a force plate. The force plate offers more valid measurements in terms of predicted weight shifts compared to the above-knee motion sensor, as it can be influenced only by weight shifts and not by movements in the vertical axis, which could be misinterpreted as forward or backward leaning, as the motion sensor does. Stins and colleagues could not (conceptually) replicate the original experiment. The participants showed no weight shifts while imagining the future or the past. These two exemplary studies show how important it is to specify the predictions made by embodied cognition approaches. Why was a small change in the design (force plate instead of motion sensor above the knee) decisive for the results? Could it also be that instead of leaning forward "toward the future," the participants in the experiment were moving in the vertical axis, that is, "kneeling in front of the future?" Systematic and potentially interdisciplinary research programs are needed to specify concrete effects and the underlying mechanisms (see ► Sect. 6.5 below in this chapter).

6.4 Movement and Perception

In addition to the embodied cognition approaches described in the Introduction, a field of research has developed in parallel that investigates the extent to which embodiment effects are already anchored at the level of perception.

In sum, both the established theories (e.g., Proffitt, 2006) and the empirical findings (for an overview, see Witt, 2011) are currently being put to the test, on the one hand theoretically (e.g., Cañal-Bruland & van der Kamp, 2012, 2015) and on the other hand empirically (Firestone & Scholl, 2015). The test includes fundamental methodological criticism. The scientific discourse is in full swing, and in our opinion, research in sport psychology can and should make a significant contribution here. In addition, sport psychology can benefit from the knowledge gained from this discourse, both for the development of sport psychology theory and for the generation of evidence-based recommendations for practice (see Cañal-Bruland & van der Kamp, 2012).

What is embodied perception? Let's begin with an example from the world of sports: Mickey Mantle, an American baseball legend, once said after a home run that the ball seemed as big as a grapefruit (see Witt & Proffitt, 2005), thus establishing a correlation between hitting performance and the perceived size of the baseball. Exactly this relationship is referred to as "action-specific effects on perception" (Witt, 2011; Witt & Proffitt, 2008).

In the following, we first explain the theoretical assumptions of the embodied perception approach (► Sect. 6.4.1). We then present empirical studies with a direct relation to sports (► Sect. 6.4.2). We end with a critical examination of theoretical assumptions and empirical methods, from which implications for future research can be derived (► Sect. 6.4.3).

6.4.1 Theoretical Background

In his embodied perception approach, Dennis Proffitt (2006, 2008) argued that the possibilities for action—so-called affordances (Gibson, 1979)—that arise when we move through our environment, whether we are climbing a mountain or shopping, are inextricably linked to visual perceptual processes. "Perceiving spatial layout combines the geometry of the world with behavioral goals and the costs associated with achieving these goals" (Proffitt, 2006, p. 110).

> Proffitt postulated that visual perception changes depending on the anticipated energetic costs (e.g., how strenuous the climb to the top of the mountain is estimated to be) and the ability to act.

Proffitt thus was describing visual perception as a constitutive element of the economy of action, placing himself on the shoulders of ecological psychology and its founder, James J. Gibson (1979). Seminal work by Proffitt and colleagues (Bhalla & Proffitt, 1999; Proffitt et al., 1995; Proffitt et al., 2003) provided the first evidence on which the embodied perception theory is based. For example, the studies cited suggested that physical exhaustion has an influence on perceived possibilities for action. Mountains were estimated to be steeper (Bhalla & Proffitt, 1999; Proffitt et al., 1995) and distances larger (Proffitt et al., 2003) when participants carried a backpack or were exhausted. Proffitt offered the following theoretical explanation for this effect: Since mountaineering with a heavy backpack generates more energetic costs (i.e., is more physically demanding), perception changes, so that the person wearing the backpack—implicitly or explicitly—makes an economic decision to act in this situation. Although the methodological critique is discussed in more detail in ► Sect. 6.4.3, it should not be left unmentioned here that a number of studies have been unable to confirm these experiments and have identified methodological weaknesses, such as experimenter bias, as an explanation for the findings (e.g., Durgin, Hajnal, et al., 2010; Durgin, Li, & Hajnal, 2010; Woods et al., 2009).

In addition to the sports-related studies that can be categorized as embodied perception research, discussed in the following section, there are numerous studies related to sports that have also investigated the relationship between perception and action but are theoretically located in embodied cognition research (for an overview see Shiffrar & Heinen, 2010; for a critical comparison of theories see Cañal-Bruland & van der Kamp, 2012). These studies include a study published in *Nature*

Neuroscience: Aglioti et al. (2008) were able to show in the abovementioned study that basketball players' motor expertise makes them better able to predict the success of a basket throw (hit or no hit) than coaches and journalists with less motor experience who had comparable visual experience. These and similar studies suggest, for example, that the outcome of observed movements that one has performed oneself can be better predicted than the outcome of the same observed movements performed by strangers (Knoblich & Flach, 2001). These findings can be theoretically assigned to one of the three theoretical embodied cognition approaches: common coding, internal model, or simulation theories (Gentsch et al., 2016). A full treatment of all approaches is beyond the scope of this chapter, so we focus here—as outlined above—on the embodied perception approach.

6.4.2 Empirical Findings in Reference to Sports

Perhaps the first work to present so-called performance-specific action effects was a study by Wesp et al. (2004), which investigated whether the hit performance in darts had an influence on the size perception of the target to be hit. Indeed, the results of the study showed that the number of throws required to hit the dart target correlated negatively with the size perception of the target. In other words, the fewer the number of throws (in other words, the better the performance), the larger the target was estimated to be. Wesp et al. (2004) argued that dart-throwing performance affects the memory for size perception.

More attention was given to a paper published a year later in *Psychological Science* by Witt and Proffitt (2005), who found performance-specific perception effects in softball (a sport similar to baseball). The experiment was amazingly simple in nature. Following a softball game, the authors asked batters to identify on a poster with circles of different sizes the circle that corresponded in size to the softball they had hit during the game. The results showed a correlation between hitting performance and the size estimation of the ball; the more successful the player, the larger the ball was estimated to be.

Witt et al. (2008) replicated this correlation in golf a little later (for contradictory findings, however, see Memmert et al., 2009).

Study Box

Further, in golf, Cañal-Bruland et al. (2011) investigated whether the alignment of visual attention to the action goal is an essential prerequisite for the effects shown (see also Cañal-Bruland & van der Kamp, 2009). In three experiments, participants played golf balls into a target circle. In the first experiment, the participants had full visibility of the target circle. In the second experiment, the participants played the ball underneath a curtain. The view of the target circle was thus blocked during the execution of the movement. For each individual experiment, the participant received feedback regarding the result of the stroke. In the third experiment, the participant had the task of first successfully passing the ball through a small goal. Hits in the target field were only scored if the ball was successfully played through the goal. The purpose of this instruction was to distribute the visual attention between the target circle and another action-relevant target. Performance-specific perception effects were found only in the first experiment. However, when the alignment of visual attention to the action goal was disrupted (Exp. 2) or visual attention was distributed (Exp. 3), the correlation between scoring performance and size perception of the action goal was absent (Cañal-Bruland et al., 2011).

In line with the assumption that visual attention processes play a significant role in the development of performance-specific perception effects, Cañal-Bruland and van der Kamp (2009) formulated the perceptual accentuation hypothesis. The hypothesis is based on the functional perception theory of Bruner (1957), a Harvard professor and one of the founders of the cognitive revolution (Bruner & Postman, 1949).

Bruner and colleagues had shown in early work that the desire for an object (e.g., a coin, see Bruner & Goodman, 1947) leads to a greater appreciation of this relevant object or to a perceptual accentuation of it. A study by Veltkamp et al. (2008) points into a similar direction. Participants rated a glass of water as larger if they were thirsty and were encouraged to drink by unconscious priming. This effect did not occur when no priming was performed to activate action. From these findings Veltkamp et al. (2008) concluded that the intention to act activates a readiness to act and by this affects basic perceptual processes. On the basis of these findings and Bruner's functional perception theory, Cañal-Bruland and van der Kamp (2009) argued that it seems likely that the perceptual accentuation of action goal objects, as reported in the case of performance-specific perception effects, serves the purpose of attentional emphasis on the action goal object. In other words, the target object appears larger because it is accentuated by other objects in the environment to serve the intended target action (functional perspective).

From the perceptual accentuation hypothesis, it follows that primary action goals should evoke performance-specific perception effects, whereas secondary or subordinate action goals should not (or not to the same extent) evoke these effects. To test this, Cañal-Bruland and van der Kamp (2009) used an original paradigm, the so-called chocolate marshmallow throwing machine (see ◘ Fig. 6.12) to study children who performed either a pure throwing task ("hit the target circle") or a throwing and catching task ("hit the target circle and, in case of a hit, catch the ball flying toward you," see ◘ Fig. 6.12). For the concrete task, the following predictions were made: Children who hit the target more often in the pure aiming task should estimate the target to be larger. On the other hand, in the throw-and-catch task, the effect should no longer occur for the target circle to be hit, but there should be a change in the assessment of the size of the ball depending on the number of balls caught. The results of the study confirmed the authors' predictions in two separate experiments and thus provided the first empirical evidence supporting the perceptual accentuation hypothesis as an explanatory approach for performance-specific perception effects.

How exactly the accentuation processes work has not yet been clarified. However, initial assumptions can be derived from sport psychology studies in particular. For example, it is assumed that gaze behavior could have a specific influence on performance-specific perception (Cañal-Bruland & van der Kamp, 2012; Cañal-Bruland et al., 2011). Numerous expert studies in sport science show that those who are trained and those who are less trained show clear differences in their gaze behavior (Mann et al., 2007). From quiet-eye research, for example, it is known that specific gaze behavior—or rather, fixation behavior (e.g., longer goal-oriented fixation before the start of a movement)—is associated with better performance (e.g., in golf, Vickers, 1992; for contradictory evidence, however, see Heinrich et al., 2020). Whether specific fixation behavior is also a significant predictor of the development of performance-specific perceptual effects must be investigated experimentally in the future.

In addition to the perceptual accentuation hypothesis and the associated assumption that attention processes play a significant role in performance-specific perceptual effects, a number of other alternative explanations have been proposed that cast doubt on a direct link between perception and action as postulated by Proffitt (2006) and Witt (2011). What these studies have in common is that although they report similar distortions of perception, these are completely independent of one's own performance. These studies show that, for example, the reputation of an observed person (Masters et al., 2010) can produce similar perceptual effects. Masters et al. showed participants videos from the pen-

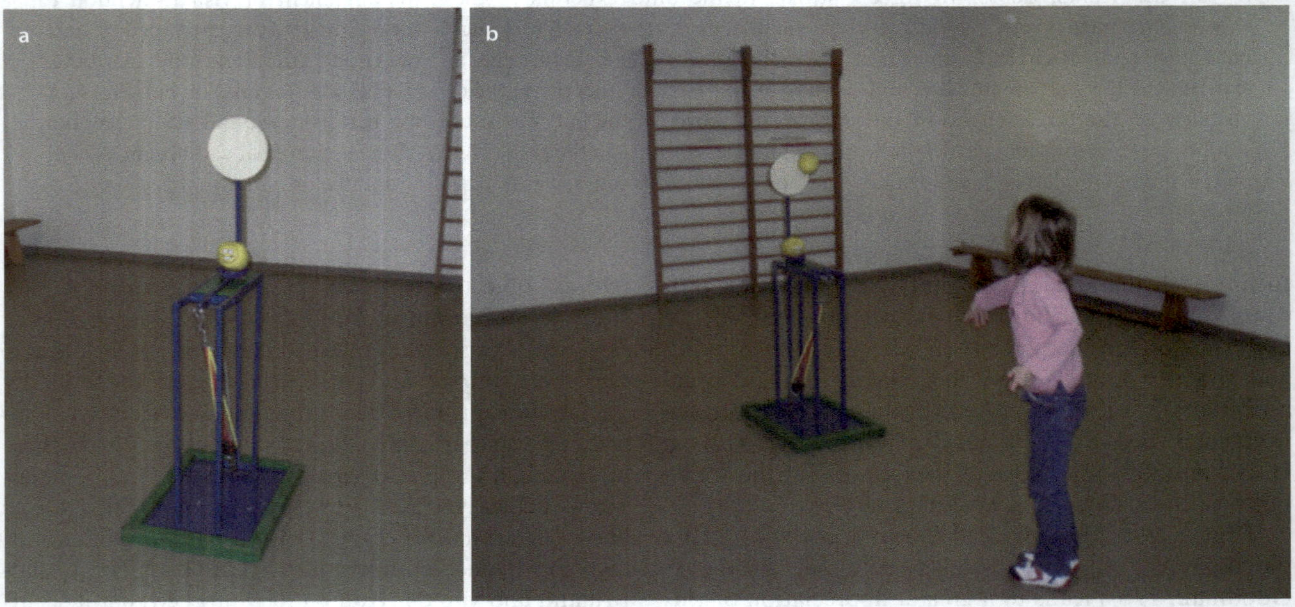

◘ **Fig. 6.12** Chocolate marshmallow throwing machine **a** and the throwing-at-target and target-and-catching task **b** (Picture: Springer)

alty shootout of the 2005 Champions League final (Liverpool FC vs. AC Milan). One group saw videos in which the then Liverpool goalkeeper (Jerzy Dudek) saved the penalties. Another group was presented with videos in which the penalty kicks were successful. Before and after watching the videos, the participants were asked to estimate the size of the goalkeeper. If participants had previously observed how the goalkeeper saved the balls, they estimated him to be taller. If participants had observed how the goalkeeper could not save the balls, they rated him smaller. This study shows that although the participants were not involved in the situation as actors but were observers, perception distortions still occurred. It follows that perception effects are not necessarily dependent on one's own performance and therefore do not necessarily have to be performance specific. If this is true, however, such alternative explanations would have to be empirically excluded for performance-specific perception effects (see Cañal-Bruland & van der Kamp, 2012); otherwise these effects could not be considered evidence supporting the embodied perception theory (Proffitt, 2006).

This and other studies, for example, by Wesp et al. (2004), seem to support Bruner's (1957) original ideas. Bruner showed that in contrast to richer children, poorer children more clearly overestimated the sizes of coins (Bruner & Goodman, 1947): For the poorer children, the coins had a higher value, so they perceived them as larger. At the time, Bruner's studies were criticized on the basis of contradictory findings and for methodological weaknesses (e.g., Klein et al., 1951). The performance-specific perception effects have been criticized as well, and this criticism should be carefully considered, given that the findings form the basis of Proffitt's (2006) embodied perception theory.

> There has been intense debate in several outstanding behavioral and neuroscientific (e.g., *Behavioral and Brain Sciences*) as well as psychology (e.g., *Perspectives on Psychological Science*) journals about the research field not only theoretically (Cañal-Bruland & van der Kamp, 2015; Firestone, 2013) but also methodologically (Firestone & Scholl, 2015), contributing to the development of theory and the validation of empirical practice and evidence.

6.4.3 Critique and Outlook

In their target article "Cognition Does Not Affect Perception: Evaluating the Evidence for 'Top-Down' Effects," published in 2016 in the journal *Behavioral and Brain Sciences*, the authors Firestone and Scholl went so far as to claim that there is not a single study that proves that cognition (including attention, action intentions, etc.) influences perception. This includes all work on embodied perception theory. Although many of the open peer reviewers (e.g., Cañal-Bruland, van der Kamp, & Gray, 2016) have expressed substantial criticism of Firestone and Scholl's basic theoretical assumptions, not only is methodological criticism welcome, but it can be regarded as a guideline for empirical work on this topic in the future. The fundamental methodological critique is based on six so-called pitfalls, and the authors argue and discuss that there is not a single article that does not fall into at least one of them. However, if—according to the authors—even just one of the pitfalls can be identified, it necessarily follows that one should not conclude that there is evidence of the influence of cognition and action on perceptual processes.

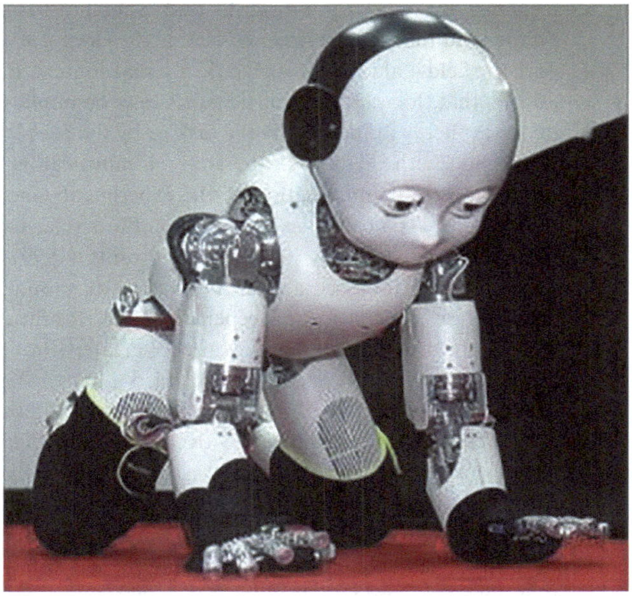

Pitfall #1	An Overly Confirmatory Research Strategy
Pitfall #2	Perception vs. Judgement
Pitfall #3	Demand and Response Bias
Pitfall #4	Low-level Differences (and Amazing Demonstrations!)
Pitfall #5	Peripheral Attentional Effects
Pitfall #6	Memory and Recognition

Methods: the six methodological pitfalls (Firestone & Scholl, 2015)

> It would go beyond the scope of this chapter to describe the discussion and pitfalls in detail, so we only briefly deal with two of the six pitfalls as examples here and refer to the article and the corresponding comments for a more in-depth examination of the topic.
> - Pitfall # 2 (perception vs. judgment) describes that an essential methodological problem of the literature is that although perception is often referred to as a dependent variable, visual perception is not necessarily measured. If we recall the study of Witt and Proffitt (2005) in softball described at the beginning of this sec-

tion, after a softball game the participants were asked to identify the circle on a poster with circles of different sizes that corresponded in size to the softball they had hit during the game. These so-called matching tasks are the basis of numerous studies on embodied perception. One of the problems associated with this is that although the participants have to estimate the size, for example, this judgment is not based exclusively on perceptual processes but relies on a number of other processes (e.g., increased self-confidence) that can also influence the judgment process. As long as methods are used that measure judgment processes (and not perceptual processes) that in turn are open to other influencing factors, it should not be concluded that we are dealing with visual distortions of perception. As a second example, consider Pitfall # 3 (demand and response bias). Here, Firestone and Scholl (2015) pointed out that an experiment—be it in the laboratory or in the field—always takes place in a social context. It follows that, for example, participants may be implicitly or explicitly influenced by the task or by the people interacting with them (e.g., the study administrator), which leads to contamination of the experiments and their results. As a catchy example, the authors refer to the backpack study by Bhalla and Proffitt (1999), which we also discussed above. As a reminder, mountains were estimated to be steeper (Bhalla & Proffitt, 1999; Proffitt et al., 1995) and distances greater (Proffitt et al., 2003) when participants carried a backpack or were exhausted. Proffitt suggested that the effect occurs because mountaineering with a heavy backpack causes more energetic costs (i.e., is more physically demanding), and therefore perception changes, so that the person wearing the backpack—implicitly or explicitly—makes an economic decision to act in this situation. Firestone and Scholl argued (with their argument empirically based on numerous studies by Durgin and colleagues; e.g., Durgin, Hajnal, et al., 2010; Durgin, Li, & Hajnal, 2010) that the participants may have shown—consciously or unconsciously—response behavior that was influenced by their guessing the purpose of the study. In other words, participants who are asked to put on a backpack and then assess the steepness of a mountain may ask themselves if the experiment is designed to explore whether wearing a backpack (and the associated increase in weight to be carried) has an effect on the perceived steepness and behave in accordance with the hypothesis. Numerous studies have proven such effects in studies on embodied perception (e.g., Woods et al., 2009). From this, numerous methodological precautions can be derived for future studies in order to avoid such distortions of results: These range from the standardized application of exit interviews to indirect measurement methods and double-blind procedures.

In summary, embodied perception is a dynamic field of research that historically rests on strong theoretical foundations. The importance of this research for sport psychology, both in terms of theory development and the generation of evidence-based recommendations for practice (see Cañal-Bruland & van der Kamp, 2012), is obvious when it comes to exploring the extent to which possibilities for action (e.g., talented vs. less talented; fatigued vs. not fatigued, etc.) are linked to or even influenced by visual perceptual processes. However, to be able to issue evidence-based recommendations, research must meet scientific quality criteria. As the methodological critique by Firestone and Scholl (2015) shows, this is not (yet) the case. At the same time, this results in the challenging task of fulfilling these methodological requirements and of establishing new methods that are capable of critically examining theory-led findings. Speculatively, it should be noted that—if the theoretical assumptions can be empirically substantiated—the bidirectionality that was discussed above for embodied cognition would also open up a meaningful research perspective for embodied perception research and sport psychology. Theoretically, not only should possibilities for action (e.g., sport motor skills) influence perception, but in return, changes in perception should lead to changes in motor control and in learning processes. For initial empirical experiments in this direction, see Chauvel et al. (2015) and Cañal-Bruland, van der Meer, and Moerman (2016).

6.5 What Does Embodied Cognition Mean for Sport Psychology?

In the broadest sense, embodied cognition research in sport psychology is applied where movements are realized. A more radical view would even relate the benefits of embodied cognition research to issues such as the termination of an athlete's career, since sensorimotor information from the body, possibly perceived unconsciously, can potentially influence the cognitive and emotional decision to retire. It is easier to investigate and theoretically deduce concrete changes in perception, for example, if different previous sensorimotor experiences are present. Above we have argued that the sensorimotor theory of perceptual experience (O'Regan & Noë, 2001) assumes that we perceive the world as we perceive it because we learn sensorimotor contingencies between our movements and the resulting perceived changes in the environment. For sport psychology this statement is applicable to all movement actions. For example, it means that when an athlete in gymnastics learns a handstand rollover over a springboard, they learn how the sensory information changes during their movement. A relevant question for sport psychology is, for example, which of the sensory changes caused by movement are decisive for the learning performance of a certain skill? In the case of a rollover, it could be that visuospatial, auditory, and kinesthetic changes contribute to the learning of the rollover to varying degrees (for an experiment investigating the significance of certain visual information such as springboard position and jumping box in the case of a handstand rollover, see Heinen et al., 2013).

In the following, we apply the findings of embodied cognition research to specific questions in sport psychology research. Instead of going into all the chapters of this textbook in detail, we ask ourselves (sorted by principles) where and how sport psychology research could be changed. An important and new position for us is that sport psychology or sports in general must not be used as a testbed for embodied cognition research; this research must be intrinsically motivated by what embodied cognition research means for theory development as well as empirical and applied practice in the field of sport psychology. This has often been called for (e.g., Beilock, 2008) and bidirectional interactions between cognitive and motor processes have been proposed (see Hohmann et al., 2010, and articles in the special issue [vol. 17, issue 4] of the *German Sport Psychology Journal*; Cappuccio, 2015). We support these calls because in sports we have the special situation of a well-structured learning environment and the tasks often have a sensorimotor component. Furthermore, the expertise and experience of athletes can be classified, and their performance can be objectified in many cases. However, this way of thinking has led to the expansion of embodied cognition research into the field of sport psychology and sports practice, without it being certain if the findings will also bring about concrete changes in sport psychology research or be of practical use in sports.

❓ We therefore recommend answering four specific questions:

- How can embodied cognition effects be specified?
- How can embodied cognition effects be quantified?
- What can embodied cognition *not* explain in sport psychology?
- How can sport psychology incorporate embodied cognition research in the future?

6.5.1 How Can Embodied Cognition Effects Be Specified?

A specification of embodied cognition effects can be made by answering the following questions: When (i.e., under what conditions or in what tasks) can effects be expected and when can they not (A.D. Wilson & Golonka, 2013)? What sensorimotor differences between individuals (e.g., in expertise research) suggest embodied cognition effects (Raab & Werner, 2017) and in what situations? Do embodied cognition effects have an influence both when movement and cognition are performed simultaneously (online effects) and when they are performed with a time lag (offline effects; Schütz-Bosbach & Prinz, 2007)?

For example, research on mental training in sports often focuses exclusively on the influence of mental training on movement (see Munzert et al., 2009). However, there is little research on the extent to which the performance of movements of the same kind improves mental imagery accuracy (de Lange et al., 2008). A field of research in sport psychology that empirically pursues this idea is still in its infancy. For example, Moreau et al. (2012) and Moreau et al. (2011) have shown that motor training has effects on mental rotational performance with different levels of sensorimotor expertise.

Another specification of embodied cognition research that might be relevant for sport psychology is whether cognitive processes in sports are influenced equally or differently depending on whether one performs the sport oneself (for an overview, see Hillman et al., 2008), realizes specific directions of movement (Löffler et al., 2018), intentionally or passively performs the movement (Hartmann & Mast, 2012), or just imagines it (Werner et al., 2019). A deeper analysis then concerns, for example, differentiating movement intensities to such an extent that, depending on the intensity, effects on cognitive processes have a facilitating or inhibiting effect (e.g., Drid et al., 2010).

Another important specification of embodied cognition research concerns the question of what movements influence cognitive functions (Raab & Werner, 2017) and what cognitive functions are specifically altered by movements (Tomporowski et al., 2008). Furthermore, it is important to examine to what extent person-related factors influence specific effects of movements on cognitive functions. For example, age-related effects are increasingly but only recently been discussed (Löffler et al., 2016; Rasmussen & Laumann, 2013).

6.5.2 How Can Embodied Cognition Effects Be Quantified?

An important task for sport psychology is the description and investigation of the part of sensorimotor processes that causes changes in cognitive processes in the sport context and thus can proportionally explain the complex behavior. Let us consider the complex behavior involved in a table tennis match. The ping-pong player has to decide in a short period of time what movement to perform (e.g., forehand or backhand stroke) and how the movement should be realized (e.g., with or without spin to the left or right corner). Classic theories describe this behavior, for example, as selecting a motor program and then applying specific parameters (Roth, 1989). Such phase models are also known from the natural decision-making literature (Klein et al., 1995), in which, for example, the situation is first analyzed in order to select a specific action, which is then implemented by sensorimotor means (Vickers, 1992). The mapping of these "what" and "how" parts of the movement to tactics and technique in a complex table tennis situation has been researched in cross-disciplinary endeavors (Raab et al., 2005). Embodied cognition research now argues against a sequential and phase-oriented description of this action. Rather, embodied cognition research predicts that the selection of the "what" decision can be influenced in advance by sensorimotor information (Raab, 2017), for example, and possibly runs in parallel (Cisek & Kalaska, 2005, for basic science studies). A statement such as "but I can't pass that far," which is the title of a research paper by Bruce et al. (2012) on Australian football, shows that tactical decisions are necessarily prespecified by sensorimotor components. In our opinion, one question that is open to sport psychology is the exact description of this relationship and a quantification of the effects, since wheelchair users without previous sensorimotor experience can also realize specific perception and action tasks (Renden et al., 2014; see also Aglioti et al., 2008).

6

> Sport psychology needs a better description and investigation of the part of sensorimotor processes that causes changes in cognitive processes so complex behavior in the sport context can be explained proportionally.

6.5.3 Why Does Sport Psychology Need Embodied Cognition?

We have argued above that theoretical embodied cognition approaches can be assigned to so-called common coding, internal model, or simulation theories (Gentsch et al., 2016). These theories are also used for explaining sensorimotor action in sport psychology research, although often for other reasons (Munzert et al., 2009). Thus, at least theoretically, and as far as movements in general are concerned, there seems to be little reason why sport psychology and embodied cognition cannot jointly describe, explain, and successfully predict actions that are relevant to sport psychology (Cappuccio, 2015). On a second glance, however, some of the goals of basic and applied research are fundamentally different, and therefore we may need to reduce our expectations somewhat. If, for example, readers of this textbook search for the keyword "embodied cognition" in the other chapters of this textbook, they will find very few explicit references. Rather, it seems that whole areas of research—on motivation, emotion, personality, and social processes in sports—can do without reference to embodied cognition. Even though we have argued above that sensorimotor processes can be fundamental for other processes, consideration of, for example, embodied emotion research (Niedenthal, 2007) in emotion research in sport psychology does not seem to take place or at least not extensively. A few studies, for example, on choking under pressure, now use the embodied cognition approach to describe unresolved phenomena of behavioral errors in sports. For example, Papineau (2015) described the so-called yips phenomenon in golf (cf. Lobinger et al., 2014) from an embodied cognition perspective, explaining why focusing on movement before and during exercise can possibly account for behavioral errors (Klämpfl et al., 2013). Similarly, this reasoning can also be applied to other areas of sport psychology. In addition to the possible different goals and possible lack of fit in certain areas of sport psychology, it may also be that embodied cognition research needs to focus on much more specific, complex actions in order to demonstrate the above specifications, quantifications, and explanations for sport psychology research.

How can sport psychology incorporate embodied cognition research in the future? Predictions about the future of research in the context of sport psychology are not new and often reach far into the future. In the context of embodied cognition research (Raab, 2017), for example, sport psychology has predicted that the topic of "mind and motion" will remain central until 2050 and will be characterized by stronger cooperation between basic research and application.

Sport psychology, in all modesty, should also assign itself the task of changing embodied cognition research in other disciplines through research accentuated in sport psychology. Sport psychology may be a good testbed that provides rich opportunities for an experimentally oriented embodied cognition approach. We would like to make a contribution to this endeavor.

Learning Control Questions

Basic:

- How do you define embodied cognition?
- What is the difference between classical cognition theories and embodied cognition approaches? What's new about it?
- Can you explain the three perspectives on embodied cognition (conceptualization, replacement, constitution (Shapiro, 2011)?
- Can you list the embodied cognition approaches and author names associated with them?
- What is your favorite embodied cognition approach? Explain why you like it the best.

Advanced:

- How do embodied cognition approaches differ from each other?
- Which study designs and methods can be used to assess the influence of movement on cognition?
- Which study designs and methods can be used to assess the influence of cognition on movement?
- How can the influence of cognition on movement be assessed?
- Can you cite empirical evidence for the relationship between movement and cognition? What study convinced you the most and why?

Experts:

- Can you describe in your own words two of the six pitfalls listed by Firestone and Scholl (2016) (see ▶ Sect. 6.4.3) and explain what can be done to counter them?
- To what extent and why could an embodied cognition perspective change sport psychology research?
- How can embodied cognition be used (or abused) in coaching to influence performance in sports?
- Can you think of a phenomenon in your favorite sport which, knowing the contents of this chapter, you see with different eyes?

References

Abrahamson, D. (2016). Learning is moving in new ways: The ecological dynamics of mathematics education. In *Proceedings of the International Conference of the Learning Sciences*. Singapoor. Retrieved from https://www.academia.edu/20180810/Learning_is_moving_in_new_ways_The_ecological_dynamics_of_mathematics_education

Aglioti, S. M., Cesari, P., Romani, M., & Urgesi, C. (2008). Action anticipation and motor resonance in elite basketball players. *Nature Neuroscience, 11*(9), 1109–1116. https://doi.org/10.1038/nn.2182

Bader, J.-P., Bühler, J., Endrass, J., Klipstein, A., & Hell, D. (1999). Muscle power and walk characteristics of depressive humans. *Der Nervenarzt, 70*(7), 613–619. https://doi.org/10.1007/s001150050486

Barsalou, L. W. (1999). Perceptual symbol systems. *Behavioral and Brain Sciences, 22*(4), 577–660.

Beilock, S. L. (2008). Beyond the playing field: sport psychology meets embodied cognition. *International Review of Sport & Exercise Psychology, 1*(1), 19–30.

Bhalla, M., & Proffitt, D. (1999). Visual-motor recalibration in geographical slant perception. *Journal of Experimental Psychology. Human Perception and Performance, 25*(4), 1076–1096.

Bornstein, M. H., Hahn, C.-S., & Suwalsky, J. T. D. (2013). Physically developed and exploratory young infants contribute to their own long-term academic achievement. *Psychological Science, 24*(10), 1906–1917. https://doi.org/10.1177/0956797613479974

Boroditsky, L. (2000). Metaphoric structuring: Understanding time through spatial metaphors. *Cognition, 75*(1), 1–28. https://doi.org/10.3389/fpsyg.2013.00142

Boroditsky, L. (2001). Does language shape thought? Mandarin and English speakers' conceptions of time. *Cognitive Psychology, 43*(1), 1–22. https://doi.org/10.1006/cogp.2001.0748

Brooks, R. A. (1991). Intelligence without representation. *Artificial Intelligence, 47*(1–3), 139–159. https://doi.org/10.1016/0004-3702(91)90053-M

Bruce, L., Farrow, D., Raynor, A., & Mann, D. (2012). *But I can't pass that far! The influence of motor skill on decision making*. ECU Publications. https://doi.org/10.1016/j.psychsport.2011.10.005

Bruner, J. (1957). On perceptual readiness. *Psychological Review, 64*(2), 123–152.

Bruner, J., & Goodman, C. C. (1947). Value and need as organizing factors in perception. *The Journal of Abnormal and Social Psychology, 42*(1), 33–44. https://doi.org/10.1037/h0058484

Bruner, J., & Postman, L. (1949). Perception, cognition, and behavior. *Journal of Personality, 18*, 14–31.

Cai, Z. G., & Connell, L. (2015). Space-time interdependence: evidence against asymmetric mapping between time and space. *Cognition, 136*, 268–281. https://doi.org/10.1016/j.cognition.2014.11.039

Cañal-Bruland, R., & van der Kamp, J. (2009). Action goals influence action-specific perception. *Psychonomic Bulletin & Review, 16*(6), 1100–1105. https://doi.org/10.3758/PBR.16.6.1100

Cañal-Bruland, R., & van der Kamp, J. (2012). Are performance-specific perceptual effects performance-specific? *Magazine for Sport Psychology*, 19, 57–69.

Cañal-Bruland, R., & van der Kamp, J. (2015). Embodied perception: A proposal to reconcile affordance and spatial perception. *I-Perception, 6*(2), 63–66. https://doi.org/10.1068/i0709jc

Cañal-Bruland, R., van der Kamp, J., & Gray, R. (2016). Acting is perceiving! *Behavioral and Brain Sciences, 39*. https://doi.org/10.1017/S0140525X15002460

Cañal-Bruland, R., van der Meer, Y., & Moerman, J. (2016). Can visual illusions be used to facilitate sport skill learning? *Journal of Motor Behavior, 48*(5), 285–389. https://doi.org/10.1080/00222895.2015.1113916

Cañal-Bruland, R., Zhu, F. F., van der Kamp, J., & Masters, R. S. W. (2011). Target-directed visual attention is a prerequisite for action-specific perception. *Acta Psychologica, 136*(3), 285–289. https://doi.org/10.1016/j.actpsy.2010.12.001

Cappuccio, M. L. (2015). Introduction: when embodied cognition and sport psychology team-up. *Phenomenology and the Cognitive Sciences, 14*(2), 213–225. https://doi.org/10.1007/s11097-015-9415-1

Carney, D. R., Cuddy, A. J. C., & Yap, A. J. (2010). Power posing: Brief nonverbal displays affect neuroendocrine levels and risk tolerance. *Psychological Science, 21*(10), 1363–1368. https://doi.org/10.1177/0956797610383437

Casasanto, D., & Boroditsky, L. (2008). Time in the mind: Using space to think about time. *Cognition, 106*(2), 579–593. https://doi.org/10.1016/j.cognition.2007.03.004

Casasanto, D., Fotakopoulou, O., & Boroditsky, L. (2010). Space and time in the child's mind: Evidence for a cross-dimensional asymmetry. *Cognitive Science, 34*(3), 387–405. https://doi.org/10.1111/j.1551-6709.2010.01094.x

Chauvel, G., Wulf, G., & Maquestiaux, F. (2015). Visual illusions can facilitate sport skill learning. *Psychonomic Bulletin & Review, 22*(3), 717–721. https://doi.org/10.3758/s13423-014-0744-9

Cisek, P., & Kalaska, J. F. (2005). Neural correlates of reaching decisions in dorsal premotor cortex: Specification of multiple direction choices and final selection of action. *Neuron, 45*(5), 801–814. https://doi.org/10.1016/j.neuron.2005.01.027

Clark, A. (2008). *Supersizing the mind: Embodiment, action, and cognitive extension*. Oxford University Press.

Cuddy, J., Wilmuth, C. A., Yap, A. J., & Carney, D. R. (2015). Preparatory power posing affects nonverbal presence and job interview performance. *Journal of Applied Psychology, 100*(4), 1286–1295. https://doi.org/10.1037/a0038543

Damasio, A. R., & Damasio, H. (1994). Cortical systems for retrieval of concrete knowledge: The convergence zone framework. In C. Koch & J. L. Davis (Eds.), *Large-scale neuronal theories of the brain* (pp. 61–74). MIT Press.

de Lange, F. P., Roelofs, K., & Toni, I. (2008). Motor imagery: A window into the mechanisms and alterations of the motor system. *Cortex, 44*(5), 494–506. https://doi.org/10.1016/j.cortex.2007.09.002

Doyen, S., Klein, O., Pichon, C.-L., & Cleeremans, A. (2012). Behavioral priming: It's all in the mind, but whose mind? *PLoS One, 7*(1), e29081. https://doi.org/10.1371/journal.pone.0029081

Drid, P., Majstorović, N., & Drapšin, M. (2010). The effects of different exercise workloads on visual perception skills in elite serbian female judokas. *Kineziologija, 42*(2), 201–207.

Durgin, F. H., Hajnal, A., Li, Z., Tonge, N., & Stigliani, A. (2010). Palm boards are not action measures: an alternative to the two-systems theory of geographical slant perception. *Acta Psychologica, 134*(2), 182–197. https://doi.org/10.1016/j.actpsy.2010.01.009

Durgin, F. H., Li, Z., & Hajnal, A. (2010). Slant perception in near space is categorically biased: evidence for a vertical tendency. *Attention, Perception & Psychophysics, 72*(7), 1875–1889. https://doi.org/10.3758/APP.72.7.1875

Fink, P. W., Foo, P. S., & Warren, W. H. (2009). Catching fly balls in virtual reality: A critical test of the outfielder problem. *Journal of Vision, 9*(13), 14–14. https://doi.org/10.1167/9.13.14

Firestone, C. (2013). How "paternalistic" is spatial perception? Why wearing a heavy backpack doesn't—and couldn't—make hills look steeper. *Perspectives on Psychological Science, 8*(4), 455–473. https://doi.org/10.1177/1745691613489835

Firestone, C., & Scholl, B. J. (2015). Cognition does not affect perception: Evaluating the evidence for "top-down" effects. *The Behavioral and Brain Sciences, 1–77*. https://doi.org/10.1017/S0140525X15000965

Firestone, C., & Scholl, B. J. (2016). Cognition does not affect perception: Evaluating the evidence for "top-down" effects. *The Behavioral and brain sciences*, 39, e229. https://doi.org/10.1017/S0140525X15000965

Fischer, J., Fischer, P., Englich, B., Aydin, N., & Frey, D. (2011). Empower my decisions: The effects of power gestures on confirmatory information processing. *Journal of Experimental Social Psychology, 47*(6), 1146–1154. https://doi.org/10.1016/j.jesp.2011.06.008

Garrison, K. E., Tang, D., & Schmeichel, B. J. (2016). Embodying power: A preregistered replication and extension of the power pose effect. *Social Psychological and Personality Science, 7*(7), 623–630. https://doi.org/10.1177/1948550616652209

Gentsch, A., Weber, A., Synofzik, M., Vosgerau, G., & Schütz-Bosbach, S. (2016). Towards a common framework of grounded action cognition: Relating motor control, perception and cognition. *Cognition, 146*, 81–89. https://doi.org/10.1016/j.cognition.2015.09.010

Gibson, J. J. (1979). *The ecological approach to visual perception*. Houghton Mifflin.

Glenberg, A. (1997). What memory is for. *The Behavioral and Brain Sciences, 20*(1), 1-19-55.

Glenberg, A., Havas, D., Becker, R., & Rinck, M. (2005). Grounding language in bodily states: The case for emotion. In D. Pecher & R. A. Zwaan (Eds.), *Grounding cognition: the role of perception and action in memory, language, and thinking*. Cambridge University Press. https://doi.org/10.1017/CBO9780511499968.006

Glenberg, A., & Kaschak, M. P. (2002). Grounding language in action. *Psychonomic Bulletin & Review, 9*(3), 558–565.

Glenberg, A., & Robertson, D. A. (2000). Symbol grounding and meaning: A comparison of high-dimensional and embodied theories of meaning. *Journal of Memory and Language, 43*(3), 379–401. https://doi.org/10.1006/jmla.2000.2714

Guillot, A., & Collet, C. (2008). Construction of the motor imagery integrative model in sport: A review and theoretical investigation of motor imagery use. *International Review of Sport and Exercise Psychology, 1*(1), 31–44. https://doi.org/10.1080/17509840701823139

Hartmann, M., & Mast, F. W. (2012). Moving along the mental time line influences the processing of future related words. *Consciousness and Cognition, 21*(3), 1558–1562. https://doi.org/10.1016/j.concog.2012.06.015

Heinen, T., Vinken, P. M., Jeraj, D., & Velentzas, K. (2013). Movement regulation of handsprings on vault. *Research Quarterly for Exercise and Sport, 84*(1), 68–78. https://doi.org/10.1080/02701367.2013.762300

Heinrich, A., Hansen, D. W., Stoll, O., & Cañal-Bruland, R. (2020). The impact of physiological fatigue and gaze behavior on shooting performance in expert biathletes. *Journal of Science and Medicine in Sport*. https://doi.org/10.1016/j.jsams.2020.02.010

Hesse, U. (2016, February 23). Thomas Müller: The modest assassin. *The Guardian*. Retrieved from https://www.theguardian.com/football/2016/feb/23/thomas-muller-modest-assassin-bayern-munich-germany

Hillman, C. H., Erickson, K. I., & Kramer, A. F. (2008). Be smart, exercise your heart: exercise effects on brain and cognition. *Nature Reviews Neuroscience, 9*(1), 58–65. https://doi.org/10.1038/nrn2298

Hochman, D. (2014, September 19). *Amy Cuddy takes a stand*. The New York Times. Retrieved from https://www.nytimes.com/2014/09/21/fashion/amy-cuddy-takes-a-stand-TED-talk.html

Hohmann, T., Heinen, T., & Raab, M. (2010). Editorial embodiment. *Zeitschrift Für Sportpsychologie, 17*(4), 105–108.

Huang, L., Galinsky, A. D., Gruenfeld, D. H., & Guillory, L. E. (2011). Powerful postures versus powerful roles—Which is the proximate correlate of thought and behavior? *Psychological Science, 22*(1), 95–102. https://doi.org/10.1177/0956797610391912

Johnson, L. G., Butson, M. L., Polman, R. C., Raj, I. S., Borkoles, E., Scott, D., et al. (2016). Light physical activity is positively associated with cognitive performance in older community

dwelling adults. *Journal of Science and Medicine in Sport, 19*(11), 877–882. https://doi.org/10.1016/j.jsams.2016.02.002
Kennedy, G., Hardman, R. J., Macpherson, H., Scholey, A. B., & Pipingas, A. (2017). How does exercise reduce the rate of age-associated cognitive decline? A review of potential mechanisms. *Journal of Alzheimer's Disease, 55*(1), 1–18. https://doi.org/10.3233/JAD-160665
Kitano, H., & Asada, M. (1998). RoboCup humanoid challenge: That's one small step for a robot, one giant leap for mankind. In *Proceedings. 1998 IEEE/RSJ international conference on intelligent robots and systems. Innovations in theory, practice and applications (Cat. No.98CH36190)* (Vol. 1, pp. 419–424). doi: https://doi.org/10.1109/IROS.1998.724655
Klämpfl, M. K., Lobinger, B. H., & Raab, M. (2013). Reinvestment—The cause of the yips? *PLoS One, 8*(12). https://doi.org/10.1371/journal.pone.0082470
Klein, G., Schlesinger, J., & Meister, D. E. (1951). The effect of personal values on perception: an experimental critique. *Psychological Review, 58*(2), 96–112.
Klein, G., Wolf, S., Militello, L., & Zsambok, C. (1995). Characteristics of skilled option generation in chess. *Organizational Behavior and Human Decision Processes, 62*(1), 63–69. https://doi.org/10.1006/obhd.1995.1031
Knoblich, G., & Flach, R. (2001). Predicting the effects of actions: Interactions of perception and action. *Psychological Science, 12*(6), 467–472. https://doi.org/10.1111/1467-9280.00387
Körner, A., Topolinski, S., & Strack, F. (2015). Routes to embodiment. *Cognition, 940*. https://doi.org/10.3389/fpsyg.2015.00940
Lakoff, G., & Johnson, M. (1980). Conceptual metaphor in everyday language. *The Journal of Philosophy, 77*(8), 453. https://doi.org/10.2307/2025464
Lakoff, G., & Johnson, M. (1999). *Philosophy in the flesh: the embodied mind and its challenge to western thought*. Basic Books.
Lemke, M. R., Wendorff, T., Mieth, B., Buhl, K., & Linnemann, M. (2000). Spatiotemporal gait patterns during over ground locomotion in major depression compared with healthy controls. *Journal of Psychiatric Research, 34*(4–5), 277–283. https://doi.org/10.1016/S0022-3956(00)00017-0
Lobinger, B. H., Klämpfl, M. K., & Altenmüller, E. (2014). We are able, we intend, we act—But we do not succeed: a theoretical framework for a better understanding of paradoxical performance in sports. *Journal of Clinical Sport Psychology, 8*(4), 357–377. https://doi.org/10.1123/jcsp.2014-0047
Löffler, J., Cañal-Bruland, R., Schröger, A., Tolentino-Castro, J. W., & Raab, M. (2018). Interrelations between temporal and spatial cognition: the role of modality-specific processing. *Frontiers in Psychology, 9*, 2609. https://doi.org/10.3389/fpsyg.2018.02609
Löffler, J., Raab, M., & Cañal-Bruland, R. (2016). A lifespan perspective on embodied cognition. *Frontiers in Psychology*. https://doi.org/10.3389/fpsyg.2016.00845
Mann, D. T. Y., Williams, A. M., Ward, P., & Janelle, C. M. (2007). Perceptual-cognitive expertise in sport: A meta-analysis. *Journal of Sport & Exercise Psychology, 29*(4), 457–478.
Masters, R., Poolton, J., & van der Kamp, J. (2010). Regard and perceptions of size in soccer: Better is bigger. *Perception, 39*(9), 1290–1295.
McBeath, M. K., Shaffer, D. M., & Kaiser, M. K. (1995). How baseball outfielders determine where to run to catch fly balls. *Science (New York, N. Y.), 268*(5210), 569–573.
Memmert, D., Blanco, M., & Merkle, V. (2009). The effects of effort, performance, and expertise on apparent size perception in golf. *International Journal of Sport Psychology, 40*(2), 270–283.
Merleau-Ponty, M. (1945). *Phénoménologie de la perception*. Gallimard.
Merleau-Ponty, M. (2002). *Phenomenology of perception*. Routledge.
Michalak, J., Mischnat, J., & Teismann, T. (2014). Sitting posture makes a difference-embodiment effects on depressive memory bias. *Clinical Psychology & Psychotherapy, 21*(6), 519–524. https://doi.org/10.1002/cpp.1890
Michalak, J., Rohde, K., & Troje, N. F. (2015). How we walk affects what we remember: Gait modifications through biofeedback change negative affective memory bias. *Journal of Behavior Therapy and Experimental Psychiatry, 46*, 121–125. https://doi.org/10.1016/j.jbtep.2014.09.004
Michalak, J., Troje, N. F., Fischer, J., Vollmar, P., Heidenreich, T., & Schulte, D. (2009). Embodiment of sadness and depression—Gait patterns associated with dysphoric mood. *Psychosomatic Medicine, 71*(5), 580–587. https://doi.org/10.1097/PSY.0b013e3181a2515c
Miles, L. K., Nind, L. K., & Macrae, C. N. (2010). Moving through time. *Psychological Science, 21*(2), 222–223. https://doi.org/10.1177/0956797609359333
Moreau, D., Clerc, J., Mansy-Dannay, A., & Guerrien, A. (2012). Enhancing spatial ability through sport practice. *Journal of Individual Differences, 33*(2), 83–88. https://doi.org/10.1027/1614-0001/a000075
Moreau, D., Mansy-Dannay, A., Clerc, J., & Guerrién, A. (2011). Spatial ability and motor performance: Assessing mental rotation processes in elite and novice athletes. *International Journal of Sport Psychology, 42*, 525–547.
Munzert, J., Lorey, B., & Zentgraf, K. (2009). Cognitive motor processes: The role of motor imagery in the study of motor representations. *Brain Research Reviews, 60*(2), 306–326. https://doi.org/10.1016/j.brainresrev.2008.12.024
Müsseler, J., & Rieger, M. (2016). *Allgemeine Psychologie* (3rd ed.). Springer.
Mussweiler, T. (2006). Doing is for thinking!: Stereotype activation by stereotypic movements. *General Psychology, 17*(1), 17–21. https://doi.org/10.1111/j.1467-9280.2005.01659.x
Newen, A., De Briun, L., & Gallagher, S. (2018). 4E cognition: Historical boots, key concepts, and central issues. In A. Newen, L. De Bruin, & S. Gallagher (Eds.), *The Oxford handbook of 4E cognition* (pp. 3–15). Oxford Press.
Niedenthal, P. M. (2007). Embodying emotion. *Science (New York, N.Y.), 316*(5827), 1002–1005. https://doi.org/10.1126/science.1136930
O'Regan, J. K., & Noë, A. (2001). A sensorimotor account of vision and visual consciousness. *The Behavioral and Brain Sciences, 24*(5), 939–973.
Paleacu, D., Shutzman, A., Giladi, N., Herman, T., Simon, E. S., & Hausdorff, J. M. (2007). Effects of pharmacological therapy on gait and cognitive function in depressed patients. *Clinical Neuropharmacology, 30*(2), 63–71. https://doi.org/10.1097/01.wnf.0000240949.41691.95
Papineau, D. (2015). Choking and the yips. *Phenomenology and the Cognitive Sciences, 14*(2) Retrieved from https://www.researchgate.net/publication/271952128_Choking_and_The_Yips
Pecher, D., van Mierlo, H., Cañal-Bruland, R., & Zeelenberg, R. (2015). The burden of secrecy? No effect on hill slant estimation and beanbag throwing. *Journal of Experimental Psychology: General, 144*, e65–e72.
Proffitt, D. (2006). Distance perception. *Current Directions in Psychological Science, 15*(3), 131–135. https://doi.org/10.1111/j.0963-7214.2006.00422.x
Proffitt, D. (2008). An action-specific approach to spatial perception. *Embodiment, Ego-Space, and Action*, 179–202.
Proffitt, D., Bhalla, M., Gossweiler, R., & Midgett, J. (1995). Perceiving geographical slant. *Psychonomic Bulletin & Review, 2*(4), 409–428. https://doi.org/10.3758/BF03210980

Proffitt, D., Stefanucci, J., Banton, T., & Epstein, W. (2003). The role of effort in perceiving distance. *Psychological Science, 14*(2), 106–112.

Raab, M. (2017). Sport and exercise psychology 2050. *German Journal of Sport Sciences*. https://doi.org/10.1007/s12662-016-0435-y

Raab, M., Masters, R. S. W., & Maxwell, J. P. (2005). Improving the "how" and "what" decisions of elite table tennis players. *Human Movement Science, 24*(3), 326–344. https://doi.org/10.1016/j.humov.2005.06.004

Raab, M., & Werner, K. (2017). Embodiment. In J. Munzert, B. Strauss, & M. Raab (Eds.), *Experimental sport psychology*. Kohlhammer.

Ranehill, E., Dreber, A., Johannesson, M., Leiberg, S., Sul, S., & Weber, R. A. (2015). Assessing the robustness of power posing: No effect on hormones and risk tolerance in a large sample of men and women. *Psychological Science, 26*(5), 653–656. https://doi.org/10.1177/0956797614553946

Rasmussen, M., & Laumann, K. (2013). The academic and psychological benefits of exercise in healthy children and adolescents. *European Journal of Psychology of Education, 28*(3), 945–962. https://doi.org/10.1007/s10212-012-0148-z

Renden, P. G., Kerstens, S., Oudejans, R. R. D., & Cañal-Bruland, R. (2014). Foul or dive? Motor contributions to judging ambiguous foul situations in football. *European Journal of Sport Science, 14*(Suppl 1), S221–S227. https://doi.org/10.1080/17461391.2012.683813

Ribbat, J. (2011). *Von space arrangement to the field of action – a cheorgraphy-project for beginners (Master thesis)*. Universität der Künste Berlin. Retrieved from http://www.musikbewegung.de/fileadmin/PDFs/DiplomarbeitJennyRibbat.pdf

Riskind, J. H., & Gotay, C. C. (1982). Physical posture: Could it have regulatory or feedback effects on motivation and emotion? *Motivation and Emotion, 6*(3), 273–298. https://doi.org/10.1007/BF00992249

Ronay, R., Tybur, J. M., van Huijstee, D., & Morssinkhof, M. (2016). Embodied power, testosterone, and overconfidence as a causal pathway to risk-taking. *Comprehensive Results in Social Psychology, 2*(1), 28–43. https://doi.org/10.1080/23743603.2016.1248081

Roth, K. (1989). *Taktik im Sportspiel : zum Erklärungswert der Theorie generalisierter motorischer Programme für die Regulation komplexer Bewegungshandlungen (1. Aufl.)*. Hofmann.

Rowlands, M. (2010). *The new science of the mind: From extended mind to embodied phenomenology*. Bradford.

Sánchez García, R., & González Álvarez, A. (2014). *Las cadenas hápticas como herramienta didáctica para la enseñanza de habilidades motrices*. Retrieved from http://abacus.universidadeuropea.es/handle/11268/3902

Schacter, D. L., Addis, D. R., & Buckner, R. L. (2007). Remembering the past to imagine the future: the prospective brain. *Nature Reviews Neuroscience, 8*(9), 657–661. https://doi.org/10.1038/nrn2213

Scherder, E., Scherder, R., Verburgh, L., Königs, M., Blom, M., Kramer, A. F., & Eggermont, L. (2014). Executive functions of sedentary elderly may benefit from walking: A systematic review and meta-analysis. *The American Journal of Geriatric Psychiatry, 22*(8), 782–791. https://doi.org/10.1016/j.jagp.2012.12.026

Schneider, I. K., Parzuchowski, M., Wojciszke, B., Schwarz, N., & Koole, S. L. (2014). Weighty data: Importance information influences estimated weight of digital information storage devices. *Frontiers in Psychology, 5*, 1536. https://doi.org/10.3389/fpsyg.2014.01536

Schubert, T. W., & Koole, S. L. (2009). The embodied self: Making a fist enhances men's power-related self-conceptions. *Journal of Experimental Social Psychology, 45*(4), 828–834. https://doi.org/10.1016/j.jesp.2009.02.003

Schütz-Bosbach, S., & Prinz, W. (2007). Perceptual resonance: action-induced modulation of perception. *Trends in Cognitive Sciences, 11*(8), 349–355. https://doi.org/10.1016/j.tics.2007.06.005

Shaffer, D. M., Krauchunas, S. M., Eddy, M., & McBeath, M. K. (2004). How dogs navigate to catch frisbees. *Psychological Science, 15*(7), 437–441. https://doi.org/10.1111/j.0956-7976.2004.00698.x

Shapiro, L. (2011). *Embodied cognition*. New York: Routledge Press.

Shiffrar, M., & Heinen, T. (2010). Die Fähigkeiten von Athleten verändern deren Wahrnehmung von Handlungen: "Embodiment" der visuellen Wahrnehmungvon menschlichen Bewegungen. *Zeitschrift für Sportpsychologie, 17*(4), 130–142. https://doi.org/10.1026/1612-5010/a000018

Slepian, M. L., & Ambady, N. (2014). Simulating sensorimotor metaphors: Novel metaphors influence sensory judgments. *Cognition, 130*(3), 309–314. https://doi.org/10.1016/j.cognition.2013.11.006

Sloman, L., Berridge, M., Homatidis, S., Hunter, D., & Duck, T. (1982). Gait patterns of depressed patients and normal subjects. *The American Journal of Psychiatry, 139*(1), 94–97. https://doi.org/10.1176/ajp.139.1.94

Sloman, L., Pierrynowski, M., Berridge, M., Tupling, S., & Flowers, J. (1987). Mood, depressive illness and gait patterns. *Canadian Journal of Psychiatry. Revue Canadienne De Psychiatrie, 32*(3), 190–193.

Stins, J., Habets, L., Jongeling, R., & Cañal-Bruland, R. (2016). Being (un)moved by mental time travel. *Consciousness and Cognition, 42*, 374–381. https://doi.org/10.1016/j.concog.2016.04.014

Thelen, E., Schöner, G., Scheier, C., & Smith, L. B. (2001). The dynamics of embodiment: a field theory of infant perseverative reaching. *The Behavioral and Brain Sciences, 24*(1)., 1-34-86.

Tomporowski, P. D., Davis, C. L., Miller, P. H., & Naglieri, J. A. (2008). Exercise and children's intelligence, cognition, and academic achievement. *Educational Psychology Review, 20*(2), 111–131. https://doi.org/10.1007/s10648-007-9057-0

Tulving, E. (2002). Episodic memory: From mind to brain. *Annual Review of Psychology, 53*(1), 1–25. https://doi.org/10.1146/annurev.psych.53.100901.135114

Varela, F. J., Rosch, E., & Thompson, E. (1992). *The embodied mind: Cognitive science and human experience*. MIT Press.

Veltkamp, M., Aarts, H., & Custers, R. (2008). Perception in the service of goal pursuit: Motivation to attain goals enhances the perceived size of goal-instrumental objects. *Social Cognition, 26*(6), 720–736. https://doi.org/10.1521/soco.2008.26.6.720

Vickers, J. N. (1992). Gaze control in putting. *Perception, 21*(1), 117–132.

Wang, W., McBeath, M. K., & Sugar, T. G. (2015). Navigational strategy used to intercept fly balls under real-world conditions with moving visual background fields. *Attention, Perception, & Psychophysics, 77*(2), 613–625. https://doi.org/10.3758/s13414-014-0797-x

Werner, K., Raab, M., & Fischer, M. H. (2019). Moving arms: the effects of sensorimotor information on the problem-solving process. *Thinking & Reasoning, 25*, 171–191. https://doi.org/10.1080/13546783.2018.1494630

6

Wesp, R., Cichello, P., Gracia, E. B., & Davis, K. (2004). Observing and engaging in purposeful actions with objects influences estimates of their size. *Perception & Psychophysics, 66*(8), 1261–1267. https://doi.org/10.3758/BF03194996

Wilson, A. D., & Golonka, S. (2013). Embodied cognition is not what you think it is. *Frontiers in Psychology, 4*(58). https://doi.org/10.3389/fpsyg.2013.00058

Wilson, R. A. (2004). *Boundaries of the mind: The individual in the fragile sciences—Cognition*. Cambridge University Press.

Witt, J. K. (2011). Action's effect on perception. *Current Directions in Psychological Science, 20*(3), 201–206. https://doi.org/10.1177/0963721411408770

Witt, J. K., Linkenauger, S. A., Bakdash, J. Z., & Proffitt, D. (2008). Putting to a bigger hole: Golf performance relates to perceived size. *Psychonomic Bulletin & Review, 15*(3), 581–585.

Witt, J. K., & Proffitt, D. (2005). See the ball, hit the ball: Apparent ball size is correlated with batting average. *Psychological Science, 16*(12), 937–938. https://doi.org/10.1111/j.1467-9280.2005.01640.x

Witt, J. K., & Proffitt, D. (2008). Action-specific influences on distance perception: A role for motor simulation. *Journal of Experimental Psychology. Human Perception and Performance, 34*(6), 1479–1492. https://doi.org/10.1037/a0010781

Woods, A. J., Philbeck, J. W., & Danoff, J. V. (2009). The various perceptions of distance: An alternative view of how effort affects distance judgments. *Journal of Experimental Psychology. Human Perception and Performance, 35*(4), 1104–1117. https://doi.org/10.1037/a0013622

Yap, A. J., Wazlawek, A. S., Lucas, B. J., Cuddy, A. J. C., & Carney, D. R. (2013). The ergonomics of dishonesty: The effect of incidental posture on stealing, cheating, and traffic violations. *Psychological Science, 24*(11), 2281–2289. https://doi.org/10.1177/0956797613492425

Zwaan, R., & Madden, C. (2005). Embodied sentence comprehension. In D. Pecher & R. Zwaan (Eds.), *The grounding of cognition: The role of perception and action in memory, language, and thinking*. Cambridge University Press.

Motivation

Contents

Motivation and Goals in the Context of Sport and Movement

Anne-Marie Elbe, Julia Schüler, Hamsini Sivaramakrishnan and Cecilie Thøgersen-Ntoumani

Contents

J. Schüler et al. (eds.), *Sport and Exercise Psychology*, https://doi.org/10.1007/978-3-031-03921-8_7

Learning Objectives

After reading this chapter, you should be able to…

Basic:

- Define motivation
- Outline the major themes of motivation research in sport

Advanced:

- Describe the phenomenon of motivation and different goals in sport
- Name and characterize different theoretical approaches to motivation

Experts:

- Critically consider measurement tools for goal orientation in sport
- Demonstrate how motivation in sport can be enhanced

7.1 Definitions and Scope

7.1.1 Motivation

If you enter the terms "motivation" and "sport" into an online search engine, you will be overwhelmed by the sheer number of entries. The popularity of the concept of motivation and the breadth of its use reflect its importance for issues relating to health, athletic performance, and general life contexts on an individual and a societal level. Light needs to be shed on the question "What motivates people to engage in sport?" and the question needs to be considered from many different perspectives. In lay language, many different synonyms are used for motivation like incentive, initiative, interest, passion, ambition, and driving force. How much of this layman's understanding is reflected in the scientific operationalizations of "motivation?" The synonyms presented above share one important aspect in common with the scientific concept of motivation: the activating or energizing component. Motivation is the driving force behind an action.

Motivation

Motivation deals with explaining the direction, persistence, and intensity of goal-directed behavior. Desired goal states and what makes them attractive are the explanatory variables and are what characterize motivation (cf. Rheinberg, 2006).

In the above definition Rheinberg describes the essential and basic elements of motivation. Goal states can be evaluated as positive and desirable, and therefore individuals strive for these goals (e.g., feeling good after a long run through the forest). If, however, pursuing the goal is evaluated negatively (e.g., profuse sweating and muscle aches while jogging), individuals will avoid these goals. Positive and negative goal states have an incentive character, which means they can either be an incentive or disincentive for subsequent behavior. Perceived or anticipated objects and events with an incentive character (i.e., that are attractive) stimulate action towards a particular goal (action goal, e.g., winning a race or enjoying a team sport activity). In ▶ Sect. 7.2.2 we return to discussing the basic direction of behavior, i.e., approaching or avoiding an action. Rheinberg's definition also considers intensity (how concentrated and effortful do I perform an action, e.g., full training intensity or half-hearted training) and persistence (e.g., how long can I keep up the training, even if it becomes strenuous? Do I resume training after a sports injury?).

7.1.2 Incentives and Affect

Let us now consider incentives in more detail. Theoretical approaches dealing with incentives see affect as the core element (McClelland, 1953; for a detailed description see Beckmann & Heckhausen, 2018). Affect has a dual role in the motivational process. On the one hand, the execution of an activity and the goal state elicit an affective response. People may feel joy when jogging through the forest and proud when they have completed the 10 km run in a good time. In this example, the affective response has a rewarding effect and thus increases the probability of similar future behavior, i.e., it encourages the person to go jogging again in the near future. The likelihood of behavior is lower if the activity or goal state is associated with negative affect (e.g., aches, muscle cramps at the finish line, unsatisfactory running time). However, actual and current experiences are not necessary to trigger motivation, but rather certain activities and goal states (which can be related to past experiences, e.g., early childhood; ▶ Chap. 9, Development of Motives) elicit a specific affective response. More precisely, it is the anticipated, i.e., the expected, imagined change of affect that acts as the incentive to engage in a specific behavior (◘ Fig. 7.1).

> Motivation is the anticipation of a change of affect. The change is caused by incentives that promise negative or positive goal states.

According to Kuhl (2001), affect has an additional function, namely, providing energy for actions. Positive affect energizes action, whereas negative affect hinders action.

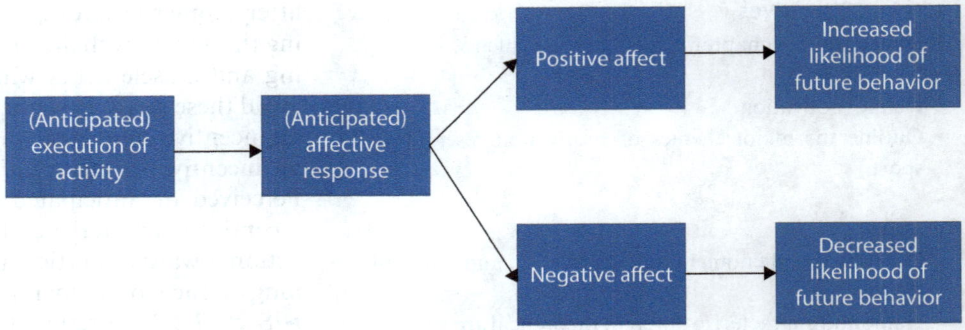

Fig. 7.1 Interplay of incentives, affect, and behavior

7

The incentives for why people engage in sports sometimes seem to be quite strong. Some people get up at 5 a.m. every morning to go jogging before work, and young elite athletes undergo strenuous daily training for years in addition to attending school and putting up with having very limited time for leisure activities. The question inevitably arises where the sources for incentives lie. It should be noted that physical activity can be rewarding in itself. The desire to move our bodies drives us to become active after phases of physical inactivity. Being active holds inherent rewards such as kinesthetic experiences. Another example includes feeling strong and experiencing a change in body position when executing a salto, which may be experienced as very pleasurable and rewarding. Such states are reflective of intrinsic motivation (► Chap. 8), and being completely absorbed in an activity is described as a flow state (Cszikszentmihalyi, 1975). Additional incentives for performing an activity may relate to the outcome of the activity, i.e., in the anticipated result. Examples of outcome-related incentives include becoming or staying healthy or to improve one's appearance/figure (details about flow and outcome- and activity-related incentives can be found in ► Chap. 8).

Abele and Brehm (1990) list ten motivation categories that reflect both outcome- and activity-related incentives. The following are particularly relevant for sport and exercise activities:

1. Health and fitness
2. Well-being (fun/feeling good, relaxing/counteracting stress)
3. Appearance (having an athletic figure, losing weight)
4. Performance (effort/training, enhancing performance, competition)
5. Kinesthetic experiences
6. Social experiences
7. Social networking (keeping in contact with old acquaintances, making new acquaintances)
8. Experiencing excitement and trying out new things in sport
9. Aesthetic experiences
10. Self-presentation

Even with strong activity incentives (e.g., for some people, though not for all (!), jogging is inherently enjoyable) and outcome incentives (e.g., wanting to lose weight for health reasons), it will sometimes be difficult to get out of bed at 5 a.m. or to resist temptations to skip behaviors needed to achieve one's goals. Kuhl (1983) suggested that additional processes must be added to the motivation process in order to ensure that an intention is translated to action and maintained until the goal is achieved. These additional processes are called volitional processes. Volitional skills are of great importance, for example, in order to maintain the decade long, extensive training required for an athlete to make it to the top but also for keeping up regular physical activity. Volition is described in detail in ► Chap. 10. The interaction of motivation and volition is theoretically anchored in the "Rubicon Model of Action Phases," which is described in more detail in ► Chap. 10 and ► Sect. 7.1.5.

7.1.3 Motivation as a Product of Person and Situation: P × S Scheme

Following from the section above one could assume that individuals anticipate that completing a challenging sport task will fill them with joy and pride, and they therefore will approach the task full of energy. However, challenging and reward promising tasks do not incentivize all people equally. There are interindividual differences in incentive preferences. Some people prefer challenges that promise pride (achievement motive), others are more strongly attracted by social reward (e.g., experiencing team spirit, building friendships) in which they feel in good hands and are happy (affiliation motive), and yet others prefer situations in which they experience power because they can lead and influence others (e.g., coach, team captain, referee; power motive; ► Chap. 9). ► Chapter 9 describes how different personality traits, the so-called implicit or explicit motives, are based on different affects. The achievement motive, for example, is based on pride; the power motive is based on feeling powerful and superior. Incentives therefore do not have the same effect on all individuals but depend on personal characteristics (e.g., motives). An individual's motivation to strive for a certain goal is determined both by personal and situational factors (Heckhausen, 1989). Personal factors include, for example, motives, needs, values, or goals. A motive (► Chap. 9) is a personality trait. A motive defines which incentives and goal states an individual strives for and also has an effect on an individual's mood (McClelland, 1987). Part A of ◘ Fig. 7.2 illustrates the person-situation-scheme (P × S scheme), a basic model of classical motivation psychology (Rheinberg, 2002). The lower part of the figure (b) applies the model to the sport performance context. Here, performance-related incentives interact with the individual's achievement motive and determines goal-oriented action via the resulting performance motivation. Part B of ◘ Fig. 7.2 also illustrates the terms "activity-related incentive" and "purpose-related incentive" and the affects associated with the activity and the result of the activity.

The motivation of a person to pursue a particular goal depends on the interaction between personal and situational factors.

7.1.4 Interaction of Desirability and Feasibility: Expectancy × Value

The P × S scheme in Part A of ◘ Fig. 7.2 can also be considered the basic principle of expectancy × value models (P × S) (cf. Beckmann & Heckhausen, 2018; Feather, 1982). The basic assumption is that people choose goals by offsetting the value, i.e., the attractiveness of the goal (e.g., success in a sporting task) against the probability of being able to achieve it (expectancy). If the incentive, e.g., the feeling of having achieved a personal best, is high and the expectancy of being able to achieve this goal is also high, training will be initiated. The formula includes a multiplication which

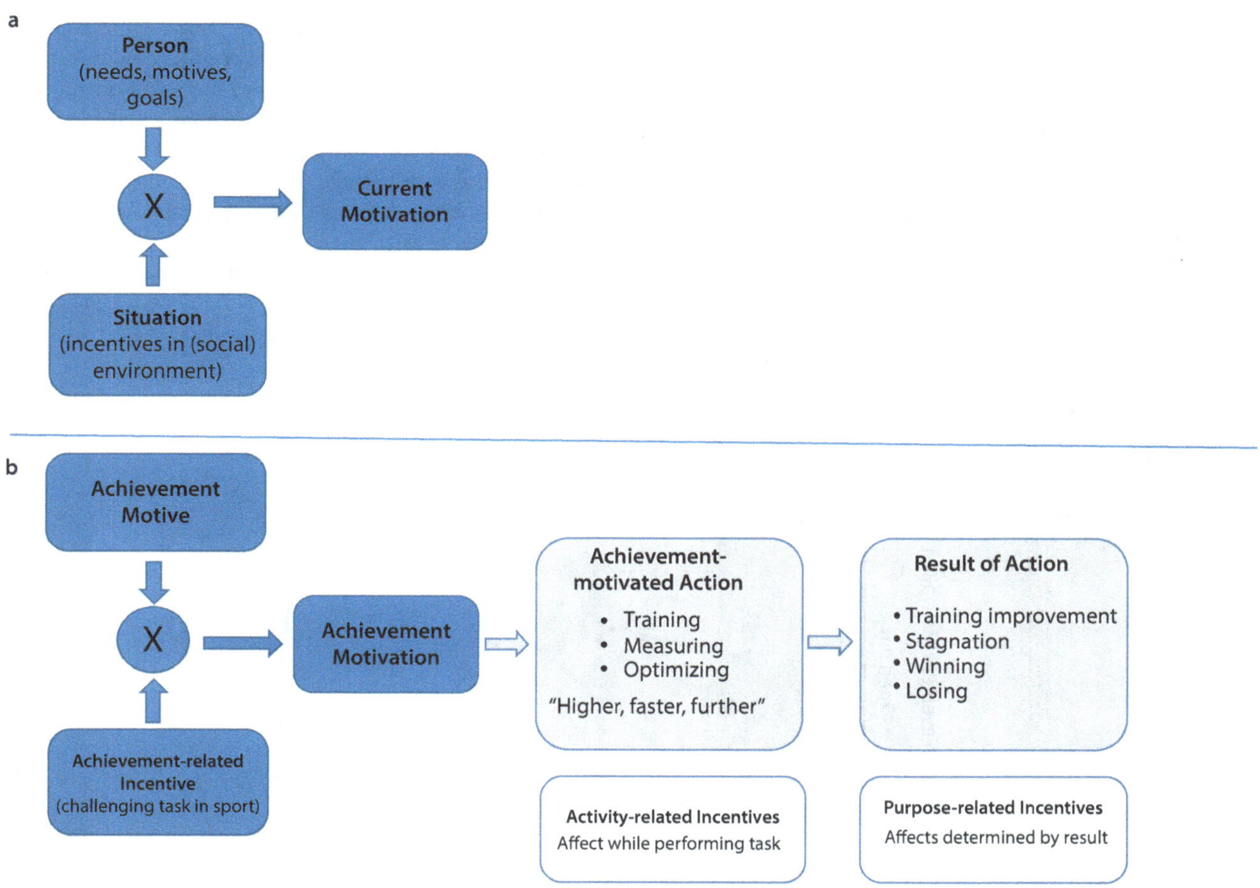

◘ **Fig. 7.2** **a** Basic model of the classical motivation psychology (according to Rheinberg, 2002). **b** An example of the achievement context. The figure also describes activity-related and purpose-related goals and affect

means that if either the expectancy or the value is zero, then the action does not take place because the product is zero. Atkinson's (1957) "risk taking model" describes the choice of goals which can be more or less "risky" in light of different failure probabilities. It thus explains the level of aspiration in setting achievement goals. Why do people, even if they have the same level of ability, still choose goals differing in difficulty? Some people choose easy goals (after 3 months of training to be able to jog 3 km without stopping), others goals with a medium difficulty (after 6 months of training to complete a half marathon), and yet others choose difficult tasks (after 6 months of training to complete a marathon in 3:15 h). Atkinson's model is a formalized model of achievement motivation, in which personal factors (the achievement motive) and situational factors (incentives and task difficulty) are taken into account. The following self-reflection task provides you with a deeper understanding of the model.

Model of Achievement Motivation

In the following, the main statements of the "model of achievement motivation" according to Atkinson (1957) are presented. Read each sentence, look for an example that personally applies to you, and then do the reasoning using ◘ Fig. 7.3. The help questions already suggest an example. Nevertheless, try to find an example that fits to you.

- The incentive for success increases with the difficulty of the task. → blue line; help question: How do you feel when you have completed a very easy task, and how do you feel when you have mastered a difficult task?
- The likelihood of success decreases with increasing task difficulty. → orange line; help question: How likely is it that you will be able to run the marathon in 3:15 h in half a year if you have not even started to train?
- Performance motivation is highest in moderately difficult tasks. This type of task has a medium incentive and a medium probability of success. → reversed U-form; help example: If you are aiming for a running time that is slightly faster than the time you have already run. The goal is demanding but feasible and will result in positive affect.

In his model, Atkinson (1957) adds a personal factor to explain the choice of tasks of varying difficulty. The left part of the ◘ Fig. 7.4 shows what already has been explained. Atkinson assumes that the relationship between the achievement motive and task difficulty only applies when individuals have high hopes for success. This refers to the approach component of the achievement motive (▸ Chap. 9). Success-motivated individuals are confident that they can succeed in tasks and want to know how good they are and how much they have improved. They therefore need a realistic reference to evaluate their performance standard. This can be done with feasible (moderately difficult) goals. On the other hand, people who are motivated by failure (or people with high fear of failure) fear being unsuccessful. They shy away from tasks that could give

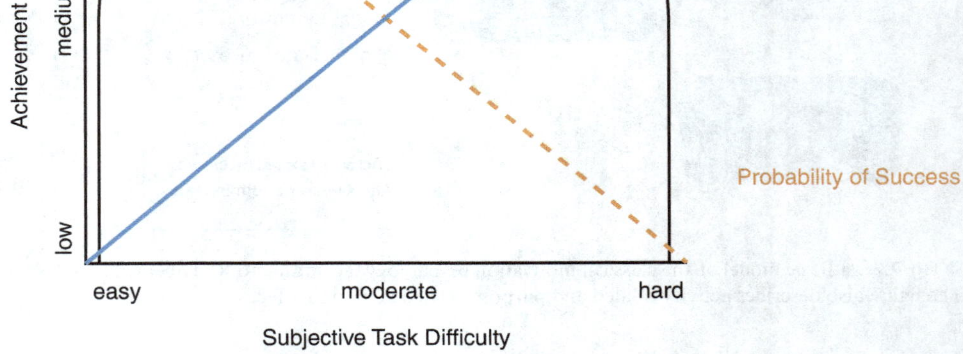

◘ **Fig. 7.3** Achievement motivation as a product of success incentive and the probability of success in differently difficult tasks (modified according to Atkinson, 1957)

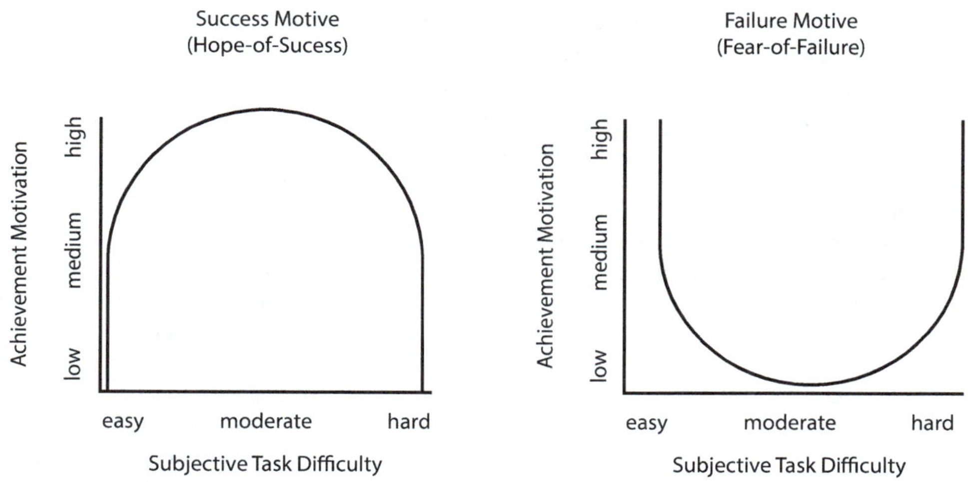

Fig. 7.4 Theoretical prediction of the risk taking model for individuals with hope for success and fear of failure (modified according to Atkinson, 1957)

them a realistic appraisal of their abilities. They choose tasks that are either too easy (these are likely to be achieved, but one does not pride oneself in their achievement) or too difficult (these are very unlikely to be achieved, but since the task was too difficult, the individual's self-esteem is not threatened: "The task was so difficult, no one could have succeeded"). This is shown in the right side of Fig. 7.4. The types of goals that individuals motivated by fear of failure choose may preserve their self-esteem, but by avoiding moderately difficult tasks it makes it impossible for them to receive a realistic appraisal of their own performance level and can also lead to suboptimal performance.

7.1.5 The Need for Motivation and Volition: The Rubicon Model of Action Phases

Once the individuals have contemplated the attraction and feasibility, and decided on a goal for action, they are likely to act. However, as Kuhl (1983) pointed out, action does not always follow these reflections. In other words, some individuals have difficulties implementing the intended action.

Key Points

Action initiation: Many people set New Year's resolutions (e.g., to lose weight) every year. However, more often than not, individuals fail to act on these goals. In other words, they experience problems translating their intentions or goals into action.

Action maintenance: Many people experience difficulties maintaining a goal-directed action over a longer period of time. Often, they fail to overcome obstacles (e.g., starting to train again after vacation, an injury, or illness).

When discussing motivation one also needs to discuss volition (choosing and evaluating the goal of an action). Due to volition's importance in the implementation of athletic goals, ► Chap. 10 focusses exclusively on this topic (► Chap. 10). Please read the detailed information about volition in sport in ► Chap. 10. Here we only briefly present the "Rubicon Model of Action Phases" by Heckhausen (Heckhausen, 1989) which describes the importance of differentiating between motivational and volitional processes (detailed presentation in ► Chap. 10). The "Rubicon Model" describes various phases and their specific function within an action. The four phases, which refer to both motivational and volitional processes, are described in detail in ► Chap. 10 (► Fig. 10.4). Here we would only like to address the terms "expectancy," "incentive," and "affect" already mentioned above. Weighing the expectancy (e.g., can I achieve the goal of going to the gym twice a week?) against the incentive (e.g., how valuable is it for me to achieve this?) leads to the formation of an intention, i.e., setting a goal (e.g., I want to go to the gym) if both expectancy and intention are positive. In order to implement this goal, volitional processes are necessary (e.g., planning the implementation of the goal, persisting even in the face of obstacles; ► Chap. 10). The evaluation of the goal (e.g., visiting the fitness studio or not) leads to certain affective responses, which in turn influence future action.

Höner and Willimczik (1998) applied the "Rubicon Model" to a variety of contexts and concluded that the model is well suited to explain numerous behaviors in sport, physical activity, and health. The model, for example, has been applied in the health context (Fuchs, 2001; example of an intention: I want to lose weight), in rehabilitation (Sudeck & Höner, 2011; example of an intention: I want to carry on with my physiotherapy exercises even after I have been discharged from the hospital), and in doping research (Kovar, 2009).

> Motivational and volitional processes need to complement each other during physical activity and in sports. Motivation determines the selection of goals and the evaluation of results. Volition helps to keep on moving towards the goals even when obstacles are encountered.

7.1.6 Goals and Goal Concepts

A very important element of any action in sport is the goal that is pursued. As the "Rubicon Model" outlines, the formation of a goal intention drives the further action. The goals, i.e., what is to be achieved or prevented, guide the action and give it direction.

Goals

According to Hacker (1998), goals are more or less conscious intentions of a person that refer to future, desired results of their actions. At the same time, goals contain cognitive representations of the desired results.

The goal concept—more precisely, the processes of goal formation (e.g., expectancy × value models, goals as an expression of motives), the analysis of structural characteristics of goals, and the goal commitment (strength of commitment to the goal)—is firmly anchored in psychological research, e.g., in social, motivation, organizational, and personality psychology (for an overview see Schüler & Brandstätter, 2010).

> **Structural Characteristics of Goals**
> The following structural characteristics of goals are of interest in psychological research, for example:
> - Direction of goals (approach vs. avoidance goals, ► Sect. 7.2.2)
> - Degree of agreement with underlying motives (motive congruence, ► Chap. 9)
> - Degree of self-determination (► Chap. 8)
> - Level of abstraction (specific goals; ► Sect. 7.5.1, goal theory)
> - Type of success criterion (► Sect. 7.5.1, learning vs. performance goals)

The goal setting theory which was originally developed in the organizational psychology context is also frequently used in sport psychology. Locke and Latham's "goal setting theory" (Locke & Latham, 1990; ► Sect. 7.5.1) defines the characteristics that a goal must have in order to be conducive to performance. The central assumption is that difficult, yet realistic, specific goals ("I want to improve my running time in the half marathon by 5 min") lead to higher performance compared to undemanding or less concrete goals ("I want to do my best!"). Specificity of goals is also central to "implementation intentions" (Gollwitzer, 1999; ► Chap. 10) and "action and coping planning" (Sniehotta et al., 2005). For example, specific goal intentions ("I want to be more physically active in order to stay fit and healthy") are better than no goals, because they create a certain goal commitment, yet they are still not sufficient to result in effective action. To result in action, goals need to be planned and a cue (e.g., time or situation) tied to the behavior (e.g., "Every Wednesday evening and Friday afternoon I will go to the gym for a one-hour aerobics class"). Coping planning helps to keep the goal on track despite encountering obstacles ("If I have to work longer on Wednesday and miss the aerobics class (obstacle), then I can jog home from work for half an hour instead"). In applied sports psychology, goal setting is an important tool to enhance self-regulation (► Chap. 20, ► Sect. 7.5.1). The following section outlines goal theories, which are frequently used in sport psychology research. In this section it will become clear that setting goals not only increases performance but also has an influence on athletes' well-being.

7.2 Performance-Motivated Actions and Goals in Sport

This section introduces the most frequently applied motivational theories and goal concepts in sports psychology.

7.2.1 Achievement Goal Theory

It is assumed that achievement-motivated individuals strive to demonstrate their abilities or competence in performance-related sport situations (Nicholls, 1984). In competitive sport, for example, the attraction is to find out who performs best and how far performance limits can be pushed (akin to the Olympic motto "faster, higher, further"). The "achievement goal theory" (Nicholls, 1984) differentiates between two distinct motivational orientations in relation to competence. On the one hand, athletes are motivated by situations where there is potential for social comparison or a competition. Success or failure is determined by comparing one's performance to that of others. This is called *performance orientation*. A performance-orientated individual wants to demonstrate his or her skills in front of others and measure himself or herself against them. If, however, the opponent's performance is better, which is very likely to happen in sport and is also uncontrollable, then this leads to disappointment, frustration, and a loss of motivation. This can also have a negative effect on feelings of competence (Duda & Hall, 2001).

Other athletes are attracted by situations in which they can learn something new or master a new task. This is called *task orientation*. The aim here is for individuals to develop competence and task mastery. Success or failure is not defined by the comparison with others but by a comparison with one's own performance. Task-oriented athletes are concerned about improving their own individual standards regardless of how they compare to others, and they then to experience less fear of failure and to perceive higher levels of competence (Table 7.1).

The "achievement goal theory" (AGC; Nicholls, 1984) distinguishes between the following:

- Performance orientation (ego orientation; focus on performance outcome and competition)
- Task orientation (mastery orientation; focus on learning and mastering a task)

It should be noted that combinations of these two orientations often exist. For example, athletes may show both a high task orientation and a high performance orientation, or both may be low. It is also possible to be high in one orientation and low in the other (Nicholls, 1984). Further support for this perspective comes from Hodge and Petlichkoff (2000) who conducted a cluster analysis of goal orientation profiles in sport. Their results revealed that groups emerged having motivational profiles that may be high on one orientation and low on the other. Additionally, according to Hanrahan and Cerin (2009), female athletes are typically more task orientated than male athletes. Individual athletes tend to be more performance oriented than team athletes.

A high level of task orientation is associated with greater enjoyment, intrinsic interest and satisfaction, lower fear of failure, greater commitment to practice and learning, and a greater willingness to invest effort. For athletes high in task orientation, cooperating with others is an important aspect of athletic success (Duda & Nicholls, 1992), and they perceive their social relations as more positive than individuals with strong performance orientations. Athletes high in performance orientation believe that it is mainly their performance that leads to success. Their reason for participating in sports is to increase their social status through being successful and achieving fame. However, performance-oriented athletes also experience greater anxiety and are less willing to invest effort when difficulties arise. For them, sport is all about comparing their performance with others and making an impression on others (Duda & Hall, 2001; Roberts, 2001). In addition, performance orientation seems to be correlated with deviant, unsportsmanlike, and antisocial behavior in sport (Kavussanu, 2006; Sage & Kavussanu, 2008; Fig. 7.5) and with a more positive attitude towards doping (Barkoukis et al., 2011).

Table 7.1 Two types of achievement goals. In addition to Nicholls (1984), other researchers have also differentiated two orientations towards achievement but named the goals that result from these orientations differently. The terms originate from different research traditions and fields of application (e.g., education, sport), yet are conceptually similar (see Ames, 1992, for details about conceptual differences)

Nicholls (1984)	Performance goals	Task-oriented goals
Elliot and Dweck (1988)	Performance goals	Learning goals
Duda (1987), Maehr and Nicholls (1980)	Ego-involvement goals	Task-involvement goals
Ames and Archer (1988), Dweck (1986)	Performance goals	Mastery goals

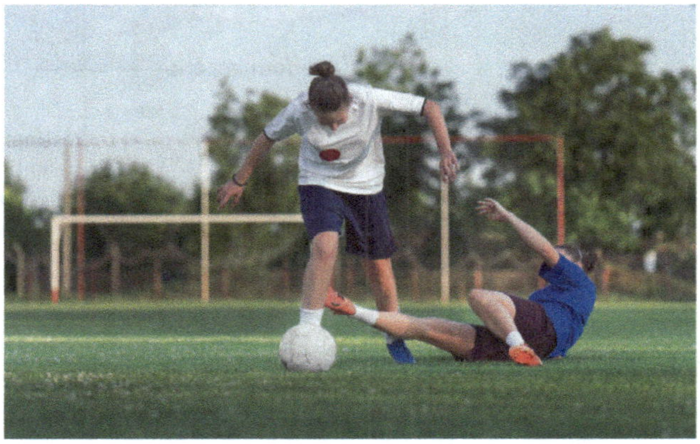

Fig. 7.5 Performance orientation (ego orientation) as one of many reasons for fouling in football

7.2.2 Approach Versus Avoidance Goals

Another aspect of the "achievement goal theory" deals with approach and avoidance goals (Elliot, 1999). It is assumed that experiencing competence is not only determined by mastery versus performance orientation but also by approach versus avoidance goals. Athletes can either focus their attention on experiencing competence (e.g., training regularly on a treadmill to improve endurance) or on avoiding incompetence (e.g., going to the gym regularly to avoid appearing unfit). Avoidance goals constantly remind athletes of the negative consequences. This can create stress and anxiety and reduce the joy of pursuing goals. Furthermore, avoidance goals can have a negative impact on self-esteem, feelings of control, and competence perceptions. On the other hand, athletes who set approach goals perceive themselves as competent and self-determined. A distinction should therefore be made between performance and mastery orientation as well as between approach and avoidance goals. Figure 7.6 shows the four categories that result when approach/avoidance is combined with performance/mastery and the assumed effects.

7

Examples of Combinations

In addition to task and performance orientation, the "achievement goal theory" distinguishes between approach and avoidance goals. This results in four combinations, which are illustrated in the following with examples:

- Mastery approach goal: "I would like to take part in the community run to improve my personal best time."
- Mastery avoidance goal: "I want to participate in the fun/community run to avoid running slower than my personal best."
- Performance approach goal: "I want to take part in the race to win and beat my competitor."
- Performance avoidance goals: "I will take part in the race and don't want to lose against my competitor."

A large number of studies have investigated the relationship between goal orientations and sport. Approach goals (both task oriented and performance oriented), for example, are positively correlated with the physical activity levels of university students (Lochbaum et al., 2013). In contrast, avoidance goals (both task-oriented and achievement-oriented goals) are correlated with a variety of negative outcomes like anxiety and amotivation (Ommundsen, 2004). If the focus is to promote performance, then the focus should lie on approach goals (Excursus: Regulation Focus Theory).

Fig. 7.6 Assumed effects of performance approach, performance avoidance, mastery approach, and mastery avoidance goals

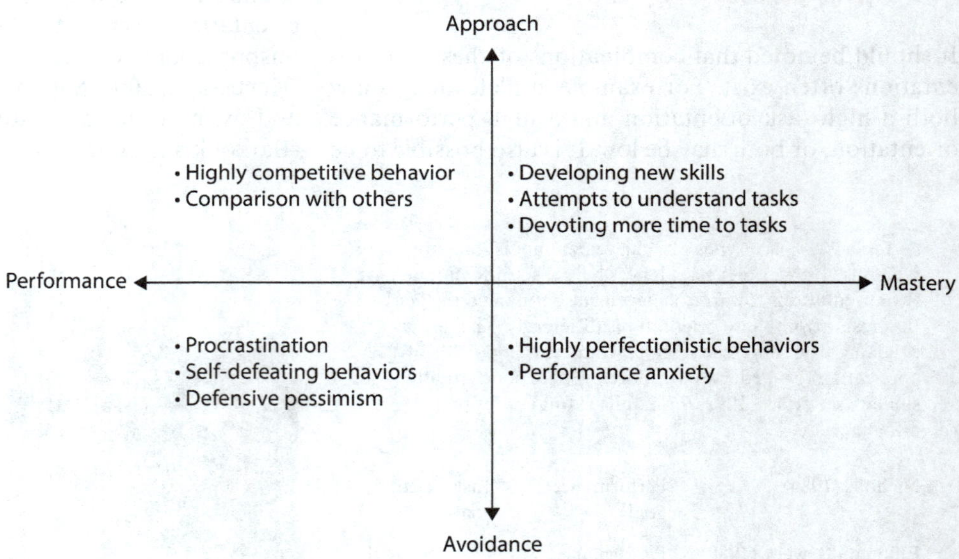

The 2 (mastery, performance) × 2 (approach, avoidance) approach (Conroy et al., 2003; Elliot & McGregor, 2001) has been expanded to a 3 × 2 approach (Elliot et al., 2011) and has been applied to sport (Mascret et al., 2015). In this approach, mastery goals have been separated into self-based and task-based categories. Self-based goals focus on how one is doing relative to one's own trajectory (e.g., degree to which one is improving in sports), whereas task-based goals focus on how one is doing relative to the absolute demands of the task or activity (i.e., to what degree the task has been accomplished).

? Examples from the 3 × 2 Achievement Goal Questionnaire for Sport (3 × 2 AGQ-S) (Mascret et al., 2015) are as follows: In my sport my aim is …

- Task approach goal: to perform well
- Task avoidance goal: to avoid performing badly.
- Self-approach goal: to do better than what I usually do
- Self-avoidance goal: to avoid having worse results than I had previously

Side Story

Although the "regulatory focus theory" ("RFT") by Higgins (1997, 2000) is not by definition an achievement motivation theory, it still warrants mentioning here because it is frequently applied in the context of performance and shows similarities with approach and avoidance goals. This motivation theory deals with the importance of self-regulation for goal achievement. The basic underlying assumption of the "regulatory focus theory" is that people approach pleasant things and tend to stay away from unpleasant things. However, people differ with regard to what they perceive to be pleasant or unpleasant and which goals they pursue. The RFT distinguishes between two types of self-regulatory foci for goal achievement, namely, promotion and prevention. When the individual is focused on promotion, attention is paid to striving for and achieving positive states. People with a promotion focus are concerned with maximizing profits in the diverse areas of life (e.g., learning new sport skills, performing successfully) and with self-fulfillment (e.g., the best possible performance development, kinesthetic experiences). Individuals with a promotion focus are active, energetic, creative, and occasionally also engage in risky behaviors. In contrast, people with a prevention focus are characterized by being responsible and acting safe. For them it is very important to act in the way others think they should. They are concerned with minimizing losses (e.g., avoiding muscle loss in old age). People with a prevention focus are more passive, cautious, and conservative (they follow the rules). It is assumed that these foci are relatively stable personality traits. They must, however, be distinguished from situational foci, which are triggered by avoidance or approach situations.

Neither focus has a performance advantage in sport in itself, but they do influence athletes' motivation and goals. Typically, athletes tend to have a chronic focus on promotion rather than prevention (Unkelbach et al., 2009). To optimize sport performance, the decisive factor seems to be whether the athlete is in a situation that is aligned with their stable (preferred) focus. This is what Higgins (2000) calls the regulatory fit (RFT). Plessner et al. (2009) showed that footballers benefited from a regulatory fit when performing penalty kicks, and in their table football studies, Memmert et al. (2015) were able to show that collective fit is also an important predictor of team success.

7.2.3 Questionnaires to Measure Goal Orientations in Sport

Several questionnaires exist to measure goal orientations in sport. In this section we will present the "Task and Ego in Sport Questionnaire" and the "Sport Orientation Questionnaire."

7.2.3.1 Task and Ego Orientation in Sport Questionnaire (TEOSQ-Sport)

The "Task and Ego Orientation in Sport Questionnaire (TEOSQ-Sport)" by Duda (1989) examines to what extent the respondents are attracted by task-oriented or competitive situations in sport. Seven items measure task orientation and six items ego orientation. Items are evaluated on a five-point scale, which ranges from "strongly agree" to "strongly disagree."

Methods Box

The Task and Ego Orientation in Sport Questionnaire (Duda, 1989)

I feel most successful in sport when…

	Strongly Disagree	Disagree	Neutral	Agree	Strongly Agree
1) I am the only one who can do the play or skill	0	1	2	3	4
2) I learn a new skill, and it makes me want to practice more	0	1	2	3	4
3) I can do better than my friends	0	1	2	3	4
4) The others cannot do as well as me	0	1	2	3	4
5) I learn something that is fun to do	0	1	2	3	4
6) Others mess up, but I do not	0	1	2	3	4
7) I learn a new skill by trying hard	0	1	2	3	4
8) I work hard	0	1	2	3	4
9) I score the most points/goals/hits, etc.	0	1	2	3	4
10) Something I learn makes me want to practice more	0	1	2	3	4
11) I am the best	0	1	2	3	4
12) A skill I learn feels right	0	1	2	3	4
13) I do my very best	0	1	2	3	4

Orange = Items that measure ego orientation
Blue = Items that measure task orientation

7

7.2.3.2 Sport Orientation Questionnaire (SOQ)

The "Sport Orientation Questionnaire" (SOQ; Gill & Deeter, 1988) is a multidimensional, sport-specific measure of individual differences in sport achievement orientations. Gill and Deeter (1988) distinguish between three motivational orientations in sport, namely, competitiveness, the desire to enter and strive for success in sport-specific situations (6 items, e.g., "I look forward to competing"); win orientation, the desire to win interpersonal competitive sporting events (13 items, e.g., "The only time I am satisfied is when I win"); and goal orientation, the desire to achieve personal goals in sport (6 items, e.g., "Reaching personal performance goals is very important to me"). Each item is rated on a scale from "1 = strongly disagree" to "5 = strongly agree."

Reflection

1. Fill out both questionnaires and calculate your values for the subscales (see coding instructions).
2. Interpret what the values suggest regarding your goals in sport.
3. Describe similarities and differences between the two questionnaires and critically consider which one is most suitable to your context.

Which inferences about sport participation can be made on the basis of the questionnaire scores? Studies applying the SOQ showed, for example, that competitiveness is higher in competitive athletes than among people who are not active in competitive sports (Elbe, 2004). In a longitudinal study with young elite Norwegian athletes, Hellandsig (1998) showed that high competitiveness and low win orientation values positively predicted future athletic performance over a period of 3 years. Höner and Feichtinger (2016) used the SOQ for talent diagnostics in the German Football Association and found that high competitiveness and a high goal orientation could positively predict football success over a period of 4 years (► Chap. 23).

Case Example: Applied Sport Psychology

During a sport psychology consultation session, a 17-year-old canoeist from the junior national team complained that he lacked motivation in training and expressed a desire to change this. His SOQ results indicated normal range values in competitiveness and win orientation. This means that he likes to measure himself against others to assess his performance and that winning was important to him. However, his goal orientation scores were in the lower norm range suggesting that comparing his performance with his own previous performance seemed rather unimportant to him. What is your suggestion for improving this athlete's motivation?

However, it is not only the athletes' individual goals that are important for keeping up regular training but also the interpersonal atmosphere in the sports or training group. Motivational climate describes the psychological atmosphere that surrounds the athlete and is created by, e.g., the coach.

7.3 Motivational Climate

The motivational climate in which a sporting activity takes place can vary. A task-oriented climate is characterized by a focus on learning, skill development, and individual performance improvement. Mistakes are seen as an important element of the learning process, and learner effort and perseverance are rewarded. On the contrary, a performance-oriented climate (also referred to as an ego-oriented climate) is characterized by a focus on winning, comparison with others, and punishment of mistakes. A systematic review of the intrapersonal correlates of motivational climates in sport and physical activity (Harwood et al., 2008) based on more than 34,000 data sets revealed that a task-oriented climate is associated with a variety of positive consequences for motivation, including the experience of competence, performance, intrinsic motivation, flow experience, and self-esteem. In contrast, a performance climate in sport is related to maladaptive strategy use, negative affect, perfectionism, extrinsic forms of motivation and amotivation, and reduced feelings of social relatedness and autonomy.

The motivational climate in sport and physical activity has an impact on achievement goal setting of participants. A task-oriented climate is associated with task-oriented goals of participants, whereas a performance-oriented climate is often associated with performance-oriented goals of participants (Duda & Hall, 2001). Wang et al. (2010) used structural equation mixture modeling and demonstrated that the nature of the motivational climate predicted the type of achievement goals, and subsequently students' enjoyment in a physical education setting.

7.3.1 Questionnaires to Measure Sport Motivational Climate

The "Perceived Motivational Climate in Sports Questionnaire" (PMCSQ) by Seifriz et al. (1992) (see also) (Fry et al., 1993) assesses the motivational climate. The questionnaire consists of two subscales, namely, mastery (or task-involving) climate ("On this team, trying hard is rewarded") and performance-oriented (ego-involving) climate ("On this team, the coach gives most of his attention to the 'stars'"). The "Motivational Climate Scale for Youth Sports" (MCSYS; Smith et al., 2008) is suitable for children and young adults and also assesses both aspects of the motivational climate.

7.3.2 How Does One Change the Motivational Climate in Sports Groups? Motivational Climate Intervention

The motivational climate influences participants' motivation and goals in sports and is strongly shaped by the leader. Leaders in the sport context can include PE teachers, trainers, and coaches. Such individuals are in a position to influence behavior by cultivating either an adaptive or maladaptive motivational climate. An unfavorable motivational climate in a sports group is characterized by instilling fear, being unempathetic, and providing performance-contingent rewards, for instance, and should be changed. Research on how to bring about changes in the motivational climate have mostly been investigated in the context of physical education and are mainly based on Ames' (1992) "TARGET model" (▪ Table 7.2). Interventions based on the TARGET model focus on the tasks, the authority behavior, the reward and recognition by the teacher, the grouping, the evaluation as well as the time allocated for certain tasks. Four of the elements of the "TARGET model" refer to how the teaching content or units should be structured. The other two elements of the model refer to the actual teaching behavior. Studies show that teachers familiar with the TARGET model are more successful at creating a more task-oriented and less performance-oriented (or

Table 7.2 Elements of an intervention applying the TARGET model (based on Ames, 1992)

Task: Task design	Content	Tasks/exercises are characterized by: • Variety • Novelty • Challenging • Meaningfulness
Authority: Decision-making process	Content	Tasks/exercises are designed to: • Enable all students/players to participate in the activities • Enable students/players to engage in own decision making (e.g., creation of own goals, designing activities)
Reward/recognition: Manner of distribution of rewards	Behavior	Teachers/coaches should reinforce and encourage: • Individual effort • Persistence
Grouping: Selection of working groups	Content	Tasks/exercises are performed in groups: • Flexible grouping arrangements during/between lessons/training sessions • Mixed groups (each group should include students/players which differ in ability/gender/ethnicity)
Evaluation: Manner of evaluation of performance standards	Behavior	Teachers/coaches should give: • Explicit and frequent information about individual progress (Private, not public)
Time: Pace of learning	Content	Tasks/exercises should provide teacher/coach with: • Time to give sound instructions for tasks to perform Tasks/exercises should provide students/players with: • Time for task completion • Time for reflection of own improvement

ego-oriented) learning environment (Perlman & Goc Karp, 2007). The "TARGET model" can be successfully applied in physical education (Braithwaite et al., 2011). Elbe et al. (2021) used the TARGET approach to change the motivational climate in PE classes that had a high proportion of pupils from a migrant background. The change in the motivational climate was expected to increase the pupils' feelings of inclusion. The results showed that the use of the "TARGET model" could reduce the performance-oriented climate in PE lessons and increase feelings of inclusion. These results are an indication that a change in the motivational climate can have a positive effect on group processes.

Smoll et al. (2007) conducted a different type of intervention to change the motivational climate in basketball teams. In a 75-min training session, they instructed coaches on how to strengthen positive behavior, encourage mistakes, formulate positive suggestions for improvement, and give understandable technical instructions. The coaches were also taught how to avoid punishing mistakes, how to create rules of behavior for the team, and how to promote prosocial behavior between players. This training at the beginning of the season led to a higher perception of the task and a lower perception of performance climate. Similarly, Ntoumanis et al. (2018) explored the efficacy of a motivationally informed antidoping intervention targeted at coaches and found that, when compared with a control condition involving standard antidoping workshops, the athletes of coaches in the intervention group were less willing to take prohibited substances and reported lower psychological need frustration. Coaches in the intervention group also perceived greater effectiveness of need-supporting behaviors, and reduced effectiveness of need thwarting behaviors, pertaining to doping-related situations. These findings highlight the potential of incorporating principles of motivation in coaching, to guide athletes towards more adaptive outcomes.

Another approach that is used to change the motivational climate is empowering coaching (Duda & Appleton, 2016), which is discussed in more detail in ► Chap. 8. This program teaches coaches how to create a task-oriented climate that simultaneously satisfies the basic psychological needs for autonomy, competence, and social relatedness. Irrespective of the motivational climate that prevails in the sports environment and athletes' personal goals, it is possible in almost all sports situations to experience either success or failure. These are central elements of motivation, which will be discussed in the following section. In addition, peer motivational climate has also shown to be of relevance in predicting adaptive outcomes (Ntoumanis et al., 2012). A longitudinal examination of adolescent athletes revealed that task-involving peer and coach climates predicted more adaptive outcomes, highlighting the need to consider peer influence in youth sport motivation (Ntoumanis et al., 2012).

7.4 Dealing with Success and Failure: Attribution Theory

Athletic success (e.g., finally mastering a difficult floor routine in gymnastics, winning the 100 m sprint) and failure (e.g., constantly falling off the balancing beam, being the last one to finish a race), which can be observed particularly well in professional sport on television, obviously result in affective reactions such as pride, euphoria, shame, or disappointment. Success and failures thus have a decisive influence on the future motivation to engage in exercise and sports. Attribution theories (Heider, 1958; Kelley, 1973; Weiner et al., 1971) are cognitive theories and are based on the assumption that individuals do not just simply accept their successes and failures but try to find explanations for them. Attribution theories describe the information that is used to explain cause-effect relationships. The various justifications for successes and failures can be described using the dimensions locus of causality (within the person: internal; outside of the person: external) and temporal stability (stable, unstable). Typical attributions for success which combine the two categories are effort (internal, unstable), ability (internal, stable), luck (external, unstable), and task difficulty (external, stable). Examples of attribution for failures include lack of effort, lack of talent, bad luck, and the task being too difficult. ◘ Figure 7.7 illustrates the different types of attribution. Robinson and Howe (1989) investigated athletes' attributions and found that they have a major influence on their subsequent affective reactions. After a competition, for example, athletes can experience pride, shame, or anger. Athletes feel proud when their success can be attributed to effort ("the athlete trained hard"). If an unexpected failure is attributed to a lack of talent, then athletes will experience shame ("not as talented for gymnastics as expected"). Joy is felt especially when the success was unexpected or occurs by chance, whereas anger is felt when unexpected failures are attributed to, for example, a task that was too difficult. These emotions in turn impact athletes' future motivational states in training and competitions. The dimension "locus of causality" (internal vs. external) determines the emotions following success or failure. ◘ Figure 7.7 also shows:

- The dimension of stability determines future expectations. If a person considers the cause of the success or failure to be stable, he or she will expect the same result in the future.
- The dimension locus of causality, on the other hand, determines affect. If a person considers himself or herself responsible for a success or failure (internal), strong positive affect occurs (e.g., pride, joy, guilt, sadness). If external causes for the failure can be found, then the affect intensity will be lower.

Two examples: Susanne experiences success in her PE lesson in gymnastics. After practicing for a long time, she manages to do a handstand on her own for the first time. If she attributes this success to a stable cause, namely, her good athletic abilities, she will expect this success to be repeated as she learns other gymnastic skills. She will be motivated and confident to face further tasks in her gymnastics lessons. She may even ask her parents if she can join a gymnastics club. However, if Tim attributes his successful salto on the trampoline to luck, he will not expect to succeed in the next jump.

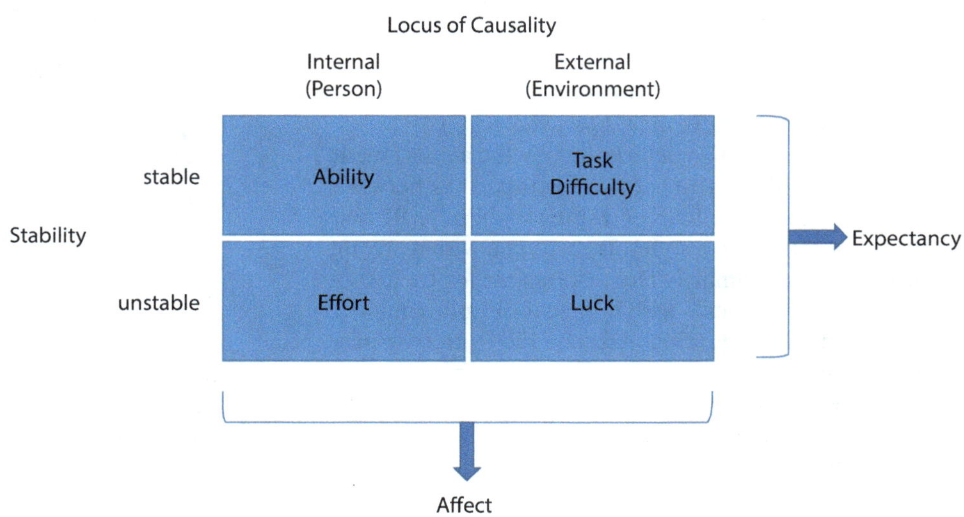

◘ **Fig. 7.7** Reasons for achievement results according to Weiner et al. (1971)

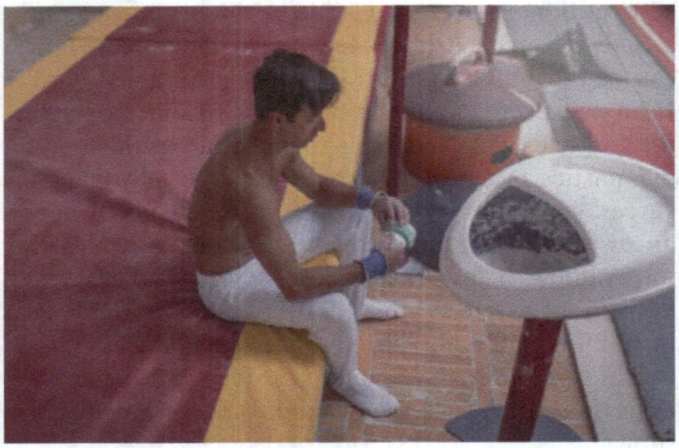

Fig. 7.8 Which attributions does this gymnast make for his unsuccessful routine on the high bar?

This successful salto will have no effect on his future motivation nor on his self-confidence. It is rather unlikely that he will develop an interest in learning more trampoline tricks or in becoming a member of the trampoline club. These examples show that the dimension "temporal stability" (stable, variable) determines expectancy of future success and failure. Expectations are important determinants of future motivation to engage in sport, in addition to affect (which result from internal or external attribution) (Fig. 7.8). However, attributions are also made after unsuccessful performances in gymnastics. Failure can also be attributed to a stable cause (e.g., low ability), which is unconducive for self-confidence and motivation. It would be preferable to attribute failure to a variable cause, since this does not have such negative consequences on the individual's self-evaluation. Blaming bad luck (variable and external) for failure is beneficial for one's self-esteem but may not be conducive for learning how to avoid failures in the future (bad luck cannot be influenced). Therefore, a variable, but internal, attribution like a "lack of effort" is more appropriate in learning contexts. Although it blames the person for the failure ("I may not have trained enough"), it gives a direction for future behavior ("If I practice more next time, I can succeed").

Attributions are also determined by the achievement motive. The achievement motive distinguishes between hope for success and fear of failure (► Chap. 9) and impacts the attribution styles. Individuals with a strong hope for success primarily feel responsible for their success, whereas individuals with high fear of failure mainly focus on their failures (Heckhausen, 1989). In case of a failure, success-motivated individuals attribute it to a lack of effort. This does not challenge their self-worth as much as a stable attribution (e.g., "I simply have no talent"), and individuals will expect to be successful in the future ("If I try harder next time, it will work out"). In other words, individuals remain confident about being successful. In contrast, failure-motivated individuals tend to blame their (stable) lack of talent for their failure ("I'm too stupid to understand that. I will never be athletic") which has negative consequences for their self-worth. This leads to negative affect and reduces future success expectations, because a stable factor cannot be changed quickly or at all. Weiner (1986) later added the dimension of controllability to the two dimensions introduced above: locus of causality and stability. Are the causes of success or failure controllable? According to Rees et al. (2005), controllability is the decisive factor when attributing failure. Irrespective of whether the cause of a failure lies inside or outside of the person, the question of whether the cause can be controlled or not is of the utmost importance for subsequent affect.

Reflection

You won a swim race. What are the reasons for this success? How do you attribute this success? You can attribute success to the following causes:

- Your swimming talent is the reason why you won (internal, stable, uncontrollable).
- You were lucky (external, variable, uncontrollable).
- You invested a lot of effort (internal, variable, controllable) in the last 10 m.
- You won because the opponents in the 50 m are weak (external, stable, uncontrollable).
- You paced the race well (internal, variable, controllable).
- Your opponents had poor endurance (external, variable, uncontrollable).

You struggle to go to the gym regularly and therefore cancel your membership. You can attribute your failure to exercise regularly to the following causes:

- You're no good at exercising (internal, stable, uncontrollable)
- The ridiculous fitness trainers who work there (external, variable, uncontrollable).
- Your back pain (internal, variable, controllable in principle).
- The gym is too far away from your home (external, stable, uncontrollable).
- Your lack of effort (internal, variable, controllable).
- The high membership fees (external, stable, uncontrollable).

Hanrahan and Cerin (2009) investigated gender, sport type, and level of participation differences in athletes' attributions. Individual sport athletes made more internal, stable, and global and less externally controllable attributions for positive events, and more internal attributions for negative events, than team sport athletes. Female competitive athletes made less global attributions for positive events than recreational athletes. This difference, however, could not be found in male athletes. Competitive individual athletes, not team athletes, made less global attributions than recreational individual athletes. These results indicate that sport psychologists might want to especially focus on team sport athletes to help them form favorable, performance-enhancing attributions. But what is a favorable, performance-enhancing attribution?

7.4.1 Self-Serving Attributional Bias

When finding reasons for one's own success and failure, a hedonistic distortion tendency can be seen, albeit more typically for Western cultures. In other words, people tend to see the causes for their successes coming from within, whereas failure is attributed to external factors. This attribution pattern, namely, to attribute success to oneself and to regard the causes for this success as stable and controllable, and to explain reasons for failure as unstable and uncontrollable, fits to peoples' general tendency to perceive themselves in an overly favorable manner. This phenomenon is called "self-serving bias" (Miller & Ross, 1975) and aims at building up or enhancing one's positive self-esteem. A cognitive technique that contributes to self-serving bias is self-serving attributions (attributing success to oneself and failure to external factors). They can be observed among individual and team sport athletes as well as among sport spectators (Allen, 2012). As already mentioned, success-motivated individuals (high in the hope-for-success component of the achievement motive) show exactly this attribution pattern.

Studies about self-serving attributions in sport show that other factors also have an influence on how frequently they occur. Male athletes more often form self-serving attributions than female athletes (Green & Holeman, 2004). This is explained by gender differences with regard to personality and indicates that women are characterized by greater conscientiousness and emotional stability (Allen et al., 2011). Furthermore, sporting experience seems to have an influence on how often self-esteem-promoting attributions are made. The longer people are involved in sport and the greater their sport abilities, the less likely they are to attribute in a self-serving manner (Grove & Prapavessis, 1995; Hamilton & Jordan, 2000). The self-serving bias has the advantage of building up or maintaining positive self-esteem. The disadvantage, however, is that learning from mistakes is hindered because only external factors are considered when explaining failure.

7.4.2 Team-Serving Attributional Bias

In team sports there is a specific type of attribution also known as group or team-serving attributional bias (Greenlees et al., 2007; Taylor & Doria, 1981). After success (e.g., winning a game), individuals are more likely to make internal, stable, and controllable attributions for the team's performance (e.g., good strategy, successful teamplay). In contrast, after failure, group members are more likely to use attributions that protect a positive image of the team. Specifically, team members are more likely to use external, unstable, and uncontrollable factors to explain poor performance (e.g., losing a game) such as unfair referees and cheating of opponents.

Individual and team sport athletes differ in their attribution style. Individual athletes tend to attribute more internally than team athletes. This means that individual athletes tend to feel solely responsible for their performance and rarely believe that external factors influenced their behavior. Instead of looking for reasons for success and failure in themselves, team athletes are likely to look for attributions in relation to the team (Allen et al. 2011; Shapcott et al., 2010). This means that team athletes make both self-serving and team-serving attributions (Sherman & Kim, 2005).

7.4.3 Attribution Training

Self-serving attributions can strengthen self-esteem, yet they can also prevent individuals from learning from their mistakes. Attributions play a key role for well-being and athletic performance (e.g., "I earned this win due to my hard work"; "I am capable of performing well"). It is worth noting that attributions are thoughts that can be altered. One method of changing attributions is attribution training. In attribution training, athletes are trained in how to change their attributions so that they have a positive effect on, for example, effort, future motivation, or success. In attribution training, athletes must first become aware of their attribution style. How do they attribute success and failure? If, for example, an athlete attributes success exclusively to external factors (e.g., luck) and failures to internal factors (e.g., "I lack talent"), this can have a negative impact on the athlete's sport motivation and self-esteem. It is therefore important to work with the athlete to ensure that success is attributed to internal factors and failure to external factors. It is particularly useful to pay attention to effort. Effort is a controllable attribution which athletes can influence and regulate themselves. If a failure is blamed on a lack of effort, then this can be improved next time. Attribution training can also be applied in team sports. Here one can work on attributing failures to controllable factors, e.g., lack of effort or a bad strategy. For teams, the recommendation is to focus on internal, controllable, and unstable attributions.

7.5 How Can Motivation for Physical Activity and Sport Be Enhanced?

One of the most important questions with regard to physical activity and sport is how to ensure that individuals remain active throughout their lifespan. Motivation is often questioned when physical activity levels are low. Within physical activity promotion the central question is how to motivate individuals to be regularly physically active (► Chaps. 10, 15, and 25). In competitive sports, the question is how athletes can stay intrinsically motivated, experience well-being, and perform their best.

7.5.1 Goal Setting Training

Goal setting is one of the most widely used motivational techniques. According to Locke and Latham's (1990) "goal setting theory" introduced above, successful goals, i.e., those that are more likely to be achieved, are characterized by being difficult, yet attainable, and specific. Setting ambitious and clearly formulated goals increases the probability of achieving them. Furthermore, setting specific and difficult goals leads to increased attention, effort, and persistence which is likely to result in better performance.

Important

The central assumptions of the "goal setting theory" were empirically tested in many studies (Locke & Latham, 2006):

- The effect of setting difficult goals: Setting difficult goals results in better performance than setting easy goals.
- The effect of setting specific goals: Setting specific goals results in better performance than the setting of vague, unspecific goals or compared to setting no goals at all.

Furthermore, one distinguishes between different types of goals, namely, outcome, performance, and process goals.

Definition

Outcome goals in the sport setting involve striving for results in a competition, e.g., a certain placement in a race or a specific rank in a league table.

Performance goals refer to striving for a performance in relation to a standard or reference level set by the athlete. Individual performance parameters refer to self-referenced standards of performance. They refer only to the athlete herself/himself. Examples include a 10-min improvement in a marathon run or an increase in the number of repetitions on the leg press to 35.

Process goals allude to how certain skills or strategies are implemented and deal with the qualitative execution of an action. Examples of process goals include a good feeling in the foot during a jump or a calm or regular steady breathing while jogging.

Research on how successful goal training is and which goals are most suitable for achieving excellence is not entirely consistent (Burton et al., 1998). However, this may be a result of contextual differences, such as training and competition situations, which have been previously neglected (Weinberg et al., 2000). Additionally, the effect of goal training is likely to vary as a function of several factors such as goal proximity, commitment, specificity, difficulty, and feedback (Kingston & Wilson, 2008). One reason for the difficulties of transferring the results of Locke and Latham's general "goal setting theory" to the sports context is that their theory was developed in organizational psychology, a field in which goals are often set externally. However, compared to the employment sector, sport is a voluntary activity, and therefore goals tend to be self-chosen (rather than externally determined).

In sport, goal setting training has proven to be a successful technique for increasing performance. It is advantageous to

- Set difficult and specific goals
- Link short and long-term goals
- Pursue a combination of different types of goals (e.g., outcome, process, and performance goals; Burton & Weiss, 2008)

An example of an advantageous goal likely to increase performance would be: I want to run a half marathon in Zurich in 6 months with a time that is less than 2 h. This

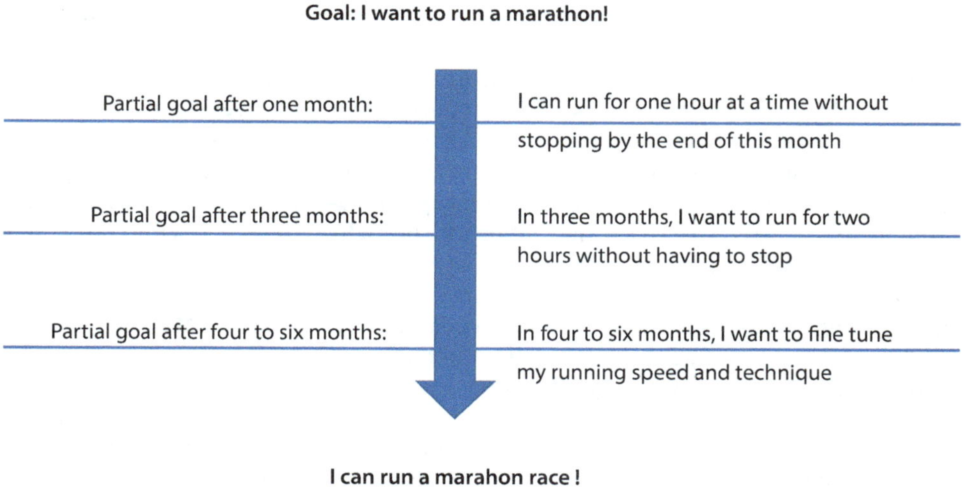
Goal: I want to run a marathon!
Partial goal after one month:
I can run for one hour at a time without stopping by the end of this month
Partial goal after three months:
In three months, I want to run for two hours without having to stop
Partial goal after four to six months:
In four to six months, I want to fine tune my running speed and technique
I can run a marahon race !

Fig. 7.9 Partial goals when planning to run a marathon

is a difficult, specific long-term goal. The achievement of this goal can be supported by formulating process goals (e.g., to develop a good running feeling during training) and result goals (e.g., to be in the midfield with my running time in Zurich). Since the overall goal is long term, its achievement can be further supported by formulating partial goals (Fig. 7.9).

Studies show that many athletes independently set at least two different types of goals (Jones & Hanton, 1996). Outcome-oriented goals can, under certain circumstances (e.g., if they only refer to the place/rank), lead to increased anxiety levels and even to withdrawal from the competition. Kingston and Hardy's (1997) study, for example, showed that golfers who formulated process goals (e.g., focus on an even swing) were better able to concentrate and control negative thoughts than golfers who had result-oriented goals (e.g., fewer strokes than my competitor). Furthermore, process goals, as opposed to outcome and performance goals, are a strong positive predictor of a psychological flow state (Kingston & Goldea, 2007), which has several benefits in terms of sport performance and well-being. Goals can also have a negative impact on performance. If the individual commits to goals that they think are unrealistic because their confidence to succeed is low, it may lead to fear of failure. In goal setting training it is therefore crucial that athletes set goals that they accept themselves and which can be internalized. Research indicates that a multi-goal strategy with a balance between outcome, performance, and process goals leads to the best performance (Filby et al., 1999). In addition, athletes must learn which type of goals are best suited at which time points and for the achievement of which goals. It is also important to divide goals into subgoals and to distinguish between short-, medium-, and long-term goals. Goals should always be set in a *SMART way*.

How SMART Is Your Goal?

SMART goals (Bull et al., 1996) are more likely to be successfully translated into behavior if they are:

- Specific (instead of inaccurate/global)
- Measurable (How do I determine goal progress?)
- Attainable (adapt it to the circumstances)
- Realistic (Are my abilities and my time budget sufficient?)
- Time-bound (deadline)

More recently, MacLeod (2012) has argued in favor of "making SMART goals SMARTER," by also making goals "engaging" (creating a sense of ownership and involvement) and "rewarding" (providing a sense of accomplishment or purpose).

7.5.2 Setting the Right Goals: Self-Concordance Model

The "self-concordance model" (Sheldon & Elliot, 1999) focuses on the significance of self-chosen goals. The "self-concordance model" describes the relationships between the selection, pursuit, and achievement of goals. The model distinguishes between self-determined and extrinsic goals. As the model is based on the "self-determination theory" (Deci & Ryan, 1985; ▶ Chap. 8), a distinction is made between intrinsically and extrinsically motivated goals. The core statement of the model is that goals fit more or less well to individuals (i.e., to the self) (hence "self-concordance"). People are more likely to choose and pursue goals that align with their fundamental interests and values. Goals that reflect a person's personal interests, desires, and needs are called self-concordant. Non-self-concordant goals can be either externally (e.g., the goal to be the best athlete on the team because parents expect it) or internally controlled (e.g., setting the goal to have big muscles to impress others). The concordance or discordance of a goal directly influences the processes of goal pursuit and achievement (e.g., joy or unhappiness when pursuing goals) and also has psychological consequences (e.g., well-being) when achieving the goal. The inception-to-attainment process describes the influence of self-concordance on goal achievement. Goals that are highly self-concordant trigger more sustained effort in the goal pursuit than a goal that is not self-concordant. As a result, self-concordant goals increase the probability of goal achievement. According to Sheldon and Elliot (1999), the pursuit of autonomous (i.e., self-determined) goals is more enjoyable and promotes the achievement of goals through a stronger commitment to goals. Controlled goals can also evoke positive intentions and a certain willingness to invest effort, but the energy for goal achievement dissipates more quickly, particularly when obstacles arise (Sheldon & Elliot, 1998). In this model, the link between goal achievement and well-being is explained by a second subprocess (attainment-to-well-being process). The achievement of self-concordant goals leads to experiencing the satisfaction of psychological needs and thus to greater well-being (◘ Fig. 7.10). This in turn increases the probability of similar future goal striving and goal achievement. Well-being is fostered when the basic psychological needs for autonomy, competence, and relatedness are satisfied (▶ Chap. 8). In contrast, controlled goals are unlikely to lead to experiences of well-being, regardless of whether they are achieved or not, because they do not satisfy the basic needs.

7

Smith et al. (2011) conducted a season-long investigation testing the assumptions of the self-concordance model in the sport context. Structural equation modeling showed that autonomous goal motives at the start of the season were associated with mid-season effort, which ultimately predicted goal attainment at the end of the season. This attainment was positively associated with changes in psychological need satisfaction and well-being. The findings also revealed that autonomous and controlled motives predicted task-oriented and disengagement-oriented coping strategies, respectively, which in turn was differentially linked with effort.

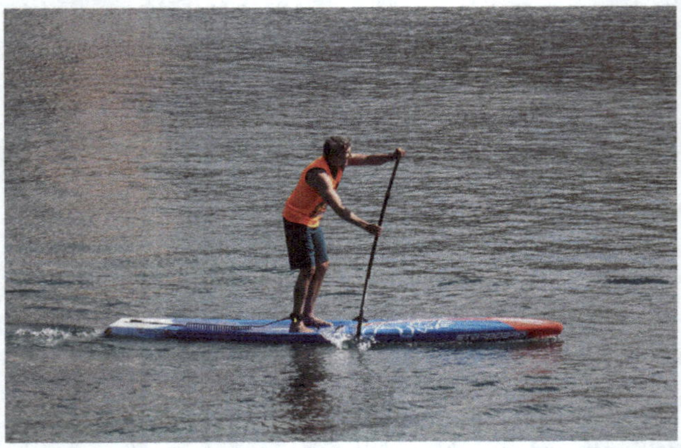

◘ **Fig. 7.10** Goals that are self-concordant lead to greater effort and increase the probability of goal achievement and well-being (Foto from: Sandra Sach)

7.5.3 Setting Team Goals

The "self-concordance model" mainly addresses individual goal setting. However, setting goals is not only important in individual sports but also in team sports. For example, the team, including the coach, can determine together which goals are to be pursued in the upcoming season. According to the "goal setting theory" (Locke & Latham, 1990), these goals should be difficult, specific, and approach oriented (i.e., not an avoidance goal in the sense of "we don't want to relegate"). Furthermore, every player can formulate his or her goals with the team and his or her goals in the team. A distinction is made between goals set by the individual (e.g., "I want to make successful passes 75% of the time/I want to assist in at least one goal scored in each game") and goals set jointly by the team (e.g., "We want to have possession of the ball for at least 60% of the game"). The former includes both individual personal goals and individual group goals; the latter includes team goals for an individual team member and team goals targeted to the team. Ultimately, especially in team sports, the setting of group goals is imperative for athletic performance because it can mobilize team spirit (van Mierlo & van Hooft, 2020). In addition, the phenomenon of "social loafing," i.e., hiding behind the team and letting others do the work, is counteracted (Burton, 1993). However, with all the positive effects goals can have, one should also be aware of potential dangers. This may include an increase in the willingness to take unnecessary risks caused by unrealistic goals. Stress can also arise if the goal is not achieved and consequently self-confidence is undermined. Setting goals that are too easy can be just as problematic as setting unrealistically high goals. If an athlete has set herself/himself the goal of reaching the semifinals at the Olympic Games, perhaps this might be a fairly easy goal for her/his capability, and she/he may be content with this performance, while she/he might actually possess the potential to win the gold medal but does not achieve this due to setting a goal too easy for her/his capabilities. Goals may also narrow one's attention so that areas unrelated to the goal are ignored. This tunnel vision can have a desired effect for goal achievement, but it can also lead to important information being missed. Essentially, athletes should be encouraged to set meaningful or self-concordant goals and to aim high but realistic. After the competition, however, the result is evaluated in a realistic, rational way in order to learn from it and develop one's skills and performance further.

7.6 When Goals Are Unattainable

Regardless of how strong the motivation for a particular goal is, there are goals that remain unattainable despite investing the greatest effort. In sport, there are many reasons for this, such as being injured or being unable to train due to illness. In addition, external factors, such as the loss of sponsors or not being drafted for the team, can play a role. Unattainable goals place a great burden on athletes. Overall, however, there has been little research to date on how to support athletes in this difficult situation. In competitive sports, letting go of a goal is often seen as a sign of weakness, because goals are set to be achieved. Athletes are constantly encouraged to reach their goals and to stretch their personal limits in order to achieve them. In particular, athletes with a high fear of failure may be very persistent in their goal pursuit, even if attainment is highly unlikely. Athletes high on fear of failure are more likely to set goals that have a very high (or very low) probability of success (▶ Sect. 7.1.4, "Risk Taking Model"). Therefore, coaches should strategically discuss with their athletes how they can best manage their limited resources and how to channel their energy. When goal pursuit seems hopeless, goals should be abandoned, and then strategies should be applied which focus on using the resources in other areas.

Motivational orientations play a key role in goal disengagement. Ntoumanis et al. (2014a, 2014b) and Smith and Ntoumanis (2014) show that it is particularly difficult to abandon autonomous, i.e., self-determined goals. Autonomous goals are pursued with more energy and stronger personal commitment, and an abandoning of autonomous goals seems to be associated with increased rumination and greater difficulties. Recent findings from Ntoumanis and Sedikides (2018) challenge previous recommendations to pursue goals relentlessly, instead suggesting that it may be important to identify when to abandon a goal and allocate resources towards a more realistic and achievable alternative goal. The ability to identify whether a goal is attainable is influenced by an individual's motivation for goal striving and a goal-regulatory technique called "mental contrasting with implementation intentions." Based on these findings, Ntoumanis and Sedikides (2018) proposed a tripartite model of goal striving encompassing goal motivation and goal regulation. However, both the active disengagement from current goals and the choice of alternative goals can have a positive effect on well-being. In summary, both goal commitment and goal disengagement have important well-being and performance consequences (Excursus: Ending a career in competitive sport).

Side Story

Career Termination in Elite Sports

An event that can be associated with great difficulties in goal disengagement is the termination of a career in elite sport. Historically, career termination has been described as a negative, sometimes even traumatic, life event (e.g., Stambulova et al., 2009). This life event requires great changes and reshaping one's own identity. Athletes have spent most of their time training and competing and have subordinated everything else in their lives to their sport goals. Studies on career termination in elite sports describe a variety of problems that can accompany this event, such as an identity crisis, emotional difficulties, and a decline in self-confidence and satisfaction. A number of studies have shown that about 15–20% of athletes experienced their career end as problematic or showed clinically relevant traumatic stress or needed psychological support (Alfermann, 2000; Lavallee et al., 2000; Wippert & Wippert, 2008). However, the severity of the problems seems to depend on when and why a career ended. For example, a distinction is often made between voluntary and involuntary reasons for termination and between planned and unplanned career termination (Alfermann et al., 2004). The personal consequences also depend on whether the reasons for the career termination lie within or outside of sport. The distinction between voluntary and involuntary career termination has received the most attention so far. Studies conclude that a planned and voluntary retirement leads to a smoother transition with fewer emotional changes and social problems than an unplanned or involuntary career end (e.g., Young et al., 2006). On the other hand, research also shows that around 80% of competitive athletes cope well with the transition out of sport in general. Indeed, Alfermann (2000) suggested that the end of a career should be seen as an opportunity for personal development. Nevertheless, competitive athletes show great interindividual differences in the phase of career termination. They should receive support in detaching themselves from their goals if, for example, the end of their career occurs unexpectedly and involuntarily, for example, due to an injury. Furthermore, competitive athletes can be supported in actively setting new goals in other life contexts.

> Goal commitment and goal disengagement are important motivational processes that impact well-being and performance.

7.7 Recommendations for Practice

This section provides recommendations for practice. It describes how to support the motivation of athletes. The tips are based on the theories presented in this chapter.

1. Choose the right goals: When selecting sport goals, "I proximity" should be taken into account, following the "self-concordance model." Goals should satisfy the basic psychological needs for autonomy, competence, and social relatedness. Selecting goals that satisfy the basic needs also promotes athletes' psychological well-being. Coaches can support athletes to set goals that are in line with their psychological needs by taking interest in athletes' welfare, and showing care and concern, as opposed to dismissing athletes' abilities, belittling them, or simply remaining unresponsive and indifferent towards their athletes (Bhavsar et al., 2019). This can be cultivated through intervention programs (Ntoumanis et al., 2018). Additionally, coaches should be careful when setting extrinsic goals. Athletes are encouraged to pursue autonomous goals. Autonomous goals are by definition meaningful, and they will be able to identify with them.
2. Setting goals: Once the overall goals have been chosen, they should be formulated in an approach rather than avoidance way. Furthermore, in accordance with the SMART principle, they should be formulated to be specific, measurable, adaptive to the respective circumstances, realistic, and time-based (Bull et al., 1996).
3. Form implementation intentions: Implementation intentions (► Chap. 10) link the desired goal state with details on the execution of an action (Gollwitzer, 1999). They describe in detail, for example, where, when, and how the goal is to be achieved (e.g., "When I get home after work today, I will put on my running shoes and go jogging in the park"). Implementation intentions help people act on their goals.
4. Pay attention to favorable attribution: Attributing failure to internal, controllable, and variable causes is associated with greater benefits for future motivation. Coaches are often familiar with athletes who do not look for the mistake in themselves but in others. Here the introduction of a "culture of mistakes," where the orientation "mistakes are good as long as they do no major damage" and "mistakes teach you faster and more," can be helpful. A mistake that is made once is unlikely to be repeated.
5. Positive coaching behavior: The motivation of athletes and the selection of suitable goals can be promoted by positive coaching behavior. An autonomy-supportive coaching style that avoids controlling behavior is to be preferred. Both an autonomy-supportive and a controlling coaching behavior have an influence on athletes' goals and promote autonomous or controlled goals (Smith et al., 2010). Autonomy-supportive behaviors respect the athletes' perspective, provide relevant information and justifications (e.g., the communication of the purpose of a training unit), offer choices, and minimize pressure. Controlling behavior is characterized by the use of commands (e.g., "You *must* win this game"), threats, and penalties (e.g., 50 pushups for each player after a lost game).
6. Supporting anxious athletes: Anxious athletes shy away from poorly defined performance situations and fear having to perform a skill in front of others that they do not perceive themselves to be competent at. Anxious athletes must therefore be given the opportunity to try out and practice new tasks on their own. It is stressful for them when they have to perform in front of a well-meaning coach if they are not 100% convinced that they can succeed. Furthermore, the comparison with others should be completely avoided, and the focus should be on the individual performance progress of each athlete. This is also called an individual reference norm orientation. The so-called principle of optimal fit states that the task difficulty is adjusted in such a way that it meets the upper end of one's abilities. Personal improvements should be praised, even if they fall short of the group's performance. These types of orientations can significantly reduce fear of failure, so that a competition is no longer perceived as stressful (see also Rheinberg & Krug, 2005).
7. Support goal disengagement when goals are unattainable and promote the formulation of new attainable goals: Coaches should support athletes in developing ways of self-assessing goal difficulties. This can be done, for example, by pointing out internal and external factors that may impair the achievement of goals (e.g., an injury) or by sharing their concern about the attainability of the desired goals with the athletes. When goals become unattainable, coaches should consider goal disengagement and focusing on alternative goals. In particular, the inability to achieve autonomous goals can be challenging for athletes. Here, the support of the social environment is of particular importance so that new goals can be identified and aspired to.

Learning Control Questions

Basic:

1. Define motivation. What role does affect play in motivation?
2. Explain the expectancy × value model?
3. How are "goals" defined?
4. What does task and performance goal orientation mean and from which theory do these two terms originate?

Advanced:

5. Which questionnaires measure goal orientation in sport?
6. What are the effects of approach and avoidance goals on well-being and performance?
7. What is the difference between a prevention focus and a promotion focus? What significance does this distinction have for performance in sport?
8. What are the consequences of a "task-oriented" or a "performance-oriented" motivational climate in sport for athletes?
9. Can the motivational climate in sports groups be changed and, if so, how?
10. Which performance attributions do Weiner et al. (1971) propose?
11. How can attributions in sport be measured?
12. What is the purpose of attribution training?
13. What is a self-serving attribution, and what are its advantages and disadvantages?

Experts:

14. What is the difference between outcome, performance, and process goals?
15. How would you define a self-concordant goal?
16. What are the consequences if goals in competitive sport cannot be achieved?

References

Abele, A., & Brehm, W. (1990). Wer ist der "typische" Fitness Sportler? Ein Beitrag zur Sportpartizipation im Erwachsenenalter [Who ist the "typical" fitness athlete? A contribution to sports participation in adulthood]. *Spektrum der Sportwissenschaft, 2*, 4–32.

Alfermann, D. (2000). Causes and consequences of sport career termination. In D. Lavallee & P. Wylleman (Eds.), *Career transitions in sport: International perspectives* (pp. 45–58). Fitness Information Technology.

Alfermann, D., Stambulova, N., & Zemaityte, A. (2004). Reactions to sport career termination: a cross-national comparison of German, Lithuanian, and Russian athletes. *Psychology of Sport and Exercise, 5*, 61–75.

Allen, M. S. (2012). A systematic review of content themes in sport attribution research: 1954–2011. *International Journal of Sport and Exercise Psychology, 10*, 1–8.

Allen, M. S., Greenlees, I., & Jones, M. V. (2011). An investigation of the five factor model of personality and coping behaviour in sport. *Journal of Sports Sciences, 29*, 841–850.

Ames, C. (1992). Classrooms: Goals, structures, and student motivation. *Journal of Educational Psychology, 84*, 261–271.

Ames, C., & Archer, J. (1988). Achievement goals in the classroom: Students' learning strategies and motivation processes. *Journal of Educational Psychology, 80*, 260–267.

Atkinson, J. W. (1957). Motivational determinants of risk-taking behavior. *Psychological Review, 64*, 359–372.

Barkoukis, V., Lazuras, L., Tsorbatzoudis, H., & Rodafinos, A. (2011). Motivational and sportspersonship profiles of elite athletes in relation to doping behavior. *Psychology of Sport and Exercise, 12*, 205–212.

Beckmann, J., & Heckhausen, H. (2018). Motivation through expectation and incentive [Motivation durch Erwartung und Anreiz]. In J. Heckhausen & H. Heckhausen (Eds.), *Motivation und Handeln* (5th ed., pp. 119–162). Springer.

Bhavsar, N., Ntoumanis, N., Quested, E., Gucciardi, D. F., Thøgersen-Ntoumani, C., Ryan, R. M., et al. (2019). Conceptualizing and testing a new tripartite measure of coach interpersonal behaviors. *Psychology of Sport and Exercise, 44*, 107–120.

Braithwaite, R., Spray, C. M., & Warburton, V. E. (2011). Motivational climate interventions in physical education: A meta-analysis. *Psychology of Sport and Exercise, 12*(6), 628–638.

Bull, S. J., Albison, J. G., & Shambrook, C. J. (1996). *The mental game plan: Getting psyched for sport*. Sports Dynamics.

Burton, D. (1993). Goal setting in sport. In R. N. Singer, M. Murphey, & L. K. Tennant (Eds.), *Handbook of research on sport psychology* (pp. 467–491). MacMillan.

Burton, D., Weinberg, R., Yukelson, D., & Weigand, D. (1998). The goal effectiveness paradox in sport: Examining the goal practices of collegiate athletes. *The Sport Psychologist, 12*, 404–418.

Burton, D., & Weiss, C. (2008). The fundamental goal concept: The path to process and performance success. In T. S. Horn (Ed.), *Advances in sport psychology*. Human Kinetics. (pp. 339–375, 470–474).

Conroy, D. E., Elliot, A. J., & Hofer, S. M. (2003). A 2 x 2 achievement goals questionnaire for sport: Evidence for factorial invariance, temporal stability, and external validity. *Journal of Sport & Exercise Psychology, 25*, 456–476.

Cszikszentmihalyi, M. (1975). *Beyond boredom and anxiety*. Jossey-Bass.

Deci, E. L., & Ryan, R. M. (1985). *Intrinsic motivation and self-determination in human behavior*. Plenum.

Duda, J.L. (1987). Toward a Developmental Theory of Children's Motivation in Sport. *Journal of Sport Psychology* 9(2), 130–145.

Duda, J. L. (1989). Relationship between task and ego orientation and the perceived purpose of sport among high school athletes. *Journal of Sport and Exercise Psychology, 11*(3), 318–335.

Duda, J. L., & Appleton, P. (2016). Empowering and disempowering coaching behaviors: Conceptualization, measurement considerations, and intervention implications. In M. Raab, P. Wylleman, R. Seiler, A.-M. Elbe, & A. Hatzigeorgiadis (Eds.), *Sport and exercise psychology research: From theory to practice* (pp. 373–388). Elsevier.

Duda, J. L., & Hall, H. (2001). Achievement goal theory in sport: Recent extensions and future directions. In R. N. Singer, H. A. Hausenblas, & C. M. Janelle (Eds.), *Handbook of sport psychology* (pp. 417–443). Wiley.

Duda, J. L., & Nicholls, J. (1992). Dimensions of achievement motivation in schoolwork and sport. *Journal of Educational Psychology, 84*, 1–10.

Dweck, C. S. (1986). Motivational processes affecting learning. *American Psychologist, 41*, 1040–1048.

Elliot, A. J., & Dweck, C. S. (1988). Goals: An approach to motivation and achievement. *Journal of Personality and Social Psychology, 54*(1), 5–12.

Elbe, A.-M. (2004). Testgütekriterien des Deutschen Sport Orientation Questionnaires [Test quality criteria of the German Sport Orientation Questionnaire]. *Spectrum der Sportwissenschaft, 16*, 96–107.

Elbe, A.-M., Sanchez, X., Otten, S., & Dankers, S. (2021). Promoting psychological integration within culturally diverse school classes: a motivational climate intervention in the physical education context. *International Journal of Sport and Exercise Psychology*, https://doi.org/10.1080/1612197X.2021.2003418

Elliot, A. J. (1999). Approach and avoidance motivation and achievement goals. *Educational Psychologist, 34*, 169–189.

Elliot, A. J., & McGregor, H. A. (2001). A 2 × 2 achievement goal framework. *Journal of Personality and Social Psychology., 80*, 501–519.

Elliot, A. J., Murayama, K., & Pekrun, R. (2011). A 3x2 achievement goal model. *Journal of Educational Psychology, 103*(3), 632–648.

Feather, N. T. (1982). *Expectations and actions: Expectancy-value models in psychology*. Erlbaum.

Filby, W. C., Maynard, I. W., & Graydon, J. K. (1999). The effect of multiple-goal strategies on performance outcomes in training and competition. *Journal of Applied Sport Psychology, 11*, 230–246.

Fry, M., Duda, J., & Chi, L.-K. (1993). The perceived motivational climate in sport questionnaire: Construct and predictive validity. *Journal of Sport & Exercise Psychology, 15*, 172–183. https://doi.org/10.1123/jsep.15.2.172

Fuchs, R. (2001). Entwicklungsstadien des Sporttreibens [Development stages of sports activities]. *Sportwissenschaft, 31*, 255–281.

Gill, D. L., & Deeter, T. E. (1988). Development of the Sport Orientation Questionnaire. *Research Quarterly for Exercise and Sport, 59*, 191–202.

Gollwitzer, P. M. (1999). Implementation intentions: Strong effects of simple plans. *American Psychologist, 54*, 493–503.

Greenlees, I., Stopforth, M., Graydon, J., Thelwell, R., Filby, W., & El-Hakim, Y. (2007). The impact of match importance and gender on the team-serving attributional bias among interdependent sports team players. *Group Dynamics: Theory, Research, and Practice, 11*(1), 54–65. https://doi.org/10.1037/1089-2699.11.1.54

Green, T. D., & Holeman, S. (2004). Athletes' attributions for team performance: A theoretical test across sports and genders. *Social Behavior and Personality: An International Journal, 32*, 199–206.

Grove, J. R., & Prapavessis, H. (1995). The effect of skill level and sport outcomes on dimensional aspects of causal attributions. *Australian Psychologist, 30*, 92–95.

Hacker, W. (1998). *Allgemeine Arbeitspsychologie. Psychische Regulation von Arbeitstätigkeiten [General organisational psychology. Psychological regulation of work activities]*. Huber.

Hamilton, P. R., & Jordan, J. S. (2000). Most successful and least successful performances: Perceptions of causal attributions in high school track athletes. *Journal of Sport Behavior, 23*, 245254.

Hanrahan, S., & Cerin, E. (2009). Gender, level of participation, and type of sport: Differences in achievement goal orientation and attributional style. *Journal of Science and Medicine in Sport, 12*, 508–512.

Harwood, C., Spray, C. M., & Keegan, R. (2008). Achievement goal theories in sport. In T. S. Horn (Ed.), *Advances in sport and exercise psychology* (3rd ed., pp. 157–185). Human Kinetics.

Heckhausen, H. (1989). *Motivation und Handeln [Motivation and action]*. Springer-Verlag.

Heider, F. (1958). *The psychology of interpersonal relations*. Wiley.

Hellandsig, E. T. (1998). Motivational predictors of high performance and discontinuation in different types of sports among talented teenage athletes. *International Journal of Sport Psychology, 29*, 27–44.

Higgins, E. T. (1997). Beyond pleasure and pain. *American Psychologist, 52*, 1280–1300.

Higgins, E. T. (2000). Making a good decision: Value from fit. *American Psychologist, 55*, 1217–1230.

Hodge, K., & Petlichkoff, L. (2000). Goal profiles in sport motivation: A cluster analysis. *Journal of Sport and Exercise Psychology, 22*(3), 256–272.

Höner, O., & Feichtinger, P. (2016). Psychological talent predictors in early adolescence and their empirical relationship with current and future performance in soccer. *Psychology of Sport and Exercise, 25*, 17–26.

Höner, O., & Willimczik, K. (1998). Mit dem Rubikon-Modell über das Handlungsloch [The Rubicon model and inaction]. *Psychologie und Sport, 5*, 56–68.

Jones, G., & Hanton, S. (1996). Interpretation of competitive anxiety symptoms and goal attainment expectancies. *Journal of Sport and Exercise Psychology, 18*, 144–157.

Kavussanu, M. (2006). Motivational predictors of prosocial and antisocial behaviour in football. *Journal of Sports Sciences, 24*, 575–588.

Kelley, H. H. (1973). The process of causal attribution. *American Psychologist, 28*, 107–128.

Kingston, K., & Hardy, L. (1997). Effects of different types of goals on processes that support performance. *The Sport Psychologist, 11*, 277–293.

Kingston, K. M. & Goldea, A. (2007). Goals and flow. Paper presented at the Annual conference of the Association for Applied Sport Psychology, Louisville, Kentucky, USA.

Kingston, K. M., & Wilson, K. M. (2008). The application of goal setting in sport. In *Advances in applied sport psychology* (pp. 85–133). Routledge.

Kovar, P. (2009). *Entstehung einer Dopingkarriere: Prädiktoren eines Phasenmodells von Kindern und Jugendlichen in Baden-Württemberg [Development of a doping career: Predictors of a phase model for children and adolescents in Baden-Württemberg]*. Südwestdeutscher Verlag für Hochschulschriften.

Kuhl, J. (1983). *Motivation, Konflikt und Handlungskontrolle [Motivation, conflict and action control]*. Springer-Verlag.

Kuhl, J. (2001). *Motivation und Persönlichkeit [Motivation and personality]*. Hogrefe.

Lavallee, D., Nesti, M., Borkoles, E., Cockerill, I., & Edge, A. (2000). Intervention strategies for athletes in transition. In D. Lavallee & P. Wylleman (Eds.), *Career transitions in sport: International perspectives* (pp. 45–58). Fitness Information Technology.

Lochbaum, M., Podlog, L., Litchfield, K., Surles, J., & Hillard, S. (2013). Stage of physical activity and approach-avoidance achievement goals in university students. *Psychology of Sport & Exercise, 14*, 161–168.

Locke, E. A., & Latham, G. P. (1990). *A theory of goal setting and task performance*. Prentice Hall.

Locke, E. A., & Latham, G. P. (2006). New directions in goal-setting theory. *Current Directions in Psychological Science, 15*, 265–268.

MacLeod, L. (2012). Making SMART goals smarter. *Physician Executive, 38*(2), 68.

Maehr, M. L., & Nicholls, J. G. (1980). Culture and achievement motivation: A second look. In N. Warren (Ed.), *Studies in cross-cultural psychology* (Vol. 3, pp. 221–267). AcademicPress.
Mascret, N., Elliot, A. J., & Cury, F. (2015). Extending the 3 x 2 achievement goal model to the sport domain: The 3 x 2 achievement goal questionnaire for sport. *Psychology of Sport and Exercise, 17*, 7–14. https://doi.org/10.1016/j.psychsport.2014.11.001
McClelland, D. C. (1953). *The achievement motive*. Appleton-Century-Crofts (Irvington/Wiley).
McClelland, D. C. (1987). *Human motivation*. Cambridge University Press.
Memmert, D., Plessner, H., Hüttermann, S., Froese, G., Peterhänsel, C., & Unkelbach, C. (2015). Collective fit increases team performances: extending regulatory fit from individuals to dyadic teams. *Journal of Applied Social Psychology, 45*(5), 274–281.
Miller, D., & Ross, M. (1975). Self-serving biases in the attribution of causality: Fact or fiction? *Psychological Bulletin, 82*, 213–225.
Nicholls, J. G. (1984). Achievement Motivation: Conceptions of ability, subjective experience, task choice, and performance. *Psychological Review, 91*, 328–346.
Ntoumanis, N., Healy, L. C., Sedikides, C., Duda, J., Stewart, B., Smith, A., & Bond, J. (2014a). When the going gets tough: The "why" of goal striving matters. *Journal of Personality, 82*(3), 225–236.
Ntoumanis, N., Healy, L. C., Sedikides, C., Smith, A. L., & Duda, J. L. (2014b). Self-regulatory responses to unattainable goals: The role of goal motives. *Self and Identity, 13*(5), 594–612.
Ntoumanis, N., Quested, E., Reeve, J., & Cheon, S. H. (2018). Need supportive communication: Implications for motivation in sport, exercise, and physical activity. *Persuasion and communication in sport, exercise, and physical activity*, 155–169.
Ntoumanis, N., & Sedikides, C. (2018). Holding on to the goal or letting it go and moving on? A tripartite model of goal striving. *Current Directions in Psychological Science, 27*(5), 363–368.
Ntoumanis, N., Taylor, I. M., & Thøgersen-Ntoumani, C. (2012). A longitudinal examination of coach and peer motivational climates in youth sport: Implications for moral attitudes, well-being, and behavioral investment. *Developmental psychology, 48*(1), 213.
Ommundsen, Y. (2004). Self-handicapping related to task and performance-approach and avoidance goals in physicaleducation. *Journal of Applied Sport Psychology, 16*, 183–197.
Perlman, D. J., & Goc Karp, G. (2007). Using TARGET to enhance preservice teachers' ability to identify and develop a motivational climate. *Physical Educator, 64*(2), 102–113.
Plessner, H., Unkelbach, C., Memmert, D., Baltes, A., & Kolb, A. (2009). Regulatory fit as a determinant of sport performance: How to succeed in a soccer penalty shooting. *Psychology of Sport and Exercise, 10*, 108–115.
Rees, T., Ingledew, D. K., & Hardy, L. (2005). Attribution in sport psychology: Seeking congruence between theory, research and practice. *Psychology of Sport and Exercise, 6*, 189–204.
Rheinberg, F. (2002). *Motivation*. Kohlhammer.
Rheinberg, F. (2006). *Motivation* (6th ed.). Kohlhammer.
Rheinberg, F., & Krug, S. (2005). *Motivationsförderung im Schulalltag [Promoting motivation in everyday school life]* (3rd ed.). Hogrefe.
Roberts, G. C. (2001). Understanding the dynamics of motivation in physical activity: The influence of achievement goals on motivational processes. In G. C. Roberts (Ed.), *Advances in motivation in sport and exercise*. Human Kinetics. (pp. 1/50).
Robinson, D. W., & Howe, B. L. (1989). Appraisal variable/affect relationships in youth sports: A test of Weiner's attributional model. *Journal of Sport & Exercise Psychology, 11*, 431–443.
Sage, L., & Kavussanu, M. (2008). Goal orientations, motivational climate, and prosocial and antisocial behaviour in youth football: Exploring their temporal stability and reciprocal relationships. *Journal of Sports Sciences, 26*, 717–732.
Schüler, J., & Brandstätter, V. (2010). Zielbildung und Zielbindung [Goal setting and goal retention]. In U. Kleinbeck & K. H. Schmidt (Eds.), *Enzyklopädie der Psychologie, Wirtschafts-, Organisations- und Arbeitspsychologie, Band 1 Arbeitspsychologie (39–88)*. Hogrefe.
Seifriz, J. J., Duda, J. L., & Chi, L. (1992). The relationship of perceived motivational climate to intrinsic motivation and beliefs about success in basketball. *Journal of Sport and Exercise Psychology, 14*, 375–391.
Shapcott, K. M., Carron, A. V., Greenlees, I., & El Hakim, Y. (2010). Do member attributions for team outcomes represent a collective belief? *Psychology of Sport and Exercise, 9*, 487–492.
Sheldon, K. M., & Elliot, A. J. (1998). Not all personal goals are personal: Comparing autonomous and controlled reasons for goals as predictors of effort and attainment. *Personality and Social Psychology Bulletin, 24*, 546–557.
Sheldon, K. M., & Elliot, A. J. (1999). Goal striving, need satisfaction, and longitudinal well-being: The self-concordance model. *Journal of Personality and Social Psychology, 7*(3), 482–497.
Sherman, D. K., & Kim, H. S. (2005). Is there an 'I' in 'team'? The role of the self in group serving judgments. *Journal of Personality and Social Psychology, 88*, 108–120.
Smith, A. L., & Ntoumanis, N. (2014). An examination of goal motives and athletes' self-regulatory responses to unattainable goals. *International Journal of Sport Psychology, 45*, 538–558.
Smith, A. L., Ntoumanis, N., & Duda, J. L. (2010). An investigation of coach behaviors, goal motives, and implementation intentions as predictors of well-being in sport. *Journal of Applied Sport Psychology, 22*, 17–33.
Smith, A. L., Ntoumanis, N., Duda, J. L., & Vansteenkiste, M. (2011). Goal striving, coping, and well-being: A prospective investigation of the self-concordance model in sport. *Journal of Sport and Exercise Psychology, 33*(1), 124–145.
Smith, R. E., Cumming, S. P., & Smoll, F. L. (2008). Development and validation of the motivational climate scale for youth sports. *Journal of Applied Sport Psychology, 20*, 116–136.
Smoll, F. L., Smith, R. E., & Cumming, S. P. (2007). Effects of a motivational climate intervention for coaches on changes in young athletes' achievement goal orientations. *Journal of Clinical Sport Psychology, 1*(1), 23–46.
Sniehotta, F. F., Schwarzer, R., Scholz, U., & Schüz, B. (2005). Action planning and coping planning for long-term lifestyle change: Theory and assessment. *European Journal of Social Psychology, 35*, 565–576.
Stambulova, N., Alfermann, D., Statler, T., & Côté, J. (2009). ISSP position stand: Career development and transitions of athletes. *International Journal of Sport and Exercise Psychology, 7*, 395–412.
Sudeck, G., & Höner, O. (2011). Volitional interventions within cardiac exercise therapy(VIN-CET): Long-Term effects on physical activity and health-related quality of life. *Applied Psychology: Health and Well-Being, 3*(2), 151–171.
Taylor, D., & Doria, J. (1981). Self-serving and group-serving bias in attribution. *The Journal of Social Psychology, 113*, 201–211.
Unkelbach, C., Plessner, H., & Memmert, D. (2009). "Fit" in sports: Self-regulation and athletic performances. In J. P. Forgas, R. F. Baumeister,

& D. M. Tice (Eds.), *Psychology of self-regulation: Cognitive, affective, and motivational processes* (pp. 93–105). Psychology Press.

van Mierlo, H., & van Hooft, E. (2020). Team Achievement Goals and Sports Team Performance. *Small Group Research: An International Journal of Theory, Investigation and Application, 51*(5).

Wang, J. C., Liu, W. C., Chatzisarantis, N. L., & Lim, C. B. (2010). Influence of perceived motivational climate on achievement goals in physical education: A structural equation mixture modeling analysis. *Journal of Sport and Exercise Psychology, 32*(3), 324–338.

Weinberg, R., Yueklson, D., Burton, D., & Weigand, D. (2000). Perceived goal setting practices of olympic athletes: An exploratory investigation. *The Sport Psychologist, 14*(3), 279–295. https://doi.org/10.1123/tsp.14.3.279

Weiner, B. (1986). *An attributional theory of motivation and emotion*. Springer-Verlag.

Weiner, B., Frieze, I. H., Kukla, A., Reed, L., Rest, S., & Rosenbaum, R. M. (1971). *Perceiving the causes of success and failure*. General Learning Press.

Wippert, P.-M., & Wippert, J. (2008). Perceived stress and prevalence of traumatic stress symptoms following athletic career termination. *Journal of Clinical Sport Psychology, 2*, 1–16.

Young, J. A., Pearce, A., Kane, R., & Pain, M. D. (2006). Leaving the professional tennis circuit: Exploratory study of experiences and reactions from elite female athletes. *The British Journal of Sports Medicine, 40*, 477–483.

7

Intrinsic Motivation in the Context of Sports

Julia Schüler, Wanja Wolff and Joan L. Duda

Contents

J. Schüler et al. (eds.), *Sport and Exercise Psychology*, https://doi.org/10.1007/978-3-031-03921-8_8

Learning Objectives

Basic:

- To describe the phenomenon of intrinsic motivation
- To differentiate intrinsic from extrinsic motivation
- To describe the "Undermining Effect" of external rewards on intrinsic motivation
- To define the flow state
- To describe the main premises of self-determination theory
- To describe what is assumed in various mini-theories under the umbrella of self-determination theory
- To be able to explain the ways intrinsic motivation is measured

Advanced:

- To understand the characteristics of intrinsically motivated behavior
- To understand the effects of intrinsic motivation and extrinsic motivation
- To describe different theoretical approaches on the nature and determinants of intrinsic motivation
- To describe determinants, characteristics, and consequences of the flow state
- To explain motivated human action from the perspective of self-determination theory
- To explain what organismic integration theory proposes
- To be aware of the instruments for measuring intrinsic motivation and their strengths and weaknesses

Experts:

- To explain processes by which behavior can transition from extrinsically motivated to intrinsically motivated
- To critically assess the merits and any drawbacks of intrinsic motivation in contrast to extrinsic motivation
- To differentiate and integrate across major theoretical approaches to intrinsic motivation
- To pull from the literature and existent theoretical approaches and explain how intrinsic motivation can be promoted via sport intervention approaches

8.1 Introduction

Athletes, coaches, parents—they all want answers to the questions: What motivates people to be physically active and to engage in sport? That is, what moves us to move and stay moving within the sporting setting? In this chapter, we focus on the driving force of action—or action regulation—that lies within oneself: intrinsic motivation.

Fun and enjoyment are characteristics that accompany intrinsic motivation. These positive experiences are reasons for participating and also likely consequences of intrinsically motivated sports participation. An activity is *intrinsically motivated* when it is carried out for its own sake, independently of extrinsic motivators. Extrinsic rewards such as winning a medal or social recognition can be present, but they are not the driving forces. When people are intrinsically motivated, they participate for the experience of joy in movement, the experience itself, the positive challenge of the activity, and/or improvement of their personal competence.

Basic Definition of Intrinsic Motivation

Behavior is intrinsically motivated if one engages in the behavior for its own sake. Motivation arises out of the person, and the activity and is independent of external factors or rewards or punishments.

Intrinsic motivation must be differentiated from extrinsic motivation. Extrinsic motivation means that the underlying reasons (or regulatory forces) for actions lie outside the person. Examples for such outside reasons are external rewards and/or constraints within the social environment. With respect to the former, medals and prize money can reward excellent performance and be a key reason why individuals engage in sport. With respect to the latter, sport engagement can lead to positive social evaluations. For example, one can attain social status and popularity via sport, and obtaining such social connection accolades may be key reasons for participation.

People can also feel pressured to participate in sport, to please others, or to avoid rejection. We will later see that extrinsic motivation is further differentiated and conceptualized within self-determination theory (see paragraph 8.2.2.3), a popular theoretical framework that includes such "introjected" reasons for sports participation.

Basic Definition of Extrinsic Motivation

Behavior is extrinsically motivated if it is driven by external incentives such as rewards, punishments, and expectations of others. This basic definition of extrinsic motivation is differentiated into different facets of extrinsic motivation in ► Sect. 8.2.2.3.

People can be motivated by intrinsic and extrinsic means to *initiate* a sport activity (e.g., a physical inactive person starts participating in a local running group) and *maintain* their behaviour over time (e.g., a grassroots level footballer stays with her sport season after season). However, a serious drawback of extrinsic motivation is that the behavior of interest (starting and staying with it!) depends on the presence of extrinsic motivators. If external rewards and punishments are removed, this also removes the reason for engaging in the behavior. If a person has only been active in sports for extrinsically motivated reasons, the removal of such 'motivators' will likely cause this person to cease participation. Another disadvantage of extrinsic motivation is that it produces high personal costs: Doing sports for extrinsic reasons requires self-control and willpower. However, people generally try to avoid applying self-control because it feels aversive.

Reflection

While we might generally really like engaging in certain activities (e.g., sports, studying, playing music), not all aspects of these activities reflect intrinsically motivated actions that we enjoy, are interested in, and that we engage in out of personal volition (see definition of intrinsic motivation). Parts of complex action sequences (e.g., necessary repetitive sequences of movement during training, considered-to-be more "boring" study contents in university, learning sheet music) may even be experienced as uninspiring or even unpleasant. Surely, readers will recognize areas in their lives in which they feel more intrinsically motivated. Where do you feel intrinsically motivated? The following questions help to identify the activities in your life which are fueled by more intrinsic motivation.

- When do you engage in an activity for its inherent enjoyment and interest and out of personal volition?
- What do you do without receiving (or not needing to receive) any kind of extrinsic reward from others?
- What do you keep coming back to after interruptions (e.g., sports injuries)?
- What would you do career-wise if you were not dependent on earning money?
- What would you do in your free time if you were independent of social obligations (e.g., partner's, family's, or social expectations)?

8.2 Theoretical Frameworks on Nature and Determinants of Intrinsic Motivation

The field of sport psychology looks to theories and models to describe, explain, and predict phenomena in sports. They are the cornerstones of our scientific thinking and professional approaches in sports practice. Thus, our theoretical understanding of intrinsic motivation not only determines the framework for our empirical work (e.g., research we do in lab experiments, behavioural observations, or surveys), but it is also the source or "idea generator" for practical applications.

There are a number of very popular theories in sport psychology which have helped us further understand the concept of intrinsic motivation and develop interventions aimed at enhancing intrinsic motivation in sport. The "theory of flow experience" (Csikszentmihalyi, 1990) focuses on a specific quality of experience that occurs when the environment provides challenges that match a person's skills. "Self-determination theory" (SDT) is a complex theory, including subtheories, that addresses the determinants and implications of intrinsic motivation and differentiates various forms of extrinsic motivation (Deci & Ryan, 1985). The "self-concordance model" (Sheldon & Elliot, 1999) and the "hierarchical model of intrinsic motivation" (Vallerand, 1997) are based on the main assumptions of SDT and provide interesting and nuanced approaches for understanding variability in sport participation and its implications.

> Important theoretical approaches to explaining intrinsic motivation are:
> - Flow theory
> - Self-determination theory
> - Self-concordance theory
> - Hierarchical model of intrinsic motivation

8.2.1 Flow Theory

The *flow theory* exemplifies a strand in psychological research called "positive psychology." Instead of investigating the causes of physical and psychological illnesses and impaired well-being, positive psychology dedicates itself to the investigation of human strengths and the causes for health, well-being, and happiness. "Flow theory" is the brainchild of Mihalyi Csikszentmihalyi (1975, 1990). He assumed that if people perceive that the (social) environment provides challenges which match the person's capacities to meet those challenges, then he or she is more likely to be in the moment to enjoy the moment. One reason for this is because when "in flow," the person is optimally stretching his or her capabilities with the likelihood of learning new skills and increasing feelings of competence and capability. With these assumptions, Csikzentmihalyi's perspective is in the tradition of earlier work by White (1959), who criticized early drive-reduction theory and psychoanalytic instinct theory for leaving something crucial unconsidered: an organism's desire and capacity to interact effectively with its environment (White, 1959). Competence cannot be fully acquired simply through behavior based on drives, but requires activities or, in other words, experiences which entail managing optimally challenging interactions with the environment. "Such activities in the ultimate service of competence must therefore be conceived to be motivated in their own right" (White, 1959, p. 329). In Csikszentmihalyi's theoretical framework, activities can be motivating in their own right and produce the experience of flow when the challenges of the activity match or, even better, "raise the game" in regard to the person's skills.

The experience of flow (see Fig. 8.1) is a prototype of intrinsic motivation, in which the activity itself and the positive quality of experience are in the foreground. Jackson and Csikszentmihalyi (1999, p. 4) asked athletes to describe their special moments in their sport and received the following answer from a swimmer:

> "When I've been happiest with my performance, I've sort of felt one with the water and my stroke and everything. … I was really tuned into what I was doing. I knew exactly how I was going to swim the race, and I just knew that I had it all under control, and I got in and was really aware of what everyone in the race was doing. … I was just totally absorbed in my stroke, and I knew I was passing them but I didn't care. I mean it's not that I didn't care; I was going, 'Oh this is cool!'. And I just swam and won, and I was totally in control of the situation. I felt really cool." (Jackson & Csikszentmihalyi, 1999, p. 4)

8

This quote illustrates important components or characteristics of the flow experience. The starting point of Csikszentmihalyi's (1975) research was the question as to why people do things that do not depend on the outcome of an activity. When people climb a mountain, they often do not experience a feeling of euphoria at the top of the mountain but rather the unpleasant realization that the joyful activity of mountaineering has now come to an end. Cost-, material-, and time-consuming water sports are further examples that people do not "calculate" rationally. Some sports even bring dangers for the participants' physical health and functioning with them but are nevertheless carried out with passion. Sports also can entail "social" costs such as the commitment to training and competing which translates into less time with family and friends. It often seems that neither the rational reasons against (e.g., expenditure of time, danger) nor for (e.g., improving one's health, affiliation) sport are central in these cases.

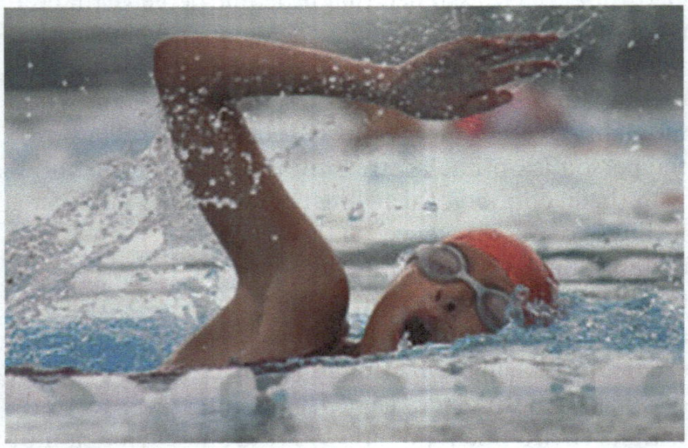

Fig. 8.1 An example for flow experience: Seemingly effortless performance of top athletes. (publication rights held by Springer)

Flow is not about the purpose(s), the result, or the instrumentality of the action but about something that lies in the activity itself. Csikszentmihalyi (1990) has made this phenomenon the object of his lifetime of research. In interviews with people acting "purposelessly" (e.g., sportsmen such as rock climbers or painters without any intention of showing or selling a picture) and later using the *experience sampling method* (participants are asked to report on their feelings, thoughts, and behaviors multiple times of day during or immediately after they've experienced them rather than evaluating them retrospectively), he identified the particular phenomenon of the "flow experience." The term is based on the characteristic feature of experiencing the activity as "flowing" (e.g., as the feelings realized when running fluently and effortlessly).

Csikszentmihalyi (1990, p. 4) defines flow as a state in which people are so involved in an activity that nothing else seems to matter. The experience during the activity is so joyful and engaging that people want to do it for its own sake.

8.2.1.1 Characteristics of Flow Experience

One of the four most important characteristics of flow experience is deep involvement in an activity. When in flow, one is fully concentrated on the execution of—and the sensations received from—the current activity. In addition, consciousness and action seem to "merge" (merging of action and awareness). Thus, one is focused on the current action, and there is no room for self-reflection (in particular, worrying about how one is doing, self-doubt). The third characteristic of flow is a feeling of strong personal control over the action. Since flow often arises during engagement in optimally challenging tasks in which one can succeed as well as fail, the feeling of control may be deceptive. However, when in flow, the individual feels like he or she is "pulling the strings." The fourth major characteristic of flow is a distorted perception of time. Flow is mostly associated with the perception of time moving faster than usual (hours pass like minutes); however, also the reverse can be true, and action sequences are perceived as if they happened in slow motion: having a flow experience while competing in a 100 m sprint.

Important characteristics of the flow experience are:

1. Being deeply involved in an activity (absorption by and in activity)
2. Merging of action and awareness (freedom from self-reflection)
3. Feeling of being in control
4. Distorted perception of time

8.2.1.2 Consequences of Flow Experience

Jackson and Csikszentmihalyi (1999) chose "The key to optimal experience and performance" as a subtitle of their book *Flow in Sport*. Other researchers too describe flow as an optimal state in at least three ways. First, it is an *optimal state of motivation* that represents a prototype of intrinsic motivation. The complete focus on the activity makes it possible to be focused on the action, even when alternative attractive activities compete for one's attention. Thus, it is not surprising that flow predicts variables such as behavioral persistence. Flow is also called *optimal experience*. The positive quality of experience acts as a reward and increases the probability that an action will be performed again: the activity becomes intrinsically motivating. The rewarding quality of flow facilitates the occurrence of positive health effects and better athletic performance through enhanced concentration and the likelihood of longer-term participation in sports. Due to the feeling of absolute personal control, flow is associated with freedom from anxiety, positive well-being, and positive self-perceptions. The result is the feeling of fully mastering a sequence of movements (feeling flow while serving in tennis) or the requirements of the sport overall (e.g., experiencing flow during a tennis match) and enjoying this feeling. It is also interesting for competitive sports that flow is associated (not equivalent to but can "set the stage for") with a state of *optimal performance*. The flow state is "… one in which an athlete or other person performs at his or her best, seemingly without effort …" (Csikszentmihalyi, 1990).

In the literature the terms *peak performance states* or *zone of optimal functioning* are often used as synonyms for flow. They are conceptually difficult to separate from the original flow concept according to Csikszentmihalyi. The state of optimal performance seems to share some characteristics (e.g., feeling of control, absolute attention on the action) but not all characteristics with flow (Jackson & Csikszentmihalyi, 1999).

Correlates of Flow Experience

Flow is associated with a positive, high-quality experience (optimal experience), behavioral persistence (optimal motivation), and high performance (peak performance state).

Side Story

The Bright and Dark Sides of Flow Experience

Flow experience does not seem to be without drawbacks. Recent studies show that people who experience flow might underestimate risks and are susceptible to becoming exercise addicted (Zimanyi et al., 2021).

Partington et al. (2009) found that most of the big wave surfers (see Fig. 8.2) they interviewed reported flow experiences. They mentioned features like deep involvement ("There is nothing else in your mind. There is nothing else that matters"), strong sense of control ("You are able to control the most uncontrollable because everything becomes slow motion and that's when you know you are surfing the best"), and distorted perception of time ("For a moment in time, time stands still") (Partington et al., 2009, p. 176). However, the authors also found statements that matched the symptoms of sports dependence (e.g., Hausenblaus & Downs, 2002). These include a feeling of addiction ("Once you get familiar with that feeling, it's an addiction"), tolerance development ("Nothing is ever enough," "After each turn, you want to accelerate faster in to the next turn"), withdrawal symptoms ("There is psychologically after all that is done, there is a depression almost"), and social conflicts ("My husband wants to have babies. I kinda don't 'cause I want to keep surfing, you know?"). It is the task of future research to examine more precisely whether the characteristics that make flow so attractive also cause its negative consequences. Does the feeling of absolute control, for example, lead to an overestimation of one's own abilities and, through this, to risky sports behavior? Is the freedom from self-reflection and fear so rewarding that the associated behavior makes one dependent?

Vallerand's dualistic model of passion (Vallerand et al., 2003) might offer a theoretical explanation for the "bright" and "dark" sides of flow experience. *Passion* is defined as a strong affinity for an activity that people enjoy and devote time and energy into. One type of passion, *harmonious passion*, leads people to choose to engage in the activity that they enjoy. In contrast, *obsessive passion* leads people to feel urged or compelled to engage in an activity, i.e.,

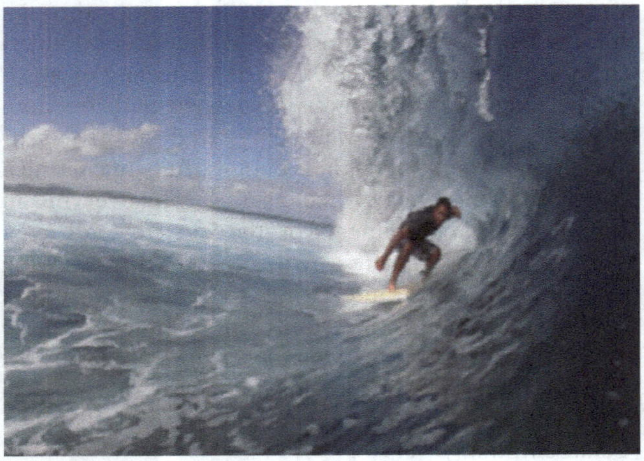

■ **Fig. 8.2** The perfect wave: A balancing act between enjoyment and risk. (publication rights held by Springer)

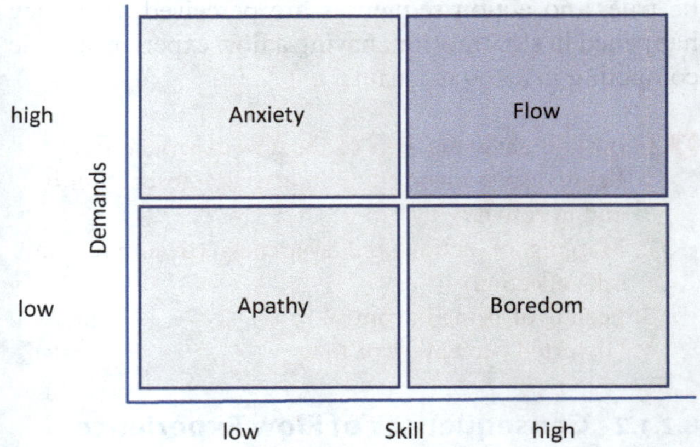

■ **Fig. 8.3** Flow quadrant model. (After Csikszentmihalyi & Csikszentmihalyi, 1988, © Cambridge University Press 1988, reproduced with permission)

8

participation feels as if it is required. Harmonious passion is based on an autonomous internalization of the activity in one's identity and positively associated with well-being, whereas obsessive passion is based on a controlled internalization (for autonomous and controlled forms of regulation, see ► Sect. 8.2.2.3) and impairs rather than fosters well-being (Vallerand et al., 2008). But what does passion have to do with flow? According to Vallerand et al. (2008), flow can be seen as a consequence of passion: The more passionate people are, the more they experience flow.

This overall assumption was supported in a study by Carpentier et al. (2012). The authors investigated the mechanisms underlying the link between passion and well-being and found that flow mediates this relationship with regard to harmonious passion only. The more harmonious passion, the more people experience flow in their favorite activity which in turn predicts higher well-being. In contrast, obsessive passion did not predict flow in the activity that one is passionate about. Rather obsessive passion predicted rumination about the passionate activity when the individual was doing another activity. Not surprisingly then, flow experiences (and associated well-being) in this other activity were compromised.

8.2.1.3 Conditions of Flow Experience

One of three central conditions of flow experience (Csikszentmihalyi et al., 2005) is the matching of a person's skills and abilities to the requirements of a task (*challenge-skill balance*). This is the case when, for example, young athletes are instructed by their coach to perform a challenging but appropriately difficult task in training. If the task would be too difficult and exceeds the abilities of the athletes, they can become anxious and afraid of failure. If the task is too easy, they are bored. Csikszentmihalyi and Csikszentmihalyi (1988) assumed that flow is more likely to occur when skills and task requirements match at a high level (e.g., challenging drill for advanced tennis players). If skills and task requirements match at a low level (e.g., simple exercises for tennis beginners), any occurrence of flow is likely to be very brief and limited in its intensity. These distinctions are assumed in the "quadrant model of flow experience" (Csikszentmihalyi & Csikszentmihalyi, 1988) (■ Fig. 8.3).

Second, flow is more likely when the individual is faced with *clear goals* (e.g., "The task is to place the tennis ball in the marked field") rather than a diffuse or vague request (e.g., "Your task is to play tennis"). Goals orient our actions and help to structure them (e.g., by using subgoals). Goals also facilitate maintaining the necessary concentration. Another facilitator of flow is receiving *direct and informing feedback* on the execution of the action. This feedback can be given by the coach ("You performed the flip great! You used your arms well when getting started on your rotation. Then you grabbed your shins just below your knees at the right moment and tucked yourself into a ball, which continued your rotation. That's why the rotation was performed so good. Very well done…."), but the feedback could also be internal to the person (e.g., kinesthetic such as the sensation that a movement simply "feels right" and fluid). Different types of feedback help to adjust actions in the direction of goal attainment and can make it more likely that flow is realized.

Important conditions of the flow experience are:
1. Challenge-skill balance
2. Clear goals
3. Immediate feedback

Researchers have continued to examine factors that promote or inhibit flow. The novelty of the task and the absence of disturbances during task execution have been identified as flow promoters in several studies. On the other hand, factors such as participating in sport in an overall demanding, unpleasant, and pressure-packed atmosphere (e.g., within a negative team climate, see ► Chap. 7) and time pressure have been found to be flow inhibitors. In a systematic review of the experience, occurrence, and controllability of flow states in elite sport in particular, Swann et al. (2012) reported some similar and additional factors that facilitate flow.

Which factors promote flow experience?
- Appropriate focus
- Effective preparation and readiness
- Optimal motivation
- Optimal arousal
- Positive thoughts and emotions
- Confidence
- Optimal environmental and situational conditions
- Positive feedback
- Starting well
- Positive team play and interaction

The authors of this meta-analysis conclude that the occurrence of flow probably results from the interaction of personal factors (e.g., concentration, activation, motivation, self-confidence, thoughts and emotions), external factors (e.g., situational and environmental conditions, e.g., weather, coach behaviours), and behavioral factors (e.g., preparation) (Swann et al., 2012). Accordingly, they recommend a multifaceted intervention to promote flow that includes psychological, physiological, and social factors instead of an intervention that only aims at changing one facet.

Side Story

Can Effort Be Intrinsically Rewarding?

According to the *law of least effort* (Hull, 1943), humans try to avoid applying effort when possible. Interestingly, sports participation often seems to be at odds with this law. Indeed, sports is sometimes performed not *despite* it being hard and requiring effort but *because* of it. To illustrate, for some recreational runners, the reason to complete an ultramarathon lies in the experience of effortfully pushing through boundaries and to still keep going. Thus, it appears that in sports, the giving of effort, in itself, can be intrinsically rewarding. This is a fascinating proposition because it decouples effort from any outcome: In most cases, giving more effort results in a higher likelihood to reach a certain goal, to acquire certain skills, play one's sport at a more enjoyable level, or to experience competence in the process. However, when effort acts as an intrinsic reward, these effort-outcome instrumentalities may not be as influential if impactful at all. In this case, a sensation that humans generally try to avoid (i.e., effort) becomes a sensation that they actively seek out. This *effort paradox* has only recently been identified as a key research topic in psychology (Inzlicht et al., 2018). The field of sports – where effort is very highly regarded – might be the most prototypical and promising domain for better understanding the conditions under which effort can be an intrinsic reward (Wolff et al., 2021).

8.2.2 Self-Determination Theory (SDT)

Self-determination theory (SDT; Deci & Ryan, 1985) is a comprehensive and multifaceted theoretical framework of human motivation and its interaction with emotion, personality, and social contexts in various areas of life. It has frequently been used by researchers and practitioners as a theoretical framework that describes, explains, and predicts sport engagement (see, e.g., Hagger & Chatzisarantis, 2007). In a nutshell, SDT proposes that self-determination is the hallmark of more high-quality motivation (which is epitomized by the quintessential intrinsic motivation) which enables well-being and personal development.

> According to "self-determination theory" (SDT; Deci & Ryan, 1985), it is important to consider how self-determined individuals are with respect to their reasons for sports participation. The most self-determined motivation for sport engagement is intrinsic motivation. The theory also makes predictions regarding the determinants of intrinsic motivation and its implications for well-being and personal development.

? The theoretical assumptions of SDT can be separated into different subtheories. Those mini-theories, which often serve as the basis for research in sport psychology, are:
- Cognitive evaluation theory
- Basic psychological needs theory
- Theory of organismic integration

8.2.2.1 Cognitive Evaluation Theory

Cognitive evaluation theory (CET; Deci, 1975) within the SDT framework assumes that people are intrinsically motivated by nature. They seek optimal challenges, are curious, want to develop their skills, and have the urge to develop personally. An example of intrinsic motivation is the playful and explorative behavior of small children. Critical for intrinsic motivation is the "cognitive evaluation" (i.e., perceived determination) of where the cause of the behavior lies. Only when the cause is perceived as being within the person, and not outside through control or constraints of the social environment, does intrinsic motivation result and be maintained.

Cognitive evaluation theory suggests that external events can affect intrinsic motivation and that this can happen in three ways. First, the social environment provides information (*informational events*), for example, on how well one is doing in a task at school, at the workplace, or in sports. This information (if positive), in turn, allows the individual to feel competent and thereby promotes intrinsic motivation (Vallerand & Reid, 1984). In contrast, *controlling events*, such as rewards (monetary incentives, praise), make people feel less self-determined and controlled by others or other things, which in turn decreases intrinsic motivation. The third way of influence is *amotivating events*, such as negative performance feedback that fosters feelings of incompetence and thereby is expected to decrease intrinsic motivation.

CET is based on seminal studies conducted by Deci (1971) on the "undermining effects" of external rewards. It has been shown that when people were rewarded with money for a task that they originally performed intrinsically motivated (e.g., solving an interesting puzzle task in Deci's experiment), they were less likely to continue this task when the extrinsic reward (money) was withdrawn compared to a group of people who were not monetarily rewarded. According to Deci (1971), people feel pressured by the social environment (directed by money) and respond quite sensitively to this restriction of autonomy (see Side Story, The Undermining Effect: Research in Process).

> **Undermining Effect**
> The undermining effect of intrinsic motivation (Deci, 1971) means that intrinsic motivation can be undermined if people receive a reward for an action, that initially was performed for its own sake, and that reward becomes the reason for the engagement. The undermining effect can also occur when negative feedback is received.

Side Story

The Undermining Effect: Research in Process

Deci's (1971) assumption regarding the undermining of intrinsic motivation by rewards was in provocative contrast to the then dominant learning-by-reward theories. These theories assumed that the probability that a desired behavior would occur again in the future was increased when that behavior had been previously rewarded. In more than four decades of research and as documented in several domains in human life (education, workplace) (for a meta-analysis see Deci et al., 1999; for an overview see Ryan & Deci, 2017), the undermining effect of extrinsic rewards on intrinsic motivation has been supported. The undermining effect mainly occurs with announced or expected rewards, but not with unannounced or unexpected rewards. Only rewards that we realize can be forthcoming and are tied to our behavior can be perceived as controlling. Meta-analytic results also indicate that the undermining effect on intrinsic motivation is weaker when people are rewarded for their performance compared to when they are only rewarded for their effort or for the completion of a task. This fits with CET's assumptions that the effects of rewards depend on whether they can be interpreted as informational (being rewarded for one's performance), or as control exercised by others to influence one's behavior (such as being rewarded for one's effort).

More recent research has shown that rewards and intrinsic motivation are not necessarily opposites or at odds but rather must be considered together (Cerasoli et al., 2014). The last half century of research has shown that, depending on the theoretical perspective, differentiation of the constructs, and meaning of the rewards (e.g., are they telling the person that he or she is competent at the activity?), the analysis of relatively simple relationships between incentives, intrinsic motivation, and performance can lead to completely different results. Even meta-analyses, which were supposed to find a "core of truth" out of a multitude of studies, deliver contradictory results that support the undermining effect or cannot find it (Cameron et al., 2001). Research is a process (that does not stop), and it is important to look at what is being studied, how, with whom, and where to understand research findings more clearly.

Cognitive evaluation theory has also been well established in sports (for a review see Frederick & Ryan, 1995). Here, the undermining effect has found the greatest resonance in the research question of whether athletic scholarships (that are regularly used by US universities to recruit and support sport talents) undermine the intrinsic motivation of college students. In fact, athletes who have the opportunity to play their sport at a high level should experience competence. Competence as a basic psychological need (see below), in turn, should lead to increased intrinsic motivation. In short, athletes on scholarships should actually report high levels of intrinsic motivation. However, studies that have been conducted on this tended to show a negative relationship between athletic scholarships and intrinsic motivation (Cremades et al., 2012; Medic et al., 2007; Ryan, 1977, 1980). Vallerand (2012) explained this seemingly contradiction so that "unfortunately, scholarship recipients may come to feel that they play more to justify the scholarship they have received than for the pleasure of the game" (p. 69). According to CET, a "controlling event" happened that makes people feel controlled by others which decreases intrinsic motivation. That the effects of scholarships depend on how they are interpreted was nicely shown by two consecutive studies by Ryan (1977, 1980).

Ryan (1977) found that college students who were rewarded for their football performance with a scholarship reported a drop in intrinsic motivation with each scholarship year. Here it was argued that the reward was perceived as controlling ("I train because I get paid for it"). For groups of athletes who were rarely awarded sports scholarships at that time (i.e., female athletes and male wrestlers), however, the informative character of the reward ("I, as a woman/as a wrestler, must really be good to receive a scholarship") appeared to be more salient, resulting in an increase in intrinsic motivation (Ryan, 1980). Thus, whether the reward is perceived as controlling or informative makes a huge difference on one's intrinsic motivation.

In a more recent study, Moller and Sheldon (2020) examined what happens to former college athletes' intrinsic motivation after college, even decades later. They found that athletes who received a scholarship (vs. no scholarship) felt stronger external motivation during college and reported less present-day enjoyment of their sport. According to this, the negative effects of scholarships seem to last much longer than previously assumed.

8.2.2.2 Basic Psychological Need Theory

Cognitive evaluation theory (CET) (Deci, 1975) points to the importance of perceptions of control and competence to understand the processes impacting intrinsic motivation (positively or negatively). Feelings of competence and whether one feels a sense of autonomy (or controlled) are important constructs in the basic psychological needs theory (BPNT; Ryan & Deci, 2002). One way that BPNT extends CET, however, it that this mini-theory assumes that there are three basic psychological needs which are held to be indispensable for intrinsic motivation, well-being, health, and personal growth (Deci & Ryan, 2000).

These three needs are the *basic need for competence*, the *basic need for autonomy*, and the *basic need for relatedness*. When one's need for *autonomy* is satisfied, the individual experiences oneself as the cause of one's own actions and not as being pushed by external constraints. Then they feel they have a voice and a choice and act in accordance with their values and interests. The basic need for *competence* is the need to experience oneself as capable and competent. People want to experience themselves as acting effectively and successfully pursuing their goals. If the need for *relatedness* is satisfied, one has a feeling of belonging to significant others or groups (e.g., friends, family, team in sport).

The three basic needs are conceptualized as being innate and essential for mental and physical well-being. It is assumed that their satisfaction or frustration has similar positive or negative consequences for all people across different cultures and situations. A plethora of studies in sports and other areas of life (e.g., family, school, work) confirm the positive effects of satisfying basic needs on, for example, intrinsic motivation, subjective well-being, physical health, and desired behavior (Adie et al., 2008; Adie et al., 2012; Alvarez et al., 2012; Gagné et al., 2003; Reinboth & Duda, 2006).

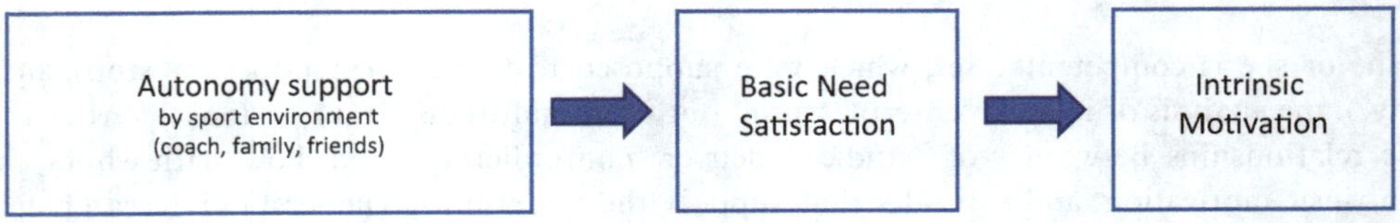

Fig. 8.4 Basic need satisfaction as a mediator in the relationship between autonomy-support and intrinsic motivation

Basic Psychological Needs

The three basic psychological needs in "self-determination theory" are the basic needs for

- Autonomy
- Competence
- Social relatedness

According to Deci and Ryan (1985), these needs are universal (innate, relevant to all people and settings), and their satisfaction fuels intrinsic motivation (and autonomous motivation overall).

If the satisfaction of basic needs is so important for intrinsic motivation, how can it be fostered? Satisfaction of the three basic needs is assumed to be impacted by the social environment (e.g., at home, in school, in sports) (Deci & Vansteenkiste, 2004). In other words, basic needs are assumed to mediate the relationship between characteristics of the perceived social environment and optimal functioning (including intrinsic motivation and well- and ill-being) (Deci & Ryan, 2000). But what or who in sport contexts determines the quality of the social environment?

A key person influencing not only sport performance but also well-being of sports participants is the coach (Duda & Balaguer, 2007). He or she determines the characteristics and quality of the coaching environment, which is perceived by the athlete and triggers motivational processes that are relevant to whether or not athletes function optimally (Adie et al., 2012). The key coach behavior to promote need satisfaction seems to be autonomy support. *Autonomy-supportive behaviors* by coaches provide athletes with choices, invite the athletes to participate in decision-making, reduce external demands as much as possible, and acknowledge their feelings and give meaningful information. An autonomy-supportive coaching/teaching style has been found to predict need satisfaction in sport (e.g., Smith et al., 2007), physical education (PE, e.g., Standage et al., 2006), dance (Quested & Duda, 2011), and exercise classes (e.g., Edmunds et al., 2007).

The mediation assumption that autonomy support leads to intrinsic motivation in sport through the satisfaction of basic needs (Fig. 8.4) has been empirically supported in the sport context (e.g., Bartholomew et al., 2011b; Fenton et al., 2014).

Coach Behavior and Athlete Motivation

Autonomy-supportive coaches foster more self-determined or autonomous forms of motivation (intrinsic and identified), while controlling coach behavior leads to less self-determined forms of motivation such as introjected and external motivation.

Autonomy Support by Coaches

Fenton et al. (2014) added two further aspects to the state of research on the potential positive effects of autonomy-supportive coach behaviors. First, in a sample of young sport participants, they examined not only the effects of autonomy support on objectively assessed sport and physical activity but also on time spent sedentary (criterion for sedentary behavior: low energy consumption of ≤1.5 MET; see Sedentary Behavior Research Network, 2012). Second, the authors tested an assumption of the "hierarchical model of intrinsic motivation" (Vallerand, 1997; see below), according to which forms of motivation can be transferred to other domains and contexts. The authors specifically tested the hypothesis that perceived autonomy support by the football coach mediates the extent of physical activity (accrued through sport and active games) and time spent sedentary via the type of motivation adopted (self-determined/autonomous vs. controlled). In their cross-sectional study of 105 young football players with an average age of about 13 years, Fenton and colleagues assessed the youth sport participants' perception of the autonomy support provided by the coach, controlling coach behaviors, and their motivation in addition to weight, height, and BMI using questionnaires.

Examples of questionnaire items are presented below.

- Perceived autonomy support by the coach: "My coach gives players choices and options."

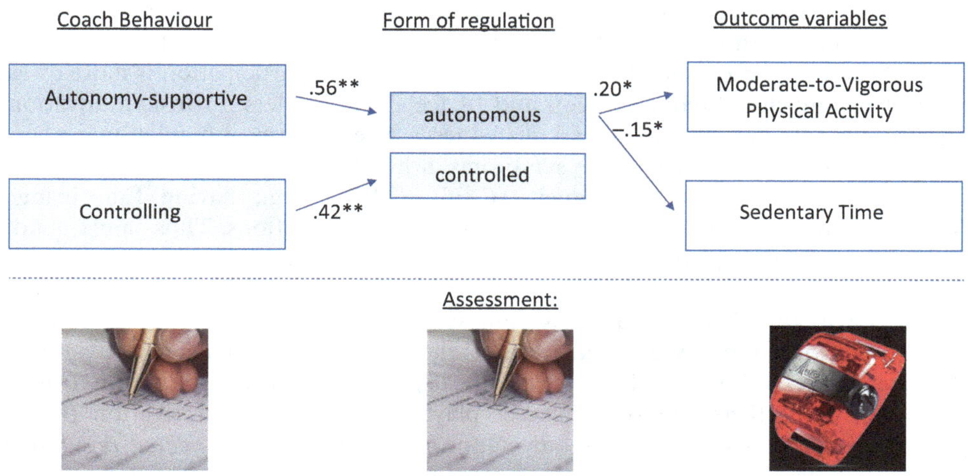

Fig. 8.5 Illustration of the results of the study by Fenton et al. (2014). Figure is adapted to Fenton et al. (2014, Fig. 2, p. 457). Only significant relationships are displayed (* $p < .05$, ** $p < .01$)

- Controlling coach behavior: "My coach threatens to punish players to keep them in line during training."
- Motivation for sports participation and physical activity: "I participate in sport and active games …
  - Intrinsic: "… because it's fun"
  - Identified: "… because I value the benefits"
  - Introjected: "… because I would feel guilty if I quit"
  - External: "… because if I don't other people will not be pleased with me"

The outcome variables physical activity and time spent sedentary were measured over a period of 7 days using an accelerometer. The activity monitors measured the time the youth sport participants spent at different activity intensities. The data were analyzed with path analyses (Fig. 8.5). Results indicated that the perceived autonomy support provided by the football coach predicted self-determined or autonomous motivation (intrinsic and identified) to engage in sport and active games, which in turn was significantly positively related to objectively assessed moderate-to-vigorous (MVPA) physical activity and negatively related to time spent sedentary. If the football coach was perceived as controlling, this was linked to greater controlled forms of motivation (introjected and external) which, however, did not make a significant contribution to explaining time spent engaged in MVPA nor time spent sedentary.

Taken together, the Fenton et al. (2014) were able to show that the autonomy-supportive or controlling coach behavior that youth athletes experienced in football training was relevant in predicting daily physical activity and sedentary activities during and outside the training setting.

It is important to note that the social environment, created by coaches and other significant others, can also have a negative impact on intrinsic motivation and well-being. The social environment can also thwart or compromise the basic needs and, as a result, undermine intrinsic motivation and well-being (Ryan & Deci, 2000). Bartholomew et al. (2011b) conceptually separated basic need thwarting from low need satisfaction by proposing that the former is qualitatively different from low need satisfaction. For example, low satisfaction of the need for competence can be experienced by an athlete who feels incompetent because he or she does not have the necessary skills to perform well (although well-supported by the coach). Here, the basic need for competence is *not satisfied*. In contrast, an athlete who feels incompetent because his or her coach perpetually gives negative feedback without meaningful information, often criticizes without giving support, or even is severely demeaning to him or her realizes an active *thwarting* of his/her need for competence and experiences competence need frustration.

The basic need for autonomy can be frustrated if the coach forces the athlete to act, think, and feel in a certain way, for instance, by excessive control, by using intimidation, and by displaying conditional regard (Bartholomew et al., 2010; Reeve, 2002). The basic need for relatedness is frustrated if the coach's behaviors are distant, cold, and dismissive (Bartholomew et al., 2011a).

Bartholomew et al. (2011b) developed the "Psychological Need Thwarting Scale" (PNTS), and its items also describe basic need thwarting behavior of coaches and teammates well: “I feel prevented from making choices with regard to the way I train” (autonomy), “There are times when I am told things that make me feel incompetent” (competence), and “I feel I am rejected by those around me” (social relatedness). Need frustration is related to depressive symptoms, a higher probability of burnout (Balaguer et al., 2012; Bartholomew et al., 2011b) in sport and exercise, and with negative affect in physical activity contexts (Gunnell et al., 2013).

Employing the PNTS and also assessing satisfaction of the needs for autonomy, competence, and relatedness, Balaguer et al. (2012) longitudinally tested the basic psychological needs theory in young soccer players. The players' perceptions of how autonomy-supportive and controlling their coaches behaved and their reported well-being (feelings of vitality) and ill-being (burnout) were also assessed over the course of a season. The coach viewed as becoming more autonomy supportive positively predicted changes in basic psychological need satisfaction (which predicted increases in reported vitality) and negatively predicted basic psychological need thwarting (which corresponded to increases in burnout). When the coach was perceived as being more controlling as the season unfolded, players reported greater frustration of their needs which linked to greater burnout over time.

> The coach's behaviors matter: An autonomy-supportive coaching style has the potential to foster intrinsic motivation, whereas a basic need thwarting coaching style can severely harm intrinsic motivation and well-being (Fig. 8.6).

8.2.2.3 Organismic Integration Theory (OIT)

Deci and Ryan (1985, 2000) go beyond a binary conceptualization of intrinsic and extrinsic motivation. Rather, in their organismic integration theory (OIT, Ryan & Deci, 2000, 2002), another mini-theory within SDT, they suggest that motivation differences are captured in athletes' answers to the question “why,” and the answers to that question can vary in the degree to which their participation is more or less self determined. SDT considers intrinsic motivation as the most self-determined form of regulation, i.e., doing sport for its own sake and out of personal choice. Incentives in the activity itself (e.g., having fun, being challenged) motivate one's actions. Thus, sport is not a means to an end, but the means has become the end.

Within the OIT, Deci and Ryan (2000) outline four different types of motivation under the broad category of “extrinsic motivation,” ranging on a continuum of self-determination from external regulation to integrated motivation (Fig. 8.7). *External regulation* and *introjected regulation* represent externally determined, controlled forms of regulation, while *identified* and *integrated motivation* are conceptualized as being self-determined or autonomous forms of regulation. *External regulation* means motivation to engage to receive rewards or avoid punishments. A good example is a young elite athlete participates because his or her parents are pushing his or her engagement in the

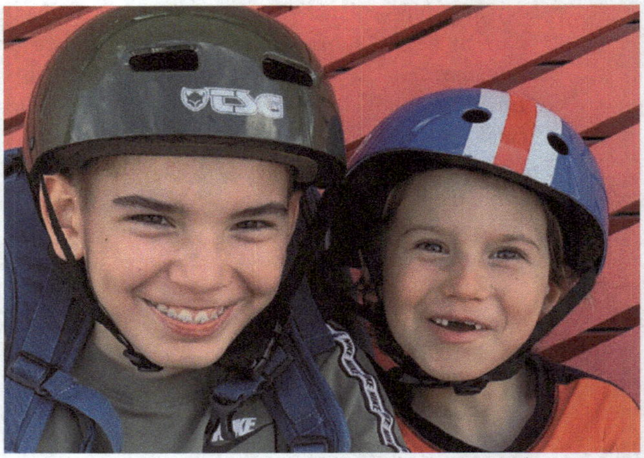

Fig. 8.6 An autonomy-supportive sport climate is assumed to enhance intrinsic motivation and well-being in youth sport. (Rights of the photo are held by the author)

Fig. 8.7 Continuum of self-determination. (Adapted from Deci & Ryan, 2002, courtesy of Boydell & Brewer)

Quality of Behavior	Nonself-determined →					Self-determined
Type of Motivation	Amotivation	Extrinsic Motivation: Controlled Motivation		Extrinsic Motivation: Autonomous Motivation		Intrinsic Motivation
Type of Regulation	Non-regulation	External regulation	Introjected regulation	Identified regulation	Integrated regulation	Intrinsic Regulation
Perceived Locus of Causality	Impersonal	External	Somewhat External	Somewhat Internal	Internal	Internal

sport. *Introjected motivation* means doing sports to avoid guilt and shame. To illustrate, a top athlete in a team sport trains hard because he/she would feel guilty not giving all for his/her team. In *identified regulation*, the sport is classified as important because it allows one to realize valued goals and objectives. Importantly, this does not imply that the person necessarily enjoys doing sports and is doing it for the joyful experience it creates. An athlete can do the hard fitness training, for example, to optimize performance in an upcoming competition. *Integrated regulation* means that sport is part of one's personal identity: it is "integrated into the self" (Deci & Ryan, 2002). This is the case when doing sports is an important part of the self-concept and sport is a part of one's life. Finally, *amotivation* is reflected in people who report no reason for engaging in the activity (autonomous or controlled) and tend to not display the behavior of interest at all, e.g., do not engage in sport or dropping out of sport if participating. However, there are much fewer studies on amotivation.

> Organismic Integration Theory (Ryan & Deci, 2000) distinguishes between controlled forms of motivation and autonomous forms of motivation. The former includes external regulation (behavior is regulated by external reward or punishment) and introjected regulation (acting to avoid guilt or fear). Among the self-determined forms of regulation are identified regulation (a person acts via volition and engages in the activity because it is consistent with his or her values and allows him or her to realize consequences which are personally important) and intrinsic motivation (engaging in the activity for its own sake, e.g., it is enjoyable).

The process of *internalization, as* assumed in OIT, means that people can learn to endorse the value of extrinsically motivated behaviors. People cannot act intrinsically motivated in all areas of life (like the aimless playing of the child) but have to adapt to requirements of life (obligations, consideration for others). Internalization means that behavioral regulation can move along the continuum of self-determination and should ideally be reflected of autonomous regulation if we want high-quality motivation to be experienced. An example is a young elite athlete who might participate in sport because the parents expect the athlete to engage in sport. After a certain time of positive experiences with sport and participation within a sports environment (experience of competence, autonomy, social relatedness), the athlete's behavioral regulation can be shifted in the direction of autonomous regulation. In this case, the person participates in sport because she considers it important, interprets it as part of her identity, and, at best, even finds pleasure and fun in participating in sport. Fostering this process of internalization through supporting basic psychological need satisfaction is one of the most challenging but very important aims in coaching. However, such efforts to engage in need supportive coaching are worthwhile: more autonomous forms of motivation are associated with more desirable cognitive, behavioral, and affective outcomes (Mossman, 2022; Ntoumanis, 2001).

8.2.3 Self-Concordance Theory

Sheldon and Elliot's (1999) "self-concordance model" is based on the organismic integration theory (OIT). The core concept is the importance of determining the degree to which people's goals fit more or less well to themselves (self-concordance). The term self-concordance describes how much a goal is in harmony with a person's fundamental interests and values. In contrast to "organismic integration theory," in the self-concordance model, the motivational types do not refer to the regulation of behavior but to a goal. What we are striving for (the goals we are pursuing, e.g., participating in training on a regular basis) could be more intrinsic (e.g., We regularly participate in training because we want to, we enjoy the sport experience) or more extrinsic (e.g., we participate in training because we feel pressured by the coach). Smith et al. (2007) and Smith et al. (2011) supported the self-concordance model (Sheldon & Elliot, 1999) as a framework for goal striving in sports. In a prospective investigation they showed, for example, that start-of-season autonomous goal motives were linked to midseason effort, which in turn predicted end-of-season goal attainment. Furthermore, goal attainment was positively related to changes in psychological need satisfaction, which, in turn, predicted changes in emotional well-being (Smith et al., 2011).

Usually, self-concordance in sport is measured by first asking participants about their personal goals in sport ("Please nominate objectives you are typically trying to attain in your sport"). Then participants rate why they were striving for each goal in terms of four reasons relating to intrinsic, identified, introjected, and external regulations (Smith et al., 2007). Seelig and Fuchs (2006) have designed a reliable and valid German-language questionnaire. Its English translation is displayed in Table 8.1.

Table 8.1 Items from the self-concordance scale for physical activity (Seelig & Fuchs, 2006, by courtesy of Hogrefe, Harald Seelig and Reinhard Fuchs. Seelig and Fuchs have checked the English translation and agreed to it). Participants indicate their agreement to each statement using a 6-point rating scale (1: completely agree, 6: completely disagree)

	I intend to be regularly active in sports in the coming weeks and months …
1	because sporting activity is simply part of my life.
2	because I simply enjoy it.
3	because I make experiences that I do not want to miss.
4	because it is good for me.
5	because the positive consequences are simply worth the effort.
6	because I have good reasons for it.
7	because otherwise I would have a bad conscience.
8	because otherwise I would have to reproach myself.
9	because I think that sometimes you have to force yourself to do something.
10	because others say I should be active in sports.
11	because otherwise I get into trouble with other people.
12	because people who are important to me urge me to do so.

The items of the illustrated questionnaire measure the self concordance of one's physical activity goal (SKK; Seelig & Fuchs, 2006). More precisely, items 1–3 represent intrinsic motivation, items 4–6 represent identified motivation, items 7–9 represent introjected motivation, and items 10–12 represent extrinsic motivation. The scores for the four forms of regulation are the means of the three corresponding items. An overall index for self-concordance can be calculated by a simple formula: (identified + intrinsic subscale) – (introjected + extrinsic subscale) (calculation according to Sheldon & Elliot, 1999). Higher positive values represent higher self concordance, indicating that a person's goals align well with his or her personal values.

8

Reflection

First complete the questionnaire on your own (see Table 8.1). Then put yourself in the shoes of a person who does significantly more or significantly less sport than you and consider how and why he or she would respond to the items.

8.2.4 Hierarchical Model of Intrinsic Motivation

Based on self-determination theory, Vallerand's (1997) "hierarchical model of intrinsic motivation" distinguishes intrinsic, extrinsic motivation, and amotivation (Fig. 8.8). He looked at these three types of motivation on three different hierarchical levels differing with respect to their generalizability from specific to more general: motivation can be linked to specific *situations*, to certain *contexts*, or it can be a relatively stable disposition that *globally* characterizes a person. Importantly, motivation on a higher hierarchical level is thought to affect lower level motivation in a top-down fashion. Thus, an athletes' global intrinsic motivation is expected to trickle down to various contexts and situations.

However, to explain why global levels of motivation can change too, Vallerand (1997) postulates that bottom-up effects can occur too. To illustrate, providing people with choices, performance feedback, and a supportive atmosphere in training (situational level) can not only increase intrinsic motivation in this very training session through the experience of autonomy, competence, and social relatedness but can also contribute to intrinsic motivation in sport in general (contextual level). Over a longer period, the next higher level (global intrinsic motivation) can also be positively influenced (Guay et al., 2003). To explain how motivation emerges on these different levels, the model makes specific predictions with respect to social environmental determi-

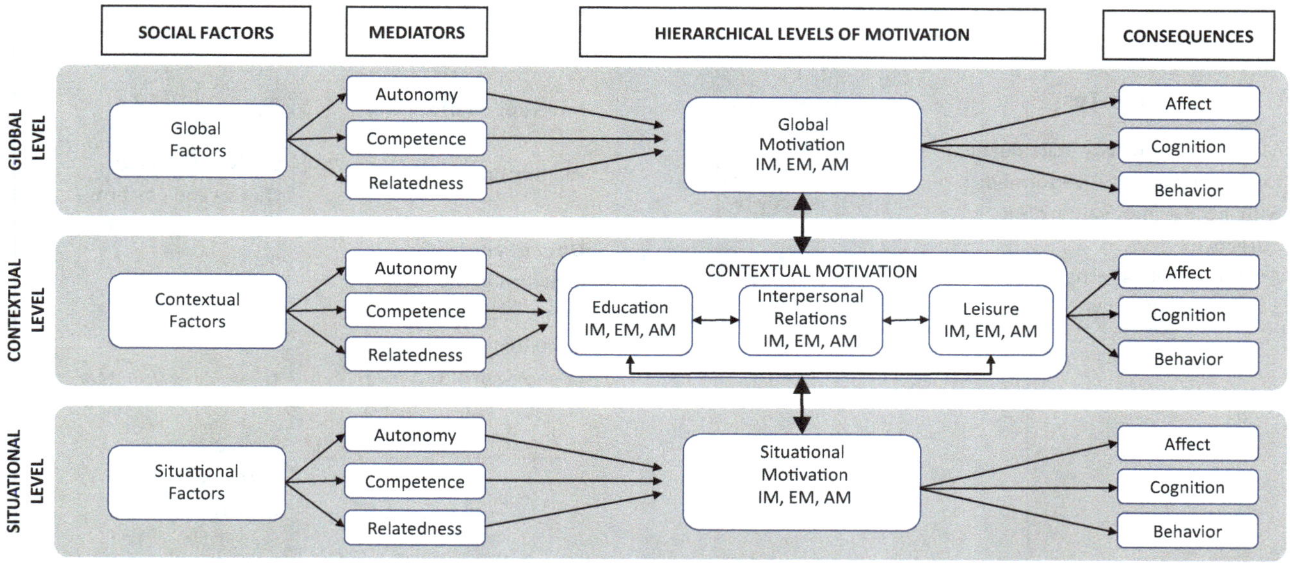

Fig. 8.8 Illustration of the hierarchical model of intrinsic motivation (adapted from Vallerand, 1997, p. 274)

nants – and mediators – that foster different types of motivation. For example, a social system that supports autonomy would be an example of a global social influencing factor that is likely to foster intrinsic motivation via satisfaction of the need for autonomy. Lastly, the model emphasizes the differential consequences different types of motivation can have for behavior, affect, and cognition

Hierarchical Model of Intrinsic Motivation of Vallerand (1997)

The hierarchical model of intrinsic motivation distinguishes between a global, contextual, and situational level, on which the three forms of motivation *intrinsic motivation*, *extrinsic motivation*, and *amotivation* exist (see Fig. 8.8).

8.3 Measuring Intrinsic Motivation

Intrinsic motivation in sport has been measured by observing behavior or by self-reports of the athletes in regard to their degree of intrinsic motivation.

8.3.1 Free Choice Paradigm

One form of behavioral observation, and the original prototype of the assessment of intrinsic motivation, is the "free choice paradigm." It was introduced by Deci (1971) and has been used in numerous follow-up studies as an operationalization of intrinsic motivation (see ▶ Methods: Free Choice Paradigm).

Methods: Free Choice Paradigm

In an experiment based on the free choice paradigm, participants first carry out an activity that was pretested to be interesting and intrinsically motivating. Then participants were told that the experimenter needs time, for example, to allegedly prepare the experimental material and that the participant can bridge this waiting time engaging with various activities. Among the attractive activities (e.g., reading journals laid out on a table), there is also the activity that was carried out before the interruption. If the study participants continue this activity unsolicitedly, and although it has no consequences for them (i.e., for its own sake), participants are deemed to act intrinsically motivated. The dependent variable is the time that the participants spend with the activity during the free choice period, which reflects the level of intrinsic motivation. The temporal procedure is described in Fig. 8.9.

Although employed in many early studies, the free choice paradigm as a standard measure of intrinsic motivation has been critically discussed (e.g., Vallerand & Fortier, 1998; Wiechman & Gurland, 2009). Most importantly, the free choice paradigm doesn't consider *why* the individual is continuing to engage in the initially intrinsically motivating activity or not. The motivation for engagement is only assumed. Further, at least two processes of the undermining effect are under-explored: (1) the duration of the free choice period (How long is enough?) (2) and the durability of the undermining effect (How long does the undermining of intrinsic motivation last?).

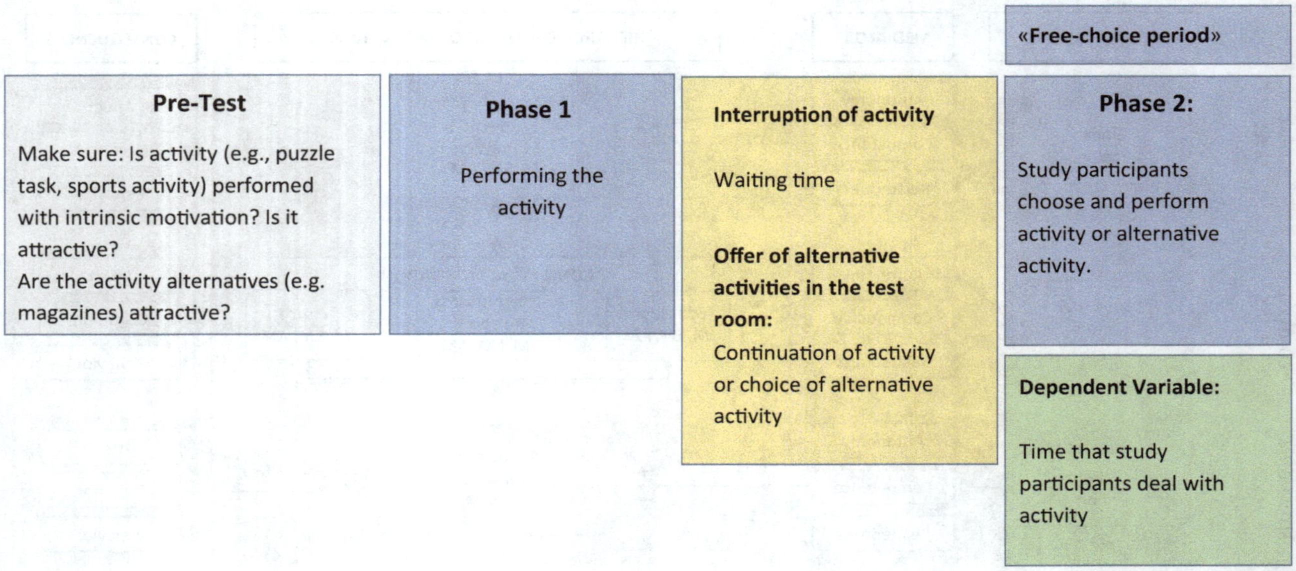

Fig. 8.9 Temporal procedure of "free choice paradigm"

> **Free Choice Paradigm**
> Intrinsic motivation is assumed to be measured by observing behavior. In the "free choice paradigm," intrinsic motivation is observed, within a certain time window, and measured how long participants engage in a task voluntarily and without influence from the experimenter. However, this paradigm is limited as the reasons or motivation behind the engagement are not considered.

8.3.2 Questionnaires Assessing Intrinsic Motivation

8.3.2.1 Intrinsic Motivation Inventory (IMI)

The Intrinsic Motivation Inventory (IMI) is a multidimensional measurement developed by a group of researchers within the framework of self-determination theory (SDT) (Ryan & Connell, 1989; Ryan et al., 1983). It aims at assessing the subjective experiences of participants during an activity and consists of the four dimensions "interest/enjoyment," "perceived competence," "perceived choice," and "pressure/tension." Contrary to what its name may imply, the IMI does not measure intrinsic motivation per se but rather captures the determinants (e.g., perceived competence) and consequences of intrinsic motivation (for more on this criticism of the IMI, see also Vallerand & Fortier, 1998). Regarding the latter, the interest/enjoyment scale can be considered as a self-report measure of one key outcome stemming from intrinsic motivation. When administering the IMI, it needs to be adjusted according to specific tasks and settings (e.g., education, sport). Its psychometric properties have also been tested and supported in the domain of sports (McAuley et al., 1989).

The seven items of the interest/enjoyment scale can be adapted to the specific sport by replacing "the task" by "playing volleyball." The items are:

1. I found the task very interesting.
2. Doing the task was fun.
3. I enjoyed doing the task very much.
4. While I was working on the task, I was thinking about how much I enjoyed it.
5. I thought the task was very boring (reversed item).
6. I thought the task was very interesting.
7. I would describe the task as very enjoyable.

8.3.2.2 Sport Motivation Scale

The "Sport Motivation Scale" and its revision (SMS II) (Pelletier et al., 2013) are based on the "organismic integration theory" (Deci & Ryan, 1985). As such, it measures intrinsic, integrated, identified, introjected, external, and amotivated regulation. Numerous studies confirmed that the SMS is a scale with high internal consistency and construct validity (Clancy et al., 2017). The antecedents and outcomes associated with different types of sport motivation, as assessed via the SMS, include persistence in sport training, practice frequency, self-esteem, positive emotions, vitality, and achievement goal orientations (see Pelletier et al., 2013 for more details).

Participants estimate the relevance of each statement to their own perspective using a 7-point Likert scale (1 = "does not apply at all"; 7 = "applies exactly"). The statements are "responses" to the question, "In general, why do you practice your sport?"

The SMS measures motivation to engage in sport at the *contextual* level (sport in general). The items reflect the different types of motivation (except integrated motivation) as assumed within SDT.

Examples:

- Intrinsic regulation: Because it gives me pleasure to learn more about my sport.
- Integrated regulation: Because participating in sport is an integral part of my life.
- Identified regulation: Because I have chosen this sport as a way to develop myself.
- Introjected regulation: Because I feel better about myself when I do.
- External regulation Because people around me reward me when I do.
- Amotivated regulation: It is not clear to me anymore; I don't really think my place is in sport.

8.3.2.3 Situational Motivational Scale (SIMS)

The Situational Motivational Scale (SIMS) (Guay et al., 2000) is a multidimensional tool that measures four types of motivation (intrinsic motivation, identified regulation, external regulation, and amotivation) on a *situational* level (e.g., a specific sport situation). Four items of each scale represent answers to the question: "Why are you currently engaged in this activity?"

- Intrinsic: Because I think that this activity is interesting.
- Identified: Because I am doing it for my own good.
- External: Because I am supposed to do it.
- Amotivation: There may be good reasons to do this activity, but personally I don't see any.

Depending on the exact wording of this questionnaire, it could be used for sport and nonsport activities (such as engagement in PE). An important characteristic of a psychological questionnaire is its measurement invariance, that is, the extent to which a measure maintains its meaning across groups (e.g., to make results of studies different groups comparable) or settings. Standage et al. (2003) showed measurement invariance for the SIMS across three physical activity samples (youth soccer players, middle school children participating in physical education, participants in college physical activity courses). Furthermore, the authors confirmed the SIMS' factorial validity in an experimental setting and therewith extend previous research based on field studies.

8.3.2.4 Behavioral Regulation in Sport Questionnaire (BRSQ)

The "Behavioral Regulation in Sport Questionnaire" (BRSQ, Lonsdale et al., 2008) consists of a 24-item questionnaire that measure 6 behavioral regulations (4 items per factor). Participants indicate their agreement to each item using a 7-point rating scale (1: "completely disagree; 7: "completely agree").

Example items for behavioral regulations as assessed via the BRSQ are:

- Amotivation: I play sports but I wonder what is the point.
- External: I practice sports because I feel pressure from other people to play.
- Introjected: I play sports because I feel obligated to continue.
- Identified: I play sports because I value the benefits.
- Integrated: I play sports because it is a part of who I am.
- Intrinsic motivation: I practice sports because I enjoy doing something to the best of my ability.

Comparing the measures to assess motivation regulations based on SDT, Rodrigues et al. (2020) concluded that the BRSQ is better suited for professional or competitive athletes, while the SMS II (Pelletier et al., 2013) is for other physical activity-related contexts.

Intrinsic Motivation Questionnaires

The Intrinsic Motivation Inventory (IMI, McAuley et al., 1989) includes subscales that capture promoters of and outcomes (e.g., interest/enjoyment) associated with intrinsic motivation in sport and other activities. Most contemporary questionnaires, which are grounded in SDT, tap the reasons for sports engagement and provide statements that capture intrinsic and extrinsic motivation (and other regulations) and amotivation. Examples of questionnaires that have been designed to tape motivation regulations at the contextual level are the "Sport Motivation Scale" ("Sport Motivation Scale"; Pelletier et al., 1995), and the "Behavioral Regulation in Exercise Questionnaire" (Mullan et al., 1997; Markland & Tobin, 2004). The Situational Motivation Scale (Guay et al., 2000) refers to the reasons for behavior in specific situations (situational level) during sport training.

8.4 Promoting Intrinsic Motivation in Sport

8.4.1 Strategies for Promoting Intrinsic Motivation

Weinberg and Gould (2015, p. 142–143) suggest strategies for promoting intrinsic motivation (terms in italics). In the following, we slightly revised and couched them according to the theories and concepts emphasized in this chapter.

1. *Provide successful and flow-conducive experiences.* Experiencing success results in experiencing competence, which represents an important basic psychological need (see SDT; Deci & Ryan, 1985). In order to be successful, the person's athletic abilities and the task difficulty have to be in a balance. A challenge-skill balance promotes flow experience. When the demands exceed the skills or vice versa, flow is less likely (see "Flow Theory" according to Csikszentmihalyi, 1990).
2. *Give feedback contingent on performance.* Feedback should be based on athletic performance, but in particular, what is controllable within that performance. If feedback is perceived as an informational about one's own performance and contributions, and not as a means to control, it can increase intrinsic motivation instead of undermining it (see SDT; Deci & Ryan, 1985).
3. *Use verbal and nonverbal praise.* Verbal praise ("well done") and nonverbal praise (thumbs up, pats on the back) motivate people who are not yet intrinsically motivated. Praise is especially powerful for people who usually get little recognition for their sport performance (e.g., people who differ from norms in sports with regard to, as examples, body weight, degree of talent). It is important though that this praise is clearly informational (aiming to enhance feelings of competence) and not manipulative or used in a way to control the person.
4. *Vary content and sequence of practice drills.* Offer variation and variety: Boredom and monotony are opponents of fun and intrinsic interest and are frequent reasons to drop out of sports programs.
5. *Involve participants in decision-making.* Invite one's athletes to participate in the design of sports lessons or in planning the strategies for the next game. Such increase the experience of autonomy. Experiencing autonomy is a basic psychological need and at the heart of Deci and Ryan's (1985) self-determination theory.
6. *Set realistic performance goals.* Help people to set realistic goals (i.e., goals that fit their skills and abilities) to make it possible to experience success and enhance feelings of competence (see also Goal Setting Strategies in High Performance Sports → ► Chaps. 7 and 20).

8.4.2 Focus: Promotion of Basic Need Satisfaction

As can be seen from these examples, most strategies to foster intrinsic motivation are based on, or could be understood via, the tenets of self-determination theory and its subtheories (see ► Sects. 8.2.2.1–8.2.2.3). According to SDT, a key to promote intrinsic motivation is satisfaction of basic needs which in turn leads to more autonomous forms of behavioral regulation (► Sect. 8.2.2.2), including the propensity for one to be intrinsically motivated. As outlined in ► Sect. 8.2.2.2, athletes' basic need satisfaction can be promoted by an autonomy-supporting coaching style, and this coaching style can be learned and developed, as has been shown in intervention studies. For example, an intervention study by Cheon et al. (2015) was based on the observation that coaches tend to adopt a controlling coaching style prior to important athletic competitions which in turn leads to a loss of self-determined motivation and further impairment in athletes. The authors tested the effects of an intervention aimed at teaching coaches an autonomy-supportive coaching style. During the preparation period for the Paralympic Games (London, 2012), they assigned 33 coaches (out of 64 athletes) to either a control group or intervention group. In terms of the latter, the autonomy-supportive intervention program consisted of a 2-h workshop focused on athletes' motivation and differential coaching styles (autonomy-supportive vs. controlling styles) (part 1 of program). Examples of autonomy-supportive coaching behavior were given (e.g., provide rationales for proposed strategies or training techniques, use of non-pressuring language, acknowledge and accepting negative affect). In the second part of the program, further information was given (e.g., how existing elements of structure that are needed for training effectiveness can be offered in an autonomy-supportive way). In a third part, each coach met the researchers so that individual questions could be answered and individual problems addressed. As expected, results revealed a decrease in self-determined motivation and functioning over time in the control group. In the intervention group, however, self-determined motivation and functioning remained intact during the competition preparation phase. There was also a positive effect in terms of performance: the athletes of the coaches in the intervention group won more Olympic medals than the athletes of the coaches in the control group.

In *For Sports Practice* a few more concrete examples of how an authority figure (coach, parent, teacher) can promote the satisfaction of all three basic needs are displayed (see also Reeve, 2002).

For Sport Practice

Ways to promote basic need satisfaction

Autonomy	Competence	Social relatedness
Aim		
Provide athletes experiences of choice in and ownership of their behavior	Promote athletes' feeling competent and efficient in dealing with the environment	Facilitate athletes feeling that they belong to (a group of) people who care about him/her and each other
Basic principle and attitude		
– Understand and take into account the perspectives of sports participants: What do they want? What do they not want? What are they feeling?	– Pay attention to the phrasing of goals – Make improvements in competence and progress tangible	Personal involvement, interest in the athlete and as a person; caring attitude
Concrete examples		
– Provide information and leeway for action – Allow exercises to be selected – Invite to participate in decisions regarding training	– Clearly define goals and expectations – Formulate goal criteria together – Provide challenge-skill balance – Give informative feedback	– Allow time for social interactions – Show feelings (personal involvement, joy) – Focus on similarities – Emphasize the qualities of each individual

8.4.3 *Empowering Coaching*™: Applying Theories Successfully for Practical Application

Self-determination theory (SDT; Ryan & Deci, 2018) provides a foundation for intervention development, providing guidance about what we can do to promote sport participants' intrinsic motivation. Based on SDT, one way to facilitate and maintain intrinsic interest is to work with those who create the motivational climate manifested in sport and develop sporting environments which are more need supportive and less likely to compromise participants' feelings of competence, autonomy, and relatedness.

Duda (Duda, 2013; Duda & Appleton, 2016) proposed a conceptualization of the motivational climate created by significant others (such as coaches, teachers, parents) which pulls from and extends the dimensions emphasized within SDT that are important to target in our intervention efforts. In particular, the features of the environment which are emphasized in achievement goal theory (Ames, 1992; Duda, 2001; Duda & Balaguer, 2007) are also considered, namely, how task involving (e.g., coach emphasizes demonstration of effort, considers mistakes as part of learning), and how ego involving (e.g., coach creates a rivalrous atmosphere and compares one athlete to another; errors are responded to punitively) is the motivational climate? In this conceptualization, sporting environments are considered more *empowering* if they are highly autonomy supportive, socially supportive, and task involving. *A disempowering* sport environment would be one in which, for example, the coach is very controlling and ego involving in his or her behaviors.

The *Empowering Coaching*™ training program (Duda, 2013; Duda & Appleton, 2016) is grounded in this conceptualization and aims to help coaches/teachers/parents understand how to be more empowering and why that approach is more adaptive. Within the training, participants have the opportunity to also reflect and become more aware of what may be existing disempowering behaviors and the costs of such in regard to sport participants' autonomous motivation, development, and well-being. More information about Empowering Coaching can be found here: ► https://empoweringcoaching.co.uk/.

Theoretical models also guide the authors of the empowering coaching program approaches to assessment. Based on the conceptualization of empowering and disempowering "coaching," ways to assess the motivational climate created by coaches via observation (Smith et al., 2015), self-reports of the athletes in that environment (Appleton et al., 2016), and the views of the coaches themselves (Solstad et al., 2020) have been developed. Using such assessment tools, the impact of *Empowering Coaching*™ has been examined. For example, this training program was evaluated in the context of youth sport (soccer) across five European countries within the Promoting Adolescent Physical Activity (PAPA) project (Duda & Appleton, 2016).

We believe that the example of *Empowering Coaching*™ provides a vivid example on how empirical and theoretical work can be adapted and utilized to create theory-driven applications for the real world. This program's success also highlights how much intrinsic motivation matters. And that in order to increase sports participation, and to make sports participation as much enjoyable as possible, further research on the processes by which intrinsic motivation can be increased is needed. As a consequence, we hope the present chapter inspires readers not only to think about how to foster intrinsic motivation in their own lives but to also think about the many open questions that remain when it comes to understanding and increasing intrinsic motivation in sports and exercise.

8

Learning Control Questions

Basic:

1. What are the main distinguishing features of intrinsic and extrinsic motivation?
2. Can effort be intrinsically rewarding?
3. What subtheories does the "self-determination theory" consist of? Name their core statements.
4. What forms of extrinsic motivation exist according to the "theory of organismic integration?" What does the "undermining effect" mean?
5. What are the three basic needs and what makes them "basic?"
6. Who is the author of the "Hierarchical Model of Intrinsic Motivation?" What do "task orientation" and "performance orientation" mean?
7. Explain the basic assumptions of "empowering coaching."

Advanced:

1. Which moderators of the relationship between positive performance feedback and intrinsic motivation do you know?
2. How can perceived autonomy support by the coach be measured?
3. What are the most important characteristics, conditions, and consequences of the flow experience?
4. What is the "free choice paradigm" and what does a typical test procedure look like?
5. Should extrinsic motivation always be avoided?
6. How is the hierarchical model of intrinsic motivation associated with self-determination theory?

Experts:

1. How can a sports teacher increase intrinsic motivation of his or her students through basic needs satisfaction?
2. When is the undermining effect most likely to occur? When is it unlikely to occur?
3. Why is the self-determination theory an umbrella theory that encompasses several mini-theories?
4. What does the general, contextual, and situational level in the "hierarchical model" refer to?
5. What tips would you give sports practitioners? Which factors promote intrinsic motivation in sport?
6. See the Empowering Coaching™ homepage and search for more information: What do you like about the concept? What could be added to such training to further promote intrinsic motivation to engage in sport?

References

Adie, J. A., Duda, J. L., & Ntoumanis, N. (2012). Perceived coach autonomy support, basic need satisfaction and the well- and ill-being of elite youth soccer players: A longitudinal investigation. *Psychology of Sport and Exercise, 13*, 51–59.

Adie, J. W., Duda, J. L., & Ntoumanis, N. (2008). Autonomy support, basic need satisfaction and the optimal functioning of adult male and female sport participants: A test of basic needs theory. *Motivation and Emotion, 32*(3), 189–199.

Alvarez, M. S., Balaguer, I., Castillo, I., & Duda, J. L. (2012). The coach-created motivational climate, young athletes' well-being, and intentions to continue sport participation. *Journal of Clinical Sport Psychology, 6*, 166–179.

Ames, C. (1992). Classrooms: Goals, structures, and student motivation. *Journal of Educational Psychology, 84*, 261–271.

Appleton, P., Ntoumanis, N., Quested, E., Viladrich, C., & Duda, J. L. (2016). Initial validation of the coach-created Empowering and Disempowering Motivational Climate Questionnaire (EDMCQ-C). *Psychology of Sport and Exercise, 22*, 53–65.

Balaguer, I., Gonzalez, L., Fabra, P., Castillo, I., Merce, J., & Duda, J. L. (2012). Coaches' interpersonal style, basic psychological needs and the well- and ill-being of young soccer players: A longitudinal analysis. *Journal of Sports Sciences, 30*(15), 1619–1629.

Bartholomew, K. J., Ntoumanis, N., Ryan, R. M., Bosch, J. A., & Thøgersen-Ntoumani, C. (2011a). Self-determination theory and diminished functioning: The role of interpersonal control and psychological need thwarting. *Personality & Social Psychology Bulletin, 37*, 1459–1473.

Bartholomew, K. J., Ntoumanis, N., Ryan, R. M., & Thogersen-Ntoumani, C. (2011b). Psychological need thwarting in the sport context: Assessing the darker side of athletic experience. *Journal of Sport and Exercise Psychology, 33*(1), 75e102.

Bartholomew, K. J., Ntoumanis, N., & Thogersen-Ntoumani, C. (2010). The Controlling interpersonal style in a coaching context: Development and initial validation of a psychometric scale. *Journal of Sport and Exercise Psychology, 32*(2), 193–216.

Cameron, J., Banko, K. M., & Pierce, W. D. (2001). Pervasive negative effects of rewards on intrinsic motivation: The myth continues. *The Behavior Analyst, 24*(1), 1–44.

Carpentier, J., Mageau, G. A., & Vallerand, R. J. (2012). Ruminations and flow: Why do people with a more harmonious passion experience higher well-being? *Journal of Happiness Studies, 13*, 501–518.

Cerasoli, C. P., Nicklin, J. M., & Ford, M. T. (2014). Intrinsic motivation and extrinsic incentives jointly predict performance: A 40-year meta-analysis. *Psychological Bulletin, 140*(4), 980–1008.

Cheon, S. H., et al. (2015). Giving and receiving autonomy support in a high-stakes sport context: A field-based experiment during the 2012 London Paralympic Games. *Psychology of Sport & Exercise, 19*, 59–69.

Clancy, R. B., Herring, M. P., & Campbell, M. J. (2017). Motivation measures in sport: A critical review and bibliometric analysis. *Frontiers in Psychology, 8*(348), 348.

Cremades, J. G., Flournoy, B., & Gomez, C. B. (2012). Scholarship status and gender differences in motivation among U.S. collegiate track and field athletes. *International Journal of Sports Science & Coaching, 7*, 333–344.

Csikszentmihalyi, M. (1975). *Beyond boredom and anxiety*. Jossey-Bass.

Csikszentmihalyi, M. (1990). *Flow: The psychology of optimal experience*. Harper & Row.

Csikszentmihalyi, M., Abuhamdeh, S., & Nakamura, J. (2005). Flow. In A. J. Elliot & C. S. Dweck (Eds.), *Handbook of competence and motivation* (pp. 598–608). Guilford Publications Inc.

Csikszentmihalyi, M., & Csikszentmihalyi, I. (1988). *Optimal experience: Psychological studies of flow in consciousness*. University Press.

Deci, E. L. (1971). Effects of externally mediated rewards on intrinsic motivation. *Journal of Personality and Social Psychology, 18*, 105–115.

Deci, E. L. (1975). *Intrinsic motivation*. Plenum.

Deci, E. L., Koestner, R., & Ryan, R. M. (1999). A meta-analytic review of experiments examining the effects of extrinsic rewards on intrinsic motivation. *Psychological Bulletin, 125*(6), 627–668.

Deci, E. L., & Ryan, R. M. (1985). *Intrinsic motivation and self-determination in human behavior*. Plenum.

Deci, E. L., & Ryan, R. M. (2000). The "what" and "why" of goal pursuits: Human needs and the self-determination of behavior. *Psychological Inquiry, 11*, 227–268.

Deci, E. L., & Ryan, R. M. (2002). *Handbook of self-determination research*. University of Rochester Press.

Deci, E. L., & Vansteenkiste, M. (2004). Self-determination theory and basic need satisfaction: Understanding human development in positive psychology. *Ricerche di Psicologia, 27*(1), 23–40.

Duda, J. L. (2001). Goal perspectives research in sport: Pushing the boundaries and clarifying some misunderstandings. In G. C. Roberts (Ed.), *Advances in motivation in sport and exercise* (pp. 129–182). Human Kinetics.

Duda, J. L. (2013). The conceptual and empirical foundations of Empowering Coaching™: Setting the stage for the PAPA project. *International Journal of Sport and Exercise Psychology, 11*(4), 311–318.

Duda, J. L., & Appleton, P. R. (2016). Empowering and disempowering coaching climates: Conceptualization, measurement considerations, and intervention implications. In M. Raab, P. Wylleman, R. Seiler, A.-M. Elbe, & A. Hatzigeorgiadis (Eds.), *Sport and exercise psychology research: From theory to practice* (pp. 373–388). Elsevier Academic Press.

Duda, J. L., & Balaguer, I. (2007). The coach-created motivational climate. In S. Jowett & D. Lavalee (Eds.), *Social Psychology of Sport* (pp. 117–130). Human Kinetics.

Edmunds, J., Ntoumanis, N., & Duda, J. L. (2007). Adherence and wellbeing in overweight and obese patients referred to an exercise on prescription scheme: a self-determination theory perspective. *Psychology of Sport and Exercise, 8*, 722–740.

Fenton, S. A. M., Duda, J. L., Quested, E., & Barret, T. (2014). Coach autonomy support predicts autonomous motivation and daily moderate-to-vigorous physical activity and sedentary time in youth sport participants. *Psychology of Sport and Exercise, 15*, 453–463.

Frederick, C. M., & Ryan, R. M. (1995). Self-determination in sport - a review using cognitive evaluation theory. *International Journal of Sport Psychology, 26*(1), 5–23.

Gagné, M., Ryan, R. M., & Bargmann, K. (2003). Autonomy support and need satisfaction in the motivation and well-being of gymnasts. *Journal of Applied Sport Psychology, 15*(4), 372–390.

Guay, F., Mageau, G. A., & Vallerand, R. J. (2003). On the hierarchical structure of self-determined motivation: A test of top-down, bottom-up, reciprocal, and horizontal effects. *Personality and Social Psychology Bulletin, 29*, 992–1004.

Guay, F., Vallerand, R. J., & Blanchard, C. (2000). On the assessment of situational intrinsic and extrinsic motivation: The situational motivation scale (sims). *Motivation and Emotion, 24*(3), 175–213.

Gunnell, K. E., et al. (2013). Psychological need satisfaction and thwarting: A test of Basic Psychological Needs Theory in physical activity contexts. *Psychology of Sport and Exercise, 14*, 599–607.

Hagger, M. S., & Chatzisarantis, N. L. D. (Eds.). (2007). *Intrinsic motivation and self-determination in exercise and sport*. Human Kinetics.

Hausenblaus, H. A., & Downs, D. S. (2002). Exercise dependence: A systematic review. *Psychology of Sport and Exercise, 3*, 89–123.

Hull, C. L. (1943). *Principles of behavior*. Appleton-Century.

Inzlicht, M., Shenhav, A., & Olivola, C. Y. (2018). The effort paradox: Effort is both costly and valued. *Trends in Cognitive Science, 1760*.

Jackson, S. A., & Csikszentmihalyi, M. (1999). *Flow in Sports. The keys of optimal experience and performance*. Human Kinetics.

Lonsdale, C., Hodge, K., & Rose, E. A. (2008). The behavioral regulation in sport questionannaire (brsq): Instrument development and initial validity evidence. *Journal of Sport and Exercise, 30*, 323–355.

Markland, D., & Tobin, V. (2004). A modification to the behavioural regulation in exercise questionnaire to include an assessment of amotivation. *Journal of Sport & Exercise Psychology, 26*(2), 191–196.

McAuley, E., Duncan, T., & Tammen, V. V. (1989). Psychometric properties of the intrinsic motivation inventory in a competitive sport setting: A confirmatory factor analysis. *Research Quarterly for Exercise and Sport, 60*, 48–58.

Medic, N., Mack, D. E., Wilson, P. M., & Starkes, J. L. (2007). The effects of athletic scholarships on motivation in sport. *Journal of Sport Behavior, 30*, 292–306.

Moller, A. C., & Sheldon, K. M. (2020). Athletic scholarships are negatively associated with intrinsic motivation for sports, even decades later: Evidence for long-term undermining. *Motivation Science, 6*(1), 43–48.

Mossman, L., H., Slemp, G. R., Lewis, K. J., Colla, R. H., & O'Halloran, P. (2022): Autonomy support in sport and exercise settings: a systematic review and meta-analysis, International Review of Sport and Exercise Psychology, https://doi.org/10.1080/1750984X.2022.2031252

Mullan, E., Markland, D., & Ingledew, D. K. (1997). A graded conceptualisation of self-determination in the regulation of exercise behaviour: Development of a measure using confirmatory factor analytic procedures. *Personality and Individual Differences, 23*(5), 745–752.

Ntoumanis, N. (2001). A self-determination approach to the understanding of motivation in physical education. *British Journal of Educational Psychology, 71*(2), 225–242.

Partington, S., Partington, E., & Olivier, S. (2009). The dark side of flow: A qualitative study of dependence in big wave surfing. *The Sport Psychologist, 23*, 170–186.

Pelletier, L., Fortier, M., Vallerand, R., Tuson, K., Brière, N., & Blais, M. (1995). Toward a new measure of intrinsic motivation, extrinsic motivation, and amotivation in sports: The sport motivation scale (SMS). *Journal of Sport and Exercise Psychology, 17*, 35e54.

Pelletier, L. G., Rocchi, M. A., Vallerand, R. J., Deci, E. L., & Ryan, R. M. (2013). Validation of the revised sport motivation scale (sms-ii). *Psychology of Sport and Exercise, 14*, 329–341.

Quested, E., & Duda, J. L. (2011). Antecedents of burnout among elite dancers: A longitudinal test of basic needs theory. *Psychology of Sport and Exercise, 12*, 159–167.

Reeve, J. (2002). Self-determination theory applied to educational settings. In E. L. Deci & R. M. Ryan (Eds.), *Handbook of self-determination research* (pp. 183–203). University of Rochester Press.

Reinboth, M., & Duda, J. L. (2006). Perceived motivationa climate, need satisfaction and indices of well-being in team sports: A longitudinal perspective. *Psychology of Sport and Exercise, 7*, 269–286.

Rodrigues, F., Macedo, R., Teixeira, D. S., Cid, L., & Monteiro, D. (2020). Motivation in sport and exercise: a comparison between the BRSQ and BREQ. *Quality and Quantity, 54*, 1335–1350.

8

Ryan, E. D. (1977). Attribution, intrinsic motivation, and athletics. In L. I. Gedvilas & M. E. Kneer (Eds.), *Proceedings of the National Association for Physical Education of College Men National Conference Association for Physical Education of College Women. National Conference* (pp. 346–353). University of Illinois at Chicago Circle.

Ryan, E. D. (1980). Attribution, intrinsic motivation, and athletics: A replication and extension. In C. H. Nadeau, W. R. Halliwell, K. M. Newell, & G. C. Roberts (Eds.), *Psychology of motor behavior and sport* (pp. 19–26). Human Kinetics.

Ryan, R. M., & Connell, J. P. (1989). Perceived locus of causality and internalization: Examining reasons for acting in two domains. *Journal of Personality and Social Psychology, 57*, 749–761.

Ryan, R. M., & Deci, E. L. (2000). Intrinsic and extrinsic motivations: Classic definitions and new directions. *Contemporary Educational Psychology, 25*, 54–67.

Ryan, R. M., & Deci, E. L. (2002). Overview of self-determination theory: An organismic dialectical perspective. In R. M. Deci & E. L. Deci (Eds.), *Handbook of self-determination research* (pp. 3–33). Rochester University Press.

Ryan, R. M., & Deci, E. L. (2017). *Self-determination theory. Basic psychological needs in motivation, development, and wellness*. Guilford Press.

Ryan, R. M., & Deci, E. L. (2018). *Self-determination Theory: Basic psychological needs in motivation, development, and wellness*. The Guilford Press.

Ryan, R. M., Mims, V., & Koestner, R. (1983). Relation of reward contingency and interpersonal context to intrinsic motivation: A review and test using Cognitive Evaluation Theory. *Journal of Personality and Social Psychology, 45*, 736–750.

Sedentary Behavior Research Network. (2012). Letter to the editor: standardized use of the terms "sedentary" and "sedentary behaviours". *Applied Physiology, Nutrition and Metabolism, 37*(3), 540–542.

Seelig, H., & Fuchs, R. (2006). Messung der sport- und bewegungsbezogenen Selbstkonkordanz. *Zeitschrift für Sportpsychologie, 13*(4), 121–139.

Sheldon, K. M., & Elliot, A. J. (1999). Goal striving, need satisfaction, and longitudinal well-being: The self-concordance model. *Journal of Personality and Social Psychology, 7*(3), 482–497.

Smith, A., Ntoumanis, N., & Duda, J. (2007). Goal striving, goal attainment, and well-being: Adapting and testing the self-concordance model in sport. *Journal of Sport & Exercise Psychology, 29*(6), 763–782.

Smith, A. L., Ntoumanis, N., Duda, J. L., & Vansteenkiste, M. (2011). Goal striving, coping, and well-being: A prospective investigation of the self-concordance model in sport. *Journal of Sport & Exercise Psychology, 33*, 124–145.

Smith, N., Tessier, D., Tzioumakis, Y., Quested, E., Appleton, P., Sarrazin, P., Papaioannou, A., & Duda, J. L. (2015). Development and validation of the multidimensional motivational climate observation system. *Journal of Sport and Exercise Psychology, 37*(1), 4–22.

Solstad, B., Stening, A., Ommundsen, Y., Wold, B., Heuze, J. P., Sarrazin, P., Castillo, I., Cruz, J., Hall, H., Papaioannou, A., & Duda, J. L. (2020). Initial psychometric testing of the coach-adapted version of the Empowering and Disempowering Motivational Climate Questionnaire: A Bayesian approach. *Journal of Sport Science, 38*(6), 626–643.

Standage, M., Duda, J. L., & Ntoumanis, N. (2006). Students' motivational processes and their relationship to teacher ratings in school physical education: A self-determination approach. *Research Quarterly for Exercise and Sport, 77*, 100–110.

Standage, M., Duda, J. L., & J. L., & Ntoumanis, N. (2003). A model of contextual motivation in physical education: Using constructs from self-determination and achievement goal theories to predict physical activity intentions. *Journal of Educational Psychology, 95*(1), 97–110.

Swann, C., Keegan, R. J., Piggott, D., & Crust, L. (2012). A systematic review of the experience, occurrence, and controllability of flow states in elite sport. *Psychology of Sport and Exercise, 13*, 807–819.

Vallerand, R. J. (1997). Toward a hierarchical model of intrinsic and extrinsic motivation. In M. P. Zanna (Ed.), *Advances in experimental social psychology* (pp. 271–360). Academic Press.

Vallerand, R. J. (2012). Intrinsic and extrinsic motivation in sport and physical activity: A review and a look at the future. In G. Tenenbaum & R. Eklund (Eds.), *Handbook of sport psychology* (3rd ed.). Wiley.

Vallerand, R. J., Blanchard, C., Mageau, G. A., Koestner, R., Ratelle, C., & Leonard, M. (2003). Les passions de l'ame: On obsessive and harmonious passion. *Journal of Personality and Social Psychology, 85*, 756–767.

Vallerand, R. J., & Fortier, M. S. (1998). Measure of intrinsic and extrinsic motivation in sport and physical activity: A review and critique. In J. L. Duda (Ed.), *Advances in sport and exercise psychology measurement* (pp. 471–483). Fitness Information Technology.

Vallerand, R. J., Mageau, G. A., Elliot, A. J., Dumais, A., Demers, M.-A., & Rousseau, F. (2008). Passion and performance attainment in sport. *Psychology of Sport and Exercise, 9*(3), 373–392.

Vallerand, R. J., & Reid, G. (1984). On the causal effects of perceived competence on intrinsic motivation: A test of cognitive evaluation theory. *Journal of Sport Psychology, 6*, 94–102.

Weinberg, R. S., & Gould, D. (2015). *Foundations of sport and exercise psychology*. Human Kinetics.

White, R. W. (1959). Motivation reconsidered: The concept of competence. *Psychological Review, 66*, 297–333.

Wiechman, B. M., & Gurland, S. T. (2009). What happens during the free-choice period? Evidence of a polarizing effect of extrinsic rewards on intrinsic motivation. *Journal of Research in Personality, 43*, 716–719.

Wolff, W., Hirsch, A., Bieleke, M., & Shenhav, A. (2021). Neuroscientific approaches to self-regulatory control in sports. Motivation and self-regulation in sport and exercise. In C. Englert & I. A. Taylor (Eds.), *Motivation and self-regulation in sport and exercise* (pp. 149–165). Routledge.

Zimanyi, Z., Wolff, W., & Schüler, J. (2021). Too much of a good thing? Exercise dependence in endurance athletes: relationships with personal and social resources. *International Journal of Environmental Research and Public Health, 18*, 2966.

Implicit Motives in Sport and Exercise

Mirko Wegner and Kerstin Brinkmann

Contents

J. Schüler et al. (eds.), *Sport and Exercise Psychology*, https://doi.org/10.1007/978-3-031-03921-8_9

9

Learning Objectives

Basic:

- Be able to describe what is meant by (implicit) motives.
- Be able to name different measurement procedures for motives and explain their measurement principle.
- Be able to distinguish implicit motives from explicit self-attributes.

Advanced:

- Be able to understand and describe the implicit motive themes (achievement, affiliation, power) and their relevance for the sport and exercise context.
- Be able to describe basic physiological associations with implicit motivational processes.
- Be able to describe considerations on the (in)congruence between implicit motives and explicit self-attributes.
- Be able to understand that one and the same action can be based on different motives.

Experts:

- Be able to reflect the evolutionary biological advantage of having two separate motivational systems.
- Be able to describe the thoughts and feelings of people with strong achievement, affiliation, and power motives in different sport contexts (e.g., competition, leisure activities).
- Be able to develop ideas on how to avoid incongruence in sports.

9.1 Definitions and Basic Assumptions

In performance and health sports, one is interested in long-term behavioral predictions. For example, a statement about the probability with which a high-performance athlete shows the drive to regard the high training and competition demands as a challenge and not as a burden up to the top of the world and maintains a performance sport behavior over many years is very valuable (see ◘ Fig. 9.1). Motives are traits of people and provide the long-term energy for action. For health sport courses, too, information about participants' personal motives can be important for program design. We already know from the classical motivation model (see ► Chap. 7) that motivation with corresponding behavioral consequences occurs primarily through the interaction of sports contexts (situation) and motives (as personal traits).

> Motives are traits of people and provide the long-term energy for action.

However, motivational psychologists noticed early on that one cannot simply ask people about their motives in order to deduce any behavioral tendencies (deCharms et al., 1955). For example, if an athlete is asked directly about his/her personal motivations for playing sports (self-report, e.g., with questionnaire), responses will be obtained that reflect what the athlete thinks about himself/herself or what the expectations are for his/her actions in a particular sporting situation/environment. For example, the father of a junior athlete, who himself was once international champion in his discipline, might expect similar performance from his son. The son would therefore be more inclined to say that achieving best performances in his sport motivates him a lot. Of course, such expectations of best performance are inherent in competitive sports. A health sport setting involves other values such as healthy eating or physical activity in everyday life. Thus, direct surveys carry the risk that people report such values in settings as their own motives for good reasons. This makes short-term predictions of behavior possible, but not predictions of long-term behavior (McClelland et al., 1989). Therefore, early work in motivational psychology addressed how to infer motives of individuals without direct questioning.

In contrast to motive characteristics, which are available from self-reports, implicit motives are inferred indi-

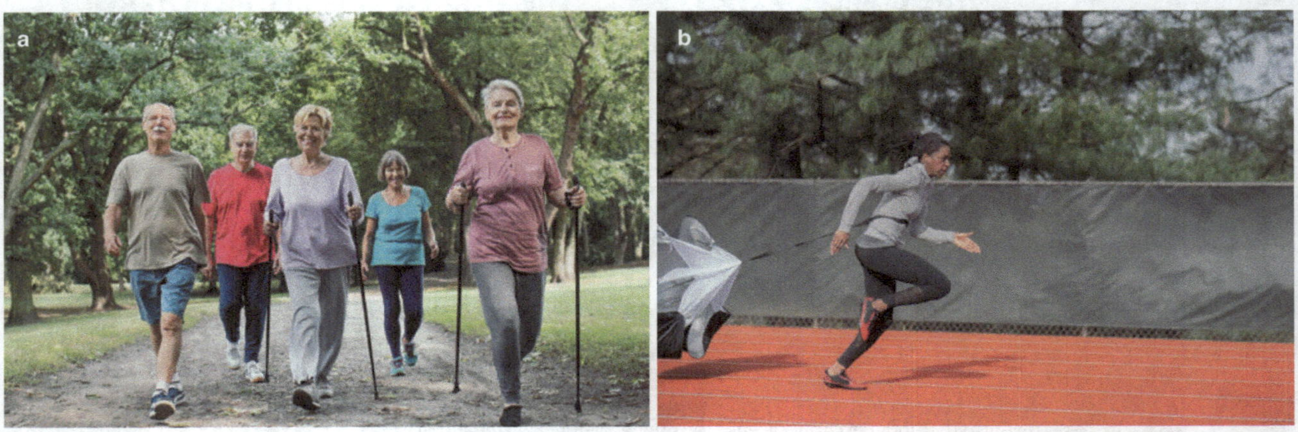

◘ **Fig. 9.1** **a**, **b** Health- and performance-oriented sports rectly, e.g., via picture story exercises, which have their origins in projective procedures (Morgan & Murray, 1935). In the context of such procedures, the way that individuals interpret certain social situations is used to infer how their own motives are expressed. More details on the measurement of implicit motives follow in ▶ Sect. 9.2.

At this point, it is important to assume that these indirectly deduced motives are not conscious for athletes. Thus, athletes are usually unaware of how their implicit motives are expressed. **Implicit motives** are defined as unconscious, enduring preferences for certain incentive classes (McClelland, 1987a, 1987b). Preferences here mean that preference is given to those situations that promise a certain affect. For example, a person with a strong achievement motive (see below) prefers challenging tasks and goals because they promise the experience of pride and competence.

Implicit motives are defined as unconscious, enduring preferences for certain incentive classes (McClelland, 1987a, 1987b).

At their core, implicit motives are thought to serve three functions:

- Implicit motives help *orient* attention toward cue stimuli that can be motive-satisfying, that is, can be incentives for a person's motive (e.g., the motive to have social interaction).
- Implicit motives provide *action energy*.
- Implicit motives *direct* behavior toward specific classes of stimuli that are relevant to motive satisfaction (McClelland, 1987a, 1987b).

Figure 9.2 illustrates these three functions (Schultheiss, 2008). Affects play a crucial role in the relationship between implicit motives and behavior. Take, for example, a female athlete with a high affiliation motive, i.e., to whom interpersonal relationships are important. A run in the woods with friends gives her a lot of pleasure—she thus experiences positive affect. When planning her next sporting activity, she is more likely to perceive a friend's offer to go running together as a relevant cue stimulus than the ad on the bulletin board of a gym where she knows no one (function of *orientation* and **selection** of cue stimuli). What is motivationally appropriate about a run in the woods with friends then also ensures that the athlete is able to run more intensively and persistently and to feel greater pleasure (**energizing** function). Motives ensure, for example, that affects are perceived more strongly in such potentially motive-relevant situations. Thus, the activity itself is more rewarding when motive and incentives match in the situation. The athlete's high affiliation motive also contributes to the fact that he/she learns better in situations that are potentially motivating, i.e., collaborative activities, and is more involved in these activities overall (**directing** function).

Incentives are situations of a prompting nature that promise an individual a positive or negative affective state. Incentives can be linked to the activity itself, the outcome of an action, or the consequences of the outcome of an action (Heckhausen & Heckhausen, 2010). For explanations of the interplay between motives and incentives, see ▶ Chap. 7.

Incentives promise an individual a positive or negative affective state. They can be linked to the activity itself (e.g., enjoying an intellectual task, enjoying time spent with other people) or to the outcome of an action (e.g., being proud because of one's mastery of a challenging task; having established a friendship).

Motive

Motive is defined as a nonconscious, nonverbally represented, affect-based preference for certain classes of incentives that orients attention toward specific cue stimuli in the environment and energizes behavior (McClelland, 1987a, 1987b).

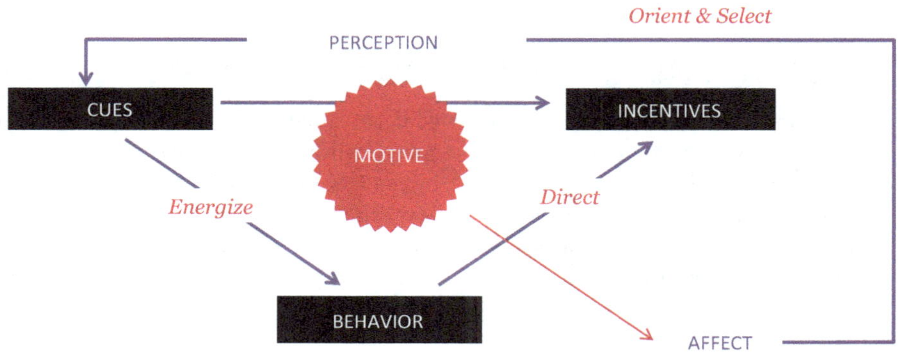

Fig. 9.2 Functions of implicit motives: (1) orienting to and selecting motive-relevant cue stimuli based on past affective experiences, (2) energizing behavior, (3) directing behavior toward specific classes of incentives. (Adapted figure from Schultheiss, 2008)

Over the past decades, motive research has focused primarily on the motive themes of **achievement**, **affiliation**, and **power**. These motives have also played a special role in sports and exercise science research. The strongest research focus was and still is on the achievement motive. The **achievement motive** is defined as an enduring preference for certain classes of incentives for the attainment of which a person wishes to increase or uphold his or her own proficiency and for which a personal standard of excellence is considered binding (Brunstein & Heckhausen, 2006; Heckhausen, 1965; McClelland et al., 1953). A typical example in sports is an athlete who wants to improve his/her best time over the 10-km running distance more and more. In the **affiliation motive**, such preferences are directed toward establishing, maintaining, or restoring positive social relationships with others (French & Chadwick, 1956; Heyns et al., 1958; Sokolowski & Heckhausen, 2010). For example, a participant in a running group with a high affiliation motive may not be greatly interested in improving his or her running performance but primarily value the contact with the nice running partners in the running group and therefore regularly participate in this sport. People with a high **power motive** prefer incentives that allow them to exert influence on other people. They want themselves to dominate and not be dominated by others (Schmalt & Heckhausen, 2010; Winter, 1973). Such influence over others may be sought on a physical, emotional, or cognitive level. For example, an athlete with a high power motive might emphasize after a high victory in a soccer game that it was important for him/her to teach his/her opponents a lesson and demonstrate his/her own strength to them. Athletes with a high power motive on the same team might find the specificity of the high victory more important than an outstanding achievement.

Achievement Motive

The **achievement motive** is the need to increase or maintain one's own proficiency in an activity in which a personal standard of excellence is considered as binding.

Affiliation Motive

The **affiliation motive** is the need to establish, maintain, or restore positive social relationships with others.

Power Motive

The **power motive** is the need to exert physical, psychological, or emotional influence over others.

Sports Practice

Individuals are motivated through all three motive themes, that is, achievement, affiliation, as well as power. However, they may strongly differ in the strength of each of these motives. If you think of a gymnast, what motive profile would benefit the strive for technical excellence in his/her sport and how may his/her motive profile differ from the motive profile of a professional soccer player?

In addition to this triad of motives, the importance of other motives for the field of sport and exercise is also discussed in recent research. One example is the autonomy motive. The implicit **autonomy motive** is understood as a person's enduring and cross-contextual preference to feel self-determined and independent of the influence of others (Schüler et al., 2016b) or, in deCharms' (1968) terms, to experience oneself as the cause of one's own action. Thus, a recreational athlete with a high autonomy motive might find it particularly important to choose the sport he or she wants to participate in to improve his or her health (for more information on the autonomy motive, see ► Side Story: Self-Determination and Autonomy Motive in Sport).

❯ In motive research three motives are typically differentiated: achievement, affiliation, and power. Some researchers have suggested to add the autonomy motive.

Side Story

Self-Determination and Autonomy Motive in Sport and Exercise

Sports environments that promote self-determination and autonomy are assumed to have a positive effect on the motivation and well-being of athletes (► Chap. 8). Such sport environments are characterized by the fact that athletes have choices between different tasks, that they can incorporate their wishes and interests in the design of training, and that trainers are less inclined to be restrictive about the content of training. However, recent studies show that not all athletes benefit in the same way from such autonomy-supporting sport environments (Schüler et al.,

2016a, 2016b). It has been shown that especially those who possess a high implicit autonomy motive benefit from autonomy-supporting sport environments. The implicit autonomy motive is defined as a stable preference for experiencing psychological freedom or autonomy and perceiving oneself as causing one's own actions across different contexts (deCharms, 1968; Schüler et al., 2016a, 2016b). These findings partially put the universality assumption of self-determination theory into perspective (Deci & Ryan, 1985), namely, that all individuals benefit equally from experiencing autonomy. Further evidence that individuals benefit from autonomy support in sport depending on the strength of their implicit autonomy motive can be found, for example, in the context of physical education (PE) in school. For example, it has been shown that students who read through a description of a sports lesson that promoted autonomy for a few minutes and pictorially placed themselves in it (so-called vignette method) showed lower levels of the stress marker and salivary enzyme alpha-amylase if they possessed a high implicit autonomy motive (Sieber et al., 2016a). Students who were measured to have a low implicit autonomy motive or who read through pure descriptions of a gym instead of autonomy-promoting instruction showed higher alpha-amylase levels, which could indicate higher stress activation. Thus, if the sports contexts (in this case, autonomy-promoting instruction) match the implicit motivational structure of the participants (in this case, a high autonomy motive), athletes benefit in well-being and motivation.

In another experiment (Sieber et al., 2016b), a physical education (PE) teacher produced either an autonomy-supporting or an autonomy-restricting sports situation in a physical education class or behaved neutrally (control condition). As expected, students with high implicit autonomy motives reported more intrinsic motivation when the PE teachers actively promoted autonomy in their lessons compared to the other two experimental conditions. All of these findings suggest that the personality of the student athlete must be taken into account if one is to optimally promote his/her motivation and well-being through appropriate sport environments.

Sports Practice

As we learnt in ▶ Chap. 7, students' motivation can be perceived as a result of a fit between a person's motives and the sport or exercise environment. When you as a possible future physical education (PE) teacher know that a person might be strongly motivated by autonomy, how would you arrange your PE class in order to foster intrinsic motivation in your students? ▶ Chapter 8 on intrinsic motivation and basic psychological needs as well as ▶ Table 7.1 on how to create a positive motivational climate might help you conceptualize your PE class.

Implicit motives direct attention toward motive-relevant cues. This is especially true for pictorial, nonverbal cue stimuli. Atkinson and Walker (1958), for example, found that individuals with a high implicit affiliation motive recognized faces better than individuals with a low affiliation motive in the presence of a rapid succession of stimulus pictures (in their study these were furniture and faces) and poor lighting. High power-motivated individuals also orient their attention more quickly toward surprised faces than toward friendly or angry faces (Hess et al., 2000) because they assume that their social efficacy (power motive) will be confirmed in the process. In addition, Schultheiss and Hale (2007) showed that nonverbal facial expressions of dominance and submissiveness are better recognized as cue stimuli by individuals with high power motives.

Motives and affect are inextricably linked. For example, motives function as affect enhancers in the attainment of motive-relevant incentives (Schultheiss, 2008). Thus, individuals with high power motives show stronger emotional (Fodor et al., 2006) and hormonal responses (Schultheiss et al., 2005a, 2005b) to power incentives than individuals with low power motives. Implicit motives are also involved in the anticipation of affective states achieved by the anticipated behavior. For example, Brunstein and Maier (2005) observed that individuals with high achievement motive anticipate more positive affect when solving a challenging task than individuals with low achievement motive.

Once a motive is stimulated by an appropriate cue stimulus that promises the achievement of certain incentives, the motive contributes to the energization of behavior. This happens, for example, through the mobilization of physiological processes or through the effective use of one's behavior (McClelland, 1987a, 1987b; Schultheiss, 2008). Classic findings on the stronger energization of physiological resources in high achievement-motivated individuals compared to low achievement-motivated individuals refer to increased muscle tension (Mücher & Heckhausen, 1962), increased skin conductance values as indicators of sympathetic nervous system activation (Raphelson, 1957), or stronger activation of the dopamine system (Bäumler, 1975) before a performance-oriented task. Recently, Mazeres et al. (2019) showed that effort-related cardiovascular parameters were also affected by the strength of the implicit achievement motive during performance of a cognitive task (see ▶ Study Box).

In addition to this physiological energization, a motive also contributes to the energization of pure behavior. Highly achievement-motivated individuals, for example, perform better in verbal and arithmetic tasks (Biernat, 1989; deCharms et al., 1955; French, 1958) and work with greater persistence on a task (Feather, 1966; Wegner & Schüler, 2014; Wendt, 1955).

Achievement Motive and Effort Mobilization

Mazeres et al. (2019) investigated the energization of behavior by the implicit achievement motive. They drew on the integrative model of effort mobilization by Wright (1996) and the observation that the impact of the sympathetic nervous system on the contractility of the heart reflects effort mobilization during cognitive tasks. Wright's model assumes that effort mobilization increases with task difficulty to a point where difficulty is either too high or not justified by success importance, in which case effort mobilization drastically drops (see ◘ Fig. 9.3a and b). The assumption of the Mazeres et al. (2019) study was that individuals with a high implicit achievement motive would invest more effort in the cognitive task than individuals with a low implicit achievement motive if the task was challenging. In contrast, the authors assumed that effort mobilization would be low and independent of implicit achievement motive strength if the task was easy or extremely difficult. Participants in Mazeres et al.'s study were confronted with an either easy or difficult mental addition task during 6 min, meanwhile their reactivity of cardiovascular parameters reflecting beta-adrenergic influences was monitored. In this context, especially the pre-ejection period—the time interval of about 100 ms between the onset of left ventricular depolarization and the opening of the left aortic valve—has proven to be a reliable and direct indicator of effort mobilization (Kelsey, 2012). Results revealed that participants with a strong implicit achievement motive had stronger pre-ejection period reactivity than participants with a weak implicit achievement motive but only when the mental addition task was difficult (see ◘ Fig. 9.4). When the task was easy, both groups of participants mobilized little effort, as would be expected by the resource conservation principle (Zipf, 1949). Similar results have been found for a memory span task and for a mental addition task when task difficulty was unknown to participants (Mazeres et al., 2021b). Interestingly, this energizing effect has also been found for the explicit achievement motive, suggesting that both implicit and explicit achievement motives can lead to more effort mobilization if aroused by specific incentives (Mazeres et al., 2021a). In addition to effort mobilization for mental activities, a strong explicit achievement motive predicts exerted physical force in a handgrip task if task difficulty is unknown to participants but not if the task is clearly easy (Richter et al., 2021). Taken together, these results indicate that a strong achievement motive indeed energizes behavior and leads to more effort mobilization but only in situations that call for high effort—like difficult tasks or tasks with unknown difficulty.

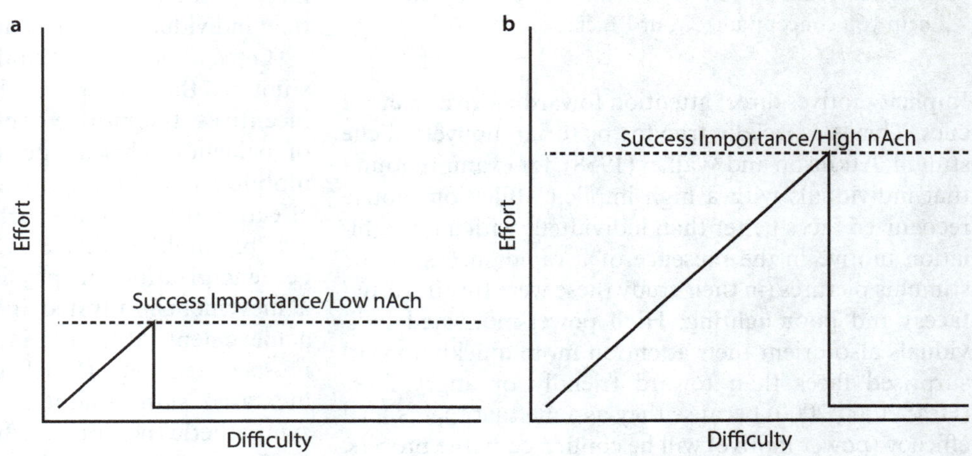

◘ **Fig. 9.3** Assumptions about the strength of effort mobilization for participants with **a** low and **b** high implicit achievement motives for tasks with clear and fixed difficulty. (Adapted from Mazeres et al., 2019)

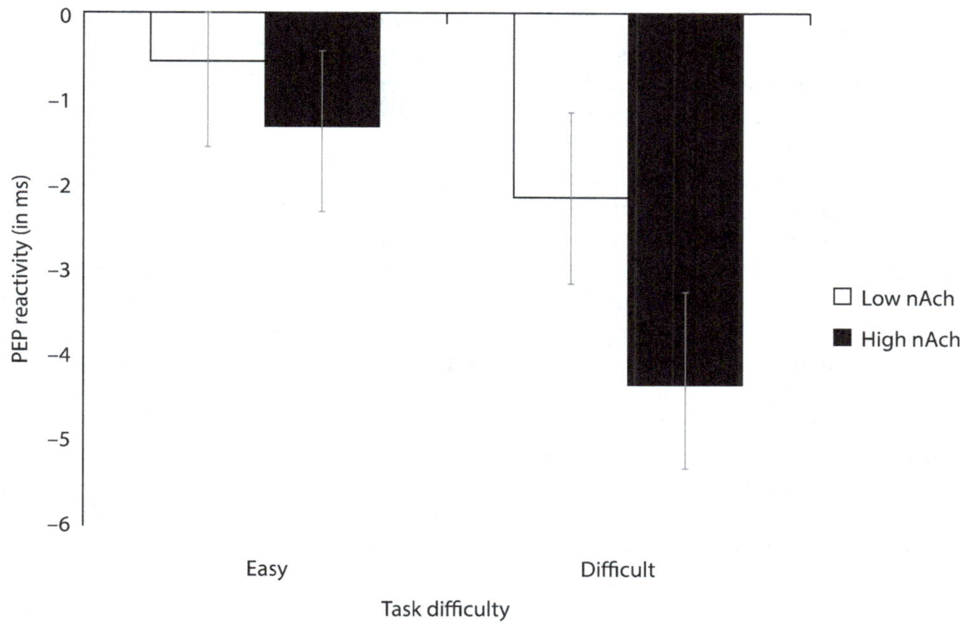

Fig. 9.4 Pre-ejection period reactivity of participants with high vs. low implicit achievement motive for easy and difficult tasks. (Adapted from Mazeres et al., 2019)

9.2 Implicit Motives in Motivation Research

Before we can understand how implicit motives help to make behavioral and experiential predictions in the field of sport and exercise, we should take a deeper look into motive research in general psychology. In doing so, we will learn what actually distinguishes implicit motives from conscious, explicit motives, which instruments are used to diagnose implicit motives, how implicit motives develop (e.g., through educational contexts), which bio-psychological explanations are used for implicit motivation processes, and which brain areas are involved in motivation.

9.2.1 Implicit and Explicit Motives

The original measurement method for implicit motives was an indirect method via picture stories, which is still used today (Morgan & Murray, 1935; Schultheiss, 2007a, 2007b). Critics of this indirect measurement method and proponents of direct measurement methods (e.g., questionnaires) cited, for example, the economy of questionnaires as an advantage. Questionnaires with predetermined response formats that only need to be ticked are much faster not only in implementation but also in analysis (e.g., Jackson, 1967; Mehrabian, 1968). Moreover, unlike picture stories, they can be evaluated unambiguously and thus correspond more closely to the psychometric quality criterion of evaluation objectivity. For many years, both measurement procedures were used in parallel under the assumption that they could measure the same motives. However, it is now known that the respective measurement procedures measure different motive systems (implicit vs. explicit) (Köllner & Schultheiss, 2014; McClelland et al., 1989; Spangler, 1992). Thus, it is useful to distinguish implicit and explicit motives not only theoretically but also in terms of measurement methodology.

As we have already learned, implicit motives are nonconscious and affectively toned preferences for certain classes of incentives. Information processing in this implicit motive system is associative, parallel, and fast (Baumann et al., 2010). In contrast, the explicit motive system involves conscious, cognitive, and evaluative self-attributions that a person thinks are expected of him or her in a given situation (Rokeach, 1973; Veroff & Smith, 1985). Thus, they tend to denote value concepts that have become part of one's self-concept (Biernat, 1989). Processing by the explicit motive system is symbolic, sequential, and slow (Schultheiss, 2001).

Implicit motives have to be differentiated from explicit motives. Whereas implicit motives are nonconscious and affectively toned preferences for certain classes of incentives, explicit motives involve conscious, cognitive, and evaluative self-attributions.

In the following it will be outlined that implicit and explicit motives…

- … differ in the incentives that arouse them
- … differ in the behavior that they predict
- … differ in the way they can be measured

Implicit and explicit motives differ in their incentives. Incentives for implicit motives typically lie in the sporting activities themselves (i.e., orientating and directing function, cf. ◘ Figure 9.2). For the implicit achievement motive, such incentives can, for example, be associated with meeting a quality standard and sporting challenges (e.g., perfecting a technique or winning a tournament). For the implicit affiliation motive, such incentives lie in positive relationships with other people (e.g., feeling pleasure when interacting with fellow athletes in a sports team). For the implicit power motive, incentives lie in athletic activities, such as when an athlete can gain fame and recognition or show dominance over other athletes. For explicit motives, incentives lie primarily in how one's current activity can meet the expectations of others in that situation, or more abstractly, the values in sport or society in general. Thus, for explicit motives, incentives are situations that promise congruence with one's self-image (e.g., being a performance-oriented person, being social, or seeing oneself as strong and influential).

Implicit and explicit motives differ in behavioral prediction. With regard to behavior (i.e., primarily energizing function, cf. ◘ Figure 9.2), a large number of studies have shown that implicit motives are more strongly associated with spontaneously exhibited, long-term, repeatedly shown behavior as well as with the effort a person shows in the context of a sporting task (McClelland, 1980). Thus, a sporting task that stimulates an athlete's motive could lead to better performance, and a suitable sport, for example, could lead to repeated performance of the activity (e.g., athletic training or going to competitions). Explicit motives are more likely to be associated with conscious choices and evaluations, especially in situations where concrete response options are available (McClelland et al., 1989). That is, an athlete with a high affiliation motive might make the decision about whether to continue a competitive athletic career more dependent on whether she perceives social interaction with others as an important value and whether her future competitive sport allows for this social interaction with, for example, parents or athlete friends. Biernat (1989) summarizes with regard to the behavioral correlates of the two motive systems that implicit motives are more strongly associated with doing, whereas explicit motives are more strongly associated with thinking.

Implicit and explicit motives differ in their measurement. Implicit motives cannot be measured directly by questionnaires. They have to be deduced indirectly. For this purpose, mainly projective and reaction-time-related methods are used. Projective procedures measure a person's learned associations to social situations given in the form of pictures as stimuli. With reaction-time-based procedures, the strength of a motive is measured by the rapid association (in the millisecond range) between, for example, the concept performance and the self ("I") or a positive category ("Good"). Explicit motives can be measured by self-statements in questionnaires. A person who considers it a high value to always try to perform well on challenging tasks will state so in questionnaires. The distinctions listed here between implicit and explicit motives (McClelland et al., 1989; Schultheiss, 2007b, 2008) at different levels are presented as an overview in ◘ Table 9.1.

Of particular relevance to the field of sport are studies linking the two motivational systems to long-term and spontaneously exhibited performance behavior (McClelland, 1980). Classic findings show, for example, that the implicit achievement motive predicts long-term prowess in business people (McClelland, 1965, 1987a), the power motive predicts success in managers over a 16-year period (McClelland & Boyatzis, 1982), and the affiliation motive predicts satisfaction in marriage over a 17-year period (McAdams & Vaillant, 1982). Questionnaire measures of corresponding explicit

◘ Table 9.1 Differences between implicit and explicit motives/self-attributes in terms of system basis, information processing, typical incentives, associated behavior, biopsychological correlates, and type of measurement. (Adapted from McClelland et al., 1989; Schultheiss, 2007b, 2008)

	Implicit motives	**Explicit motives**
Basis	Affective, hormonal	Cognitive, self-attributes
Information processing	Associative, parallel, fast, nonconscious	Sequential, slow, conscious
Incentives	Challenges **(achievement)** Social closeness **(affiliation)** Dominance **(power)**	Social desirability
Behavior	Long-term, effort	Conscious decisions
Biopsychological correlates	**Achievement:** vasopressin, dopamine **Affiliation:** progesterone, immune activity (+), parasympathetic activity **Power:** testosterone, immune activity (−), sympathetic activity	None
Measurement	Indirect (e.g., OMT, PSE)	Direct (e.g., AMS, PRF)

Note: OMT = Operant Motive Test, PSE = Picture Story Exercise, AMS = Achievement Motive Scale, PRF = Personality Research Form, (+) = Increase, (−) = Decrease motive themes, on the other hand, had no predictive value for long-term behavior in these studies. In sport, certain desired effects, such as health effects or increased athletic performance, also occur only after a longer period. Thus, measures such as the implicit achievement motive are needed that predict long-term behavior.

Studies comparing the predictive value of implicit and explicit motives are still rare. For example, individuals with a high achievement motive have been shown to perform better in a task that is intrinsically challenging (i.e., has task-inherent incentives) than individuals with a low implicit achievement motive (McClelland, 1987b). However, in tasks set by individuals from the social environment (external demands on performance quality), individuals with a high explicit achievement motive perform better than those with a low explicit achievement motive (Patten & White, 1977).

Impressive findings exist regarding the comparison of the implicit and explicit achievement motive in academic contexts: For example, Brunstein and Hoyer (2002) report that students with a high implicit achievement motive perform better in actual performance (reaction times) on a concentration test than do individuals with a low implicit achievement motive (similar findings in a d2 concentration task and an anagram task are found in Brunstein and Maier (2005) and deCharms et al. (1955)). In contrast, the explicit achievement motive did not predict this concentration performance. However, when it came to deciding whether to continue this concentration task, those with a high explicit achievement motive chose to do so more often than individuals with a low explicit achievement motive. In contrast, the implicit achievement motive had no influence on the decision to continue the task. In a school project, it was also shown that children with a high implicit achievement motive worked more intensively on a project than children with a low implicit achievement motive. However, the decision whether the children wanted to participate in the school project at all was influenced by the explicit and not by the implicit achievement motive (Dahme et al., 1993; ► Study Box: Implicit vs. Explicit Achievement Motive and Feedback).

Implicit vs. Explicit Achievement Motive and Feedback

In an experiment by Brunstein and Maier (2005), 22-year-old psychology students ($N = 96$) worked on a d2 concentration test (Brickenkamp, 2002) on a computer. The task was to mark as quickly as possible (measuring reaction times) only the ds that had two dashes (i.e., in ◻ Fig. 9.5, only the right, outer d). The other ds and ps served as distractors. The d2 test is a measure of perceptual speed and selective attention. Participants first processed two series of 80 characters as a control condition and 6 of these series as a test condition. In the test condition, they received either fake feedback on their own performance (individual reference norm) or fake normative feedback as a comparison to other participants in the form of a graph (► Chap. 7 on motivational climate in sports contexts). This falsified feedback illustrated either an increase in performance (points scored from 726 to 790) or a decrease in points (790–726) over the six test series. After the total of eight series, participants could decide whether to continue with this task or to work on an aesthetic evaluation task. The ◻ Fig. 9.6a and b show the different predictions by the implicit and explicit achievement motives. Students with a high implicit achievement motive showed better performance in the concentration task with increasingly positive individual feedback than students with a low implicit achievement motive or with feedback on decreasing performance (◻ Fig. 9.6a). The explicit achievement motive had no predictive value for actual concentration performance (reaction times). The situation was different for the decision to continue the concentration task (◻ Fig. 9.6b): Here, only the strength of the explicit (and not the implicit) achievement motive influenced the decision to continue the task. Students with a high explicit achievement motive were more likely to decide to continue the task when they received feedback on decreasing performance compared to students with a low explicit achievement motive or in the condition with feedback on increasing performance.

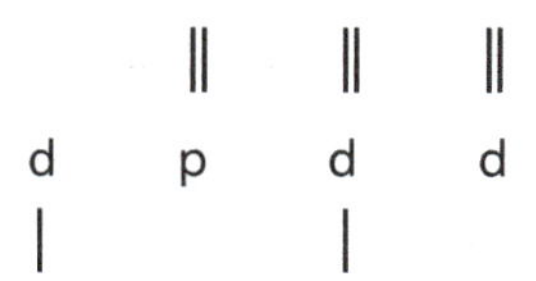

◻ **Fig. 9.5** Examples for stimulus material in the d2 concentration test

It becomes obvious that the problem with explicit performance motivation is that the external social incentives are not always present. That is, coaches, parents, or friends cannot be there all the time to spur athletes to peak performance or training diligence. Rather, it is cru-

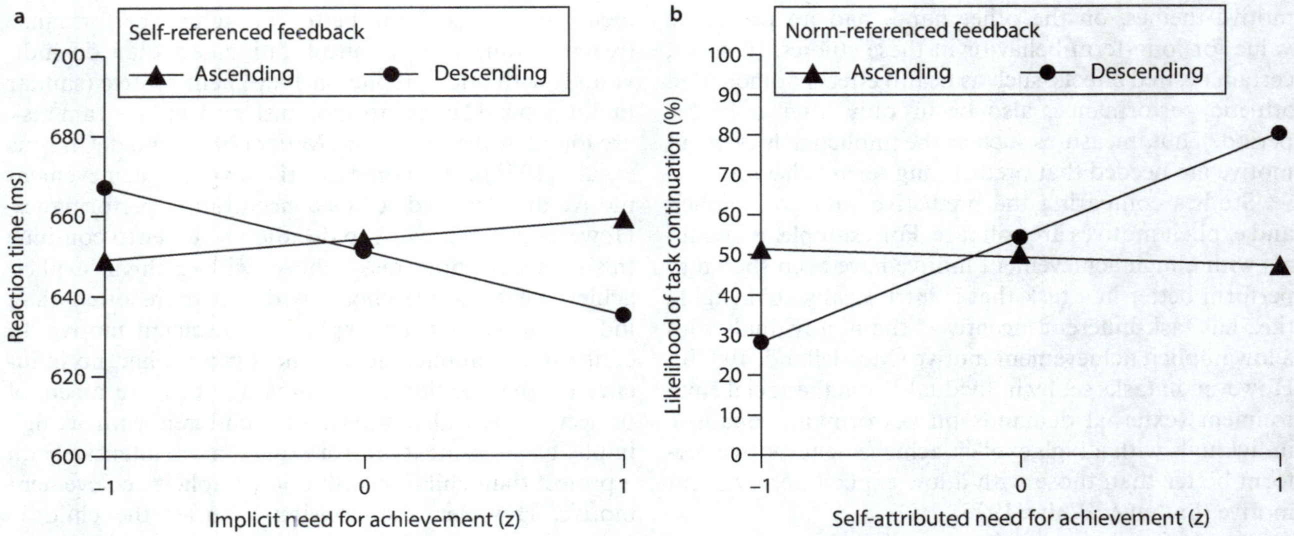

Fig. 9.6 Influence of implicit and explicit achievement motive on **a** performance in a concentration test and **b** the decision to continue with the task. (Figure adapted, Brunstein & Maier, 2005)

cial to be able to generate strong motivation from the inherent incentives of the athletic task itself. Thus, if athletes cannot simply be asked about their motives (explicit motives), i.e., values resulting from the athletes' self-reflection, one must address the question of how implicit, unconscious motives can be measured in any meaningful way at all.

9.2.2 Measuring Implicit Motives

This question of how best to measure motives was already intensively discussed by motivational psychologists in the 1930s. At that time, Morgan and Murray (1935) proposed the "Thematic Apperception Test" (TAT), a measurement procedure for extracting motives from people's fantasy stories. Over the following decades, various research groups (Atkinson, 1958; Heckhausen, 1963; Kuhl & Scheffer, 1999; Ramsay & Pang, 2013; Schultheiss, 2007a, 2007b; Winter, 1994) worked on optimizing the measurement of unconscious motives from such written stories based on Morgan and Murray's basic idea. Meanwhile, an up-to-date standardized procedure for measuring implicit motives, which is a further development of Morgan and Murray's (1935) procedure, is the "Picture Story Exercise" (PSE) described by Schultheiss and Pang (2007) (see ▸ Methods Box: Measuring Implicit Motives Using the "Picture Story Exercise").

? Researchers have sought different ways to measure implicit motives:
- Picture Story Exercise (PSE)
- Multi-Motive Grid (MMG)
- Operant Motive Test (OMT)
- Implicit Association Test (IAT)

Measuring Implicit Motives Using the *"Picture Story Exercise"*

The Picture Story Exercise (PSE) is a standardized procedure for measuring implicit motives (Schultheiss & Pang, 2007). It is a further development of the "Thematic Apperception Test," which was developed as a personality test (TAT; Morgan & Murray, 1935). Underlying these picture story procedures is the idea that individuals incorporate their learned associations to social situations into their interpretation of pictures. Persons differ, then, in terms of their motive-specific views of the picture set. The pictures are deliberately kept ambiguous to allow for a variety of interpretations. In the frequently used version, persons are presented with a total of six pictures (an example is Fig. 9.7). The pictures are presented for 10–15 s to avoid participants describing too much detail in the pictures. The respondents are then asked to write a short, imaginative story about this picture presentation with a beginning, middle, and end. To help them invent the stories, there are sample questions, even though they do not have to be answered directly (Atkinson, 1958): "What is happening? Who are the characters portrayed? What happened before? How did the story begin? What are the characters portrayed thinking, feeling, or wanting? What happens next? How does the story end?" The written text is then often coded by experienced coders using Winter's (1994) coding system. Here, the **achievement motive** is coded whenever the text positively evaluates goals or achievements, e.g., with appropriate adjectives (e.g., "being better than"), mentions wins or competitions, mentions unique achievements (e.g., "winning the World Cup"), or mentions lack of excellence or failures. The **affiliation motive** is coded when positive, friendly feelings toward others are mentioned, when negative feelings about separation are expressed, and when companionate or interactive activities or friendly, caring actions are described. The **power motive** is coded whenever strong, powerful actions, controlling or regulating others, influencing, persuading, or arguing are described, when advice or support is given even though it was not asked for, when a person is described as caring about prestige and recognition or when a person evokes strong emotional reactions in others. The coding system can be seen as a fixed set of rules that increases the objectivity of the evaluation. Since the number of words written can vary from person to person and the probability of naming a motive naturally increases with each sentence written, the motive score is relativized to the number of words for further statistical processing.

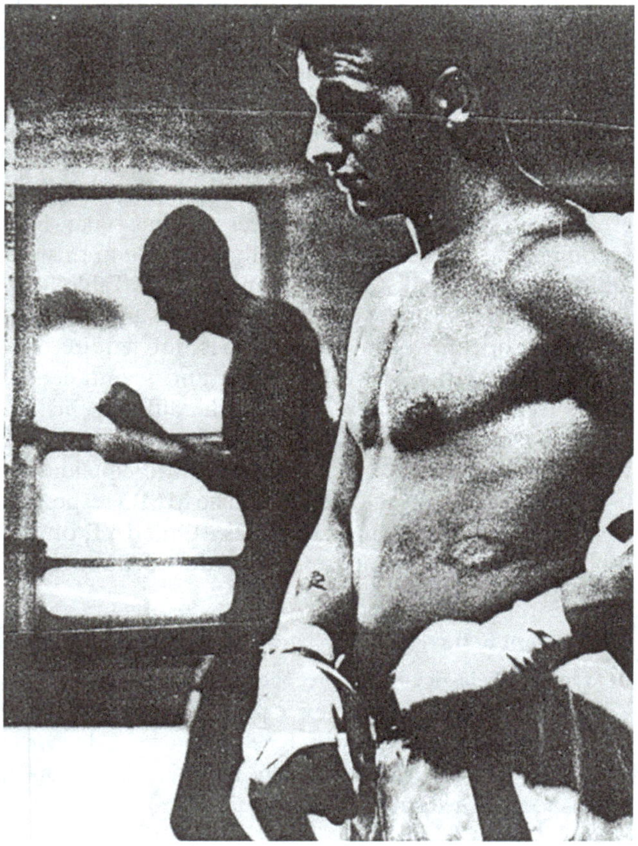

Fig. 9.7 The boxer from the TAT picture set (Smith, 1992)

Reflection

Look at the picture illustrated in Fig. 9.7 for not more than 15 s. Then turn the page and on a separate piece of paper write a short story with a beginning, a main part, and an ending for maximum 5 min. In the short story please provide answers to the following questions: "What is happening? Who are the characters portrayed? What happened before? How did the story begin? What are the characters portrayed thinking, feeling, or wanting? What happens next? How does the story end?"

After finishing your writing try to find instances in your story in which goals or achievements are evaluated positively, in which wins or competitions are mentioned, unique achievements (e.g., "winning the World Cup") are described, or the lack of excellence or failures are displayed.

Although researchers working on implicit motives appreciate the advantages of implicit motives in predicting operant behavior, i.e., behavior in relatively open situations, and the link to neurobiological processes (Schultheiss & Wirth, 2008; Stanton & Schultheiss, 2009), these advantages are bought with a time-consuming measurement. In order to elicit a person's implicit motives, subjects have to complete an approximately 30-min picture story exercise (high effort for study participants). In addition, an evaluation effort of about 15–20 min per participant is required for skilled coders (high effort for researchers). For these reasons, various efforts have been made to develop other methods in addition to this classic method of indirect motive measurement.

The advantage of the Picture Story Exercise (PSE) is that it allows to indirectly (via writing stories to pictures) measure implicit motives that a person may not necessarily be aware of. The disadvantage is the high expenditure of time and personnel in coding the stories.

One direction that has been taken in this regard combined respondent-based answering behavior, as found when filling out a questionnaire, with the presentation of picture stimuli. The so-called Multi-Motive Grid (MMG; Sokolowski et al., 2000) presents the respondent with a selection of four to ten prefabricated descriptions of thoughts, feelings, and modes of experience per picture that a person may experience in the depicted situations. For this, the respondent then only has to check "Yes" or "No" if, in his or her opinion, the description applies to the situation in the picture. Hereby, Sokolowski et al. achieve a strong reduction of the time needed for both the respondent and the person evaluating the questionnaire. A critical discussion of the MMG as an implicit motive measurement tool can be found in Schüler et al. (2015).

Another method for measuring implicit motives is the "Operant Motive Test" (OMT; Kuhl & Scheffer, 1999; Scheffer et al., 2003). Here, with the help of pictures, not only motive themes (e.g., achievement, affiliation, power) are measured but also accompanying affects to the motive themes, e.g., whether someone associates an achievement action with positive emotions such as pride or negative emotions such as shame in case of failure. They can give an indication of the way in which the motive in question is integrated in the self. The advantage over the PSE here is that the respondents have to answer in bullet points to four short picture-related questions only and do not have to write imaginative short stories.

Another way to optimize the elaborate measurement of implicit motives is to use the "Implicit Association Test" (IAT; Brunstein & Schmitt, 2004; Slabbinck et al., 2013). The IAT, which is primarily used to survey attitudes (Greenwald et al., 1998), measures associations between different concepts (e.g., achievement orientation and self/other) using millisecond response rates. In one study, Brunstein and Schmitt (2004) had participants assign different words (e.g., "competent") to a combination of the categories (1) achievement ("achievement-oriented" vs. "nonachievement-oriented") and (2) self ("self" vs. "other"). If participants were able to repeatedly assign achievement-oriented words to the category "achievement-oriented" and "self" more quickly than to the category "achievement-oriented" and "other," this can be interpreted as attributing achievement orientation to self ("self") rather than to other people ("other"). Thus, a stronger association, a stronger neural linkage, and thus proximity of the two concepts "self" and "achievement orientation" are assumed for the person. Brunstein and Schmitt (2004) found that the IAT measure of achievement orientation behaved similarly to an implicit measure of achievement motive, namely, it predicted actual performance on a concentration test and was uncorrelated with the explicit measure of achievement orientation. Slabbinck et al. (2011) also used stimulating imagery for the power motive in their IAT version. By making this change, i.e., including pictures instead of words as stimulus material, they were able to increase the validity of the power IAT in predicting operant power behavior and achieve greater agreement with the classic measure of power motive via PSE (Slabbinck et al., 2013).

The previously mentioned measurement instruments for implicit motives do show variation in determining the strength of implicit motives, even when completed by the same person (Schüler et al., 2015). Thus, it is suggested that such differences are due to the fact that the instruments (1) differ in the stimulus material. In the IAT, words or pictures are presented. In PSE, photographs with higher detail density are used, whereas MMG and OMT use abstracted drawings without recognizable faces. In addition, the instruments (2) differ in the extent to which respondent behavior is measured. Whereas answers are formulated very freely in the PSE stories, responses to questions are made in keyword form in the OMT. In the MMG and IAT, participants respond only to prompts provided by the stimulus material. In strongly responding behavior, people's decisions are based on deliberation processes that take into account what they consider socially desirable in this situation (stronger link to explicit motives; ◘ Table 9.1). Implicit motives, on the other hand, are assumed to predict more operant behavior that does not require prolonged deliberation, is self-initiated and spontaneous, and is frequently repeated. Finally, the different instruments (3) vary with respect to the scoring of responses. In the OMT and PSE, text responses are categorized using coding systems that do differ. The MMG responses cover few of these coding categories. In the IAT, on the other hand, only response times are accounted for (Schüler et al., 2015).

Operant Behavior

Operant behavior is not preceded by lengthy deliberations. It is self-initiated by a person and is demonstrated spontaneously and repeatedly over a longer period of time (e.g., repeatedly returning to performance-oriented sports over one's life span).

Respondent Behavior

Respondent behavior is deliberately weighed and is the reaction to people's expectations or to circumstances of a situation (e.g., playing competitive sports because one is currently in a sporting circle of friends). These are usually decisions or evaluations that are seen as socially desirable and result from thoughtful deliberation processes (McClelland, 1980).

9.2.3 Developmental Aspects of Implicit and Explicit Motives

Regarding the ontogenesis of implicit motives, it is assumed that early childhood affective experiences are crucial, especially before language acquisition (McClelland et al., 1989). In addition, implicit motives are thought to be partially genetically predisposed (Weinberger & McClelland, 1990). Implicit motives are thus distinguished from explicit motives, which are thought to be shaped primarily by verbal transmission of values and goals by parents, coaches, teachers, or peers. Language acquisition is necessary for this. Very few studies have looked at the ontogenesis of motives. One exception is McClelland and Pilon's (1983) study in which they examined the strength of implicit and explicit motives of 31-year-olds and related them to their parents' early childhood child-rearing practices ($N = 76$). Twenty-six years earlier, parents of then 5-year-olds were surveyed about their child-rearing practices (Sears et al., 1957). For the implicit achievement motive, for example, the authors show significant correlations with fixed mealtimes and with toilet training in very early childhood. Thus, it seems to be important for the expression of the implicit achievement motive that children learn to control their needs. These findings are interesting in light of studies showing that achievement-motivated children are able to delay gratification and resist temptations (Mischel & Gilligan, 1964). This type of control of nearbody needs appears to have been trained in early childhood. In contrast, parental practices that impose early performance demands on children are shown to be conducive to the development of the explicit achievement motive. Such normative demands are increasingly placed on children during the school years.

Because the achievement motive has been identified in early motive research as particularly relevant to the productivity of a society (McClelland, 1961), e.g., because it fosters entrepreneurial success (Collins et al., 2004), attempts have been made to develop training programs for the achievement motive (see ▶ Methods Box: Can Implicit Motives Be Changed?).

Failure of the mother to respond to the child's crying is significantly associated with high implicit affiliation motive in the child at age 31 (McClelland & Pilon, 1983). McClelland et al. (1989) suggest that this finding may be due to the proportion of the fear component of the implicit affiliation motive. Such behavior on the part of the mother could result in a stronger expression of fear of rejection in the child. Other study results also point in the direction that deprivation of warmth and cohesion favored a stronger expression of the affiliation motive, e.g., in second-born children who receive less attention and warmth than first-born children (Connors, 1963) or in children raised in institutions (Youngleson, 1973). In contrast, when the mother frequently told the children to be nice to others and not to retaliate in arguments, the children in their early 30s showed a more pronounced explicit affiliation motive.

Parenting behaviors that allowed aggressive and sexual impulses on the part of the child were positively associated with the implicit power motive. Children's early experiences of assertive aggression, i.e., experiencing social efficacy, seem to favor the development of the implicit power motive. Scheffer (2001) primarily names maternal compliance with the child's impulses, which are normally suppressed, and the father's absence or low involvement in parenting as a prerequisite for the development of the implicit power motive. General punishment as well as punishment for aggressiveness by parents, on the other hand, are positively related to the explicit power motive. Thus, among the 31-year-olds, those who describe themselves as dominant were more likely to have been physically punished as children, especially when they were hostile to their parents.

Overall, these patterns of findings support the assumptions that implicit motives are more likely to be shaped by nonverbal affective experiences in early childhood, whereas explicit motives are more likely to be consolidated later, namely, after language acquisition, through frequent verbal repetition and strong social stimuli. Nevertheless, it can be stated that the available studies are very sparse and should be interpreted with caution.

> Implicit motives are assumed to be shaped by nonverbal affective experiences in early childhood, whereas explicit motives are assumed to be consolidated later in childhood (after language acquisition) through frequent verbal repetition and strong social stimuli.

Can Implicit Motives Be Changed?

The first attempts to change implicit motives through training were made in the 1960s (McClelland & Winter, 1969). The idea was that productivity and entrepreneurship in emerging economies could be effectively stimulated by improving the achievement motive of entrepreneurs. Indeed, it was known from previous studies that successful entrepreneurs exhibit higher achievement motives than other employment groups (McClelland, 1961; Collins et al., 2004). Achievement-motivated individuals exhibit behaviors that could help successful businesses: They are always looking for ways to optimize processes and operations, are willing to take controlled risks, and proactively seek feedback on their own entrepreneurial actions for which they feel personally accountable. Within a 2-week training program, McClelland et al. sought to (1) expand and strengthen the affective network of the achievement motive, (2) make it more clearly perceivable and identifiable, (3) link it to everyday experiences and behaviors, and (4) align it with higher-level personal values and cultural norms (McClelland & Winter, 1969). Thus, participants learned to *think*, *feel*, *talk*, and *act* like someone with a strong achievement motive (Rheinberg & Engeser, 2010). The economic effects of the study were very promising. Program participants were more industrious, invested more, and created more new jobs compared to a control group. In addition, after 2 years, one-third more jobs were created in the region from which the participants came than in a comparable control region. However, the changeability of the implicit achievement motive was contrary to McClelland's own theoretical assumptions that it is a stable personality trait that is partly genetically determined (Weinberger & McClelland, 1990). In a reanalysis of McClelland's data, Heckhausen and Krug (1982) later found that the implicit achievement motive had indeed changed and that these changes were also related to subsequent entrepreneurial activity. The authors looked at the directions of action tendencies contained in achievement motive stories (hope for success vs. fear of failure). They found that individuals with fear of failure, in particular, had changed more toward hope for success over the course of the program. That this change in the direction of the achievement motive appears to be related to entrepreneurial success was also shown in a replication study (Varga, 1977). In summary, the achievement motive appears to be relatively stable but modifiable by experience (e.g., through training).

9.3 Biopsychological Approaches for Implicit Motivational Processes

A distinctive feature of implicit motives is that they are closely linked to biopsychological processes. In the following section, brain areas involved in core motivational processes are first described. Subsequently, findings on endocrinological and physiological correlates of the achievement, affiliation, and power motives are explained with transfer to the sport and exercise context. For an in-depth review of these processes, see Schultheiss and Wirth (2008).

Biopsychological Approaches

Biopsychological approaches to motivation explain behavior and experience with the help of functions of the brain/central nervous system. In this context, findings from experiments with animals of related species are often used and transferred to the functioning of the human brain (Schultheiss & Wirth, 2008).

9.3.1 Motivational Brain Areas

Here, the brain areas involved in most motivational processes will be briefly mentioned. Readers should nevertheless keep in mind that different motivational processes lead to different functional associations of brain areas and neurophysiological processes. Thus, it is a complex process that cannot be detailed here in brief. The amygdala, the mesolimbic dopamine system, the orbitofrontal cortex, and the lateral prefrontal cortex are involved in many basic motivational processes (◘ Fig. 9.8; Cardinal et al., 2002; Schultheiss & Wirth, 2008).

The **amygdala** in the medial temporal lobe is part of the limbic system and provides the initial emotional and motivational evaluation of a stimulus based on stimulus-response patterns. For example, in young children, after only a few learning experiences, a soccer ball may be associated with joy and play within a fraction of a second. Stimuli associated with motive satisfaction are automatically evaluated positively because they promise motive-specific affect. For example, it is known from imaging techniques (functional magnetic resonance imaging) that the amygdala in humans is responsible for emotionally encoding human facial expressions (Adolphs, 2002; Adolphs et al., 1995), and this is without individuals being aware of it (Whalen et al., 1998). In addition, the amygdala provides an affective-impulsive response to sensory stimuli. Depending on the learning experiences of a fouled soccer player, an arm perceived out of the corner of the eye, for example, may be perceived as an apology gesture or as repeated unsportsmanship. Schultheiss and Wirth (2008) refer to this feature of the amygdala as the **motivational knee jerk**. The amygdala also ensures that emotional aspects of a piece of information are better remembered (Cahill, 2000) and that primarily affectively relevant information is selected during stimulus perception (Vuilleumier et

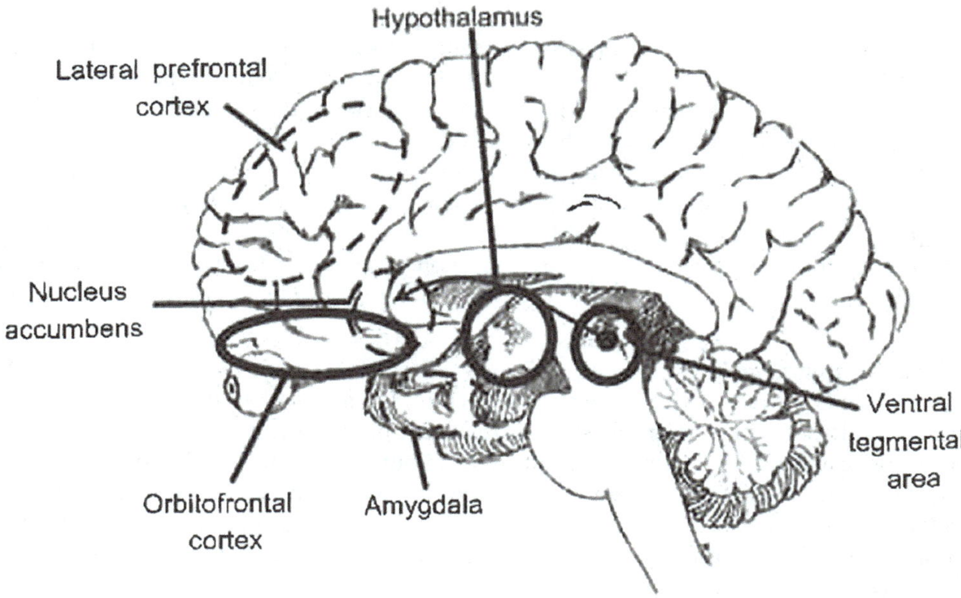

Fig. 9.8 Areas of the motivational brain (sagittal section). Areas visible through the section are marked with a solid black line, areas not visible with a dashed line. The nucleus accumbens and the ventral tegmental area belong to the mesolimbic system. (Adapted representation from Schultheiss & Wirth, 2008)

al., 2004). From lesion studies, two areas of the amygdala can be assigned to different functions: The central nucleus primarily influences emotional response and, through its connection to the hypothalamus and brainstem, results in increased sympathetic activation (e.g., heart rates, blood pressure, skin conductance) and production of stress hormones (e.g., cortisol) and neurotransmitters (e.g., nor-/epinephrine). The basolateral nucleus shows connections to the nucleus accumbens and influences motivated actions as in a stimulus-response chain.

The **mesolimbic dopamine system** comprises neuronal connections extending from the ventral tegmentum of the upper brainstem to the nucleus accumbens and prefrontal cortex. Portions of the mesolimbic dopamine system can be viewed as a kind of interface for incoming sensory information from the amygdala and orbitofrontal cortex, which is relayed to the basal ganglia for preparation of motor responses (Mogenson et al., 1980). Appropriate stimuli cause dopamine to be released in the nucleus accumbens and prefrontal cortex, which may lead to an increase of synaptic transmission (Schultz, 1998). An increase in dopamine activity in the nucleus accumbens then leads to stronger goal-directed behavior, that is, the targeted stimulus is more strongly wanted. Figuratively speaking, dopamine thus acts like a magnet here (Schultheiss & Wirth, 2008). For example, a recreational athlete in whom the dopamine system is very active might show strong, goal-directed training for her first marathon. However, this does not mean that stronger dopamine activity also makes the stimulus more liked (see ► Study Box: Study on the Difference Between "Wanting" and "Liking" by Ikemoto & Panksepp, 1996). Activity of the mesolimbic system is associated with active avoidance behavior in addition to the reinforcement of approach behavior.

Study on the Difference Between "Wanting" and "Liking" by Ikemoto and Panksepp (1996)

In the study by Ikemoto and Panksepp, rats had the chance to run along a track and drink a sucrose solution in a target area, which is perceived by rats as pleasant, that is, what they like. During the first training session, the rats completed five runs in which they drank the sucrose solution for 60 s per run when the target was reached. The speed at target approach and the amount of sucrose solution drunk were measured. The rats were then injected with either 1, 5, or 25 μg of a dopamine receptor antagonist (flupenthixol) for an additional five runs each. With the strongest dose of the dopamine receptor antagonist (25 μg), the speed in cm/s at target approach (wanting) decreased significantly (Fig. 9.9, left panel). At the same time, however, sucrose preference (liking) did not change, that is, the rats still drank as much of the sucrose solution as in the control condition or when they had been injected with only small amounts of the dopamine receptor antagonist (▣ Fig. 9.9, right panel). This finding powerfully illustrates how the dopamine system is more responsible for goal-directed behavior than for rendering a goal more affectively positive. Thus, goal attainment is more important than the reward stimulus associated with it. Although these are results from animal experiments, a transfer to the sports world can be made if one thinks, for example, of extreme endurance athletes (e.g., marathon runners) for whom the goal of finishing the marathon is far more important than possible financial or affective incentives. In this case, this strong activity of the dopamine system and the associated goal obsession are so strong that many hours of training per week and sometimes the alignment of the entire life with the sporting activity take place.

The **orbitofrontal cortex** is located in the ventral part of the prefrontal cortex above the eyes. The orbitofrontal cortex is attributed to the limbic system because it plays a role primarily in the evaluation of rewards and punishments. This is where the representation of the **emotional value** of incoming information (e.g., visual, auditory, olfactory) and the sensory integration of this information occur. However, the orbitofrontal cortex is also involved in the formulation of decisions and expectations, in planning behavior (considering reward and punishment), and in the regulation of emotions (Bechara et al., 1994; Kringelbach & Rolls, 2004). In this context, not only the true strength of the reward of a stimulus but also the expected strength of the reward and the positive evaluation of a set of associations connected with the trigger stimulus appear to be stored in the orbitofrontal cortex (Kringelbach, 2005; Rolls, 2000). Thus, for a striker in soccer, the view of a wide-meshed net (goal) might already be associated with positive feedback from fans after a goal is scored. Here, the medial parts of the orbitofrontal cortex are more likely to be associated with reward stimuli (e.g., happy faces; Monk et al., 2003), whereas the lateral parts are associated with punishment stimuli (e.g., angry faces; Blair et al., 1999), which should prompt behavior change. However, the orbitofrontal cortex is also involved in disengagement from a stimulus. When the motivational needs of the organism are met, a low level of activation of the orbitofrontal cortex leads to disengagement from a stimulus (Hall et al., 2010; Rolls et al., 1989). Everyone is familiar with the term "cabin fever" at a training camp. To be sure, the community experienced may go a long way toward satisfying the affiliation or power motive. However, after several days of forced community, one or another player will also seek out individual retreats. That is, a strong activation of this area is only observable and functional as long as the trigger stimulus is rewarding (Schultheiss & Wirth, 2008).

The **lateral prefrontal cortex** extends behind the forehead to the temples and is one of the brain areas that acquires its full functionality comparatively late in life, in early adulthood (Fuster, 2001). The lateral prefrontal cortex is where goals are represented and plans on how to achieve them (e.g., the goal of getting through the marathon). It supports the retrieval and storage of content in working memory, for example, and is further

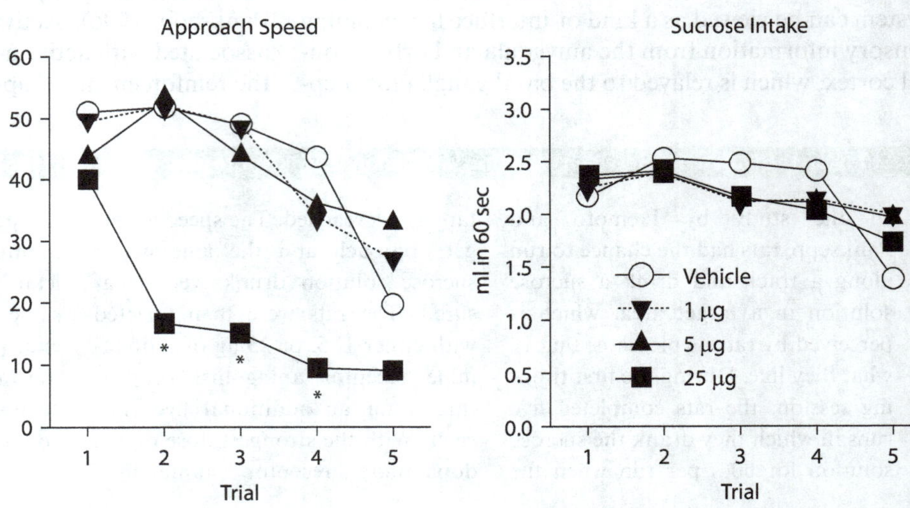

▣ **Fig. 9.9** Approach speed in cm/s (left, "wanting") of rats and amount of sucrose solution drunk (right, "liking") during five runs to reach sucrose solution in a control condition and after injection of 1, 5, or 25 µg of a dopamine receptor antagonist

involved in motor control and language control. More importantly, the lateral prefrontal cortex can regulate the activation of other motivational brain areas (e.g., the amygdala) (e.g., the impulse to give up and relax can be resisted). In particular, this part of the cortex is involved in complex actions that require volitional support and an interlocking of verbal processes, memory content, and motor control (Luria, 1992). The lateral prefrontal cortex is also involved in the (self-)control of motivational needs and impulses and supports the choice of one of several motivational tendencies. For example, this part of the brain is involved when an athlete goes to the weight room to complete her stabilization exercises despite the tempting offer to play tennis with a friend.

The following section provides specific findings on biopsychological correlates of the three basic motive themes of achievement, affiliation, and power.

> The brain areas that are strongly involved in motivational processes are the amygdala, the mesolimbic dopamine system, the orbitofrontal cortex, and the lateral prefrontal cortex.

9.3.2 The Achievement Motive and Physiological Processes

While the physiological correlates of the affiliation and power motives have been well studied (see below), there are few studies on the achievement motive. The achievement motive is associated with physiological parameters that indicate greater sympathetic activation, e.g., increased muscle tone at rest (Mücher & Heckhausen, 1962). In addition, higher uric acid levels have been found in achievement-motivated individuals (Kasl, 1974; Mueller et al., 1970). The research group of McClelland (1995) was able to confirm the relationship of the achievement motive with urinary volume in several studies. For example, the amount of urine passed was lower in individuals with a high achievement motive than in individuals with a low achievement motive. These effects were also obtained when the achievement motive was experimentally stimulated. The antidiuretic peptide hormone (ADH) vasopressin, which helps regulate human water balance through its vasoconstrictor action, is thought to be responsible for this (Robertson, 2006; Schrier, 2006; Stricker & Verbalis, 2002). Vasopressin is produced in the hypothalamus and stored in the pituitary gland. There, it also intervenes in hormonal stress regulation, for example, through its involvement in cortisol release (Torpy et al., 1994). Furthermore, increased dopamine activity has been shown in individuals with high achievement motivation scores (Bäumler, 1975; Schultheiss & Brunstein, 2005). However, Hall et al. (2010) point out that explorations of these findings, particularly at the neural level, have been lacking to date.

> The empirical link between the achievement motive and physiological processes is less strong than for the affiliation and power motives (see below). Some studies suggest, however, that the achievement motive is associated with physiological parameters that indicate greater sympathetic activation and the release of vasopressin.

9.3.3 The Affiliation Motive and Physiological Processes

In contrast to the achievement motive, the affiliation motive is more strongly associated with parasympathetic activation (Jemmott, 1987; McClelland, 1989). Thus, individuals with high affiliation motive exhibit a stronger immune system. For example, affiliation-motivated individuals show higher levels of endogenous killer cell activity (Jemmott et al., 1990). In addition, they respond with a stronger release of immunoglobulin-A (s-IgA) when stressful situations arise (Jemmott et al., 1983; McClelland et al., 1985), as well as when affiliation-themed stimuli are presented (McClelland & Kirshnit, 1988). Such affiliation-themed stimuli are followed by not only increased immune activity but also higher dopamine concentrations in individuals with high affiliation motives (McClelland et al., 1987). In addition, affiliation-motivated individuals show chronically lower blood pressure levels over a 20-year period (McClelland, 1979). The affiliation motive has also been associated with the activity of the steroid hormone progesterone. For example, Schultheiss et al. showed that women who used contraceptives (birth control pills) and thus showed higher levels of progesterone had stronger affiliation motives than women with normal menstrual cycles (Schultheiss et al., 2003). This was also confirmed by experimental stimulation of the affiliation motive or social proximity, which led to higher progesterone levels in both women and men (Brown et al., 2009; Schultheiss et al., 2004). Wirth and Schultheiss (2006) argue that progesterone releases in the brain have an anxiety-reducing effect to attenuate flight or aggressive behavioral responses and initiate affiliative behaviors (Taylor, 2006; Taylor et al., 2000). Other work has also described that affiliation-oriented behavior increases in the presence of threats (Gump & Kulik, 1997) and that social interactions (Heinrichs et al.,

2003) and the implicit affiliation motive (Wegner et al., 2014b) have stress-reducing effects, which is also reflected in low cortisol responses, for example. In this context, it can be speculated that the link between progesterone and affiliation motivation might be mainly due to the activity of the bonding hormone oxytocin (Hall et al., 2010; Insel & Young, 2001).

> The affiliation motive is associated with a stronger immune system and higher levels of progesterone and oxytocin.

9.3.4 The Power Motive and Physiological Processes

Much of the research on physiological correlates of the power motive has focused on the steroid hormones testosterone (Schultheiss et al., 2003) and estradiol (especially in women) (Hall et al., 2010; Schultheiss & Wirth, 2008, for a review). The power motive is more strongly stimulated when image stimuli involve aggressive or dominance behavior, such as scenes from a power-themed mafia movie (Schultheiss et al., 2004). However, individuals with high implicit power motives also respond with higher testosterone release to a non-sports-related competition in which, for example, they must connect ascending number sequences as quickly as possible (Schultheiss et al., 1999, 2005a, 2005b). Study participants also showed similar testosterone responses when they imagined a competition. Schultheiss and Rhode (2002) showed that the power motive was associated with testosterone releases after victories, but only in participants with low impulse control (activity inhibition). Testosterone increases dopamine transmission in the nucleus accumbens (Packard et al., 1998) and is thus involved in primary motivational processes in the brain (Cardinal et al., 2002). Testosterone thus has a rewarding, stimulus-reinforcing effect (Alexander et al., 1994). Because testosterone is much lower in females, power-motivated females show a stronger link to estradiol activity (Stanton & Schultheiss, 2007). The rewarding effect of estradiol in women after victories in competitions behaves similarly to the effect of testosterone in men. This may lead to stronger activation of motivational brain areas and thus to increased dopamine releases (Hu & Becker, 2003; Russo et al., 2003).

> The power motive is associated with steroid hormones such as testosterone for men and estradiol for women.

Unconscious Impulse Control ("Activity Inhibition")

Unconscious impulse control refers to a person's ability to inhibit involuntary impulses to act in various situations (McClelland et al., 1972).

Overall, victories in dominance competitions, in which social status is vied for, seem to lead to stronger adrenaline and noradrenaline releases. This results in greater activity of the steroid hormones testosterone and estradiol accompanied by greater aggression, competitive orientation, and supply to many muscle groups (Schultheiss, 2007a; Stanton & Schultheiss, 2007). This mechanism also leads to stronger dopamine activity in the corresponding brain regions. Defeats in such competitive situations, on the other hand, tend to lead to cortisol releases and a blockade of the gonadal steroid hormones testosterone and estradiol and thus do not show positive motivational effects (◘ Fig. 9.10). Wirth et al. (2006), for example, showed that the strength of the power motive is negatively associated with cortisol releases of winners but positively associated with those of losers. Similar findings were secured in a study with

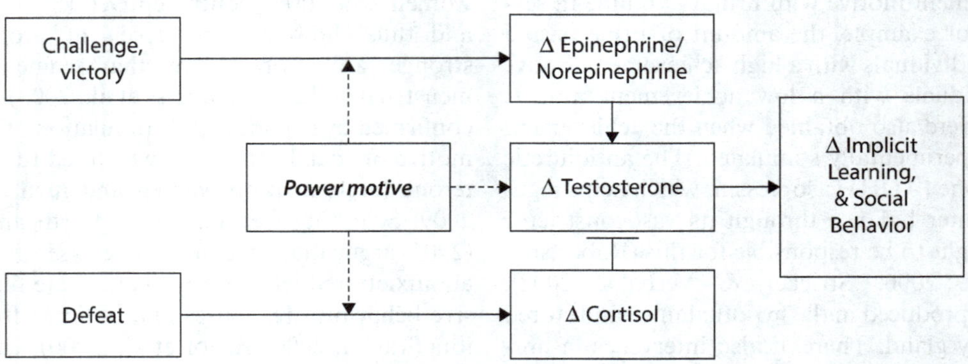

◘ **Fig. 9.10** Model assumptions about biological substrates of the power motive in men. Solid arrows symbolize the pathway of activity, dashed arrows represent moderation, and orthogonal end lines represent inhibition of activity. (Adapted figure from Stanton & Schultheiss, 2009)

adolescents (Wegner et al., 2015a). Here, students with a high power motive responded with higher cortisol levels to psychosocial stress than participants with a lower power motive.

9.3.4.1 Chronic Health Effects of the Power Motive

It is not only in experimentally induced or short-term situational contexts that the physiological correlates of the power motive are evident. Since power-motivated individuals tend to have stronger sympathetic activation, negative chronic health effects are not surprising. Thus, it has been shown that the health of highly power-motivated individuals suffers particularly under stress. Students during exam periods or prisoners reporting particularly high levels of stress then showed lower immune activity (measured with immunoglobulin-A, s-IgA) when they were highly power motivated (Jemmott et al., 1983; McCelland et al., 1982). Similarly, endogenous killer cell activity is lower in power-motivated individuals under stress, indicating low immune activity (Jemmott et al., 1990). McClelland et al. attribute this lower immune system activity to chronic activation of the sympathetic nervous system, which is also reflected, for example, in more frequent and severe reports of symptoms of illness (McClelland et al., 1982; McCelland et al., 1980; McClelland & Jemmott, 1980). Wirth et al. (2006) additionally cite chronically elevated cortisol levels. Regarding increased sympathetic activation, previous studies found that power-motivated individuals respond to stress with higher blood pressure (Fontana et al., 1987; McClelland, 1979), increased muscle tone (Fodor, 1985), and increased adrenaline and noradrenaline production (McCelland et al., 1980; McClelland et al., 1985).

9.4 Behavioral Correlates of Implicit Motives in Sport Science Research

We already know from non-sport-related research on the achievement motive that implicit motives are associated with actual performances that are spontaneous, repeated, and shown over a longer period of time, whereas explicit motives are more strongly associated with conscious decision-making processes and values (Brunstein & Hoyer, 2002; McClelland, 1987a; Patten & White, 1977; overview in ◘ Table 9.1). ◘ Figure 9.11 systematizes the assumed influences of implicit and explicit motives in the course of action. Whereas implicit motives are activated more strongly by situations that fit the motive and lead to an energization of behavior primarily through incentives inherent in the action, the results of an action and its consequences are especially important for the activation of explicit motives. For example, a highly implicitly achievement-motivated athlete will work long hours on learning a new technique, forget about time, and become completely absorbed in the process if she has not previously known the technique and finds it challenging. A highly explicitly power-motivated climber, on the other hand, will look more at how to use a new climbing technique to be better than his climbing peer (◘ Fig. 9.11).

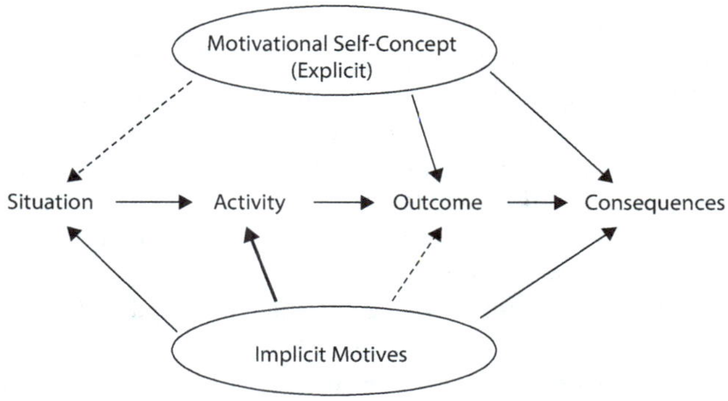

◘ **Fig. 9.11** Influences of implicit and explicit motives in the course of action. (Adapted figure from Rheinberg & Engeser, 2010)

9.4.1 Achievement Motive

The implicit achievement motive was already studied in swimmers in the 1970s by Gabler (1972). He was able to show that swimmers in the high-performance range achieved higher values in an implicit motive test than swimmers at a lower performance level. Concomitantly, higher scores in the implicit achievement motive were also associated with greater training volumes. This relationship between implicit achievement motive and training volumes was found among recreational athletes in university sports as well as amateur and high-performance athletes (Gröpel et al., 2016). The difference in the expression of the implicit achievement motive between competitive and recreational sport participants shown by Gabler is also found in other technique-oriented individual sports such as apparatus gymnastics, track and field, or climbing (Study 1; Gröpel et al., 2015). These results suggest that performance sport contexts and performance sport training have a strong incentive character for individuals with a high implicit achievement motive and potentially satisfy their motive. In another study with high performance tennis players, it was shown that they compete longer and play longer rallies when they have a high implicit achievement motive (Wegner & Schüler, 2014). Because an equally strong opponent in particular leads a tennis player to play a longer match, the findings confirm assumptions that achievement motivation is particularly strong for individuals with a high approach-oriented achievement motive at intermediate task difficulty (► Chap. 7; Atkinson, 1957).

In addition to these links of the achievement motive to athletes' willingness to exert effort, recent findings also show that highly achievement-motivated individuals become more absorbed in an achievement-oriented task and experience, for example, more flow, which is a special form of intrinsic motivation (see ► Chap. 8 in this book). In the case of recreational badminton players, for example, it has been shown that they experience more flow when they feel they receive feedback on their performance progress in their sports environments, i.e., when they can perceive themselves as competent (Schüler & Brandstätter, 2013). Similar findings on improved flowering were evident in a volleyball experiment where the focus was on one's own performance improvement and learning, and there was an opportunity to feel pride in one's performance (Study 2). Findings also point in the same direction for extreme endurance athletes (Schüler et al., 2014). Thus, a fit between situations that stimulate the achievement motive and the strength of one's motive can lead to an optimization of performance and experience in sport. In the sport studies reported here, the explicit achievement motive did not have predictive power for the behavioral parameters examined (Wegner & Teubel, 2014; ► Study Box: Implicit and Explicit Achievement Motive and Behavior in Sport). In summary, this study shows that the implicit achievement motive more strongly predicts actual, repeatedly demonstrated performance in complex game situations, whereas the explicit achievement motive is associated with decision behavior in sporting situations with a social evaluation character.

9

> The achievement motive is associated with better sports performance, higher willingness to invest effort, and more frequent flow experience during sports.

Implicit and Explicit Achievement Motive and Behavior in Sport (Wegner & Teubel, 2014)

The aim of this study was to investigate different behavioral predictions by the implicit and explicit achievement motive. It was hypothesized that the implicit achievement motive would be associated with repeatedly demonstrated behavior in complex athletic situations, whereas the explicit achievement motive would be more associated with decision-making behavior in situations of a social evaluation nature. In this study, the strength of the implicit achievement motive was measured in sport students ($N = 42$) using an indirect procedure (OMT; Kuhl & Scheffer, 1999). The strength of the explicit achievement motive was assessed with the sport-related achievement motive scale (AMS; Elbe et al., 2005). The study was conducted in four team sports: basketball, soccer, handball, and volleyball. Students participated in two parts of an experiment: in the first experiment, for example, they performed a throwing task in basketball. This was based on the ring throw paradigm of Atkinson (1960). Lines were marked on the hall floor at intervals of one meter (◘ Fig. 9.12). With ten throwing attempts, the students were to score as many points as possible and thus improve their position in a ranking list. It was assumed that the decision to throw a certain distance to the target was predicted by the social comparison with other students through the explicit achievement motive. In contrast, performance in the second experiment was to be predicted by the implicit achievement motive. Here, students played four-on-four in a free basketball tournament. In total, participants completed eight rounds each. In each round, which lasted 8 min, participants played in a randomly assembled new team of four. In each round, the participants collected points for their personal points account. For a win, the participants received the number of points earned by their own team plus ten points, for a draw the number of points plus five points, and for a defeat only the number of points "earned." The results of these two studies confirmed the assumptions: Only the implicit achievement motive could significantly predict actual performance in the complex team tournament over several rounds, but not the explicit achievement motive. Thus, even for athletic performance, long-term prediction of real performance seems to be more strongly determined by the implicit motive. In contrast, the decision for distances to the target (e.g., basketball hoop) from the first experiment could only be significantly predicted by the explicit achievement motive. Conscious decision behavior in a social-evaluative pressure situation seems to be more strongly related to the explicit motive system.

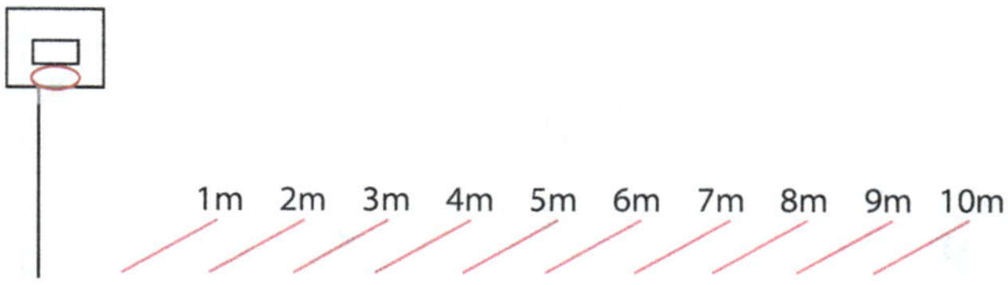

Fig. 9.12 Example basketball throwing task: the sports students decided on a distance to the target and got more points if the distance was greater

9.4.2 Affiliation Motive

The affiliation motive is often described as less beneficial in performance contexts (Krug & Kuhl, 2006; Schmalt & Heckhausen, 2008). However, the work that has examined the affiliation motive in sport shows that the affiliation motive can also become effective in performance sport contexts. This seems to be especially the case when the contexts facilitate positive social interaction. A classic finding for this comes from Sorrentino and Sheppard (1978). They were able to show that highly implicitly affiliation-motivated athletes swam faster in group competitions, in which they could contribute to their team's performance, than when they were asked to perform individually in competition with others. Similar findings were seen in a study of physical education students who were asked to complete qualitatively well-performed pushups. Compared to a control condition, students with a high implicit affiliation motive completed more and better pushups when they were told that they were completing the pushups for their team, i.e., for a team performance (Schüler et al., 2016a, 2016b). Thus, the affiliation motive can certainly lead to high performance if the right affiliation-themed incentives are provided. In addition to the findings on performance achieved, affiliation-motivated students in the team condition also reported positive emotions more often and negative emotions less often during the task. Similar findings on the experience of flow in implicitly affiliation-motivated students in athletic settings that promise social inclusion are also found in other studies (Schüler & Brandstätter, 2013). In addition to such performance and experience predictions in sport, the distinction between unconscious and conscious motivational systems can also be used to make predictions about different social behaviors in sport. For example, in a real competition in backstroke sports (e.g., badminton, tennis, table tennis), nonverbal behavior (e.g., avoiding behavior that provokes the opponent) can be attributed to the strength of the implicit affiliation motive, but the frequency of verbal exchanges with one's team members can be attributed to the explicit affiliation motive (Wegner et al., 2014a). Thus, the implicit affiliation motive seems to be reflected in such social behavior that is not consciously reflected. Highly implicit affiliation-motivated athletes, for example, make their opponents wait less long when changing sides and are more likely to avoid disputes about referee decisions.

> The affiliation motive is also beneficial for sports performance, when the performance context is embedded in a social context that promises to satisfy the affiliation motive (e.g., winning for the team).

If we additionally look at findings on the explicit affiliation motive in sports, a distinction between hope and fear components of the affiliation motive makes sense. For example, Teubel (2012) was able to show that the strength of the fear component of the affiliation motive (fear of rejection) worsens athletes' performance for a team in coordinative tasks. Thus, if an athlete has high fear of rejection, his or her performance in a team coordinative task will tend to deteriorate. This study of the explicit affiliation motive in sport confirms early findings on the fear component of the implicit affiliation motive by deCharms (1957), in which corresponding individuals were found to be less productive in a group condition (Fig. 9.13).

9.4.3 Power Motive

The power motive can be of great importance for athletic competition in sports, in which athletic performance is primarily determined by a direct interaction event (Kuhl & Krug, 2006). Such interactive sports include tennis, judo, and soccer. Unlike, for example, a swimmer whose world-class performance makes it impossible for the other athletes to take away a victory in the competition, in interaction sports the performance level of the opponents and their chosen tactics play a decisive role in how well an athlete will perform in the competition. In such interactional competitions, the power motive can help, for example, to identify emotional states of the opponent (Schultheiss & Hale, 2007) or to learn one's own behaviors during the competition that promise to prevail in the competition against an opponent (Schultheiss et al., 2005a, 2005b). From their many years of coaching high-performance athletes from interactive sports, Krug and Kuhl (2006) report that the power motive is on average more pronounced in these athletes than the achievement or affiliation motives. This

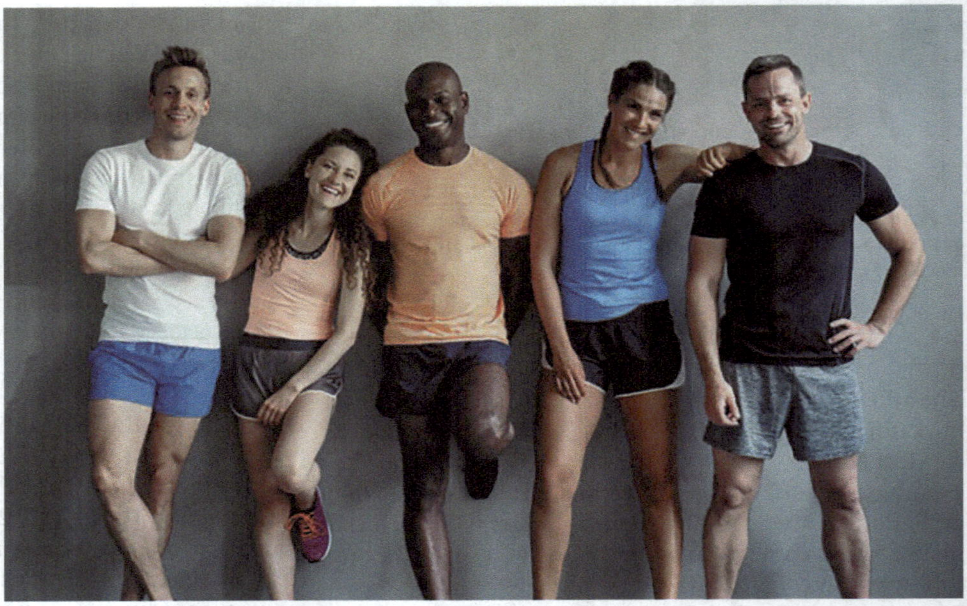

Fig. 9.13 Sport offers many incentives for the affiliation motive

observation has since been empirically confirmed (Study 2; Gröpel et al., 2015). Thus, the power motive seems to be functional in high-performance sports when it comes to a direct interaction with an athletic opponent. Furthermore, in the interaction sports of karate and tennis, it has been shown that male and female athletes with high implicit power motive report higher training volumes than male and female competitive athletes with low implicit power motive (Wegner et al., 2015a, 2015b). Interestingly, it is the avoidance component of the power motive, that is, a fear of losing control, that is associated with training volumes. That is, karateka and tennis players who had a higher fear of loss of control (high implicit power motive) trained at greater durations than male and female athletes with low power motive. The authors hypothesized that fear of defeat in competition, which is equivalent to loss of power, moved athletes to higher training volumes.

> The power motive unfolds its effects on performance in contexts that are determined by a direct interaction event (e.g., one against one battle).

The findings presented here in the area of sport and exercise make it clear that, for example, trainers in competitive sport, course leaders in health sport, or physical education teachers can create sport- and exercise-related contexts that help athletes improve their performance, feel more comfortable, experience flow, and be more motivated overall. Table 9.2 provides examples of such sport-related contexts that are expected to produce motive satisfaction for the various motive themes (Duda & Nicholls, 1992). In addition, examples are given of affects that have been associated with corresponding motive satisfaction in previous work (Bolger & Amarel, 2007; Job et al., 2012; McClelland, 1985b).

Table 9.2 Appropriate sport contexts and accompanying affect expressions for the implicit motives of achievement, affiliation, and power

	Achievement	Affiliation	Power
Suitable sport contexts	Possibility of improving one's own performance, e.g., through feedback; individual engagement with a task; little time pressure and pressure to compare oneself with others; varied, joyful tasks; sports tasks that I can cope with	Cooperative organizational forms; familiar social environments; for individuals with high fear of rejection, cooperative settings lead to poorer performance	Helping others, supporting them, guiding them (e.g., in skill acquisition); gaining prestige, direct comparison, competition with others
Affect expressions associated with motive satisfaction	Pride, efficiency	Joy, calm, relaxation, harmony	Strength, excitement, enthusiasm

9.5 Implicit Motives and Interaction with Explicit Motives and Goals

9.5.1 Motive Incongruence

Implicit and explicit motives are thought to play different roles in action control (Biernat, 1989; McClelland, 1985a). Implicit motives are more responsible for energizing the actual action and influence the seeking out of certain situational contexts, whereas explicit motives influence the action more by focusing on the expected outcome of an action and its consequences in the context of the demands of the social environment (◘ Fig. 9.11). It has been noted, however, that a person's explicit and implicit motives may have different thematic orientations (McClelland et al., 1989). For example, a junior athlete, because he or she is on a regional squad and his or her parents are former high-performance athletes, may set the goal of making the national team (explicit achievement goal). At the same time, however, this junior athlete has a strong implicit affiliation motive and less strong implicit achievement or power motives. Such incongruencies of explicit and implicit motives may act as hidden stressors (Baumann et al., 2005; Schüler et al., 2009) in the long run and worsen health on a psychological and physical level. In the example given, the athlete may have his sights firmly set on playing for the national team. Meeting the expectations of his coach or parents additionally promises him valuable prospects as positive consequences of his athletic actions. In daily life, however, the athlete will lack the energy/drive for the laborious daily training routine. He is more likely to experience this supportive energy in meetings with friends or family, which he experiences as more emotionally satisfying than the "torture" he feels in training and competition.

> Implicit and explicit motives can strongly overlap (= motive-congruence) or can be more or less disconcordant (= motive incongruence). The latter leads to trouble in terms of reduced performance and well-being.

9.5.1.1 Mediation Processes Between Implicit and Explicit Motives

The discrepancy between consciously set (i.e., explicit) athletic goals and implicit motives must be compensated by increased self-control, i.e., the athlete must show a stronger will (e.g., cutting short or canceling time together with friends or family) to suppress/control these impulses of the implicit affiliation motive (Schüler et al., 2019). For example, in a study with managers, Kehr (2004) showed that volitional processes mediate the influence of incongruence between implicit and explicit motives on well-being. Motive incongruencies lead to volitional strength being depleted, which in turn has an impact on a person's subjective well-being.

Motive Congruence

Motive congruence refers to the thematic fit of explicit motives (e.g., high explicit achievement motive) or explicit goals (e.g., an achievement goal such as becoming a national champion) to a person's dominant implicit motive (here, correspondingly, a high implicit achievement motive). The non-fit is referred to as motive incongruence (Brunstein et al., 1995).

However, self-regulation processes can also help to explain congruencies between implicit and explicit motives. As already mentioned in ► Sect. 9.2, implicit and explicit motives often turn out to be uncorrelated (Spangler, 1992). However, if one additionally looks at the volitional ability of action and state orientation of persons (► Chap. 10 on volitional traits) whose implicit and explicit motives have been surveyed, one can observe that action-oriented persons (i.e., persons with good access to the self and their own needs; Kuhl, 2001) are more likely to set explicit goals that fit well with their implicit motives (Brunstein, 2001). In contrast, individuals with low self-access (situation-oriented) are more likely to choose explicit goals that do not match their implicit motives. Kuhl (2001) suggests that positive affect states are required for access to the self. Action-oriented individuals are good at downregulating negative affect, such as that resulting from frustrations caused by athletic failure, in order to gain access to the self. State-oriented individuals remain stuck in negative affect states for a long time after such failures and often do not consider their own implicit needs when forming explicit goals. Instead, they tend to adopt the goals of others (e.g., coaches, parents) and interpret them as self-set (Kuhl & Kazén, 1994). In addition to the possibility of improving self-access by upregulating positive affect, goal imagery can lead to more congruence between explicit goals and implicit motives. In the context of such goal imagery, a person translates a verbal goal (e.g., being allowed to play for the national team) into an experiential format, thus attempting to visualize the goal pursuit and realization for him- or herself and "prefeeling" the emotions in the visualization (Schultheiss & Brunstein, 1999). Such goal imagery can help preprocess the non-explicit, less socially desirable aspects of an action to test for self-fit. In junior swimming, for example, it has been shown that self-access control (operationalized here as unconscious impulse control) limits the energizing function of the achievement motive (Sieber & Mempel, 2015). The achievement motive was related to improvement in athletic performance (crawl time) over a 3-year period only among those junior athletes that did not inhibit their achievement motive. Such inhibitions can arise, for example, in a team when one does not want to be considered too ambitious.

Goal Imagery in Sports

Imagine you were a leisure runner who enjoys going for a run in the woods. One day, a friend runner tells you about an upcoming marathon and suggests you enroll for that sports challenge. You think of yourself as a sportive person, and you think you should prove yourself in your sports activity. Therefore, you agree to participate in a marathon race. In order to know whether this explicit goal (i.e., making a good time in that competition) fits your implicit motivation, you make the following exercise:

> "Try to imagine the day of the marathon as vividly as possible. Imagine yourself running the long distance, imagine having difficult times in the second half of the run, imagine passing these difficult moments, and imagine you finally finishing the marathon. How do you feel during the entire run? How does it feel for you when you pass the difficult moments? What are your feelings when you finally finish the marathon? Do you feel pride about your performance?"

Making this exercise can help you to "prefeel" the emotions that you might experience during the marathon. Positive emotions (e.g., pride) might signal that your explicit goal (i.e., making a good time in the marathon) matches your implicit motivation. Negative emotions (e.g., frustration), on the other hand, might signal that your explicit goal does not perfectly match your implicit motivation and that the competitive situation might not be a perfect situation to satisfy your implicit needs.

Goal Imagery

Goal imagery refers to a simulation of the pursuit and realization of a potential goal that provides a perception (cognition, including emotions) as similar as possible to an action that is actually realized (Schultheiss & Brunstein, 1999).

9.6 Implications for the Field of Sport and Physical Activity

That eliciting unconscious motives has additional explanatory value for behavior and experience in different contexts has been well described in motivational psychology for several decades. The present chapter highlights the value of research on implicit motives in sport psychology. Previous studies on implicit motives in sport describe their value primarily in three areas (Wegner & Schüler, 2015):

First, implicit motives allow for experiential and behavioral predictions in sport that are not possible with traditional direct questionnaire instruments. Not only do implicit motives differentiate between competitive and recreational athletes, but their strength also appears to be associated with indicators of competitive sport success (e.g., training volumes). Moreover, implicit motives are associated with repeatedly demonstrated performance in complex athletic situations. Explicit motives seem to have stronger relevance for decision-making or goal-setting behavior in sports.

Second, depending on the implicit motive characteristics, individuals react sensitively to situational incentives that address their dominant motives. Here, studies exist for all three major motives—achievement, affiliation, and power—in sports. Meanwhile, studies in sport also find that autonomy support is particularly beneficial for individuals with high autonomy motives.

Third, clear (neuro-)physiological associations emerge especially for implicit motives. Incentives that satisfy the motive seem to lead to lower stress responses (e.g., measurable in the hormone cortisol) or lead to better social learning (e.g., mediated by the hormone testosterone). However, this is also associated with long-term health impairments: for example, if an affiliation-motivated person frequently seeks out positive social interactions, this has positive health consequences. A power-motivated person who repeatedly seeks out confrontations in order to be able to demonstrate dominance will suffer long-term health impairments (e.g., of the cardiovascular system), especially if the power motive encounters resistance.

Research on implicit motives in sport is still emerging. However, the findings to date are promising, and it is worthwhile to study this motive system, which has been relatively costly to measure. Future research on implicit motives in sport should address the hypothesized long-term predictions of real-world competitive and training behavior in sport in true longitudinal studies. While such studies are costly and time-consuming, they are certainly justified in light of the effectiveness of health sport programs or the costly promotion of young talents in competitive sport. However, the specifics of the respective sport and its relevance to motives should be taken into account.

In addition to such longitudinal studies with strong proximity to the field of competitive and health sports, research on implicit motives also needs well-controlled experimental studies that test mechanisms of action in sports-relevant contexts. Such studies already exist to some extent, namely, where clear controlled competition conditions are examined in the laboratory (e.g., Schultheiss & Rhode, 2002).

Because the explicit achievement motive is an intensely researched area in sport, future studies should also clearly contrast the dissociation of implicit and explicit motives and their different predictors of experience and behavior. This may help to make the respective concepts, with their strengths, most useful for the sport and exercise domain.

Moreover, few studies in sport have so far addressed incongruencies between implicit and explicit motives and the role that self-regulatory processes play in this relationship. Especially if one wants to make long-term complex behavioral predictions, the inclusion of different motive systems and different self-regulatory aspects is desirable and could be a substantial contribution to the development of this research field.

Finally, there are efforts in various research groups to simplify and optimize the laborious measurement of implicit motives (e.g., Schultheiss, 2013; Schultheiss & Pang, 2007; Slabbinck et al., 2013). In order for the concept of implicit motives to become an even greater subject of future research, research activities that simplify the coding process or speed up the assessment process are valuable.

Learning Control Questions

Basic:

1. What are the most important implicit motive topics in motivation research? Define the terms in each case.
2. What physiological processes are associated with the major motivational themes (achievement, affiliation, power)?
3. What is activity inhibition? Why is it relevant to sports practice?

Advanced:

4. Why are implicit motives important for behavior and experience in sports?
5. What differential predictions can be obtained from implicit motives and explicit self-images in the context of sport? To what extent do these findings reflect theoretical assumptions about the two motivational systems?
6. How is the picture story exercise (PSE) conducted? Briefly describe the procedure and evaluation. Are test scores on the PSE more strongly associated with operant or responding behavior?
7. What motivational brain areas are you aware of? For which processes in the course of motivation and action are these brain areas responsible in each case?
8. What psychological processes are thought to promote congruence between implicit motives and explicit self-images? What are the benefits of this congruence for practice in sport and exercise contexts?

Experts:

9. What four core components of a training program to change the implicit achievement motive do McClelland and Winter (1969) describe? What aspect of the achievement motive seemed to have changed most in this training program?
10. Describe how an affective need, such as the implicit affiliation motive, influences behavior and experience in sport.
11. What sports do you know in which the power motive influences performance? Why would the power motive be relevant there?

References

Adolphs, R. (2002). Recognizing emotion from facial expressions: Psychological and neurological mechanisms. *Behavioral and Cognitive Neuroscience Reviews, 1*, 21–61.

Adolphs, R., Tranel, D., Damasio, H., & Damasio, A. R. (1995). Fear and the human amygdala. *The Journal of Neuroscience, 15*(9), 5879–5891.

Alexander, G. M., Packard, M. G., & Hines, M. (1994). Testosterone has rewarding affective properties in male rats: Implications for the biological basis of sexual motivation. *Behavioral Neuroscience, 108*(2), 424–428.

Atkinson, J. W. (1957). Motivational determinants of risk-taking behavior. *Psychological Review, 64*(6), 359–372.

Atkinson, J. W. (1958). *Motives in fantasy, action, and society: A method of assessment and study*. Van Nostrand.

Atkinson, J. W., & Litwin, G. H. (1960). Achievement motive and test anxiety conceived as motive to approach success and motive to avoid failure. *The Journal of Abnormal and Social Psychology, 60*(1), 52–63. https://doi.org/10.1037/h0041119

Atkinson, J. W., & Walker, E. L. (1958). The affiliation motive and perceptual sensitivity to faces. In J. W. Atkinson (Ed.), *Motives in fantasy, action, and society: A method of assessment and study* (pp. 360–366). Van Nostrand.

Baumann, N., Kaschel, R., & Kuhl, J. (2005). Striving for unwanted goals: Stress dependent discrepancies between explicit and implicit achievement motives reduce subjective well-being and

increase psychosomatic symptoms. *Journal of Personality and Social Psychology, 89*(5), 781–799.
Baumann, N., Kazén, M., & Kuhl, J. (2010). Implicit motives: A look from personality systems interaction theory. In O. C. Schultheiss & J. C. Brunstein (Eds.), *Implicit motives* (pp. 375–403). Oxford University Press.
Bäumler, G. (1975). Beeinflussung der Leistungsmotivation durch Psychopharmaka: I. Die 4 bildthematischen Hauptvariablen [The effects of psychoactive drugs on achievement motivation: I. The four motive scales]. *Zeitschrift für Experimentelle und Angewandte Psychologie, 22*, 1–14.
Bechara, A., Damasio, A. R., Damasio, H., & Anderson, S. W. (1994). Insensitivity to future consequences following damage to human prefrontal cortex. *Cognition, 50*, 7–15.
Biernat, M. (1989). Motives and values to achieve: Different constructs with different effects. *Journal of Personality, 57*(1), 69–95.
Blair, R. J., Morris, J. S., Frith, C. D., Perrett, D. I., & Dolan, R. J. (1999). Dissociable neural responses to facial expressions of sadness and anger. *Brain, 122*(Pt. 5), 883–893.
Bolger, N., & Amarel, D. (2007). Effects of social support visibility on adjustment to stress: Experimental evidence. *Journal of Personality and Social Psychology, 92*(3), 458–475.
Brickenkamp, R. (2002). *Test d2 Aufmerksamkeits-Belastungs-Test*. Hogrefe.
Brown, S. L., Fredrickson, B. L., Wirth, M. M., Poulin, M. J., Meier, E. A., & Heaphy, E. D. (2009). Social closeness increases salivary progesterone in humans. *Hormones and Behavior, 56*(1), 108–111.
Brunstein, J. C. (2001). Persönliche Ziele und Handlungs- vs. Lageorientierung: Wer bindet sich an realistische und bedürfniskongruente Ziele? [Personal goals and action versus state orientation: Who builds a commitment to realistic and need-congruent goals?]. *Zeitschrift für Differentielle und Diagnostische Psychologie, 22*(1), 1–12.
Brunstein, J. C., & Heckhausen, H. (2006). Leistungsmotivation. In J. Heckhausen & H. Heckhausen (Eds.), *Motivation und Handeln* ((3 ed., pp. 143–192). Springer.
Brunstein, J. C., & Hoyer, S. (2002). Implizites versus explizites Leistungsstreben: Befunde zur Unabhängigkeit zweier Motivsysteme [Implicit versus explicit achievement motivation: Findings on the independence of two motivational systems]. *Zeitschrift für Pädagogische Psychologie, 16*(1), 51–62.
Brunstein, J. C., Lautenschlager, U., Nawroth, B., Pöhlmann, K., & Schultheiss, O. C. (1995). Persönliche Anliegen, soziale Motive und emotionales Wohlbefinden [Personal goals, social motives, and emotional well-being]. *Zeitschrift für Differentielle und Diagnostische Psychologie, 16*(1), 1–10.
Brunstein, J. C., & Maier, G. W. (2005). Implicit and self-attributed motives to achieve: Two separate but interacting needs. *Journal of Personality and Social Psychology, 89*(2), 205–222.
Brunstein, J. C., & Schmitt, C. H. (2004). Assessing individual differences in achievement motivation with the Implicit Association Test. *Journal of Research in Personality, 38*, 536–555.
Cahill, L. (2000). Modulation of long-term memory in humans by emotional arousal: Adrenergic activation and the amygdala. In J. P. Aggleton (Ed.), *The amygdala: A functional analysis* (pp. 425–446). Oxford University Press.
Cardinal, R. N., Parkinson, J. A., Hall, J., & Everitt, B. J. (2002). Emotion and motivation: The role of the amygdala, ventral striatum, and prefrontal cortex. *Neuroscience & Biobehavioral Reviews, 26*(3), 321–352.
Collins, C. J., Hanges, P. J., & Locke, E. A. (2004). The relationship of achievement motivation to entrepreneurial behavior: A meta-ana- lysis. *Human Performance, 17*, 95–117.
Connors, C. K. (1963). Birth order and needs for affiliation. *Journal of Personality, 31*(3), 408–416.
Dahme, G., Jungnickel, D., & Rathje, H. (1993). Güteeigenschaften der Achievement Motives Scale (AMS) von Gjesme und Nygard (1970) in der deutschen Übersetzung von Göttert und Kuhl: Vergleich der Kennwerte norwegischer und deutscher Stichproben [Validation data for the Achievement Motives Scale (AMS) by Gjesme and Nygard (1970) in the German version by Göttert and Kuhl: Comparison of the data from the Norwegian and the German samples]. *Diagnostica, 39*(3), 257–270.
deCharms, R. (1957). Affiliation motivation and productivity in small groups. *The Journal of Abnormal and Social Psychology, 55*(2), 222–226.
deCharms, R. (1968). *Personal causation*. Academic Press.
deCharms, R., Morrison, H. W., Reitman, W., & McClelland, D. C. (1955). Behavioral correlates of directly and indirectly measured achievement motivation. In D. C. McClelland (Ed.), *Studies in motivation* (pp. 414–423). Appleton-Century-Crofts.
Deci, E. L., & Ryan, R. M. (1985). *Intrinsic motivation and self-determination in human behavior*. Plenum Press.
Duda, J. L., & Nicholls, J. G. (1992). Dimensions of achievement motivation in schoolwork and sport. *Journal of Educational Psychology, 84*(3), 290–299.
Elbe, A.-M., Wenhold, F., & Müller, D. (2005). Zur Reliabilität und Validität der Achievement Motive Scale-Sport [On the reliability and validity of the Achievement Motive Scale-Sport]. *Zeitschrift für Sportpsychologie, 12*(2), 57–68.
Feather, N. T. (1966). The relationship of persistence at a task to expectation of success and achievement-related motives. In J. W. Atkinson & N. T. Feather (Eds.), *A theory of achievement motivation* (pp. 117–133). Wiley.
Fodor, E. M. (1985). The power motive, group conflict, and physiological arousal. *Journal of Personality and Social Psychology, 49*(5), 1408–1415.
Fodor, E. M., Wick, D. P., & Hartsen, K. M. (2006). The power motive and affective response to assertiveness. *Journal of Research in Personality, 40*(5), 598–610.
Fontana, A. F., Rosenberg, R. L., Marcus, J. L., & Kerns, R. D. (1987). Type A behavior pattern, inhibited power motivation, and activity inhibition. *Journal of Personality and Social Psychology, 52*(1), 177–183.
French, E. G. (1958). Some characteristics of achievement motivation. In J. W. Atkinson (Ed.), *Motives in fantasy, action, and society* (pp. 270–277). Van Nostrand.
French, E. G., & Chadwick, I. (1956). Some characteristics in affiliation motivation. *Journal of Abnormal and Social Psychology, 52*(3), 296–300.
Fuster, J. M. (2001). The prefrontal cortex—An update: Time is of the essence. *Neuron, 30*(2), 319–333.
Gabler, H. (1972). *Leistungsmotivation im Hochleistungssport [Achievement motivation in high-performance sport]*. Hofmann.
Greenwald, A. G., McGhee, D. E., & Schwartz, J. L. K. (1998). Measuring individual differences in implicit cognition: The Implicit Association Test. *Journal of Personality and Social Psychology, 74*(6), 1464–1480.
Gröpel, P., Schöne, L., & Wegner, M. (2015). Implizite und explizite Motive von Leistungs- und Freizeitsporttreibenden [The implicit and explicit motives of high-performance and recreational athletes]. *Zeitschrift für Sportpsychologie, 22*(1), 6–19.
Gröpel, P., Wegner, M., & Schüler, J. (2016). Achievement motive and sport participation. *Psychology of Sport & Exercise, 27*, 93–100.
Gump, B. B., & Kulik, J. A. (1997). Stress, affiliation, and emotional contagion. *Journal of Personality and Social Psychology, 72*(2), 305–319.
Hall, J. L., Stanton, S. J., & Schultheiss, O. C. (2010). Biopsychological and neural processes of implicit motivation. In O. C. Schul-

theiss & J. C. Brunstein (Eds.), *Implicit motives* (pp. 279–307). Oxford University Press.

Heckhausen, H. (1963). *Hoffnung und Furcht in der Leistungsmotivation [Hope and fear components of achievement motivation]*. Anton Hain.

Heckhausen, H. (1965). Leistungsmotivation. In H. Thomae (Ed.), *Handbuch der Psychologie* (Vol. II, pp. 602–702). Hogrefe.

Heckhausen, H., & Heckhausen, J. (2010). *Motivation und Handeln*. Springer.

Heckhausen, H., & Krug, S. (1982). Motive modification. In A. J. Stewart (Ed.), *Motivation and society* (pp. 274–318). Jossey-Bass.

Heinrichs, M., Baumgartner, T., Kirschbaum, C., & Ehlert, U. (2003). Social support and oxytocin interact to suppress cortisol and subjective responses to psychosocial stress. *Biological Psychiatry, 54*(12), 1389–1398.

Hess, U., Blairy, S., & Kleck, R. E. (2000). The influence of facial emotion displays, gender, and ethnicity on judgments of dominance and affiliation. *Journal of Nonverbal Behavior, 24*, 265–283.

Heyns, R. W., Veroff, J., & Atkinson, J. W. (1958). A scoring manual for the affiliation motive. In J. W. Atkinson (Ed.), *Motives in fantasy, action, and society: A method of assessment and study*. Princeton.

Hu, M., & Becker, J. B. (2003). Effects of sex and estrogen on behavioral sensitization to cocaine in rats. *Journal of Neuroscience, 23*(2), 693–699.

Ikemoto, S., & Panksepp, J. (1996). Dissociations between appetitive and consummatory responses by pharmacological manipulations of reward-relevant brain regions. *Behavioral Neuroscience, 110*, 331–345.

Insel, T. R., & Young, L. J. (2001). The neurobiology of attachment. *Nature Reviews: Neuroscience, 2*(2), 129–136.

Jackson, D. N. (1967). *Personality Research Form manual*. Research Psychologists Press.

Jemmott, J. B. (1987). Social motives and susceptibility to disease: Stalking individual differences in health risks. *Journal of Personality, 55*(2), 267–298.

Jemmott, J. B., Borysenko, J. Z., Borysenko, M., McClelland, D. C., Chapman, R., & Meyer, D. (1983). Academic stress, power motivation, and decrease in secretion rate of salivary secretory immunoglobulin A. *The Lancet, 8339*, 1400–1402.

Jemmott, J. B., Hellman, C., McClelland, D. C., Locke, S. E., Kraus, L., & Williams, R. M. (1990). Motivational syndromes associated with natural killer cell activity. *Journal of Behavioral Medicine, 13*(1), 53–73.

Job, V., Bernecker, K., & Dweck, C. S. (2012). Are implicit motives the need to feel certain affect? Motive-affect congruence predicts relationship satisfaction. *Personality and Social Psychology Bulletin, 38*(12), 1552–1565.

Kasl, S. V. (1974). Are there any promising biochemical correlates of achievement behavior and motivation? The evidence for serum uric acid and serum cholesterol. *Review of Educational Research, 44*(4), 447–462.

Kehr, H. M. (2004). Implicit/explicit motive discrepancies and volitional depletion among managers. *Personality and Social Psychology Bulletin, 30*(3), 315–327.

Kelsey, R. M. (2012). Beta-adrenergic cardiovascular reactivity and adaptation to stress: The cardiac pre-ejection period as an index of effort. In R. A. Wright & G. H. E. Gendolla (Eds.), *How motivation affects cardiovascular response: Mechanisms and applications* (pp. 43–60). American Psychological Association.

Köllner, M. G., & Schultheiss, O. C. (2014). Meta-analytic evidence of low convergence between implicit and explicit measures of the needs for achievement, affiliation, and power. *Frontiers in Psychology: Personality and Social Psychology, 5*, 826.

Kringelbach, M. L. (2005). The human orbitofrontal cortex: Linking reward to hedonic experience. *Nature Reviews: Neuroscience, 6*(9), 691–702.

Kringelbach, M. L., & Rolls, E. T. (2004). The functional neuroanatomy of the human orbitofrontal cortex: Evidence from neuroimaging and neuropsychology. *Progress in Neurobiology, 72*, 341–372.

Krug, J. S., & Kuhl, U. (2006). Motivausprägung und Erfolg im Spitzensport oder—Reicht Sportlern ein hohes Leistungsmotiv zum Erfolg? [Motive characteristics and success in elite sports or—Is a high achievement motive enought for athletes?]. In J. S. Krug & U. Kuhl (Eds.), *Macht, Leistung, Freundschaft: Motive als Erfolgsfaktoren in Wirtschaft, Politik und Spitzensport [Power, achievement, friendship: Motives as factors of success in economy, politics, and elite sports]* (pp. 126–138). Kohlhammer.

Kuhl, J. (2001). *Motivation und Persönlichkeit: Interaktion psychischer Systeme [Motivation and personality: Interaction of mental systems]*. Hogrefe.

Kuhl, J., & Kazén, M. (1994). Self-discrimination and memory: State orientation and false self-ascription of assigned activities. *Journal of Personality and Social Psychology, 66*, 103–115.

Kuhl, J., & Scheffer, D. (1999). *Der Operante Multi-Motiv-Test (OMT): Manual [The Operant Multimotive Test (OMT): Manual]*. University of Osnabrück.

Kuhl, U., & Krug, S. (2006). Macht erfolgreich? Macht erfolgreich! Die Rolle des Machtmotivs im Spitzensport [Is power a prerequisite of success? Power is a prerequisite of success!]. *Leistungssport, 36*(5), 5–10.

Luria, A. (1992). *Das Gehirn in Aktion [The brain in action]*. Rowohlt.

Mazeres, F., Brinkmann, K., & Richter, M. (2019). Implicit achievement motive limits the impact of task difficulty on effort-related cardiovascular response. *Journal of Research in Personality, 82*, 103842. https://doi.org/10.1016/j.jrp.2019.06.012

Mazeres, F., Brinkmann, K., & Richter, M. (2021a). Explicit achievement motive strength determines effort-related myocardial beta-adrenergic activity if task difficulty is unclear but not if task difficulty is clear. *International Journal of Psychophysiology, 169*, 11–19. https://doi.org/10.1016/j.ijpsycho.2021.08.004

Mazeres, F., Brinkmann, K., & Richter, M. (2021b). Motivated but not engaged: The implicit achievement motive requires difficult or unclear task difficulty conditions to exert an impact on effort. *Journal of Research in Personality., 94*, 104145.

McAdams, D. P., & Vaillant, G. E. (1982). Intimacy, motivation and psychological adjustment: A longitudinal study. *Journal of Personality Assessment, 46*, 586–593.

McCelland, D. C., Alexander, C., & Marks, E. (1982). The need for power, stress, immune function, and illness among male prisoners. *Journal of Abnormal Psychology, 91*(1), 61–70.

McCelland, D. C., Floor, E., Davidson, R. J., & Saron, C. (1980). Stressed power motivation, sympathetic activation, immune function, and illness. *Journal of Human Stress, 6*, 11–19.

McClelland, D. C. (1961). *The achieving society*. Van Nostrand.

McClelland, D. C. (1965). N achievement and entrepreneurship: A longitudinal study. *Journal of Personality and Social Psychology, 1*, 389–392.

McClelland, D. C. (1979). Inhibited power motivation and high blood pressure in men. *Journal of Abnormal Psychology, 88*(2), 182–190.

McClelland, D. C. (1980). Motive dispositions: The merits of operant and respondent measures. In L. Wheeler (Ed.), *Review of personality and social psychology* (Vol. 1, pp. 10–41). Sage.

McClelland, D. C. (1985a). How motives, skills, and values determine what people do. *American Psychologist, 40*(7), 812–825.

McClelland, D. C. (1985b). *Human motivation*. Scott, Foresman & Co.

McClelland, D. C. (1987a). Characteristics of successful entrepreneurs. *Journal of Creative Behavior, 3*, 219–233.
McClelland, D. C. (1987b). *Human motivation*. Cambridge University Press.
McClelland, D. C. (1989). Motivational factors in health and disease. *American Psychologist, 44*(4), 675–683.
McClelland, D. C. (1995). Achievement motivation in relation to achievement-related recall, performance, and urine flow, a marker associated with release of vasopressin. *Motivation and Emotion, 19*(1), 59–76.
McClelland, D. C., Alexander, C., & Marks, E. (1982). The need for power, stress, immune function, and illness among male prisoners. *Journal of Abnormal Psychology, 91*(1), 61–70.
McClelland, D. C., Atkinson, J. W., Clark, R. A., & Lowell, E. L. (1953). *The achievement motive*. Appleton-Century-Crofts.
McClelland, D. C., & Boyatzis, R. E. (1982). The leadership motive pattern and long term success in management. *Journal of Applied Psychology, 67*, 737–743.
McClelland, D. C., Davis, W. N., Kalin, R., & Wanner, E. (1972). *The drinking man*. Free Press.
McClelland, D. C., & Jemmott, J. B. (1980). Power motivation, stress and physical illness. *Journal of Human Stress, 6*(4), 6–15. https://doi.org/10.1080/0097840X.1980.9936101
McClelland, D. C., & Kirshnit, C. (1988). The effect of motivational arousal through films on salivary immunoglobulin A. *Psychology and Health, 2*(1), 31–52.
McClelland, D. C., Koestner, R., & Weinberger, J. (1989). How do self-attributed and implicit motives differ? *Psychological Review, 96*(4), 690–702.
McClelland, D. C., Patel, V., Stier, D., & Brown, D. (1987). The relationship of affiliative arousal to dopamine release. *Motivation and Emotion, 11*(1), 51–66.
McClelland, D. C., & Pilon, D. A. (1983). Sources of adult motives in patterns of parent behavior in early childhood. *Journal of Personality and Social Psychology, 44*(3), 564–574.
McClelland, D. C., Ross, G., & Patel, V. (1985). The effect of an academic examination on salivary norepinephrine and immunoglobulin levels. *Journal of Human Stress, 11*(2), 52–59.
McClelland, D. C., & Winter, D. G. (1969). *Motivating economic achievement*. Free Press.
Mehrabian, A. (1968). Male and female scales of the tendency to achieve. *Educational and Psychological Measurement, 28*(2), 493–502.
Mischel, W., & Gilligan, C. (1964). Delay of gratification, motivation for the prohibited gratification, and responses to temptation. *Journal of Abnormal and Social Psychology, 69*(4), 411–417.
Mogenson, G. J., Jones, D. J., & Yim, C. Y. (1980). From motivation to action: Functional interface between the limbic system and the motor system. *Progress in Neurobiology, 14*, 69–97.
Monk, C. S., McClure, E. B., Nelson, E. E., Zarahn, E., Bilder, R. M., & Leibenluft, E. (2003). Adolescent immaturity in attention-related brain engagement to emotional facial expressions. *NeuroImage, 20*(1), 420–428.
Morgan, C., & Murray, H. A. (1935). A method for investigating fantasies: The Thematic Apperception Test. *Archives of Neurology and Psychiatry, 34*, 289–306.
Mücher, H. P., & Heckhausen, H. (1962). Influence of mental activity and achievement motivation on skeletal muscle tonus. *Perceptual and Motor Skills, 14*, 217–218.
Mueller, E. F., Kasl, S. V., Brooks, G. W., & Cobb, S. (1970). Psychosocial correlates of serum urate levels. *Psychological Bulletin, 73*(4), 238–257.
Packard, M. G., Schroeder, J. P., & Alexander, G. M. (1998). Expression of testosterone conditioned place preference is blocked by peripheral or intra-accumbens injection of α-flupenthixol. *Hormones and Behavior, 34*(1), 39–47.
Patten, R. L., & White, L. A. (1977). Independent effects of achievement motivation and overt attribution on achievement behavior. *Motivation and Emotion, 1*(1), 39–59.
Ramsay, J. E., & Pang, J. S. (2013). Set ambiguity: A key determinant of reliability and validity in the picture story exercise. *Motivation and Emotion, 37*(4), 661–674.
Raphelson, A. C. (1957). The relationship among imaginative, direct verbal, and physiological measures of anxiety in an achievement situation. *Journal of Abnormal and Social Psychology, 54*, 13–18.
Rheinberg, F., & Engeser, S. (2010). Motive training and motivational competence. In O. C. Schultheiss & J. C. Brunstein (Eds.), *Implicit Motives* (pp. 510–548). Oxford University Press.
Richter, M., Mazeres, F., & Brinkmann, K. (2021). Clarity of task difficulty moderates the impact of the explicit achievement motive on physical effort in hand grip tasks. *PLoS One, 16*, e0252713.
Robertson, G. L. (2006). Regulation of arginine vasopressin in the syndrome of inappropriate antidiuresis. *The American Journal of Medicine, 119*(7A), S36–S42.
Rokeach, M. (1973). *The nature of human values*. Free Press.
Rolls, E. T. (2000). The orbitofrontal cortex and reward. *Cerebral Cortex, 10*(3), 284–294.
Rolls, E. T., Sienkiewicz, Z. J., & Yaxley, S. (1989). Hunger modulates the responses to gustatory stimuli of single neurons in the caudolateral orbitofrontal cortex of the macaque monkey. *European Journal of Neuroscience, 1*(1), 53–60.
Russo, S. J., Festa, E. D., Fabian, S. J., Gazi, F. M., Kraish, M., & Jenab, S. (2003). Gonadal hormones differentially modulate cocaine-induced conditioned place preference in male and female rats. *Neuroscience, 120*(2), 523–533.
Scheffer, D. (2001). *Entwicklungsbedingungen impliziter Motive: Bindung, Leistung & Macht [Developmental conditions of implicit motives: Affiliation, Achievement, & Power]*. (Doctoral Thesis). Universität Osnabrück.
Scheffer, D., Kuhl, J., & Eichstaedt, J. (2003). Der Operante Motiv-Test (OMT): Inhaltsklassen, Auswertung, psychometrische Kennwerte und Validierung [The Operant Motive Test (OMT): Contents, scoring, psychometric values, and validation]. In J. Stiensmeier-Pelster & F. Rheinberg (Eds.), *Diagnostik von Motivation und Selbstkonzept [Diagnostic of motivation and self-concept]* (pp. 151–180). Hogrefe.
Schmalt, H.-D., & Heckhausen, H. (2008). Power motivation. In J. Heckhausen & H. Heckhausen (Eds.), *Motivation and action* (pp. 202–226). Cambridge University Press.
Schmalt, H.-D., & Heckhausen, H. (2010). Machtmotivation. In J. Heckhausen & H. Heckhausen (Eds.), *Motivation und Handeln* (4th ed., pp. 211–236). Springer.
Schrier, R. (2006). Water and sodium retention in edematous disorders: Role of vasopressin and aldosterone. *The American Journal of Medicine, 119*(7A), S47–S53.
Schüler, J., & Brandstätter, V. (2013). How basic need satisfaction and dispositional motives interact in predicting flow experience in sport. *Journal of Applied Social Psychology, 43*(4), 687–705.
Schüler, J., Brandstätter, V., Wegner, M., & Baumann, N. (2015). Testing the convergent and discriminant validity of three implicit motive measures: PSE, OMT, and MMG. *Motivation and Emotion, 39*(6), 839–857.
Schüler, J., Guidon, L., Hofstetter, D., Suter, T., Sieber, V., & Wegner, M. (2016a). Affiliation-related goal instructions by coaches—The secret of success for affiliation-motivated individuals. *International Journal of Sport Psychology, 47*, 1–10.
Schüler, J., Job, V., Fröhlich, S. M., & Brandstätter, V. (2009). Dealing with a hidden stressor: Emotional disclosure as a coping

9

strategy to overcome the negative effects of motive incongruence on health. *Stress and Health, 25*(3), 221–233.

Schüler, J., Sheldon, K. M., Prentice, M., & Halusic, M. (2016b). Do some people need autonomy more than others? Implicit dispositions toward autonomy moderate the effects of felt autonomy on well-being. *Journal of Personality, 84*(1), 5–20.

Schüler, J., Wegner, M., & Knechtle, B. (2014). Implicit motives and basic need satisfaction in extreme endurance sports. *Journal of Sport & Exercise Psychology, 36*(3), 293–302.

Schüler, J., Zimanyi, Z., & Wegner, M. (2019). Paved, graveled, and stony paths to high performance: Theoretical considerations on self-control demands of achievement goals based on implicit and explicit motives. *Performance Enhancement & Health, 7*, 100146. https://doi.org/10.1016/j.peh.2019.100146

Schultheiss, O. C. (2001). An information processing account of implicit motive arousal. In M. L. Maehr & P. Pintrich (Eds.), *Advances in motivation and achievement* (New directions in measures and methods) (Vol. 12, pp. 1–41). JAI Press.

Schultheiss, O. C. (2007a). A biobehavioral model of implicit power motivation arousal, reward, and frustration. In E. Harmon-Jones & P. Winkielman (Eds.), *Social neuroscience: Integrating biological and psychological explanations of social behavior* (pp. 176–196). Guilford.

Schultheiss, O. C. (2007b). A memory-systems approach to the classification of personality tests: Comment on Meyer and Kurtz (2006). *Journal of Personality Assessment, 89*(2), 197–201.

Schultheiss, O. C. (2008). Implicit motives. In O. P. John, R. W. Robins, & L. A. Pervin (Eds.), *Handbook of personality: Theory and research* (3rd ed., pp. 603–633). Guilford Press.

Schultheiss, O. C. (2013). *Are implicit motives revealed in mere words?* Frontiers in Psychology. https://doi.org/10.3389/fpsyg.2013.00748

Schultheiss, O. C., & Brunstein, J. C. (1999). Goal imagery: Bridging the gap between implicit motives and explicit goals. *Journal of Personality, 67*, 1–38.

Schultheiss, O. C., & Brunstein, J. C. (2005). An implicit motive perspective on competence. In A. J. Elliott & C. S. Dweck (Eds.), *Handbook of competence and motivation* (pp. 31–51). Guilford.

Schultheiss, O. C., Campbell, K. L., & McClelland, D. C. (1999). Implicit power motivation moderates men's testosterone responses to imagined and real dominance success. *Hormones and Behavior, 36*(3), 234–241.

Schultheiss, O. C., Dargel, A., & Rohde, W. (2003). Implicit motives and gonadal steroid hormones: Effects of menstrual cycle phase, oral contraceptive use, and relationship status. *Hormones and Behavior, 43*(2), 293–301.

Schultheiss, O. C., & Hale, J. A. (2007). Implicit motives modulate attentional orienting to facial expressions of emotion. *Motivation and Emotion, 31*, 13–24.

Schultheiss, O. C., & Pang, J. S. (2007). Measuring implicit motives. In R. W. Robins, R. C. Fraley, & R. Krueger (Eds.), *Handbook of research methods in personality psychology* (pp. 322–344). Guilford.

Schultheiss, O. C., Pang, J. S., Torges, C. M., Wirth, M. M., & Treynor, W. (2005a). Perceived facial expressions of emotion as motivational incentives: Evidence from a differential implicit learning paradigm. *Emotion, 5*(1), 41–54.

Schultheiss, O. C., & Rhode, W. (2002). Implicit power motivation predicts men's testosterone changes and implicit learning in a contest situation. *Hormones and Behavior, 41*(2), 195–202.

Schultheiss, O. C., & Wirth, M. M. (2008). Biopsychological aspects of motivation. In J. Heckhausen & H. Heckhausen (Eds.), *Motivation and action* (pp. 247–271). Cambridge University Press.

Schultheiss, O. C., Wirth, M. M., & Stanton, S. J. (2004). Effects of affiliation and power motivation arousal on salivary progesterone and testosterone. *Hormones and Behavior, 46*(5), 592–599.

Schultheiss, O. C., Wirth, M. M., Torges, C. M., Pang, J. S., Villacorta, M. A., & Welsh, K. M. (2005b). Effects of implicit power motivation and men's and women's implicit learning and testosterone change after social victory or defeat. *Journal of Personality and Social Psychology, 88*(1), 174–188.

Schultz, W. (1998). Predictive reward signal of dopamine neurons. *Journal of Neurophysiology, 80*(1), 1–27.

Sears, R. R., Maccoby, E. E., & Levin, H. (1957). *Patterns of child rearing*. Row Peterson.

Sieber, V., & Mempel, G. (2015). Der prognostische Wert von impliziten Motiven für die Talentdiagnostik im Schwimmsport: Die moderierende Rolle unbewusster Impulskontrolle [The prognostic value of implicit motives for the talent diagnostics in swimming: The moderating role of activity inhibition]. *Zeitschrift für Sportpsychologie, 22*(1), 46–56.

Sieber, V., Schüler, J., & Wegner, M. (2016a). The effects of autonomy on salivary alpha-amylase: The role of individual differences. *Psychoneuroendocrinology, 74*, 173–178.

Sieber, V., Wegner, M., & Schüler, J. (2016b). Autonomie als Prädiktor intrinsischer Motivation im Schulsport: Eine Person x Situation-Perspektive. *Zeitschrift für Gesundheitspsychologie, 24*(3), 1–7. https://doi.org/10.1026/0943-8149/a000166

Slabbinck, H., De Houwer, J., & Van Kenhove, P. (2011). A pictorial attitude IAT as a measure of implicit motives. *European Journal of Personality, 25*(1), 76–86.

Slabbinck, H., De Houwer, J., & Van Kenhove, P. (2013). Convergent, discriminant, and incremental validity of the Pictorial Attitude Implicit Association Test and the Picture Story Exercise as measures of the implicit power motive. *European Journal of Personality, 27*, 30–38.

Smith, C. P. (1992). *Motivation and personality: Handbook of thematic content analysis*. Cambridge University Press.

Sokolowski, K., & Heckhausen, H. (2010). Soziale Bindung: Anschluss- motivation und Intimitätsmotivation. In J. Heckhausen & H. Heckhausen (Eds.), *Motivation und Handeln* (4th ed., pp. 193–210). Springer.

Sokolowski, K., Schmalt, H.-D., Langens, T. A., & Puca, R. M. (2000). Assessing achievement, affiliation, and power motives all at once: The Multi-Motive Grid (MMG). *Journal of Personality Assessment, 74*(1), 126–145.

Sorrentino, R. M., & Sheppard, B. H. (1978). Effects of affiliation-related motives on swimmers in individual versus group competition: A field experiment. *Journal of Personality and Social Psychology, 36*(7), 704–714.

Spangler, W. D. (1992). Validity of questionnaire and TAT measures of need for achievement: Two meta-analyses. *Psychological Bulletin, 112*(1), 140–154.

Stanton, S. J., & Schultheiss, O. C. (2007). Basal and dynamic relationships between implicit power motivation and estradiol in women. *Hormones and Behavior, 52*, 571–580.

Stanton, S. J., & Schultheiss, O. C. (2009). The hormonal correlates of implicit power motivation. *Journal of Research in Personality, 43*(5), 942–949.

Stricker, E. M., & Verbalis, J. G. (2002). Hormones and ingestive behaviors. In J. B. Becker, S. M. Breedlove, & D. Crews (Eds.), *Behavioral endocrinology* (2nd ed., pp. 451–473). MIT Press.

Taylor, S. E. (2006). Tend and befriend: Biobehavioral bases of affiliation under stress. *Current Directions in Psychological Science, 15*(6), 273–277.

Taylor, S. E., Klein, L. C., Lewis, B. P., Gruenewald, T. L., Gurung, R. A., & Updegraff, J. A. (2000). Biobehavioral responses to stress in females: Tend-and-befriend, not fight-or-flight. *Psychological Review, 107*(3), 411–429.

Teubel, T. (2012). *Das Anschlussmotiv zur Erklärung sportlicher Leistungen [The affiliation motive as a predictor for sports performance]*. Verlag Dr. Kovac.

Torpy, D. J., Grice, J. E., Hockings, G. I., Walters, M. M., Crosbie, G. V., & Jackson, R. V. (1994). Alprazolam attenuates vasopressin-stimulated adrenocorticotropin and cortisol release: Evidence for synergy between vasopressin and corticotropin-releasing hormone in humans. *The Journal of Clinical Endocrinology and Metabolism, 79*(1), 140–144.

Varga, K. (1977). Who gains from achievment motivation training? Vikalpa (The Journal for Decision Making), 2(3), 187–200. https://doi.org/10.1177/0256090919770301.

Veroff, J., & Smith, D. A. (1985). Motives and values over the adult years. In D. Kleiber & M. Maehr (Eds.), *Advances in motivation and achievements* (pp. 1–53). JAI Press.

Vuilleumier, P., Richardson, M. P., Armony, J. L., Driver, J., & Dolan, R. J. (2004). Distant influences of amygdala lesion on visual cortical activation during emotional face processing. *Nature Neuroscience, 7*(11), 1271–1278.

Wegner, M., Bohnacker, V., Mempel, G., Teubel, T., & Schüler, J. (2014a). Explicit and implicit affiliation motives predict verbal and nonverbal social behavior in sports competition. *Psychology of Sport and Exercise, 15*, 588–595.

Wegner, M., & Schüler, J. (2014). The implicit achievement motive and general life stress affect time spent on competitive matches in racquets sports. In C. Mohiyeddini (Ed.), *Contemporary topics and trends in the psychology of sports* (pp. 153–176). Nova Science.

Wegner, M., & Schüler, J. (2015). Implizite Motive—Perspektiven im Kontext Sport und Bewegung. *Zeitschrift für Sportpsychologie, 22*(1), 2–5.

Wegner, M., Schüler, J., & Budde, H. (2014b). The implicit affiliation motive moderates cortisol responses to acute psychosocial stress in high school students. *Psychoneuroendocrinology, 48*, 162–168.

Wegner, M., Schüler, J., Scheuermann, K. S., Machado, S., & Budde, H. (2015a). The implicit power motive and adolescents' salivary cortisol responses to acute psychosocial stress and exercise in school. *CNS & Neurological Disorders Drug Targets, 14*(9), 1219–1224.

Wegner, M., & Teubel, T. (2014). The implicit achievement motive predicts match performances and the explicit motive predicts choices for target distances in team sports. *International Journal of Sport Psychology, 45*(6), 621–638.

Wegner, M., Wieland, A., & Mempel, G. (2015b). The implicit fear of power motive is associated with practice time in elite karateka and tennis players. *International Journal of Sport and Exercise Psychology, 15*(3), 258–272.

Weinberger, J., & McClelland, D. C. (1990). Cognitive versus traditional motivational models: Irreconcilable or complementary? In E. T. Hig- gins & R. M. Sorrentino (Eds.), Handbook of motivation and cognition: Bd. 2. foundations of social behavior (S. 562–597). : Guilford.

Wendt, H.-W. (1955). Motivation, effort, and performance. In D. C. McClelland (Ed.), *Studies in motivation* (pp. 448–459). Appleton-Century-Crofts.

Whalen, P. J., Rauch, S. L., Etcoff, N. L., McInerney, S. C., Lee, M. B., & Jenike, M. A. (1998). Masked presentations of emotional facial expressions modulate amygdala activity without explicit knowledge. *Journal of Neuroscience, 18*(1), 411–418.

Winter, D. G. (1973). *The power motive*. The Free Press.

Winter, D. G. (1994). *Manual for scoring motive imagery in running text (Version 4.2)*. University of Michigan.

Wirth, M. M., & Schultheiss, O. C. (2006). Effects of affiliation arousal (hope of closeness) and affiliation stress (fear of rejection) on progesterone and cortisol. *Hormones and Behavior, 50*(5), 786–795.

Wirth, M. M., Welsh, K. M., & Schultheiss, O. C. (2006). Salivary cortisol changes in humans after winning or losing a dominance contest depend on implicit power motivation. *Hormones and Behavior, 49*(3), 346–352.

Wright, R. A. (1996). Brehm's theory of motivation as a model of effort and cardiovascular response. In P. M. Gollwitzer & J. A. Bargh (Eds.), *The psychology of action: Linking cognition and motivation to behavior* (pp. 424–453). Guilford Press.

Youngleson, M. L. (1973). The need to affiliate and self-esteem in institutionalized children. *Journal of Personality and Social Psychology, 26*(2), 280–286.

Zipf, G. K. (1949). *Human behavior and the principle of least effort*. Addison-Wesley Press.

Volition in Sport and Exercise

Chris Englert, Ian Taylor and Alex Bertrams

Contents

J. Schüler et al. (eds.), *Sport and Exercise Psychology*, https://doi.org/10.1007/978-3-031-03921-8_10

Learning Objectives

Basic:

- Being able to describe the phenomenon of volition.
- Understanding the differences between motivation and volition.
- Knowing how volition in sport and exercise can be measured using questionnaires.
- Summarizing in your own words the main points of the Rubicon model of action phases, the theory of action control, and the strength model of self-control.

Advanced:

- Showing what different approaches to volition exist and what distinguishes them.
- Showing why volition is of central importance in the context of sport and exercise.
- Showing how volitional competencies can be strengthened.

Experts:

- Identifying criticisms of the above theoretical approaches and consider which studies might be used to rebut them.
- Putting yourself in the perspective of a sports practitioner (e.g., coach) and develop theory-based ideas about how to strengthen athletes' volition.

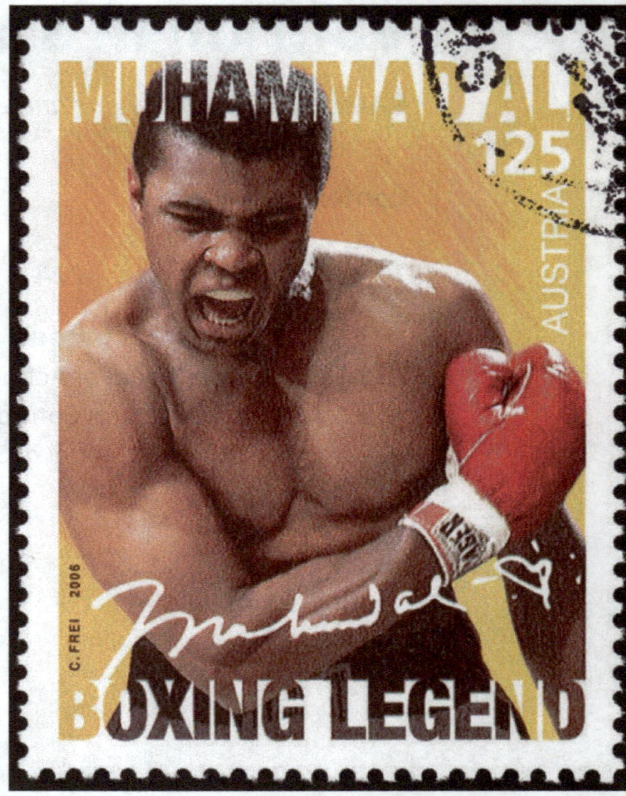

Fig. 10.1 Muhammad Ali's iron will and his successes in a high performance context

10.1 Introduction

> Champions aren't made in gyms. Champions are made from something they have deep inside them—a desire, a dream, a vision. They have to have the skill. But the will must be stronger than the skill (Muhammad Ali, 1942–2016).

Muhammad Ali (1942–2016; Fig. 10.1) was one of the greatest boxers of all time, known for his "iron will." This chapter deals with the concept of will as it is used in current research on volition.

The awareness that regular physical activity can have beneficial effects on health and subjective well-being is widespread in society (Lamprecht et al., 2014). Many individuals have the intention to play sports regularly in order to optimize their fitness and health. However, they often fail to put their intentions into practice, for example, if an alternative is perceived as more pleasant in a given situation than the originally intended sporting activity (e.g., Höner & Willimczik, 1998; Rhodes et al., 2008). Imagine an amateur sportsperson who has decided to go jogging for an hour three times a week. In the beginning, the person may find it relatively easy to go running, but after a while unforeseen temporary temptations may jeopardize the implementation of the respective action, making it more attractive to spend the evening at the cinema with friends rather than running in rainy weather conditions.

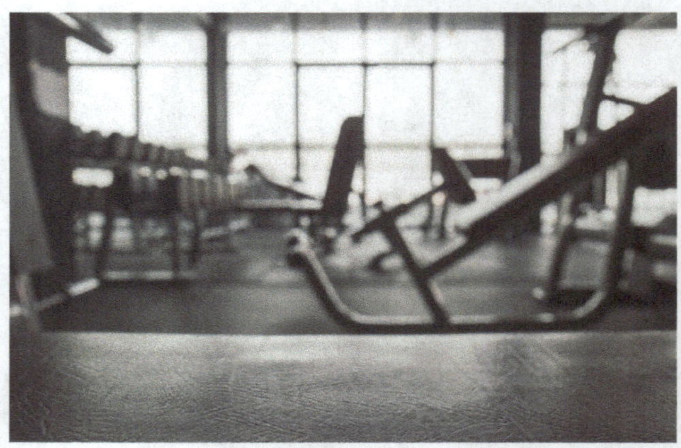

Fig. 10.2 Empty gyms: Exercise intentions are often not translated into action

Classical motivation theories (see ▶ Chap. 7) are limited to the process of intention formation and are less suitable for explaining why it is sometimes so difficult for us to put good intentions into practice on a permanent basis (e.g., Hagger et al., 2002; Sniehotta et al., 2014; Fig. 10.2). The fact that intentions can't always be translated into long-lasting behavior is called the *intention-behavior gap* (Sheeran, 2002). Attempts to explain this gap often refer to a lack of motivation. However, a motivational deficit is not sufficient to explain the intention-behavior gap, since even individuals who are motivated often fail to follow their intentions (e.g., Hagger, 2010; Schwarzer & Luszczynska, 2008). Despite goal formation (e.g., "I want to exercise regularly") and strong goal commitment (e.g., "I am determined to achieve my goal"), the implementation of the intended behavior might fail. It seems that there are two different processes at work. In the 1980s, a distinction was therefore made between processes that contribute to the formation of intentions and processes that are involved in the implementation of intentions (e.g., Heckhausen & Gollwitzer, 1987; Kuhl, 1984). Kuhl (1984, 1987), for example, notes that human behavior is insufficiently explained by motivational processes and that volitional processes for predicting behavior should be integrated also. Motivation must therefore be supplemented by volition.

> The intention-behavior gap cannot be fully explained by a lack of motivation. Even individuals who are motivated to exercise often fail to realize their intentions. They fall into the gap between intention and behavior (intention-behavior gap).

According to this distinction, *motivational processes* support the formation of intentions to act (*goal setting*), whereas *volitional processes* make it possible to implement these intentions, even if more attractive alternatives (e.g., watching television instead of exercising) or barriers (e.g., fatigue after a hard day at work) are present (*goal striving*; Achtziger & Gollwitzer, 2010). Kuhl describes volition as a class of psychological functions that "mediate the coordination of a large number of individual subfunctions (…) such as perception, attention, cognition, emotion, motivation, activation and movement control (…) based on a uniform control principle that we call 'intention' or 'goal'" (Kuhl, 1996, p. 678). Consequently, volition refers to the pursuit of goals (e.g., Beckmann, 1999) and to the control of disruptive factors that may impede or prevent the implementation of these goals (Achtziger & Gollwitzer, 2010; Kuhl & Beckmann, 1994). Disruptive factors can occur internally (e.g., fatigue, aversion) and externally (e.g., the bus to the gym is cancelled, more attractive action alternatives; e.g., Kuhl, 1983, 1987). This definition makes it clear that in the context of sport and exercise, volition has a very special significance, not only to health-oriented sports but also to competitive sports. In competitive situations, for example, it is necessary to control one's own nervousness deliberately (e.g., Beilock & Gray, 2007; Englert & Bertrams, 2012), or a racing cyclist must "force" himself to continue riding despite the pain in order to reach the finish line (e.g., Englert & Wolff, 2015; Taylor et al., 2020; Wagstaff, 2014).

> **Supporting Volitional Processes**
> - The initiation of an intended action (e.g., the scheduled start of training).
> - The persistent implementation of an intended action (e.g., successfully implementing the training over a longer period of time).
> - The persistent implementation of an intended action, even if possible obstacles could make implementation difficult (e.g., a possible meeting with the peer group during the intended training period; Elbe et al., 2005).

In summary, volition can be defined as a collective term for self-regulatory functions that support the realization of intentions to act, in which strong competing motivational tendencies must be controlled deliberately (volitionally) in order to achieve overarching goals (Brandstätter & Gollwitzer, 2005; Brandstätter et al., 2013). With reference to the initial example, the aforementioned amateur sportsperson would have to deliberately suppress the competing desire to go to the cinema because of the rain in order to implement the original intention to go running.

Volition

Volition serves as a collective term for self-regulatory functions that enable the initiation and maintenance of a target intention, even when obstacles and barriers to action occur.

> **Motivation** supports the formation of action intentions (*goal setting*), whereas **volition** refers to the implementation of the action intentions (*goal striving*).

Reflection

Many individuals decide to exercise regularly for their health. But this intention and other health-related intentions often fail to be implemented despite a high level of motivation. In addition to motivation, volition also plays a decisive role in the implementation of target intentions. What is your view on the **intention-behavior gap**? The following questions should help you find answers.

- In which areas do I find it particularly difficult to achieve a certain goal behavior? In which areas, on the other hand, do I find it easy?
- Which intentions do I usually implement, no matter what obstacles should stand in my way?
- Which obstacles do I often face when implementing my goal intentions?
- What do I do in order to implement a goal intention (e.g., exercising regularly) if there is an alternative action that currently seems more attractive and less strenuous (e.g., going to the cinema)?

- Do I know a person with an "iron will" who can usually always put his/her intention into practice? Why do I think this person usually succeeds in the implementation?

10.2 Theoretical Embedding of Volition

The first studies in the field of **volition** research took place in the early twentieth century, when Narcissus Ach (1905, 1935) was interested in the processes that made the implementation of intentions more likely (cf. Beckmann et al., 2009). In sport and exercise psychology, the construct of volition is an integral part of past and current research efforts (e.g., Beckmann & Strang, 1991; Fuchs, 1997, 2006; Höner & Willimczik, 1998). In the following sections, we will present the volition theories that are particularly important in sport and exercise psychology, namely, the "Rubicon model of action phases" (e.g., Heckhausen, 1989), the "theory of action control" (e.g., Kuhl, 1983; Kuhl & Beckmann, 1994), and the "strength model of self-control" (e.g., Baumeister et al., 1994; Baumeister et al., 2007; ► Side Story: The Marshmallow Test).

Theoretical Approaches to Volition

Important theoretical approaches to volition include:
- The Rubicon model of action phases (Heckhausen, 1989).
- The theory of action control (Kuhl, 1983; Kuhl & Beckmann, 1994).
- The strength model of self-control (Baumeister et al., 1994, 2007).

Side Story

The Marshmallow Test

Early studies on volition from the perspective of developmental psychology were conducted by Walter Mischel. The ability to resist temptation and immediate rewards was investigated in several studies in the context of Mischel's research on *delay of gratification* (e.g., Mischel, 1974). Today, Mischel's work is mainly associated with the so-called marshmallow test (Fig. 10.3). In Mischel's classic studies, preschool children had the choice between an immediate but smaller reward (i.e., a marshmallow) and a larger reward, which they receive later (i.e., two marshmallows). During the experiment, the children sat at a table with the first potential reward. The experimenter then left the room and informed the children that they would receive a larger reward if they did not eat the smaller reward until the experimenter returned. Video recordings clearly show how much effort it took for the children to follow the instructions.

The individual latency period, i.e., how long a child can resist the smaller reward, serves as a predictor for various health- and performance-related criteria in these studies. For example, longitudinal studies show that even years after the marshmallow test had been carried out, longer waiting times were associated with social competence, stress reactivity, or a healthy body weight (e.g., Mischel et al., 1989; Schlam et al., 2013). These findings indicate that volitional competences are developed in early childhood and that well-functioning volitional strategies are associated with positive outcomes in various areas of life. However, a recent replication study (Watts et al., 2018) found weaker relationships between *delay of gratification* and behavioral measures in adolescence than those originally reported by Shoda et al. (1990).

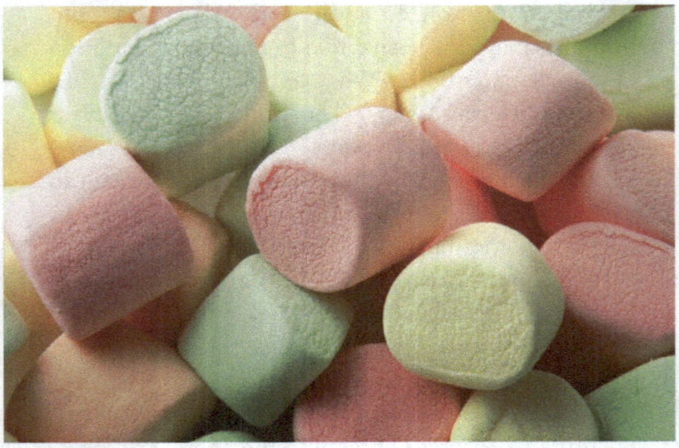

Fig. 10.3 The marshmallow test of Mischel (1974) was one of the first investigations in the field of volition research. Can you imagine that children found it difficult to resist this temptation?

10.2.1 Rubicon Model of Action Phases

The "Rubicon model of action phases" (Fig. 10.4; ► Chap. 7) was developed by Heinz Heckhausen, who was one of the first researchers to postulate that motivational processes can explain how intentions for action are formed (choice of goals), but cannot provide a satisfactory explanation of why the implementation of an action (achievement of goals) can sometimes fail (Heckhausen, 1989; Heckhausen et al., 1987). For this reason, the "Rubicon model" integrates both motivational and volitional processes that are functionally interrelated, i.e., mutually dependent and not acting independently of each other (Heckhausen & Gollwitzer, 1987). The validity of the "Rubicon model" has been repeatedly demonstrated in the context of sport and

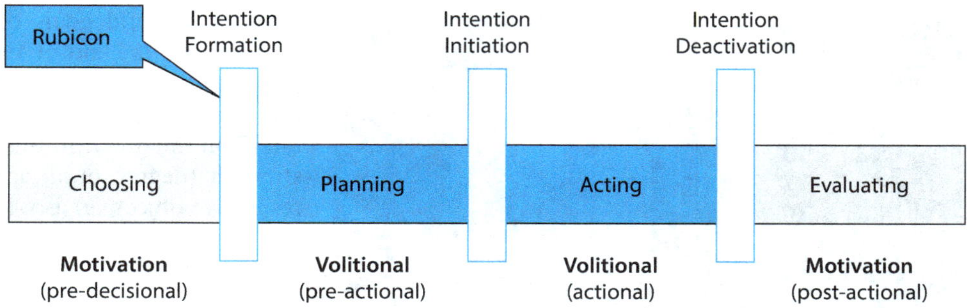

Fig. 10.4 The "Rubicon model of action phases" (based on Heckhausen & Gollwitzer, 1987)

exercise (e.g., Fuchs, 1997; Höner, 2006; Höner & Willimczik, 1998). The structural and functional model divides the course of action into four successive, discrete phases. In each phase, different requirements must be fulfilled in order to move on to the next phase. Each of the four phases is accompanied by a specific cognitive orientation or *mindset* (Achtziger & Gollwitzer, 2009), which serves to meet the requirements of the respective phase (Gollwitzer, 2012). These four phases are described in more detail in the following sections.

Mindset

Mindset describes a cognitive orientation, which is associated with each phase of the course of action.

The "Rubicon model" divides the course of action from goal formation to goal attainment into four phases, which differ in terms of the tasks they set for the person acting. Each phase is accompanied by a specific level of consciousness that enables the transition to the next phase.

10.2.1.1 Predecisional Phase

The **predecisional phase** is at the beginning of the course of action and describes a motivational phase that is associated with a deliberative mindset (Heckhausen, 1989). A person usually has several different needs and motives in a given situation, which compete with each other and cannot be implemented simultaneously (e.g., playing sports vs. meeting friends; Gollwitzer, 1996). Some of these needs promise immediate positive consequences (e.g., going to the cinema), whereas other action alternatives promise more long-term success (e.g., weight loss if you exercise regularly over a longer period). Consequently, in the predecisional phase, the feasibility or accessibility and the desirability or expected value of the individual alternatives must first be weighed against each other. In this context, feasibility describes a subjective assessment of whether one's own actions lead to a desired result (e.g., "Does regular jogging lead to weight reduction?"), whereas desirability represents the value of the expected result of the action (e.g., "How much is weight loss worth to me?"; Gollwitzer, 1996). If a person has the expectation that he/she cannot achieve a possible goal of action with his/her own efforts or considers the potential goal of action to be unattractive, then the person in question is unlikely to form a corresponding intention of action. This is where expectation and value interact (see also expectation × value models in ▶ Chap. 7). The so-called **facit (concluding) tendency** ensures that the weighing up of options does not take too long and that a person decides on a course of action at the end of the predecisional phase (Heckhausen, 1989). The action option, which appears particularly desirable and at the same time feasible, is now transformed into a concrete action goal, i.e., the person forms a binding goal and metaphorically transcends the "Rubicon" (cf. Gollwitzer, 1996). Heckhausen et al. (1987) refer to a heritage according to which Julius Caesar, after weighing the pros and cons of crossing the Rubicon river for a long time, decided to cross it, knowing fully well that a crossing would trigger a civil war (▶ Side Story: Alea iacta est). This step across the Rubicon is the basis for the formation of the will and initiates the volitional phase. A sense of *commitment to* achieve the intended goal is now developing.

Side Story

Alea iacta est

An essential component of Heckhausen's "Rubicon model" (1989) is the Rubicon, a small river in Italy south of Ravenna. When Julius Caesar (Fig. 10.5) had ended his campaigns in Gaul in 49 BC, the members of the Roman Senate feared his return and wanted to deprive him of his power. So they ordered him to disband his army. Caesar was aware that crossing the Rubicon would trigger a civil war. After careful consideration of what to do next, he decided to cross the river and move to Rome. In this context, the famous words "alea iacta est" (Latin for "the die is cast") were used. Thus, in Heckhausen's model, the Rubicon symbolizes the boundary between the phase of consideration and planning of the concrete behavior to achieve the goal intention.

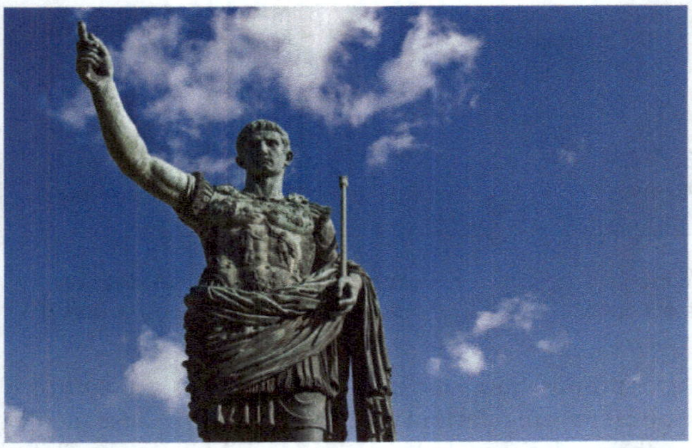

Fig. 10.5 The name of the "Rubicon model" refers to the river Rubicon, which was crossed by Julius Caesar and his army in 49 BC. The crossing of the Rubicon symbolizes the formation of intention, which initiates the realization of the goal. As can be seen in the figure, it points decisively in the direction of the goal

Facit (Concluding) Tendency

The **facit (concluding) tendency** describes the endeavor to reach a decision after a certain time of considering between different action alternatives.

10

Volitional Strength

Volitional strength is a positive function of the expected value and the degree of feasibility of a target intention. The higher the value and the higher the feasibility, the higher the volitional strength of a target intention.

> In the **predecisional phase,** individuals weigh up the feasibility and expected value of different action options against each other. At the end of this phase, the Rubicon is metaphorically crossed, and a binding target intention is formed.

10.2.1.2 Preactional Phase

The **preactional phase** is a volitional phase in which a person has an implemental (planning) mindset and thinks about how the intended action can be initiated and sustained. However, in most cases, an action goal cannot be achieved immediately, so that a suitable situation must occur in order to initiate appropriate action to achieve the goal. Different situations can be suitable for achieving several goals of action (cross-competition), for example, the end of the working day could make it possible to achieve the goal of "physical fitness" on the one hand but also the goal of "maintaining social contacts" on the other. In this case, the degree of volitional strength (degree of desirability and feasibility of the respective objective) as well as the propitiousness of the given situation is decisive for the final objective to be pursued, which is known as the **fiat tendency.**

Fiat Tendency

The level of a **fiat tendency is determined by** the volition strength of a target intention and the favorable nature of the present situation. The target intention with the highest fiat tendency is realized.

Gollwitzer (1999) refers to the usefulness of so-called implementation intentions, which can be helpful in the implementation of the generated action plans. These implementation intentions aim to persuade a person not to form unspecific intentions (e.g., "I would like to do more sport") but to formulate precisely where, when, and in what way he or she would like to implement this intention (e.g., "When I get home tonight, I will go jogging in the forest for 30 minutes"; Hagger & Luszczynska, 2014). In other words, an anticipated situation is linked to a concretely intended behavior, and a cognitive association is formed. If the situation occurs, the behavior is (automatically) triggered and a prior weighing of different action alternatives is not necessary (Brandstätter et al., 2001; Gollwitzer & Oettingen, 2011). Numerous studies indicate that implementation intentions can support successful intention implementation (e.g., Achtziger et al., 2008; Gollwitzer & Sheeran, 2006; Höner, 2005; ► Study Box: The Use of Implementation Intentions in Rehabilitation).

Implementation Intentions

Implementation intentions describe precisely where, when, and in what way a target intention is to be realized. They support the successful implementation of a target intention.

> In the **preactional phase,** a person gives concrete thought to how a goal intention can be initiated and maintained.

Study Box

The Use of Implementation Intentions in Rehabilitation

After serious illness or surgery, many patients decide to adopt a healthier lifestyle in the future (e.g., more physical activity). However, numerous studies show that this good intention is often no longer put into action after only a few months (cf. van Elderen et al., 1994). In her study, Luszczynska (2006) tested in a 2-week inpatient rehabilitation program whether the use of implementation intentions supports patients after a heart attack in regularly implementing the training plans presented in the rehabilitation program. The patients were randomly assigned to a control group (no formation of implementation intentions) or a training group (formation of implementation intentions) and asked 6 months after the end of the rehabilitation program whether they had successfully implemented their training plan on a regular basis. In the training group, the participants were instructed to specify in writing exactly when, where, and how they would like to carry out their training plans in the future, which took about 15 min. In the control group, the subjects did not receive any instructions. The *follow-up measurement* after 6 months showed that the patients in the training group implemented their training plan significantly more often than the patients in the control group. A brief 15-min intervention thus led them to develop and maintain a healthier, more physically active lifestyle.

10.2.1.3 Actional Phase

The **actional phase** is a volitional phase with an actional mindset in which the action plan selected in the preactional phase is initiated to achieve the goal specified in the predecisional phase. Here the behavior is finally expressed, e.g., exercising. In this phase, the degree of willingness to make an effort to persistently pursue a goal is again determined by the volitional strength of the target. The action phase ends when the goal is achieved or when the action is terminated prematurely (Heckhausen et al., 1987).

10.2.1.4 Postactional Phase

The final **postactional phase** takes place after the completion of the goal-oriented actions (e.g., at the end of the training session) and describes a motivational phase in which the person shows an evaluative mindset. In this phase, the person compares the achieved result with the expected or desired result (e.g., "Do I feel better?", "Did I enjoy it?", "Was it worth the effort?"). When the desired result has been achieved, the action goal is deactivated and considered to be completed. A positive evaluation of this sequence of actions can also lead to the setting of similar goals (rewards increase the probability of behavior occurring). However, if the intended result has not been achieved (e.g., weight loss not within the desired range, agony instead of pleasure), the person may be able to initiate alternative actions to achieve the goal (e.g., instead of jogging, the person could go to a gym or adjust the training plan) or lower the level of ambition and thus deactivate the goal (e.g., accept a weight loss of 5 kilograms instead of the previously intended 10 kilograms). Beckmann et al. (2009) emphasize, however, that the deactivation of a goal is not always achieved, so that this goal "may persist as a 'degenerated intention' and repeatedly enters consciousness in the form of disturbing thoughts (intrusions)" (Beckmann et al., 2009, p. 549).

Key Point

In the **actional phase,** the implementation of the target intention is initiated, whereby the volitional strength of the respective target intention determines the persistence in its implementation.

In the **postactional phase,** a person carries out an actual/target comparison after the end of the targeted behavior. If a goal is reached, the goal is deactivated, and if it is not reached, the goal intention or the strategies to reach the goal can be adjusted. However, unsuccessfully implemented target intentions can also persist as "degenerated intentions."

10.2.1.5 Concluding Remarks

Heckhausen's division into motivational and volitional phases during the course of action has had a decisive influence on psychological research and has inspired volitional research to a large extent (Achtziger & Gollwitzer, 2009). This also applies to research in sport and exercise psychology. Nevertheless, it is critical that, especially in team sports, the so-called shielding and interruption dilemma (Höner, 2006; see also Goschke, 1997, 2008) is not given enough consideration. According to Heckhausen (1989), individuals at the end of the predecisional phase form a goal intention and feel obliged to implement this intention. As a result, this intention is shielded in the actional phase against potentially irrelevant, disruptive stimuli. This may, however, make it difficult to adapt to new circumstances flexibly, e.g., an adjustment of objectives or strategy due to changing conditions (cf. Goschke, 2008). In football, for example, an attacker might overlook a better-positioned teammate if he had previously made up his mind to take the shot himself (Höner, 2006). Future research efforts should therefore focus on how the balance between flexibility and persistence can be regulated dynamically as well as context-dependent processes (see Dreisbach & Goschke, 2004).

The **shielding-interruption dilemma** states that the deliberate shielding of a target intention in the actional phase can lead to not perceiving relevant information that might suggest a change in behavior and rigidly continuing with the original behavior.

10.2.2 Theory of Action Control

The "theory of action control," like the "Rubicon model" (Heckhausen, 1989), is interested in volitional processes which support the realization of action goals, even when distractions, obstacles, or situational supposedly more desirable alternatives exist (Kuhl, 1983). In order to measure various skills and deficits in the area of volition, Wenhold et al. (Wenhold et al., 2009a, 2009b) developed the sport-specific questionnaire "volitional components in sport" (VKS; ▶ Sports Practice: Measuring Skills and Deficits in the Area of Volition). For the amateur sportsperson who wants to go jogging for an hour, three times a week, competing action alternatives must be deliberately resisted. In addition, negative thoughts after failures must be suppressed in order to successfully implement the intention (Kuhl & Beckmann, 1994). The so-called action control strategies (Table 10.1) can support the implementation of intentions by regulating cognitions, impulses, or internal and external resistance that are irrelevant to the situation (Achtziger & Gollwitzer, 2010; Kuhl, 1983). In this context, Kuhl and Beckmann (1994) differentiate between self-control and self-regulation. The authors understand **self-control** as a conscious use of action control strategies to shield the target intention. In this case, a person acts on extrinsic motivation (e.g., jogging to reduce weight and not because jogging is fun). Self-control is often associated with willpower, which is by definition a rather strenuous property, so that a person, for example, has to force himself or herself to exercise (Beckmann et al., 2009). This form of self-control is often described as an "authoritarian form" of will (Kuhl, 2001). **Self-regulation**, on the other hand, takes place unconsciously and occurs primarily in actions that are intrinsically motivated. In this case, "the action-regulating processes interlock harmoniously, the needs and experiences of the person are taken into account as well as the requirements of the environment; one could say that the person follows an inner compass that shows him or her the right path, seemingly without effort" (Brandstätter et al., 2013, p. 121). Therefore, Kuhl (2001) also describes this mode of self-regulation as the "democratic form" of will.

Table 10.1 Action control strategies (based on Kuhl, 1983)

Action control strategy	Description	Example
Environmental monitoring	Environment is structured in such a way that the implementation of an intention can be realized	Do not keep sweets in the apartment during preparation for a boxing competition in a certain weight category
Attention control	Focusing attention on stimulus information that promotes the implementation of an intention and blanking out obstructive stimulus information	Hide heckling from the audience during a competition
Encoding control	Stimulus information that is relevant for the implementation of intentions is preferred and encoded in greater depth	During a competition, look for positive reactions from the spectators instead of negative reactions
Emotion control	Strengthening of emotions that are conducive to the implementation of an intention	Regulation of the fear of condition in a competition situation
Motivation control	Focus on the positive incentives of the target (imagination)	Focus on the positive long-term consequences during strenuous training

Sports Practice

Measuring Skills and Deficits in the Area of Volition

In order to measure skills and deficits in the area of volition, Wenhold et al. (Wenhold et al., 2009a, 2009b) developed the sport-specific questionnaire "Volitional Components in Sport" (VKS), which is also used in talent diagnostics (e.g., Höner & Feichtinger, 2016). This diagnostic tool consists of a total of 60 items, which are divided into the skill factor self-optimization (SO; 29 items; example item: "In almost everything I do in sports, I feel that I do it voluntarily.") and the deficit factors self-blocking (SB; 9 items; example item: "When I get in a bad mood during sport, it's hard to get out of it."), lack of activation (AM; 13 items; example item: "I usually only start a strenuous training session when it can no longer be postponed."), or loss of focus (FV; 9 items; example item: "During training, I often have to think about things that have nothing to do with what I'm doing at the moment."). The items are each answered on four Likert scales (0 = "does not apply at all," 1 = "applies somewhat," 2 = "applies predominantly," 3 = "applies decidedly"). Higher scores on the self-optimization skill factor indicate higher volitional skills, while higher scores on the deficit factors indicate that there is still room for improvement.

Self-Control

According to Kuhl and Beckmann (1994), **self-control** refers to a conscious use of action control strategies and is also referred to as an "authoritarian form" of the will.

Self-Regulation

Self-regulation takes place unconsciously, is less strenuous, and is also called the "democratic form" of will.

10.2.2.1 State vs. Action Orientation

The "theory of action control" (▶ Chap. 19) differentiates between two types of action control after failure: *action orientation* and *state orientation* (see Kuhl, 2001, 2010). With an **action orientation**, a person is focused on quickly realizing a goal intention. It concentrates on the situational aspects that are relevant for the execution of an action (e.g., if a basketball player misses a shot, he immediately concentrates on the next move) and allows for better coping with setbacks (Kuhl & Beckmann, 1994). In contrast, under **state orientation**, one tends to deal with negative thoughts (e.g., thinking about the negative consequences of losing a point after a miss; Kuhl & Beckmann, 1994; ◻ Fig. 10.6). Cognitive activities are directed less toward the information relevant for the realization of the target intention but rather toward the analysis of past, present, or future states or "situations" (e.g., one's own state of mind, feeling bad, incapable or guilty when a misthrow occurs; Brand, 2010). Consequently, a person's current state of control determines whether he or she tries to put his or her intentions into practice and initiate appropriate action control

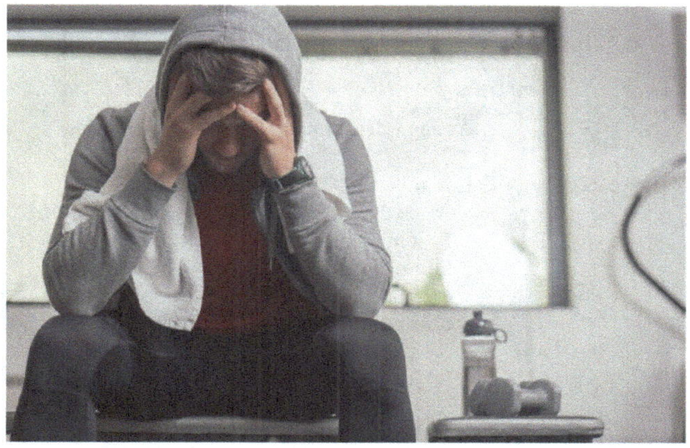

◻ **Fig. 10.6** Under state orientation, one tends to think and brood over negative thoughts after failure

strategies to achieve the goal or whether he or she tends to be more passive and ruminating (Goschke, 2008).

Whether a person in a particular situation is more action-oriented or state-oriented partly depends on the characteristics of the situation. For example, most individuals will lapse into a state orientation in the event of a personal setback and will reflect on the circumstances of the situation (Brandstätter et al., 2013; Conzelmann et al., 2013). In addition, the individual disposition for one of the two control states is also of importance (e.g., Beckmann et al., 2009). This is because individuals differ at the dispositional level in the type of action control they tend to have, which can be diagnosed, for example, with the help of the "Action Orientation Questionnaire Sport" (HOSP; Beckmann & Wenhold, 2008) (▶ Sports Practice: Measuring the Individual Control State). Some individuals are therefore chronically state-oriented across different situations (e.g., failure in sports, in studies), while others tend to be more action-oriented across different areas of life.

Three types of dispositional action/state orientations can be distinguished, namely, the prospective, the failure-related, and the activity-related (Beckmann et al., 2009; ◻ Table 10.2). Prospective state orientation is characterized by hesitation to put intentions into practice and thinking through the various possibilities for implementation (e.g., "Should I play the ball or should I throw the ball?"). In contrast, a prospective action orientation is characterized by individuals showing initiative and trying to realize an action as quickly as possible (e.g., "throw again at the next opportunity"; Kuhl, 1982). In a failure-related state orientation, individuals ponder over a negative emotional experience that can no longer be changed and find it difficult to regulate their negative affect, which is also known as **preoccupation** (e.g., "I failed and missed. Should I change my sport? What will my teammates say afterward?", etc.). In contrast, individuals with a failure-related action orientation can more easily check off negative experiences, devote them-

Table 10.2 Characteristics of action and state orientation (based on Kuhl, 1994)

	Action orientation	State orientation
Prospective	Initiative – Quick decision – Fast implementation of intentions – Mobilization of positive affects	Hesitation – Postponement of the implementation of the intention – Lack of mobilization of positive affects – Negative thoughts
Activity-related	Persistence – Ability to perform an activity with perseverance – Focus on implementation of intentions	Volatility – Problems in focusing attention on relevant information – Distractibility
Failure-related	Disengagement – Replacement of unachieved goals (disengagement) – Ability to devote oneself to new intentions – Affect regulation ability	Preoccupation – Brooding over irreversible, negative events – Lack of control of negative affect

selves more quickly to new tasks and are more adept to regulate negative affect (e.g., "I didn't hit. New game, new opportunity"; Kuhl & Beckmann, 1994). However, brooding over unfinished tasks or failure requires cognitive resources that are consequently not available for subsequent tasks (Beckmann et al., 2009). Individuals with an activity-related state orientation often pay attention to things and thoughts that are not important for the actual current action (e.g., thinking about things that are not related to the immediate game). Individuals with an activity-related action orientation, on the other hand, are completely absorbed in an action and do not allow themselves to be distracted by irrelevant stimuli or inner thoughts (e.g., they are fully involved in the game). According to Beckmann (1987), an activity-related action orientation is of central importance, especially for the maintenance of training as well as for top athletic performance.

Action Orientation

Action orientation makes it possible to direct all mental processes toward the mastering of situational challenges with the aim of realizing an intention as quickly as possible. It also enables faster processing of possible failures.

State Orientation

State orientation reflects a tendency to deal with negative thoughts that relate to past, present, or future events (preoccupation), rather than focusing attention on the concrete implementation of a target intention.

Whether an action or state orientation is activated is determined by the interaction between situational characteristics and personal disposition. Thus, situational and personal characteristics interact here as in many other areas known in psychology (see P × S scheme in ► Chap. 7).

Sports Practice

Measurement of the Individual Control Status

The "Action Orientation Questionnaire Sport" (HOSP; Beckmann, 2003; Beckmann & Wenhold, 2008, 2009) is a sport-specific adaptation of the "Questionnaire for the Assessment of Action Versus State Orientation" (HAKEMP 90; Kuhl, 1990) and is based on Kuhl's "theory of action control" (1983). The questionnaire measures the action and state orientation by means of 36 items, each offering two possible answers. Twelve of the 36 items can be assigned to one of the following subscales: action and state orientation after failure (HLOM; example item: "If I lose a competition because I could not find the right attitude, I quickly manage to check off this defeat."), prospective action and state orientation (HLOP; example item: "When I am faced with the question of whether or not to participate in a competition, I usually decide for or against it without difficulty."), as well as activity-related action and state orientation (HLOT; example item: "When I prepare for a competition, I get so involved in the preparation that I stay with it for a long time."). A maximum value of 12 can be achieved on each of the three subscales, with higher values representing a higher action orientation.

10

10.2.2.2 Empirical Findings in Sport

In the context of sport and exercise, the overall findings indicate that individuals with a state orientation perform worse than those with an action orientation (cf. Gabler, 2004). For example, Strang et al. (1987) were able to show that experience of failure in an initial task affected performance in a subsequent motor task to a greater extent in state-oriented sport students than in action-oriented sport students. The authors assume that the experience of failure in the first task led to increased preoccupation in the state-oriented sport students, which blocked cognitive resources that would have been necessary for the complex motor follow-up task. The action-oriented sport students, on the other hand, were able to process the failure more quickly and were able to mobilize cognitive resources for the complex motor follow-up task. A study by Sahre (1991) with basketball players comes to a similar conclusion: Action-oriented players performed better in the decisive phases of a game than players with a state orientation.

However, it should be noted that an action orientation is not necessarily superior to a state orientation in all situations. Beckmann et al. (2009), for example, postulate that state orientation favors peak performance in disciplines where short-term maximum power output is important (e.g., weightlifting; Beckmann et al., 2009). In other domains (e.g., endurance sports), on the other hand, a state orientation is rather obstructive (cf. Beckmann, 1987).

Furthermore, Roth (1991) was able to show that individuals with a state orientation are more likely to follow their trainer's instructions than individuals with an action orientation. This is in line with the findings of Kuhl (1994), who was able to show that state orientation is accompanied by an increased tendency to accept and follow given rules rather rigidly. However, under psychological and physical stress, the opposite effect occurs, so that action-oriented individuals are better able to follow instructions. Beckmann et al. (2009) explain this pattern of findings by the fact that the probability of setbacks and failures under stress is higher than in neutral situations. Since state-oriented individuals tend to brood when failing, they have less cognitive capacity for the follow-up task, in this case for following given instructions.

> Generally, in sport and exercise settings, action orientation is superior to state orientation in many areas. In certain contexts, such as sports that require maximum short-term performance, state orientation seems to be associated with better performance.

10.2.2.3 Concluding Remarks

Various practical implications for the sports sector can be derived from the "theory of action control" (self-regulation in competitive sports, for a detailed account ▶ Chap. 20). On the one hand, knowledge about a person's dispositional orientation provides important indications of how resilient they are in high pressure situations (cf. Beckmann et al., 2009). For example, a coach might be more likely to select players with an action orientation for a critical penalty kick in football. In addition, individuals can select certain sports depending on their dispositional orientation, as outlined in the study presented earlier by Beckmann et al. (2009), which showed that a state orientation is particularly advantageous in those disciplines where short-term maximum strength performance is important. Similarly, the individual orientation could help to assign athletes to a "suitable" position in certain types of game sports (Beckmann & Trux, 1991; Sahre, 1991). In this context, Raab and Johnson (2004) found that action-oriented basketball players tend to move to the basket more often, whereas state-oriented basketball players are more likely to pass the ball to their teammates.

10.2.3 The Strength Model of Self-Control

In the "strength model of self-control," it is assumed that all volitional processes, i.e., self-control-related actions, are energized by a central metaphorical resource (e.g., Baumeister et al., 1994, 2007). In contrast to Kuhl and Beckmann (1994), Baumeister and colleagues use the terms "self-regulation" and "self-control" synonymously and understand them to mean a deliberate regulation of dominant action tendencies or impulses in order to be able to achieve higher-level goals (Baumeister et al., 1994). There are interindividual differences in the capacity of this strength (*trait self-control*), which means that some individuals are better at controlling themselves than others (Bertrams & Dickhäuser, 2009; Tangney et al., 2004). There are also differences in how much self-control a person has in a particular situation (*state self-control*; Baumeister et al., 1994). The ability to control oneself can be temporarily exhausted after a self-control action, which can result in poorer performance in subsequent self-control actions: This state of situational exhaustion of self-control is called *ego depletion* (Baumeister et al., 1994). The effect of *ego depletion* is not domain-specific, so that Baumeister et al. (1994, 2007) assume that this strength energizes all kinds of self-control (e.g., emotion regulation, attention regulation, thought control). This also implies that a primary self-control action (e.g., voluntary attentional regulation in a cognitive self-control task) can impair performance in a secondary self-control task that apparently places different demands on the individual in terms of content (e.g., emotion regulation during the execution of a motor self-control task; e.g., Bray et al., 2012). A classic example of this would be a working day full of adverse tasks reducing the self-control strength required for evening golf.

❓ Tasks that, according to Baumeister et al. (2007), require self-control include:
- Attention control (e.g., ignoring irrelevant stimuli).
- Emotion control (e.g., regulation of fear in competition).
- Cognitive control (e.g., not thinking about a possible failure during a free throw).
- Impulse control (e.g., regulating an early sprint start in the 100-m run).
- Choice between different attractive action alternatives (e.g., exercising vs. going to the cinema).
- Persistence (e.g., continuing to run a marathon despite fatigue).
- Complex cognitive operations (e.g., complex mathematical tasks).

Strength Model of Self-Control

The **strength model of self-control** states that all self-control actions are controlled by a global metaphorical resource with limited capacity. There are interindividual differences in the capacity of the self-control strength at *trait level* (*trait self-control*). Furthermore, there seem to be inter- and intraindividual differences in temporarily available self-control strength (*state self-control*).

Ego Depletion

"Ego depletion" describes a temporary exhaustion of self-control strength after a primary self-control action. Under "ego depletion," subsequent self-control actions are performed less effectively. The strength does not regenerate immediately after a self-control action.

In order to investigate the effects of *ego depletion* experimentally, the so-called two-task paradigm is often used (see Baumeister et al., 1998; ► Methods: The "Two-Task Paradigm"). Here, one group of participants completes a first task that requires self-control (e.g., watching a sad video, but during which no

Methods: The "Two-Task Paradigm"

In the Stroop test (Stroop, 1935), several colored words appear one after another on a computer screen (◘ Figs. 10.7 and 10.8). They can either be written in the color of the word (e.g., "green" in green font color; congruent trial), or the color word can appear in a different font color (e.g., "green" in red color; incongruent trial). The task of the test subjects is to name the color in which the respective color word is written as quickly and accurately as possible, ignoring the semantic content of the color word. Numerous studies have shown that the processing of a series of incongruent Stroop trials can lead to an exhaustion of self-control strength (*ego depletion*) available in a given situation (e.g., Bray et al., 2011). In the context of sport and exercise, for example, it was shown that individuals performed an endurance task on a bicycle ergometer less persistently after completing incongruent Stroop trials than after completing a series of congruent Stroop trials (Englert & Wolff, 2015). A similar finding was observed when the second task required participants to hold a physical demanding posture for as long as possible (i.e., a wall sit; Boat & Taylor, 2017).

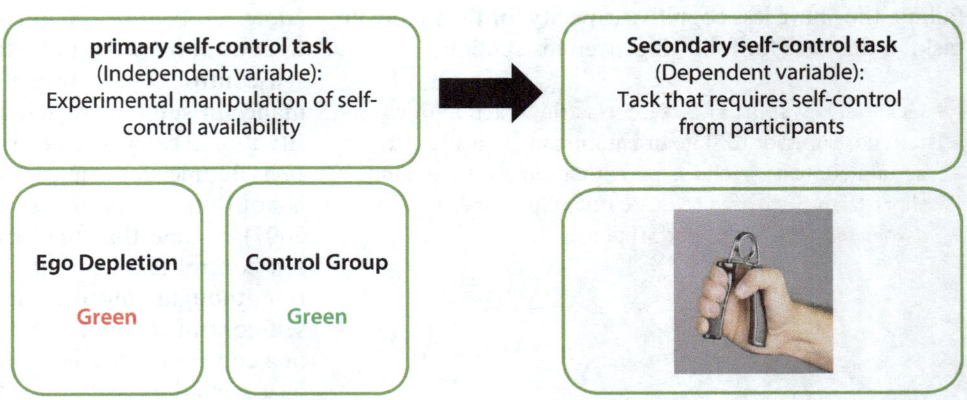

◘ **Fig. 10.7** Representation of the "two-task paradigm"

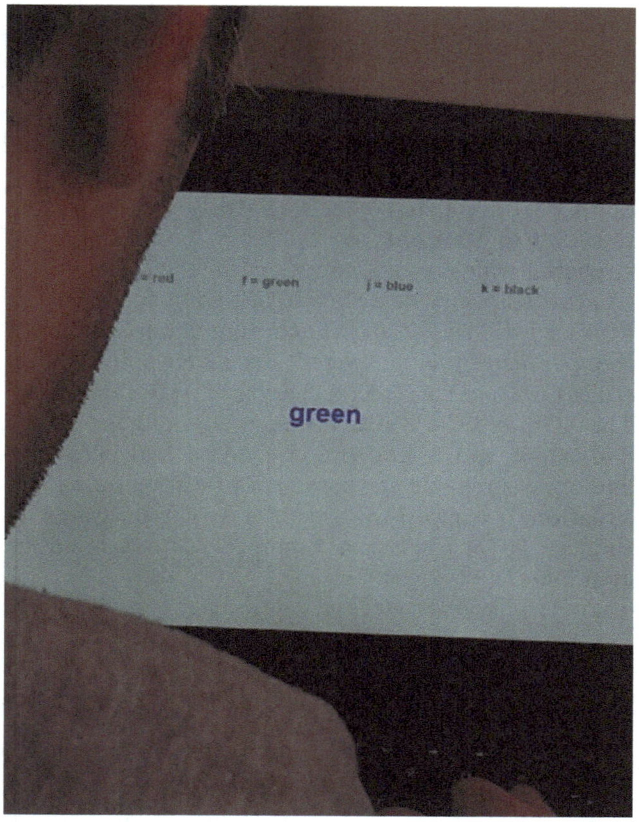

Fig. 10.8 The Stroop test (incongruent trial; Stroop, 1935)

emotions may be shown), while another group of participants completes a similar task that does not require self-control (e.g., watching the same video, but the subjects are allowed to show their emotions; Muraven et al., 1998). Subsequently, all participants complete a second task that requires the exercise of self-control (e.g., squeezing a hand trainer as long as possible, which requires self-control due to the increasing effort; see Bray et al., 2012; for an example ► Study Box: The "Two-Task Paradigm" in Sports Psychological Research). According to the assumptions of the "strength model," participants who exercised self-control in the first task should perform worse in the second self-control task than participants who did not have to exercise self-control in the first task (Baumeister et al., 1998). The results of a meta-analysis by Hagger et al. of 83 studies showed a medium-to-large effect of *ego depletion* on secondary self-control actions (Hagger et al., 2010).

To **measure dispositional self-control strength**, Tangney et al. (2004) developed the "Self-Control Scale" (SCS). The long version of this one-dimensional scale comprises a total of 36 items, while the frequently used brief version consists of 13 items, each of which can be

Study Box

The "Two-Task Paradigm" in Sport and Exercise

Dorris et al. (Dorris et al., 2012) aimed to answer the question of whether *ego depletion* can affect the performance of professional athletes in well-practiced physical exercises. In Experiment 1, Irish rowers were tested at two times of measurement (*within-subjects design*). In a first task, the currently available self-control strength of the rowers was experimentally manipulated (independent variable) by asking the participants to count backward from 1000 in steps of 7 and to balance a spirit level. This activity required the exercise of self-control and should consequently lead to a state of *ego depletion* (cf. Webb & Sheeran, 2003). At a second time of measurement, the subjects performed a comparable task, but this did not require the exercise of self-control and therefore should not induce an *ego-depletion state* (counting backward in steps of 5 from 1000 without any additional balancing task). As a secondary self-control task within the "two-task paradigm," the participants performed as many push-ups as possible at both times of measurement. The number of push-ups was the dependent variable in this experiment. Even supposedly simple physical exercises become painful and strenuous from a certain point on, which is why self-control must be invested in order to "force yourself to continue" (cf. Englert & Wolff, 2015). The results were in line with expectations: The rowers performed fewer press-ups if they had previously exercised self-control in a primary task (counting backward in steps of 7 and balancing) compared to the time of measurement when no self-control (counting backward in steps of 5 without balancing) had to be invested during the performance of the primary task. This result is particularly impressive, as the authors have chosen a *within-subjects design*: The *same* subjects performed significantly worse in a supposedly simple physical task if they had previously worked on a strenuous cognitive task.

In Experiment 2, the pattern was replicated in a sample of semiprofessional rugby and hockey players: The subjects performed fewer *sit-ups* at the time of measurement at which they had to exercise self-control in a primary task (counting backward in steps of 7 and balancing) compared with the time of measurement at which they did not have to invest self-control in a primary task (counting backward in steps of 5 without balancing).

Table 10.3 Items of the brief version of the Self-Control Scale for measuring *trait self-control* (SCS; Tangney et al., 2004). The possible answers range from 1 = "not at all" to 5 = "very much." The following items need to be recoded: 2, 3, 4, 5, 6, 7, 8, 10, 11

To what extent do the following questions generally apply to you?		1	2	3	4	5
1	I'm good at resisting temptation					
2	I have hard time breaking bad habits					
3	I am lazy					
4	I say inappropriate things					
5	I do certain things that are bad for me, if they are fun					
6	I wish I had more self-discipline					
7	Pleasure and fun sometimes keep me from getting work done					
8	I have trouble concentrating					
9	I am able to work effectively toward long-term goals					
10	Sometimes I can't stop myself from doing something even though I know it is wrong					
11	I often act without thinking through all the alternatives					
12	I refuse things that are bad for me					
13	People would say that I have iron self-discipline					

Table 10.4 Items of the 5-Item Brief State Self-Control Capacity Scale (SMS-5; Lindner et al., 2019). The following items need to be recoded: 1, 3, 5

How much do the following questions apply to you at the moment?		1	2	3	4	5	6	7
1	I feel drained							
2	I feel calm and rational							
3	I feel lazy							
4	I feel sharp and focused							
5	I feel like my willpower is gone							

answered from 1 = "not at all" to 5 = "very much" (sample item: "I am good at resisting temptation"; Table 10.3). Higher values indicate higher trait self-control-strength.

In addition to the SCS, Lindner and colleagues (Lindner et al., 2019) developed the 5-Item Brief State Self-Control Capacity Scale (SMS-5) for measuring the level of momentarily available state self-control strength, which is an adoption of the "State Self-Control Capacity Scale" (SSCCS; Ciarocco, Twenge, Muraven, & Tice, 2007). Each item (sample item: "I feel drained.") is answered on seven-point Likert scales (1 = "not true" to 7 = "very true") (Table 10.4). The SCS and the SSCCS have been validated in the context of sports and exercise on several occasions and allow a reliable measurement of dispositional and situational self-control strength (e.g., Bertrams & Englert, 2013; Englert & Rummel, 2016; Schöndube et al., 2017).

Reflection

1. First fill out the two questionnaires for yourself (Tables 10.3 and 10.4).
2. Then put yourself in the place of a person who is clearly good/bad at putting their intentions into practice. How would this person respond to these items?

The "strength model of self-control" has been successfully used in sport and exercise contexts for some years now (for an overview, see Audiffren & André, 2015; Englert, 2016, 2019). In various studies, subjects in a state of *ego depletion* performed fewer sit-ups and push-ups (Dorris et al., 2012; Study Box: The "Two-Task Paradigm" in Sports Psychological Research) and invested less effort in physically tiring activities (e.g., Boat & Taylor, 2017; Boat et al., 2016; Bray et al., 2008, 2011; Englert & Wolff, 2015; Wagstaff, 2014). In the following two sections, the effects of *ego depletion* on the anxiety-performance relationship and on the intention-behavior gap will be examined more closely.

10.2.3.1 Performance Under Pressure

In pressure situations (e.g., the penalty kick in football), athletes often experience increased anxiety (e.g., Gucciardi et al., 2010). Increased anxiety makes voluntary attention regulation more difficult. The ability to regulate attention is often necessary for precision tasks in sports (e.g., Beilock & Gray, 2007). A basketball player, for example, needs to ignore distracting stimuli (e.g., interjections from the audience) during a free throw and instead focus on the basket. In a study by

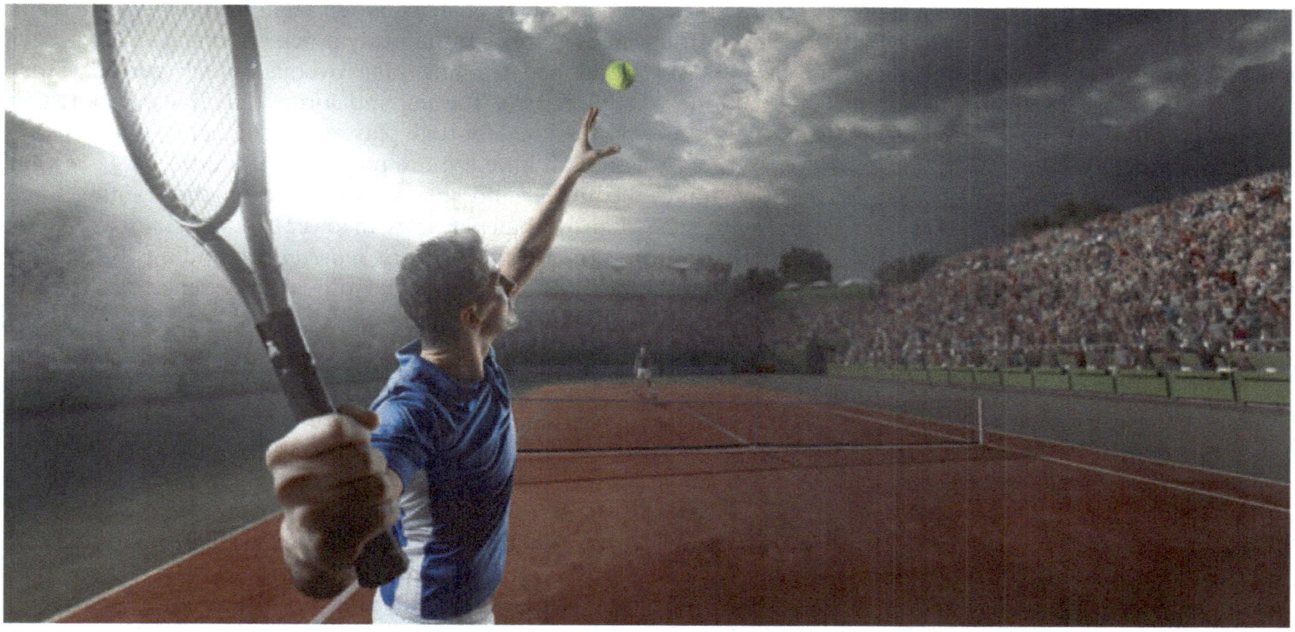

Fig. 10.9 In pressure situations (e.g., during a sporting competition), individuals often experience increased anxiety, which can impair their sporting performance

Wilson et al. (Wilson et al., 2009), individuals who experienced increased anxiety were less adept at focusing their attention on the basketball hoop and were less successful at free throws than individuals with lower anxiety (attention was recorded by *eye tracking*; Fig. 10.9).

However, the findings on the anxiety-performance relationship in sport contexts are heterogeneous, so that some studies assume a negative anxiety-performance relationship (e.g., Nibbeling et al., 2012), whereas in other studies no negative relationships between anxiety and performance could be found (e.g., Craft et al., 2003; Woodman & Hardy, 2003; see ► Chap. 12). This inconsistent pattern of findings can, among other things, be explained with the help of the "strength model of self-control" (Englert & Bertrams, 2015): Voluntary attention regulation is to be understood as a volitional process that depends on the current availability of self-control strength (Schmeichel & Baumeister, 2010). A number of studies have shown that a negative anxiety-performance relationship was only present if a person's self-control strength was experimentally depleted in a previous task (Englert & Bertrams, 2012, 2013, 2015). Subjects who did not have to exercise self-control strength before the respective sporting task were able to maintain their performance despite increased anxiety. Subjects with increased state anxiety in a state of *ego depletion* scored fewer free throws and performed worse in a dart-throwing task than subjects with increased state anxiety who were not in a state of ego depletion (Englert & Bertrams, 2012). Similarly, Englert et al. were able to show by means of gaze measurements that anxious subjects not ego-depleted were more adept at controlling their visual attention than anxious subjects in a state of *ego depletion* (Englert, Zwemmer, et al., 2015; see also Englert, Bertrams, et al., 2015). Taken together, the current findings indicate that state self-control strength can compensate for the negative effects of state anxiety on attention control and athletic performance.

The Importance of "Ego Depletion" for Performance Under Pressure

The heterogeneous anxiety-performance relationship in sport can be explained, among other things, by the level of temporarily available self-control strength. Individuals with higher levels of state self-control strength are more likely to maintain their performance in pressure situations than individuals in a state of "ego depletion."

10.2.3.2 Regular Physical Activity

As mentioned in the introductory example, individuals often fail to implement their good intentions to engage in regular physical activity (e.g., Rhodes et al., 2008). Attractive action alternatives (e.g., spending time with friends) must be deliberately resisted, and instead the less attractive action that was originally intended must be carried out (e.g., going for a run despite the bad weather). Findings from basic research in (sports) psychology suggest that the intention-behavior gap (Sheeran, 2002) can be explained with the help of the "strength model of self-control" (Ntoumanis, 2014). For example, Vohs and Heatherton (2000) report that obese patients are less adept at continuously implementing their diet plans when they are in a state of *ego depletion*. According to Martin Ginis and Bray (2010), self-control must also be invested in the implementation of an exercise schedule in order to resist situational action alternatives and achieve the overall goal of physical fitness (see also Iso-Ahola, 2013).

At the dispositional level, it has been shown that individuals with higher *trait self-control* strength are more likely to achieve their exercise goals (Bertrams & Englert, 2013). This pattern is consistent with the findings of Stork et al. who found that *trait self-control* could predict how continuously a person would follow a self-developed training plan over a 4-week period (Stork et al., 2016). Toering and Jordet (2015) also report that professional football players with higher *trait self-control* strength have a more professional lifestyle (e.g., regular bedtimes) and spend more time on the training pitch than football players with lower *trait self-control strength*.

In addition to *trait self-control*, findings by Englert and Rummel (2016) provide evidence that state self-control strength also appears to play an important role in the implementation of training plans. In this study, the subjects were instructed to perform a series of physical exercises (e.g., push-ups) every day for 1 week, which were part of a training plan. In addition, the state self-control strength was measured by means of a questionnaire in the evening. Participants were less likely to implement their training plans on days with lower levels of state self-control than on days with higher levels of state self-control strength. The findings of Schöndube et al. (2017) point in a similar direction, so that in their 20-day study, individuals were more likely to implement their training plan on days when they had more state self-control than on days when they had less state self-control.

Side Story

Science Communication

It is sometimes difficult to translate complex theoretical principles into language that nonscientists understand and can apply to their daily lives. An example of communicating scientific evidence in straightforward language can be found in this video: ► https://www.youtube.com/watch?v=cXn68fepGaU. Dr. Ian Taylor provides tips to help individuals achieve their fitness and healthy eating goals. Many of the tips are underpinned by theories of volition and related constructs, such as self-control, even though the theories are not mentioned in the video. For example, Dr. Taylor suggests trying to avoid using willpower (i.e., a colloquial term for self-control) as a primary source of motivation because willpower is associated with increasing negative affect and, therefore, increasingly hard to maintain (Inzlicht & Legault, 2014). In addition, Dr. Taylor advises to plan ahead, think about when self-control might be low, and avoid exercise at these times. This tip is based on evidence that willpower strength is typically lower when the individual is stressed or tired (e.g., Englert & Rummel, 2016).

Another suggestion for exercise beginners is to make the activity as easy as possible to implement. Simply having your running shoes ready at the door, for example, requires less effort, compared to having them stored away in a cupboard. Humans have a propensity to avoid effort (Inzlicht et al., 2018), so simple strategies like these make exercise more likely. Dr. Taylor also suggests focusing on immediate, rather than delayed, incentives. The motivation strength of immediate rewards like enjoyment and fun becomes associated with the activity itself. In contrast, delayed rewards (e.g., health benefits) do not transfer their motivational power to the activity because of the length of time between the activity and incentive (Woolley & Fishbach, 2016).

The communication of scientific evidence to the general population is an important skill to develop for researchers and is essential for research to have a real-world impact.

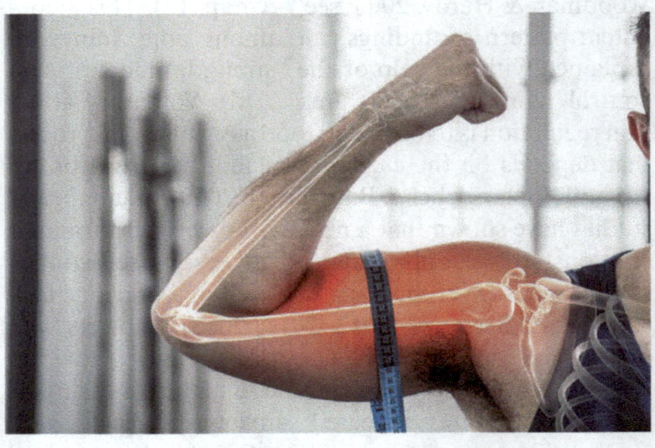

Fig. 10.10 According to Baumeister et al. (1998), the self-control strength can be compared to a muscle that can be trained

> **The Importance of "Ego Depletion" for the Implementation of Training Plans**
>
> The ability to regularly implement training plans seems to be influenced by *trait self-control* and the self-control strength available in a given situation.

10.2.3.3 Concluding Remarks

Baumeister et al. (1998) compare self-control strength with a human muscle: Strength can be temporarily exhausted after an initial self-control action and does not regenerate immediately after the self-control action is completed. In addition, strength can be improved by performing certain exercises, just like a muscle, which should lead to a "growth" in strength and in the long run to better self-control performance (Baumeister et al., 2006; ► Study Box: Training of Self-Control; ◘ Fig. 10.10).

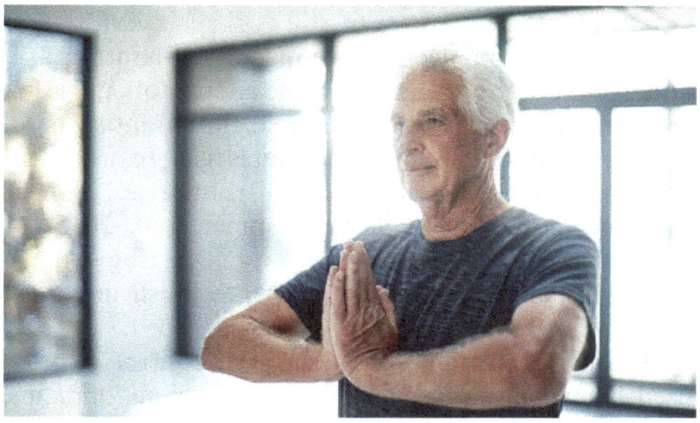

◘ **Fig. 10.11** Relaxation and yoga techniques can lead to a faster regeneration of depleted self-control strength

Study Box

Self-Control Training

In one of their studies, Bray et al. (Bray et al., 2015) tested the assumption that self-control strength can be improved through regular exercising of self-control (Baumeister et al., 2006) in sport and exercise contexts. The test subjects first carried out an endurance test on a bicycle ergometer, after they had previously been put into a state of *ego depletion* through an initial self-control task. In the following 2 weeks, the subjects of a training group were asked to squeeze a hand trainer twice a day for as long as possible. According to the authors, this activity requires self-control, because at a certain point in time one has to force oneself to keep the hand trainer pressed despite the increasingly severe pain (see also Bray et al., 2008). The control group, on the other hand, did not participate in any special self-control training. After 2 weeks, the subjects of the training and control group again performed the endurance test in a state of *ego depletion*. The subjects in the training group performed significantly better at the second time of measurement than at the first time of measurement, whereas the performance in the endurance test did not change significantly in the control group. These results therefore indicate that regular self-control exertion (i.e., use of the hand trainer) positively influenced performance in a task with a different content (i.e., endurance test).

In psychological experiments, for example, subjects were instructed to perform everyday actions with their nondominant hand over a period of 2 weeks, which the authors believe should require self-control (cf. Baumeister et al., 2006). In *follow-up* measurements, subjects who had participated in this training scored significantly higher in various self-control tasks (e.g., Stroop test; ► Methods: The "Two-Task Paradigm") than subjects who had not participated in this training (see also Gailliot et al., 2004; Muraven, 2010). In addition to training that improves self-control strength, there are also techniques to regenerate depleted self-control more quickly. In this context, relaxation techniques (e.g., Englert & Bertrams, 2016; Tyler & Burns, 2008), mindfulness, or even yoga exercises (Friese et al., 2012), which were performed after an initial self-control action, have shown to be valuable tools (◘ Fig. 10.11).

A central problem of research on the "strength model of self-control" is the external validity of the model. This raises the question of which actions or situations actually require self-control during a sporting competition and can evoke *ego-depletion states.* This question is not easy to answer experimentally. In one of their studies, Gröpel et al. (Gröpel et al., 2014) instructed subjects in a first self-control task to complete a 15-min physically demanding training session. The training led to ego depletion on the part of the test subjects and impaired performance in a secondary self-control task. Other situations and actions in the context of sport that require self-control are, for example, the voluntary regulation of undesirable emotional states (e.g., fear of competition; Englert & Bertrams, 2012), the regulation of one's own attention (Englert, Zwemmer, et al., 2015), or the voluntary suppression of slowly occurring exhaustion in order to be able to reach the finish line (e.g., Wagstaff, 2014).

Even if the "strength model of self-control" is often used to explain volitional deficits in various domains, criticism of the validity of the model has been growing for some years now (e.g., Schmeichel & Macrae, 2014; see also Englert et al., 2019; Wolff et al., 2018). In a large-scale replication study, the *ego-depletion* effect could not be replicated (Hagger et al., 2016). Similarly, the findings of Carter et al. suggest that the extent of the *ego-depletion* effect may have been overestimated in previous studies and meta-analyses (Carter et al., 2015). Therefore, future studies should aim to test the validity of the "strength model of self-control" in sport and exercise.

Learning Control Questions

Basic:

1. What is the difference between motivation and volition?
2. What is the intention-behavior gap?
3. What is the "marshmallow test"?
4. What are the characteristic features of the phases of the "Rubicon model of action phases"?

Advanced:

5. How can implementation intentions be used in sport contexts?
6. Why does the shielding-interruption dilemma play a role in sport contexts?
7. According to Kuhl, what are the differences between self-regulation and self-control?
8. What practical implications can be derived for the context of sports from the knowledge of whether an athlete is more action- or state-oriented?

Experts:

9. Can it be concluded that in the context of sport and exercise, an action orientation is generally superior to a state orientation?
10. How can the effect of ego depletion on subsequent performance be investigated in sport and exercise settings?
11. With reference to the "strength model of self-control," how can the volitional competences of an athlete be promoted?
12. Why does it not matter within the "two-task paradigm" whether the primary task is sport-specific or not?
13. What advice would you give to sports practitioners? How can volitional competences in sport be increased?

References

Ach, N. (1905). *Über die Willenstätigkeit und das Denken*. Göttingen: Vandenhoeck & Ruprecht.

Ach, N. (1935). Analyse des Willens. In E. Aberhalden (Hrsg.), *Handbuch der biologischen Arbeitsmethoden* (Bd. VI). Berlin: Urban und Schwarzenberg.

Achtziger, A., & Gollwitzer, P. M. (2009). Rubicon model of the action phases. In V. Brandstätter & J. H. Otto (Eds.), *Handbuch der Allgemeinen Psychologie—Motivation und Emotion* (pp. 150–156). Hogrefe.

Achtziger, A., & Gollwitzer, P. M. (2010). Motivation and volition in the course of action. In J. Heckhausen & H. Heckhausen (Eds.), *Motivation and action* (pp. 309–335). Springer.

Achtziger, A., Gollwitzer, P. M., & Sheeran, P. (2008). Implementation intentions and shielding goal striving from unwanted thoughts and feelings. *Personality and Social Psychology Bulletin, 34*, 381–393.

Audiffren, M., & André, N. (2015). The strength model of self-control revisited: Linking acute and chronic effects of exercise on executive functions. *Journal of Sport and Health Science, 4*, 30–46.

Baumeister, R. F., Bratslavsky, E., Muraven, M., & Tice, D. M. (1998). Ego depletion: Is the active self a limited resource? *Journal of Personality and Social Psychology, 74*, 1252–1265. https://doi.org/10.1037/0022-3514.74.5.1252

Baumeister, R. F., Gailliot, M., DeWall, C. N., & Oaten, M. (2006). Self-regulation and personality: How interventions increase regulatory success, and how depletion moderates the effects of traits on behavior. *Journal of Personality, 74*, 1773–1802.

Baumeister, R. F., Heatherton, T. F., & Tice, D. M. (1994). *Losing control: How and why people fail at self-regulation*. Academic Press.

Baumeister, R. F., Vohs, K. D., & Tice, D. M. (2007). The strength model of self-control. *Current Directions in Psychological Science, 16*, 351–355.

Beckmann, J. (1987). Maximum performance as a result of failed self-regulation. In J. P. Jansen, W. Schlicht, & H. Strang (Eds.), *Handlungskontrolle und Soziale Prozesse im Sport*. bps-Verlag.

Beckmann, J. (1999). Volition and sporting action. In D. Alfermann & O. Stoll (Eds.), *Motivation and Volition in Sports from Planning to Action* (pp. 13–26). bps-Verlag.

Beckmann, J. (2003). *HOSP*. Unpublished questionnaire.

Beckmann, J., Fröhlich, S. M., & Elbe, A.-M. (2009). Motivation and Volition. In W. Schlicht & B. Strauß (Eds.), *Encyclopedia of psychology: Sport psychology. Volume I—Fundamentals of sport psychology* (pp. 511–562). Hogrefe.

Beckmann, J., & Strang, H. (1991). *Activity control in sports. Sports psychology, 5*, 5–10.

Beckmann, J., & Trux, J. (1991). Who do I get to play where? personality traits and suitability for certain positions in sports teams. *Sports psychology, 5*, 18–21.

Beckmann, J. & Wenhold, F. (2008). HOSP: Questionnaire for recording the activity orientation in sport. Retrieved December 17, 2016, from www.bisp.de.

Beckmann, J., & Wenhold, F. (2009). *Activity Orientation in Sport (HOSP)—Manual*. Sports publisher Strauß.

Beilock, S. L., & Gray, R. (2007). Why do athletes choke under pressure? In G. Tenenbaum & R. C. Eklund (Eds.), *Handbook of sport psychology* (pp. 425–444). John Wiley & Sons.

Bertrams, A., & Dickhäuser, O. (2009). Measurement of dispositional self-control capacity: A German adaptation of the short form of the Self-Control Scale (SCS-KD). *Diagnostica, 55*, 2–10.

Bertrams, A., & Englert, C. (2013). Implementation of subjective sports frequency standards—On the role of dispositionally available self-control power. *Sports science, 43*, 276–282.

Boat, R., & Taylor, I. M. (2017). Prior self-control exertion and perceptions of pain during a physically demanding task. *Psychology of Sport & Exercise, 33*, 1–6.

Boat, R., Taylor, I. M., & Hulston, C. (2016). Self-control exertion and glucose supplementation prior to endurance performance. *Psychology of Sport & Exercise, 29*, 103–110. https://doi.org/10.1016/j.psychsport.2016.12.007

Brand, R. (2010). *Sports psychology*. VS publishing house for social sciences.

Brandstätter, V., & Gollwitzer, M. (2005). Motivation and volition. In S. Lautenbacher, H. Lelg, & A. Schütz (Eds.), *Psychology: An introduction to its fundamentals and fields of application* (pp. 201–216). Kohlhammer.

Brandstätter, V., Lengfelder, A., & Gollwitzer, P. M. (2001). Implementation intentions and efficient action initiation. *Journal of Personality and Social Psychology, 81*, 946–960.

Brandstätter, V., Schüler, J., Puca, R. M., & Lozo, L. (2013). *Textbook motivation and emotion*. Springer.

Bray, S. R., Graham, J. D., Martin Ginis, K. A., & Hicks, A. L. (2012). Cognitive task performance causes impaired maximum force production in human hand flexor muscles. *Biological Psychology, 89*, 195–200.

Bray, S. R., Graham, J. D., & Saville, P. D. (2015). Self-control training leads to enhanced cardiovascular exercise performance. *Journal of Sports Sciences, 33*, 534–543. https://doi.org/10.1080/02640414.2014.949830

Bray, S. R., Martin Ginis, K. A., Hicks, A. L., & Woodgate, J. (2008). Effects of self-regulatory strength depletion on muscular performance and EMG activation. *Psychophysiology, 45*, 337–573.

Bray, S. R., Martin Ginis, K. A., & Woodgate, J. (2011). Self-regulatory strength depletion and muscle-endurance performance: A test of the limited-strength model in older adults. *Journal of Aging and Physical Activity, 19*, 177–188.

Carter, E., Kofler, L., Forster, D., & McCullough, M. (2015). A series of meta-analytic tests of the depletion effect: Self-control does not seem to rely on a limited resource. *Journal of Experimental Psychology: General, 144*, 796–815.

Conzelmann, A., Hänsel, F., & Höner, O. (2013). Individual and action—Sports psychology. In A. Güllich & M. Krüger (Eds.), *Sport—Das Lehrbuch für das Sportstudium* (pp. 271–337). Springer.

Ciarocco, N. J., Twenge, J. M., Muraven, M., & Tice, D. M. (2007). Measuring state self-control: Reliability, validity, and correlations with physical and psychological stress. Unpublished manuscript.

Craft, L. L., Magyar, T. M., Becker, B. J., & Feltz, D. L. (2003). The relationship between the Competitive State Anxiety Inventory-2 and sport performance: A meta-analysis. *Journal of Sport and Exercise Psychology, 25*, 44–65.

Dorris, D. C., Power, D. A., & Kenefick, E. (2012). Investigating the effects of ego depletion on physical exercise routines of athletes. *Psychology of Sport and Exercise, 13*, 118–125.

Dreisbach, G., & Goschke, T. (2004). How positive affect modulates cognitive control: Reduced preservation at the cost of increased distractibility. *Journal of Experimental Psychology: Learning, Memory, and Cognition, 30*, 343–353.

Elbe, A. M., Szymanski, B., & Beckmann, J. (2005). The development of volition in young elite athletes. *Psychology of Sport and Exercise, 6*, 559–569.

Englert, C. (2016). The strength model of self-control in sport and exercise psychology. *Frontiers in Psychology, 7*.

Englert, C. (2019). The self-regulation of human performance: A critical discussion and future directions for self-control research. *Performance Enhancement and Health, 6*, 156–157. https://doi.org/10.1016/j.peh.2019.04.001

Englert, C., & Bertrams, A. (2012). Anxiety, ego depletion, and sports performance. *Journal of Sport and Exercise Psychology, 34*, 580–599.

Englert, C., & Bertrams, A. (2013). Too exhausted for Operation? Anxiety, depleted self-control strength, and perceptual-motor performance. *Self and Identity, 12*, 650–662.

Englert, C., & Bertrams, A. (2015). Integrating attentional control theory and the strength model of self-control. *Frontiers in Psychology, 6*, 824. https://doi.org/10.3389/fpsyg.2015.00824

Englert, C., & Bertrams, A. (2016). Active relaxation counteracts the effects of ego depletion on performance under evaluative pressure in a state of ego depletion. *Sportwissenschaft, 46*, 110–115.

Englert, C., Bertrams, A., Furley, P., & Oudejans, R. R. D. (2015). Is ego depletion associated with increased distractibility? Results from a basketball free throw task. *Psychology of Sport and Exercise, 18*, 26–31.

Englert, C., Koroma, D., Bertrams, A., & Martarelli, C. (2019). Testing the validity of the attention control video: An eye-tracking approach. *PlosOne, 14*(1), e0211181. https://doi.org/10.1371/journal.pone.0211181

Englert, C., & Rummel, J. (2016). I want to keep on exercising but I don't: The negative impact of momentary lacks of self-control on exercise adherence. *Psychology of Sport and Exercise, 26*, 24–31.

Englert, C., & Wolff, W. (2015). Ego depletion and persistent performance in a cycling task. *International Journal of Sport Psychology, 46*, 137–151.

Englert, C., Zwemmer, K., Bertrams, A., & Oudejans, R. R. D. (2015). Ego depletion and attention regulation under pressure: Is a temporary loss of self-control strength indeed related to impaired attention regulation? *Journal of Sport and Exercise Psychology, 37*, 127–137.

Friese, M., Messner, C., & Schaffner, Y. (2012). Mindfulness meditation counteracts self-control depletion. *Consciousness and Cognition, 21*, 1016–1022.

Fuchs, R. (1997). *Psychology and physical exercise*. Hogrefe.

Fuchs, R. (2006). Motivation and volition in leisure and health sports. In M. Tietjens & B. Strauß (Eds.), *Handbook on sport psychology* (pp. 270–278). Hofmann.

Gabler, H. (2004). Motivational aspects of sporting activities. In H. Gabler, J. R. Nitsch, & R. Singer (Eds.), *Introduction to sport psychology. Part 1: Basic topics* (pp. 197–245). Hofmann.

Gailliot, M. T., Plant, E. A., Butz, D. A., & Baumeister, R. F. (2004). Increasing self-regulatory strength can reduce the depleting effect of suppressing stereotypes. *Personality and Social Psychology Bulletin, 33*, 281–294.

Gollwitzer, P. M. (1996). The Rubicon model of the action phases. In J. Kuhl & H. Heckhausen (Eds.), *Encyclopaedia of Psychology.*

Volume C/IV/4: Motivation, volition and action (pp. 531–582). Hogrefe.

Gollwitzer, P. M. (1999). Implementation intentions. Strong effects of simple plans. *Journal of Personality and Social Psychology, 73*, 186–197.

Gollwitzer, P. M. (2012). Mindset theory of action phases. In P. Van Lange, A. W. Kruglanski, & E. T. Higgins (Eds.), *Handbook of theories of social psychology* (pp. 526–545). Sage.

Gollwitzer, P. M., & Oettingen, G. (2011). Planning promotes goal striving. In K. D. Vohs & R. F. Baumeister (Eds.), *Handbook of self-regulation. Research, theory, and applications* (pp. 162–185). Guilford Press.

Gollwitzer, P. M., & Sheeran, P. (2006). Implementation intentions and goal achievement: A meta-analysis of effects and processes. *Advances in Experimental Social Psychology, 38*, 69–119.

Goschke, T. (1997). On the functional analysis of the will: Integration of cognitive, motivational and neuropsychological perspectives. *Psychological contributions, 39*, 375–412.

Goschke, T. (2008). Volition and cognitive control. In J. Müsseler (Ed.), *General psychology* (pp. 232–293). Springer.

Gröpel, P., Baumeister, R. F., & Beckmann, J. (2014). Action versus state orientation and self-control performance after depletion. *Personality and Social Psychology Bulletin, 40*, 476–487.

Gucciardi, D. F., Longbottom, J. L., Jackson, B., & Dimmock, J. A. (2010). Experienced golfers' perspectives on choking under pressure. *Journal of Sport and Exercise Psychology, 32*, 61–83.

10

Hagger, M. S. (2010). Self-regulation: An important construct in health psychology research and practice. *Health Psychology Review, 4*, 57–65.

Hagger, M. S., Chatzisarantis, N. L., & Biddle, S. J. (2002). A meta-analytic review of the theories of reasoned action and planned behavior in physical activity: Predictive validity and the contribution of additional variables. *Journal of Sport and Exercise Psychology, 24*, 3–32.

Hagger, M. S., Chatzisarantis, N. L. D., Alberts, H., Anggono, C. O., Batailler, C., Birt, A. R., et al. (2016). A multilab preregistered replication of the ego-depletion effect. *Perspectives on Psychological Science, 11*, 546–573.

Hagger, M. S., & Luszczynska, A. (2014). Implementation intention and action planning interventions in health contexts: State of the research and proposals for the way forward. *Applied Psychology: Health and Well Being, 6*, 1–47.

Hagger, M. S., Wood, C., Stiff, C., & Chatzisarantis, N. L. D. (2010). Ego depletion and the strength model of self-control: A meta-analysis. *Psychological Bulletin, 136*, 495–525. https://doi.org/10.1037/a0019486

Heckhausen, H. (1989). *Motivation and action*. Springer.

Heckhausen, H., & Gollwitzer, P. M. (1987). Thought contents and cognitive functioning in motivational versus volitional states of mind. *Motivation and Emotion, 11*, 101–120.

Heckhausen, H., Gollwitzer, P. M., & Weinert, F. E. (1987). *Beyond the Rubicon: The will in the human sciences*. Springer.

Höner, O. (2005). *Decision-making in the game of football—An analysis in the light of the Rubicon theory*. Hofmann.

Höner, O. (2006). The shielding-interruption dilemma in sport games. *Journal of Psychology, 214*, 173–184.

Höner, O., & Feichtinger, P. (2016). Psychological talent predictors in early adolescence and their empirical relationship with current and future performance in soccer. *Psychology of Sport and Exercise, 25*, 17–26.

Höner, O., & Willimczik, K. (1998). Closing the action gap with the Rubicon model—On the explanatory value of motivational and volitional model conceptions for sporting actions. *Psychology and Sports, 5*, 56–68.

Inzlicht, M., & Legault, L. (2014). No pain, no gain: How distress underlies effective self-control (and unites diverse social psychological phenomena). In J. P. Forgas & E. Harmon-Jones (Eds.), *Sydney symposium of social psychology. Motivation and its regulation: The control within* (pp. 115–132). Psychology Press.

Inzlicht, M., Shenhav, A., & Olivola, C. Y. (2018). The effort paradox: Effort Is both costly and valued. *Trends in Cognitive Sciences, 22*(4), 337–349. https://doi.org/10.1016/j.tics.2018.01.007

Iso-Ahola, S. E. (2013). Exercise: Why it is a challenge for both the non-conscious and conscious mind. *Review of General Psychology, 17*, 93–110.

Kuhl, J. (1982). Action control as metacognitive mediator between intention and action: Leisure activities for secondary school students. *Journal of Developmental and Educational Psychology, 14*, 141–148.

Kuhl, J. (1983). *Motivation, conflict and action control*. Springer.

Kuhl, J. (1984). Motivational aspects of achievement motivation and learned helplessness: Toward a comprehensive theory of action control. In B. A. Maher & W. B. Maher (Eds.), *Progress in experimental personality research* (Vol. 13, pp. 99–171). Academic Press.

Kuhl, J. (1987). Motivation and control of action: Without good will it is not possible. In H. Heckhausen, P. M. Gollwitzer, & F. E. Weinert (Eds.), *Jenseits des Rubikon: Der Wille in den Humanwissenschaften* (pp. 101–120). Springer.

Kuhl, J. (1990). *Questionnaire for the recording of action control: HAKEMP 90, unpublished questionnaire*. University of Osnabrück.

Kuhl, J. (1994). Motivation and volition. In G. d'Ydevalle, P. Bertelson, & P. Eelen (Eds.), *Current advances in psychological science: An international perspective*. Erlbaum.

Kuhl, J. (1996). Will and experience of freedom. Forms of self-regulation. In J. Kuhl & H. Heckhausen (Eds.), *Encyclopedia of Psychology. Series IV, Volume 4: Motivation, volition and action* (pp. 665–765). Hogrefe.

Kuhl, J. (2001). *Motivation and personality*. Hogrefe.

Kuhl, J. (2010). Individual differences in self-control. In J. Heckhausen & H. Heckhausen (Eds.), *Motivation and action* (4th ed., pp. 337–363). Springer.

Kuhl, J., & Beckmann, J. (1994). *Volition and personality: Action versus state orientation volition and personality*. Hogrefe.

Lamprecht, M., Fischer, A., & Stamm, H. P. (2014). *Sport Switzerland 2014: Sports activity and sports interest of the Swiss population*. Federal Office for Sport FOSPO.

Lindner, C., Lindner, M. A., & Retelsdorf, J. (2019). Measuring self-control depletion in achievement situations: A validation of the 5-item brief state self-control capacity scale. *Diagnostica, 65*(4), 228–242.

Luszczynska, A. (2006). An implementation intentions intervention, the use of a planning strategy, and physical activity after myocardial infarction. *Social Science and Medicine, 62*, 900–908.

Martin Ginis, K. A., & Bray, S. R. (2010). Application of the limited strength model of self-regulation to understanding exercise effort, planning, and adherence. *Psychology and Health, 25*, 1147–1160. https://doi.org/10.1080/08870440903111696

Mischel, W. (1974). Processes in delay of gratification. *Advances in Experimental Social Psychology, 7*, 249–292.

Mischel, W., Shoda, Y., & Rodriguez, M. L. (1989). Delay of gratification in children. *Science, 244*, 933–938.

Muraven, M. (2010). Building self-control strength: Practicing self-control leads to improved self-control performance. *Journal of Experimental Social Psychology, 46*, 465–468.

Muraven, M., Tice, D. M., & Baumeister, R. F. (1998). Self-control as a limited resource: Regulatory depletion patterns. *Journal of*

Personality and Social Psychology, 74, 774–789. https://doi.org/10.1037/0022-3514.74.3.774

Nibbeling, N., Oudejans, R. R. D., & Daanen, H. A. M. (2012). Effects of anxiety, a cognitive secondary task, and expertise on gaze behavior and performance in a far aiming task. *Psychology of Sport and Exercise, 13*, 427–435.

Ntoumanis, N. (2014). The strength model of self-control. In R. C. Eklund & G. Tenenbaum (Eds.), *Encyclopaedia of sport and exercise psychology* (pp. 714–717). Sage.

Raab, M., & Johnson, J. G. (2004). Individual differences of action orientation for risk taking in sports. *Research Quarterly for Exercise and Sport, 75*, 326–336.

Rhodes, R. E., Plotnikoff, R. C., & Courneya, K. S. (2008). Predicting the physical activity-intention behavior profiles of adopters and maintainers using three social cognition models. *Annals of Behavioral Medicine, 36*, 244–252.

Roth, K. (1991). Decision behavior in the sports game. *Sports science, 21*, 229–246.

Sahre, E. (1991). *Action control in basketball*. Meyer and Meyer.

Schlam, T. R., Wilson, N. L., Shoda, Y., Mischel, W., & Ayduk, O. (2013). Preschoolers' delay of gratification predicts their body mass 30 years later. *The Journal of Pediatrics, 162*, 90–93.

Schmeichel, B. J., & Baumeister, R. F. (2010). Effortful attention control. In B. Bruya (Ed.), *Effortless attention: A new perspective in the cognitive science of attention and action* (pp. 29–49). MIT Press.

Schöndube, A., Bertrams, A., Sudeck, G., & Fuchs, R. (2017). Self-control strength and physical exercise: An ecological momentary assessment study. *Psychology of Sport and Exercise, 29*, 19–26.

Schwarzer, R., & Luszczynska, A. (2008). How to overcome health-compromising behaviors: The Health Action Process Approach. *European Psychologist, 13*, 141–151.

Sheeran, P. (2002). Intention—Behavior relations: A conceptual and empirical review. *European Review of Social Psychology, 12*, 1–36.

Shoda, Y., Mischel, W., & Peake, P. K. (1990). Predicting adolescent cognitive and self-regulatory competencies from preschool delay of gratification: Identifying diagnostic conditions. *Developmental Psychology, 26*, 978–986.

Sniehotta, F. F., Presseau, J., & Araújo-Soares, V. (2014). Time to retire the theory of planned behavior. *Health Psychology Review, 8*, 1–7.

Stork, M. J., Graham, J. D., Bray, S. R., & Martin Ginis, K. A. (2016). Using self-reported and objective measures of self-control to predict exercise and academic behaviors among first-year university students. *Journal of Health Psychology, 22*(8), 1056–1066.

Strang, H., Wegner, M., & Schwarze, p. (1987). Overcoming experiences of failure. *Sports psychology, 1*, 22–25.

Stroop, J. R. (1935). Studies of interference in serial verbal reactions. *Journal of Experimental Psychology, 18*, 643–662.

Tangney, J. P., Baumeister, R. F., & Boone, A. L. (2004). High self-control predicts good adjustment, less pathology, better grades, and interpersonal success. *Journal of Personality, 72*, 271–324.

Taylor, I. M., Smith, K., & Hunte, R. (2020). Motivational processes during physical endurance tasks. *Scandinavian Journal of Medicine & Science in Sports, 30*(9), 1769–1776. https://doi.org/10.1111/sms.13739

Toering, T., & Jordet, G. (2015). Self-control in professional soccer players. *Journal of Applied Sport Psychology, 27*, 335–350.

Tyler, J. M., & Burns, K. C. (2008). After depletion: The replenishment of the self's regulatory resources. *Self and Identity, 7*, 305–321.

van Elderen, T. M. L., Maes, S., & van den Broek, Y. (1994). Effects of a health education programme with telephone follow-up during cardiac rehabilitation. *British Journal of Clinical Psychology, 33*, 367–378.

Vohs, K. D., & Heatherton, T. F. (2000). Self-regulatory failure: A resource depletion approach. *Psychological Science, 11*, 249–254. https://doi.org/10.1111/1467-9280.00250

Wagstaff, C. (2014). Emotion regulation and sport performance. *Journal of Sport and Exercise Psychology, 36*, 401–412.

Watts, T. W., Duncan, G. J., & Quan, H. (2018). Revisiting the marshmallow test: A conceptual replication investigating links between early delay of gratification and later outcomes. *Psychological Science, 29*(7), 1159–1177. https://doi.org/10.1177/0956797618761661

Webb, T. L., & Sheeran, P. (2003). Can implementation intentions help to overcome ego-depletion? *Journal of Experimental Social Psychology, 39*, 279–286.

Wenhold, F., Elbe, A.-M., & Beckmann, J. (2009a). *Volitional Components in Sport (VKS)—Manual*. Sports publisher Strauß.

Wenhold, F., Elbe, A.-M., & Beckmann, J. (2009b). Test quality criteria of the VKS questionnaire for the recording of volitional components in sport. *Journal of Sports Psychology, 16*, 91–103.

Wilson, M. R., Vine, S. J., & Wood, G. (2009). The influence of anxiety on visual attentional control in basketball free throw shooting. *Journal of Sport and Exercise Psychology, 31*, 152–186.

Wolff, W., Baumann, L., & Englert, C. (2018). Self-reports from behind the scenes: Questionable research practices and rates of replication in ego depletion research. *PLoS One, 13*(6), e0199554. https://doi.org/10.1371/journal.pone.0199554

Woodman, T., & Hardy, L. (2003). The relative impact of cognitive anxiety and self-confidence upon sport performance: A meta-analysis. *Journal of Sports Sciences, 21*, 443–457.

Woolley, K., & Fishbach, A. (2016). For the fun of it: Harnessing immediate rewards to increase persistence in long-term goals. *Journal of Consumer Research, 42*(6), 952–966. https://doi.org/10.1093/jcr/ucv098

Emotion

Contents

Emotions in Sport

Philip Furley, Sylvain Laborde, Claudio Robazza and Andrew Lane

Contents

J. Schüler et al. (eds.), *Sport and Exercise Psychology*, https://doi.org/10.1007/978-3-031-03921-8_11

Learning Objectives

Basic:
- To be able to describe emotions
- To understand the contribution of nature and nurture for emotional expression
- To understand mind-body interaction using emotions as examples

Advanced:
- To be able to describe interindividual and intraindividual functions of emotions
- To be able to describe the influence of emotions in sport
- To be able to describe emotion regulation
- To understand emotional intelligence and its influence on athletic performance

Experts:
- To learn about methods to induce emotions and moods
- To gain knowledge about instruments measuring emotions, emotional intelligence, and mood

11.1 Introduction

Emotions play an important role in sport. The desire to experience or not to experience an emotion motivates a lot of behavior in humans. It helps explain why millions of spectators at major sporting events are spellbound in front of the television or flock to large sports arenas and live public viewing events. Think, for example, of the moment when in the USA, Michael Jordan scored the last shot in the fourth game of the 1998 National Basketball Association (NBA) final series against the Utah Jazz. This iconic moment has recently been covered in the widely viewed documentary "The Last Dance" which vividly captured the intense emotional reactions the event caused all over the world with players and spectators jumping with joy and creating a good mood among Chicago Bulls fans even days later. However, if you were a supporter of the Utah Jazz in the final, the identical situation most likely had a different effect on you as the numerous pictures of crying and mourning players and fans in the media showed. Although intense emotions like the ones described tend to be more memorable, more subtle forms of emotions are omnipresent in sports for everyone involved. For instance, athletes and spectators might be annoyed or angry when the referee decides against their own team. Or think about how you might feel when watching a super slow-motion picture of an athlete getting injured (e.g., breaking a leg). Further, athletes and fans are probably familiar with feeling nervous tension in anticipation of an important match or competition. Interestingly, most research on emotions in sports is conducted on the last example, that is, on anxiety and stress. Therefore, this textbook contains a separate chapter on the topic of anxiety and stress in sports.

The influential emotion researcher Richard Lazarus (2000) criticizes that stress/anxiety research and research on emotions, in general, have been conducted in relative isolation from each other:

> "In the past, two almost separate research literatures have grown up, one centered on stress and coping, the other on emotion. […] This is illogical and counterproductive." (p. 231)

The reason that anxiety or the stress process has received a lot of attention in sport psychology has to do with two historically important publications (Martens, 1977; Martens et al., 1990a) that provided a theory and tool to examine sport-specific anxiety, and thereby providing a major thrust for research. As research evolved, it became clear these emotions are commonly experienced. It also became clear that the influence of anxiety on sports performance was complicated; some people thrive when feeling anxious, while others perform poorly (Neil & Woodman, 2019).

Reflection

Try to remember emotional experiences that you have had while doing or watching sports.

What emotions do you remember in this context?

In everyday life, we often get asked how we are feeling or how we are doing. Usually, we answer this question without much thought with relatively empty statements like "good," "It is going well," or "It could be worse," without giving much detail on our complex inner world of experiencing and feeling. Although feelings and emotions seem to be so central to human psychology, there is hardly any other topic within psychology that has led to such great controversy (e.g. Beck, 2015). This is exemplified by a recent review article entitled *What Scientists Who Study Emotion Agree About* published by the prominent emotion psychologist Paul Ekman (Ekman, 2016). The controversy on emotions in psychology is also expressed by the fact that most standard textbooks in the applied field of sport psychology do not contain a chapter on emotions in sport but usually only deal with anxiety and the stress process in sport. Even though most people have an intuitive understanding of what is meant by the term "emotions" or "moods," this understanding differs considerably from person to person (Ekman, 2016), which complicates both research and applied interventions targeting emotions. Emotions in everyday life are usually thought to be merely a feeling (e.g., "I am happy" or "I am angry with my colleague"). However, common psychological theories define emotions more broadly.

> **Emotions**
>
> **Emotions** describe a complex pattern of physical and mental changes in response to a triggering situation perceived as personally significant. These changes include physiological arousal, feelings, cognitive processes, expression, and behavior. We are usually emotional about something or someone, and these feelings are intense and relatively short.

> **Moods**
>
> **Moods** are distinguished from emotions primarily by the fact that emotions are considered to be reactions to specific events that are short term and intense. Moods are usually less intense, do not have a specific antecedent or cause that an individual can identify, and can last for several hours or days. There is a weaker relationship between moods and their triggering events.

11.2 Universal Emotions and Culture: Darwin's Observations on the Connection Between Emotions and Evolution

When we travel to foreign countries and cultures, communication is impeded by our relative inability to master the different languages. In contrast, Charles Darwin (◘ Fig. 11.1) noted that the experience and expression of emotional states seems to be relatively universal and cross-culturally recognized, thereby facilitating intercultural communication beyond language. In his book *The Expression of the Emotions in Man and Animals*, Darwin (1872/1998), describes that emotions have developed hand in hand with other important structures and functions of living beings. Darwin regarded emotions as adaptive mechanisms representing highly specific, coordinating operations of the brain. These operations had the purpose of preparing a living being for certain categories of reoccurring situations/stimulus patterns in the environment and in the body. They also help them to respond adaptively to recurring problems and opportunities in their environment (e.g., threat, disgust, or feelings of sexual arousal). Darwin saw emotions as inherent, specialized physiological programs that increase the chances of living beings to pass on their genes to the next generation. Or as de Waal (2019) puts it, "emotions help us navigate a complex world that we don't fully comprehend."

According to Darwin's theoretical considerations, physiological processes and muscle movements associated with emotions generally fulfill two functions: 1) preparing the organism for adaptive actions in reoccurring stimulus constellations and 2) communicating important social cues.

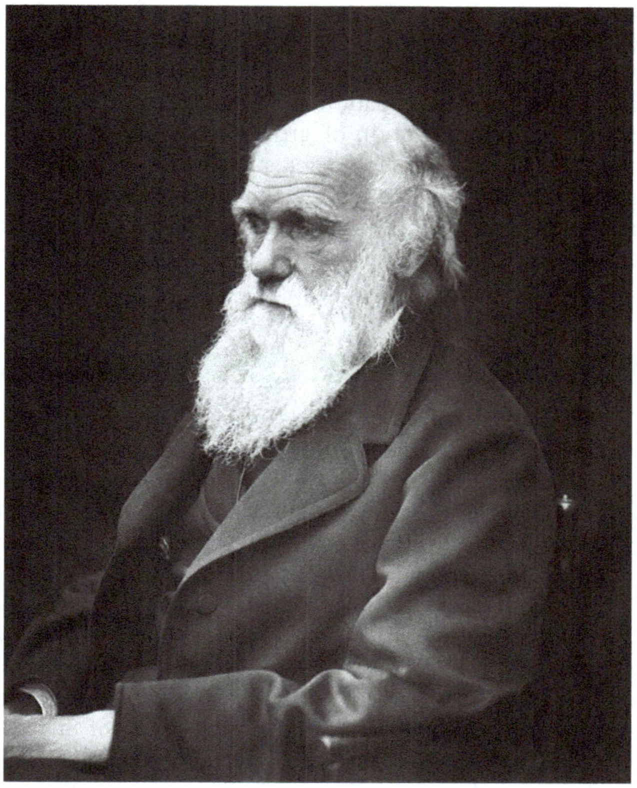

◘ **Fig. 11.1** Charles Darwin

? How can the main ideas of Darwin's "theory of emotional expression" be summarized?

- Emotional expressions developed hand in hand with other physiological reactions to prepare an organism for adaptive actions (e.g. fight or flight). These emotional expressions also signal to others that adaptive actions are likely.
- If emotional signals are useful to the individual (i.e., increased reproductive fitness), the communicative function might become more important than the physiological function. In turn, evolutionary selection pressure would lead to exaggerated expressions, and physiological functions might become vestiges. As a consequence, contrary messages (e.g., pride and shame) are often expressed by opposing movements and postures to make them better recognizable by observers (e.g., pride takes up more place in space, whereas the expression of shame makes you collapse and take up less place in space; principle of antithesis).

A recent theory has taken up these considerations and integrated them into the "two-step model of emotional expression" (see for an overview Shariff & Tracy, 2011). In this two-step model, it is suggested that internal physiological regulation drives the intensity of emotional expressions (e.g., dilated pupils in anxiety to identify the source of a possible threat). Later in the process, however, social communication is more important, since the efficient organization of groups leads to a range of adaptational advantages (e.g., signaling to the social group through dilated pupils that danger was imminent). Another example illustrative of Darwin's theoretical considerations is the evolution of display behaviors and threatening gestures. Behaviors such as staring at an enemy, flaring and standing up, tensing muscles, and displaying one's weapons were used to prepare for a fight. All these behaviors could be interpreted by an observer or rival as signs of imminent aggression and danger. The signaling and interpretation of aggressive or dominant behavior gave both parties a survival advantage, as the probability of a life-threatening fight decreased (► Study Box: "This Is What Winners Look Like": Can Spectators Judge the Score Based on Body Language?; ► Side Story: Body Language and Emotions in Sport).

Case Study Box

"The Expression of Winning": Can Spectators Judge the Score Based on Body Language?

From Darwin's theory on the evolution of display behavior follows that people in confrontational situations should display nonverbal behavior that provides information about who is superior or inferior (see Furley, 2021, for an evolutionary account of emotions and applications in the sport context). Furley and Schweizer (2014a, 2014b) based a study on this hypothesis, examining it in athletic competitions and whether people can distinguish between leading and trailing athletes based on their nonverbal behavior.

In Study 1, participants viewed short video recordings of basketball and table tennis players playing in competition. The actual score at the time of the recordings varied from "trailing by far" to "leading by far" for the player shown. For each video recording, participants assessed how far the athletes were leading or trailing on a continuous scale.

Study 2 investigated developmental differences by comparing the results of Study 1 with one group of children aged 4–8 years and a second group of children aged 9–12 years.

Study 3 served to replicate Study 1 with new stimulus material (recordings of handball players) and investigate if domain-specific sports knowledge moderated the effect. Participants were either experienced handball players or handball laymen or laywomen.

The results of these three studies showed that participants were able to distinguish between leading and trailing athletes. The effect size was consistently high by statistical convention. Interestingly, participants with sport-specific experience were not more accurate in their assessments, and so knowledge of the sport and its culture were not influential. Although children were also able to distinguish between leading and trailing athletes, the effect was more pronounced in adults.

Side Story

Body Language and Emotions in Sports

There is hardly a television broadcast in sports in which the commentator does not mention the body language of the athletes (see Furley & Schweizer, 2020 for a recent review on body language in sports). Statements such as "You can see the team has given up" or "The player is bursting with self-confidence" are commonplace in sports like football.

Charles Darwin observed and documented in detail that certain emotional states are communicated uniformly. Therefore, it is not surprising that we are so familiar with body language and can interpret it reliably. After all, language developed late in evolutionary history, and our ancestors were dependent on nonverbal communication (see Fridlund, 1994, for an alternative explanatory approach, arguing that nonverbal communication has the adaptive advantage of communicating social motives and behavioral intentions rather than just emotions).

A particularly important category of nonverbal behavior, especially among primates, is the communication of dominance and submissiveness to quickly and efficiently convey information about rank and status (Furley, 2019) and, thus, prevent possible life-threatening attacks. In this context, studies have made the remarkable observation that winning or losing in competition leads to changes in blood hormone levels (Booth et al., 1989; Edwards & Casto, 2018) associated with dominant or submissive behavior. Against this background, the frequent comments on body language in football also make sense. Recent studies show that individuals are extremely efficient at assessing the correct score tendency based solely on nonverbal signals (Furley & Schweizer, 2016) and that even children with autism spectrum disorder are capable of doing so (Ryan et al., 2016).

Of greater practical relevance are studies showing that dominant and submissive nonverbal behavior have an important influence on the opponent (Furley & Dicks, 2012; Furley et al., 2012a). The experiments demonstrate that a dominant body language is unconsciously associated with positive characteristics such as self-confidence and competence. Conversely, a submissive body language is associated with negative characteristics such as insecurity or fearfulness. Even the slightest signals of dominance or submissiveness activate stored schemata. For example, submissive body language leads opponents to assess them negatively and then to strengthen their perception of being able to counter them successfully. Numerous studies on self-efficacy show that the belief to perform successfully is closely related to performance (Budden et al., 2020; Feltz & Öncü, 2014). Conversely, doubts about success often lead to failure of the action (Furley & Schweizer, 2014a). Theoretically, it would, therefore, be conceivable that an athlete's nonverbal behavior could be part of a vicious (or virtuous) circle. For example, a team trailing in a competition might, in turn, show submissive body language. This is perceived by the opponent who in return grows in self-confidence and so is more convinced in his ability to beat the opponent. This might result in the opponent actually playing more successfully and again displaying more dominant body language.

Sport Practice

How Do I Hide My Nervousness During the Penalty Kick and Increase My Chances of Success?

Two studies provide some insight into this question by showing a connection between emotions and nonverbal behavior (Jordet & Hartman, 2008; Jordet, 2009). These studies show that football players tend to display certain nonverbal avoidance behaviors during very important penalties. More specifically, they tend to turn their backs to the goalkeeper and spend less time between the referee's whistle and the start of their run-up, possibly because they want to get the important penalty kick over as quickly as possible or it could be that the players are hiding from the stressors, albeit nonconsciously. Such behavior has been shown to have a negative influence on the shooter's probability of success. It is argued that this shows that the emotion fear/anxiety is associated with poorer performance (▶ Chap. 12). It could also partly be due to the extent to which the goalkeeper has learned from observing such preperformance nonverbal behavior. Research has shown that goalkeepers feel more confident in saving the penalty kick when they perceive the striker is uncertain on where to place the shoot and believe they can adapt their behavior accordingly—i.e., by waiting longer until they initiate their movement (Furley et al., 2012b). Interestingly, it is precisely those nations showing this avoidance behavior most frequently that have been less successful in penalty shootouts in the past (e.g., England!!!!!).

Taken together, evidence-based recommendations for penalty takers could be as follows: (1) show high self-confidence by how you pick up the ball, (2) establish good eye contact with the goalkeeper, (3) place the ball on the spot, (4) look at the goalkeeper when running back to the starting point, (5) take a deep breath after the referee's whistle and allow yourself 2 s (possibly count "21, 22"), and (6) initiate the run-up.

A straightforward hypothesis that can be derived from Darwin's theoretical considerations is that certain emotional reactions should occur universally irrespective of cultural origin of a person; emotions are universal and it was the same adaptive processes that shaped them over generations of evolution. Various researchers have tested this universality hypothesis by comparing the emotional responses of newborns and the consistency of facial expressions across cultures. If Darwin's theory was supportable, children all over the world should show comparable emotional responses (Izard, 1994). The first psychologist to provide evidence for this assumption was Silvan Tomkins (1962, 1981). He was able to show comparable, unlearned emotional responses in infants when loud sounds elicited fear. These results were interpreted as a kind of neural "hardware program" in response to a certain kind of triggering stimulus patterns. Certain environmental stimuli lead to neuronal response patterns that are automatically interconnected to brain areas and effector organs leading to an emotional response that is universal enough to fit a wide range of situational conditions. Comparative cultural research confirms this theorizing by providing evidence that some emotional responses in young children are very similar (Camras, 1992; Camras et al., 1992; ▶ Case Study Box: Do Infants Show Comparable Emotional Reactions?).

Case Study Box

Do Infants Show Comparable Emotional Reactions?

Five and 12-month-old infants from the USA and Japan reacted very similarly when the experimenter grasped the children's wrists and fixed them to their stomachs. The children's reactions were all recorded on video and compared with each other using a coding system. Both the children's facial expressions and behavior were highly comparable between Japanese and American children (Camras et al., 1992).

However, this finding was not supported by a later study led by the same author (Camras et al., 1998). In this study, 11-month-old infants from China reported less intense emotional expressions than their Japanese and the American peers. This finding could be interpreted that culture might be having an early influence on the emotional hardware program of children, and clearly further evidence is needed.

Various studies on **universal expressions** of emotions suggest that the interpretation and recognition of emotional expressions has also an evolutionary innate component. For example, 4- to 6-month-old infants could reliably distinguish between surprise, fear, and anger (Serrano et al., 1992). In addition, infants show more approach behavior and smile more often in response to looking at happy facial expressions. Infants show avoidance behavior and frowning in response to looking at angry facial expressions (Serrano et al., 1995). Infants, therefore, seem to be able to distinguish not only basic emotional expressions but also show an early understanding of their meaning.

Probably the most prominent proponent of this **basic emotion approach** is Paul Ekman, who was the only psychologist to be named as 1 of the 100 most influential people by Time Magazine in 2009. In his detailed intercultural studies, Ekman (1984, 1992, 1994) has shown what Darwin first suspected—that is, the existence of a kind of universal emotional language (at least for some facial expressions), which presumably is an innate component of the human evolutionary heritage.

? Thanks to Paul Ekman and his work on facial expression, emotion, and deception, we have a better understanding of how the expressions and gestures we display on the surface are a direct reflection of what is going on in the neurocircuitry deep inside our brains (Quote from the laudation of the Time Magazine from 30th April, 2009).

Specifically, it has been demonstrated that the emotional facial expressions of joy, anger, disgust, fear, and sadness (and possibly also surprise and contempt, depending on the study) are shown and reliably recognized all over the world (Ekman & Friesen, 1986, ◘ Fig. 11.2). Regarding basic emotions, it is important to mention that not all emotional expressions are universally recognized. This has only been shown for the five emotions: joy, anger, disgust, fear, and sadness (although there is still debate here). According to Ekman (2007), all other facial expressions are composed of a mixture of these primary facial expressions (see Gendron et al., 2018, for a recent critique of this theory).

? Based on his many years of research on emotional expressions, Paul Ekman and his daughter Eve Ekman have launched the online Atlas of Emotions in 2016 (► http://atlasofemotions.org/). The goal of this interactive tool is to sensitize and improve the emotional awareness of people. This, in turn, aims to help people recognize how emotions affect their lives. The atlas is based on the "neurocultural theory of emotion" (Ekman, 1994) and assumes there are (at least) five universal emotions all people can recognize and express, regardless of their origin or social background. The Atlas of Emotions is summarized in ◘ Table 11.1.

? What does it mean to assume emotions as basic?
The adjective basic contains two main characteristics regarding emotions (Ekman & Cordaro, 2011):

One is that these emotions are discrete, meaning they can be clearly distinguished from other emotions. Differentiation criteria include facial expressions, the voice, the physiology of the autonomic nervous system, and the triggers initiating the emotion.

Second, emotions are an evolutionary product of our adaptation to the environment. Although humans are incredibly versatile in their behavior, they embody biological mechanisms that allow them to deal with basic life tasks (e.g., loss, frustration, success). Every basic (universal) emotion guides human behavior in a certain direction that has proven to be superior to other directions in the course of evolution (see Gendron et al., 2018, for a critique of this view).

In regard to the popular nature vs. nurture debate, it should be noted that the basic emotion approach does not argue that emotions are 100% nature and 0% nurture.

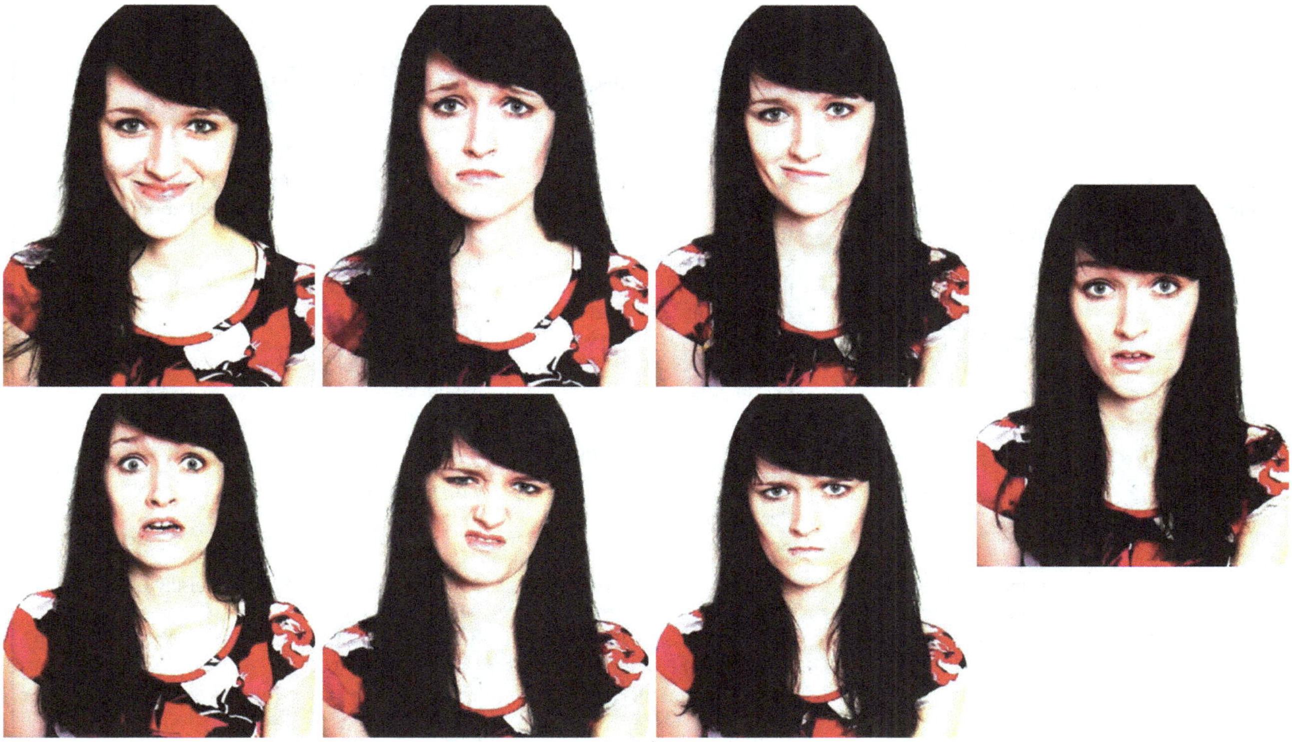

Fig. 11.2 Evaluation of emotional facial expressions (Author: Icerko Lýdia). Assign these seven emotional terms to the faces shown: fear, disgust, joy, surprise, contempt, anger, and sadness

Table 11.1 Ekman's Atlas of Emotions

Emotion	Experience	Condition (sorted by intensity)	Response	Trigger	Moods
Anger	We get angry when something blocks us or when we think we're being treated unfairly	Annoyance Frustration Exasperation Argumentativeness Bitterness Vengefulness Fury	Dispute Be passive-aggressive Insult Quarrel Scream/yell Simmer/brood Suppress Use physical force Undermine	Interference with locomotion Interference with action Rejection by a loved one Inefficiency or bureaucracy Being put down by an authority figure Encountering Offensive beliefs Being wrongfully accused	Irritable: predisposed to becoming angry, easily provoked

(continued)

Table 11.1 (continued)

Emotion	Experience	Condition (sorted by intensity)	Response	Trigger	Moods
Enjoyment	Enjoyment describes the many good feelings that arise from experiences both novel and familiar	Sensory pleasure Rejoicing Compassion/joy Amusement Schadenfreude Relief Peace Fiero Pride Naches Wonder Excitement Ecstasy	Exclaim Engage/connect Gloat Indulge Maintain Savor Seek more	Sensory experience of nature Helping others Social interaction Playing sports Places associated with enjoyable memories The taste of something nice Spending time with loved ones	Elated: a long-lasting, generalized good feeling
Disgust	Feeling disgusted by what is toxic helps us to avoid being poisoned, physically or socially	Dislike Aversion Distaste Repugnance Revulsion Abhorrence Loathing	Avoid Dehumanize Vomit Withdraw	Anything coming out of the body Rotting or decay Fans of opposing sport teams Unfamiliar religious customs Eating insects or raw meat	Sour: generally repulsed
Fear	Our fear of danger lets us anticipate threats to our safety and, thus, ensures security and well-being	Trepidation Nervousness Anxiety Dread Desperation Panic Horror Terror	Avoid Freeze Hesitate Ruminate Scream/yell Withdraw Worry	Imminent bodily impact Sudden loss of gravity Threat to safety snake-like shapes Threat of losing job Thunder Public speaking	Apprehensive: anxious that something bad will happen, on edge
Sadness	Sadness is a response to loss, and feeling sad allows us to take a timeout and show others that we need support	Disappointment Discouragement Distraughtness Resignation Helplessness Hopelessness Misery Despair Grief Sorrow Anguish	Feel ashamed Mourn Protest Ruminate Seek comfort Withdrawal	Being rejected by someone important Losing a loved one Perceiving a loss of status Not being invited to a party Losing a treasured belonging	Dysphoric (or feeling blue): an enduring feeling of discouragement or disappointment

The interactive Atlas of Emotions with more detailed descriptions can be found at ► http://atlasofemotions.org/

Ekman (1994) claims in his "**neurocultural theory of emotion**" that both evolution (through the pre-connection of neural circuits in the brain) and culture influence emotional programs and their expression.

The influence of culture on emotional programs occurs via social learning and socialization, which teaches the appropriate handling of emotion according to the social situation. In this way, social rules or cultural norms are established about when and to what extent certain emotions are expressed or lived out (Mesquita & Frijda, 1992; Ratner, 2000).

The zoologist Ernst Mayr's (1974) distinction between open and closed genetic programs is helpful in understanding the relative influences of nature and nurture on emotions. In a closed genetic program, no "add-ons" through experience are possible, whereas open genetic programs can integrate additional input through experience. Mayr argues that organisms with long developmental periods of parental care have more time to learn and adapt to varying environmental conditions and therefore have a selection advantage through open genetic programs (see Sterelny, 2012, for a detailed argumentation on this). In this context, Ekman and Cordaro (2011) argue emotions belong to the open genetic developmental programs since humans need to learn to adapt their universal emotional programs to their living conditions through experience.

According to this view, universal emotion programs evolve in the process of ontogenesis by the interconnection of sensory cells, neuron groups and effector organs (e.g. muscles), but can be influenced by experiential input.

Reflection

Am I Laughing Because I'm Happy, or Am I Happy Because I'm Laughing?

Research suggests that there is evidence for both and that our facial expressions influence our emotional experience (▫ Fig. 11.3, Adelmann & Zajonc, 1989). To test this so-called facial feedback hypothesis (Strack et al., 1988), participants were instructed to show different facial expressions while viewing a series of photographic slides (Rutledge & Hupka, 1985). The results showed that participants reported that the slides made them happier or less annoyed when they made a happy facial expression compared to an angry expression.

Try it yourself: Pull your eyebrows down and together at the same time. Lift your upper eyelids, tighten your lower eyelids, make your lips narrow, and press them together. If you hold this expression for a while and notice you feel slightly upset, you have just experienced the effect of facial feedback.

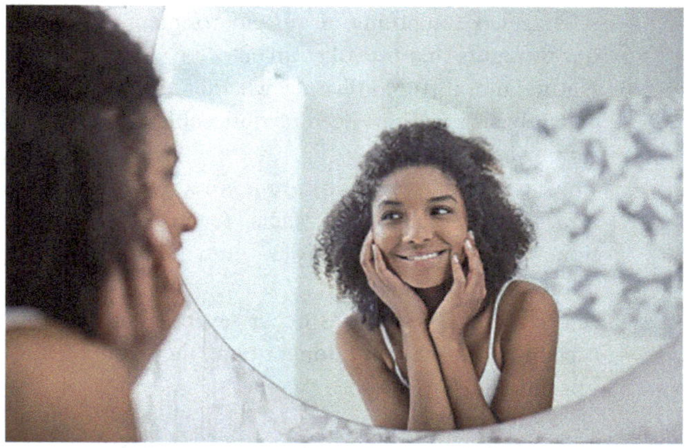

▫ **Fig. 11.3** Laughing/smiling can lift your mood

The "Try it yourself example" on facial feedback shows that we can control our facial expressions at will and the human facial expression is not just a display that shows others what evolutionary emotional program is currently running. Thus, humans can consciously put on facial expressions and suppress automatic, "real" facial expressions, as predicted by **dual-process models** (Furley et al., 2015b, for an overview in sports). For example, you can put on a fake smile to hide a lie. However, some cues allow for distinguishing real expressions from fake ones (Ekman, 2007). Ekman was able to show that fake emotions are often interrupted by very short facial expressions (**micro-expressions**) of the true emotion. Such micro-expressions usually last about 0.05 s, but with appropriate training, they can be recognized without technical aids.

Besides micro-expressions, other cues allow to distinguish between real and staged expressions. In 1862 the French anatomist Duchenne claimed a real smile could be distinguished from a fake smile by looking at the two muscles contracted during a real smile: the musculus orbicularis oculi, which surrounds the eyes, and the musculus zygomaticus major, which lifts the corners of the mouth. According to Duchenne, people do not have any problems to arbitrarily contract the zygomaticus major muscle to lift the lips, whereas most people cannot contract the orbicularis oculi muscle purposefully. With a real smile, both eyes and mouth laugh, whereas with a fake smile, usually only the mouth laughs. Therefore, the real smile was called a Duchenne smile (Ekman & Davidson, 1993).

Universal emotions and culture

- Universal emotions serve a specific purpose and help people deal with a range of reoccurring situations.
- Universal emotions vary in the intensity by which they are experienced.
- We react to our universal emotions with certain actions or action tendencies.

- A trigger is something in our environment and in our thoughts that provokes an emotion.
- Nature and nurture influence whether and to what extent basic emotions become noticeable in expression or behavior.
- Emotions and expressions are in a reciprocal relationship with each other (facial feedback): Emotions influence expressions and expressions influence emotions.
- If certain basic emotions occur several times in a certain period or over a longer time, they influence our mood.

So far, research has been covered showing that some physiological responses to emotional events have a genetic origin but can be influenced by social learning. Based on these findings, we now turn to emotion theories explicitly dealing with the interaction of physiological and psychological processes.

11.3 Physiology of Emotions

Everyone knows the feeling of experiencing a strong emotion: For example, you notice your heart beats faster, your breathing becomes faster, your muscles become tense, and your mouth begins to dry. Many further physiological processes can accompany emotional reactions that do not necessarily have to be consciously noticed. All these physiological reactions evolved to mobilize the organism to respond adaptively to the current environmental conditions (Kalat, 2019).

In this process, the **autonomic nervous system** plays a key role in preparing the body for adaptive reactions by orchestrating the activity of the parasympathetic and sympathetic components. The activity ratio of the respective parasympathetic and sympathetic systems depends on the quality and intensity of the triggering stimuli.

In the present chapter, we give a schematic overview of the most important general physiological principles of emotions rather than enter into the highly complex discussion on the physiological processes of emotions in detail. It is generally accepted that the sympathetic nervous system directs its activating effect by releasing the hormones adrenaline and noradrenaline from the adrenal gland and thus controls a cascade of other physiological processes, which, for example, stimulates other internal organs, increases blood sugar, or increases sweat production. In contrast, the parasympathetic system is considered to have a deactivating or calming role, for example, by inhibiting the release of activating hormones into the bloodstream. Comparative cultural studies suggest that the autonomic nervous system is an important component of our innate emotional hardware preparing people for a wide range of reoccurring emotional situations (Levenson et al., 1992 for more detail). Research results have also shown that participating in a sport competition have a measurable impact on hormone levels in athletes (Edwards & Casto, 2018).

In addition to the autonomic nervous system, the central nervous system needs to be briefly discussed to enable a comprehensive understanding of the physiological hardware of emotions. The **hypothalamus** and the **limbic system** are responsible for the interaction of hormonal and neural aspects of emotions. At the center of neuronal emotion research is the **amygdala**, which is part of the limbic system (Pinel & Barnes, 2018). Metaphorically, the amygdala is often described as the "gate of emotions" and as a kind of "filter for memory." In this sense, the amygdala "colors" information from the environment and memory in a way that gives it emotional meaning or valence (i.e., pleasure or displeasure). This process metaphorically describes the mechanism by which experience influences the open basic emotional programs of humans.

The cortex, the seat of many memories, has also been shown to be involved in emotional experiences. Metaphorically speaking, sensory impressions are emotionally colored and stored as the foundation for future behavior. This process points to a close interconnection of cognition and emotion, which is also increasingly anchored in the literature (e.g. Damasio, 1994: "Somatic Marker Hypothesis"; Slovic et al., 2007: affect heuristics). In his *Somatic Marker Hypothesis*, Damasio argues that perceptual events—imagined or generated by one's actions—are related to certain somatic reactions of the body and are stored in memory together with these somatic/emotional reactions. This means that recalling certain memories automatically activates somatic representations that were active when experiencing (or encoding) the memorized event. This gives perceptual events and anticipated perceptual events a certain valence, which is transmitted via emotional reactions (for Seligman et al., 2016, the emotional coloring of imagined prospective actions could even be the central role of emotions since the direct influence of emotions on behavior is often difficult to prove).

As a result, when making decisions and planning our behavior, we can draw on emotional valence information and thus adapt our decision-making and anticipation behavior effectively to the environment. In other words, people seem to attribute emotional valence to different action alternatives, which help us to choose between these alternatives. People who lose this function due to brain lesions have great problems to regulate themselves in everyday life, as shown in the case of Phineas Gage (► Side Story: The Case of Phineas Gage and How It Changed Previous Thinking About Emotions).

Side Story

The Case of Phineas Gage and How It Changed Previous Thinking About Emotions

The young railway worker Phineas Gage was the victim of a tragic industrial accident in 1848. During a blowup, he was shot through his face, skull, and brain with a 3-cm-thick, 90-cm-long ramming iron. This caused a lesion in the orbitofrontal and prefrontal cortex. Miraculously, Gage survived the accident. However, he appeared to be a different person thereafter. Previously, Gage was described as a responsible, intelligent, and social person and was very popular with friends and colleagues. After he recovered from his accident, Gage appeared to be as intellectually and physically capable as before, but both his personality and his emotional world had changed completely. Above all, his disrespect, vulgarity, and impulsiveness were noticeable. As a result, he lost his job and was no longer able to take on a position involving responsibility. He became a vagabond who wandered the country in the San Francisco area until his death. Although Gage was buried along with the ramming iron that had injured him, neurologist John Harlow received permission to examine Gage's body and the ramming iron 5 years after the funeral. Today, the skull and the ramming iron are exhibited in a museum at Harvard University, and Gage's condition is now called frontal brain syndrome since the frontal brain performs important functions in terms of self-control, impulse control, and executive functions.

The cortex can thus be seen as a kind of archive in which associations are stored that connect psychological experience with physical reactions. In this context, some researchers have suggested that emotions lead to two distinct behavioral tendencies: **approach and avoidance behavior** or **approach and avoidance motivation** (Davidson et al., 2000). In this context, Davidson et al. (2000) speak of two different perceptual-action systems that are governed by emotions and are responsible for approach- and avoidance-related reactions.

Physiology of Emotions

- The autonomic nervous system prepares the body for emotional reactions using the parasympathetic and sympathetic components in order to adapt.
- The hypothalamus and the limbic system are responsible for hormonal and neuronal interactions of emotion.
- Via the limbic system/amygdala, incoming information and memory content receive emotional valence.
- Emotional valence stored in networks involving the cortex influences information processing and behavior (*somatic marker* hypothesis, affect heuristics).
- Basically, a distinction can be made between an approach-related and an avoidance-related emotional system.

11.4 The Connection Between the Physiology and the Psychology of Emotions

The previous section summarized evidence that the human organism, through evolution and learning, shows a variety of rapid physiological reactions to reoccurring, meaningful events, called emotions. All these rapid reactions serve the purpose of enabling adaptive behavior. In the following, we will briefly present basic theories on the origin of emotions integrating the interaction of physiological responses, cognitive evaluations, and behavioral tendencies.

11.4.1 James-Lange Theory

Aristotle already assumed that a psychological feeling sets in after the body has reacted to a situation. The founding father of American psychology, William James, also assumed this sequence: physiological reaction followed by psychological emotion (James, 1890). This view of emotions coming from physical feedback has become known in the psychological literature as the "**James-Lange theory of emotion**" (Carl Lange was a Danish psychologist who formulated a similar theory at the same time). According to this theory, the perception of a situation leads to somatic reactions, which in turn leads to the experience of a psychological emotion.

11.4.2 Cannon-Bard Theory

The American physiologist Walter Cannon (as well as another physiologist: Philip Bard) rejected the theory of "James Lange" due to empirical evidence not being consistent with the theory (Leventhal, 1980, for an overview). Furthermore, it had been argued that the reactions of the autonomic nervous system are too slow to be the cause of the rapidly developing psychological emotions. According to Cannon, the thalamus registers incoming information, which is then transmitted in parallel to different areas. They simultaneously cause emotional experience and further somatic reactions. According to this theory, an emotional stimulus is at the same time the trigger for physical arousal and subjective experience of the emotion. A central hypothesis of this theory implies that physical arousal and emotional experience are not mutually dependent. However, more recent cognitive assessment theories suggest that this does not seem to be true.

11.4.3 Appraisal Theory (Lazarus-Schachter Theory)

In many situations, internal states of arousal are very similar, even when emotions are different. Therefore, there is a risk of ambiguity and confusion in the physiological excitation pattern. For this reason, Schachter and Singer (1962) postulated that the psychological experience of emotions is a joint effect of physiological arousal and cognitive assessment. Physiological arousal is only the first step in the emotional chain. This physical arousal is assessed (typically unconsciously) by the person in terms of its significance. Another supporter of the central role of cognitive assessment in the emergence of emotions was Richard Lazarus (Lazarus, 1991; Lazarus & Lazarus, 1994). He argued that emotions cannot be fully understood through physiological processes, but rather they result from the dynamic interaction of the person with the environment, which is continually being evaluated nonconsciously and consciously.

? Are there discrete emotions or do emotions differ only in terms of a few dimensions?

- A lengthy controversy within emotion research concerns the question of whether there are different discrete emotions (Ekman & Cordaro, 2011, for an overview) or whether emotions are better characterized as a two-dimensional (or multidimensional) construct that varies on the dimensions valence (pleasant vs. unpleasant) and activation (high vs. low) (e.g., Russell et al., 1989).
- This controversy continues and cannot be clearly resolved in favor of one or the other perspective at this time.
- Without going too deeply into this debate (see Gendron et al., 2018, for an up-to-date overview), both the supporters of the discrete emotion approach (e.g. Ekman, 2016; Lazarus, 2000) and the supporters of the dimensional approach (Crivelli & Fridlund, 2018, for an up-to-date overview) provide conclusive arguments in favor of the respective theory.
- First studies (e.g., Cowen & Keltner, 2017) have meanwhile made promising progress in integrating the two theoretical approaches.

Even though there is plenty of empirical evidence for the important role of cognitive evaluation processes in the experience of emotions (Lazarus, 1991, 2000, for an overview), this theory is not without criticism (e.g. Zajonc, 2000), since studies suggest certain emotions cannot result from evaluation processes. Taken altogether, however, it can be said that cognitive evaluations can make an important contribution to emotional experience but are not the only source (Izard, 1993). In some situations, emotional experience appears to be controlled of innate, evolutionary "programming" of the human nervous system occurring independently of cognitive assessment. These different sources of emotional experience might be indicative that emotions fulfill different functions in humans. The assumed functions of emotions will be discussed in the next section.

Psychology of Emotions

- James Lange Theory: Experiencing emotions arises from physical/somatic feedback.
- Cannon-Bard Theory: Incoming information is registered by the thalamus and simultaneously influences physical arousal and emotional experience.
- Lazarus-Schachter Theory: Experiencing emotions is a joint effect of physiological arousal and cognitive evaluation.
- Discrete emotion approaches assume qualitatively different emotions, whereas dimensional approaches distinguish between pleasant and unpleasant states with different activation levels.

11.5 Functions of Emotions

Throughout this chapter, it was argued that emotions play an important role in the evolution of humans and other animals by preparing them to react adaptively in reoccurring, important situations. The next section will elaborate on the assumed adaptive functions of emotions.

11.5.1 Motivation and Attention

Emotions are often the driving force for action, as is evident in everyday expressions such as "I yelled at the referee because I was angry at him." Therefore, emotions have motivational character by encouraging people to act in a certain way based on a previous experienced or imagined event or an anticipated prospect in the future. In this respect, emotions often inform the direction and intensity of behavior toward a certain goal (see the action tendencies in ◘ Table 11.1).

In addition to this motivational effect of emotions on observable behavior, emotions also influence the orientation of attention. Humans can only process a small fraction of the incoming information. Attention processes ensure that the most relevant information is processed in detail and irrelevant information is faded out. Emotions help to adjust this attentional filter to ensure that currently relevant information is processed. Thus, emotions concentrate the limited attentional resources on information that is congruent with the current emotional state of the individual. As Janelle et al. (2020) have pointed out, recent evidence suggests that the motivational intensity of an emotion may moderate the influence of affective valence (i.e., pleasantness or unpleasantness) on attentional focus. For example, unpleasant emotions high in avoidance motivation, such as anxiety and fear, tend to narrow the attentional focus and promote actions to escape threats or perceived danger. Unpleasant emotions low in avoidance motivational intensity, such as sadness, do not necessitate action and tend to broaden the attentional focus. Similar effects on attentional focus have been observed for pleasant emotions. More elaborate processing of emotion-congruent objects or events further leads to better memory recall of these object or events. Studies inside (Wilson et al., 2009) or outside of sport (e.g., Öhman et al., 2001) indicate that discrete emotions have an influence on setting of the attention filter and thus influence which information is processed elaborately and which is not.

11.5.2 Cognition

Emotions influence not only attention allocation but also numerous other cognitive processes such as learning, memory, judgment and decision-making, and creative performance (Forgas, 2006, for an overview). In general, emotions have been shown to influence the important processes of organizing and categorizing our experience. In this respect, studies have shown that an emotion or a mood is stored in memory together with the accompanying events as a global schema (Bower, 1981, 1991a, 1991b). These associative memory representations are evident in findings of mood-congruent processing and mood-dependent memory. Studies on mood-congruent processing indicate that people show a selective sensitivity to stimuli that match their current moods. For example, Gilligan and Bower (1983) have shown that stimuli that are congruent with a person's prevailing mood (e.g., images of a spider when anxious) are more likely to be noticed, attended to, and processed more elaborately. A related body of research has provided evidence for mood-dependent memory recall. People find it easier to recall certain events from memory if their current mood is congruent with their mood when they first remembered/stored an event (Eich, 1995; Eich & Macaulay, 2000; Terry et al., 2005). Studies also suggest that positive feelings lead to more efficient and creative thinking and problem-solving than negative feelings (Isen, 1987).

11.5.3 Social Functions of Emotions

A growing body of literature shows that emotions fulfill not only intrapersonal but also interpersonal functions (see Friesen et al., 2013a for a review). Interpersonal perspectives in sport provide information on the ways in which athletes' emotions and emotion regulation operate interdependently in influencing sports performance and relationships between athletes and their teammates, coaches, and parents. According to this perspective, emotions make an essential contribution to the regulation of social interactions. For example, emotions help organizing groups by binding some individuals together and distancing them from other individuals. If a person is "boiling with anger," we would probably tend to keep our distance from that person, whereas we would probably be more likely to seek contact with a smiling person (▶ Side Story: Dunbar's "Social Brain Hypothesis"). Friesen et al. (2013b) illustrate how emotion regulation of others and self can operate in the context of a team environment.

Side Story

Dunbar's "Social Brain Hypothesis"

Cozolino (2006) proposed a memorable analogy to describe the nonverbal communication of emotions within "social synapse theory." Cozolino compared nonverbal communication between individuals with the neurochemical communication of nerve cells. Accordingly, people constantly send out signals into the social synapse (the space between people) which are picked up by the sensory organs of other people and transformed into electrochemical signals that influence the thoughts and behavior of the recipients, which are again communicated over the social synapse. Cozolino (2006, p. 24) claims that the nonverbal emotional communication has an important adaptation advantage because it has allowed the organization into increasingly larger groups: "It appears that social communication has been chosen by natural selection to be of greater survival value than disguising our intentions and feelings, so much so that we even have ways of unintentionally 'outing' ourselves to others."

In this context, Dunbar (1993) was able to demonstrate an impressive correlation between brain size and group size of living beings. This correlation has been interpreted as evidence for the coevolution of increasing computational power (i.e., larger brains) that is required to coordinate increasing complexity of life in larger groups. One aspect of this is interpreting and acting upon the emotional signals sent out by group members.

An influential model assigning central importance to the social function of emotions is the "EASI model" (Emotions As Social Information; van Kleef, 2009). This model originated from the social-functional perspective of emotions (Parkinson, 1996) and is based on the premise that emotions serve to communicate important social information to other people: "Emotion is not just a feeling. Emotion is for influence" (Van Kleef et al., 2011, p. 154, see also Friesen et al., 2021; Friesen et al., 2013a, 2013b for extensions to sport). The "EASI model" assumes two specific mechanisms of how emotional expressions influence observers: via (1) inferential processes and (2) affective processes. Inferential processes describe how observers extract information from emotional signals and use it to better assess the situation and adapt their behavior accordingly (e.g., someone is angry because I was late, so I better apologize). Affective processes refer to a direct path through which observed emotional expressions influence one's own emotional reactions (e.g., when one automatically has to laugh when another person laughs; for this reason, e.g., background laughter is used in comedy series). This process is commonly referred to as **emotional contagion** in the literature (Emotional Contagion; Hatfield et al., 1993; ► Study Box: Facial Expressions and Emotional Contagion?).

11

Study Box

Facial Expressions and Emotional Contagion?

Dimberg et al. (2000) provided evidence that people tend to imitate other people's facial expressions even if they are not conscious about what they see. The participants were shown either a happy or an angry face for only 30 ms, immediately masked by a neutral face. None of the participants could report the emotional face presented because it was not consciously perceived. Nevertheless, facial muscles (measured by facial EMG) revealed that the participants who had been presented with a happy face showed a slightly happy expression, whereas those who had been shown a slightly angry expression reacted with a slightly more angry expression.

The relative influence of whether an observed emotional expression leads to more inferential or affective processing depends on moderating circumstances, e.g., whether the observed person is in a cooperative or competitive relationship with you. Competing relationships are more likely to be related to inferential processes, whereas cooperative relationships are more likely to lead to emotional contagion (van Kleef, 2009). The predictions of the "EASI model" were tested and confirmed in a study in sport (◘ Fig. 11.4; Furley et al., 2015a). This study demonstrated that the emotional expressions of pride and shame in the context of penalty shootouts have a variety of effects on opponents and teammates.

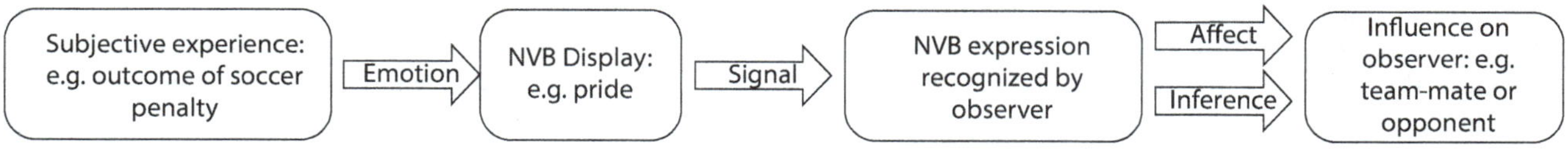

Fig. 11.4 Schematic presentation of the "EASI model" in sport following Furley et al. (2015a)

Sport Practice

Show Your Joy and Pride After a Successful Sporting Performance!

Moll et al. (2010) analyzed all penalties taken during World and European football championships. Not surprisingly, they were able to show that athletes expressed different emotional behavior depending whether a penalty was successful or not. More noteworthy was the finding that certain emotional expressions were related to the subsequent success or failure of the players and opponents. Players who expressed pride after a penalty kick increased the probability of their team winning the penalty shootout. This further increased the probability that the following competitor missed his penalty kick. More specifically, it was twice as likely that an opponent would miss his penalty if he had seen a proud emotional expression from the opposing team right before his penalty kick, compared to a player who did not celebrate his success. Although the authors of the study explain these results via the mechanism of emotional contagion, Furley et al. (2015a) pointed out that the results by Moll and colleagues are likely explained by both inferential processing (in the opponent) and emotional contagion (in teammates). An earlier study by Totterdell (2000) provided initial evidence that longer-lasting moods can also be transmitted via emotional contagion during long cricket matches and impact on a team's performance (Fig. 11.5).

Functions of Emotions

- Emotions motivate to act.
- Emotions influence information processing, decisions, and behavior.
- Current theories point to important social functions of emotions in the field of communication.
- Emotions can be "contagious."

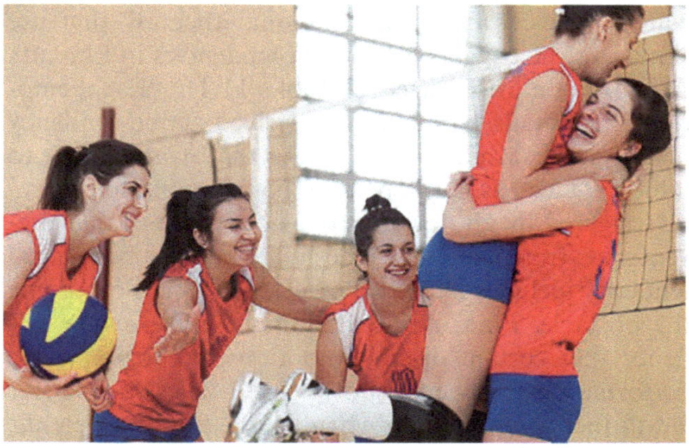

Fig. 11.5 Emotional contagion in sports

11.6 Emotions and Athletic Performance

Explaining or predicting performance in sports across situations is an exceptionally difficult task. In this regard, the emotion-performance relationship seems to be particularly complicated (see Hanin, 2000; Ruiz & Robazza, 2020). Systematic investigations on the effects of discrete emotions on specific behaviors and performance in sport are rare in the literature. Nevertheless, several meta-analyses indicate a connection between sport-related performance and emotions. However, this relationship has primarily been established for anxiety or stress and athletic performance (Craft et al., 2003; Jokela & Hanin, 1999). Since ► Chap. 12 deals with anxiety and athletic performance, anxiety is not discussed in detail here. Lazarus (2000, p. 231) criticizes that stress/anxiety research and research on emotions, in general, have been conducted in relative isolation from each other:

> Stress is important in its own right, but emotion encompasses all of the important phenomena of stress. I believe that emotions provide a far richer understanding of the adaptation struggles of human and infrahuman animals.

Few studies have tested Lazarus's "cognitive-motivational theory of emotions" (1991, 2000) in sport to approach the complex relationship between discrete emotions and specific performance (where again the majority of studies are in the area of stress and anxiety). Similar to Ekman's considerations, Lazarus assumes that discrete emotions of an athlete are associated with certain "core relational themes" that are similar to the triggers and action tendencies in Ekman's Atlas of Emotions (see ◘ Table 11.1). "Each emotion also entails a biologically derived action tendency or impulse that may be so strong that it is difficult to inhibit" (Lazarus, 2000, p. 243). For example, anger can be triggered by an obstacle (object or person) that prevents you from achieving a desired goal. The behavioral tendency includes increased muscle tension to overcome the obstacle. First, isolated studies could provide evidence that certain discrete emotions led to improved performance in specific sport-related tasks, e.g., anger led to increased strength when lifting, holding weights, or throwing (Rathschlag & Memmert, 2013; Woodman et al., 2009).

Self-Reflection

Remember personal emotional experiences in sports. Try to think of as many different emotional experiences (joy, pride, shame, anger, relief, etc.) as possible and answer the following questions as accurately as possible:

- How would you describe the trigger of the emotional experience?
- Was this experience linked to any action tendencies or thought processes? If so, to which ones?
- What else do you associate this emotional experience with?

The emotion-performance relationship in sport is moderated by interindividual appraisal styles and **coping** strategies of athletes (Hanin, 2007). For this reason, the first textbook on emotions in sport (Hanin, 2000) postulates a highly individualized approach (individual zones of optimal functioning, IZOF) for understanding emotions in sport. Twenty years later, a second textbook has been published (Ruiz & Robazza, 2021) summarizing contemporary knowledge on a wide range of emotion and emotion-related feeling states in sport through a multidisciplinary perspective. Although largely expanded and integrated, Hanin's emphasis and contribution on individual performance states, experiences, and emotion self-regulation strategies are still valid today.

? What does IZOF mean?

- Emotion-performance relationships in sport are very complex. Simple models are likely inadequate (e.g., inverted-U hypothesis, ▶ Chap. 12).
- The influence of emotions on athletic performance can only be understood as an individualized person-environment interaction.
- Person-environment interactions describe the relationship between task characteristics and the resources of a person.
- Research on emotions in sport should relate the optimal and suboptimal emotional experiences of an athlete to their successful and unsuccessful performances.
- IZOF envisages five dimensions of emotions: form, content, intensity, time, and context.
- Athletes should use their own labels to describe emotions before, during, and after competition since common measurement instruments do not include about 80% of the idiosyncratic emotion labels used by athletes (Ruiz & Hanin, 2004; Syrjä & Hanin, 1998).

11.7 Emotion Regulation

Emotion Regulation

Emotion regulation describes the process of how people influence what emotions are experienced, when they occur, and how they are experienced and expressed (Gross, 1998).

Emotion regulation can be distinguished from the term "coping," as coping is always related to a stressor and can be problem-focused or emotion-focused. Emotion regulation differs in that people regulate to a standard and, therefore, engage in regulation strategies when they perceived a discrepancy between current and desired emotions. Emotion regulation is not always stress related; people can engage in emotion regulation strategies to remain happy or try to feel happier, for example. A dominant model of emotion regulation (Gross, 1998, 2014) is the process model. In this model, there are five families of emotion regulation: (a) situation selection, (b) situation modification, (c) attention orientation, (d) modification of cognition, and (e) suppression of emotions (see Lane et al., 2012a, for a review of emotion regulation in sport).

By seeking out or avoiding certain situations, (a) people can influence their emotional experience. Athletes who feel nervous and possibly ashamed during public television interviews can influence their emotional experience, for example, by avoiding giving television interviews. However, they could also modify this situation (b) by not giving an interview immediately after a match and waiting until they have calmed down and rested. Through attention orientation (c), athletes can control which aspects of a situation they focus on. For example, if basketball players focus on the situation in which they felt they were being treated unfairly by the referee, this will have different emotional consequences than if they focus their attention on their own performance. Analogous to attention orientation, athletes can modify the cognitive assessment of a situation (d). If a handball penalty is assessed as a threat due to the chance of letting one's team down, this will probably have different emotional consequences than if the situation is assessed as a challenge in helping one's own team. All these examples illustrate how the emotional experience can be regulated at different points in time and thus lead to different emotional reactions (experience and physiological reactions) and associated behavioral tendencies. The last point of emotion suppression (e) describes how athletes can suppress emotions to regulate emotions. To return to the example of the football penalty kick, penalty shooters often show the behavioral tendency to get out of a penalty situation as quickly as possible in stressful conditions and do not take their time to prepare for the penalty kick (Furley et al., 2012b). When there is not a clear opportunity to change or modify the situation, alter attention, or think differently about the situation, and knowing this can lead to negative performance (Jordet & Hartman, 2008), penalty shooters can instruct themselves to take two deep breaths after the referee's whistle before initiating the run-up.

The different points in the emotional regulation process can be more or less automatic or controlled as well as nonconscious or conscious. Through learning processes or sport psychological interventions, conscious, controlled emotional regulation processes can be trained and become increasingly autonomous (e.g., Furley et al., 2015b). In this way, the emotional experience of a person can be intentionally changed and stabilized.

11.8 Emotional Intelligence

In the previous sections, emotions have been treated as transient states. However, it is also possible to investigate the stable aspects of an individual's emotional experience (Lazarus, 2000). The most prominent concept reflecting these relatively stable emotional characteristics has been termed **emotional intelligence (EI)**

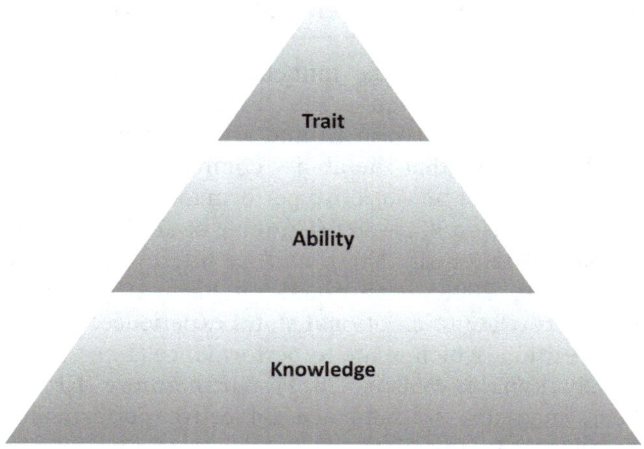

Fig. 11.6 Illustration of the "three-part model of emotional intelligence" (Nelis et al., 2009)

(Petrides & Furnham, 2003; Salovey & Mayer, 1990). Since the emergence of the concept in the 1990s, there has been much debate on EI, especially regarding the conception of EI as a trait or as an ability. The "tripartite model of EI" (Fig. 11.6) embraced the trait and ability models by assuming there are different components of EI that perform important functions: (1) a knowledge component, (2) an ability component, and, (3) trait component (Nelis et al., 2009).

> **Emotional Intelligence**
>
> **Emotional intelligence** describes the relatively stable aspects of an individual's emotional experience and actions. It is divided into knowledge, ability, and trait components. Emotional intelligence is relatively stable but can be improved via training (Laborde et al., 2021).

The **knowledge level** refers to the complexity and range of emotional knowledge. It describes the emotional knowledge of a person and how this knowledge is used to deal with emotionally charged situations.

The **ability level** refers to applying emotional knowledge in an emotional situation and using strategies for how to act. The focus here is not on what people know, but on how they can act.

The **trait level** refers to emotional dispositions, namely, the tendency to behave in a certain way in emotional situations. The focus here is not on what people know or can do, but on what they habitually do.

These three levels of EI are loosely connected: "Knowledge is not always immediately transformed into abilities, which in turn are not always put into practice" (Nelis et al., 2009, p. 36).

11.8.1 Emotional Intelligence in Sport

A review paper on the influence of EI on athletic performance (Laborde et al., 2016a) showed a positive correlation between EI and athletic performance. Studies suggest that the ability component of EI has a positive effect on objective performance criteria over an entire season in cricket (Crombie et al., 2009), basketball (Zizzi et al., 2003), and ice hockey (Perlini & Halverson, 2006). Emotional intelligence has been found to relate to emotional states experienced before competition, which relate to performance (Lane et al., 2012b; Lane & Wilson, 2011). Furthermore, EI has been suggested to influence subjective performance happiness. In this context, stress perception, coping strategies, and the assessment of situations as challenging rather than threatening were identified as mechanisms (Laborde et al., 2014a). Moreover, EI is found to make people more resistant to pressure and severe stress. Athletes with a high trait EI were able to perform better under pressure by using more efficient coping strategies (Laborde et al., 2012) and were found to have superior physiological stress resistance (Laborde et al., 2011, 2014b, 2015b).

11

EI is important not only for athletes but also for coaches (Hopkins et al., 2011; Thelwell et al., 2008). In general, coaches with higher EI have been shown to coach more effectively, for example, by exhibiting a more efficient management style and by paying more attention to athletes' needs.

With regard to physical activity and exercise, a positive relationship between trait EI and an active lifestyle has been documented, which has significant benefits for both **health and well-being**. Trait EI is believed to promote an active lifestyle through motivational mechanisms that play a role in initiating and maintaining physical activity behavior (Saklofske et al., 2007a,b; Solanki & Lane, 2010). Consequently, trait EI goes hand in hand with an active and healthy personality (Laborde et al., 2017).

11.8.2 Training of EI in and Through Sport

EI training has already been implemented in a variety of sports including cricket (Crombie et al., 2011), netball (Barlow & Banks, 2014), and rugby (Campo et al., 2016). An overview article on EI training (Campo et al., 2015) recommends that successful EI training should ideally be based on the tripartite model of EI (Nelis et al., 2009). The organization of such training aims to increase both the emotional knowledge and ability component to initiate changes at the trait level of EI. Successful EI training programs have demonstrated positive long-term consequences on the psychological and physiological level (Kotsou et al., 2011; Nelis et al., 2011).

Emotional Intelligence
- EI describes how a person deals with emotions in different situations.
- EI is subdivided into a knowledge, ability, and trait level.
- EI has a positive influence on athletes and coaches in sports and exercise.
- EI can be trained.

11.9 Measurement of Emotions and Emotional Intelligence

11.9.1 Measurement of Emotions

The controversies in emotion research addressed in the introduction are particularly evident in the scientific investigation and measurement of emotions. As a result, no standard paradigm for the investigation and measurement of emotions has been established so far.

Why is the scientific study of emotions a real challenge?

A quotation from Alan Fridlund vividly illustrates the problem (Beck, 2015): "At the heart of 'emotion' is the experience of emotion, and this can't be measured. Recorded, maybe, but not measured. This leaves scientists studying 'emotion' trying instead to measure everything around it."
- Emotions are multidimensional **constructs**.
- Exploring them requires a **multi-methodological approach**.
- Inducing emotions under standardized conditions is a challenge.
- Intense emotional states are ethically hardly feasible in the laboratory.

11.9.1.1 Inducing Emotions

Different approaches have been used in emotion research to induce and investigate emotional states (Table 11.2; Coan & Allen, 2007; Quigley et al., 2014; for overviews; Wetherell et al., 2018, for an overview of techniques of inducing stress).

Table 11.2 Selected emotion induction techniques (based on Quigley et al., 2014)

Method	Stimulus material and references	Advantages	Disadvantages
Images	Bradley et al. (2001) International Affective Picture System (IAPS) (Lang et al., 2008)	Easy presentation Economical	Do not include all emotions or are not suitable for all
Videos	Gross and Levenson (1995) Philippot (1993) Schaefer et al. (2010)	Easy presentation Economical More emotional information compared to pictures	Familiarity of the content can cause variability
Faces	Ekman and Friesen (1978) Matsumoto and Ekman (1988) Beaupré and Hess (2005)	Easy presentation Economical Faces have high emotional valence	Not clear whether faces trigger emotions or activate concepts
Sounds/voices	IADS (Bradley & Lang, 2007) Bliss-Moreau et al. (2010) Simon-Thomas et al. (2009)	Easy presentation Economical	Not well researched whether emotions are actually induced
Music	Eich and Metcalfe (1989)	Easy presentation Can preserve emotional states over a long period	Not suitable to evoke discrete emotions (rather valence)
Words	Bradley and Lang (1999) Stevenson et al. (2007)	Simple presentation Relatively low effect strength	Not clear whether words trigger emotions or activate concepts
Imagination techniques and recall	Wilson-Mendenhall et al. (2011) Olatunji et al. (2009) Velten (1968) Carter et al. (2002)	External validity Can be ideographically manipulated	Great interindividual variability in ability of imagination
Movement and posture: facial (body) feedback paradigm	Strack et al. (1988) Duclos et al. (1989) Stepper and Strack (1993)	Relatively implicit method to induce emotions	Needs good cover story to avoid demand effects
Staged interactions	Cohen et al. (1996) DeSteno et al. (2006)	External validity	Complicated Needs good cover story and actors
In situ observation and motivated performance tasks	TSST (Kirschbaum et al., 1993) Akinola and Mendes (2008) Teachman (2007) Castanier et al. (2011)	External validity	Complicated Expensive Ethical concerns
Virtual reality	Riva et al. (2007)	External validity in combination with experimental control	Complicated Expensive
Physiological and pharmacological manipulation	z.B. epinephrine-injections (Schachter & Singer, 1962) Oxytocin injections (Norman et al., 2011) Sport (Ekkekakis et al., 2011)	High impact	Medical expertise needed Expensive Ethical concerns Needs good cover story

This list represents measures from the entire scientific spectrum. The sports reference is made in the measurement section

How can emotions be induced and investigated?
- Presentation of standardized stimuli material with validated emotional content (pictures, films, faces, sounds/voices, music, words)
- Imagination techniques and memories
- Movement and posture: facial (bodily) feedback paradigm
- Staged interactions
- In situ observation and motivated performance tasks
- Virtual reality
- Physiological (e.g., sports) and pharmacological (e.g., drugs) manipulation

11.9.1.2 Measuring Induced States

Depending on the author, there are substantial differences in how many dimensions should be distinguished in the measurement of emotions. According to Scherer (2005), there are five dimensions of emotions: cognitive, neuropsychological, motivational, motor-expressive, and subjective emotional component (◘ Fig. 11.7).

It is important to note that the various components of emotions can function separately from one another (Scherer, 2005). It is therefore advisable to measure several components at the same time (Mauss & Robinson, 2009). It should be emphasized, however, that the assessment of all the different components is difficult to realize and therefore this should not be made a standard procedure. We aim to inform sports scientists and sport psychologists about the possibilities of measuring different emotional components so that they can make an informed choice about appropriate measurement tools to answer their research question.

▪ Cognitive Component

The cognitive component refers to the appraisal of objects, events, and situations. To evaluate the cognitive assessment component, a contemporary questionnaire in sport, the "precompetitive appraisal measure" (PAM; Wolf et al., 2015), was developed. The PAM is based on the "cognitive-motivational-relational theory" (Lazarus, 1999) and records the primary (How do I assess the situation?) and secondary assessment processes (How do I assess my resources to cope with the situation?) of a person. It aims to determine what generates precompetitive emotions.

▪ Neurophysiological Component

The most important neurophysiological parameters related to emotions and athletic performance are electrodermal activity, heart rate, heart rate variability, hormone concentrations, and brain measurements. The collection of neurophysiological parameters in sport can be problematic, since these parameters change not only in relation to emotions but also in relation to movement and physical activity.

▪▪ Electrodermal Activity

The electrodermal activity of the skin coincides with affective, motivational, and attention processes of the central nervous system (LaCaille et al., 2013). The electrodermal activity of the skin can be divided into a tonic and a phasic category.

The tonic value of skin resistance (also known as conductance) is the absolute degree of resistance or conductance at a given moment in the absence of a measurable phasic reaction. This value is known as skin conductance. In tonic measurements, rest conditions prevail, whereas in phasic measurements, certain stimuli are used to induce activation in the subject (Dawson et al., 2000).

Electrodermal activity is used as an indicator of arousal (intensity), but not of the valence of the emotion. The skin conductance response correlates positively with emotional arousal regardless of valence (Bradley & Lang, 2000). It is assumed that the skin conductance response is regulated exclusively by the sympathetic nervous system (Venables & Christie, 1980). The sympathetic innervations of the sweat glands induce changes in skin conductivity (Gutrecht, 1994), which is associated with emotional arousal in a variety of situations (Dawson et al., 2000). In sports, skin conductance response has rarely been used as a measure of emotion, as it is strongly associated with physical activity (for exceptions, see Collet et al., 2003; Rada et al., 1995).

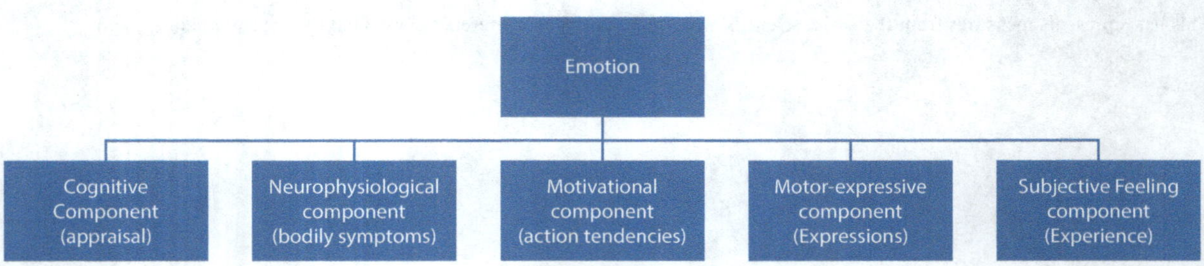

◘ **Fig. 11.7** The five relevant components for measuring emotions according to Scherer (2005)

Heart Rate

To a certain extent, **heart rate** can indicate the valence and intensity of an emotion. Bradley and Lang (2000) demonstrated that emotional images led to systematic changes in the classic three-phase pattern—an initial delay, an acceleration component, and a secondary delay—of heart rate. More specifically, it was shown that affective valence contributed to the extent of initial deceleration and acceleration activity, with unpleasant stimuli producing a stronger initial deceleration and pleasant stimuli producing a stronger peak acceleration.

There are however many other variables that influence heart rate, such as posture, breathing, and physical constitution. These variables may obscure an affective influence on heart rate (Bradley & Lang, 2000). Nevertheless, it might be possible to measure the effect of affective valence on heart rate when the processing context is appropriately controlled. Although physical activity complicates the interpretation of heart rate as an emotional indicator in sport, some studies in sport have demonstrated association between heart rate and anxiety in climbing (Oudejans & Pijpers, 2010) and gymnastics (Tremayne & Barry, 1988).

Heart Rate Variability

Heart rate variability (HRV) can be calculated from the time intervals between the R-R peaks of the ECG. HRV is never constant but varies from beat to beat and corresponds to the variability of RR intervals (i.e., intervals between successive R-R peaks; Niskanen et al., 2004).

HRV reflects the interaction between the sympathetic and parasympathetic branches of the autonomic nervous system (Malik, 1996). Both sympathetic and parasympathetic branches of the autonomic nervous system are involved in emotions (Levenson, 2003); therefore, HRV can be considered an objective measure of emotional response (Appelhans & Luecken, 2006). Of the two branches, HRV can only indicate the activity of the parasympathetic nervous system regulating cardiac functioning, also known as cardiac vagal activity (Malik, 1996). This is of particular interest for the sports domain since it has been postulated that resting cardiac vagal activity has a positive relationship to cognitive functions, emotion regulation, and health according to the "neurovisceral integration model" (Thayer et al., 2009).

In sport, athletes who show a lower decrease in cardiac vagal activity under pressure show better decision-making performance (Laborde & Raab, 2013; Laborde et al., 2014c) and memory performance (Laborde et al., 2015a), which is consistent with the "neurovisceral integration model" (Thayer et al., 2009). Emotional intelligence has also been associated with higher resting cardiac vagal activity and lower cardiac vagal activity reduction under pressure (Laborde et al., 2011, 2015b), which is indicative of a biological basis of more adaptive emotional dispositions.

Hormonal Measurement

Measurement of **hormones,** in particular cortisol, can serve as indicators of anxiety or stress (Denson et al., 2009a, 2009b). **Cortisol** measurement in saliva is particularly helpful because it is noninvasive, painless, and thus ethically justifiable. It can be carried out without medical expertise (Kirschbaum & Hellhammer, 2000).

In athletic competition, an increase in cortisol levels often coincides with an individual's stress experience (Filaire et al., 1996, 1999, 2001). Research has, for example, shown that the closer a competitive encounter approaches, the higher the cortisol level is (Strahler et al., 2010). The cortisol response of athletes to stressful encounters has been shown to be less important at the highest-performance level compared to low-performance levels (Moya-Albiol et al., 2001). However, a growing number of studies suggests that there is a negative correlation between cortisol and athletic performance (Lautenbach et al., 2014, 2015a, 2015b).

Measurement of Brain Activity

Measurements of brain activity are a promising new development in the field of emotion and performance (see Bertollo et al., 2020, for a recent overview). In sports, for example, **functional magnetic resonance imaging (fMRI)** has been used to investigate the effect of cognitive interventions on coping with sports failure at the neurophysiological level (Davis et al., 2008). A further study combined fMRI with neuroendocrine measurements to investigate the correlates of neuronal activation with cortisol and testosterone (Davis et al., 2012). A challenge for researchers is adapting athletic emotional tasks to the particularities of fMRI (Daamen & Raab, 2012) since a large number of observations is required to derive reliable brain activation patterns.

Another method for measuring brain activity with a higher time resolution is **electroencephalography (EEG)**. Although electroencephalography has been extensively used in sports to study attention processes (e.g., Sanchez-Lopez et al., 2016), this method has rarely been used to study emotional processes in sports and needs to be further established (for an exception, see Ring et al., 2016).

First studies suggest that neurofeedback may be a useful applied tool to improve performance under pressure (Ring et al., 2014). The development of mobile EEG methods might provide a promising perspective to improve the understanding of emotions in sports (Park et al., 2015).

■ Motivational Component

The motivational component within the measurement of emotions reflects the action tendencies associated with discrete emotions (Ekman & Cordaro, 2011; Lazarus, 2000). The motivational component can affect behavior by interrupting or inhibiting current behavior and generating new goals and plans (Scherer, 2005). The motivational component of emotions is based on circuits in the brain that respond to appetitive and aversive stimuli (Lang & Bradley, 2010). Most commonly the motivational component is assessed via self-report or behavioral observation. Another possibility to investigate the motivational component of emotions is the use of EEG and event-related potentials. This method has been used, for example, to demonstrate the influence of emotions on risk preference and outcome assessment during a decision task (Zhao et al., 2016).

■ Motor-Expressive Component

According to Bradley and Lang (2000), behavioral events can be assessed either by direct actions (e.g., emotional expressions, approach, avoidance, flight, attack, defensive reflexes) or indirect indicators (e.g., response latency, amplitude; ► Study Box: Winning Athletes Show Discrete Emotional Expression After a Triumph).

Study Box

Winning Athletes Show Discrete Emotional Expression After a Triumph

Matsumoto and Hwang (2012) recorded the spontaneous reactions of successful judoka at the 2004 Olympics. Detailed evaluation of the nonverbal behaviors of the athletes showed that the emotional expressions after success or failure were different from known emotional expressions like pride. This was confirmed in a second study where trained coders evaluated the behavior. The authors argued that certain expressions of superiority and triumph have developed over the course of evolution (◘ Fig. 11.8), which help to establish status and dominance in social groups and thus establish hierarchies. This line of argumentation was further confirmed by the finding that the expressions of superiority and triumph were also shown by athletes at the Paralympics who were blind from birth and therefore could not have learned these expressions (Tracy & Matsumoto, 2008).

11

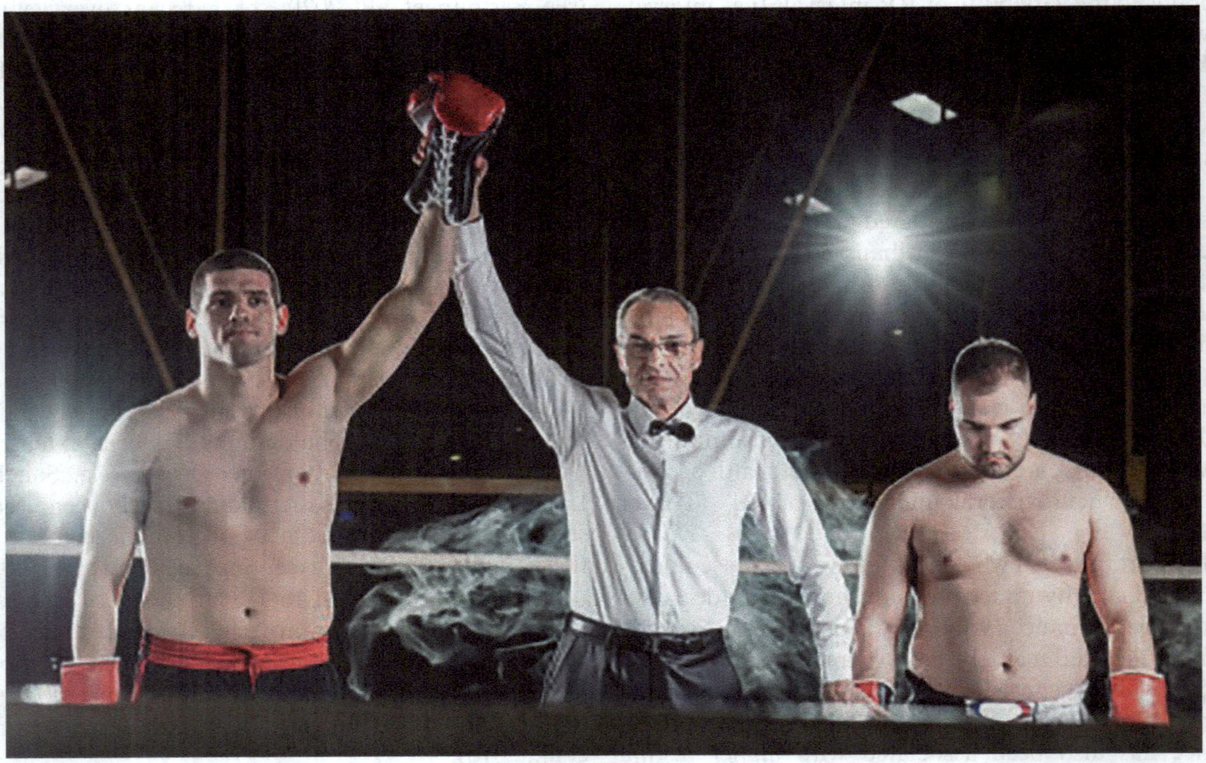

◘ **Fig. 11.8** Athletes show a discrete emotional expression after a success

The effects of emotions on muscle activity and movement behavior can be evaluated by controlled monitoring of changes in movement patterns and muscle tension (Pijpers et al., 2003, 2005). These studies show that it is possible to use electromyographic data to assess qualitative differences in muscle tension and movement patterns as a function of emotional state. It has also been shown that emotions influence the speed and initiation time of targeted movements (Beatty et al., 2016).

The influence of emotions on physical performance was demonstrated in various sport-related tasks, such as the strength of the finger muscles, jump height of a countermovement jump, the speed of a thrown ball (Rathschlag & Memmert, 2013), and sprint performance (Rathschlag & Memmert, 2014; ◘ Fig. 11.9). Furthermore, it has been demonstrated that changes in performance under pressure are mediated by emotionally induced changes in muscle activity and kinematic parameters (Cooke et al., 2010; ► Side Story: What Do Movements Say About Emotions in Sport?).

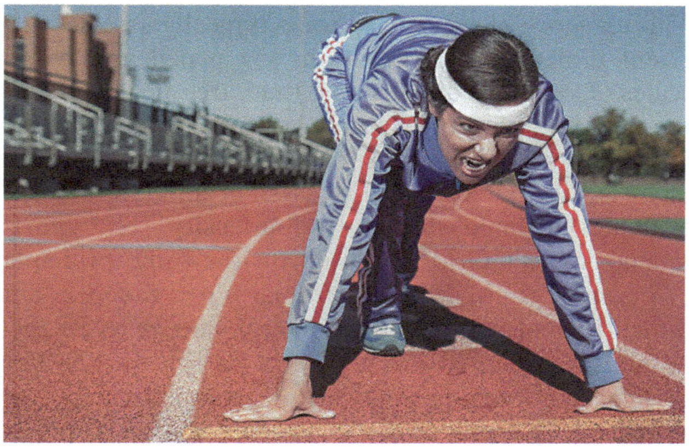

◘ **Fig. 11.9** Emotions can influence sprint performance, for example (Rathschlag & Memmert, 2014)

Side Story

What Do Movements Say About Emotions in Sport?
Motion recordings can make an important contribution to the analysis of the motor component of emotions in sports, even though there is a controversial discussion about whether it is possible to reliably draw conclusions about emotional states based on movement (Castellano et al., 2007). First studies show that it is possible to identify discrete emotions through movement (Li et al., 2016; Vernazza-Martin et al., 2015, ◘ Fig. 11.10).

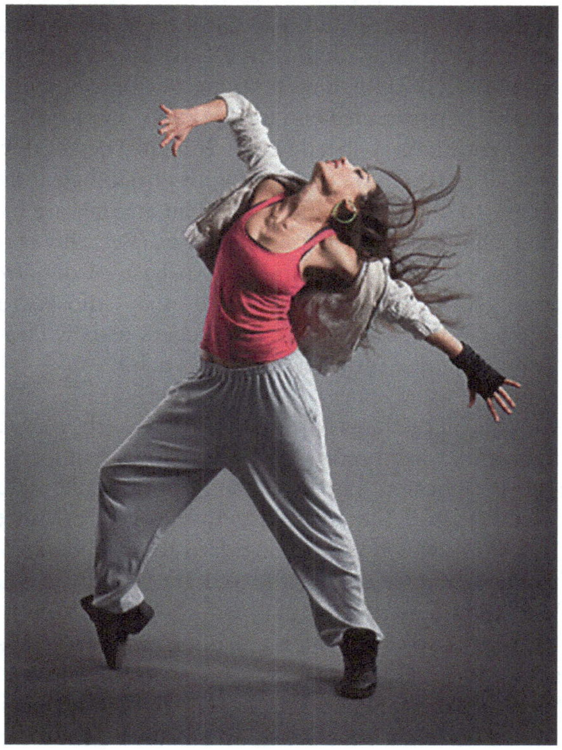

◘ **Fig. 11.10** Expression of emotions in sports

Subjective Emotional Component

There are two main methods for obtaining self-evaluations of emotional experiences: the discrete emotion approach and the dimensions approach (Scherer, 2005).

Discrete Emotions

There are two approaches for measuring discrete emotions: individualized (**idiosyncratic**) and group-oriented (**nomothetic**).

Idiosyncratic The individualized approach was initiated by the work of Hanin and his colleagues with the IZOF (Hanin, 2000; Jokela & Hanin, 1999). An individualized approach allows scientists to get closer to the experienced emotions of athletes and to grasp their idiosyncratic nature for each individual athlete. To allow for group analysis of IZOF data, a method has been proposed that combines performance-enhancing and performance-reducing emotions (Laborde et al., 2016b). The IZOF was further developed and combined with physiological measurements to allow predictions of when athletes are in an optimal emotional performance range (Bertollo et al., 2012). Since theory testing and the synthesis of data from different studies is difficult with this idiosyncratic approach (Jones et al., 2005), researchers usually choose the group-oriented (nomothetic) approach.

Nomothetic For the group-oriented approach, there are several standardized sport-specific measures that focus on one specific emotion, e.g., fear. These, for example, include the "Competitive State Anxiety Inventory-2" (Martens et al., 1990b), which has been revised to an updated version (Martinent et al., 2010), and the "Sport Anxiety Scale-2" (Smith et al., 2006).

Non-sport-specific scales are often used to assess a broader range of affective states: the Profile of Mood States (POMS; McNair et al., 1971; although it refers to moods rather than emotions), the Brunel Mood Scale (BRUMS: Terry et al., 2003), and the Positive Affect and Negative Affect Schedule (PANAS; Watson et al., 1988). The POMS and BRUMS assess anger, tension, depression, fatigue, confusion, tension, and vigour.

Even though the POMS and the PANAS have been used in athletic contexts, they were not designed to assess emotions in sport. Therefore, the sport-specific questionnaire "Sport Emotion Questionnaire" (SEQ: Jones et al., 2005) was developed. It contains 22 emotion adjectives from five different dimensions (anger, anxiety, dejection, excitement, and happiness) and has been validated to measure emotions before a competition. The SEQ correlates very closely to the BRUMS, and the resultant measure was very similar to the model developed initially for clinical use. As emotions are universal, one might wonder why specific emotions might arise in certain contexts, and rather than seek different emotions, it is more reasonable to expect the intensity of emotions to vary by context. Thus we expect anxiety to be high before competition and low after competition. Further instruments measuring emotion-related feelings in sport ("Psychobiosocial States Scale, Trait Version", PBS-ST, and Psychobiosocial Experience Semantic Differential scale in sport, PESD-Sport) were developed by Robazza et al. (2016, 2021; see Ruiz et al., 2019, for a state version of the questionnaire).

The Competitive Aggressiveness and Anger Scale (CAAS; Maxwell & Moores, 2007) was used to reveal correlations between certain emotions and illegal aggressive behavior in rugby (Maxwell & Visek, 2009). In addition, picture tests have been used to measure people's attitudes toward participating in physically and emotionally challenging tasks in physical education (Bortoli & Robazza, 1994) and high-risk sports (Robazza et al., 2006; ◘ Fig. 11.11).

Dimensional Approach

This category of measuring tools typically assesses different dimensions of emotions via pencil and paper scales. Common dimensions that are measured are the **hedonic valence** (pleasant vs. unpleasant) and the activation level (i.e., arousal). A frequently used instrument is the "Affect Grid" (Russell et al., 1989) which evaluates **hedonic valence** and **intensity**. The sport-related "Affect Grid" is based on the same principle (Woodman et al., 2009). It evaluates two independent dimensions of affect: activation and valence (pleasantness). It is presented as a 9 × 9 grid (◘ Fig. 11.12): The vertical axis evaluates activation (from extremely low to extremely high), and the horizontal axis evaluates hedonic valence (from unpleasant feeling to pleasant feeling).

Another popular instrument is the "activation-deactivation checklist" (Thayer, 1989). It records the activation dimension and was used to assess affective sensation after physical activity (Ekkekakis et al., 2005). The "Affect Scale" (Hardy & Rejeski, 1989) is a bipolar evaluation scale used to assess emotional reactions during training.

The "Visual Analog Scale" is a biaxial orthogonal grid (200 mm axes with the poles "not at all" and "very much") that has been used to measure the arousal and hedonic valence dimensions. The scale is frequently used as a quick and effective measure to control emotional manipulations (Davis et al., 2010).

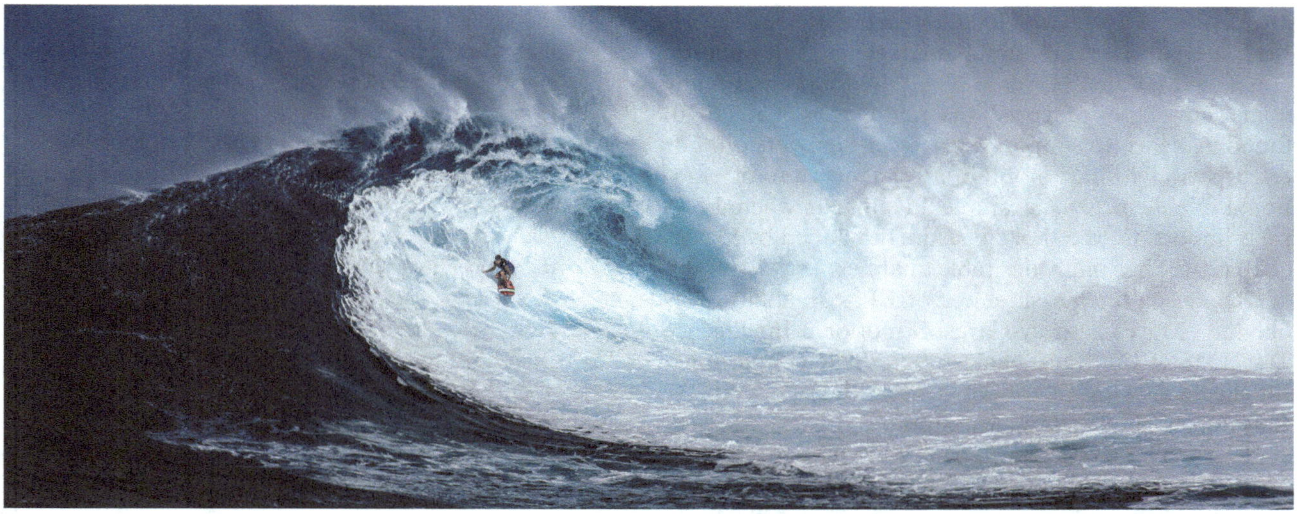

Fig. 11.11 In big wave surfing, the athletes expose themselves to an enormous risk

Fig. 11.12 "Sport Affect Grid." Participants are asked to mark a section of the grid with an X that represents the current emotional state. The score for activation and the hedonic valence of feelings are calculated separately by converting the position of the X on each axis to a value from 1 to 9 (Woodman et al., 2009)

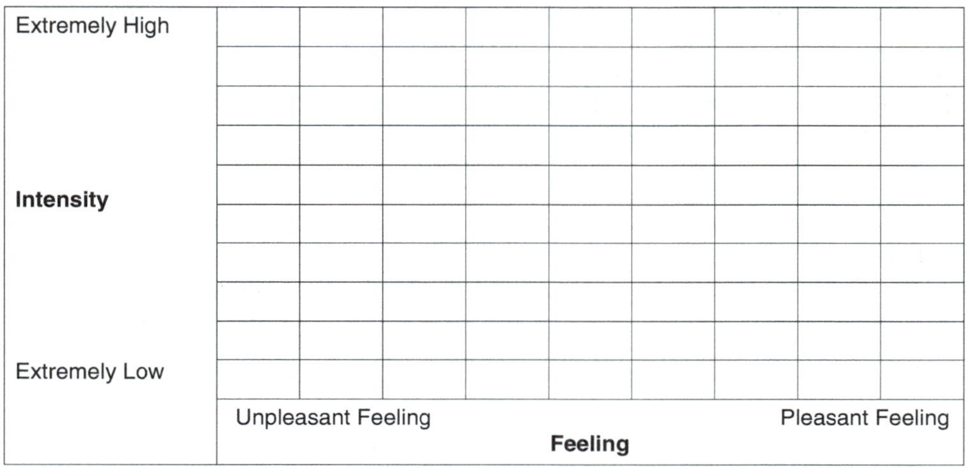

In general, dimensional measures provide less information than inventories assessing discrete emotions but can be helpful for quick affective assessments.

Measuring Emotions

Measuring emotions is complex. The following indicators provide information about a person's emotional states:

- Cognitive component
- Neuropsychological component
- Motivational component
- Motor-expressive component
- Subjective emotional component

11.9.2 Measuring Emotional Intelligence

Emotional intelligence as a **personality trait** is usually measured with personality questionnaires, while EI as an ability is measured with emotional intelligence tests (Petrides, 2009a). Regarding the measurement of EI as a personality trait, nine different questionnaires have been used in the sport context (Laborde et al., 2016a). A full description of all these questionnaires is beyond the scope of this chapter, so we will limit ourselves here to the description of the emotional intelligence questionnaire (Petrides, 2009b).

This questionnaire shows the best psychometric properties (Petrides, 2009a) and the highest external validity. Furthermore, the questionnaire showed associations with physiological and hormonal responses (Laborde et al., 2011, 2014a, 2014b, 2014c, 2015a, 2015b). The questionnaire contains 153 terms that can be used to calculate 15 subscales included in 4 factors (i.e., well-being, self-control, emotionality, and sociability) and a global EI score. This factor structure has been replicated using a sample of sportsmen and women (Laborde et al. 2014a, 2014b, 2014c).

In sport, Lane et al. (2009) examined the validity of the frequently used emotional intelligence scale (Schutte et al., 1998). Lane, Meyer et al. (2009) found that many items showed poor face validity, and Davies et al. (2010) found evidence to support a brief ten-item version. For researchers wishing to obtain a brief measure of emotional intelligence, for example, in contexts where brevity is important, the short measure developed by Davies et al. (2010) has many desirable qualities.

Regarding the measurement of EI as an ability, tests like the "Mayer-Salovey-Caruso Emotional Intelligence Test" (MSCEIT; Mayer et al., 2002), "Test of Emotional Intelligence" (TEMINT; Blickle et al., 2011), and "Ability Emotional Intelligence Measure" (AEIM; Warwick et al., 2010) have been developed (Warwick et al., 2010).

The MSCEIT is the most commonly used ability EI test and the only one used in sport (Crombie et al., 2009, 2011). It evaluates four emotional dimensions: the ability (1) to perceive emotions, (2) to use emotions to facilitate thoughts, (3) to understand emotions, and (4) to control emotions. The four dimensions are assessed with 141 items. Although this measure has been criticized (Fiori et al., 2014), it currently represents the most widely used measure in the field of sport.

Learning Control Questions

Basic:

1. What is an emotion? How does an emotion differ from a mood?
2. What is the main statement of Darwin's "theory of emotional expression" and why are emotional expressions central to understanding emotions?
3. What are the findings on Darwin's theoretical assumptions in sport? Describe them and discuss their significance for sport practice.
4. What do the studies dealing with emotional expressions say about the influence of nature and nurture in the field of emotions?
5. What does facial feedback mean? Discuss the significance of these findings for emotional experience and behavior.

Advanced:

6. Describe Ekman's "neurocultural theory of emotions" in your own words.
7. What is meant by characterizing emotions as universal?
8. What emotions are described as universal/basic? Describe their assumed function, states, triggers, behavioral tendencies, and associated moods.
9. Describe the most important anatomical structures and the associated physiological processes related to emotions.
10. How are emotional physiological processes related to information processing, decision-making, and behavior?
11. Name the three theoretical approaches to describe the connection between physiology and emotional experience.
12. How does the discrete emotion approach differ from the dimensional approach? What are the arguments for the discrete emotion approach?
13. What are the functions of emotions?
14. Which findings support the interpersonal functions of emotions?

Experts:

15. Describe the "EASI model" and discuss the significance of the model for sports.
16. What is the relationship between emotions and sports performance? Outline key assumptions and findings.
17. What are the five aspects that can be addressed by emotion regulation?
18. What is emotional intelligence? What is the relationship between emotional intelligence and sports performance?
19. List different ways to induce emotions.
20. Which dimensions can be distinguished when measuring emotions in sport?

References

Adelmann, P. K., & Zajonc, R. B. (1989). Facial efference and the experience of emotion. *Annual Review of Psychology, 40*, 249–280.

Akinola, M., & Mendes, W. B. (2008). The dark side of creativity: Biological vulnerability and negative emotions lead to greater artistic creativity. *Personality and Social Psychology Bulletin, 34*, 1677–1686.

Appelhans, B. M., & Luecken, L. J. (2006). Heart rate variability as an index of regulated emotional responding. *Review of General Psychology, 10*, 229–240. https://doi.org/10.1037/1089-2680.10.3.229

Barlow, A., & Banks, A. P. (2014). Using emotional intelligence in coaching high-performance athletes: A randomised controlled trial. *Coaching: An International Journal of Theory, Research and Practice, 7*, 132–139. https://doi.org/10.1080/17521882.2014.939679

Beatty, G. F., Cranley, N. M., Carnaby, G., & Janelle, C. M. (2016). Emotions predictably modify response times in the initiation of human motor actions: A meta-analytic review. *Emotion, 16*(2), 237–251. https://doi.org/10.1037/emo0000115

Beaupré, M. G., & Hess, U. (2005). Cross-cultural emotion recognition among Canadian ethnic groups. *Journal of Cross-Cultural Psychology, 36*, 355–370.

Beck, J. (2015). Hard feelings: Science's struggle to define emotions. The Atlantic. Retrieved from http://www.theatlantic.com.

Bertollo, M., Doppelmayr, M., & Robazza, C. (2020). Using brain technologies in practice. In G. Tenenbaum & R. C. Eklund (Eds.), *Handbook of sport psychology* (4th ed., pp. 666–693). Wiley. https://doi.org/10.1002/9781119568124.ch32

Bertollo, M., Robazza, C., Falasca, W. N., Stocchi, M., Babiloni, C., Del Percio, C., et al. (2012). Temporal pattern of pre-shooting psycho-physiological states in elite athletes: A probabilistic approach. *Psychology of Sport and Exercise, 13*, 91–98. https://doi.org/10.1016/j.psychsport.2011.09.005

Blickle, G., Momm, T., Liu, Y., Witzki, A., & Steinmayr, R. (2011). Construct Validation of the Test of Emotional Intelligence (TEMINT). *European Journal of Psychological Assessment, 27*, 282–289. https://doi.org/10.1027/1015-5759/a000075

Bliss-Moreau, E., Owren, M. J., & Barrett, L. F. (2010). I like the sound of your voice: Affective learning about vocal signals. *Journal of Experimental Social Psychology, 46*, 557–563.

Booth, A., Shelley, G., Mazur, A., Tharp, G., & Kittok, R. (1989). Testosterone and winning and losing in human competition. *Hormones and Behavior, 23*, 556–571.

Bortoli, L., & Robazza, C. (1994). The motor activity anxiety test. *Perceptual & Motor Skills, 79*(1 Part 1), 299–305.

Bower, G. H. (1981). Mood and memory. *American Psychologist, 36*, 129–148.

Bower, G. H. (1991a). Mood congruity of social judgments. *Emotion and Social Judgments*, 31–53.

Bower, G. H. (1991b). Mood congruity of social judgments. In J. P. Forgas (Ed.), *Emotion and social judgments* (pp. 31–53). Pergamon Press.

Bradley, M. M., & Lang, P. J. (1999). Affective norms for English words (ANEW): Instruction manual and affective ratings. University of Florida: The Center for Research in Psychophysiology.

Bradley, M. M., & Lang, P. J. (2000). Measuring emotion: Behavior, feeling and physiology. In R. Lane & L. Nadel (Eds.), *Cognitive neuroscience of emotion* (pp. 242–276). Oxford University Press.

Bradley, M. M., & Lang, P. J. (2007). *The International Affective Digitized Sounds (2nd Edition; IADS-2): Affective ratings of sounds and instruction manual.* University of Florida.

Bradley, M. M., Codispoti, M., Cuthbert, B. N., & Lang, P. J. (2001). Emotion and motivation I: Defensive and appetitive reactions in picture processing. *Emotion, 1*, 276–298.

Budden, T. J. H., Jackson, B., & Dimmock, J. A. (2020). Self-efficacy. In D. Hackfort & R. J. Schinke (Eds.), *The Routledge international encyclopedia of sport and exercise psychology* (Theoretical and methodological concepts) (Vol. 1, pp. 584–594). Routledge.

Campo, M., Laborde, S., & Mosley, E. (2016). Emotional intelligence training in team sports. *Journal of Individual Differences, 37*(3), 152–158. https://doi.org/10.1027/1614-0001/a000201

Campo, M., Laborde, S., & Weckemann, S. (2015). Emotional Intelligence training: Implications for performance and health. In A. M. Colombus (Ed.), *Advances in psychology research* (pp. 75–92). Nova Publishers.

Camras, L. A. (1992). Expressive development and basic emotions. *Cognition & Emotion, 6*, 269–283.

Camras, L. A., Oster, H., Campos, J. J., Miyake, K., & Bradshaw, D. (1992). Japanese and American infants' responses to arm restraint. *Developmental Psychology, 28*, 578–583.

Camras, L. A., Oster, H., Campos, J., Campos, R., Ujiie, T., Miyake, K., Wang, L., & Meng, Z. (1998). Production of emotional facial expressions in European American, Japanese, and Chinese infants. *Developmental Psychology, 34*, 616–628.

Carter, L. E., McNeil, D. W., Vowles, K. E., Sorrell, J. T., Turk, C. L., Ries, B. J., & Hopko, D. R. (2002). Effects of emotion on pain reports, tolerance and physiology. *Pain Research & Management, 7*, 21–30.

Castanier, C., LeScanff, C., & Woodman, T. (2011). Mountaineering as affect regulation: The moderating role of self-regulation strategies. *Anxiety, Stress, and Coping, 24*, 75–81.

Castellano, G., Villalba, S. D., & Camurri, A. (2007). Recognising human emotions from body movement and gesture dynamics. In A. C. R. Paiva, R. Prada, & R. W. Picard (Eds.), *Affective computing and intelligent interaction: Lecture notes in computer science* (Vol. 4738, pp. 71–82). https://doi.org/10.1007/978-3-540-74889-2_7

Coan, J. A., & Allen, J. J. B. (Eds.). (2007). *Handbook of emotion elicitation and assessment* (Vol. 13). Oxford University Press.

Cohen, D., Nisbett, R. E., Bowdle, B. F., & Schwarz, N. (1996). Insult, aggression, and the southern culture of honor: An "experimental ethnography". *Journal of Personality and Social Psychology, 70*, 945–960.

Collet, C., Guillot, A., Bolliet, O., Delhomme, G., & Dittmar, A. (2003). Correlats neurophysiologiques des processus mentaux enregistres en situation reelle par micro-capteurs non invasifs [Neurophysiological correlates of mental processes through non invasive micro-sensors recording in the field]. *Science & Sports, 18*, 74–85. https://doi.org/10.1016/S0765-1597(03)00081-9

Cooke, A., Kavussanu, M., McIntyre, D., & Ring, C. (2010). Psychological, muscular and kinematic factors mediate performance under pressure. *Psychophysiology, 47*, 1109–1118. https://doi.org/10.1111/j.1469-8986.2010.01021.x

Cowen, A. S., & Keltner, D. (2017). Self-report captures 27 distinct categories of emotion bridged by continuous gradients. *Proceedings of the National Academy of Sciences, 114*, E7900–E7909. https://doi.org/10.1073/pnas.1702247114

Cozolino, L. (2006). *The neuroscience of human relationships: Attachment and the developing social brain.* WW Norton & Co.

Craft, L. L., Magyar, T. M., Becker, B. J., & Feltz, D. L. (2003). The relationship between the Competitive State Anxiety Inventory-2 and sport performance: A meta-analysis. *Journal of Sport & Exercise Psychology, 25*, 44–65.

Crivelli, C., & Fridlund, A. J. (2018). Facial Displays Are Tools for Social Influence. Trends in cognitive sciences, 22(5), 388–399. https://doi.org/10.1016/j.tics.2018.02.006.

Crombie, D., Lombard, C., & Noakes, T. D. (2009). Emotional intelligence scores predict team sports performance in a national cricket competition. *International Journal of Sports Science & Coaching, 4*, 209–224. https://doi.org/10.1260/174795409788549544

Crombie, D., Lombard, C., & Noakes, T. D. (2011). Increasing emotional intelligence in cricketers: An intervention study. *International Journal of Sports Science & Coaching, 6*, 69–86.

Daamen, M., & Raab, M. (2012). Psychological assessments in physical exercise functional neuroimaging in exercise and sport sciences.

Damasio, A. R. (1994). *Descartes' error: Emotion, reason, and the human brain*. Vintage.

Darwin, C. (1998). *The expression of the emotions in man and animals* (3rd ed.). John Murray. (Original work published 1872).

Davidson, R. J., Jackson, D. C., & Kalin, N. H. (2000). Emotion, plasticity, context, and regulation: Perspectives from affective neuroscience. *Psychological Bulletin, 126*, 890–909.

Davies, K., Lane, A. M., Devonport, T., & Scott, J. (2010). Validity and reliability of a Brief Emotional Intelligence Scale: The BEIS-10. *Journal of Individual Differences, 31*, 198–208.

Davis, H., Liotti, M., Ngan, E. T., Woodward, T. S., Snellenberg, J. X., Anders, S. M., et al. (2008). fMRI BOLD signal changes in elite swimmers while viewing videos of personal failure. *Brain*

Imaging and Behavior, 2, 84–93. https://doi.org/10.1007/s11682-007-9016-x

Davis, H., van Anders, S., Ngan, E., Woodward, T. S., Snellenberg, J. X. V., Mayberg, H. S., & Liotti, M. (2012). Neural, mood, and endocrine responses in elite athletes relative to successful and failed performance videos. *Journal of Clinical Sport Psychology, 6*, 6–21.

Davis, P. A., Woodman, T., & Callow, N. (2010). Better out than in: The influence of anger regulation on physical performance. *Personality and Individual Differences, 49*, 457–460. https://doi.org/10.1016/j.paid.2010.04.017

Dawson, M. E., Schell, A. M., & Filion, D. L. (2000). The electrodermal system. In J. T. Cacioppo, L. G. Tassinary, & G. G. Berntson (Eds.), *Handbook of psychophysiology* (2nd ed., pp. 200–223). Cambridge University Press.

Denson, T. F., Spanovic, M., & Miller, N. (2009a). Cognitive appraisals and emotions predict cortisol and immune responses: A meta-analysis of acute laboratory social stressors and emotion inductions. *Psychological Bulletin, 135*, 823–853.

Denson, T. F., Spanovic, M., & Miller, N. (2009b). Stress and specificity: Reply to Miller (2009). *Psychological Bulletin, 135*, 857–858.

DeSteno, D., Valdesolo, P., & Bartlett, M. Y. (2006). Jealousy and the threatened self: Getting to the heart of the green-eyed monster. *Journal of Personality and Social Psychology, 91*, 626–641.

de Waal, F. (2019). *Mama's last hug. Animal emotions and what they can tell us about ourselves*. W. W. Norton & Company.

Dimberg, U., Thunberg, M., & Elmehed, K. (2000). Unconscious facial reactions to emotional facial expressions. *Psychological Science, 11*, 86–89.

11

Duclos, S. E., Laird, J. D., Schneider, E., Sexter, M., Stern, L., & Van Lighten, O. (1989). Emotion-specific effects of facial expressions and postures on emotional experience. *Journal of Personality and Social Psychology, 57*, 100–108.

Dunbar, R. I. (1993). Coevolution of neocortical size, group size and language in humans. *Behavioral and Brain Sciences, 16*, 681–694.

Edwards, D. A., & Casto, K. V. (2018). The social neuroendocrinology of athletic competition. In O. C. Schultheiss & P. H. Mehta (Eds.), *Routledge international handbook of social neuroendocrinology* (pp. 730–746). Routledge.

Eich, E. (1995). Searching for mood dependent memory. *Psychological Science, 6*, 67–75.

Eich, E., & Macaulay, D. (2000). Are real moods required to reveal mood-congruent and mood-dependent memory? *Psychological Science, 11*, 244–248.

Eich, E., & Metcalfe, J. (1989). Mood dependent memory for internal versus external events. *Journal of Experimental Psychology, 15*, 443–455.

Ekkekakis, P., Hall, E. E., & Petruzzello, S. J. (2005). Evaluation of the circumplex structure of the Activation Deactivation Adjective Check List before and after a short walk. *Psychology of Sport and Exercise, 6*, 83–101. https://doi.org/10.1016/j.psychsport.2003.10.005

Ekkekakis, P., Parfitt, G., & Petruzzello, S. J. (2011). The pleasure and displeasure people feel when they exercise at different intensities: Progress towards a tripartite rationale for exercise intensity prescription. *Sports Medicine, 41*, 641–671.

Ekman, P., & Davidson, R. J. (1993). Voluntary smiling changes regional brain activity. *Psychological Science, 4*, 342–345.

Ekman, P., & Friesen, W. V. (1986). A new pan-cultural facial expression of emotion. *Motivation and Emotion, 10*, 159–168.

Ekman, P. (1984). Expression and the nature of emotion. In Scherer, K. & Ekman, P. (Eds.), *Approaches to Emotion* (pp. 319–343). Hillsdale, NJ: Lawrence Erlbaum.

Ekman, P. (1992). An argument for basic emotions. *Cognition & Emotion, 6*, 169–200.

Ekman, P. (1994). Strong evidence for universals in facial expression: A reply to Russell's mistaken critique. *Psychological Bulletin, 115*, 268–287.

Ekman, P. (2007). *Emotions revealed: Recognizing faces and feelings to improve communication and emotional life*. St. Martin's Griffin.

Ekman, P. (2016). What scientists who study emotion agree about. *Perspectives on Psychological Science, 11*, 31–34.

Ekman, P., & Cordaro, D. (2011). What is meant by calling emotions basic. *Emotion Review, 3*, 364–370.

Ekman, P., & Friesen, W. V. (1978). *The facial action coding system (FACS): A technique for measurement of facial movement*. Consulting Psychologists Press.

Feltz, D. L., & Öncü, E. (2014). Self-confidence and self-efficacy. In A. G. Papaioannou & D. Hackfort (Eds.), *Routledge companion to sport and exercise psychology: Global perspectives and fundamental concepts* (pp. 417–429). Routledge.

Filaire, E., Duché, P., Lac, G., & Robert, A. (1996). Saliva cortisol, physical exercise and training: Influences of swimming and handball on cortisol concentrations in women. *European Journal of Applied Physiology and Occupational Physiology, 74*, 274–278.

Filaire, E., Le Scanff, C., Duche, F., & Lac, G. (1999). The relationship between salivary adrenocortical hormones changes and personality in elite female athletes during handball and volleyball competition. *Research Quarterly for Exercise and Sport, 70*, 297–302.

Filaire, E., Maso, F., Sagnol, M., Ferrand, C., & Lac, G. (2001). Anxiety, hormonal responses, and coping during a judo competition. *Aggressive Behavior, 27*, 55–63.

Fiori, M., Antonietti, J. P., Mikolajczak, M., Luminet, O., Hansenne, M., & Rossier, J. (2014). What is the Ability Emotional Intelligence Test (MSCEIT) good for? An evaluation using item response theory. *PLoS One, 9*, 1–11. https://doi.org/10.1371/journal.pone.0098827

Forgas, J. (2006). *Affect in social thinking and behavior*. Psychology Press.

Fridlund, A. J. (1994). *Human facial expression: An evolutionary view*. Academic.

Friesen, A. P., Lane, A. M., Devonport, T. J., Sellars, C. N., Stanley, D. M., & Beedie, C. J. (2013a). Emotion in sport: Considering interpersonal regulation strategies. *International Review of Sport and Exercise Psychology, 6*(1), 139–154. https://doi.org/10.1080/1750984X.2012.742921

Friesen, A. P., Devonport, T. J., Sellars, C. N., & Lane, A. M. (2013b). A narrative account of decision-making and interpersonal emotion regulation using a social-functional approach to emotions. *International Journal of Sport and Exercise Psychology, 11*, 203–214. https://doi.org/10.1080/1612197X.2013.773664

Friesen, A. P., Wolf, S. A., & van Kleef, G. A. (2021). The social influence of emotions within sports teams. In M. C. Ruiz & C. & Robazza (Eds.). Feelings in sport: Theory, research, and practical implications for performance and well-being (pp. 49–57). : Routledge.

Furley, P. (2019). What modern sports competitions can tell us about human nature. *Perspectives on Psychological Science, 14*, 138–155. https://doi.org/10.1177/1745691618794912

Furley, P. (2021). An evolutionary approach to emotions in sports. In M. C. Ruiz & C. Robazza (Eds.), *Feelings in sport: Theory, research, and practical implications for performance and well-being* (pp. 27–36). Routledge.

Furley, P., & Dicks, M. (2012). "Hold your head high". The influence of emotional versus neutral nonverbal expressions of dominance and submissiveness in baseball. *International Journal of Sport Psychology, 43*, 294–311.

Furley, P., & Schweizer, G. (2014a). "I'm pretty sure that we will win!" The influence of score-related nonverbal behavioral changes on the confidence in winning a basketball game. *Journal of Sport and Exercise Psychology, 35*, 316–320.
Furley, P., & Schweizer, G. (2014b). The expression of victory and loss: Estimating who's leading or trailing from nonverbal cues in sports. *Journal of Nonverbal Behavior, 38*, 13–29.
Furley, P., & Schweizer, G. (2016). In a flash: Thin slice judgment accuracy of leading and trailing in sports. *Journal of Nonverbal Behavior, 40*, 83–100.
Furley, P., & Schweizer, G. (2020). Body language in sport. In G. Tenenbaum & R. C. Eklund (Eds.), *Handbook of sport psychology* (4th ed., pp. 1201–1219). Wiley.
Furley, P., Dicks, M., & Memmert, D. (2012a). Nonverbal behavior in soccer: The influence of dominant and submissive body language on the impression formation and expectancy of success of soccer players. *Journal of Sport and Exercise Psychology, 34*, 61–82.
Furley, P., Dicks, M., Stendtke, F., & Memmert, D. (2012b). "Get it out the way. The wait's killing me." Hastening and hiding during soccer penalty kicks. *Psychology of Sport and Exercise, 13*, 454–465.
Furley, P., Moll, T., & Memmert, D. (2015a). Put your hands up in the air? The interpersonal effects of pride and shame expressions on opponents and teammates. *Frontiers in Psychology, 6*, 1361. https://doi.org/10.3389/fpsyg.2015.01361
Furley, P., Schweizer, G., & Bertrams, A. (2015b). The two modes of an athlete: Dual-process theories in the field of sport. *International Review of Sport and Exercise Psychology, 8*, 106–124.
Gendron, M., Crivelli, C., & Barrett, L. F. (2018). Universality reconsidered: Diversity in making meaning of facial expressions. *Current Directions in Psychological Science, 27*(4), 211–219. https://doi.org/10.1177/0963721417746794
Gilligan, S. G., & Bower, G. H. (1983). Reminding and mood-congruent memory. *Bulletin of the Psychonomic Society, 21*, 431–434.
Gross, J. J. (1998). The emerging field of emotion regulation: An integrative review. *Review of General Psychology, 2*, 271–299.
Gross, J. J. (2014). Emotion regulation: Conceptual and empirical foundations. In J. J. Gross (Ed.), *Handbook of emotion regulation* (2nd ed., pp. 3–20). The Guilford Press.
Gross, J. J., & Levenson, R. W. (1995). Emotion elicitation using films. *Cognition & Emotion, 9*, 87–108.
Gutrecht, J. A. (1994). Sympathetic skin response. *Journal of Clinical Neurophysioly, 11*, 519–524.
Hanin, Y. (2000). *Emotions in sport*. Human Kinetics.
Hanin, Y. L. (2007). Emotions in sport: Current issues and perspectives. In G. Tenenbaum & R. C. Eklund (Eds.), *Handbook of sport psychology* (3rd ed., p. 3358). Wiley.
Hardy, C. J., & Rejeski, W. J. (1989). Not what, but how one feels: The measurement of affect during exercise. *Journal of Sport & Exercise Psychology, 11*, 304–317.
Hatfield, E., Cacioppo, J. T., & Rapson, R. L. (1993). Emotional contagion. *Current Directions in Psychological Science, 2*, 96–99.
Hopkins, M. M., Hanin, Y., Chan, J. T., & Mallett, C. J. (2011). The value of emotional intelligence for high performance coaching. *International Journal of Sports Science & Coaching, 6*, 333–336.
Isen, A. M. (1987). Positive affect, cognitive processes, and social behavior. *Advances in Experimental Social Psychology, 20*, 203–253.
Izard, C. E. (1993). Four systems for emotion activation: Cognitive and noncognitive processes. *Psychological Review, 100*, 68–90.
Izard, C. E. (1994). Innate and universal facial expressions: Evidence from developmental and cross-cultural research. *Psychological Bulletin, 115*, 288–299.
Janelle, C. M., Fawver, B., & Beatty, G. F. (2020). Emotion and sport performance. In G. Tenenbaum & R. C. Eklund (Eds.), *Handbook of sport psychology* (4th ed., pp. 254–298). Wiley.
James, W. (1890). *The principles of psychology*. Holt.
Jokela, M., & Hanin, Y. (1999). Does the individual zones of optimal functioning model discriminate between successful and less successful athletes? A meta-analysis. *Journal of Sports Sciences, 17*, 873–887. https://doi.org/10.1080/026404199365434
Jones, M. V., Lane, M., Bray, S., Uphill, M., & Catlin, J. (2005). Development and validation of the sport emotion questionnaire. *Journal of Sport & Exercise Psychology, 27*, 407–431.
Jordet, G. (2009). Why do English players fail in soccer penalty shootouts? A study of team status, self-regulation, and choking under pressure. *Journal of Sports Sciences, 27*, 97–106.
Jordet, G., & Hartman, E. (2008). Avoidance motivation and choking under pressure in soccer penalty shootouts. *Journal of Sport and Exercise Psychology, 30*, 450–457.
Kalat, J. W. (2019). *Biological psychology* (13rd ed.). Cengage.
Kirschbaum, C., & Hellhammer, D. H. (2000). Salivary cortisol. In G. Fink (Ed.), *Encyclopedia of stress* (pp. 379–383). Academic Press.
Kirschbaum, C., Pirke, K. M., & Hellhammer, D. H. (1993). The "Trier Social Stress Test"—A tool for investigating psychobiological stress responses in a laboratory setting. *Neuropsychobiology, 28*, 76–81.
Kotsou, I., Nelis, D., Grégoire, J., & Mikolajczak, M. (2011). Emotional plasticity: Conditions and effects of improving emotional competence in adulthood. *Journal of Applied Psychology, 96*, 827–839.
Laborde, S., & Raab, M. (2013). The tale of hearts and reason: The influence of mood on decision making. *Journal of Sport & Exercise Psychology, 35*, 339–357.
Laborde, S., Brüll, A., Weber, J., & Anders, L. S. (2011). Trait emotional intelligence in sports: A protective role against stress through heart rate variability? *Personality and Individual Differences, 51*, 23–27. https://doi.org/10.1016/j.paid.2011.03.003
Laborde, S., Dosseville, F., & Allen, M. S. (2016a). Emotional intelligence in sport and exercise: A systematic review. *Scandinavian Journal of Medicine & Science in Sports, 26*, 862–874. https://doi.org/10.1111/sms.12510
Laborde, S., Dosseville, F., Guillén, F., & Chávez, E. (2014a). Validity of the trait emotional intelligence questionnaire in sports and its links with performance satisfaction. *Psychology of Sport and Exercise, 15*, 481–490. https://doi.org/10.1016/j.psychsport.2014.05.001
Laborde, S., Dosseville, F., Wolf, S., Martin, T., & You, M. (2016b). Consequences and antecedents of debilitative precompetitive emotions. *Psychologie Française, 61*(4), 303–317. https://doi.org/10.1016/j.psfr.2016.05.002
Laborde, S., Eyre, J., Akpetou, J., Engler, A.-C., Hofmann, F., Klanderman, J., et al. (2021). Emotional competences training. In M. C. Ruiz & C. Robazza (Eds.), *Feelings in sport: Theory, research, and practical implications for performance and well-being* (pp. 93–106). Routledge.
Laborde, S., Furley, P., & Schempp, C. (2015a). The relationship between working memory, reinvestment, and heart rate variability. *Physiology & Behavior, 139*, 430–436. https://doi.org/10.1016/j.physbeh.2014.11.036
Laborde, S., Guillén, F., & Watson, M. (2017). Trait emotional intelligence questionnaire full-form and short-form versions: Links with sport participation frequency and duration and type of sport practiced. *Personality and Individual Differences, 108*, 5–9. https://doi.org/10.1016/j.paid.2016.11.061
Laborde, S., Lautenbach, F., & Allen, M. S. (2015b). The contribution of coping-related variables and heart rate variability to visual

search performance under pressure. *Physiology & Behavior, 139*, 532–540. https://doi.org/10.1016/j.physbeh.2014.12.003

Laborde, S., Lautenbach, F., Allen, M. S., Herbert, C., & Achtzehn, S. (2014b). The role of trait emotional intelligence in emotion regulation and performance under pressure. *Personality and Individual Differences, 57*, 43–47. https://doi.org/10.1016/J.Paid.2013.09.013

Laborde, S., Raab, M., & Kinrade, N. P. (2014c). Is the ability to keep your mind sharp under pressure reflected in your heart? Evidence for the neurophysiological bases of decision reinvestment. *Biological Psychology, 100C*, 34–42. https://doi.org/10.1016/j.biopsycho.2014.05.003

Laborde, S., You, M., Dosseville, F., & Salinas, A. (2012). Culture, individual differences, and situation: Influence on coping in French and Chinese table tennis players. *European Journal of Sport Science, 12*, 255–261. https://doi.org/10.1080/17461391.2011.566367

LaCaille, L., Patino-Fernandez, A. M., Monaco, J., Ding, D., Upchurch Sweeney, C. R., Butler, C. D., et al. (2013). Electrodermal Activity (EDA). In M. D. Gellman & J. R. Turner (Eds.), *Encyclopedia of behavioral medicine* (pp. 666–669). Springer. https://doi.org/10.1007/978-1-4419-1005-9_13

Lane, A. M., Beedie, C. J., Jones, M. V., Uphill, M., & Devonport, T. J. (2012a). The BASES Expert Statement on emotion regulation in sport. *Journal of Sports Sciences, 30*(11), 1189–1195. https://doi.org/10.1080/02640414.2012.693621. Based on the BASES expert statement. Retrieved from www.bases.org.uk/BASES-Expert-Statements.

Lane, A. M., Devonport, T. J., & Beedie, C. J. (2012b). Can anger and tension be helpful? Relationships between emotions and emotional intelligence during optimal performance. *Athletic Insight, 14*, 187–198.

Lane, A. M., Meyer, B. B., Devonport, T. J., Davies, K., Thelwell, R., Gill, G. S., Diehl, C., Wilson, M., & Weston, N. (2009). Validity of the Emotional Intelligence Scale for use in Sport. *Journal of Sports Science and Medicine, 8*, 289–295.

Lane, A. M., & Wilson, M. (2011). Emotions and emotional intelligence among ultra-endurance runners. *Journal of Science and Medicine in Sport, 14*, 358–362.

Lang, P. J., & Bradley, M. M. (2010). Emotion and the motivational brain. *Biological Psychology, 84*, 437–450. https://doi.org/10.1016/j.biopsycho.2009.10.007

Lang, P. J., Bradley, M. M., & Cuthbert, B. N. (2008). International affective picture system (IAPS): Affective ratings of pictures and instruction manual. Technical report A-8.

Lautenbach, F., Laborde, S., Achtzehn, S., & Raab, M. (2014). Preliminary evidence of salivary cortisol predicting performance in a controlled setting. *Psychoneuroendocrinology, 42*, 218–224.

Lautenbach, F., Laborde, S., Klampfl, M., & Achtzehn, S. (2015a). A link between cortisol and performance: An exploratory case study of a tennis match. *International Journal of Psychophysiology, 98*, 167–173. https://doi.org/10.1016/j.ijpsycho.2015.10.002

Lautenbach, F., Laborde, S., Mesagno, C., Lobinger, B. H., Achtzehn, S., & Arimond, F. (2015b). Nonautomated pre-performance routine in tennis: An intervention study. *Journal of Applied Sport Psychology, 27*(2), 123–131. https://doi.org/10.1080/10413200.2014.957364

Lazarus, R. S. (1991). Progress on a cognitive-motivational-relational theory of emotion. *American Psychologist, 46*, 819–834.

Lazarus, R. S. (1999). *Stress and emotion: A new synthesis*. Springer.

Lazarus, R. S. (2000). How emotions influence performance in competitive sports. *The Sport Psychologist, 14*, 229–252.

Lazarus, R. S., & Lazarus, B. N. (1994). *Pasion and reason: Making sense of our emotions*. Oxford University Press.

Levenson, R. W. (2003). Blood, sweat, and fears—The autonomic architecture of emotion. *Annals of the New York Academy of Sciences, 1000*, 348–366. https://doi.org/10.1196/annals.1280.016

Levenson, R. W., Ekman, P., Heider, K., & Friesen, W. V. (1992). Emotion and autonomic nervous system activity in the Minangkabau of West Sumatra. *Journal of Personality and Social Psychology, 62*, 972–988.

Leventhal, H. (1980). Toward a comprehensive theory of emotion. *Advances in Experimental Social Psychology, 13*, 139–207.

Li, S., Cui, L., Zhu, C., Li, B., Zhao, N., & Zhu, T. (2016). Emotion recognition using Kinect motion capture data of human gaits. *PeerJ, 4*, e2364. https://doi.org/10.7717/peerj.2364

Malik, M. (1996). Heart rate variability. Standards of measurement, physiological interpretation, and clinical use. Task Force of the European Society of Cardiology and the North American Society of Pacing and Electrophysiology. *European Heart Journal, 17*, 354–381.

Martens, R. (1977). *Sport Competition Anxiety Test*. Human Kinetics Publishers.

Martens, R., Vealey, R. S., & Burton, D. (1990a). *Competitive anxiety in sport*. Human Kinetics Publishers.

Martens, R., Vealey, R. S., Burton, D., Bump, L., & Smith, D. E. (1990b). Development and validation of the Competitive Sports Anxiety Inventory-2. In R. Martens, R. S. Vealey, & D. Burton (Eds.), *Competitive anxiety in sport* (pp. 127–173). Human Kinetics.

Martinent, G., Ferrand, C., Guillet, E., & Gautheur, S. (2010). Validation of the French version of the Competitive State Anxiety Inventory-2 Revised (CSAI-2R) including frequency and direction scales. *Psychology of Sport and Exercise, 11*, 51–57.

Matsumoto, D., & Ekman, P. (1988). Japanese and Caucasian facial expressions of emotion and neutral faces (JACFEE and JACNeuF). Human Interaction Laboratory, University of California, San Francisco, 401.

Matsumoto, D., & Hwang, H. S. (2012). Evidence for a nonverbal expression of triumph. *Evolution and Human Behavior, 33*, 520–529.

Mauss, I. B., & Robinson, M. D. (2009). Measures of emotion: A review. *Cognition and Emotion, 23*(2), 209–237. https://doi.org/10.1080/02699930802204677

Maxwell, J. P., & Moores, E. (2007). The development of a short scale measuring aggressiveness and anger in competitive athletes. *Psychology of Sport and Exercise, 8*, 179–193. https://doi.org/10.1016/j.psychsport.2006.03.002

Maxwell, J. P., & Visek, A. (2009). Unsanctioned aggression in rugby union: Relationships among aggressiveness, anger, athletic identity, and professionalization. *Aggressive Behavior, 35*(3), 237–243. https://doi.org/10.1002/ab.20302

Mayer, J. D., Salovey, P., & Caruso, D. R. (2002). *Mayer-Salovey-Caruso Emotional Intelligence Test (MSCEIT): User's Manual*. Multi-Health Systems Inc.

Mayr, E. (1974). Behavior programs and evolutionary strategies. *American Scientist, 62*, 650–659.

McNair, D. M., Lorr, M., & Droppleman, L. F. (1971). *Profile of Mood State manual*. Educational and Industrial Testing Service.

Mesquita, B., & Frijda, N. H. (1992). Cultural variations in emotions: A review. *Psychological Bulletin, 112*, 179–204.

Moll, T., Jordet, G., & Pepping, G.-J. (2010). Emotional contagion in soccer penalty shootouts: Celebration of individual success is associated with ultimate team success. *Journal of Sports Sciences, 28*, 983–992.

Moya-Albiol, L., Salvador, A., Costa, R., Martínez-Sanchis, S., González-Bono, E., Ricarte, J., & Arnedo, M. (2001).

Psychophysiological responses to the Stroop Task after a maximal cycle ergometry in elite sportsmen and physically active subjects. *International Journal of Psychophysiology, 40*, 47–59.
Neil, R., & Woodman, T. (2019). Performance anxiety, arousal, and coping in sport. In T. Horn & A. Smith (Eds.), *Advances in sport and exercise psychology* (4th ed., pp. 211–227). Human Kinetics.
Nelis, D., Kotsou, I., Quoidbach, J., Hansenne, M., Weytens, F., Dupuis, P., & Mikolajczak, M. (2011). Increasing emotional competence improves psychological and physical well-being, social relationships, and employability. *Emotion, 11*, 354–366. https://doi.org/10.1037/a0021554
Nelis, D., Quoidbach, J., Mikolajczak, M., & Hansenne, M. (2009). Increasing emotional intelligence: (How) is it possible? *Personality and Individual Differences, 47*, 36–41. https://doi.org/10.1016/j.paid.2009.01.046
Niskanen, J. P., Tarvainen, M. P., Ranta-Aho, P. O., & Karjalainen, P. A. (2004). Software for advanced HRV analysis. *Computer Methods and Programs in Biomedicine, 76*, 73–81. https://doi.org/10.1016/j.cmpb.2004.03.004
Norman, G. J., Hawkley, L. C., Cole, S. W., Berntson, G. G., & Cacioppo, J. T. (2011). Social neuroscience: The social brain, oxytocin, and health. *Social Neuroscience, 7*, 18–29.
Öhman, A., Flykt, A., & Esteves, F. (2001). Emotion drives attention: Detecting the snake in the grass. *Journal of Experimental Psychology: General, 130*, 466–478.
Olatunji, B. O., Babson, K. A., Smith, R. C., Feldner, M. T., & Connolly, K. M. (2009). Gender as a moderator of the relation between PTSD and disgust: A laboratory test employing individualized script-driven imagery. *Journal of Anxiety Disorders, 23*, 1091–1097.
Oudejans, R. R., & Pijpers, J. R. (2010). Training with mild anxiety may prevent choking under higher levels of anxiety. *Psychology of Sport and Exercise, 11*, 44–50. https://doi.org/10.1016/j.psychsport.2009.05.002
Park, J. L., Fairweather, M. M., & Donaldson, D. I. (2015). Making the case for mobile cognition: EEG and sports performance. *Neuroscience and Biobehavioral Reviews, 52*, 117–130. https://doi.org/10.1016/j.neubiorev.2015.02.014
Parkinson, B. (1996). Emotions are social. *British Journal of Psychology, 87*, 663–683.
Perlini, A. H., & Halverson, T. R. (2006). Emotional intelligence in the National Hockey League. *Canadian Journal of Behavioural Science, 38*, 109–119. https://doi.org/10.1037/cjbs2006001
Petrides, K. V. (2009a). Psychometric properties of the Trait Emotional Intelligence Questionnaire (TEIQue). In C. Stough, D. H. Saklofske, & J. D. A. Parker (Eds.), *Assessing emotional intelligence: Theory, research, and applications* (pp. 85–101). Springer Science.
Petrides, K. V. (2009b). *Technical manual for the Trait Emotional Intelligence Questionnaire (TEIQue)*. London Psychometric Laboratory.
Petrides, K. V., & Furnham, A. (2003). Trait emotional intelligence: Behavioural validation in two studies of emotion recognition and reactivity to mood induction. *European Journal of Personality, 17*, 39–57. https://doi.org/10.1002/per.466
Philippot, P. (1993). Inducing and assessing differentiated emotion-feeling states in the laboratory. *Cognition & Emotion, 7*, 171–193.
Pijpers, J. R., Oudejans, R. R., & Bakker, F. C. (2005). Anxiety-induced changes in movement behaviour during the execution of a complex whole-body task. *The Quarterly Journal of Experimental Psychology A, Human Experimental Psychology, 58*, 421–445. https://doi.org/10.1080/02724980343000945
Pijpers, J. R., Oudejans, R. R., Holsheimer, F., & Bakker, F. C. (2003). Anxiety-performance relationships in climbing: A process-oriented approach. *Psychology of Sport and Exercise, 4*, 283–304.
Pinel, J. P. J., & Barnes, S. J. (2018). *Biopsychology* (10th ed.). Pearson Education.
Quigley, K. S., Lindquist, K. A., & Barrett, L. F. (2014). Inducing and measuring emotion: Tips, tricks, and secrets. In H. T. Reis & C. M. Judd (Eds.), *Handbook of research methods in social and personality psychology* (pp. 220–250). Cambridge University Press.
Rada, H., Dittmar, A., Delhomme, G., Collet, C., Roure, R., Vernet-Maury, E., & Priez, A. (1995). Bioelectric and microcirculaiton cutaneous sensors for the study of vigilance and emotional response during tasks and tests. *Biosensors and Bioelectronics, 10*, 7–15.
Rathschlag, M., & Memmert, D. (2013). The influence of self-generated emotions on physical performance: An investigation of happiness, anger, anxiety, and sadness. *Journal of Sport & Exercise Psychology, 35*, 197–210.
Rathschlag, M., & Memmert, D. (2014). Self-generated emotions and their influence on sprint performance: An investigation of happiness and anxiety. *Journal of Applied Sport Psychology, 27*(2), 186–199. https://doi.org/10.1080/10413200.2014.974783
Ratner, C. (2000). A cultural-psychological analysis of emotions. *Culture & Psychology, 6*, 5–39.
Ring, C., Cooke, A., Kavussanu, M., McIntyre, D., & Masters, R. (2014). Investigating the efficacy of neurofeedback training for expediting expertise and excellence in sport. *Psychology of Sport and Exercise.* https://doi.org/10.1016/j.psychsport.2014.08.005
Ring, C., Kavussanu, M., & Willoughby, A. (2016). Pain thresholds, pain-induced frontal alpha activity and pain-related evoked potentials are associated with antisocial behavior and aggressiveness in athletes. *Psychology of Sport and Exercise, 22*, 303–311. https://doi.org/10.1016/j.psychsport.2015.09.003
Riva, G., Mantovani, F., Capideville, C. S., Preziosa, A., Morganti, F., et al. (2007). Affective interactions using virtual reality: The link between presence and emotions. *CyberPsychology and Behavior, 10*, 45–56.
Robazza, C., Bortoli, L., Carraro, A., & Bertollo, M. (2006). "I wouldn't do it; it looks dangerous": Changing students' attitudes and emotions in physical education. *Personality and Individual Differences, 41*, 767–777. https://doi.org/10.1016/j.paid.2006.03.020
Robazza, C., Bertollo, M., Ruiz, M. C., & Bortoli, L. (2016). Measuring psychobiosocial states in sport: Initial validation of a trait measure. *PLoS One, 11*(12), e0167448. https://doi.org/10.1371/journal.pone.0167448
Robazza, C., Ruiz, M. C., & Bortoli, L. (2021). Psychobiosocial experiences in sport: Development and initial validation of a semantic differential scale. *Psychology of Sport and Exercise, 55*, 101963. https://doi.org/10.1016/j.psychsport.2021.101963
Ruiz, M. C., & Hanin, Y. L. (2004). Metaphoric description and individualized emotion profiling of performance related states in high-level karate athletes. *Journal of Applied Sport Psychology, 16*, 1–16.
Ruiz, M. C., & Robazza, C. (2020). Emotion regulation. In D. Hackfort & R. J. Schinke (Eds.), *The Routledge international encyclopedia of sport and exercise psychology* (Applied and practical measures) (Vol. 2, pp. 263–280). Routledge.
Ruiz, M. C., & Robazza, C. (Eds.). (2021). *Feelings in sport: Theory, research, and practical implications for performance and well-being*. Routledge.
Ruiz, M. C., Robazza, C., Tolvanen, A., & Hanin, J. (2019). The Psychobiosocial States (PBS-S) scale: Factor structure and reliability. *European Journal of Psychological Assessment, 35*, 658–665. https://doi.org/10.1027/1015-5759/a000454

Russell, J. A., Weiss, A., & Mendelsohn, G. A. (1989). Affect grid: A single-item scale of pleasure and arousal. *Journal of Personality and Social Psychology, 57*, 493–502.

Rutledge, L. L., & Hupka, R. B. (1985). The facial feedback hypothesis: Methodological concerns and new supporting evidence. *Motivation and Emotion, 9*, 219–240.

Ryan, C., Furley, P., & Mulhall, K. (2016). Judgments of nonverbal behaviour by children with high-functioning Autism Spectrum Disorder: Can they detect signs of winning and losing from brief video clips? *Journal of Autism and Developmental Disorders, 46*, 16–23.

Saklofske, D. H., Austin, E. J., Galloway, J., & Davidson, K. (2007a). Individual difference correlates of health-related behaviours: Preliminary evidence for links between emotional intelligence and coping. *Personality and Individual Differences, 42*, 491–502. https://doi.org/10.1016/j.paid.2006.08.006

Saklofske, D. H., Austin, E. J., Rohr, B. A., & Andrews, J. J. W. (2007b). Personality, emotional intelligence and exercise. *Journal of Health Psychology, 12*, 937–948. https://doi.org/10.1177/1359105307082458

Salovey, P., & Mayer, J. D. (1990). Emotional Intelligence. *Imagination, Cognition, and Personality, 9*, 185–211.

Sanchez-Lopez, J., Silva-Pereyra, J., & Fernandez, T. (2016). Sustained attention in skilled and novice martial arts athletes: A study of event-related potentials and current sources. *PeerJ, 4*, e1614. https://doi.org/10.7717/peerj.1614

Schachter, J., & Singer, J. E. (1962). Cognitive, social, and physiological determinants of emotional state. *Psychological Review, 69*, 379–399.

Schaefer, A., Nils, F., Sanchez, X., & Philippot, P. (2010). Assessing the effectiveness of a large database of emotion-eliciting films: A new tool for emotion researchers. *Cognition & Emotion, 24*, 1153–1172.

Scherer, K. R. (2005). What are emotions? And how can they be measured? *Social Science Information, 44*, 695–729. https://doi.org/10.1177/0539018405058216

Schutte, N. S., Malouff, J. M., Hall, L. E., Haggerty, D. J., Cooper, J. T., Golden, C. J., & Dornheim, L. (1998). Development and validation of a measure of emotional intelligence. *Personality and Individual Differences, 25*, 167–177.

Seligman, M. E., Railton, P., Baumeister, R. F., & Sripada, C. (2016). *Homo prospectus*. Oxford University Press.

Serrano, J. M., Iglesias, J., & Loeches, A. (1992). Visual discrimination and recognition of facial expressions of anger, fear, and surprise in 4-to 6-month-old infants. *Developmental Psychobiology, 25*, 411–425.

Serrano, J. M., Iglesias, J., & Loeches, A. (1995). Infants' responses to adult static facial expressions. *Infant Behavior and Development, 18*, 477–482.

Shariff, A. F., & Tracy, J. L. (2011). What are emotion expressions for? *Current Directions in Psychological Science, 20*, 395–399.

Simon-Thomas, E. R., Keltner, D., Sauter, D., Sinicropi-Yao, L., & Abramson, A. (2009). The voice conveys specific emotions: Evidence from vocal burst displays. *Emotion, 9*, 838–846.

Slovic, P., Finucane, M. L., Peters, E., & MacGregor, D. G. (2007). The affect heuristic. *European Journal of Operational Research, 177*, 1333–1352.

Smith, R. E., Smoll, F. L., Cumming, S. P., & Grossbard, J. R. (2006). Measurement of multidimensional sport performance anxiety in children and adults: The sport anxiety scale-2. *Journal of Sport and Exercise Psychology, 28*, 479–501.

Solanki, D., & Lane, A. M. (2010). Relationships between exercise as a mood regulation strategy and trait emotional intelligence. *Asian Journal of Sports Medicine, 1*, 195–200.

Stepper, S., & Strack, F. (1993). Proprioceptive determinants of emotional and nonemotional feelings. *Journal of Personality and Social Psychology, 64*, 211–220.

Sterelny, K. (2012). *The evolved apprentice*. MIT press.

Stevenson, R. A., Mikels, J. A., & James, T. W. (2007). Characterization of the affective norms for English words by discrete emotional categories. *Behavior Research Methods, 39*, 1020–1024.

Strack, F., Martin, L. L., & Stepper, S. (1988). Inhibiting and facilitating conditions of the human smile: A nonobtrusive test of the facial feedback hypothesis. *Journal of Personality and Social Psychology, 54*(5), 768–777. https://doi.org/10.1037/0022-3514.54.5.768

Strahler, K., Ehrlenspiel, F., Heene, M., & Brand, R. (2010). Competitive anxiety and cortisol awakening response in the week leading up to a competition. *Psychology of Sport and Exercise, 11*, 148–154. https://doi.org/10.1016/j.psychsport.2009.10.003

Syrjä, P., & Hanin, Y. (1998). Individualized and group-oriented measures of emotion in sport: A comparative study. *Journal of Sports Sciences, 16*, 398–399.

Teachman, B. A. (2007). Evaluating implicit spider fear associations using the Go/No-go Association Task. *Journal of Behavior Therapy and Experimental Psychiatry, 38*, 156–167.

Terry, P. C., Lane, A. M., & Fogarty, G. J. (2003). Construct validity of the profile of mood states—Adolescents for use with adults. *Psychology of Sport and Exercise, 4*, 125–139.

Terry, P. C., Stevens, M. J., & Lane, A. M. (2005). Influence of response time frame on mood assessment. *Anxiety, Stress and Coping, 18*, 279–285.

Thayer, J. F., Hansen, A. L., Saus-Rose, E., & Johnsen, B. H. (2009). Heart rate variability, prefrontal neural function, and cognitive performance: The neurovisceral integration perspective on self-regulation, adaptation, and health. *Annals of Behavioral Medicine, 37*, 141–153. https://doi.org/10.1007/s12160-009-9101-z

Thayer, R. E. (1989). *The biopsychology of mood and arousal*. Oxford University Press.

Thelwell, R. C., Lane, A. M., Weston, N. J. V., & Greenlees, L. A. (2008). Examining relationships between emotional intelligence and coaching efficacy. *International Journal of Sport & Exercise Psychology, 6*, 224–235.

Tomkins, S. S. (1962). *Affect, Imagery, Consciousness: Vol. 1. The positive affects*. Springer.

Tomkins, S. S. (1981). The quest for primary motives: Biography and autobiography of an idea. *Journal of Personality and Social Psychology, 41*, 306–329.

Totterdell, P. (2000). Catching moods and hitting runs: Mood linkage and subjective performance in professional sport teams. *Journal of Applied Psychology, 85*, 848–859.

Tracy, J. L., & Matsumoto, D. (2008). The spontaneous expression of pride and shame: Evidence for biologically innate nonverbal displays. *Proceedings of the National Academy of Sciences, 105*, 11655–11660.

Tremayne, P., & Barry, R. J. (1988). An application of psychophysiology in sports psychology: Heart rate responses to relevant and irrelevant stimuli as a function of anxiety and defensiveness in elite gymnasts. *International Journal of Psychophysiology, 6*(1), 1–8.

Van Kleef, G. (2009). How Emotions Regulate Social Life: The Emotions as Social Information (EASI) Model. *Current Directions in Psychological Science, 18*, 184–188.

Van Kleef, G. A., Van Doorn, E. A., Heerdink, M. W., & Koning, L. F. (2011). Emotion is for influence. *European Review of Social Psychology, 22*, 114–163.

Velten, E. (1968). A laboratory task for induction of mood states. *Behaviour Research and Therapy, 6*, 473–482.

Venables, P. H., & Christie, M. J. (1980). Electrodermal activity. In I. Martin & P. H. Venables (Eds.), *Techniques in psychophysiology* (pp. 3–67). Wiley.

Vernazza-Martin, S., Longuet, S., Damry, T., Chamot, J. M., & Dru, V. (2015). When locomotion is used to interact with the environment: Investigation of the link between emotions and the two-fold goal-directed locomotion in humans. *Experimental Brain Research, 233*(10), 2913–2924. https://doi.org/10.1007/s00221--015-4361-2

Warwick, J., Nettelbeck, T., & Ward, L. (2010). AEIM: A new measure and method of scoring abilities-based emotional intelligence. *Personality and Individual Differences, 48*, 66–71. https://doi.org/10.1016/j.paid.2010.03.020

Watson, D., Clark, L. A. A., & Tellegen, A. (1988). Development and validation of brief measures of positive and negative affect: The PANAS scales. *Journal of Personality and Social Psychology, 54*, 1063. https://doi.org/10.1037/0022-3514.54.6.1063

Wetherell, M. A., Craw, O., & Smith, M. A. (2018). Techniques for inducing stress: Problems and opportunities. In P. N. Murphy (Ed.), *The Routledge international handbook of psychobiology* (pp. 109–124). Routledge. https://doi.org/10.4324/9781315642765

Wilson, M. R., Vine, S. J., & Wood, G. (2009). The influence of anxiety on visual attentional control in basketball free throw shooting. *Journal of Sport and Exercise Psychology, 31*, 152–168.

Wilson-Mendenhall, C. D., Barrett, L. F., Simmons, W. K., & Barsalou, L. W. (2011). Grounding emotion in situated conceptualization. *Neuropsychologia, 49*, 1105–1127.

Wolf, S. A., Evans, M. B., Laborde, S., & Kleinert, J. (2015). Assessing what generates precompetitive emotions: Development of the precompetitive appraisal measure. *Journal of Sports Sciences, 33*(6), 579–587. https://doi.org/10.1080/02640414.2014.951873

Woodman, T., Davis, P. A., Hardy, L., Callow, N., Glasscock, I., & Yuill-Proctor, J. (2009). Emotions and sport performance: An exploration of happiness, hope, and anger. *Journal of Sport & Exercise Psychology, 31*, 169–188.

Zajonc, R. B. (2000). *Feeling and thinking: Closing the debate over the independence of affect*. Cambridge University Press.

Zhao, D., Gu, R., Tang, P., Yang, Q., & Luo, Y. J. (2016). Incidental emotions influence risk preference and outcome evaluation. *Psychophysiology, 53*(10), 1542–1551. https://doi.org/10.1111/psyp.12694

Zizzi, S. J., Deaner, H. R., & Hirschhorn, D. K. (2003). The relationship between emotional intelligence and performance among college basketball players. *Journal of Applied Sport Psychology, 15*, 262–269. https://doi.org/10.1080/10413200305390

Anxiety in Sport

Felix Ehrlenspiel and Christopher Mesagno

Contents

J. Schüler et al. (eds.), *Sport and Exercise Psychology*, https://doi.org/10.1007/978-3-031-03921-8_12

Learning Objectives

Basic:

- Distinguishing anxiety from similar constructs and describing anxiety as a situation-specific state that depends on attention and appraisal processes
- Naming the internal and external factors that influence these processes and describing the relevant models and theories

Advanced:

- Imagining and examining the anxiety reaction with its physiological, experiential and behavioural components and demonstrating how to measure these components
- Naming effects of anxiety in sports, identifying the relationship between anxiety and performance in sport and explaining the mechanisms of this relationship

Experts:

- Demonstrating how anxiety can be regulated and managed in sport
- Explaining how sport can contribute to the regulation and management of anxiety

12.1 Introduction

Sport is associated with different emotions for everyone involved—whether the athlete "on the pitch", whether the coach on the sideline or even the spectators in the stands. However, one emotion sticks out among athletes: anxiety. The beach volleyball player who serves for the match ball in the Olympic final, the climber at base before a free solo ascent on El Capitan, the student in the gymnastics lesson who is standing in line and waiting to jump over the vaulting horse or the parachutist just before jumping out of the plane at 4000 m—they are all likely to feel anxiety at this moment. If we take a closer look at these and similar situations, the question arises whether the experience of anxiety in these situations can explain the person's behaviour (e.g. the faking of an injury in the gymnastics lesson, the serving mistake in the Olympic final, the intensive preparation at the foot of El Capitan or the joy on the ground after a successful parachute landing). In fact, one of the central questions in sport psychology is the connection between anxiety and performance. Other questions relate to how and why anxiety actually arises in sport situations as people usually approach these voluntarily. Furthermore, we have to establish the meaning of the term anxiety—is it the volleyball player's sweaty hand, the worried look of the climber, the student's worry about an injury or the skydiver's weak stomach?

In the "Emotion" chapter, various approaches to research on emotion have already been presented. Several models can explain the development of emotions, their expression and their effects in sport. To provide an insight into anxiety in sport and the currently discussed theories, models and findings, this chapter takes a very pragmatic approach. Therefore, the presentation and understanding of anxiety in sport is based on the Consensual Modal Model of Emotion (Gross, 2008; Mauss & Robinson, 2009). This model corresponds to a lay understanding of emotion, but also—if simplified—to most of the theoretical approaches and empirical findings currently being discussed.

> A core topic for both applied sport psychology and research is the connection between anxiety and sport performance.

Within this Consensual Modal Model, an emotion develops over time, triggered by a situation that initiates an evaluation (or appraisal) process by the person. Depending on how the situation is evaluated, a complex emotional reaction develops, which has a physiological and behavioural component in addition to the subjective experience. This reaction can in turn be the basis for the next emotional episode, but it also has other effects on the behavioural and physiological level (Fig. 12.1).

Along the lines of the Consensual Modal Model, this chapter explains which characteristics of situations in sport trigger anxiety and how cognitive processes of attention and of situational appraisal lead to an anxiety reaction, which components make up this anxiety reaction and what effect anxiety has on behaviour in sport. The Consensual Modal Model also allows us to illustrate the effects that the characteristics of people in this process have and, finally, the strategies that exist for coping with, or regulating, anxiety, in sport. Interestingly, sport itself can contribute to changing the experience of anxiety.

What Is Anxiety?

When people talk about anxiety in everyday life, they usually talk about the manifestation or experience of the feeling of anxiety rather than the process leading to this experience. The experience, which is explained in more detail in ► Sect. 12.4, is usually the central component of the anxiety reaction when it comes to defining anxiety. Definitions, or rather descriptions, of anxiety usually revolve around three facets: Anxiety (1) is a temporary state, usually perceived as unpleasant, which (2) arises as a reaction to a threat in a situation and (3) is characterized by changes at the physiological, experiential and behavioural levels. Anxiety ultimately arises from an expectation about the progress of a situation, i.e. from the anticipated consequences of a situation or action. It is thus temporally preceding an event.

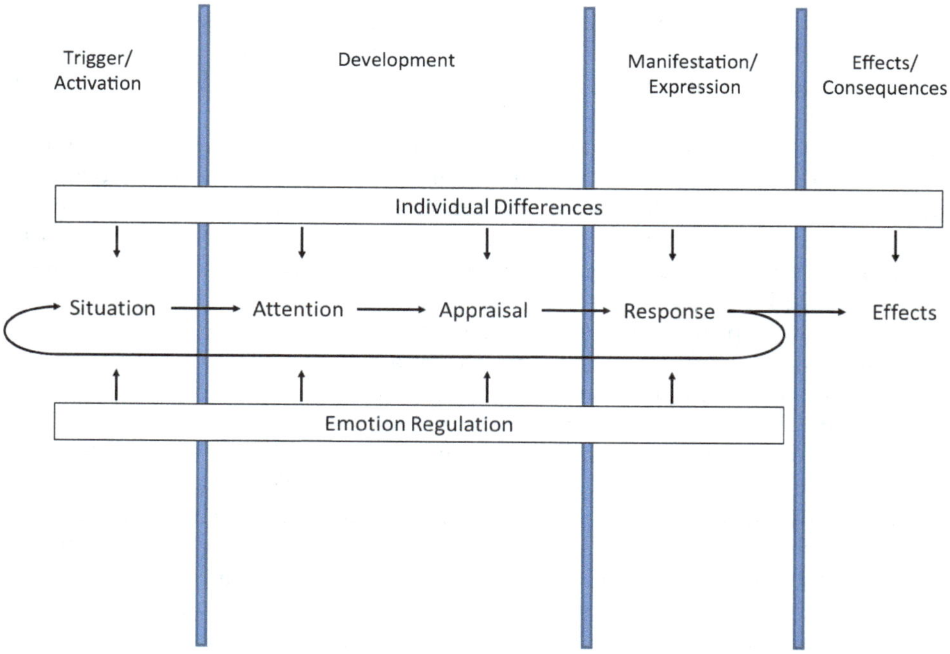

Fig. 12.1 Extended representation of the "Consensual Modal Model" of Emotion (Gross, 2008). It depicts emotions as a process and thus allows the structured presentation of findings on anxiety in sport. In sport, these findings relate primarily to the triggering situation of competition

As a construct, anxiety should serve to explain and predict individual behaviour and experiences. Anxiety is therefore often distinguished from other constructs such as fear, arousal and stress, although this distinction is difficult and sometimes controversial. In particular, the triggering conditions and reactions would have to be distinguished in a meaningful way in order to be able to speak of different constructs.

> Anxiety is a temporary state that is usually perceived as unpleasant and is characterized by changes at the physiological, experiential and behavioural levels. It arises from an undefined outset and the uncertain anticipation about future threat and is thus temporally preceding an event.

Anxiety and Fear

Fear and anxiety are both revolving around threat and share an unpleasant state of activation and negative feelings. Yet, fear is considered to be more object-related regarding a fairly well-defined (imminent) danger and is therefore a more short-term reaction to a single event. Because fear thus is also more concrete than anxiety, its functionality consists of showing immediate defensive behaviour ("fight/flight"). In contrast, anxiety is usually understood as a somewhat vague, objectless emotion, which can also last longer and is more oriented towards expected future environmental conditions. Therefore, anxiety should motivate information processing and even planning behaviour (Öhman, 2008). On the physiological level, specific reactions are also postulated—for example, different hormonal reactions; in addition, anxiety, fear and their respective reactions are associated with different subcortical brain regions. Thus, the amygdala appears to be the central switch point for fear, and the nucleus stria terminalis is likely the central switch point for anxiety (LeDoux & Pine, 2016). In practice, it is difficult to clearly assign fear to a situation in sport. If there is an immediate (real or perceived) threat of physical (or psychological) harm in a situation, for example, the student's first look at the gymnastics vaulting horse, fear could be the main emotion. Nevertheless, the normally uncertain or vague outset, the "not knowing" what will happen, ▶ Sect. 12.2, is the trigger for anxiety (and not fear) in sport.

> Fear can be described as a short-term, object- and present-related reaction that motivates immediate defence or escape behaviour.

Anxiety and Arousal

It is obvious that emotions are always associated with a physiological response, and for a long time, understanding the role of physiological responses in the development of emotions was important (see Chap. 10: Emotion). This physiological reaction is referred to as arousal, especially in the context of anxiety research. The underlying idea is that humans or organisms are in a state of energy at all times, which can vary between complete rest (e.g. in deep sleep) and complete arousal (e.g. in panic). This state of energy or physiological excitement is functionally connected to emotions: The arousal that accompanies anxiety is supposed to energize the organism. That way the organism is ready to flee or fight and able to protect itself. In some studies, arousal is not only seen as a part of anxiety but is equivalent to anxiety, for example, in models about the relationship between anxiety and performance. However, this equation is problematic for many reasons. An increased or even high level of arousal is associated not only with anxiety but also with other unpleasant (anger) and pleasant (joy) emotions. Moreover, arousal does not seem to be a one-dimensional construct, but rather different dimensions or facets can be distinguished. Arousal can take place centrally (i.e. in the brain or more precisely in the cortex) or peripherally, for example, through the activity of the autonomous nervous system. Many studies also use the term "activation", which is sometimes understood synonymously but could be different. For example, arousal is understood as the activation of the sensory organs and all afferent information processing, while the actual activation refers to the effector organs and the efferences. Arousal is also seen as a "tonic" level of activation, whereas activation is phasic (i.e. a reaction to a stimulus). Activation could then even be understood as an increase in arousal (Barry et al., 2005). Arousal then might be characterized by the activity of the autonomic nervous system, while activation expresses the activity of the central nervous system. Cognitive processes control both the energy intensity and its direction and are thus able to control peripheral (excitation) processes (cf. Beckmann & Rolstad, 1997).

> Arousal refers to the more general level of activation of the organism, characterized by the energy of the autonomous nervous system and related to the processing of afferent information (i.e. the perception of stimuli).

> Activation can be understood as a consequence of task-related activity of the central nervous system, which occurs as a result of stimuli and events and refers primarily to the (efferent) energy of effector organs.

Only very rarely is a differentiation of the concept of arousal made in sport psychology literature. This makes a summarized description of different works difficult. In this chapter, the term activation is used throughout, regardless of whether the respective literature refers to arousal (which is probably more frequent) or activation. This unification is based on the assumption that the physiological response measured in the context of anxiety in sport is an expression of cognitive processes based on an (anticipated) situation. Furthermore, the physiological response is usually also related to the preparatory activation in order to act—it is therefore activation rather than arousal.

> Anxiety is associated with an energy state of activation that is at least originally functional ("fight/flight").

Anxiety and Stress

If you asked the gymnastics student preparing for the vault or the skydiver in the plane about how they feel, they might not say that they are afraid but rather that they are stressed or experiencing stress. In fact, the distinction between anxiety and stress is not easy. One reason for this is the use of the term stress—stress is sometimes understood as the state of the organism, sometimes as the process of stress development and sometimes as the reaction of the body. Depending on the theoretical approach, stress is also considered from different perspectives. From a reaction-oriented perspective, stress is seen as a reaction to a stressor, for example, in the form of increased activity of the autonomic nervous system in response to an acute threat. From a stimulus-oriented perspective, stress is also a reaction to stimuli, but these are defined more broadly, so that all stimuli and stimulus constellations requiring adaptation are stressors. These stressors can then even be ordered hierarchically according to the need for adaptation. Finally, cognitive approaches are interested in the subjective view and in the evaluation processes that lead to the experience of stress—but this also makes stress more of a process (see Chap. 27 for an overview of theories and approaches). Common to all approaches, however, is the idea that stress is an imbalance (or a reaction to it) between demands on an organism or a person and his or her capacity to cope with the demands.

From these perspectives, the emotion of anxiety is difficult to separate from stress (cf. Weinberg & Gould, 2018). Anxiety is accompanied by physiological activation, especially of the autonomic nervous system. Situations and stimulus constellations can be identified that trigger anxiety (▶ Sect. 12.2), which can hardly be separated from stress-triggering ones. Anxiety is said to arise as a consequence of appraisal processes—the perception of threat and lack of coping options. The decisive difference is therefore likely to lie in the temporal extension (cf. Scherer, 1985): Anxiety represents a state in a situation, an acute reaction to an (anticipated) threat. Stress, on the other hand, is subject to the same mechanisms of development, but the system is out of balance in the long term or repeatedly (McEwen, 1998) and stress may last correspondingly longer. In this respect, the student in gymnastics lessons may indeed be more likely to experience stress—because he has already been exposed to the situation repeatedly—and the skydiver may show a physiological stress reaction but may also experience anxiety. This difference becomes decisive when it comes to the question of how to deal with anxiety and stress—stress as a long-term process must then be coped with, but anxiety as a state must be regulated (see ► Sect. 12.6).

Anxiety and stress are related constructs, which differ mainly in that anxiety is experienced rather in the short term and before an event and stress is rather longer term and is a reaction to an event.

Trait and State Anxiety: Global or Domain-Specific?

Finally, it is important to separate anxiety, as a momentary experience, as a state, from trait anxiety. Trait anxiety can be understood as a personality trait that expresses a person's tendency or disposition to experience anxiety (Spielberger, 1966). People differ in the extent of their trait anxiety—in situations in which they experience anxiety, how quickly anxiety develops and how pronounced the anxiety state is.

The constructs trait and state anxiety are supposed to serve to explain and predict behaviour. However, since behaviour takes place in situations, psychological research soon asked the question whether situations can be grouped into classes or domains for which domain-specific anxiety can then be assumed and measured. People could then, for example, be minimally anxious in general but feel more anxious in examination situations, for example. If anxiety is then assessed in a specific domain, e.g. academic exams or tests, the prediction of behaviour should also be more accurate.

State anxiety is a momentary and temporary feeling, while trait anxiety expresses the general tendency to experience anxiety in different situations.

Even within the domain of sport, domain-specific anxieties have been assumed. An (early) approach of anxiety research in sport (and especially in Germany) was the assumption of "sport anxiety": Individuals should differ in the extent to which they feel anxiety in different situations in sport, largely independent of (general) anxiety. In these conceptions, the fear (or anxiety) of injury represents an important facet. Next to this is social anxiety—people evaluate their own performance and their appearance. This facet of evaluation is the focus of two domains of anxiety in sport that are now playing a greater role in research: competitive anxiety and social physique anxiety. Whereas competitive anxiety actually refers to one domain of situations—namely, competitions—social physique anxiety is concerned with how others perceive and evaluate the external body appearance. This concern can occur in various situations but is more prevalent in situations where the body is visible, such as swimming or physical education. Sport psychology research is particularly interested in anxiety in competition and its relation to performance. Therefore, the majority of the considerations in this chapter will be related to competitive anxiety.

In sport, social anxiety plays a particularly important role, which is expressed in specific domains as competitive anxiety and social physique anxiety.

Self-Reflection: My Own Experience of Anxiety in Sport

When and if we experience anxiety is rather individualistic and subjective. Make a list of three concrete situations in which you have experienced anxiety in sports—e.g. in sports lessons, at a competition and in the gym. Try to remember each situation vividly. Then, for each situation, describe (1) what might have triggered the feeling in that situation, (2) what you noticed or felt when you were anxious and (3) the short- or long-term consequences of the anxiety experience.

The construct anxiety can thus be differentiated from other related constructs such as fear, stress or activation. However, the distinction is difficult and sometimes controversial. Theoretically, these constructs may by definition differ from one another. In concrete situations, however, a mixture of many of these emotions occurs, so that it seems practical to use anxiety as an umbrella term. This chapter will use anxiety under this umbrella meaning. Whenever it is necessary to differentiate, specific terms will be used.

12.2 Trigger of Anxiety in Sports

The situations described in the introduction are exemplary, perhaps even prototypical of situations in which people experience anxiety in sport. To understand anxiety and develop interventions for dealing with anxiety in sport, it is also helpful to know which situations or characteristics of situations can trigger anxiety in detail. An important research approach is to first generate lists of stress- or anxiety-inducing situations or situation characteristics using qualitative methods. We may then assign these characteristics to topics or categories. A second approach originates from social psychology and mostly experimental research on the connection between anxiety and performance or the phenomenon of "choking under pressure". Characteristics of a "pressure situation" are defined, which can then be systematically manipulated and examined against their effect on performance. Both approaches again essentially focus on anxiety before or during a competition.

12.2.1 Sport Psychological Approach

Hackfort (1986) probably offers the most detailed analysis of anxiety in the context of sport and the specific characteristics of the person-environment relationship that leads to this anxiety (referred to as "sources"). For Hackfort, the central point is that people in competitive sports are particularly concerned about the uncertainty of the situation. This feeling of uncertainty manifests in four types of fear: fear of (1) failure, (2) the unknown, (3) negative social evaluation and (4) injury or physical harm. This means that apparently an essential characteristic of competitive sports, namely, the openness of the outcome of the competition, is a significant source of anxiety! This openness results first and foremost from the fact that both success and failure are possible (fear of failure). Secondly, openness is linked to the observation that the outcome is only partly under the control of the person acting but is also dependent on external factors such as the opponents or the weather and material conditions (fear of the unknown). The outcome of competitions is also closely linked to self- and external evaluations: Failure can lead to a feeling of incompetence or inadequacy. People in sport worry what others (e.g. trainers, family and friends) think about their performance and fear a negative evaluation (fear of negative social evaluation). Finally, the fourth source of fear is physical: Athletes fear injuring themselves or getting injured by others during competitions (◘ Fig. 12.2). This differentiation (Hackfort, 1986) is supported by empirical results. In a study with a group of young wrestlers, 33 different sources of stress were named, but these are only assigned to three factors (Gould et al., 1983): fear of failure/feeling of inadequacy, external control/blame and social evaluation. Gould and Weinberg (1985) further found that wrestlers were particularly concerned with their expected performance and its evaluation. A similar list of characteristics of stress-/anxiety-inducing situations is provided by Lazarus and Folkman (1984) in the context of the transactional stress model (► Sect. 12.3.2), which can be supplemented by two sport-specific characteristics (Thatcher & Day, 2009).

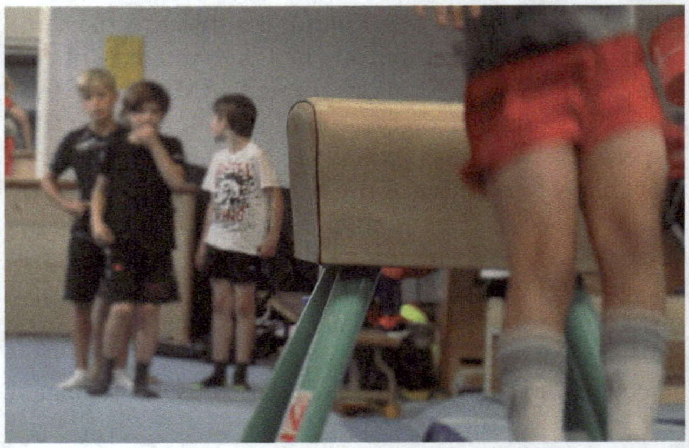

◘ **Fig. 12.2** A classic anxiety situation: queuing for the jump over the vaulting horse and the fear of pain and injury should be in the foreground

12

> Sport psychology studies show that anxiety is characterized by fear of:
> - Failure
> - The unknown
> - Negative evaluation by others
> - Injuries

What characteristics of situations cause stress and anxiety (in sport)? If:

- The event is new and unknown.
- The progression of the situation is not predictable or only predictable with difficulty.
- It is not certain whether the event will actually occur and when.
- The situation persists.
- The situation is unclear in itself and there is insufficient information or knowledge to assess it.
- The timing of the event coincides with other significant events
- A direct comparison with others in terms of performance-related characteristics (e.g. technical execution) is possible.
- The athlete is underprepared physically for the competition.

Preparation for a competition refers to the preparation in training yet also to the circumstances immediately before a competition. Conversely, the circumstances immediately before a competition influence a person's preparedness. For example, athletes that report poor sleep before competitions may feel increased anxiety regarding the competition (Ehrlenspiel et al., 2018a).

Finally, qualitative studies in competitive sports show that expectations—about your own performance and the performance of others—lead to anxiety (Hill et al., 2010). However, the interaction of own and other people's expectations seems unclear. Although it would be plausible to assume that the expectations of others increase the concern to make a good impression, which presumably leads to (social) anxiety, this mechanism has not yet been explicitly investigated.

12.2.2 Social-Psychological Approach

Social-psychological research in the 1960s and 1970s investigated the effect of situational characteristics on different performances and especially how "pressure situations" affected motor performance. Baumeister (1984) defined a "pressure situation" as "any factor or combination of factors that increases or enhance the importance of good performance during special occasions" (p. 610). These factors, which were later called situational incentives for optimal performance (Baumeister & Showers, 1986), are characterized as external characteristics (i.e. the environment and the situation) and internal characteristics (i.e. individual perceptions or states). Baumeister and Showers (1986) identified central pressure-generating factors including observation by spectators, the contingency of reward and punishment, competition and the personal importance of the task. Research on the relationship between anxiety and performance provides evidence for the anxiety-inducing effect of these factors. They are therefore often used in experimental research to design pressure situations under laboratory conditions.

> From a social-psychology perspective, "pressure" in sport arises from situational incentives for optimal performance, which may include (but are not limited to) observation by spectators, the contingency of reward and punishment, competition and the personal importance of the task.

12.2.2.1 Audience Effects

It is impossible to imagine sport, at least competitive sport, without spectators, and it is easy to see that spectators (can) create pressure and cause anxiety (◘ Fig. 12.3). The presence of spectators is therefore suitable to create pressure in an experimental, mostly laboratory situation. Essential characteristics of the audience are directly related to the perceived pressure, with a supportive, large and educated audience increasing the athlete's performance pressure. If performing in front of a supporting audience, this may create "impression management" issues and the (perceived) need to "look good" arises. Butler and Baumeister (1998) compared the performance in a task performed in front of a supporting, hostile or neutral audience. A supportive audience leads to not only increased anxiety but also a decrease in accuracy performance. This effect was found even with people stating they would be happy to have the encouragement of the (supporting) audience when performing.

In experimental research investigating the relationship between anxiety and performance, video cameras are also widely used to increase perceived pressure. Even among experienced golfers, a video camera increased state anxiety during a golf putt task (Linder et al., 1999). However, when using video cameras to manipulate pressure, instructions must be followed carefully. These should relate primarily to the impression the person is expected to make on others and threaten the person's self-concept (e.g. as a successful sportsman; Mesagno et al., 2011).

> The direct (spectators) or indirect (video cameras) observation in sports leads to anxiety, especially if it increases the necessity to leave a good impression on others.

12.2.2.2 Contingencies

Rewards or punishments are usually contingent on performance in competition situations—a first free solo ascent of a route on El Capitan, for example, leads to great media coverage and worldwide recognition. Contingencies lead to a perception of pressure. In experimental studies, financial incentives are often used, mostly in the sense of positive contingencies (possible profit), occasionally in combination with negative contingencies (loss of expected payment; see Masters, 1992). In these studies, it was indeed shown that anxiety increases and performance suffers (Baumeister, 1984; Beilock & Carr, 2001; Linder et al., 1999; Masters, 1992). However, in the progression of these studies, other characteristics were usually manipulated, for example, the personal importance ("ego relevance") of the tasks or video cameras or spectators was used. Although such combined study designs can be used to manipulate anxiety well, it is impossible to determine whether the financial incentive or, for example, the expected evaluation by an expert is the cause of anxiety and the associated loss of performance. Only one study with experienced golfers (Gucciardi & Dimmock, 2008), using a performance-based financial incentive but without further ego-relevant or social pressure manipulation, found a significant increase in state anxiety from a practice to a test situation in golf. Thus, it appears that although financial incentives can motivate people to perform better, they do not necessarily instil anxiety and therefore tend to have a performance-enhancing effect (Mesagno et al., 2011).

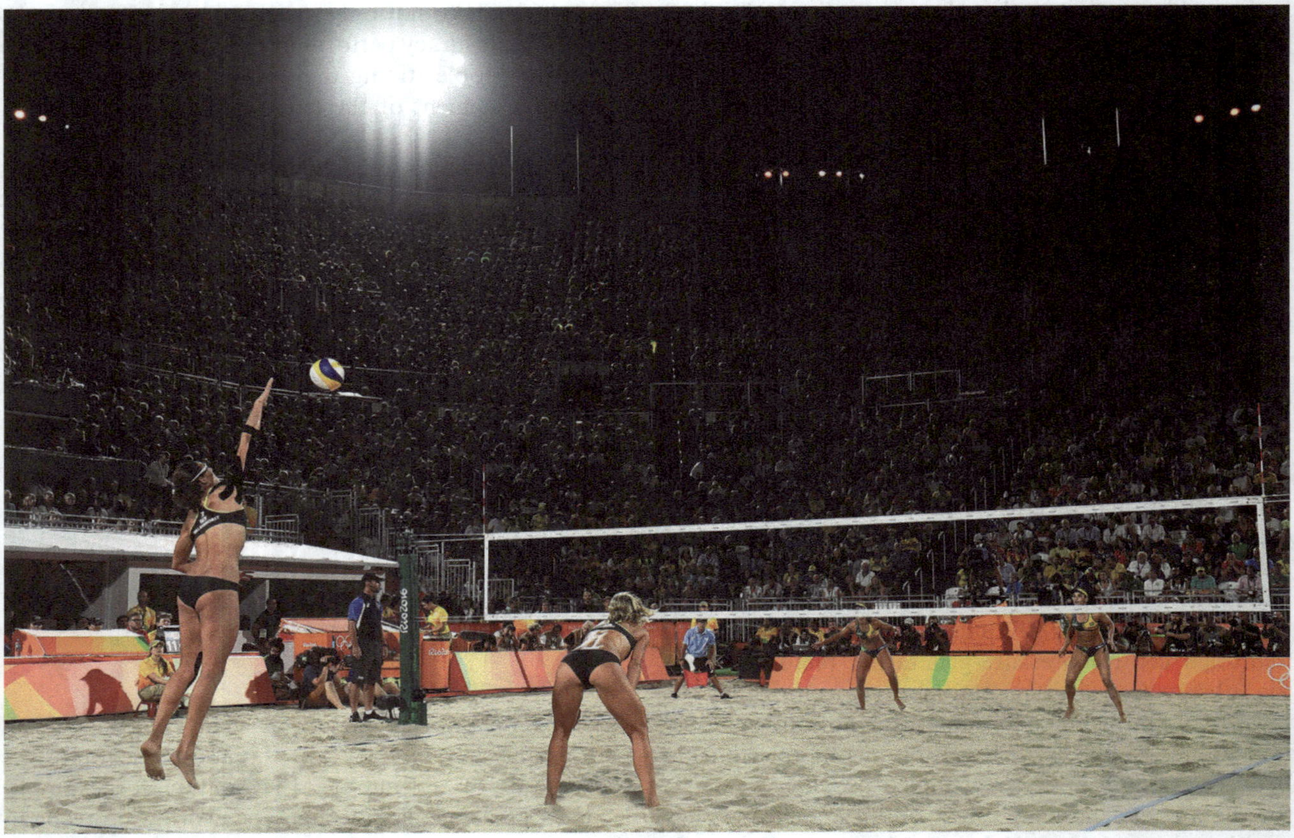

12

Fig. 12.3 Serve in the Olympic final (LEON NEAL/AFP/Getty Images)

> Financial incentives in pressure situations probably increase motivation above all without necessarily creating anxiety.

12.2.2.3 Competition

Sport is usually characterized by competition. Whether during a scrimmage at the end of a practice, or the Olympic Games, it is usually about comparing the performance of one person (or a group of people) to another and finding a winner. Competition does not even have to exist formally or explicitly. An (implicit) competition is created when you tacitly want to perform better than another person during voluntary training. Apparently, competitions lead to the perception of pressure and often poor performance (Baumeister & Showers, 1986).

In applied sport psychology, the main focus is on overcoming competitive anxiety and thus supporting athletes and achieving optimal performance in competitive situations. In the context of psychological skill training, attempts have been made to integrate characteristics of competition into daily training. In addition to the characteristics already described (e.g. spectators, or positive/negative contingencies), other characteristics (e.g. limited number of attempts) often specific to a particular sport are also incorporated into training (e.g. Low et al., 2021).

? What are the most anxiety-inducing characteristics of competitions in sport?

- An audience is present.
- Consequences are contingent upon the outcome of the competition.
- A direct comparison of performance with other persons or groups.
- The relevant action is attempted only once (e.g. penalty kicks) or is attempted only to a limited extent (e.g. a maximum of three attempts).
- The timing of the competition is uncontrollable (e.g. starting time is fixed) or even unpredictable (starting time of tennis match fluctuates due to match length on competition day).

12.2.2.4 Importance of the Event

A problem in laboratory-based, experimental research is that the experimental situation itself is usually not very important for the participants being tested. Many findings show that the importance of a situation—usually competitions or competition simulations—is positively associated with increased (competitive) anxiety

(Marchant et al., 1998; Martens et al., 1990a). The importance of a performance situation can result from the context of the situation itself (e.g. training vs. competition) or the possible consequences (e.g. win or loss). The extent to which the importance aspects contribute to anxiety depends primarily on a person's motivational orientation. If the task performed is closely linked to a person's self-esteem, this will lead to more anxiety. Thus, people who feel successful when they perform better than others ("ego orientation") are more likely to report anxiety in competitive situations than those who improve their own performance based on mastery of the skill ("task orientation"; Hall et al., 1998). In a study in golf, the effect of incentives of different levels (consequences; Marchant et al., 1998) was examined. Golfers with a low handicap (i.e. at a fairly high level of expertise) were divided into pairs and completed a golf chipping task. The prizes for winning were either golf balls (low importance) or golf shoes (high importance). It was found that people involved in the high importance, compared to low importance, incentive indicated a higher level of anxiety. The importance of the consequences was therefore a strong positive predictor of anxiety.

> Only in important performance situations in sport does anxiety arise; this importance arises both from the context of the actor's situation and from the consequences of the action.

Experimental Comparison of the Effect of Pressure Conditions

The self-presentation model (▶ Sect. 12.3) aims to explain how anxiety and poor performance can occur in competitive situations. The model assumes that situational and personal characteristics influence self-presentation and anxiety. In an initial study (Mesagno et al., 2011) of the self-presentation model of choking under pressure (more discussion of choking under pressure later), hockey players were asked to take penalty shots under normal "training" conditions or under "high pressure." For the "high pressure" condition, the participants were randomly assigned to different manipulations. The "self-presentation" condition involved a social evaluation situation, where the penalty shots were taken in front of spectators or under video observation where the camera was focused on the performer and participants were told their performance would be scrutinized by their coach. In a "motivational" pressure condition, participants were able to earn money depending on their performance, or the video camera was focused on the target to ensure accurate recording of scores. Results indicated that the self-presentation condition reported higher anxiety and also showed decreased performance under pressure than the motivational pressure manipulation. This indicates a connection between self-presentation, increased anxiety and choking under pressure.

Reflection: Competition Preparation

In psychologically oriented training, an attempt is made to make everyday training "psychologically valuable." For example, the training conditions can be adapted as closely as possible to the conditions of the competition or these can be simulated. In this way, it is possible to practice dealing with conditions that trigger anxiety. For "your" sport, think about which aspects of a competition you could incorporate into a typical final training session (and how).

12.3 How Anxiety Arises in Sport

Various external situations and internal states can thus be described as outsets for anxiety. These outsets are only possible, perhaps even necessary conditions for the development of anxiety in sport, but certainly insufficient. Whether anxiety develops from objective situations must therefore depend on other factors. In the Consensual Modal Model (Gross, 2008), these are attention and appraisal processes.

> Whether anxiety arises from specific characteristics of situations in sport, such as a competition, depends on attention and appraisal processes.

12.3.1 Attention Processes

It seems plausible that in a given situation an emotion—in this case anxiety—only arises when corresponding emotionally relevant features are perceived. There is some evidence of a connection between emotions and a corresponding distortion of attention towards the emotionally relevant characteristics of the situation ("emotion-related attentional bias"). Empirically, this distortion of attention phenomenon is often investigated by means of two reaction-time paradigms: the emotional Stroop test (Williams et al., 1996) and the dot probe test (MacLeod et al., 1986) (see ◘ Figs. 12.4 and 12.5 in the Methods Box). In each test, emotionally related stimuli (e.g. words) attract attention and are processed more quickly, thereby inhibiting other processes simultaneously and facilitating subsequent appropriate processes.

List 1	List 2
blue	Relegation Fight
green	Front Runner
red	Endurance
blue	Sports Jacket
yellow	Ball Loss
red	Final Victory

◘ **Fig. 12.4** Stroop test: The task is to name the printed colour of the displayed words as quickly and accurately as possible

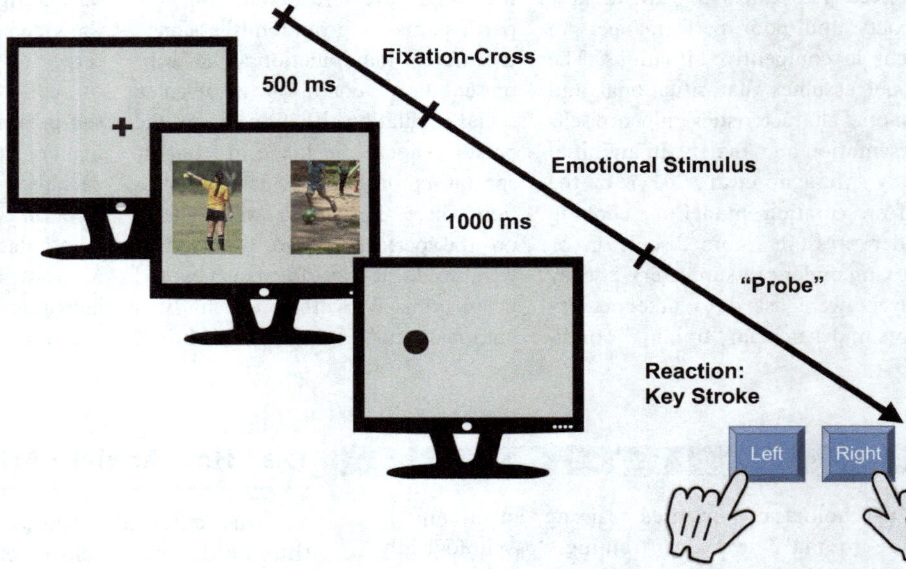

◘ **Fig. 12.5** Dot probe test: stimuli with emotional content attract attention—this leads to shorter reaction times if the "dot probe" appears at the location of the emotional stimulus

[Paradigms: Emotional Stroop Test and Dot Probe Test]

The Stroop test is a classic test for measuring attentional processes. Participants are presented with a list of words (originally words of colours), printed in different colours (see list 1). The task is to name the printed colour of the words as quickly and accurately as possible. John Ridley Stroop reported in 1935 in his classic study that there is interference of the word meaning with the naming of the printed colour. If word meaning and printed colour match, the answers are quicker and more correct than if they are different. The emotional Stroop test is designed to determine whether the emotional content of a word attracts attention and whether there is interference. A person who suffers from anxiety in competitions may therefore take a little longer to name the colour ("yellow" or "red") for the "negative" words in list 2 ("relegation fight", "ball loss").

The dot probe test is used to record selective attention to emotional, especially threatening, stimuli. Participants look at a monitor on which a fixation cross appears to ensure that the person is actually looking at the monitor. Then, for a predetermined time, images are shown to the left and right of the fixation cross: one "neutral" (e.g. "playing children") and one with emotional stimuli (e.g. "referee shows a yellow card"). Then a dot appears at the position of one of the two images (i.e. right or left), and the task is to press a corresponding button (i.e. "left"/"right") as quickly as possible when the dot appears. The special processing of emotional stimuli or the "attentional bias" is then shown with shorter reaction times to dots that appear at the position of the emotional stimulus. The attention was therefore already drawn to the dot by the emotional stimulus and was not distributed equally.

Both paradigms provide clear evidence of attentional bias towards threat or anxiety-related stimuli in individuals with high anxiety and anxiety disorders (Bar-Haim et al., 2007). Both conscious, top-down, and unconscious, bottom-up, processes (see definitions information below) contribute to this distortion of attention. It is controversial whether people with anxiety disorders usually draw attention to threatening stimuli or whether a preferred perception of threatening stimuli may lead to an anxiety disorder.

In sports, this anxiety-related distortion of attention has rarely been investigated. Moreover, the few findings are not entirely consistent. With the help of a version of the emotional Stroop test adapted to competitive sports, Lautenbach et al. (2016) showed that athletes seem to gravitate towards negative, threatening sports-related stimuli independently of the "pressure" prevailing within a situation. In a dot probe test, however, Chuang et al. (2015) could not find any behavioural distortion of attention to negative, threatening stimuli in archers.

Bottom-Up Process

When events or stimuli "automatically" attract attention, we speak of bottom-up processes, for example, the reactions to a loud bang.

Top-Down Process

If attention is consciously and intentionally directed to selected events or stimuli, we speak of top-down processes.

Attentional processes are also often accessed through the analysis of eye movements. Thus, indirect indications of the connection between attention and competitive anxiety are found in research on gaze behaviour, where pressure situations influence eye movement behaviour. In a study on free-throw basketball, a pressure situation led to a reduction in a "quiet eye" period (e.g. the final fixation of the target with task-related and external attentional focus; see Methods Box), an increase in fixations and a decrease in fixation duration (Wilson et al., 2009). Apparently, pressure leads to an impairment, perhaps an interruption, of cognitive processing of task-related processes—an indication, in turn, of preferred processing of anxiety-related stimuli.

Method: Quiet Eye

Usually we control our movements by processing visual stimuli, for example, when a volleyball is to be played over a net or a small rock ledge is to serve as the next footing in climbing. With the help of eye movement cameras, the eye movements necessary for the perception of visual stimuli can be recorded and examined. The "last look" before the beginning of a movement plays a key role in the processing of visual information—a topic to which Joan Vickers has devoted extensive research time and gave it the name "quiet eye" (QE) (see Vickers, 2016). QE is defined as the last fixation of an eye movement before the start of the final movement (e.g. stretching the arm in volleyball, stretching the legs when climbing). The fixation is understood as the lingering of the gaze within an angle of vision of 3° around a location or an object for a time of at least 100 ms.

The quiet eye period likely leads to better motor performance due to effective motor programming. The significance of QE for motor performance is deduced by comparing experts or top athletes with people who are less successful in their sport or have only been doing it for a short time. Furthermore, QE can be compared between successful and unsuccessful performances. Meanwhile, there are also studies in which the duration of QE has been experimentally manipulated (Klostermann et al., 2013). These studies show that the length of QE is directly related to success in different motor tasks, with the general rule: The longer QE, the better performance. Successful athletes not only fixate longer—they usually succeed by fixing earlier—they are also more constant in their QE. However, motor tasks make specific demands on the optimal duration of QE. The QE can also be trained.

Which personality and personal characteristics influence anxiety-related attention processes in sports?

- When experiencing anxiety, people who interpret anxiety as performance-inhibiting generally process ambiguous stimuli more intently (Eubank et al., 2002).
- People with high competitive anxiety tend to avoid anxiety-related stimuli, i.e. tend to divert their attention (Chuang et al., 2015).
- QE training leads to pressure situations being interpreted less as a threat and instead more as a challenge (Moore et al., 2013b).

12

12.3.2 Appraisal Processes

Fundamental to all approaches within the Consensual Modal Model (Gross, 2008) is the assumption that the (objective) characteristics of a situation do not directly lead to the (subjective) experience of anxiety. Rather, these characteristics are first assessed in terms of their meaning/significance for the individual and, in the case of anxiety, the situational appraisal as "threatening." The most prominent and also first explicit theoretical idea about these cognitive appraisal processes was formulated by Richard Lazarus (1966) in his transactional stress model.

12.3.2.1 Transactional Stress Model

While stress research after the Second World War was still strongly behaviourist and interested in the direct effects of stress conditions on behaviour, Richard Lazarus observed that characteristics of the person seem to have an influence on this effect. He therefore assumed that there is a bidirectional, transactional relationship between the individual and the situation or environment, in which cognitive processes mediate whether (subjective) stress is actually triggered by an (objective) stressor. These cognitive processes should essentially be about appraising the significance and characteristics of the situation and events in this transactional relationship (Lazarus & Folkman, 1984). This appraisal (see Fig. 12.6) includes how significant the situation is for a person ("primary appraisal") and whether the individual has the resources to cope with the demands of

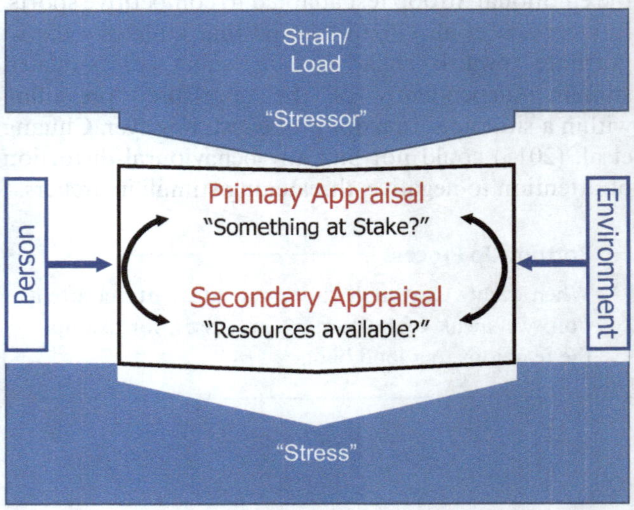

Fig. 12.6 Schematic representation of the transactional stress model

the situation ("secondary appraisal"). In principle, an event or situation can be cognitively appraised as irrelevant, benign-positive or stress-relevant. If the situation is appraised as a stressor, the individual would have to adapt to the situation. This need for adaptation can be perceived as a challenge, a loss/harm or a threat. A perception of loss or harm clearly refers to a situation in the past, whereas a perception of threat refers to possible loss or damage in the future—which then leads to stress. The term secondary appraisal seems to imply a hierarchical or sequential process. However, Lazarus and Folkman (1984) postulate that the appraisal of whether the person has possibilities for coping with the need for adaptation—such as corresponding own competences, social support or other resources—runs rather parallel and interacts with the primary, situational appraisal.

The transactional stress theory was further developed by Lazarus into an emotion theory, the "cognitive-motivational-relational theory" (Lazarus, 1991), in which the two appraisal processes still play the central role. The "primary appraisal" now includes not only what relevance an event has for the achievement of personal goals but also how much it is in line with personal goals and what consequences the event has for the self (e.g. self-worth, own values). In the "secondary appraisal", it is a question of not only whether behaviour can be generated to cope with the situation but also what causes (or "causers") can be found for an event and how the situation likely develops regarding one's goals. According to Lazarus (1991), emotions are linked to specific appraisal patterns. Therefore, anxiety should arise from the appraisal that a situation or an event has high importance for the achievement of one's goals, whereby one's goals are rather threatened and one's self-esteem must be protected.

Key Points

Stressors (situations, events) are not always and, for everyone, equal triggers for stress/anxiety.

In between, there are appraisal processes of a situation ("Is something at stake?") and of coping resources ("Can I do it?").

Appraisal processes are dependent on environmental and personal characteristics.

The "core theme" of anxiety is the expectation of an uncertain, existential threat.

Effect of Stressors in Sport

Even if the transactional stress model is difficult to test as a whole, there are many indications of the validity of its core assumptions in sport. For example, there are interindividual differences in which events and situations are experienced as anxiety-inducing. This can be seen in the lists of anxiety-triggering situations obtained by interviewing athletes and that there is little agreement between individuals about which situations trigger anxiety. A study of former female figure skaters, for example, revealed five major sources or "triggers" of stress in sport, including the anxiety-relevant area of "negative aspects of competition" (cf. Scanlan et al., 1991). However, only one stressor ("worries about competition") met with the approval of at least half of the respondents. Furthermore, it was shown that the same event (e.g. "performing in front of an audience") labelled by some as a "stressor" was labelled by others as "enjoyment".

Situational and Resource Appraisal in Sport

The perception of a threat also proves to be decisive for the development of anxiety in sport. In a qualitative study with athletes from different sports, anxiety arose from the perception of threat or insecurity in the context of a competitive situation. However, appraisal processes convey not only *whether* anxiety arises in sport situations but also *how strongly* the anxiety is expressed (Cerin & Barnett, 2011; Hammermeister & Burton, 2001). For example, the more the opponent is perceived as strong, or the competition is perceived as important, thus as a threat, the higher the anxiety intensity. With coping or resource appraisal, it shows that perceived resources, especially emotional support, are associated with low anxiety in competition. Furthermore, factors of competition situations over which little control is experienced (e.g. weather) are associated with higher anxiety, and increased perceived situational control is associated with lower anxiety. However, coping appraisal seems less relevant for *triggering* competitive anxiety. It is likely to play a central role in *intensifying* the emotional experience of anxiety in the sense of a spiral of anxiety rather than an initial precursor to it. For example, a table tennis player reports: "I was anxious. I did not play well. I perceived that I was not able to play better. And this situation further increased my anxiety" (Martinent & Ferrand, 2015, p. 60).

Situational (demand) and resource (coping) appraisal in competition are apparently related primarily to the intensity (and the increase) of the cognitive component (or worry) of competitive anxiety.

Personal and Environmental Characteristics as Moderators of Anxiety in Competition

The extent to which environmental and personal characteristics actually play a moderating role between stressors and anxiety experiences has hardly been investigated directly, for example, by means of moderation analysis (Cerin & Barnett, 2011). However, there is a whole range of indirect evidence: If one assumes that competition or other anxiety-triggering situations are *objectively* the same for all people, then differences in *subjective* anxiety experience must be due to the influence of moderators. Among those, primarily personal and less environmental have been examined.

In sports and especially competitive situations, for example, men usually report lower levels of anxiety intensity than women (Jones et al., 1990, cf. also lower norms in the corresponding diagnostic instruments, e.g. Ehrlenspiel et al., 2009). It is assumed that age and experience are associated with low anxiety—but research findings are contradictory and mostly indicate that age, experience and performance level play a limited role. Even within a group of people who had competed at least nationally, age had no effect on anxiety, but experience (> 10 years) and a current top competition level were associated with lower competitive anxiety (Hanton et al., 2008b). Thus, it is probably competition experience that leads to a more favourable coping appraisal and thus lower anxiety. Correspondingly, cross-sectional studies (Fletcher & Hanton, 2001) and intervention studies (Ehrlenspiel & Elbe, 2008) show that the possession of psychological skills such as relaxation or imagery ability—which are acquired during basic sport psychological or skill training (Beckmann & Elbe, 2015)—can reduce anxiety experiences.

It is mainly the experience with competition, rather than age or practice of the sporting disciplines or techniques, that leads to low anxiety in competition.

On which personal and environmental characteristics does the degree of anxiety of competition depend?

Factors associated with higher anxiety:

- Female gender (Jones et al., 1990).
- Neuroticism (Cerin & Barnett, 2011).
- Perfectionism (Hall et al., 1998).
- Competitive trait anxiety (Hanton et al., 2002).
- Strong identification with the role as athlete ("athletic identity"; Mesagno et al., 2011).
- "Performance" vs. "mastery" goals (Kaye et al., 2015), with female athletes affected more by performance approach goals than male athletes (Stenling et al., 2014).
- An "entity mindset" vs. a "growth mindset" (Stenling et al., 2014).
- Gross (rugby) vs. fine motor (golf) sports (Mellalieu et al., 2004).
- Parental behaviour including being very directive (Fink et al., 2013) or initiating a low mastery or high ego motivational climate (O'Rourke et al., 2011).
- Red vs. blue uniform of the opponent (Recours & Briki, 2015).
- Individual sports (Martin & Hall, 1997; Flowers & Brown, 2002). Nevertheless, aggravating effects of team sports have been found as well (Cooke et al., 2013).

Factors associated with lower anxiety:

- "Hardiness"/resilience (Hanton et al., 2013)
- Training climate that promotes mastery vs. performance goals (Smith et al., 2007)
- Perceived cohesion in a team (Borrego et al., 2012)
- Home competition (Wolf et al., 2015)

12.3.2.2 Theory of Challenge and Threat States in Athletes

A further framework for understanding the emergence of anxiety is provided by the theory of challenge and threat states in athletes (TCTSA, Jones et al., 2009). The TCTSA (see Fig. 12.7) also fits well into the Consensual Modal Model (Gross, 2008). Similar to Lazarus (1966), the core assumption is that a person appraises a situation within a goal-oriented performance action either as a challenge or a threat (Blascovich, 2008). This (cognitive) appraisal process includes both the evaluation of situational demands and individual resources for coping (Blascovich & Mendes, 2000).

The evaluation of the situational demands results in the perception of the significance of a situation, for example, when hazards are perceived, uncertainty prevails or a great deal of effort will be required. The evaluation of one's resources then determines whether a person perceives the demands and the situation as a challenge or a threat. The situation is perceived as challenging if the person assesses that he or she has sufficient resources to cope with the situational demands and perceived as threatening if the person assesses insufficient resources to cope with the situation. These possible resources include abilities and skills and knowledge but also dispositional (i.e. stable) characteristics of the person such as self-efficacy and perception of control or goal orientation but also external support (Blascovich et al., 2003). In addition, Skinner and Brewer (2004) assume that a perception as challenge occurs when the situation offers sufficient prospects of success and the opportunity to acquire or develop one's competencies. This, in turn, should increase confidence that the situational demands can ultimately be met. Conversely, a perception of threat should arise when a person assesses that the demands threaten his or her own self-esteem and he or she has little confidence in own abilities to cope with the demands. Challenge and threat are understood in the model as motivational states that indicate how a person deals with a personally significant situa-

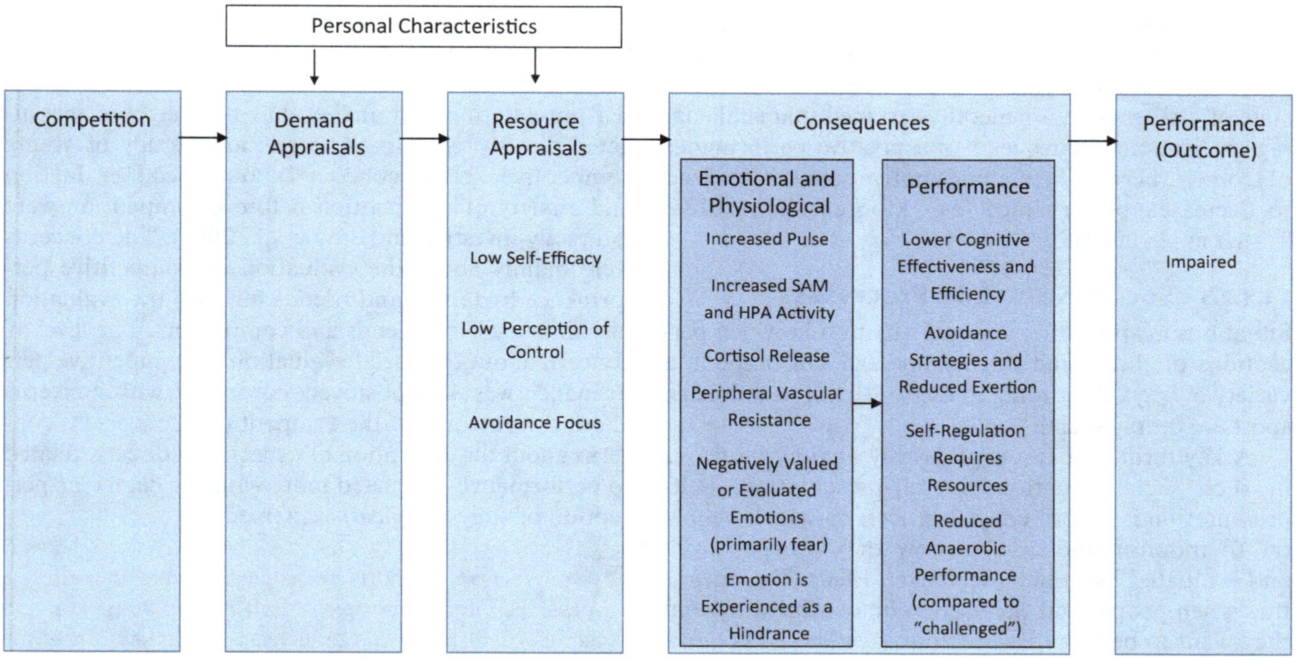

Fig. 12.7 Theory of challenge and threat states in athletes: the state of threat (after Jones et al., 2009)

tion (Blascovich & Mendes, 2000). For athletes, sport and competitions in general are likely "personally meaningful", which is why states of challenge or threat—and, in the latter case, anxiety—arise very quickly.

> Situations in sport are more likely to be seen as challenging if coping with them is also associated with a gain, such as the acquisition of skills.

As a biopsychosocial model, TCTSA is somewhat more explicit in its assumption of the resulting reactions than the transactional stress model: The challenge or threat perception of a situation results in corresponding physiological and emotional reactions. As motivational states, both perceptions lead to an activation of the organism, but two "routes" of activation can be distinguished: the activation of the so-called sympathetic-adreno-medullary system (SAM), as well as the parallel activation of hypothalamic-pituitary-adrenal axis (HPA) (see Table 12.1).

The TCTSA further assumes that the emotions associated with the motivational states can become the subject of evaluation or rather interpretation processes and that these interpretations then (retroactively) influence the currently activated motivational state (Mendes et al., 2008).

Table 12.1 Comparison of reactions to situations that are perceived as threats or challenges (Blascovich & Tomaka, 1996)

Challenge	Threat
Activation of the sympathetic-adreno-medullary system (SAM) - Activation of the sympathetic nervous system - Release of nor/-adrenaline	Activation of the sympathetic-adreno-medullary system (SAM)
Coordinated cardiovascular response - Increased cardiac output - Reduced peripheral vascular resistance - Increased blood flow - Efficient energy consumption	Parallel activation of the hypothalamic-pituitary-adrenal axis (HPA) - Inhibition of nor-/adrenalin release - (Slight) increase in vascular resistance - Blood pressure rises - Inappropriate energy consumption
Joy, hope	Fear, anxiety

> Negative emotions (e.g. anxiety)—usually associated with a motivational state of threat—can also lead to the perception of a challenge if they are interpreted as helpful for overall performance.

Studies in sports show that a state of threat is associated with a stronger perception of anxiety, which is also interpreted as impairing performance compared to a state of challenge. It is generally assumed that challenging motivational states lead to a positive performance outcome, whereas threatening motivational states lead to decreased performance (e.g. Moore et al., 2013a; Turner et al., 2012).

12.3.2.3 Social Evaluation Processes

Situations in sport offer a social situation in which perceptions of threat and threat appraisal can occur in a variety of ways. According to Leary (1992), situations in sport are deeply social.

A key term that can explain why anxiety increases in such social situations is self-presentation. Self-presentation is described as a process in which people try to monitor and control how they are perceived and evaluated by others (Schlenker, 1980). This means that when people find themselves in a social situation, they want to behave in a way that they leave a positive impression on others. As a result of self-presentation, corresponding thoughts or concerns can arise ("self-presentation concerns"), in particular the anxiety of being evaluated by others. These thoughts and concerns in turn influence how people continue to behave in this situation. As a result of self-presentation, athletes may have concerns about their current form or fitness or about their own (lack of) ability. Doubts may also arise as to whether they can cope with pressure situations at all (e.g. Williams et al., 1999; Wilson & Eklund, 1998).

> Self-presentation means to monitor and control how you are perceived and evaluated by others.

In a qualitative study, self-presentation proved to be a source of anxiety in competitions focusing on the importance of the competition itself or the presence of family and friends (James & Collins, 1997). Furthermore, 67% of the 48 sources of anxiety and stress around a competition could be attributed to the topic of self-presentation—a strong indication that these concerns about observing and evaluating oneself are widespread in sport. Research also shows a clearly positive correlation between self-presentation (or the thoughts and worries that follow from it) and state and trait anxiety (e.g. Hudson & Williams, 2001; Wilson & Eklund, 1998). Despite the knowledge of these apparently positive connections between self-presentation, anxiety and sources of stress in sports, the connection between self-presentation and anxiety has not yet been investigated directly. In a small correlational study of young competitive skiers, concerns about social evaluation and anxiety of competition before a competition were indirectly investigated (Bray et al., 2000). The concerns were mainly about the evaluation of competitive performance by family and friends but also the evaluation of skiing itself by friends and competitors. The level of concern about the social evaluation of competitive performance was also positively correlated with concerns about the outcome of the competition. Conversely, concerns about the evaluation of aspects not directly related to performance correlated more with the degree of perception of (physiological) excitement.

> Many people in sports are concerned that they are observed and evaluated ("self-presentation concerns"), which can lead to increases in anxiety.

As shown earlier in this chapter in the analysis of the sources of stress in sport study, observation by video cameras or spectators alone is not always sufficient to cause anxiety. This insight can also be well integrated into more comprehensive theoretical concepts ("social evaluative threat theory", e.g. Rohleder et al., 2007), which define five necessary elements for the perception of social threat (see Question box below). It is assumed that people react to social threats in a similar way as to physical threats. Sporting competition situations are used to test predictions of the theory, for example, in dance sports. Furthermore, there are approaches to integrate the five elements into the design of training conditions in order to better prepare people for competitions and, in particular, to reduce anxiety (Argelaguet Sanz et al., 2015).

Under what conditions does the perception of social threat arise?

- The situation involves a goal that is important to the person.
- A skill or personal attribute (e.g. "strength") must be demonstrated that is important to the person.
- This skill or attribute is evaluated by others.
- A negative evaluation results in the loss of recognition or social status.
- Factors affecting goal achievement are perceived as insufficiently or as not at all controllable.

12.4 The Core: The Anxiety Response in Sport

Now we know characteristics of situations in sport that can trigger anxiety, and we know that attention and evaluation processes take place in these situations, which ultimately lead to the anxiety experienced. But how do we know that we are afraid? How can anxiety be described? If you asked the gymnastics student before his attempted vault, he would probably answer that he is quite excited, maybe a little shaky, and that he is worried that everyone will be watching and laughing at him if he makes a mistake. The student experiences and feels anxiety quite subjectively, without outsiders being able to judge it. Nevertheless, anxiety can also become visible to others, for example, when the teacher feels the student's cold hands or looks into his worried face while helping. The anxiety reaction can therefore be described—like any emotional reaction—as a multidimensional construct with reactions on different levels. A distinction is usually made between an experiential, a physiological and a behavioural component (Mauss & Robinson, 2009; Hackfort & Schwenkmezger, 1989). In principle, "anxiety" can be measured by means of all three components, although it is generally shown that there is little agreement between the measurements of the components—all three components therefore each represent something specific (Mauss & Robinson, 2009).

> Anxiety as a reaction is expressed in subjective experiences, physiological responses and behaviour.

12.4.1 Experiential Component

The experiential component makes up the actual "feeling" (i.e. the phenomenal and conscious experience) and its accompanying thoughts. It comprises everything that a person consciously experiences and "has in his/her head" in a situation. It is the level of reaction that probably has the fundamental meaning for the person, which includes feelings of tension, fear and arousal. In sport psychology studies, this reaction component is also in the forefront, especially when it comes to the question what effect anxiety has on sporting performance (▶ Sect. 12.5.1). Although there are approaches that assume anxiety as a unidimensional reaction (Spielberger, 1966), two facets of the anxiety experience are predominantly discussed in sport, namely, emotionality and worry (Liebert & Morris, 1967). Emotionality (also known as "somatic anxiety") is the *subjective* perception of physical bodily experiences. This is different to the actual physiological reactions of a situation where arousal changes. In fact, the two facets of reaction do not even have to be related (Mauss & Robinson, 2009). Emotionality is therefore the perception of how much excitement and tension a person feels, for example, the perception of a racing heart or the perception of "butterflies in the stomach". The worry facet, conversely, encompasses the pure thought content, which in an anxiety situation mainly comprises worries and negative expectations but also negative thought loops, ruminations about oneself, the current situation or event and possible consequences (Morris et al., 1981). However, there are also indications that the distinction between somatic and cognitive anxiety experience can also be distinguished neurophysiologically. Apparently, somatic anxiety (as "anxious arousal") and cognitive anxiety (as "anxious apprehension") are based on the activation of different specific networks (e.g. Burdwood et al. 2016).

> Emotionality refers to the perception of physiological symptoms of anxiety, such as the queasy feeling in the stomach. It is also known as somatic anxiety.

> Worry is the cognitive component of anxiety, which is expressed in worries, apprehensions and negative thought loops. It can be referred to as cognitive anxiety.

Measuring the experience of trait or state anxiety is important for researchers to understand the interaction between anxiety and performance. The experiential component of anxiety can only be determined by asking the individual about the content of his or her emotion. This is of course possible by asking open questions (qualitative approach) or by using standardized measuring methods, namely, questionnaires (quantitative approach). For qualitative inquiry into competitive anxiety, mostly semi-structured interviews have been used but also analyses of diaries, open questions in questionnaires or recordings of think-aloud verbalizations (Neil et al., 2009). While there is a whole range of instruments for measuring trait anxiety in different sports contexts, there are only a few instruments for measuring state anxiety (see Methods Box and ◘ Table 12.2).

Table 12.2 Questionnaires for assessing trait anxiety and state anxiety, which are frequently used for research studies but also in counselling practice in sport

Questionnaire	Introduction/item-stem	Subscales	Example for item content
State-Trait Anxiety Inventory (Trait)	Answer which best describes how you **usually** feel	–	I'm worried about a possible mishap
State-Trait Anxiety Inventory (State)	Give the answer which seems to describe your **present feelings** best	–	I am perturbed
Sport Anxiety Scale (Trait)	[Answer] how you *usually* feel before or while you compete in sports **Before or while I compete in sports:**	Somatic anxiety	…I feel tense in the stomach
		Cognitive anxiety	…I worry that I will not play well
		Concentration disruption	…I cannot think clearly during the game
Competitive State Anxiety Inventory-2	… choose the answer which describes your feelings **right now**	Somatic anxiety	…my heart is racing
		Cognitive anxiety	…I'm concerned about performing poorly
		Self-confidence	…I'm confident I can meet the challenge

What methods are available for measuring trait anxiety and state anxiety in sport?

Trait anxiety

- Physical Activity and Sport Anxiety Scale(PASAS; Norton et al., 2004)
- Sport Anxiety Scale (SAS; Smith et al., 1990; Revised Form: Smith et al., 2006; translations and adaptations into French, German, Norwegian, Spanish and other languages)
- Sport Competition Anxiety Test (SCAT; Martens et al., 1990b)
- Sport Injury Anxiety Scale (SIAS; Rex & Metzler, 2016)
- Sport Injury Trait Anxiety Scale (SITAS; Kleinert, 2002)
- Social Physique Anxiety Scale (SPAS; Hart et al., 1989)
- Trait version of the State-Trait Anxiety Inventory (STAI, Spielberger et al., 1983; translations into many other languages)

State anxiety

- State version of the STAI (Spielberger et al., 1983; translations into many other languages)
- Competitive State Anxiety Inventory-2 (Martens et al., 1990a; new version Cox et al., 2003; translations and adaptations into Brazilian, French, Greek, Swedish, and other languages)
- Mental Readiness Form (Krane, 1994)
- Retrospectively through direct questioning in an interview (e.g. Mesagno et al., 2009).

12

For the situations described in the introduction, there are many indications of increased anxiety reaction in the experiential component. For example, it was shown that competition-related somatic anxiety and also cognitive anxiety in the period of 4 days before a competition increase towards the day of the competition, with a greater increase in somatic anxiety (Hanton et al., 2002). There is evidence that climbers report higher levels of somatic and cognitive anxiety using the CSAI-2R in the ascent than in the descent (Draper et al., 2008). When people skydive for the first time, they report higher levels of state anxiety when waiting in the airplane for their jump than when they fill out the questionnaire after the jump (Hare et al., 2013).

12.4.2 Physiological Component

Emotions are always associated with activation states of the body, which are accompanied by changes in the different physiological systems operated by the brain or the autonomic nervous system. These represent functional changes in response to the perception of a threat. The core of the physiological reaction component of anxiety is an activation of the organism—especially the autonomic nervous system—and thus a change in the activity of the sympathetic and parasympathetic nervous systems. This leads to measurable physiological changes in the various systems. Hackfort and Schwenkmezger (1989) have tried to categorize these changes into three different classes: respiratory-cardiovascular, electrophysiological and biochemical changes. Psychophysiology provides methods of detecting these changes. A general problem with measuring anxiety in sport via the physiological component is that sporting activity in itself causes physiological changes.

Table 12.3 Physiological indicators of anxiety and methods of measuring them (Hackfort & Schwenkmezger, 1989)

Indicator	Physiological change	Measurement method
Respiratory-cardiovascular	Blood pressure rises Heart rate increases Heart rate variability Respiratory frequency increases Depth of breath increases Peripheral vasoconstriction	Sphygmomanometer Heart rate monitor Electrocardiogram (ECG) Respiration sensor (chest/abdominal belt) Photoplethysmography
Electrophysiological	Skin conductance increases Muscle tone increases Cortical spontaneous activity changes	Electrodermal activity (EDA) Electromyogram (EMG) Electroencephalogram (EEG)
Biochemical	Adrenaline release Cortisol release Alpha-amylase increase Lactate increase	Plasma, urine samples Plasma, saliva samples Saliva sample Blood sample

An increased pulse rate before the 100 m run, for example, is probably largely due to the warm-up programme. Table 12.3 gives an overview of physiological indicators of anxiety and how to measure them.

Methods for measuring changes in the cardiovascular system as well as electrophysiological changes are often used in laboratory studies for a so-called manipulation check (Manipulation check). Thus, "pressure situations" can be detected in the laboratory by increased heart rate (e.g. Masters, 1992), increased sweating (measured via electrodermal activity, e.g. Tremayne & Barry, 1990), an increase in muscle tone (e.g. Caruso et al., 1990) or altered neurophysiological processes (e.g. Murray & Janelle, 2007).

In contrast, biochemical or neuroendocrine indicators are often used in field studies. Many neuroendocrine indicators or "markers" can now be easily collected using saliva samples and evaluated in the laboratory (Strahler & Klumbies, 2012) (Fig. 12.8).

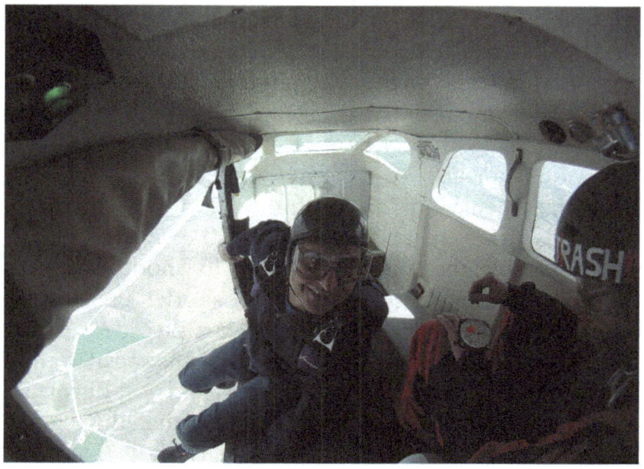

Fig. 12.8 Parachutist shortly before exiting the airplane

Manipulation Check

In psychological experiments, one would like to determine the effect of a condition on a dependent variable, for example, the effect of anxiety on the performance of a sporting task. To do this, an experimental manipulation is first carried out to create this condition in the laboratory. Anxiety is to be created, for example, by a simulated competition situation. In order to be able to trace changes in the dependent variable (here, execution of movement) back to the condition (here, anxiety of competition), this condition must have been proven to exist. It is easy to imagine that "competitive anxiety" cannot be generated in a psychological laboratory immediately. Therefore, it is important to test the effectiveness of the manipulation of conditions (e.g. by spectators or the threat of punishment) independently of the effect (e.g. changed, shaky execution of movements). In experiments on the phenomenon of choking under pressure, therefore, it is usually first checked whether the participants were "under pressure", e.g. by means of an anxiety questionnaire (e.g. Ehrlenspiel et al., 2010) or by means of changes in physiological variables such as heart rate (e.g. Masters, 1992). Only when this proof has been successful can changes in the dependent variable be meaningfully attributed to the experimental manipulation. In the experiments of Ehrlenspiel et al. (2010), for example, only the data of people who actually reported higher anxiety in the "pressure condition" were therefore evaluated.

12.4.3 Behaviour Component

Since emotions have evolved, presumably to produce adaptive behaviour, emotions are also associated with behaviour or behavioural tendencies. Depending on the conception, the behavioural component comprises only expressive behaviour (e.g. facial expressions and gestures) or information processing processes (e.g. attention) or even behavioural willingness and tendencies (e.g. approach or avoidance behaviour).

12.4.3.1 Expressive Behaviour

How anxiety in sport is reflected in expressive behaviour has not yet been explicitly investigated. But the results of studies on non-verbal expressive behaviour in football (e.g. Furley et al., 2012) can be interpreted in such a way that the so-called submissive behaviour of, for example, a penalty kicker—lowered gaze, avoidance of eye contact, drooping shoulders—gives goalkeepers the impression that the kicker experiences anxiety. It is also suspected that penalty shooters who hurry to prepare their shot and may even turn away from the goalkeeper to take a run-up are also expressing anxiety (Jordet & Hartman, 2008). This behaviour can also be interpreted as escape or at least avoidance behaviour—a central behavioural tendency associated with anxiety. Because actual escape behaviour is not possible, for example, in a penalty shootout, escapist tendencies might include a final, shorter preparation time or avoiding eye contact to at least provide a quick, albeit short-term relief from anxiety and the social evaluation situation. However, analyses of World and European Championship penalty shootouts show that this behaviour also tends to lead to missed penalty shots (Jordet & Hartman, 2008). It remains unclear in these studies on expressive behaviour and behavioural willingness whether and to what extent they are really related to anxiety or even express anxiety. It is obvious to assume anxiety in the case of a penalty shooter. Surveys of participants in a penalty shootout at a European Championship confirm this impression (Jordet & Elferink-Gemser, 2012), but in the studies themselves anxiety was not recorded or even deliberately manipulated.

12

> Anxiety in sport is expressed at the behavioural level in the form of submissive (e.g. lowered gaze) or avoidance behaviour (e.g. turning away from the goalkeeper).

12.4.3.2 Information Processing

The altered cognitive processes associated with anxiety are also blamed for the often unfavourable effects of anxiety on behaviour—such as on athletic performance in competition (▶ Sect. 12.5). The focus is on altered attention processes, and there is also evidence of altered decision-making processes. The latter have so far been studied mainly in referees (e.g. Neil et al., 2013). It can be assumed that anxiety is also associated with altered processes, for example, in individual or group tactical decisions. While the self-report of English referees (Neil et al., 2013) did not indicate any effect of pressure characteristics (such as spectator behaviour) on their decisions in the game, an experimental study was able to prove such an influence (Balmer et al., 2007). In the evaluation of controversial video scenes of a football match, noise from the spectators led to a preferential treatment of the home team. This tendency to judge was stronger the more the experienced referees reported cognitive anxiety.

> Anxiety also expresses itself in changed and rather unfavourable attention processes and decision-making behaviour.

More extensive are the findings on altered attention processes, which play a major role in explaining performance deficits under pressure. In theory, the altered cognitive processes can be classified in the Attentional Control Theory: Sports (Eysenck & Wilson, 2016).

Side Story

[Attentional Control Theory: Sports]

If one wants to explain how anxiety leads to poor performance (▶ Sect. 12.5), information processing and especially attention processes play a major role. According to the attentional control theory (Eysenck et al., 2007), anxiety is associated with a lower processing efficiency of information processing, although this is not necessarily reflected in performance effectiveness. This distinction thus allows to explain why pressure situations do not necessarily lead to worse performance. Additional effort and motivation can compensate for the reduced processing efficiency and maintain performance. The theory also distinguishes two attention systems: a targeted, intentional "top-down" system of "proactive control" and a stimulus-driven "bottom-up" system of "reactive control" that responds to sensory stimuli. Under pressure, proactive control is disturbed. Especially central executive functions such as "inhibition" (i.e. of stimuli and reactions) and "shifting" (i.e. changing of attention) should be impaired. Stimulation (and thus bottom-up attention) is thus given greater importance, but a person would also be more easily distracted from the actual task.

The extension to Attentional Control Theory: Sports (ACTS; Eysenck & Wilson, 2016) takes into account the specific conditions of performance situations in sports compared to the cognitive performance usually investigated. Thus, the current anxiety state probably plays a more important role. According to ACTS, this arises primarily from distorted attention control and a distorted appraisal of the situation (Sect. 12.3). In a sport performance situation ("pressure"), threat-relevant stimuli (e.g. the opponent) are perceived and ambiguous stimuli (e.g. spectators) are perceived as threatening, which increases anxiety. These cognitive distortions are also accompanied by increased "error monitoring"—people compare the execution of tasks with a target and are more likely to perceive mistakes. This can create a vicious circle in sport situations: The increased perception of errors also leads to a perception of failed execution or even failure, which is likely to result in increased anxiety and increased selective attention to threatening stimuli and their interpretation. Sporting situations with their mostly immediate performance feedback and the "costs" associated with failure represent special conditions in this respect. However, the ACTS explicitly assumes that inadequate attention control occurs only rarely and only under particularly high levels of anxiety, for example, when serving in the Olympic final or after a particularly unsuccessful attempt. However, in order for the targeted and proactive control system to remain activated even in cases of anxiety, either special motivation or at least additional processing resources and self-control are required.

Anxiety seems to be primarily associated with the fact that distracting or disturbing thoughts are harder to suppress ("inhibition", Attentional Control Theory: Sports) and that the focus of attention is unfavourably changed ("shifting", Attentional Control Theory: Sports). That disturbing thoughts appear in anxiety situations can be shown by qualitative methods. Correspondingly, a quarter of the statements of top athletes on thought content during competitions could be assigned to the categories "distraction" or "disturbance", whereby the recording was thus again based on the experience component (Oudejans et al., 2011).

> Anxiety in sport is expressed in the fact that distracting thoughts are harder to control and the focus of attention is directed to threat-relevant stimuli.

More objectively and actually on the behavioural component, attention processes can be inferred by recording eye movements. The "quiet eye" (Methods Box Quiet Eye) is particularly relevant here (i.e. the final fixation) in the course of movement. The quiet eye requires attention control in terms of orientation and shielding from other stimuli (Eysenck & Wilson, 2016). Accordingly, anxiety should affect the duration of the quiet eye and the number of fixations. And indeed, a study on free-throw basketball (Wilson et al., 2009) showed that under anxiety the duration of the quiet eye decreased and at the same time the number of (further) fixations increased—an indication of impaired inhibition and greater distractibility by external stimuli. Attentional control can also be trained, for example, by means of simple visual search tasks on a monitor. After such attention training, tennis players in a pressure situation showed longer final fixations and more stable scoring performance compared to a control group without attention training (Ducrocq et al., 2016).

> Anxiety is expressed in the gaze behaviour by numerous and restless eye movements and a short last fixation ("quiet eye").

Sports Practice

In football, the penalty kick represents the greatest possible pressure situation for shooters. In addition to the situation as such, the goalkeeper's behaviour has a strong influence on the penalty kick and thus causes further uncertainty among the players. When it was still one of the truths in football—or at least a felt truth—that English teams in particular lose in important penalty kicks, this was one of the reasons why the British Association of Sport and Exercise Sciences invited experts to compile the most important findings on psychological preparation for a penalty kick and to communicate them in an understandable way in an "expert statement" (Wilson et al., 2013).

While it is difficult to imitate in training the tension of a penalty kick during a World Cup final, the action strategies of penalty takers can be trained. Such strategies can be derived from many research findings and should be developed jointly in team meetings. Penalty takers show more precise performance when they choose their target independently of the goalkeeper. A hard and precise penalty kick is difficult to "save" anyway. So work should be done to constantly convert shots from the penalty spot into all four corners of the goal. In order to increase the difficulty of the exercise and the pressure, the goalkeeper can even be told the shot direction in advance. The sequence of action steps during the penalty, from the placing of the ball on the penalty spot to the cheering after the goal, can also be stabilized by rituals. The individually rehearsed routines help players to achieve maximum performance in extreme situations such as the World Cup final.

In competition, it is important that players trust their own learned skills, set the goal in advance and focus on it. In addition, it is crucial to maintain temporal consistency throughout the course of the action to avoid rushed shots and unsuccessful performance. For example, players were more successful if they took more time when placing the ball and after the referee's whistle (Jordet & Hartman, 2008). Finally, penalty kicks are not only about doing your own job, but also about keeping your teammates on the ball. Cheers and openly displayed emotions after a goal is scored are conducive to encouraging those who follow and intimidating the opposing team.

Finally, tactical measures can also be used; it is a psychological advantage to start in a penalty shootout with the first penalty kick. If you take a penalty kick that promotes your team's victory, you are more likely to succeed than if you take a penalty kick to avoid defeat (i.e. you are currently behind).

12.5 Effects of Anxiety in Sport

The question of the effects of anxiety in sport, especially on athletic performance, is one of the core questions in sport psychology research and consulting. Anxiety is often seen as the cause of failure in competition or of apparent avoidance behaviour in physical education. Research first attempts to clarify the relationship between anxiety and behaviour and especially performance in sport (see ◘ Fig. 12.9). From this personality psychological "state perspective" (Ehrlenspiel et al., 2018b), the connection between anxiety and performance is quantified, for example, by correlating values in an anxiety questionnaire with sporting performance. Research also attempts to elucidate the mechanisms of this relationship and to establish generally valid rules. From this "general psychological" perspective, cognitive processes, especially of attention control during movement but also of motivation, are suspected and tested. Finally, research attempts to identify stable characteristics of people (and situations) that have an influence on this relationship (the "trait perspective"). In addition to the effect of anxiety on performance in sport situations, anxiety has other effects such as preventive actions, but these have rarely been studied.

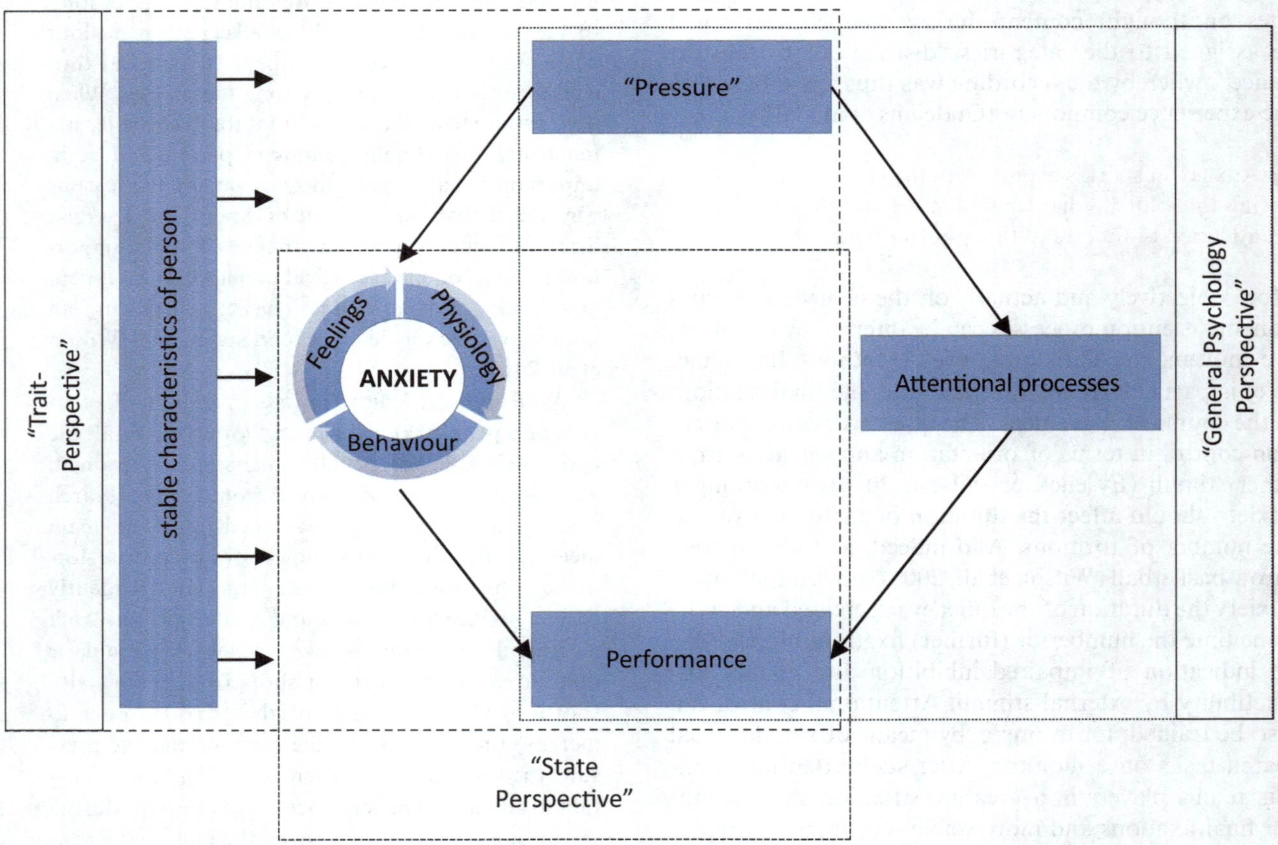

◘ **Fig. 12.9** Perspectives on the relationship between anxiety and performance

12.5.1 Anxiety and Athletic Performance

Intuitively, the relationship between anxiety and sporting performance might be that anxiety has a negative effect on sporting performance and that this becomes even stronger with an increase in anxiety intensity. However, research over the last 100 years shows that this relationship is by no means simple.

12.5.1.1 Drive

An early conceptual anxiety-performance relationship was Hull's drive theory and the expansion of Spence's approach (Hull, 1952; Spence & Spence, 1966). In essence, this is a motivation theory which assumes that energy activation of the organism occurs when especially primary and thus mostly physiological needs are threatened or unstable (so-called drive). With increasing drive, the activation ("arousal") also increases, which in turn increases effort, emotions and motivation. The greater the drive or activation, the better the sporting performance should be. However, perhaps also on the basis of personal experience, one can doubt whether an increased level of activation in all sports is purposeful and results in optimal performance. Golfers, for example, do not usually hype themselves up before they tee off or putt; they want to be calm. And (only) in this way they are able to consistently achieve their best performance in these situations. Hull's theory is therefore not particularly successful in predicting athletic performance under conditions of increased activation. Moreover, as a motivation theory, it cannot explain important phenomena—such as the motivational effect of money, which does not satisfy any physiological need. But it is the basis for a more general psychological extension, which assumes that differences in activation stimulate different cognitive processes.

12.5.1.2 Inverted-U Hypothesis

A better-known anxiety and performance assumption is an initially positive effect of increased (anxiety-related) activation but, rather than linear, an inverted U-shaped connection between anxiety (or, more precisely, activation) and performance. This assumption, also known as the "Yerkes-Dodson hypothesis", states that when activation increases, (athletic) performance also increases until an optimal activation level is reached. Once the optimal activation level is reached, however, a further increase in activation leads to decreased performance. This means that moderate activation levels create optimal performance. Low or high activation levels, conversely, can result in poorer performance. This assumption is based on a study of mice by Yerkes and Dodson (1908). The mice learned to orient themselves in a labyrinth and were punished with electrical shocks of different currents when they made mistakes. Mice that were punished with a medium current needed the least learning attempts; at very high or very low currents, the mice learned much slower.

> The inverted-U hypothesis` means that a medium activation level is most effective for optimal performance.

The inverted-U hypothesis offers an intuitive and easy answer about the anxiety-performance relationship (Krane, 1992), and some empirical evidence of its validity can also be found. For example, an inverted U-shaped relationship between competitive anxiety and performance was found in female basketball players (Sonstroem & Bernardo, 1982) when comparing three games. In the game, the players indicated a medium level of competitive anxiety, and the best performance was also shown.

? What are the criticisms of the so-called inverted-U hypothesis?

- Some researchers suggest that the theory, by its simplicity, is not able to describe what happens when performance drops dramatically and abruptly.
- Optimal performance does not occur in all sports or all athletes at a moderate level of activation.
- Research on the inverted-U hypothesis takes a one-dimensional perspective. In essence, it refers only to the physiological aspect, the activation, but not to the experience.
- In many empirical studies, however, the physiological aspect is then only investigated by means of questionnaires and the recording of emotionality.

12.5.1.3 Multidimensional Anxiety Theory

With the development of a multidimensional understanding of anxiety with the components worry and emotionality, the idea of the connection between anxiety and performance also changed. The focus of the multidimensional anxiety theory (MAT; Burton, 1988; Martens et al., 1990a) is no longer physiological activation but the subjective experience of anxiety with its components. For both components, different specific correlations with performance are postulated.

For cognitive anxiety, the hypothesis is that it is linearly negatively related to performance. Performance decreases with an increase in cognitive anxiety because essential resources are consumed by cognitive anxiety and therefore no further attention capacity is available to support task performance (Wine, 1971). The MAT assumes the relationship between somatic anxiety and performance has an inverted-U relationship, whereby optimal performance can be expected with moderate somatic anxiety. Performance slumps, however, can occur when the optimal level of somatic anxiety is not achieved or is exceeded. In addition, the MAT indicates that self-confidence has a moderating influence on the anxiety-performance relationship. Self-confidence is conviction in the ability to successfully perform an action or behaviour. In general, the more self-confidence a person has, the less anxiety he or she feels. Self-confidence and performance have a positive linear relationship. With increasing confidence, performance is also enhanced.

> According to multidimensional anxiety theory, cognitive anxiety is negatively related, and emotionality is inversely U-shaped, to performance.

Only a few studies have explicitly tested the inverted-U relationship between somatic anxiety and performance. Burton (1988) found an inverted-U relationship between somatic anxiety and performance in various swimming competitions and a negative linear relationship between cognitive anxiety and performance. However, this negative linear correlation seems to be only slight. This is shown by meta-analyses (Craft et al., 2003; Woodman & Hardy, 2003), and these also fail to agree on the influence of gender or competitive level on this correlation (Ehrlenspiel et al., 2018b). The correlation between self-confidence and performance seems to be a strong positive correlation (i.e. confidence leads to better performance). One might say that it is not anxiety that leads to poor performance but the absence of anxiety that leads to good performance.

> In summary, the MAT assumes that the best possible performance is achieved when there is high self-confidence, a moderate level of somatic anxiety and low cognitive anxiety.

12.5.1.4 Catastrophe Theory

A major criticism of the MAT is that it cannot explain why a significant sudden drop in performance can occur even though, for example, an athlete has shown a good competitive performance up to that point. These sudden drops in performance are the beginning of the "catastrophe theory". It is based on a multidimensional understanding of anxiety and assumes an interaction, a mutual influence of somatic and cognitive anxiety (Hardy, 1990).

The catastrophe theory predicts that when cognitive anxiety is low, the relationship between physiological activation (arousal) and performance changes depending on the level of cognitive anxiety. In principle, the catastrophe theory assumes an inverted-U shape between arousal and performance. Moderate arousal leads to optimal performance; too low or too high arousal can impair performance. Increasing cognitive anxiety now results in a more pronounced inverted-U relationship. With increases in cognitive anxiety, increasing physiological arousal increases performance to an optimal point. A further increase in arousal (under higher cognitive anxiety) beyond this point results in "drastic" performance losses, a "catastrophe" (Hardy & Parfitt, 1993). This catastrophe is also reflected in a hysteresis effect: When a catastrophe occurs, a significant reduction in arousal is necessary to restore the previous performance level.

> According to catastrophe theory, the effect of arousal on performance is also inversely U-shaped, but increasing cognitive anxiety leads to a more pronounced correlation and therefore tends to lead to drastic performance losses.

The dramatic course, the "catastrophe", between anxiety increase and performance is, for example, presented in a qualitative study (Edwards et al., 2002): The athletes from very different sports complained about a sudden but also an unstoppable drop in performance. In quantitative studies, however, there was often no evidence of the hysteresis effect (Hardy et al., 1994). Presumably, self-confidence could have a buffering effect on the relationship (Hanton et al., 2008a). For example, athletes with strong self-confidence may be able to tolerate increased arousal before a drastic drop in performance occurs.

> Once sporting performance has collapsed under high cognitive anxiety due to too much arousal, a significant relaxation is required before performance can be maintained or increase again.

The merit of the catastrophe theory lies first in that at least two components of anxiety are no longer only considered independently of each other (as in the MAT) but that they (obviously) interact. However, the postulated nonlinear relationship is difficult to test empirically (cf. Krane, 1992). And in terms of content, it remains controversial whether this is actually arousal (i.e. the physiological) or whether the somatic anxiety (i.e. the experiential component) is not actually the more relevant factor.

12.5.2 Anxiety and Movement Control

Based on the anxiety-performance relationship discussed thus far, one might question what processes are responsible for declines in performance as a result of increased anxiety. From a general psychological perspective, we try to uncover generally valid mechanisms that can explain *how* anxiety leads to poor performance. Important explanatory approaches were initially based on the ideas of the drive theory already discussed (Hull, 1952), which focused primarily on physiological arousal. Currently, however, mainly attention processes are discussed, partly in connection with working memory.

The first theoretical approaches to the mechanisms of the anxiety-performance relationship originate from a diametrically opposed research approach, the research on social facilitation. Beginning with the observation by Norman Tripplett (1898) that cyclists in his laboratory rode faster when other cyclists were present, attempts were made to investigate the (beneficial) effect of spectators or those present on (athletic) performance. With increasing research, there were increasing indications of a "paradoxical" effect (Baumeister & Showers, 1986), namely, failure under pressure—known as choking under pressure (i.e. choking). It seems important to note that for choking to occur, the increase in perceived anxiety and a decrease in performance below the individual's normal performance level are essential (Mesagno & Hill, 2013).

Choking under pressure is the acute and significant decline in skill and performance caused by increased anxiety under perceived pressure, even if one's own performance expectations were actually achievable (Mesagno & Hill, 2013).

Optimal performance in sport is characterized by the direction of attentional focus towards task-related information and simultaneous ignoring of irrelevant information (Moran, 1996). For example, a student queuing to perform a gymnastics vault might concentrate on a specific point on the vaulting horse (task-related information) rather than focusing on the painful experiences of previous attempts over the apparatus (irrelevant information). Focusing on a specific point would help the student to successfully complete the task. Under increased anxiety, however, unfavourable attentional shifts may occur, and in the case of choking it is discussed whether anxiety leads to distraction (Distraction Model) or to increased self- or movement-related attention (Self-Focus Model) (see ◘ Fig. 12.10).

12.5.2.1 Distraction

In sport, the so-called distraction models of choking show that athletes are more easily distracted by task-irrelevant information when their anxiety increases (Mesagno & Beckmann, 2017). This leads to a shift in attention away from task-relevant information. Choking occurs mainly because the processing of task-irrelevant information (e.g. also anxiety, explicit self-instructions) exceeds a certain level of attention capacity and thus reduces the potential space of attention that would be necessary for optimal performance. Evidence of the validity of the "distraction" assumption is derived from qualitative studies on the experience of "pressure" by competitive athletes and from experimental studies, especially on perception and eye movements. In a qualitative, interview-based study, experienced competitive athletes stated that in decisive situations (i.e. "pressure situations") they focused primarily on worries and negative thoughts and thought little about the execution of movements (Oudejans et al., 2011). In addition, they often expressed the desire to choose a positive internal-personal attention focus, which could be used for motivation or concentration control. If one examines eye

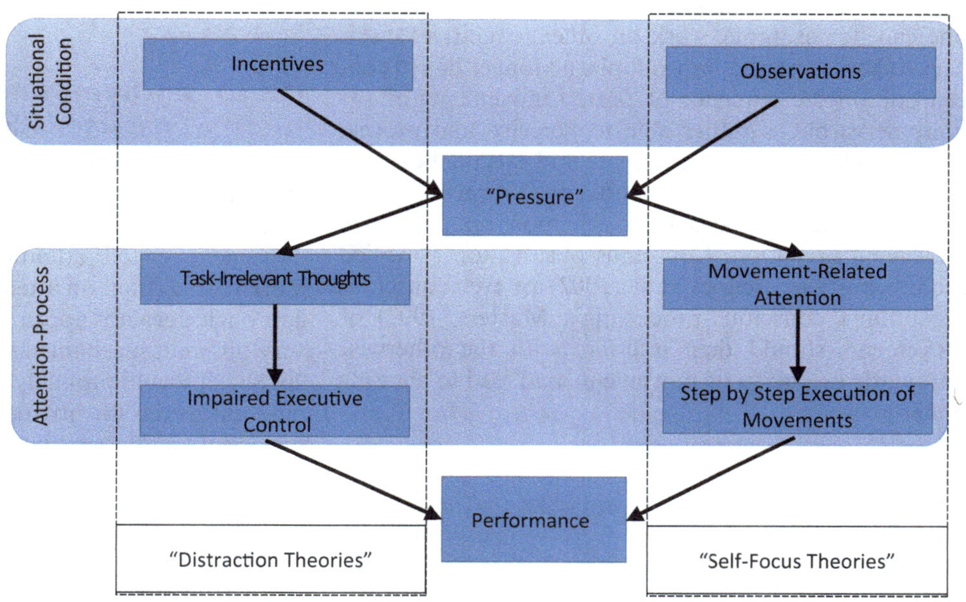

◘ **Fig. 12.10** Contrast of the two most discussed approaches to explain the phenomenon of choking under pressure

movements under pressure, athletes tend to look at more places, more briefly, and, in particular, focus on the target more briefly, than under no anxiety (e.g. Vickers & Williams, 2007; Wilson et al., 2009).

> Distraction models assume that under pressure, task-irrelevant information is processed and therefore attention resources are missing.

One mechanism is explicitly postulated by the attentional control theory ▶ Sect. 12.3.1 of Eysenck et al. (2007), which assumes that anxiety impairs working memory functions. As a result, more task-irrelevant internal and external stimuli are processed, and the capacity of working memory decreases further. This deficient information processing can, however, be compensated by increased effort, and experiments have shown evidence of impaired attention processes (in the EEG; Murray & Janelle, 2007 or in eye movements; Alder et al., 2016) while maintaining the same effectiveness (i.e. performance). However, these compensation strategies can also be ineffective (Eysenck & Calvo, 1992).

12.5.2.2 Movement Focused Attention

Advocates of the so-called self-focus models (e.g. Baumeister, 1984; Beilock & Carr, 2001; Masters, 1992) assume that choking occurs because attention is focused on the execution of movement when anxiety increases. The origins for self-focus models are theories of motor learning (e.g. Fitts & Posner, 1967). These theories assume that, at least in explicit (i.e. conscious) motor learning processes, movements are initially performed step by step, consciously and in a controlled manner. With increasing skill level, the execution no longer requires constant conscious control. From a moderate skill level and above, movements are automated and one can, for example, work on other (cognitive) tasks. The volleyball player, for example, no longer has to concentrate on the sequence of partial movements of the jump serve but is rather able to perceive and process the tactical signs of her teammate and execute her serve accordingly. With increased anxiety, however, people may involuntarily focus their attention on their own movement execution. Conscious observation ("explicit monitoring"; see Beilock et al., 2002) or even conscious execution ("conscious processing"; Masters, 1992) of movements should then interfere with the otherwise automatic execution of movements and lead to choking under pressure.

> Self-focus models assume that attention is drawn to the movement under pressure, which impairs the "automatic" fluid execution.

Beilock and Carr (2001) showed that pressure can lead to performance-impairing attempts at conscious control and a step-by-step execution of movements, even if these are otherwise already executed automatically. Normally fluid movements, which are necessary for the successful execution of movements, are thus prevented. In this way the volleyball player could become aware of the steps required for a serve, and through this conscious control, mistakes could arise, for example, at transitions between partial movements.

Masters (1992) furthermore suggested that under "pressure" explicit knowledge about movement is reinvested (i.e. becomes conscious and is used to control movements). This knowledge is usually used at the beginning of motor learning processes and also traditionally at the heart of skill instruction. Controlled execution, as it takes place at the beginning of learning, should then lead to poor performance. In his study, masters' participants were supposed to learn golf putts—by explicit (explicit instructions on how to execute movements) or implicit movement learning (without explicit instructions, with additional task). The golf putts were then to be executed under low and high stress. Masters was able to prove that the performance of participants who had acquired the skills through explicit movement learning deteriorated under stress. In contrast, those participants who had learned the skills implicitly were able to maintain their performance. People who learn movements implicitly should therefore be able to automatically retrieve their performance under stress, as they do not have explicit information available to them, which may be detrimental under stress.

> Learning processes in sport are often designed in such a way that a lot of explicit knowledge about movement is generated. However, implicit learning, for example, via analogies or metaphors, could prevent choking.

12.5.2.3 Environmental and Personal Characteristics as Moderators

There are attempts to reconcile the two different approaches (see Mesagno et al., 2015), with "distraction" and "self-focus" as two sides of the same coin—movement-related attention would then be nothing more than a drain on attention resources. However, this approach does not appear to be effective in view of the very different mechanisms of action (Ehrlenspiel et al., 2018b). It would probably be more beneficial to look for moderators (i.e. for situation or personal characteristics) that could influence the relationship between anxiety and performance.

On the situational side, there are indications that distraction is more likely to be effective in cognitive performance (e.g. arithmetic tasks). Attentional resources are then no longer available for executive functions such as planning. In the case of procedural performances such as sport, movement-related attention should interfere with otherwise automatic execution. The type of "pressure" is discussed as a further situation characteristic. If "pressure" results mainly from incentives or the avoidance of negative consequences ("outcome pressure"), this should lead to distracting thoughts. If, however, "pressure" results from the expectation of an evaluation of the person ("monitoring pressure"), self-monitoring and conscious task execution arise (see Beilock & Carr, 2001).

People also differ in their inclination to certain attention or information processing processes, especially when they are under pressure. In the research literature, two very close constructs are discussed: tendency to reinvest and state orientation. The "theory of reinvestment" (Masters & Maxwell, 2008) states that individuals have a predisposition to focus on the execution of movement, whereby they can retrieve knowledge about the components of the skill. Reinvestment thus describes the tendency of people in sport to make declarative knowledge of movement sequences conscious and to control them, even though they are already well mastered. Indeed, this tendency to conscious attention control seems to be related to failure under pressure (Masters & Maxwell, 2008).

Similarly, state-oriented people, especially in assessment situations (Kuhl, 1992), tend to maintain cognitive, affective and attention-related states—for example, to ruminate—even if this is accompanied by impaired performance. By contrast, action-oriented people are able to change these states in order to optimize their performance. In fact, it has been shown that state-oriented people perform worse in pressure situations than action-oriented people, e.g. in basketball free throws (Gröpel, 2016). Apparently, it is more difficult for state-oriented people under pressure to change their focus of attention and divert it away from themselves.

> The risk of choking under pressure increases for people who tend to think intensively about the way they move and/or their current condition.

Mediation Versus Moderation

Psychological research attempts in particular to make statements about which characteristics of a person or a situation have an effect on the behaviour and experience—for example, whether the presence of spectators leads to poor performance in a competition. However, people are usually more complex than such simple cause-and-effect relationships would suggest. Either another characteristic can influence the cause-and-effect relationship (moderation), or the cause does not act directly, but via another variable (mediation). For example, the more persons think intensively about how they present themselves in public and what other people think about them, the more likely and stronger it is that the presence of spectators will lead to poor performance. There is therefore an interaction between the situation characteristic of the presence of spectators and the person characteristic of "self-awareness". Analyses of variance examine the interaction effects of two independent *discrete* variables or characteristics on a dependent variable. By means of a moderation analysis, the interaction of continuous variables can be examined; self-awareness would then be the moderator. Mediation analyses, on the other hand, examine paths of effects: The presence of spectators leads to self-monitoring and attention being focused on the execution of movements, which in turn leads to altered execution of movements and ultimately to poor performance. A mediator such as attention control is thus simultaneously a dependent variable (on the presence of spectators) and an independent variable (it affects performance).

The Self-Presentation Model Empirically Tested

A subsequent study shows that these connections are moderated by personal characteristics. Here, the effect of pressure manipulation on the performance of basketball players was examined, who showed a low or high degree of fear of negative evaluation (Mesagno et al., 2012). Participants attempted basketball free throws in a normal or pressure condition, where pressure was generated by a combination of cash incentives, a video camera and the presence of other players. Both the anxiety state and the free-throw performance were recorded. Athletes with a pronounced fear of negative evaluation had higher anxiety levels and showed weaker performance under pressure than those with a low fear of negative evaluation. In fact, people with a low fear of negative evaluation did not experience an increase in anxiety and were even able to improve their performance under pressure—clear indications of resilience. Mediation analyses also showed that the personality trait of fear of negative evaluation not only had a direct effect on performance but that this effect was also partly mediated by cognitive anxiety. Performance apparently declines under pressure because the fear of negative evaluation causes worry and doubt.

12.5.3 Other Effects of Anxiety in Sport

Sport and anxiety is—as seen—mainly considered from the perspective of sport or motor performance. Accordingly, both the theoretical considerations of the connection and the empirical findings are extensive and detailed. As our initial examples show, we encounter anxiety in sport outside the performance context, and anxiety has other additional effects and functions, yet only limited research has been done on these other effects.

12.5.3.1 Physical Activity and Exercise

For example, anxiety in sport has been associated with the level of participation in physical education or physical activity in general. However, with regard to social physique anxiety, no clear connection can be deduced from the research (Sabiston et al., 2014). Studies show that increased social physique anxiety is associated with less effort in physical education and even absenteeism (Cox et al., 2011). Other studies show that social physique anxiety is not directly related to sports (Melbye et al., 2007) or even to increased physical effort in sports (Aşçı et al., 2006). In fact, social physique anxiety is also associated with excessive exercise (i.e. exercise dependence) or even sports addiction (Cook et al., 2015).

> Studies show that anxiety in the form of concerns about one's appearance can lead to both increased or decreased physical activity.

Personal and situational characteristics are blamed for these at least apparently contradictory findings, and it is assumed that social physique anxiety is not directly related to sporting activity but primarily influences motivational variables (Sabiston et al., 2014). For example, social physique anxiety is more likely to be observed in individuals—predominantly women—with high self-presentation concerns (► Sect. 12.3.2). It is also found among people who feel less recognized by their environment and those who do sports mainly because of their own appearance. Social physique anxiety therefore may also lead to less sporting activity if one's own figure (or that of other participants) becomes more visible during sport—for example, through mirrors or figure-hugging clothing (Crawford & Eklund, 1994). There is also evidence that social physique anxiety is associated primarily with lower intrinsic motivation to engage in sports and a more controlled regulation of motivation (Cox et al., 2011). However, a major problem with research on sporting activity and social physique anxiety remains that studies predominantly use cross-sectional designs. Therefore, one can only make statements about correlations, but not inferences about causalities. It is quite conceivable that sporting activity leads to a confrontation with the body, from which anxiety could arise.

12.5.3.2 Risk and Safety Behaviour

From our introductory examples from climbing and skydiving, it is clear that anxiety in sport can also arise from a real danger. In such sports, which are also known as high-risk sports, serious injury or even death must be expected as an inherent part of the sport (Barlow et al., 2015).

People who engage in these risky sports often do so in search of intense emotional experiences. In other words, they are virtually searching for the anxiety experiences associated with risky sports. Anxiety is then not necessarily experienced as unpleasant, but as pleasant and rewarding. People probably expose themselves to such anxiety experiences in sport for two different motives: the pure constant search for unusual, new and intense experiences—what is also called "sensation-seeking" (Zuckerman, 2007)—and the search for experiences to determine how to handle emotions and cope with them. In order to further strengthen the intense experiences, people with a need for sensation-seeking often try to further increase danger and the risk of physical injury through special risky behaviour (e.g. not wearing protective equipment). Experiencing anxiety thus leads to risky behaviour (■ Fig. 12.11).

> Sensation-seekers—people in search of unusual, intense experiences—increase their anxiety experiences through risky behaviour. Anxiety is perceived as pleasant.

Another motivation for engaging in risky sports activities is that people are looking for ways to handle emotions and cope with them because they tend to have a rather shallow emotional experience in everyday life (Barlow et al., 2013). Their outdoor activities therefore differ from other common activities of sensation-seekers such as dangerous driving or skydiving. Rather, the chosen risky sports such as rock climbing, expeditions in the perpetual ice of the Antarctic or round-the-world single-handed sailboat trips always involve great efforts both in preparation and execution. These then offer the opportunity to experience a strong and concrete emotion such as anxiety and to see how this is heightened by the activity but also how it can be "brought under control" through behavioural measures. The risky sport then serves the experience of emotion regulation.

Correspondingly, sensation-seekers tend to deliberately provoke risks and put themselves in danger, while people who are motivated to engage in risky sports with the opportunity to regulate their emotions tend to act

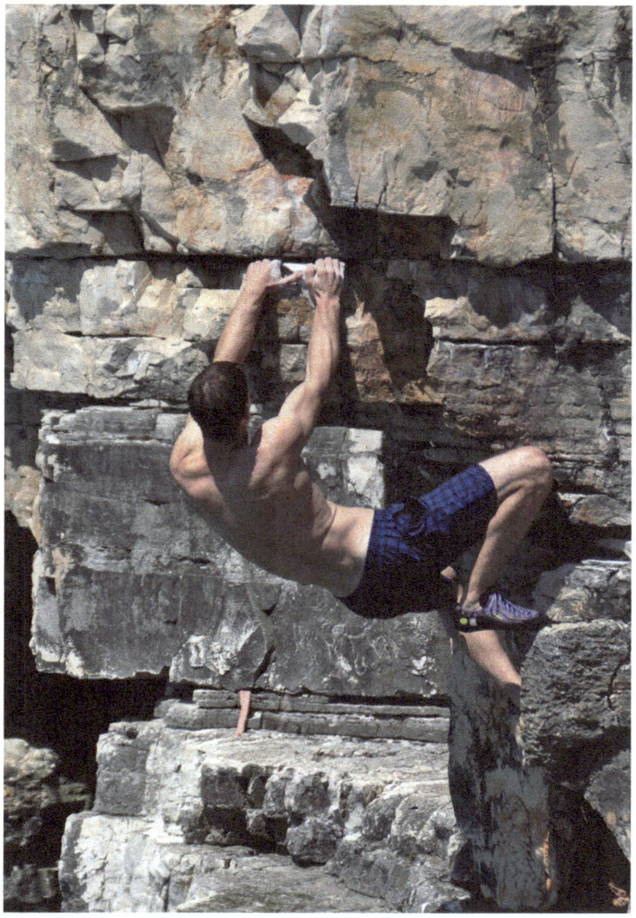

Fig. 12.11 Free solo climbing: risky sport with intensive emotional experiences

cautiously and with precautionary. Risks in sports and the associated experience of anxiety can therefore lead to both risky and protective behaviour—depending on overarching personality traits.

> For many people who practice dangerous outdoor sports, the focus is not on the anxiety experience but on coping with anxiety—which then also leads to preventive safety behaviour.

Question

Reinhold Messner, one of the most famous mountaineers, who among other things was the first person to summit all 14 eight-thousanders without supplementary oxygen, once said: "Stress, anxiety, the cold and the state between life and death are such powerful experiences that we need them again and again. We become addicted. Strangely enough, we try hard to get back home safely, but at home we want nothing more than to return to danger" (Reinhold Messner in Coffey, 2005, p. 17).

Think about what type of motivation might be the main focus for Reinhold Messner. Also do some research on his attitudes towards mountaineering with aids (such as bottled oxygen) or on how he dealt with the death of his brother on Nanga Parbat.

12.6 Managing Anxiety in Sport

Our initial examples from beach volleyball, climbing, gymnastics lessons and skydiving have shown that we encounter anxiety in many sport situations. Since anxiety is a condition that is usually perceived as unpleasant and is often closely related to poor performance, it seems sensible to consider how to manage it. Attempts at managing anxiety, however, do not necessarily have to lead to a reduction in anxiety to have positive effects on performance. It seems more important that the individual attempts to reach an emotional state that allows to master the task in the respective sporting situation. Although this idea of an (individual) "zone of optimal functioning" (Hanin, 2000) takes into account various positive and negative emotions, reaching an adaptive, a functional level of anxiety is pertinent to reach optimal performance.

> Coping with anxiety in sport means that a person achieves a state that is functional for him or her and that is conducive to coping with the task in the sporting situation.

Managing anxiety can be viewed from two temporal perspectives: anticipation and compensation. Anxiety often arises in anticipation and is an expression of the perception of a threat from a future situation. Thus, anxiety may occur when putting on gym clothes or when warming up for the Olympic finals. From a compensation perspective, which is temporally prior to an event, it is primarily about managing the situation and preventing the feeling of anxiety from arising in the first place. These coping efforts can be particularly well anchored in the transactional stress model (Lazarus & Folkman, 1984), where they are also referred to as "coping". However, compensatory strategies are also necessary if anxiety is to be regulated in a situation, for example, immediately before jumping out of an airplane or while climbing a rock (see Tenenbaum & Sacks, 2007).

In this context, coping with anxiety is understood to mean the preventive and rather long-term preparation for the situation, whereas anxiety regulation is aimed at the immediate change in the anxiety experienced during a certain situation.

While coping efforts are usually aimed at reducing negative emotions or conditions such as stress, emotion regulation can also serve to intensify or transfer emotions into others. Negative emotions such as anxiety can also be intentionally amplified if this is functional in the situation, for example, to increase energy (or arousal) before a 100 m run. Emotion regulation can be well described within the Consensual Modal Model (Gross, 2008). An attempt is made to assign strategies and techniques of anxiety regulation in sport to the individual phases of the emotional process. Many of the techniques of anxiety regulation can also be understood as coping techniques.

> Anxiety regulation does not only mean the reduction of anxiety but possibly also the increase of anxiety or the change to another emotion.

12.6.1 Coping with Anxiety

In ► Sect. 12.3.2, the transactional stress model (Lazarus & Folkman, 1984) was described, whereby anxiety should arise from a threat perception, the perception may indicate the situational importance, and a limited ability to cope with the stressor is determined. Coping or stress management is therefore understood by Lazarus (1999) as a process consisting of coping with a stressor. It includes efforts on the cognitive, affective and behavioural levels. Such a stress would be, for example, the unimaginably large audience in the stadium and behind television screens around the world when serving in the Olympic beach volleyball final.

Coping efforts can have different functions and can therefore be assigned to different categories. Lazarus and Folkman (1984) generally distinguish at least strategies that directly deal with the problem and the situation ("problem-focused coping") from those that are more aimed at alleviating the effects of the stress ("emotion-focused coping"). In the breaks between the sets of a beach volleyball match, for example, the players could try to block out the spectators by pulling towels over their heads, or they could do relaxation exercises. Both strategies mentioned here could also be assigned to another common category, namely, avoidance coping (Roth & Cohen, 1986).

> Problem-focused coping with anxiety tries to directly change the situation or behaviour, whereas emotion-focused coping attempts to alleviate the stress and its associated experiences.

To avoid such conceptual overlaps between possible categories, a three-factorial system has been proposed (Nicholls et al., 2016), which distinguishes between "mastery" coping, "internal regulation" and "goal withdrawal". Mastery coping includes all attempts to bring the situation under control and/or to remove the stress or anxiety trigger. This includes, for example, methods of goal-setting or targeted preparation. "Internal regulation" attempts to control the internal, psychological and physiological stress or anxiety reaction, for example, by relaxing or blocking out the environment with a towel. Finally, "goal withdrawal" aims at overcoming stress and anxiety by not pursuing the goal of the action or by lowering expectations. Furthermore, an effective strategy for coping with anxiety of competition seems to be "self-handicapping" (Coudevylle et al., 2008). Berglas and Jones (1978) defined self-handicapping as "any action or choice of performance setting that enhances the opportunity to externalize (or excuse) failure and to internalize (reasonably accept credit for) success" (p. 406). An example of self-handicapping before a competition might be an athlete suggesting that an alleged, or actual, bad sleep may affect performance. This coping strategy might decrease anxiety because it may decrease the importance of the event, but it is sometimes counterproductive to sport performance.

Long-term stress management in sport, however, includes not only measures that relate to behaviour but also those that intend to change conditions. Based on the transactional stress model, the idea is not only to change appraisal processes or to regulate the stress response, but stressors can be reduced and conditions for successful coping can be created. For example, by seeking social support or by setting tasks differently (real training breaks for recovery), this can then also be called stressor management (Beckmann & Ehrlenspiel, 2018).

For physical education research on interventions is lacking. Schack (1997) presents a comprehensive intervention for overcoming anxiety. This aims at a (re-)establishment of action control. Here, different approaches are combined, for example, regulation of tension through breathing and counting exercises or imagination. In the course of the intervention, the school age students are taught what functional benefits anxiety can have. For example, anxiety signifies possible actual dangers and ensures caution. In this way it should no longer be perceived as a "foe" to be overcome, but as a helpful friend.

> In order to cope with anxiety, it helps to become aware that anxiety can be helpful, for example, it leads to preventive behaviour (◘ Fig. 12.12).

12

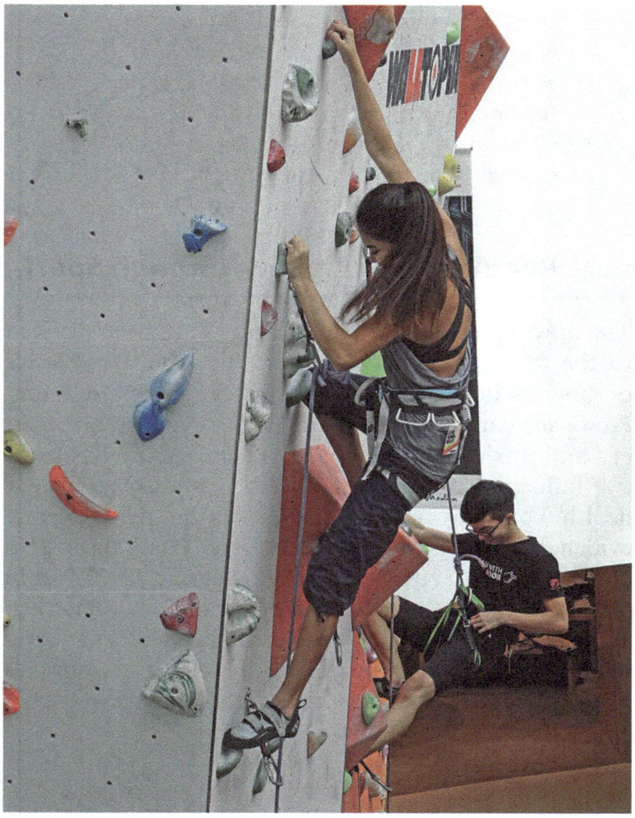

Fig. 12.12 Climbers in a secured lead: Anxiety can help to ensure that safety measures are taken

12.6.2 Anxiety Regulation

Based on the Consensual Modal Model (Gross, 2008), strategies of emotion regulation can be explained. A distinction must be made between strategies that aim to prevent the development of emotions ("antecedent-focused") and those that tend to change the experience and expression of emotions ("response-focused"). In an interview study, table tennis players were asked about their emotion regulation strategies (Martinent et al., 2015). Players stated they did not try to regulate in any way (intentionally) some emotions. However, whenever they experienced anxiety, they did regulate anxiety intentionally. The strategies mentioned can be assigned to the stages in the Consensual Modal Model.

> Emotion regulation refers to "processes by which individuals influence what emotions they have, when they have them and how they experience and express these emotions" (Gross, 1998, p. 275).

> Emotion regulation can refer both to the development of the emotion and to its change in experience and expression over time.

12.6.2.1 Situation

The triggers of anxiety described in ▶ Sect. 12.2 can also be the start of the regulation of anxiety in sport. Here, one can distinguish, albeit somewhat overlapping, strategies that involve the selection of situations, from strategies that involve the modification of a situation. Avoidance behaviour would be a classic form of anxiety regulation through selection. Sitting on the bench while others have to jump over the vaulting horse feels good. Situations cannot be avoided permanently in competitive sports, but they can be changed to a certain extent. Situation modification refers to the change of the external environment, not the internal experience. In the Olympic final, one strategy for regulating anxiety could be to bring friends or the coach into the stadium. And the tense situation of the skydivers in the airplane shortly before jumping could be eased (and thereby changed) by "cracking" a few jokes.

12.6.2.2 Attention

Situations provide stimuli that offer information about the existence of a threat. These stimuli then come to the forefront, are given preferential treatment and promote the development of anxiety (see ▶ Sect. 12.3.1). The intentional control of attention therefore effectively influences the development of emotions. While the table tennis players in the study by Martinent et al. (2015) did not name a situation-related regulation strategy, attentional strategies were the most frequently used. The players expressed above all an increased concentration on the game in order to be able to fade out anxiety and anxiety-relevant stimuli. Other strategies consisted in the targeted planning of actions, for example, by designing tactical measures. Finally, the table tennis players reported that they specifically tried to stop negative thoughts and focus on the current game situation. Such thought-stopping techniques, such as actually imagining a stop sign, can be learned well and is the subject of "mental skill training" (Beckmann & Elbe, 2015).

12.6.2.3 Appraisal

Even if a potentially threatening situation such as gymnastics lessons or the Olympic final cannot be avoided or at least changed and the relevant stimuli such as the gymnastics vaulting horse or the many spectators are perceived, anxiety only arises from appraisal processes. In this respect, conscious and intentional appraisals can prevent the "natural" course of anxiety development.

A central strategy of emotion regulation therefore consists of "reframing", in a reappraisal, in which the situation is evaluated under a new light. For this purpose, the table tennis players mainly used self-talk with either rational or positive contents. Rational self-talk is about seeing things reasonably and logically regarding other criteria. In the Olympic beach volleyball finals, such self-talk could include that this match point is what I have been training so hard for to this stage. The student could also rationally say to himself before the vaulting horse attempt that the injured knee during the last football match probably hurt more than the possible fall into the mat might hurt. Positive self-talk includes more optimistic content and positive memories. A climber could talk about the climbs he has already mastered and the skydiver could talk about the adrenaline that is about to come. But self-talk can simply have self-encouraging content in the sense of "I can do it!".

12.6.2.4 Anxiety Response

Finally, the last form of emotion regulation is to change the emotional response. All three components are available for this: experience, physiology and behaviour. The table tennis players (Martinent et al., 2015) regulated anxiety mainly through behaviour but also through the regulation of their physiological reaction. For example, they slowed down the time between rallies or points, or they tried to follow a very conscious routine. In fact, pre-performance routines (also called pre-shot routines) are often taught in sport psychology training. A pre-performance routine is any systematic cognitive and behavioural preparation strategy that an athlete engages in prior to performance execution (Cotterill, 2010). Routines specify behavioural patterns that run in a certain order and are thus intended to prevent the experience of anxiety because they convey a feeling of security and controllability. Pre-performance routines are effective in stabilising performance under pressure (Gröpel & Mesagno, 2019).

Since anxiety is associated with increased arousal, strategies are used to reduce arousal. For example, breathing exercises or relaxation techniques may help in reducing anxiety, which is one reason why teaching relaxation competence is a core component of basic sport psychology training (Beckmann & Elbe, 2015).

Methods of Regulating Anxiety in Sport
- Aim at the prevention of anxiety ("antecedent-focused").
- Change the experience and the anxiety reaction ("response-focused").
- This may include:
  - Avoiding or changing the situation before a competition
  - Focusing attention on less anxiety-inducing stimuli
  - Reappraising of the situation
  - Changing the emotional response, for example, through relaxation exercises or routines

12.7 Regulation of Anxiety Through Sport

The previous sections of this chapter have been devoted to the topic of anxiety in sport from the perspective of how anxiety arises in and affects sport situations. However, can sport be used to help cope with anxiety and anxiety disorders? In general, sport has positive influences not only on physical but also on mental health. For many facets of mental health, there is strong evidence for the positive effects of sport and, more generally, physical activity (Ekkekakis et al., 2013)—from quality of life to the reduction of mental disorders such as depression and aging successfully. There are also a number of empirical studies on the effect of sport on anxiety as well as surveys and meta-analyses (Utschig et al., 2013).

The health effects of sport go beyond physical effects; sport also has a positive impact on mental health and can help people to cope with anxiety and anxiety disorders.

12.7.1 Studies About the Efficacy of Sport on Anxiety

The empirical studies on the impact and effectiveness of sports follow different research approaches, which are based on different groups of people and use different success criteria. However, this diversity of studies makes it difficult to draw firm conclusions on effectiveness even when using meta-analyses.

12.7.1.1 Reduction of Anxiety in Healthy Populations

In cross-sectional studies, usually epidemiological studies covering a large sample, a negative correlation between physical activity and anxiety is often found. In a study of almost 20,000 Dutch twins, for example, those who were moderately active for about 4 h a week reported lower anxiety and neuroticism scores than those who did not engage in any sporting activity (De Moor et al., 2006). However, this correlation could also be because anxious people are less likely to engage in sport. It is therefore necessary to prove the causal relationship between physical activity and anxiety by means of experimental studies. To do this, at least one experimental group that participates in sport or physical activity as a treatment or intervention must be compared with a control group that receives no intervention or at least no intervention with sport participation (see ▶ Study Box). Overall, the experimental findings show (despite some methodological weaknesses) that an increase in physical activity leads to a reduction in anxiety experiences and a reduced risk of developing an anxiety disorder in people who do not otherwise complain about physical impairments or mental disorders (Herring et al., 2014).

Epidemiological and experimental studies show that sport and physical activity lead to less state anxiety and trait anxiety.

Similar Patterns of Change in Physiological and Mood Parameters as a Result of an Exercise Intervention

In a first controlled experiment, DiLorenzo et al. (1999) investigated the effects of exercise on anxiety. Participants were randomly assigned either to an intervention ($n = 82$) or a "wait list control" group ($n = 29$). Participants received training on a bicycle ergometer four times a week for 12 weeks (intervention group) or had to wait for participation in the intervention ("wait list control" group). Participants went through assessment and testing before the intervention period, immediately post and 3, 6 and 12 months' post intervention. The assessment consisted first of a battery of psychological questionnaires on anxiety, depression and mood. Importantly, the study controlled for the fitness effects of the intervention. Thus, secondly a functional fitness test (bicycle ergometer test) was also applied at all times of measurement. Only participants that did show (intervention group) or did *not* show (control group) an increase in fitness were used for analyses. These revealed a remarkable decrease in anxiety levels immediately after the exercise intervention in the intervention compared to the control group. Anxiety slightly increased within 3 months' follow-up but remained lower compared to before the intervention over a period of 1 year. Similar patterns of change were found for the other mood-related outcomes (e.g. depression) but also fitness outcomes (submaximal heart rate, body weight). Although this study provides strong experimental evidence of the benefit of exercise for anxiety and depression, it does not reveal the underlying mechanisms. As the authors conclude, the benefits could be explained, for example, by any or a combination of the following factors: the weight loss and subsequent more positive body image, the experience of social interaction and support during the group intervention, that exercise simply provided a distraction from worries and elevated levels of biochemicals such as serotonin associated with better mood. Unfortunately, the authors also do not report correlations between changes in fitness level or physiological data and psychological outcomes.

12.7.1.2 Sport, Physical Activity and Anxiety Disorders

But is physical activity or sport participation also suitable as a treatment for people who already suffer from an anxiety disorder? Anxiety disorders such as panic disorder, generalized anxiety disorder or phobias are among the most common mental disorders. They are characterized by a pronounced and chronic experience of anxiety, which is often associated with high levels of physical arousal and which leads to avoidance behaviour, for example, social withdrawal (Utschig et al., 2013). A large-scale representative cohort study in the United States showed that almost 25% of women and 12% of men had been diagnosed with an anxiety disorder within the last 12 months. However, the probability of this diagnosis was drastically reduced in people who were regularly physically active. In fact, there was even a dose-response relationship: The more active people were, the less likely they were to be diagnosed with an anxiety disorder (Goodwin, 2003; see Fig. 12.13). Experimental studies, however, do not provide clear evidence of the effectiveness of physical activity for the treatment of anxiety disorders. For example, in a study of 75 people with panic disorder, 4 treatment methods were compared (Wedekind et al., 2010). The interventions over 10 weeks consisted of either running or relaxation training, each of which was supplemented by either drug therapy or placebo therapy. For all four groups, improvements were found in specific symptoms—with stronger improvements in those who had received the drug. Only for the general clinical assessment was there a small advantage for the groups that had received running training over the relaxation groups.

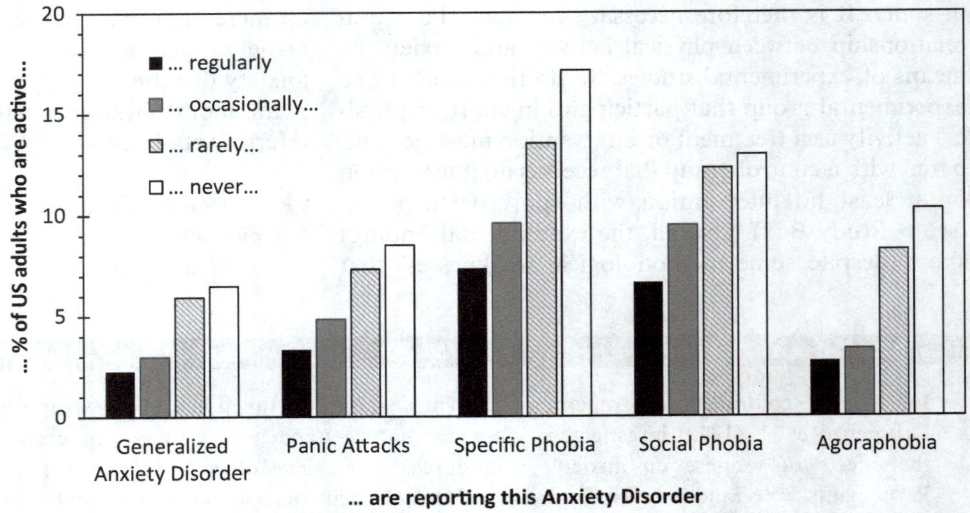

Fig. 12.13 Dose-response relationship between self-reported frequency of physical activity. Anxiety disorders in adults in the United States: Groups of people with higher physical activity levels have a lower prevalence. (According to Goodwin, 2003)

Overall, meta-analyses have concluded that experimental studies provide evidence that physical activity is a beneficial and practical treatment for anxiety disorders yet a number of methodological shortcomings are listed that make a reliable assessment difficult (Stonerock et al., 2015; Stubbs et al., 2017).

While epidemiological studies show that physical activity is also a treatment for anxiety disorders, controlled experimental studies do not provide clear evidence.

12

What shortcomings have meta-analyses identified in studies on the effectiveness of physical activity in the treatment of anxiety disorders?

- Low test strength ("power") due to small number of participants
- Participants and study management insufficiently "blinded" with regard to study purposes and group allocation
- Scope and intensity of sport insufficiently recorded
- Physiological effects not investigated
- Too many different measures (acute vs. chronic, subjective vs. objective…)
- Unclear mechanisms—psychological (e.g. about self-efficacy?) or physiological models (e.g. about serotonin neurotransmitter system)

Meta-analysis

In a meta-analysis, the results of empirical studies on a research question are not only summarized but also statistically evaluated. The idea behind this is that although the results of each individual study are associated with a certain error, the combination of several studies allows a more precise estimate of a "true effect". Today, meta-analyses follow standardized rules, as do systematic reviews, in which the results are evaluated in terms of content but not statistically (Moher et al., 2009). Initially, all empirical studies on a particular issue (e.g. anxiety-reducing effects of sport) are researched in databases and then evaluated according to inclusion and exclusion criteria (e.g. intervention design with control group) and, if necessary, excluded. Hedges' *g*, which is a measure of the size of the estimated "true" effect, is then often calculated from the various mean differences between the studies. Meta-analyses of experimental studies (called *randomized controlled trials*, RCTs) on a treatment method are necessary, for example, to establish this as an "evidence-based method". Although meta-analyses are important for the evaluation of a research field or a treatment method, they are also viewed critically. A major problem is the possible systematic distortion of the results of meta-analyses. Thus, the selection of studies included in a meta-analysis is ultimately subjective, even if objective criteria are mentioned. A further distortion can arise from the fact that usually empirical studies are more likely to be published if they show effects, but non-significant or negative results tend to remain in the proverbial drawer of a researcher's "filing cabinet". A meta-analysis then overestimates the effect, because negative or zero effects may not be included in the analysis. Although there are methods to identify possible distortions (e.g. "funnel plot"), even these may be controversial.

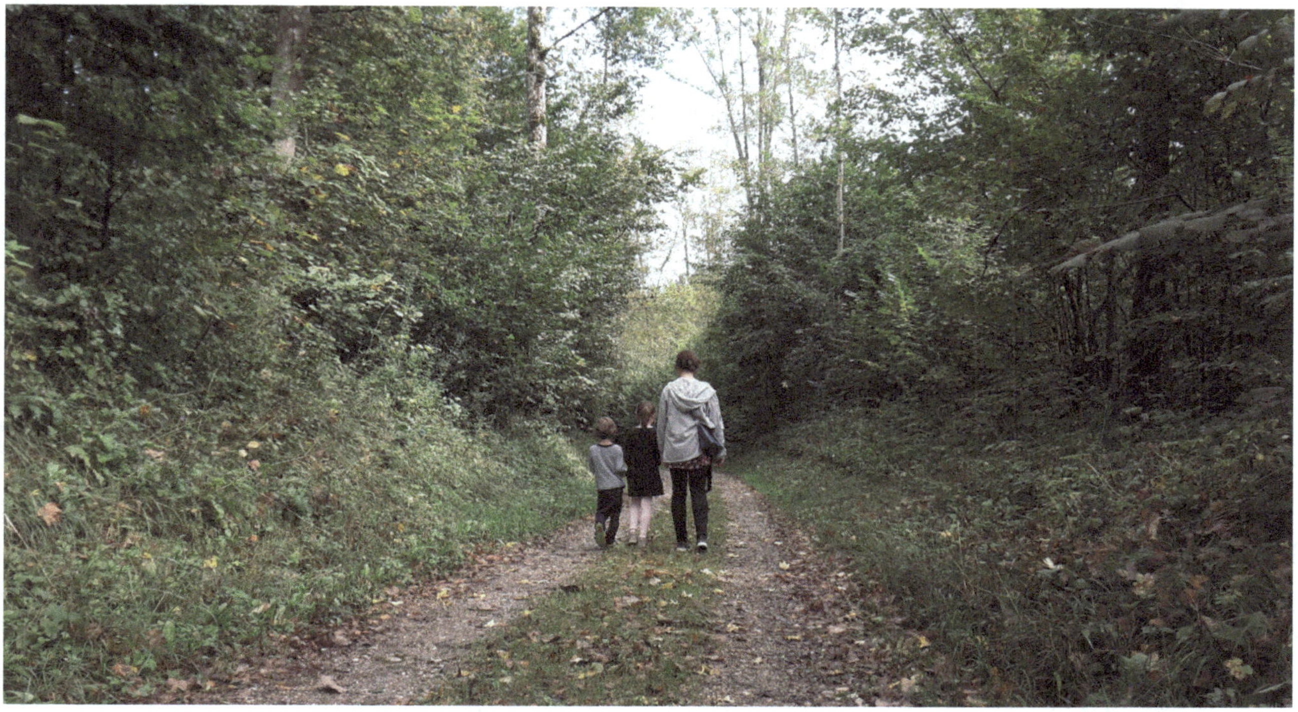

Fig. 12.14 Green exercise—experiencing nature can enhance the health effects of sport or physical activity such as hiking

12.7.2 Implication for Practice

It is neither certain to what extent physical activity and sport have an effect on anxiety and anxiety disorders, nor is it clear how sport affects them. Nevertheless, from the many studies and meta-analyses, some recommendations can be derived—at least cautiously—on the duration, type and intensity of physical activity and the setting of treatment. The setting of physical activity may have an effect on anxiety reduction. The gym may not be the best place to do physical activity for "anxiolytic effects" (anxiety-reducing effects) since studies have shown that "green exercise" (training outdoors) has a greater psychological effect (Mackay & Neill, 2010). Moreover, the potential of (high-)risk sports such as mountaineering or climbing, which are likely to further intensify the experience of nature, has not yet been tapped for targeted use in the treatment of anxiety and anxiety disorders. As seen, an important motive for participating in such risky sports seems to be the ability to regulate and manage intense emotions (Fig. 12.14).

What characteristics should a sports programme with long-term effects (reduction of anxiety, anxiety disorders) have (see Schwerdtfeger, 2012)?

- According to general health recommendations for physical activity at least two to three training sessions per week
- Over a period of at least 9 weeks
- Moderate intensity to increase aerobic endurance (from at least 50% maximum heart rate or, for example, a brisk walk)
- In the form of an institutionalized intervention (as part of a programme, facility or fitness studio)
- Change in physical activity as the main focus of the programme, not simultaneously addressing other health behaviour (e.g. nutrition)

Learning Control Questions

Basic:

1. Does an athlete that constantly shows superior performance in practice but fails under pressure more likely have a state anxiety or a trait anxiety problem?
2. What is meant by "social physique anxiety"? Explain how social physique anxiety may be related to the sources of uncertainty found for competitive anxiety.
3. What empirical evidence is there that shows that even in competition our attention is biased towards the perception of threatening, anxiety-inducing stimuli?
4. Which basic strategies for coping with stress can be distinguished?
5. Before jumping out of the plane, a skydiver tells a lot of jokes. Which strategy for regulating emotions and to which stage in the process of developing anxiety can this be assigned?

Advanced:

6. Compare the characteristics of anxiety-triggering situations in sport, as defined from the sport psychological and social psychological approaches. Which essential facet of anxiety in sport is probably missing in the social-psychological approach?
7. Imagine yourself serving in the Olympic beach volleyball finals. For this situation, formulate a "primary appraisal" that leads to a stress perception and a "primary appraisal" that does not lead to stress.
8. Think about the situation of the student before the vaulting horse attempt and think of a "secondary appraisal" from which stress arises and of a "secondary appraisal" from which no stress would arise.
9. A climber is in a critical position on the rock face. According to the theory of challenge and threat states in athletes, how could we tell whether the climber perceives this situation as a threat or a challenge?
10. You are training a young athlete and want to prepare her optimally for the upcoming championships. What methods could you use to determine whether she is afraid in competitions?
11. Is there anything good to be gained from anxiety in sport?

Experts:

12. A female footballer tells you about the new sport psychologist, who primarily conducts relaxation training. He explains that the players are then less excited before matches. Think about and describe whether or to what extent relaxation before a game is actually beneficial for performance. Why? Why not?
13. Compare and contrast the two currently discussed theories for explaining choking under pressure and consider whether they are not mutually exclusive.
14. Why can the evidence for the effectiveness of sport in treating anxiety disorders not be interpreted clearly?

References

Alder, D., Ford, P. R., Causer, J., & Williams, A. M. (2016). The effects of high-and low-anxiety training on the anticipation judgments of elite performers. *Journal of Sport and Exercise Psychology, 38*, 93–104.

Argelaguet Sanz, F., Multon, F., & Lécuyer, A. (2015). A methodology for introducing competitive anxiety and pressure in VR sports training. *Frontiers in Robotics and AI, 2*, 10.

Aşçı, F. H., Tüzün, M., & Koca, C. (2006). An examination of eating attitudes and physical activity levels of Turkish university students with regard to self-presentational concern. *Eating Behaviours, 7*, 362–367.

Balmer, N. J., Nevill, A. M., Lane, A. M., & Ward, P. (2007). Influence of crowd noise on soccer refereeing consistency in soccer. *Journal of Sport Behavior, 30*, 130–145.

Bar-Haim, Y., Lamy, D., Pergamin, L., Bakermans-Kranenburg, M. J., & van Ijzendoorn, M. H. (2007). Threat-related attentional bias in anxious and nonanxious individuals: A meta-analytic study. *Psychological Bulletin, 133*, 1–24.

Barlow, M., Woodman, T., Chapman, C., Milton, M., Stone, D., Dodds, T., & Allen, B. (2015). Who takes risks in high-risk sport?: The role of alexithymia. *Journal of Sport and Exercise Psychology, 37*, 83–96.

Barlow, M., Woodman, T., & Hardy, L. (2013). Great expectations: Different high-risk activities satisfy different motives. *Journal of Personality and Social Psychology, 105*, 458–475.

Barry, R. J., Clarke, A. R., McCarthy, R., Selikowitz, M., & Rushby, J. A. (2005). Arousal and activation in a continuous performance task. *Journal of Psychophysiology, 19*, 91–99.

Baumeister, R. F. (1984). Choking under pressure: Self-consciousness and paradoxical effects of incentives on skillful performance. *Journal of Personality and Social Psychology, 46*, 610–620.

Baumeister, R. F., & Showers, C. J. (1986). A review of paradoxical performance effects: Choking under pressure in sports and mental tests. *European Journal of Social Psychology, 16*, 361–383.

Beckmann, J., & Ehrlenspiel, F. (2018). Strategien der stressregulation im leistungssport. In R. Fuchs & M. Gerber (Eds.), *Handbuch stressregulation und sport* (pp. 417–433). Springer.

Beckmann, J., & Elbe, A. M. (2015). *Sport psychological interventions in competitive sports*. Cambridge University Press.

Beckmann, J., & Rolstad, K. (1997). Aktivierung, selbstregulation und leistung: Gibt es so etwas wie übermotivation? *Sportwissenschaft, 27*, 23–37.

Beilock, S. L., & Carr, T. H. (2001). On the fragility of skilled performance: What governs choking under pressure? *Journal of Experimental Psychology: General, 130*, 701–725. https://doi.org/10.1037/0096-3445.130.4.701

Beilock, S. L., Carr, T. H., MacMahon, C., & Starkes, J. L. (2002). When paying attention becomes counterproductive: impact of divided versus skill-focused attention on novice and experienced performance of sensorimotor skills. *Journal of Experimental Psychology: Applied, 8*, 6–16.

Berglas, S., & Jones, E. E. (1978). Drug choice as a self-handicapping strategy in response to noncontingent success. *Journal of Personality and Social Psychology, 36*, 405–417.

Blascovich, J. (2008). Challenge and threat. In A. J. Elliot (Ed.), *Handbook of approach and avoidance motivation* (pp. 431–445). Psychology Press.

Blascovich, J., & Mendes, W. B. (2000). Challenge and threat appraisals: The role of affective cues. In J. Forgas (Ed.), *Feeling and thinking: The role of affect in social cognition* (pp. 59–82). Cambridge University Press.

Blascovich, J., Mendes, W. B., Tomaka, J., Salomon, K., & Seery, M. (2003). The robust nature of the biopsychosocial model challenge and threat: A reply to Wright and Kirby. *Personality and Social Psychology Review, 7*, 234–243.

Blascovich, J., & Tomaka, J. (1996). The biopsychosocial model of arousal regulation. *Advances in Experimental Social Psychology, 28*, 1–51.

Borrego, C. C., Cid, L., & Silva, C. (2012). Relationship between group cohesion and anxiety in soccer. *Journal of Human Kinetics, 34*, 119–127.

Bray, S. R., Martin, K. A., & Widmeyer, W. N. (2000). The relationship between evaluative concerns and sport competition anxiety among youth skiers. *Journal of Sports Sciences, 18*, 353–361.

Burdwood, E. N., Infantolino, Z. P., Crocker, L. D., Spielberg, J. M., Banich, M. T., Miller, G. A., & Heller, W. (2016). Resting–state functional connectivity differentiates anxious apprehension and anxious arousal. *Psychophysiology, 53*, 1451–1459. https://doi.org/10.1111/psyp.12696

Burton, D. (1988). Do anxious swimmers swim slower? Re-examining the elusive anxiety-performance relationship. *Journal of Sport and Exercise Psychology, 10*, 45–61.

Butler, J. L., & Baumeister, R. F. (1998). The trouble with friendly faces: Skilled performance with a supportive audience. *Journal of Personality and Social Psychology, 75*, 1213–1230.
Caruso, C. M., Dzewaltowski, D. A., Gill, D. L., & McElroy, M. A. (1990). Psychological and physiological changes in competitive state anxiety during noncompetitive and competitive success and failure. *Journal of Sport and Exercise Psychology, 12*, 6–20.
Cerin, E., & Barnett, A. (2011). Predictors of pre- and post-competition affective states in male martial artists: A multilevel interactional approach. *Scandinavian Journal of Medicine and Science in Sports, 21*, 137–150.
Chuang, L., Huang, C., & Hung, T. (2015). Effects of attentional training on visual attention to emotional stimuli in archers: A preliminary investigation. *International Journal of Psychophysiology, 98*, 448–454.
Coffey, M. (2005). *Where the mountain casts its shadow: The dark side of extreme adventure*. Macmillan.
Cook, B., Karr, T. M., Zunker, C., Mitchell, J. E., Thompson, R., Sherman, R., et al. (2015). The influence of exercise identity and social physique anxiety on exercise dependence. *Journal of Behavioural Addictions, 4*, 195–199.
Cooke, A., Kavussanu, M., McIntyre, D., & Ring, C. (2013). The effects of individual and team competitions on performance, emotions, and effort. *Journal of Sport and Exercise Psychology, 35*, 132–143.
Cotterill, S. (2010). Pre-performance routines in sport: Current understanding and future directions. *International Review of Sport and Exercise Psychology, 3*, 132–153. https://doi.org/10.1080/1750984X.2010.488269
Coudevylle, G. R., Ginis, K. A. M., Famose, J.-P., & Gernignon, C. (2008). Effects of self-handicapping strategies on anxiety before athletic performance. *The Sport Psychologist, 22*, 304–315.
Cox, A. E., Ullrich-French, S., Madonia, J., & Witty, K. (2011). Social physique anxiety in physical education: Social contextual factors and links to motivation and behaviour. *Psychology of Sport and Exercise, 12*, 555–562.
Cox, R. H., Martens, M. P., & Russell, W. D. (2003). Measuring anxiety in athletics: The revised competitive state anxiety inventory–2. *Journal of Sport and Exercise Psychology, 25*, 519–533.
Craft, L. L., Magyar, T. M., Becker, B. J., & Feltz, D. L. (2003). The relationship between the competitive state anxiety inventory-2 and sport performance: A meta-analysis. *Journal of Sport and Exercise Psychology, 25*, 44–65. https://doi.org/10.1123/jsep.25.1.44
Crawford, S., & Eklund, R. (1994). Social physique anxiety, reasons for exercise, and attitudes toward exercise settings. *Journal of Sport & Exercise Psychology, 16*, 70–82.
De Moor, M. H. M., Beem, A. L., Stubbe, J. H., Boomsma, D. I., & De Geus, E. J. C. (2006). Regular exercise, anxiety, depression and personality: A population-based study. *Preventive Medicine, 42*, 273–279.
DiLorenzo, T. M., Bargman, E. P., Stucky-Ropp, R., Brassington, G. S., Frensch, P. A., & LaFontaine, T. (1999). Long-term effects of aerobic exercise on psychological outcomes. *Preventive Medicine, 28*, 75–85.
Draper, N., Jones, G. A., Fryer, S., Hodgson, C., & Blackwell, G. (2008). Effect of an on-sight lead on the physiological and psychological responses to rock climbing. *Journal of Sports Science and Medicine, 7*, 492–498.
Ducrocq, E., Wilson, M., Vine, S. J., & Derakshan, N. (2016). Training attentional control improves cognitive and motor task performance. *Journal of Sport and Exercise Psychology, 38*, 521–533.
Edwards, T., Hardy, L., Kingston, K., & Gould, D. (2002). A qualitative analysis of catastrophic performances and the associated thoughts, feelings, and emotions. *The Sport Psychologist, 16*, 1–19. https://doi.org/10.1123/tsp.16.1.1
Ehrlenspiel, F., Brand, R., & Graf, K. (2009). Das Wettkampfangst—Inventar—State. In R. Brand, F. Ehrlenspiel, & K. Graf (Eds.), *Das Wettkampfangst—Inventar. Manual zur komprehensiven Eingangsdiagnostik von Wettkampfangst, Wettkampfängstlichkeit und Angstbewältigungsmodus im Sport* (pp. 71–100). Bundesinstitut für Sportwissenschaft.
Ehrlenspiel, F., & Elbe, A.-M. (2008). Reduktion der Wettkampfangst mittels sportpsychologischen Grundlagentrainings. *Leistungssport, 38*(4), 25–28.
Ehrlenspiel, F., Erlacher, D., & Ziegler, M. (2018a). Changes in subjective sleep quality before a competition and their relation to competitive anxiety. *Behavioural Sleep Medicine, 16*, 553–568.
Ehrlenspiel, F., Geukes, K., & Beckmann, J. (2018b). Stress, angst und leistung im leistungssport. In R. Fuchs & M. Gerber (Eds.), *Handbuch stressregulation und sport* (pp. 391–416). Springer.
Ehrlenspiel, F., Wei, K., & Sternad, D. (2010). Open-loop, closed-loop and compensatory control: Performance and improvement under pressure in a rhythmic task. *Experimental Brain Research, 201*, 729–741.
Ekkekakis, P. E., Cook, D. B., Craft, L. L., Culos-Reed, S., Etnier, J. L., Hamer, M. E., et al. (2013). *Routledge handbook of physical activity and mental health*. Routledge.
Eubank, M., Collins, D., & Smith, N. (2002). Anxiety and ambiguity: It's all open to interpretation. *Journal of Sport and Exercise Psychology, 24*, 239–253.
Eysenck, M. W., & Calvo, M. G. (1992). Anxiety and performance: The processing efficiency theory. *Cognition and Emotion, 6*, 409–434.
Eysenck, M. W., Derakshan, N., Santos, R., & Calvo, M. G. (2007). Anxiety and cognitive performance: Attentional control theory. *Emotion, 7*(2), 336–335.
Eysenck, M. W., & Wilson, M. R. (2016). Sporting performance, pressure and cognition: Introducing attentional control theory: Sport. In D. Groome & M. W. Eysenck (Eds.), *An introduction to applied cognitive psychology* (pp. 341–362). Psychology Press.
Fink, A., Fischler, K., Raschner, C., Hildebrandt, C., Ledochowski, L., & Kopp, M. (2013). Association between parenting practices and competitive trait anxiety in female gymnasts. *International Journal of Sport Psychology, 44*, 515–530.
Fitts, P. M., & Posner, M. I. (1967). *Human performance*. Brooks/Cole.
Fletcher, D., & Hanton, S. (2001). The relationship between psychological skills usage and competitive anxiety responses. *Psychology of Sport & Exercise, 2*, 89–101. https://doi.org/10.1016/S1469-0292(00)00014-5
Flowers, R. A., & Brown, C. (2002). Effects of sport context and birth order on state anxiety. *Journal of Sport Behaviour, 25*, 41–56.
Furley, P., Dicks, M., & Memmert, D. (2012). Nonverbal behaviour in soccer: The influence of dominant and submissive body language on the impression formation and expectancy of success of soccer players. *Psychology of Sport and Exercise, 34*, 61–82.
Goodwin, R. D. (2003). Association between physical activity and mental disorders among adults in the United States. *Preventive Medicine, 36*, 698–703.
Gould, D., Horn, T., & Spreeman, J. (1983). Competitive anxiety in junior elite wrestlers. *Journal of Sport Psychology, 5*, 58–71. https://doi.org/10.1123/jsp.5.1.58
Gould, D., & Weinberg, R. S. (1985). Sources of worry in successful and less successful intercollegiate wrestlers. *Journal of Sport Behaviour, 8*, 115–127.
Gröpel, P. (2016). Self-focused attention and motor skill failure: The moderating role of action orientation. *Sport, Exercise, and Performance Psychology, 5*(3), 206.
Gröpel, P., & Mesagno, C. (2019). Choking interventions in sports: A systematic review. *International Review of sport and exercise psychology, 12*(1), 176–201. https://doi.org/10.1080/1750984X.2017.1408134

Gross, J. J. (1998). The emerging field of emotion regulation: an integrative review. *Review of General Psychology, 2*, 217–299. https://doi.org/10.1037/1089-2680.2.3.271

Gross, J. J. (2008). Emotion regulation. In M. Lewis, J. M. Haviland-Jones, & L. F. Barrett (Eds.), *Handbook of emotions* (pp. 497–512). Guilford.

Gucciardi, D. F., & Dimmock, J. A. (2008). Choking under pressure in sensorimotor skills: Conscious processing or depleted attentional resources? *Psychology of Sport and Exercise, 9*, 45–59.

Hackfort, D. (1986). *Theorie und Analyse sportbezogener Ängstlichkeit: Ein situationsanalytischer Ansatz*. Hofmann.

Hackfort, D., & Schwenkmezger, P. (1989). Measuring anxiety in sports: Perspectives and problems. In D. Hackfort & C. D. Spielberger (Eds.), *Anxiety in sports: An international perspective* (pp. 55–74). Hemisphere.

Hall, H. K., Kerr, A. W., & Matthews, J. (1998). Precompetitive anxiety in sport: The contribution of achievement goals and perfectionism. *Journal of Sport and Exercise Psychology, 20*, 194–217.

Hammermeister, J., & Burton, D. (2001). Stress, appraisal, and coping revisited: Examining the antecedents of Competitive State Anxiety with Endurance Athletes. *The Sport Psychologist, 15*, 66–90.

Hanin, Y. L. (2000). Successful and poor performance and emotions. In Y. L. Hanin (Ed.), *Emotions in sport* (pp. 157–187). Human Kinetics.

Hanton, S., Mellalieu, S. D., & Hall, R. (2002). Re-examining the competitive anxiety trait-state relationship. *Personality and Individual Differences, 33*, 1125–1136.

Hanton, S., Neil, R., & Evans, L. (2013). Hardiness and anxiety interpretation: An investigation into coping usage and effectiveness. *European Journal of Sport Science, 13*, 96–104.

Hanton, S., Neil, R., & Mellalieu, S. (2008a). Recent developments in competitive anxiety direction and competition stress research. *International Review of Sport and Exercise Psychology, 1*, 45–57.

Hanton, S., Neil, R., Mellalieu, S., & Fletcher, D. (2008b). Competitive experience and performance status: An investigation into multidimensional anxiety and coping. *European Journal of Sport Science, 8*, 143–152.

Hardy, L. (1990). A catastrophe model of anxiety and performance. In J. G. Jones & L. Hardy (Eds.), *Stress and performance in sport*. Wiley.

Hardy, L., & Parfitt, G. (1993). A catastrophe model of anxiety and performance. *British Journal of Psychology, 82*, 163–178.

Hardy, L., Parfitt, G., & Pates, J. (1994). Performance catastrophes in sport: A test of the hysteresis hypothesis. *Journal of Sports Sciences, 12*, 327–334.

Hare, O. A., Wetherell, M. A., & Smith, M. A. (2013). State anxiety and cortisol reactivity to skydiving in novice versus experienced skydivers. *Physiology & Behaviour, 118*, 40–44.

Hart, E. A., Leary, M. R., & Rejeski, W. J. (1989). The measurement of social physique anxiety. *Journal of Sport and Exercise Psychology, 11*, 94–104.

Herring, M. P., Lindheimer, J. B., & O'Connor, P. J. (2014). The effects of exercise training on anxiety. *American Journal of Lifestyle, 8*, 388–403.

Hill, D. M., Hanton, S., Matthews, N., & Fleming, S. (2010). Choking in sport: A review. *International Review of Sport and Exercise Psychology, 3*, 24–39.

Hudson, J., & Williams, M. (2001). Associations between self-presentation and competitive A-Trait: A preliminary investigation. *Social Behaviour and Personality: An International Journal, 29*, 1–10.

Hull, C. L. (1952). *A behavior system; an introduction to behavior theory concerning the individual organism*. Yale University Press.

James, B., & Collins, D. (1997). Self-presentational sources of competitive stress during performance. *The Journal of Sport and Exercise Psychology, 19*, 17–35.

Jones, G., Swain, A., & Cale, A. (1990). Antecedents of multidimensional competitive state-anxiety and self-confidence in elite intercollegiate middle-distance runners. *The Sport Psychologist, 4*, 107–118.

Jones, M. V., Meijen, C., McCarthy, P. J., & Sheffield, D. (2009). A theory of challenge and threat states in athletes. *International Review of Sport and Exercise Psychology, 2*, 161–180.

Jordet, G., & Elferink-Gemser, M. (2012). Stress, coping, and emotions on the world stage: The experience of participating in a Major Soccer Tournament Penalty Shootout. *Journal of Applied Sport Psychology, 24*, 73–91.

Jordet, G., & Hartman, E. (2008). Avoidance motivation and choking under pressure in soccer penalty shootouts. *Journal of Sport & Exercise Psychology, 30*, 450–457.

Kaye, M. P., Frith, A., & Vosloo, J. (2015). Dyadic anxiety in youth sport: The relationship of achievement goals with anxiety in young athletes and their parents. *Journal of Applied Sport Psychology, 27*, 171–185.

Kleinert, J. (2002). An approach to sport injury trait anxiety: Scale construction and structure analysis. *European Journal of Sport Science, 2*(3), 1–12.

Klostermann, A., Kredel, R., & Hossner, E.-J. (2013). The "quiet eye" and motor performance: Task demands matter! *Journal of Experimental Psychology: Human Perception and Performance, 39*, 1270–1278.

Krane, V. (1992). Conceptual and methodological considerations in sport anxiety research: From the inverted-U hypothesis to catastrophe theory. *Quest, 44*, 72–87.

Krane, V. (1994). The mental readiness form as a measure of competitive state anxiety. *The Sport Psychologist, 8*, 189–202.

Kuhl, J. (1992). A theory of self-regulation: action versus state orientation, self-discrimination, and some applications: Self-regulation. *Applied Psychology, 41*, 97–129.

Lautenbach, F., Laborde, S. J. P., Putman, P., Angelidis, A., & Raab, M. (2016). Attentional distraction by negative sports words in athletes under low-and high-pressure conditions: Evidence from the sport emotional Stroop task. *Sport, Exercise, and Performance Psychology, 5*, 296–307.

Lazarus, R. S. (1966). *Psychological stress and the coping process*. McGraw-Hill.

Lazarus, R. S. (1991). *Emotion and adaption*. Oxford University Press.

Lazarus, R. S. (1999). *Stress and emotion: A new synthesis*. Springer.

Lazarus, R. S., & Folkman, S. (1984). *Stress, appraisal, and coping*. Springer Pub. Co.

Leary, M. R. (1992). Self-presentational processes in exercise and sport. *Journal of Sport and Exercise Psychology, 14*, 339–351.

LeDoux, J. E., & Pine, D. S. (2016). Using neuroscience to help understand fear and anxiety: A two-system framework. *American Journal of Psychiatry, 173*, 1083–1093.

Liebert, R. M., & Morris, L. W. (1967). Cognitive and emotional components of test anxiety: A distinction and some initial data. *Psychological Reports, 20*, 975–978.

Linder, D. E., Lutz, R., Crews, D., & Lochbaum, M. (1999). Who chokes and when? Situational and dispositional factors in failure under pressure. In M. R. Farrally & A. J. Cochran (Eds.), *Proceedings of the world scientific congress of golf* (pp. 207–212). Human Kinetics.

Low, W. R., Sandercock, G. R. H., Freeman, P., Winter, M. E., Butt, J., & Maynard, I. (2021). Pressure training for performance domains: A meta-analysis. *Sport, Exercise, and Performance Psychology, 10*(1), 149–163.

Mackay, G. J., & Neill, J. T. (2010). The effect of "green exercise" on state anxiety and the role of exercise duration, intensity, and greenness: A quasi-experimental study. *Psychology of Sport and Exercise, 11*, 238–245.

MacLeod, C., Mathews, A., & Tata, P. (1986). Attentional bias in emotional disorders. *Journal of Abnormal Psychology, 95*, 15–20.
Marchant, D. B., Morris, T., & Anderson, M. B. (1998). Perceived importance of outcome as a contributing factor in competitive state anxiety. *Journal of Sport Behaviour, 21*, 71–91.
Martens, R. S., Burton, D., Vealey, R. S., Bump, L. A., & Smith, D. E. (1990a). Development and validation of the competitive state anxiety inventory-2. In R. Martens, R. S. Vealey, & D. Burton (Eds.), *Competitive anxiety in sport* (pp. 117–190). Human Kinetics.
Martens, R. S., Vealey, R. S., & Burton, D. (1990b). *Competitive anxiety in sport*. Human Kinetics.
Martin, K. A., & Hall, C. (1997). Situational and intrapersonal moderators of sport competition state anxiety. *Journal of Sport Behaviour, 20*, 435–447.
Martinent, G., & Ferrand, C. (2015). A field study of discrete emotions: Athletes' cognitive appraisals during competition. *Research Quarterly for Exercise and Sport, 86*, 51–62.
Martinent, G., Ledos, S., Ferrand, C., Campo, M., & Nicolas, M. (2015). Athletes regulation of emotions experienced during competition: A naturalistic video-assisted study. *Sport, Exercise, and Performance Psychology, 4*, 188–205.
Masters, R., & Maxwell, J. (2008). The theory of reinvestment. *International Review of Sport and Exercise Psychology, 1*, 160–183.
Masters, R. S. W. (1992). Knowledge, knerves and know-how: The role of explicit versus implicit knowledge on the breakdown of a complex motor skill under pressure. *British Journal of Psychology, 83*, 334–358.
Mauss, I. B., & Robinson, M. D. (2009). Measures of emotion. *A review. Cognition and Emotion, 23*, 209–237.
McEwen, B. S. (1998). Stress, adaptation, and disease: Allostasis and allostatic load. *Annals of the New York Academy of Sciences, 840*, 33–44.
Melbye, L., Tenenbaum, G., & Eklund, R. (2007). Self-objectification and exercise behaviours: The mediating role of social physique anxiety. *Journal of Applied Biobehavioural Research, 12*, 196–220.
Mellalieu, S., Hanton, S., & O'Brien, M. (2004). Intensity and direction of competitive anxiety as a function of sport type and experience. *Scandinavian Journal of Medicine and Science in Sports, 14*, 326–334.
Mendes, W. B., Major, B., McCoy, S., & Blascovich, J. (2008). How attributional ambiguity shapes physiological and emotional responses to social rejection and acceptance. *Journal of Personality and Social Psychology, 94*, 278–291.
Mesagno, C., & Beckmann, J. (2017). Choking under pressure: Theoretical models and interventions. *Current Opinion in Psychology, 16*, 170–175.
Mesagno, C., Geukes, K., & Larkin, P. (2015). Choking under pressure: A review of current debates, literature, and interventions. In S. D. Mellalieu & S. Hanton (Eds.), *Contemporary advances in sport psychology: A review* (pp. 148–174). Routledge.
Mesagno, C., Harvey, J. T., & Janelle, C. M. (2011). Self-presentation origins of choking: Evidence from separate pressure manipulations. *Journal of Sport & Exercise Psychology, 33*, 441–459.
Mesagno, C., Harvey, J. T., & Janelle, C. M. (2012). Choking under pressure: The role of fear of negative evaluation. *Psychology of Sport and Exercise, 13*, 60–68. https://doi.org/10.1016/j.psychsport.2011.07.007
Mesagno, C., & Hill, D. M. (2013). Definition of choking in sport: Re-conceptualization and debate. *International Journal of Sport Psychology- Performance under Pressure, 4*, 267–277.
Mesagno, C., Marchant, D., & Morris, T. (2009). Alleviating choking: The sounds of distraction. *Journal of Applied Sport Psychology, 21*, 131–147. https://doi.org/10.1080/10413200902795091
Moher, D., Liberati, A., Tetzlaff, J. M., & Altman, D. G. (2009). Preferred reporting items for systematic reviews and meta-analyses: The PRISMA statement. *Open Medicine, 3*, 123–130.
Moore, L. J., Vine, S. J., Freeman, P., & Wilson, M. R. (2013b). Quiet eye training promotes challenge appraisals and aids performance under elevated anxiety. *International Journal of Sport and Exercise Psychology, 11*, 169–183.
Moore, L. J., Wilson, M. R., Vine, S. J., Coussens, A. H., & Freeman, P. (2013a). Champ or Chump?: Challenge and threat states during pressurized competition. *Journal of Sport and Exercise Psychology, 35*(6), 551–562.
Moran, A. P. (1996). *The psychology of concentration in sports performers: A cognitive analysis*. Psychology Press.
Morris, L., Davis, D., & Hutchings, C. (1981). Cognitive and emotional components of anxiety: Literature review and revised worry-emotionality scale. *Journal of Educational Psychology, 73*, 541–555.
Murray, N. P., & Janelle, C. M. (2007). Even-related potential evidence for the processing efficiency theory. *Journal of Sports Sciences, 25*, 161–171.
Neil, R., Bayston, P., Hanton, S., & Wilson, K. (2013). The influence of stress and emotions on association football referees' decision-making. *Sport & Exercise Psychology Review, 9*, 22–41.
Neil, R., Mellalieu, S. D., & Hanton, S. (2009). The contribution of qualitative inquiry towards understanding competitive anxiety and competition stress. *Qualitative Research in Sport and Exercise, 1*, 191–205.
Nicholls, A. R., Taylor, N. J., Carroll, S., & Perry, J. L. (2016). The development of a new sport-specific classification of coping and a meta-analysis of the relationship between different coping strategies and moderators on sporting outcomes. *Frontiers in Psychology, 7*, 1674.
Norton, P. J., Hope, D. A., & Weeks, J. W. (2004). The physical activity and sport anxiety scale (PASAS): Scale development and psychometric analysis. *Anxiety, Stress & Coping, 17*(4), 363–382.
O'Rourke, D. J., Smith, R. E., Smoll, F. L., & Cumming, S. P. (2011). Trait anxiety in young athletes as a function of parental pressure and motivational climate: Is parental pressure always harmful? *Journal of Applied Sport Psychology, 23*(4), 398–412.
Öhman, A. (2008). Fear and anxiety: Overlaps and dissociations. In M. Lewis, J. M. Haviland-Jones, & L. F. Barrett (Eds.), *Handbook of emotions* (pp. 709–729). Guilford.
Oudejans, R. R. D., Kuijpers, W., Kooijman, C. C., & Bakker, F. C. (2011). Thoughts and attention of athletes under pressure: Skill-focus or performance worries? *Anxiety, Stress, and Coping, 24*, 59–73.
Recours, R., & Briki, W. (2015). The effect of red and blue uniforms on competitive anxiety and self-confidence in virtual sports contests. *Revue Européenne de Psychologie Appliquée, 65*, 67–69.
Rex, C. C., & Metzler, J. N. (2016). Development of the sport injury anxiety scale. *Measurement in Physical Education and Exercise Science, 20*(3), 146–158.
Rohleder, N., Beulen, S. E., Chen, E., Wolf, J. M., & Kirschbaum, C. (2007). Stress on the dance floor: The cortisol stress response to social-evaluative threat in competitive ballroom dancers. *Personality and Social Psychology Bulletin, 33*, 69–84.
Roth, S., & Cohen, L. J. (1986). Approach, avoidance, and coping with stress. *American Psychologist, 41*, 813–819.
Sabiston, C. M., Pila, E., Pinsonnault-Bilodeau, G., & Cox, A. E. (2014). Social physique anxiety experiences in physical activity: A comprehensive synthesis of research studies focused on measurement, theory, and predictors and outcomes. *International Review of Sport and Exercise Psychology, 7*, 158–183.
Scanlan, T. K., Stein, G. L., & Ravizza, S. (1991). In-depth study of former elite figure skaters: III. Sources of stress. *Journal of Sport and Exercise Psychology, 13*, 103–120.

Schack, T. (1997). *Ängstliche Schüler im Sport: Interventionsverfahren zur Entwicklung der Handlungskontrolle*. Hofmann.

Scherer, K. R. (1985). Stress und emotion: Ein Ausblick. In K. R. Scherer, H. G. Wallbott, F. J. Tolkmitt, & G. Bergmann (Eds.), *Die stressreaktion: Physiologie und verhalten* (pp. 195–205). Hogrefe.

Schlenker, B. R. (1980). *Impression management: The self-concept, social identity and interpersonal relations*. Brooks/Cole.

Schwerdtfeger, A. (2012). Sportliche aktivität und angst. In R. Fuchs & W. Schlicht (Eds.), *Seelische gesundheit und sportliche aktivität* (pp. 186–207). Hogrefe.

Skinner, N., & Brewer, N. (2004). Adaptive approaches to competition: Challenge appraisals and positive emotion. *Journal of Sport and Exercise Psychology, 26*, 283–305. https://doi.org/10.1123/jsep.26.2.283

Smith, R. E., Smoll, F. L., & Cumming, S. (2007). Effects of a motivational climate intervention for coaches on young athletes' sport performance anxiety. *Journal of Sport & Exercise Psychology, 29*, 39–59.

Smith, R. E., Smoll, F. L., Cumming, S. P., & Grossbard, J. R. (2006). Measurement of multidimensional sport performance anxiety in children and adults: The Sport Anxiety Scale-2. *Journal of Sport and Exercise Psychology, 28*, 479–501.

Smith, R. E., Smoll, F. L., & Schutz, R. W. (1990). Measurement and correlates of sport-specific cognitive and somatic trait anxiety: The sport anxiety scale. *Anxiety Research, 2*, 263–280.

Sonstroem, R. J., & Bernardo, P. (1982). Intraindividual pregame state anxiety and basketball performance: A reexamination of the inverted-U curve. *Journal of Sport and Exercise Psychology, 4*, 235–245.

Spence, J. T., & Spence, K. W. (1966). The motivational components of manifest anxiety: Drive and drive stimuli. In C. D. Spielberger (Ed.), *Anxiety and behaviour* (pp. 291–326). Academic Press.

Spielberger, C. D. (1966). Theory and research on anxiety. In C. D. Spielberger (Ed.), *Anxiety and behaviour* (pp. 3–19). Academic Press.

Spielberger, C. D., Gorsuch, R. L., Lushene, R., Vagg, P. R., & Jacobs, G. A. (1983). *Manual for the state-trait anxiety inventory*. Consulting Psychologists Press.

Stenling, A., Hassmén, P., & Holmström, S. (2014). Implicit beliefs of ability, approach-avoidance goals and cognitive anxiety among team sport athletes. *European Journal of Sport Science, 14*, 720–729.

Stonerock, G. L., Hoffman, B. M., Smith, P. J., & Blumenthal, J. A. (2015). Exercise as treatment for anxiety: Systematic review and analysis. *Annals of Behavioural Medicine, 49*, 542–556.

Strahler, J., & Klumbies, E. (2012). Foundations in psychoneuroendocrinology. In F. Ehrlenspiel & K. Strahler (Eds.), *Psychoneuroendocrinology of sport and exercise: Foundations, markers, trends* (pp. 20–39). Routledge.

Stroop, J. R. (1935). Studies of interference in serial verbal reactions. *Journal of Experimental Psychology, 18*, 643–662.

Stubbs, B., Vancampfort, D., Rosenbaum, S., Firth, J., Cosco, T., Veronese, N., Salum, G. A., & Schuch, F. B. (2017). An examination of the anxiolytic effects of exercise for people with anxiety and stress-related disorders: A meta analysis. *Psychiatry Research, 24*, 102–108.

Tenenbaum, G., & Sacks, D. N. (2007). Die emotionale Seite der sportlichen Höchstleistung. In N. Hageman, M. Tietjens, & B. Strauß (Eds.), *Psychologie der sportlichen Höchstleistung: Grundlagen und Anwendungen der Expertiseforschung im Sport* (pp. 118–139). Hogrefe.

Thatcher, J., & Day, M. C. (2009). Re-appraising stress appraisals: The underlying properties of stress in sport. *Psychology of Sport and Exercise, 9*, 318–335.

Tremayne, P., & Barry, R. J. (1990). Repression of anxiety and its effects upon psychophysiological responses to relevant and irrelevant stimuli in competitive gymnasts. *Journal of Sport and Exercise Psychology, 12*, 327–352.

Turner, M. J., Jones, M. V., Sheffield, D., & Cross, S. L. (2012). Cardiovascular indices of challenge and threat states predict performance under stress in cognitive and motor tasks. *International Journal of Psychophysiology, 86*, 48–57.

Utschig, A. C., Otto, M. W., Powers, M. B., & Smits, J. A. J. (2013). The relationship between physical activity and anxiety and its disorders. In P. Ekkekakis, D. B. Cook, L. L. Craft, S. N. Culos-Reed, J. L. Etnier, M. Hamer, K. A. Martin Ginis, J. Reed, J. A. J. Smits, & M. Ussher (Eds.), *Routledge handbooks. Routledge handbook of physical activity and mental health* (pp. 105–116). Routledge.

Vickers, J. N. (2016). Origins and current issues in Quiet Eye research. *Current Issues in Sport Science, 1*, 101.

Vickers, J. N., & Williams, A. M. (2007). Performing under pressure: The effects of physiological arousal, cognitive anxiety, and gaze control in biathlon. *Journal of Motor Behaviour, 39*, 381–394.

Wedekind, D., Broocks, A., Weiss, N., Engel, K., Neubert, K., & Bandelow, B. (2010). A randomized, controlled trial of aerobic exercise in combination with paroxetine in the treatment of panic disorder. *The World Journal of Biological Psychiatry, 11*, 904–913.

Weinberg, R., & Gould, D. (2018). *Foundations of sport and exercise psychology* (7th ed.). Human Kinetics.

Williams, J. M., Mathews, A., & MacLeod, C. (1996). The emotional Stroop task and psychopathology. *Psychological Bulletin, 120*, 3–24.

Williams, M., Hudson, J., & Lawson, R. (1999). Self-presentation in sport: Initial development of a scale for measuring athlete's competitive self-presentation concerns. *Social Behaviour and Personality: An International Journal, 27*, 487–502.

Wilson, M., Wood, G., & Jordet, G. (2013). The BASES expert statement on the psychological preparation for football penalty shootouts. The Sport and Exercise Scientist, 38, 8–9.

Wilson, M. R., Vine, S. J., & Wood, G. (2009). The influence of anxiety on visual attentional control in basketball free throw shooting. *Journal of Sport & Exercise Psychology, 31*, 152–168.

Wilson, P., & Eklund, R. (1998). The relationship between competitive anxiety and self-presentational concerns. *Journal of Sport and Exercise Psychology, 20*, 81–97.

Wine, J. (1971). Test anxiety and direction of attention. *Psychological Bulletin, 76*, 92–104.

Wolf, S. A., Eys, M. A., & Kleinert, J. (2015). Predictors of the precompetitive anxiety response: Relative impact and prospects for anxiety regulation. *International Journal of Sport and Exercise Psychology, 13*, 344–358.

Woodman, T., & Hardy, L. (2003). The relative impact of cognitive anxiety and self-confidence upon sport performance: A meta-analysis. *Journal of Sports Sciences, 21*, 443–457.

Yerkes, R. M., & Dodson, J. D. (1908). The relation of strength of stimulus to rapidity of habit-formation. *Journal of Comparative Neurology and Psychology, 18*, 459–482.

Zuckerman, M. (2007). *Sensation seeking and risky behaviour*. American Psychological Association.

Personality and Development

Contents

Person, Situation, and Person-Situation Interaction in Sports

Katharina Geukes, Stephanie J. Hanrahan and Mitja D. Back

Contents

Supplementary Information The online version contains supplementary material available at https://doi.org/10.1007/978-3-031-03921-8_13.

J. Schüler et al. (eds.), *Sport and Exercise Psychology*, https://doi.org/10.1007/978-3-031-03921-8_13

Learning Objectives

Basic:

- To define psychological states, personality, and situations and to describe corresponding approaches to their measurement
- To describe effects of the person and effects of the situation on psychological states and to understand corresponding empirical findings

Advanced:

- To describe the interplay of person and situation (person-situation interaction effects) and to distinguish their three forms
- To describe stable individual profiles of psychological states across situations (stable situation profiles, if… then… rules)

Experts:

- To explain the level and fluctuations of individual psychological states and to differentiate between two types of individual state fluctuations (within contexts and across contexts)
- To describe the relationships between the introduced concepts
- To understand the challenges and implications for research and practical application

13.1 Introduction

The aim of sport psychology is to describe and explain human experiences and behaviors in the context of health-related physical activity or in competitive sports (cf. Aidmann & Schofield, 2004; ◘ Fig. 13.1). Experience is a summary term for thoughts (cognitions), feelings (emotions), and strivings (motivations). Behavior refers to *what* and *how well* people do things and what is—at least potentially—observable (behavior and performance).

The focus of this chapter is the description and explanation of momentary experiences and behaviors (i.e., states). What is a person thinking, how is she feeling, what is she striving for, and how is she behaving? In everyday life, as well as in sport and physical activity, humans are continually experiencing and behaving. Psychology, above all, is interested in differences in these states—in differences between individuals, that is, *interindividual* differences (e.g., Do the states of Aisha and Céline differ?), and in differences within individuals, that is, *intraindividual* differences (e.g., Do Aisha's (Céline's) states differ in two different situations?).

The explanation of states or differences in states targets the identification of causes for momentary experiences and behaviors. Because each single state refers to a

13

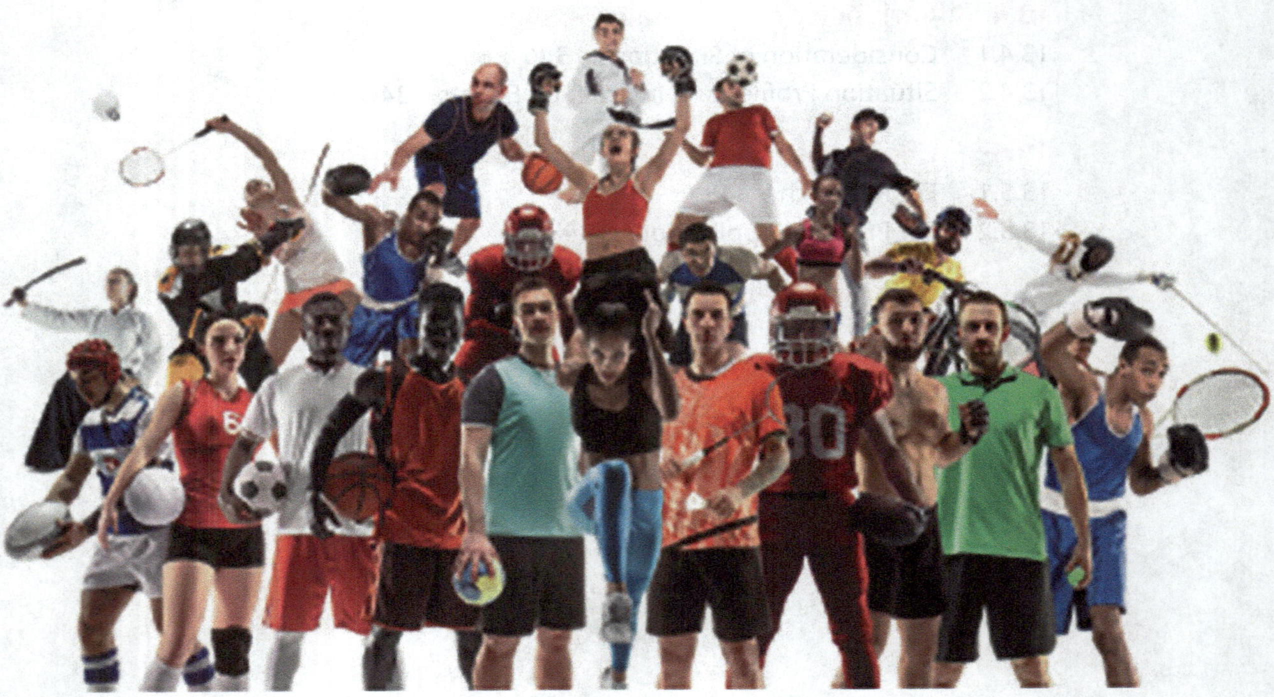

◘ **Fig. 13.1** Persons in contexts of sports

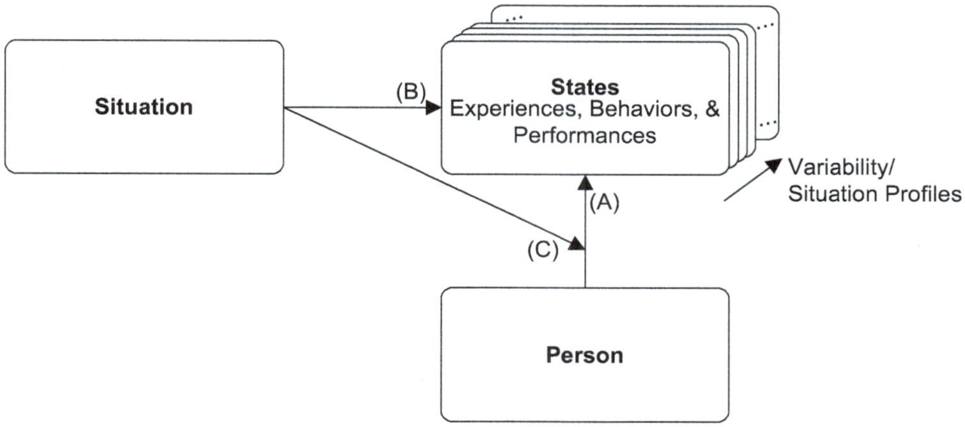

Fig. 13.2 Person, situation, and states

person in a given *situation*, these causes are assumed to be (a) characteristics of the person who experiences or shows a state, (b) characteristics of the situation in which a state is experienced or shown, and (c) the interplay of person and situation (Fig. 13.2). In this chapter, we first address the conception and assessment of psychological states.

13.1.1 States: Conception and Assessment

What Are States?

States refer to momentary experiences (thoughts, feelings, strivings) and behaviors in a given situation.

The focus of this chapter is on experiences and behaviors: What are people thinking, feeling, and striving for, and how are they behaving at a particular point in time, in the moment? Or more specifically, what are Aisha and Céline thinking, feeling, and striving for in training and in competition? And how are they behaving, respectively? Table 13.1 provides potential states of Aisha and Céline in training and in competition.

When assessing states, the goal is to *quantify* experiences and behaviors by translating individual cognitions, emotions, motivations, and behaviors into corresponding scores that adequately reflect interindividual and intraindividual differences.

States can be assessed in the laboratory as well as in the field (Table 13.2). Either separately or in combination, different approaches can be used as follows:

- Questionnaires
  (e.g., "Right now, I am anxious" on a rating scale from 1 = *not at all*, to 7 = *very much so)*
- Physiological measures
  (e.g., heart rate, skin conductance level, or hormonal responses; these somatic reactions serve as approximations of psychological states)
- Behavioral observations and measurements
  (e.g., global ratings—"This person behaves anxiously" on a rating scale from 1 = *not at all*, to 7 = *very much so*— or specific codings: frequency/duration/intensity of "This person fidgets"/"This person fiddles with her uniform"/"This person bites her lip.")

Behavioral observations and measurements can be understood as performance observations and measurements when they concern behavioral dimensions that

Table 13.1 Examples of different experiences and behaviors in training and competition

	Training		**Competition**	
	Aisha	**Céline**	**Aisha**	**Céline**
Experiences				
Thoughts	Asks herself whether she is going to be in the starting 11	Thinks about what she will eat after training	Thinks about her competition result	Imagines her big victory
Feelings	Is a bit nervous	Looks forward to physical activity	Becomes anxious	Feels joyful anticipation
Strivings	Wants to show her coach that she can do it	Wants to have fun	Wants to give her best	Only wants the convincing triumph
Behaviors	Gives everything	Is the center of attention as the team clown	Is jittery	Jokes around with her coach

Table 13.2 Assessment methods of states and their limitations in the laboratory and in the field

	Laboratory	Field
Questionnaires	Paper-pencil or computer-based questionnaires	Paper-pencil or computer-based questionnaires as well as smartphone-based questionnaires (apps)
Limitations	Represent a subjective perspective on states	As in the lab plus difficult to do during activity/competition
Physiological measurements	For example, heart rate, skin conductance level, or hormonal responses	For example, heart rate, skin conductance level, or hormonal responses
Limitations	Only reflect physiological responses, not necessarily the psychological relevance of states	As in the lab plus confounded with changes in bodily reactions due to physical activity
Behavior observation and measurement	Video-based, general ratings or specific codings	Video-based, general ratings or specific codings
Limitations	Requires opportunity for video recording, interrater agreement should be high	As in the lab plus possibly difficult to measure before and after competitions

13

represent *normative* (as good, important, or desirable) skills. In the context of biathlon, for instance, the measurement of skiing speed and shooting accuracy can be considered as performance assessment, because high speeds and accurate shots are normative, desirable behaviors in biathlon. Smiling and letting hard effort looks effortless are not performance indicators in biathlon. In figure skating, however—at least within the score

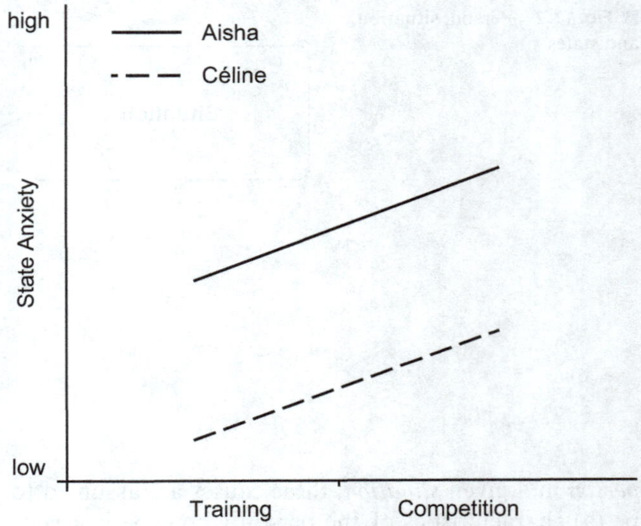

Fig. 13.3 Aisha's and Céline's anxiety during training and competition

relating to artistry and presentation—these behaviors have definite performance-related meaning.

As can be seen in Table 13.1, Aisha and Céline underwent an extensive assessment of their state anxiety during training and competition. Averaging (aggregating) across indicators of momentary thoughts, feelings, strivings, and behaviors resulted in the following summary (Fig. 13.3).

Based on this figure, one can easily conclude that Aisha and Céline differ during training and competition: Aisha is more anxious than Céline during both training and competition (influence of the person), and both of them are more anxious during competition than during training (influence of the situation).

The focus of the following sections is on the conceptions and assessments of the person and the situation, before comprehensively targeting the explanation of states through the person (person effects, effects of personality), the situation (situation effects), as well as the interplay of person and situation (their interaction).

Side Story

Absolute vs. Relative Assessment of States: Raw Scores vs. Z-Scores

Because raw scores only allow absolute statements (e.g., Aisha's raw score, 5; Céline's raw score, 2), researchers typically refer to *z*-scores to interpret differences between persons (e.g., Aisha and Céline) in relation to a sample. *Z*-scores result from a simple transformation in which the difference between a raw score (*R*) of a person (i) and the sample mean (*M*) is divided by the standard deviation (*SD*) of the sample:

$$z_i = \frac{R_{\text{Person}_i} - M_{\text{Sample}}}{SD_{\text{Sample}}}$$

When all raw scores of a sample get transformed into *z*-scores, the resulting distribution is a standard normal distribution with a mean of 0 and a standard deviation of 1 (Fig. 13.4).

This distribution has the advantage that the absolute information captured by the raw score can be interpreted relative to the distribution within the sample, as a multiple of the sample's standard deviation. To calculate Aisha's and Céline's *z*-scores, one needs the sample mean

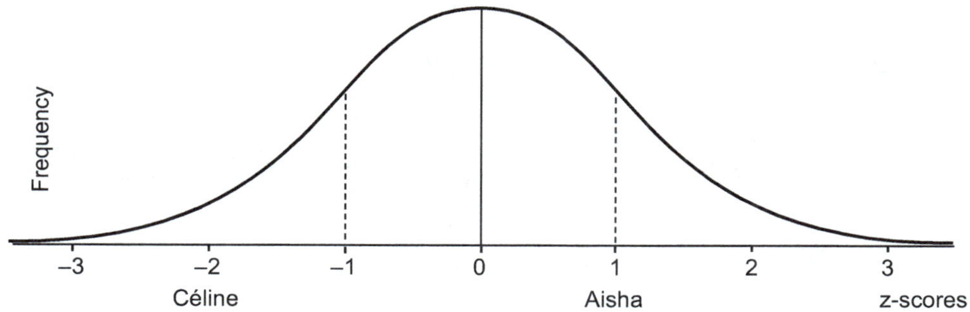

Fig. 13.4 Standard normal distribution

(e.g., $M = 4$) and sample standard deviation (e.g., $SD = 1$):

$$z_{\text{Aisha}} = \frac{5-4}{1} = 1 \; z_{\text{Céline}} = \frac{2-4}{1} = -2$$

Aisha has a *z*-score of 1 and Céline of −2. Thus, Aisha's and Céline's anxiety scores lie one and two standard deviations above and below the sample mean, respectively. So we know that Aisha's score is still average but above the sample's mean, whereas Céline's score is well below the sample's average.

13.1.2 Person: Conception and Assessment

The question concerning how to describe a person addresses her uniqueness in experiences (thoughts, feelings, and strivings) and behaviors. It is a person's individuality that distinguishes her from others. One commonly refers to this uniqueness, being different from others, as the *personality* of a person: the unique, individual structure of personality characteristics (i.e., *traits*).

Personality Traits?

Personality traits describe relatively stable differences between individuals in how they think, feel, strive, and behave.

Synonyms are terms such as "personality characteristic," "personality disposition," "personality dimension," and "character trait."

Even though there have been repeated attempts to assign individuals to personality types, the most prominent perspective on personality traits in psychology is a dimensional perspective (e.g., Allport (1927, 1937)) to describe personality as a whole. According to the dimensional perspective, the assumption is that persons possess all traits, but they differ in the strength of the expression of the different personality traits.

Side Story

Personality Types

Historically, there were many attempts to identify a relatively small number of distinct personality or character types to classify and describe individuals based on their physical or psychic features.

The history of personality types is long and dates back to ancient Greek philosophy. Attempts were made to identify personality types based, for example, on the four elements and corresponding humors (Hippocrates) or on four temperaments (Galen, Table 13.3).

Further attempts were made to assign individuals to personality types based on bodily features such as the physiological features of the head, the face (physiognomy and phrenology, for example, Aristotle, Lavater, and Gall), or the body (study of human constitution; Kretschmer, Sheldon; cf. Asendorpf, 2011).

Researchers have again and again tried to identify personality types (e.g., Jung's typology, Myers-Briggs Type Indicator). An established typology for

Table 13.3 Personality types according to Hippocrates and Galen

Hippocrates		Galen	Example: How does someone with this personality type behave when confronted with an obstacle?
Element	Humor	Temperament	
Air	Blood	Sanguine	She jumps over it.
Fire	Yellow bile	Choleric	She is in a rage.
Earth	Black bile	Melancholic	She sadly puts up with the obstacle.
Water	Phlegm	Phlegmatic	She stays well clear from the obstacle.

young adults, for example, incorporates three types: the resilient, the overcontrolled, and the under-controlled (Asendorpf et al., 2001). Asendorpf (2003) directly tested this typology against the dimensional approach and found that this typology, compared to dimensional operationalizations of personality, was inferior with regard to its predictive validity. Accordingly, approaches based on personality types are still the target of criticism (e.g., Asendorpf (2003); McCrae and Costa (1989); Pittenger (2004)).

Even though typologies are intuitive and plausible and are therefore well suited for communication to the general public, their broad applied and especially commercial success is not justified from a scientific perspective.

Within the trait paradigm, one uses dimensionally regarded personality traits to describe a person's unique individual experiences and behaviors. Accordingly, *all* individuals possess the descriptive traits, but they differ in the degree of *how strongly* each trait is pronounced. Differences between persons (interindividual differences) do not result from one person possessing trait X and another person not possessing it (personality types) but from one person holding a *higher or lower* expression of trait X than another person. Even though expressions of traits, or personalities as a whole, are conceptualized as having relative temporal stability, personality traits and personalities change and develop across the entire life span.

13

13.1.2.1 Global Personality Traits

It remains unclear *which* and *how many* personality traits are necessary for a comprehensive (as many traits as needed) but sufficient (as few traits as possible) description of a person. Researchers have gotten closer to achieving an exact description of personality by using a lexical approach. Acting on the assumption that meaningful differences between persons should necessarily manifest in everyday language, researchers have investigated adjectives that are used to describe persons and their idiosyncrasies. This process has happened worldwide. In English-speaking countries (mainly the USA), Allport and Odbert (1936) collected person-descriptive adjectives in four different lists and achieved the impressive numbers of 3682–5226 adjectives per list.

Reflection

Use Allport and Odbert's (1936) approach to create a single list. You need a sheet of paper, a black pen, and several colored pens:

- Take 10 min. With the black pen, write down all adjectives that describe individuals or their personalities that come to your mind. You can write them anywhere on the sheet of paper; just try to write down as many adjectives as possible. Even when two adjectives appear to be similar, write down both of them.
- Now try to group the adjectives according to their content with the help of the color pens. Adjectives that describe something similar should go in the same group. Use as many groups as needed and as few groups as possible.
- Create a label for each of the groups.
- How many groups did you find? What labels do they have?

Such adjective lists (which were of course created on the basis of dictionaries instead of the memory and creativity of researchers) were the foundation of a subsequent study in which many people were asked to rate themselves on these adjectives. The data from these self-assessments were then, by means of factor analyses, used to identify meaningful groups. Adjectives on which persons ascribed themselves similar scores (e.g., anxious and nervous, sociable and talkative) were grouped to establish as many groups as necessary and as few groups as possible.

Around the world, researchers found, more often than expected simply by random chance, exactly five adjective groups. These five groups are the basis for the widely used Big Five personality model (e.g., McCrae and Costa (1987)). These five groups were labeled *neuroticism*, *extraversion*, *openness*, *agreeableness*, and *conscientiousness* and serve as the current consensus for a comprehensive but sufficient personality description.

Table 13.4 presents typical adjectives for low and high expressions of these five dimensions.

Accordingly, persons differ in how neurotic, extraverted, open, agreeable, and conscientious they are, with each person having her own individual Big Five profile.

Reflection

Think of yourself. Try—with the help of the adjectives provided in Table 13.4—to create your own Big Five profile. Place a cross on each double arrow in Fig. 13.5 to indicate (somewhere between low, moderate, and high) what, according to your self-view, describes you best. Connect these crosses from the top to bottom to produce a profile.

Think of a person you know well (e.g., friend, parent, sibling). Develop, as described above, a Big Five profile for this person from your perspective (informant report). Choose a different color than you have used for your own profile. Repeat this procedure for two other people you know well.

How similar are the resulting Big Five profiles? On which dimension (or on which dimensions) are the profiles most similar? On which dimension (or on which dimensions) do they differ most?

Individuals' Big Five personality profiles, in raw scores or *z*-scores, are typically assessed by using *self-report questionnaires*. One can use brief screening instruments (e.g., Ten Item Personality Inventory, TIPI (Gosling et al., 2003), Big Five Inventory-2-S, BFI-2-S, or Big Five Inventory-2-XS, BFI-2-XS, with 30 or 15 items, respectively (Soto and John (2017a)) or longer and more comprehensive instruments (e.g., the Big Five Inventory-2 (BFI-2) with 60 items (Soto and John (2017b) or the NEO-group: NEO-FFI with 60 items (Costa & McCrae, 1989) and NEO-PI-R with 240 items (Costa & McCrae, 1992)) that allow more differentiated, reliable, and valid assessments of personality. Besides self-reports, one can also use *informant reports* to assess individuals' personalities (obtained from family mem-

Table 13.4 Adjectives for low and high expressions of the Big Five dimensions

	Low expressions	High expressions
Neuroticism	Unconcerned, relaxed, calm, placid, optimistic, carefree, stress-resistant	Anxious, worried, touchy, frustrated, pessimistic, vulnerable, fragile
Extraversion	Reserved, reclusive, cautious, calm, inactive, quiet, submissive	Warm-hearted, friendly, sociable, assertive, dominant, active, happy, cheerful
Openness	Pragmatic, uncreative, factual, conservative, tangible, conventional, traditional	Imaginative, creative, visionary, intellectual, abstract, tolerant, liberal
Agreeableness	Suspicious, egocentric, careful, antagonistic, aggressive, competitive, cautious	Trustworthy, honest, altruistic, cooperative, empathetic, modest, sensitive
Conscientiousness	Unorganized, chaotic, unreliable, laid-back, planless, spontaneous, indifferent	Organized, systematic, reliable, ambitious, planned, tidy, success-oriented

Fig. 13.5 Example of Big Five profiles

	Low Manifestation — Moderate Manifestation — High Manifestation
Neuroticism	←→
Extraversion	←→
Openness	←→
Agreeableness	←→
Conscientiousness	←→

bers, friends, partners, ex-partners, etc.) or behavioral observations.

13.1.2.2 Specific Personality Traits

Using the Big Five dimensions, one achieves a relatively broad description of persons' experiences and behaviors, which is why these traits are referred to as *global traits*. Each of these global traits, however, can be further divided into facets. Within the BFI-2 (Soto & John, 2017b), for example, each Big Five dimension is assessed with three facets and within the NEO-PI-R (Costa & McCrae, 1992; ◘ Table 13.5) with six facets. In contrast to the superordinate global traits, these facets can be regarded as *conceptually specific traits*.

Other forms of conceptually specific traits are those that (a) lie on the conceptual intersection of two Big Five traits (e.g., perfectionism combines aspects of conscientiousness and neuroticism; narcissism combines aspects of extraversion and (dis)agreeableness) and (b) are identified on the basis of theoretical models (e.g., self-consciousness, resilience, or mental toughness).

Finally, one can distinguish situation-specific traits. These traits describe global or conceptually specific personality dispositions in specific situations (e.g., work-related conscientiousness, test or competition anxiety, or sport-related perfectionism).

Whether global or specific personality traits are used to describe individuals' personalities is usually dependent on the scientific or applied diagnostic question one seeks to answer. Thus, the Big Five model serves as a central and parsimonious framework to globally conceptualize personality. An even more comprehensive psychological description, however, could also involve intelligence (e.g., fluid and crystallized intelligence), abilities (e.g., motor and cognitive abilities), temperaments (e.g., emotionality and sociability) or emotions (e.g., joy, sadness, fear, anger, surprise, disgust), motives (e.g., achievement, power, affiliation), self-concepts (e.g., self-esteem, appearance, and ability attributes), interpersonal styles (e.g., dominance, warmth), and values (e.g., self-determination, tradition, hedonism, security). In the history of sport psychology, the focus often has been on one or *several specific aspects of personality*. The Big Five only played a minor role.

13.1.3 Situation: Conception and Assessment

The question of how to describe a situation targets, according to Kurt Lewin (1936), the *current characteristics of the environment*. Surprisingly, current characteristics of the environment have only rarely been investigated systematically.

What Is a Situation?

A situation is the entirety of the current characteristics of the environment with which a person is confronted and that may be psychologically meaningful.

In many classic studies in social and sport psychology, researchers typically created sufficiently different situations (conditions) in which to assess, observe, and com-

13

◘ **Table 13.5** Two examples of facets (conceptually specific traits) within the Big Five global traits

	Neuroticism	Extraversion	Openness	Agreeableness	Conscientiousness
BFI-2					
1	Anxiety	Sociability	Intellectual curiosity	Compassion	Organization
2	Depression	Assertiveness	Aesthetic sensitivity	Respectfulness	Productiveness
3	Emotional volatility	Energy level	Creative imagination	Trust	Responsibility
NEO-PI-R					
1	Anxiety	Warmth	Fantasy	Trust	Competence
2	Hostility	Gregariousness	Aesthetics	Modesty	Self-discipline
3	Depression	Assertiveness	Feelings	Compliance	Achievement striving
4	Self-consciousness	Activity	Actions	Altruism	Dutifulness
5	Impulsiveness	Excitement seeking	Ideas	Straightforwardness	Order
6	Vulnerability	Positive emotions	Values	Tender-mindedness	Deliberation

pare individuals (▶ Chaps. 16 and 17). Examples in sport psychology include the following:

- The comparison of situations with and without the presence of an audience (Bond & Titus, 1983; Strauss, 2002)
- The comparison of situations with and without the presence of competitive pressure (Baumeister, 1984; Baumeister & Showers, 1986; Mesagno et al., 2015; Otten, 2009)
- The comparison of home and away games (Baumeister & Steinhilber, 1984; Jamieson, 2010)

This procedure (i.e., to compare distinct situations) can be labeled as a *categorical approach* to the description of situations where situations are assigned to *classes of situations*. These situation classes do not need to refer only to experimental situations, but they can also describe everyday situations. Prominent examples of the categorical approach to situations include the following:

- Work vs. leisure-time situations (Diener et al., 1984)
- Social vs. nonsocial situations (Lucas & Diener, 2001)
- Situations of pleasure vs. situations of individual adversity vs. situations of interpersonal conflict vs. situations of social demand (Ten Berge & De Raad, 2002)

In recent research on the description of situations, researchers have also used *dimensional approaches*. Within the Big Eight DIAMONDS model (Rauthmann et al., 2014; Rauthmann & Sherman, 2016), for example, situations are differentiated along eight dimensions (◘ Table 13.6) to comprehensively and sufficiently describe them.

◘ **Table 13.6** Big Eight DIAMONDS

Dimension	Question
Duty	Does something need to be done?
Intellect	Is deep (cognitive) information processing required?
Adversity	Is someone threatened by external forces?
Mating	Can (potential) mates be attracted or courted?
POsitivity	Does the situation have pleasurable aspects?
Negativity	Could the situation entail negative emotions?
Deception	Is deception or mistrust an issue?
Sociality	Is (meaningful) social interaction important?

Just as the Big Five provide a global and parsimonious framework for personality, the Big Eight DIAMONDS provide such a framework for situations.

At the most basic level, the assessment of situations, be it categorically or dimensionally, can be realized in two ways: via *subjective and objective measurements* of situation information. On the one hand, individuals whose states are of interest can be asked how they experienced the given situation. They can subjectively evaluate the class (category) of a situation or the qualities of the situation on different dimensions. On the other hand, objective measurements—or at least *more* objective measurements—of situations are also possible. In this case, several independent individuals who are not part of the situation themselves are asked to evaluate the class or qualities of a situation. The average of these evaluations (i.e., consensus) serves as an (more) objective situation assessment.

13.2 Effects of the Person and/or Effects of the Situation?

Social and personality psychologists have long been tackling the question of whether the person or the situation has effects on states—and if so, how strong these effects are.

Based on the intuitive assumption that individuals' experiences and behaviors are consistent across situations, researchers have assumed strong *person effects*. Aisha, who is the most anxious athlete during training, is likely to be the most anxious athlete during competition, too. Céline, in contrast, who is quite relaxed during training, will presumably be relatively relaxed during competitions.

Similarly intuitive, however, is the assumption that individuals' experiences and behaviors consistently change from one situation to the next, meaning that there are strong *situation effects*. In this sense, Aisha and Céline are both presumably more anxious during competitions than during training (◘ Fig. 13.3).

13.2.1 Effects of the Person

The central assumption is that the personality of a person predicts her current experiences and behaviors and accordingly also her current sport-related actions and performances. The expression of *states* is a function of the person: *States* = f(Person).

In empirical studies, it is consistently found that the prediction of single states is successful; however, the established correlations are disappointingly small. On the basis of these findings, it was long believed that a correlation of a personality trait with a state cannot be higher than .30 (perhaps .40). This "magical" upper limit of possible correlations received the label *personality coefficient*.

When testing these relationships within meta-analyses (i.e., within studies that statistically combine findings of multiple single studies), it was revealed that strong relationships are possible between personality traits and states. Fleeson and Gallagher (2009), for example, found correlations between .53 and .68 between the Big Five traits and self-reported behaviors. These findings are a clear indication that the assumption that personality can predict current experiences and behaviors is justified because the prediction of average states is successful. In this meta-analysis, however, self-reported traits were correlated with self-reported states so that, due to the common data source (i.e., common method variance), correlations were expected to be rather strong and the "true correlation" might have been overestimated. Nevertheless, these findings support the idea of correlations of .30 (or .40) between traits and objective behaviors.

Side Story

Use of Aggregates

When predicting states—be it through the person or through the situation—researchers are interested in whether (and how well) states can be predicted. Therefore, researchers have investigated whether state values combined in meaningful aggregates could be more accurately predicted than single state values.

These aggregates can be calculated in two ways: First, they can regard states in similar situations (e.g., the average anxiety value of repeated assessments during competitions). Second, they can regard several state assessments within one situation (e.g., the average of different anxiety items: sweaty hands, butterflies in the stomach, being worried). Of course, these methods of aggregation can also be combined so that values are aggregated across items and situations.

The *prediction* of aggregated states is more successful than the prediction of single states. A single state is less representative of *typical* momentary experiences and behaviors, because it contains more measurement error and is more prone to random fluctuations than aggregates of states. Aggregated scores, thus, reduce the influence of measurement error and of random fluctuations so that they provide a better representation of the typical individual characteristics, which is exactly the intention of the trait assessment to measure typical individual characteristics.

13

13.2.1.1 Person Effects in Sport

The significance of aggregation is also evident within the investigation and prediction of motor performance through personality traits. Researchers have identified only weak, or even no, personality effects on single states (Morgan, 1980; Rogulj et al., 2006). When sport-related behaviors or performances were aggregated across longer stretches of time (e.g., level of competition, elite status, successful vs. unsuccessful career paths), however, significant effects of personality were found, which help to answer the following important sport psychology questions:

1. Does *the* athlete personality exist?

Reflection

Develop average Big Five profiles for the subsequent groups of people (see Fig. 13.5):

1. People who do not exercise at all
2. People who exercise three times a week
3. People who play recreational volleyball
4. People who are part of the national Olympic team:

- For which dimensions did you think the evaluation of trait expressions was easy? For which did you think it was difficult?
- For which dimensions do you expect between-group differences? For which dimensions do you not expect such differences?
- What do you think is/are the most important personality dimension(s) to be successful as an elite athlete?

Meta-analytic findings to answer the question of whether there is a distinct athlete personality show that athletes are characterized by high values on extraversion and conscientiousness as well as low values on neuroticism. Regarding openness and agreeableness, no differences have been found between groups of athletes and nonathletes (Rhodes & Smith, 2006).

2. Does *the* elite athlete's personality exist?

Similarly, athletes who compete on a national or international level are typically found to be more extraverted and less neurotic than those competing at

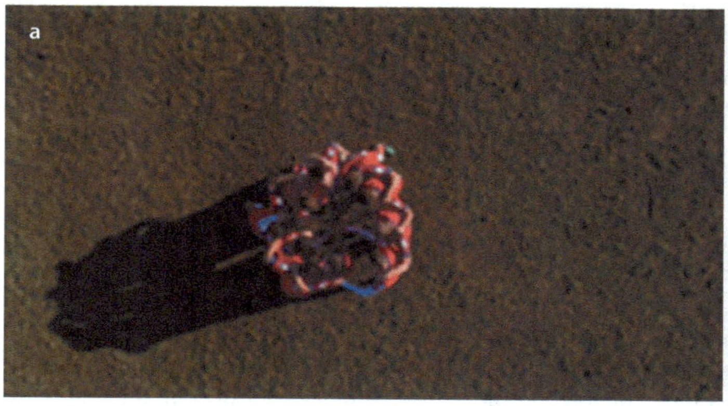

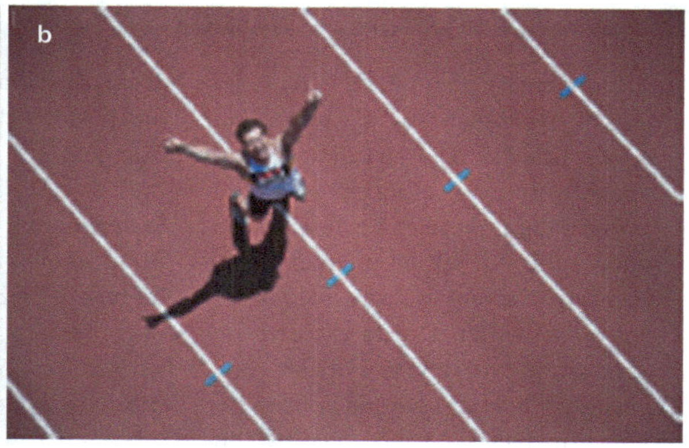

Fig. 13.6 **a**, **b** Team- vs. individual sports (**a**: © miodrag ignjatovic/Getty Images/iStock; **b**: © Paul Bradbury/Getty Images/iStock)

lower levels. In some studies, additional differences in conscientiousness and agreeableness were identified. Better athletes were found to be more conscientious and more agreeable (Allen et al., 2011; Egloff & Jan Gruhn, 1996; Kirkcaldy, 1982a; Williams & Parkin, 1980).

3. Are there personality differences between athletes who engage in different types of sports?

   Findings of studies that targeted this question showed that, typically, athletes do not differ according to the type of sport (Johnson & Morgan, 1981; Lackie, 1962; O'Sullivan et al., 1998) but according to broader classifications of types of sports (e.g., between team and individual sports, Fig. 13.6). Team athletes describe themselves as being more extraverted and conscientious than do individual athletes (Allen et al., 2011; Eagleton et al., 2007), and athletes who engage in high-risk sports describe themselves as comparably more extraverted and less conscientious compared to athletes who participate in low-risk sports (Castanier et al., 2010; Rhea & Martin, 2010; Tok, 2011).

4. Are there personality differences within team sports depending on the players' positions?

   There is weak empirical evidence for attacking players being more extraverted than defending players (Kirkcaldy, 1982b), but another study did not find such differences (Cameron et al., 2012).

For all these studies, it is important to consider that they, by design, cannot determine whether athletes already had these personality profiles before starting careers in their sports and became successful because of it (*selection hypothesis*) or whether athletes developed these personality profiles through participation in their sports (*socialization hypothesis*). To test these hypotheses against each other, one needs to analyze longitudinal data with the first measurement taken before entering a sport. These data are obviously rare.

Coming back to the example of Aisha and Céline (Fig. 13.3), the most plausible personality effect that could be investigated would be the one of neuroticism, because anxiety is an aspect of neuroticism. An online survey assessment identified a neuroticism score of 5 for Aisha; Céline, in contrast, had a score of 1. Thus, we identified a person effect because higher values on neuroticism predict higher values in state anxiety. The rank order of traits corresponds to the rank order of states: Aisha > Céline.

Because Aisha's and Céline's scores differ during training and during competition, it is obviously not the person or the personality alone influencing states but also the situation.

13.2.2 Effects of the Situation

When investigating situation effects, the central assumption is that the situation predicts a person's momentary experiences and behaviors and accordingly her momentary sport-related actions and performances. The expression of states is a function of the situation: States = f(Situation).

Within social and personality psychology, numerous studies have been conducted to investigate these associations. As already stressed regarding the measurement of situations, these studies were largely based on the comparison of states in different situations or conditions. The following situation effects were found in three classic social psychological experiments (Funder, 2015):

Three Classic Social Psychological Experiments Testing Situation Effects

Experiment 1

In an experiment by Festinger and Carlsmith (1959), participants were first involved in a boring and time-consuming experiment. Subsequently, they were to tell participants who were still waiting to participate in this experiment that it is an exciting and interesting experiment. For this statement, participants earned either $1 or $20. Finally, they were asked by confederates how they actually found the experiment. The counterintuitive finding showed that those participants who only earned $1 for their wrong statement reported that the experiment had indeed been exciting and interesting. In contrast, those participants who had received $20 told the identical (white) lie but evaluated the experiment as boring and uninteresting (Festinger & Carlsmith, 1959).

This experiment is one of the first demonstrations of the *cognitive dissonance* effect. The small reward of $1 for a wrong statement produced cognitive dissonance, because the behavior contradicted one's own attitude and could not be attributed to the financial reward. Participants retrospectively adjusted their attitudes to again establish cognitive consonance. In the $20 condition, participants could attribute their behavior to the high reward so that no dissonance occurred and there was no need to adjust one's own attitude. Converted into the metric of correlations, the association was −.36 (i.e., the smaller the reward, the greater the attitude change).

Experiment 2

In experiments by Darley and colleagues (1968, 1973), participants were students of theology. They first worked on a task in one building and were then sent into another building—either in a hurry or not. On the way to the other building, they walked past a man who laid crouched, coughing, and groaning at the entrance. Participants were less likely to stop when more spectators were present and when they were in a hurry (Darley & Batson, 1973; Darley & Latané, 1968).

This experiment targeted the *bystander effect* and identified diffusion of responsibility (feeling less responsible oneself when many people could feel responsible) as an explanation for not helping in emergency situations. Converted into the metric of correlations, associations were −.38 for the number of spectators (i.e., the more spectators present, the less likely participants were to stop and help) and −.38 for hurry (i.e., the greater the hurry, the less likely participants were to stop and help).

Experiment 3

In a famous experiment, Milgram (1975) investigated whether and when participants follow authoritative instructions—even if they are in conflict with their conscience. Participants were more likely to follow instructions to apply electric shocks to an innocent victim when the commander was in the same room and when they could not see or hear the victim. By implication, they were more likely to refuse the commands when the commander was not in the same room and the victim was out-of-sight and hearing distance (Milgram, 1975). No one actually received an electric shock within the famous Milgram experiment.

Converted into the metric of correlations, associations were −.36 for the proximity of the commander (i.e., the closer the commander, the less likely the refusal of the authoritative instruction) and 0.42 for the proximity of the victim (i.e., the closer the victim, the more likely the refusal).

These classic experiments highlight the important influence of the situation on momentary experiences and behaviors. The disadvantage of relying on classic experiments lies in the fact that they are typically particularly successful experiments (i.e., those experiments that have shown large situation effects). The average social psychological situation effect is a correlation of .21. With a standard deviation of .15, this correlation means that two-thirds of all studies have identified a situation effect between .06 and .36 (Richard et al., 2003).

13

13.2.2.1 Situation Effects in Sports

Situation effects have also been frequently assumed and investigated in sport science and sport psychology (► Chaps. 16 and 17). Examples include (a) the influence of the presence (vs. absence) of others, (b) the influence of the presence (vs. absence) of pressure, and (c) the influence of home vs. away games:

1. With regard to the influence of the presence (vs. absence) of others on motor performance, findings draw a complex picture. Depending on the task, motor performance becomes either facilitated (*social facilitation*) or hindered (*social inhibition*) in comparison to a situation without spectators. In cases where the task is simple or purely depending on endurance or strength (e.g., sprint or weight lifting), performance improves. The correlation is .16. In cases where the task is complex and involves coordination (e.g., shooting basketball free throws), deteriorated performance is the result compared to a situation in which no one watches ($r = -.18$; Bond & Titus, 1983; Strauss, 2002).
2. A similar hypothesis has been tested for the comparison of situations that differ in the presence vs. absence of performance pressure. Based on anecdotal evidence for the metaphorically labeled phenomenon “choking under pressure” (Baumeister, 1984; Baumeister & Showers, 1986), it has been assumed that athletes execute poorer performances when

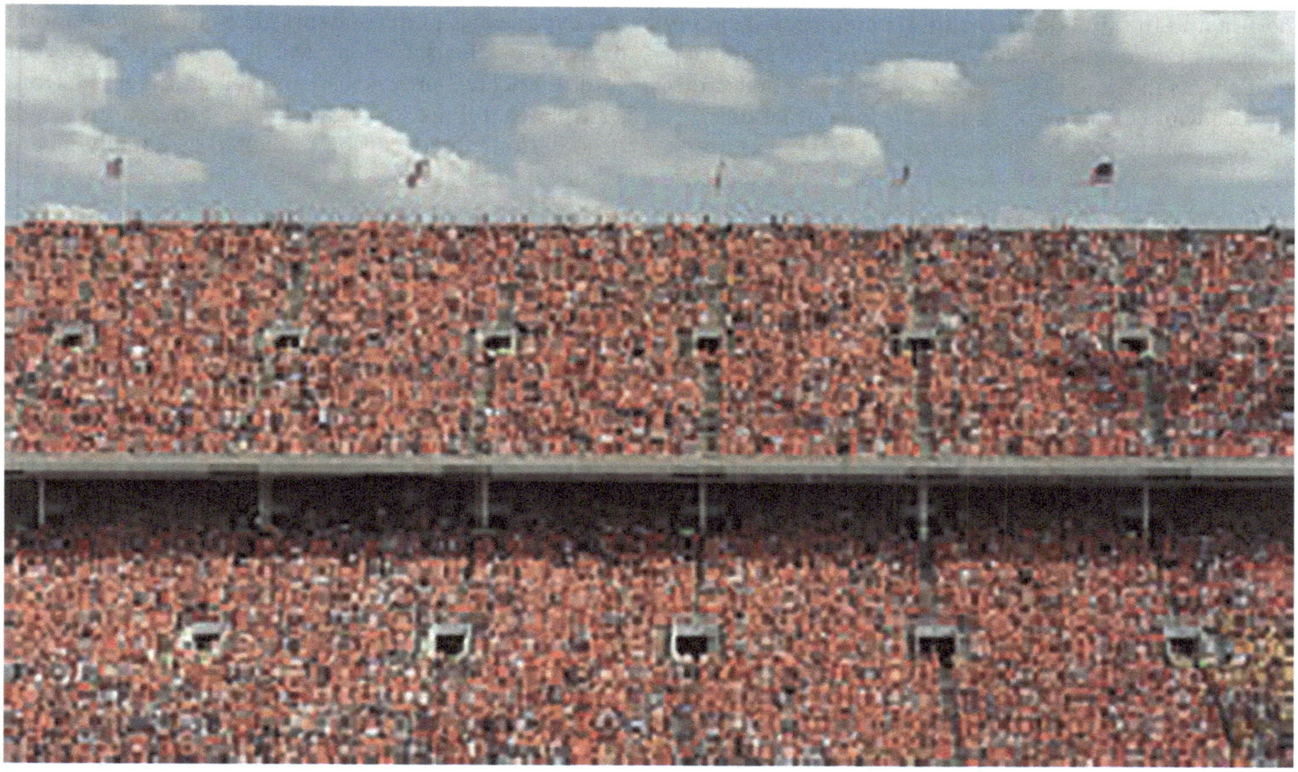

Fig. 13.7 Home advantage or home disadvantage?

under pressure than when not under pressure. However, the opposite hypothesis has also been formulated where athletes show better performances when it counts (excelling under pressure; Otten (2009)). Empirically, findings are inconsistent: comparing groups, researchers sometimes find choking, sometimes find excelling, and sometimes find no differences at all between the performances in the two conditions (e.g., Baumeister and Showers (1986); Geukes et al. (2013a, 2013b); Otten (2009)).

3. Regarding the influence of home vs. away games (see Fig. 13.7), a meaningful home advantage has been identified. In a meta-analysis, Jamieson (2010) showed that in 60% of games, home athletes or home teams won. Many sport journalists as well as athletes and coaches believe in the home advantage. This advantage, however, seems to reverse in particularly important games (Baumeister & Steinhilber, 1984; Wright et al., 1991). In decisive competitions or games, home athletes or home teams tend to show comparatively weaker performances in front of their home crowds.

These examples illustrate that situations have a considerable influence on performances of athletes. Much stronger than the influence on performance, however, is the influence on momentary experiences and behaviors (e.g., excitement, nervousness, anxiety, self-confidence; Woodman and Hardy (2003)). Aisha's and Céline's (Fig. 13.3) story is quite similar; both are more anxious during competition than during training, which nicely summarizes a strong situation effect.

13.2.3 Effects of the Person and Effects of the Situation

In the example of Aisha and Céline, we have identified a strong person effect and a strong situation effect. Aisha is more anxious than Céline on average (person effect), and both are more anxious during competition than during training (situation effect). Accordingly, person and situation effects can occur simultaneously. But which of those effects is more important?

Surprisingly, researchers have only rarely directly compared the relative influence of person effects and situation effects. An important exception is the study by Leikas et al. (2012), which aimed to make this exact comparison. Within dyadic interactions of individuals with actors, Leikas et al. showed that the relative influence of person and situation varied with the behavior of interest. Some behaviors were particularly well predicted by the person (e.g., number of smiles/laughs or gestures), other behaviors were particularly well predicted by the situation (e.g., number of questions or mutual gaze frequency), and still other behaviors were predicted by the person and the situation (e.g., total amount of speaking or nods). One could similarly compare person and situation effects in the sports context with studies that target the behaviors of many persons in various situations.

To summarize the abovementioned studies, both variables, the person and the situation, predict momentary experiences and behaviors. The correlations found for person effects are—as the personality coefficient would indicate—around .30 and .40 and can be stronger when states are aggregated. The correlations found for situation effects can be evaluated as equally meaningful.

Side Story

Person-Situation Debate or Consistency Debate

Within the research on the effects of persons and situations and their relative influences, a long and intensive debate had unfolded: the person-situation or consistency debate. Ultimately, the debate revolved around the question of which influence on states is stronger: effects of the person or effects of the situation?

This complex debate began with a publication by Walter Mischel (1968), in which he claimed:

> "... highly generalised behavioral consistencies have not been demonstrated, and the concept of personality traits as broad dispositions is thus untenable"

The starting point of Mischel's rationale was the observation that the behavior of individuals across situations is not consistent (a lack of *trans-situational consistency*), because behavior is, above all, situation-dependent. When behavior is inconsistent and situation-dependent, Mischel concluded that personality cannot play an important role. Mischel even went so far to put the existence of personality traits into question.

It is unsurprising that other psychologists vigorously contradicted Mischel's pointed statement, especially those who had long worked on personality traits. In this way, the debate evolved.

Two contrary positions were facing each other: the situationists on Mischel's side and the personists who defended the existence of personality as a meaningful psychological concept. The personists rebutted the harsh criticism of the situationists using conceptual and methodological clarifications. These clarifications involved the important distinction between absolute and relative trans-situational inconsistency (see below) and the significance of aggregation, which we already introduced in the section regarding person effects.

The end of the consistency debate, to which Mischel himself significantly contributed, dates back to the 1990s. Psychologists found a consensus in the assumption that person and situation effects are not contradictory but both effects can exist simultaneously and independently. Currently, the consistency debate no longer plays a major role, because a compromise was found within the interactionist perspective.

13

13.3 Interactionism

Interactionism is the perspective within social and personality psychology that considers the interplay of persons and situations.

Interactionism

Interactionism is a perspective within personality psychology in which momentary human experiences and behaviors (states) are explained by characteristics of the person, characteristics of the situation, and the interplay of characteristics of the person and characteristics of the situation.

Let us consider an extended example (Fig. 13.8), not only Aisha and Céline but also Beth.

In the training situation, Beth's anxiety score is between those of Aisha and Céline. In the competition situation, however, Beth is the most anxious of the three. Both the absolute (comparison of raw scores) and the relative trans-situational consistencies (comparison of z-scores) across the situations are reduced when Beth's scores are added.

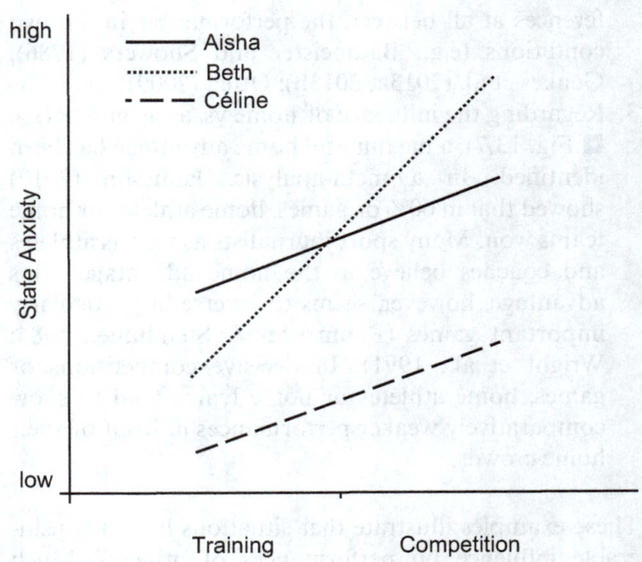

Fig. 13.8 Aisha's, Beth's, and Céline's anxiety during training and competition

Side Story

Absolute vs. Relative Trans-situational Consistency

Imagine we had measured individuals' anxiety values in ten different situations (e.g., at the cinema box office (1), during training (3), on a first data (5), during competition (8), shortly before a bungee jump (10)). Now, have a look at ◘ Fig. 13.9. You see three coordinate systems in which situations are plotted on the x-axis and anxiety values on the y-axis using raw scores (left and center panel) or z-scores (right panel).

The left panel (**a**) of ◘ Fig. 13.9 illustrates (perfect) absolute trans-situational consistency using data from four fictitious individuals. To be able to talk about absolute trans-situational consistency, the observed anxiety scores need to be identical across situations. Thus, the anxiety profiles across situations are parallel lines. This absolute trans-situational consistency is, of course, not really the case. That is why we used fictitious data for this illustration.

More realistic is the illustration in the panel in the center (**b**) of ◘ Fig. 13.9, in which real anxiety data of four individuals has been plotted. When regarding each person separately, one can easily recognize that each individual reports different anxiety values in each situation. All four of them increase in their anxiety from situation 1 to situation 10 (situation effects). For example, all of them are much more anxious shortly before doing a bungee jump than at the cinema box office.

Comparing the four individuals' anxiety profiles, one recognizes that Person 1, in each of the situations, is more anxious than Person 2, who is more anxious than Person 3, and Person 4 always is the least anxious person. The rank order of the individuals in anxiety remains identical across the ten situations (person effects). This ranking is visible in the fact that the lines that connect the anxiety values of each person, respectively, do not cross each other. Relative trans-situational consistency is evident when the rank order of individuals is identical or at least similar across situations.

In the right panel of this figure (**c**), z-scores, instead of raw scores, are plotted. Here, it becomes evident that the lines do not cross each other, speaking for relative trans-situational consistency. Additionally, this figure provides the relative information of z-scores. Because all four lines are approximately horizontal and parallel lines, the z-scores of the individuals remain almost identical across all situations. Although absolute trans-situational consistency is unlikely, relative trans-situational consistency is realistic and has strong empirical support in many studies.

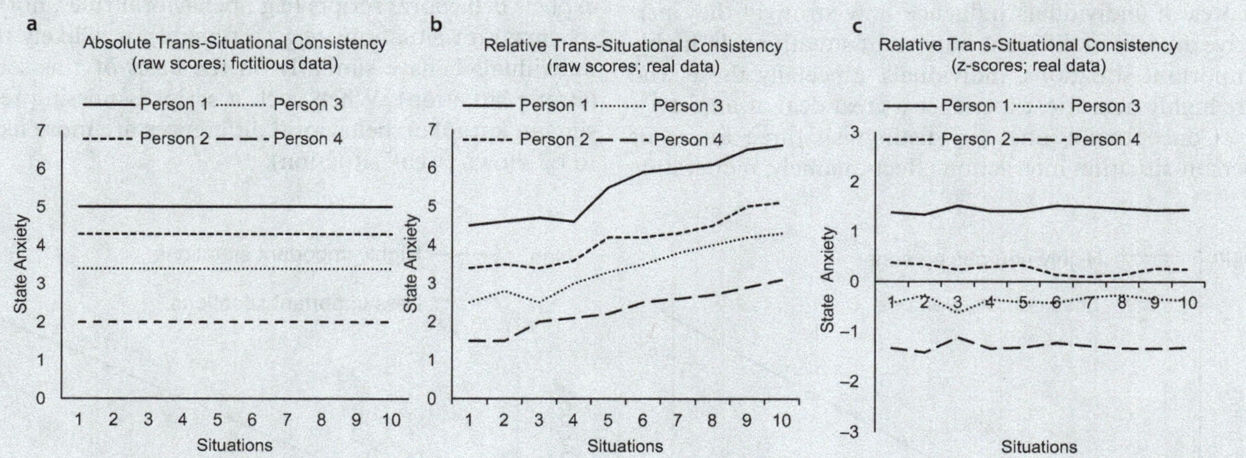

◘ **Fig. 13.9** Trans-situational consistency

In the case of missing or only weak relative trans-situational consistency (in the example including Beth), simple person and situation effects are insufficient to explain state anxiety. Beth's high state anxiety in competitive situations can be explained by the interplay of the person (Beth) and the situation (training/competition).

13.3.1 Effects of the Interaction of Person and Situation

These interaction effects of person and situation incorporate the assumption that specific associations between personality traits and states are dependent on the situation. Thus, the expressions of states are a function of the person, the situation, and the interaction of the person and the situation: States = f(Person, Situation, Person * Situation).

What Are Interaction Effects of Person and Situation?

The influence of a person (i.e., a personality trait) on a state (momentary experience and behavior) is differently strong in different situations.

Figure 13.10 summarizes two different illustrations of the identical interaction effect. In the left part of the figure, the importance of the situation is plotted on the x-axis, and state anxiety is plotted on the y-axis. The two lines represent individuals with high values (solid line) and low values (dotted line) on the trait of neuroticism.

It is evident that the slopes of the two lines are considerably different. The importance of the situation, thus, influences how strongly (more, solid line, or less, dotted line) neurotic individuals experience anxiety. Highly neurotic individuals experience a high level of anxiety, especially in important situations.

In the right part of the figure, the trait of neuroticism is plotted on the x-axis, with anxiety again plotted on the y-axis. The two lines represent highly important (solid line) and less important (dotted line) situations. Again, the slopes of the two lines are different. The neuroticism scores of individuals influence how strongly they perceive anxiety in different important situations. In highly important situations, individuals, especially those who are highly neurotic, experience a great deal of anxiety.

13

Conceptually, one can distinguish three forms of person-situation interaction effects, namely, moderating effects of situation strength, trait relevance, and situation-specific person effects.

13.3.1.1 Moderating Effects of the Strength of a Situation

The strength of a situation refers to its characteristic or capability of provoking individual differences in experiences and behaviors. Strong situations do not, or only weakly, provoke such differences, whereas weak situations are well capable of producing such differences.

The situation strength is a continuum that ranges from weak to strong. Even though situation strength influences experiences as well as behaviors, the explanation of this concept is easier when considering behaviors, because behaviors are more easily observable from the outside. For example, when in the locker room celebrating the latest win, large behavioral differences can be observed (weak situation). Athletes may be joking with their coach, sitting calmly listening to music, searching for the physiotherapist, or heading to the shower. In direct race preparation (i.e., immediately before the starting signal), behavioral differences are only barely visible (strong situation). All athletes are busy preparing for the imminent start (see Fig. 13.11).

The clarity of the task is an important factor determining the strength of a situation. A related factor is the normativity of the situation. When there are clear and explicit behavioral scripts (e.g., behavioral rules, norms, schemas) for situations (e.g., a funeral), it is likely that individuals behave similarly on the basis of this script (strong situation). When such a script is missing (e.g., singing karaoke), behavioral differences are more likely to be shown (weak situation).

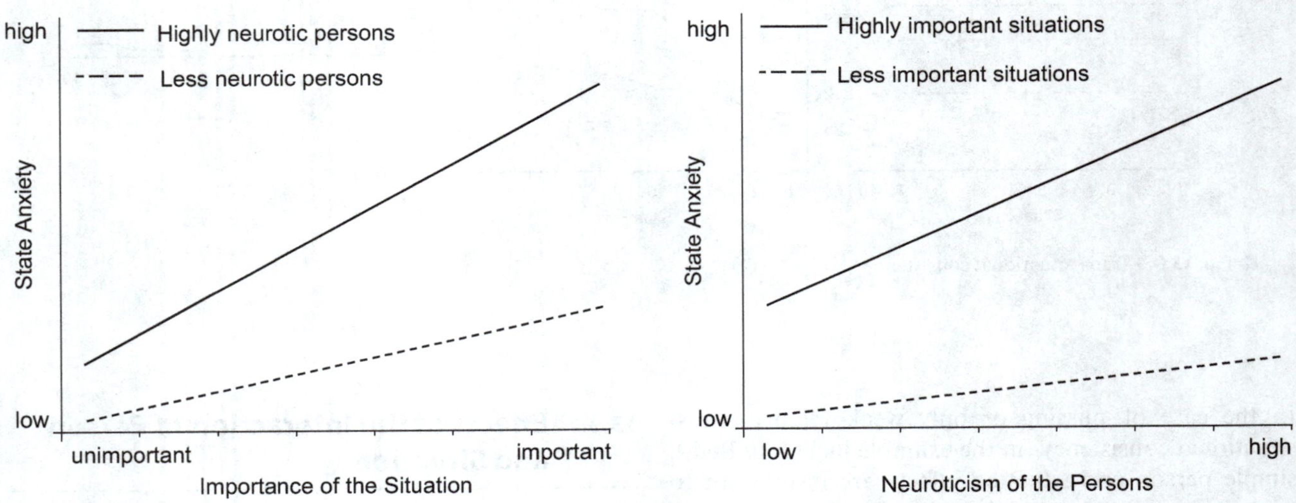

Fig. 13.10 Interaction effect of person and situation

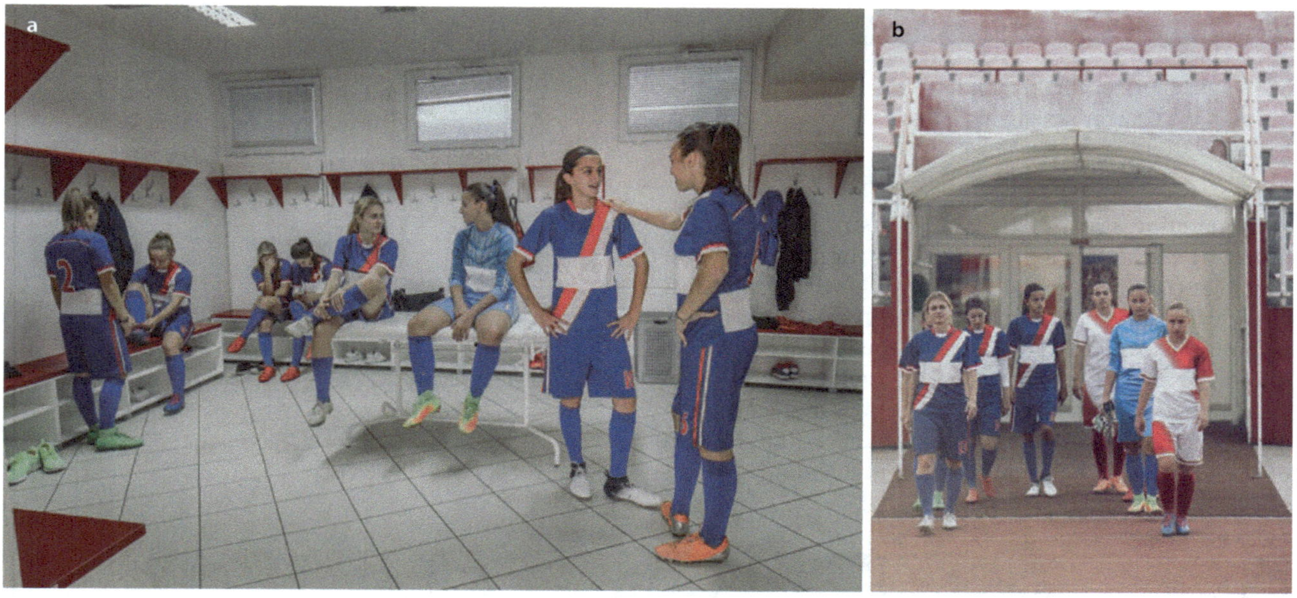

■ **Fig. 13.11** **a**, **b** Weak and strong situation (© skynesher/Getty Images/iStock)

Reflection

For each of the different contexts, please think of examples of a weak and a strong situation, respectively, and fill in ■ Table 13.7.

■ **Table 13.7** Situation strength in five contexts

Context	Weak situation	Strong situation
At the university		
With family		
With friends		
During training		
During competition		

A moderating effect of situation strength is found when the strength of an association between two variables (i.e., person and state) is influenced by a third (i.e., situation strength). Personality traits are capable of predicting behavioral differences in weak situations (locker room, significant correlation) but not in strong situations (direct start preparation, null correlation). The strength of a situation influences the strength of an association between personality trait and state (e.g., neuroticism and state anxiety).

13.3.1.2 Moderating Effects of the Trait Relevance of the Situation

Trait relevance refers to the conceptual match of the investigated personality trait and the investigated situation. The foundation of this idea is the theoretical principle of trait activation (Tett & Guterman, 2000). This principle states that a personality trait will successfully predict a state only when it is relevant in the investigated situation, that is, when it becomes activated.

For example, when the aim is to predict momentary experiences and behaviors through neuroticism, neuroticism should be relevant in that situation. Within the sport context, such relevance can be found in competitive situations. Because competitive situations incorporate aspects of performance pressure and the presence of an audience, they have the potential to evoke anxiety and worry, and individuals react with different amounts of anxiety, nerves, or worry. If we investigated a situation that does not activate this trait (e.g., a games night with friends), neuroticism should be irrelevant and remain unactivated (see ■ Fig. 13.12). If our interest was in sociability, however, trait relevance would be reversed; it would be high for the games night but rather low for the competition.

Reflection

For each of the Big Five traits, please think of examples of a trait-irrelevant and a trait-relevant situation, respectively, and fill in Table 13.8.

Table 13.8 Trait (ir)relevance in five contexts

	Trait-irrelevant situation	Trait-relevant situation
Neuroticism		
Extraversion		
Openness		
Agreeableness		
Conscientiousness		

A moderating effect of the situation's trait relevance is found when the strength of an association between two variables (i.e., person and state) is influenced by a third (i.e., trait relevance). In a competitive situation, for instance, neuroticism is capable of predicting individual differences in states (significant correlation), whereas this prediction is unsuccessful in a games night situation (null correlation). Trait relevance influences the strength of an association between a trait and a state (e.g., neuroticism and state anxiety).

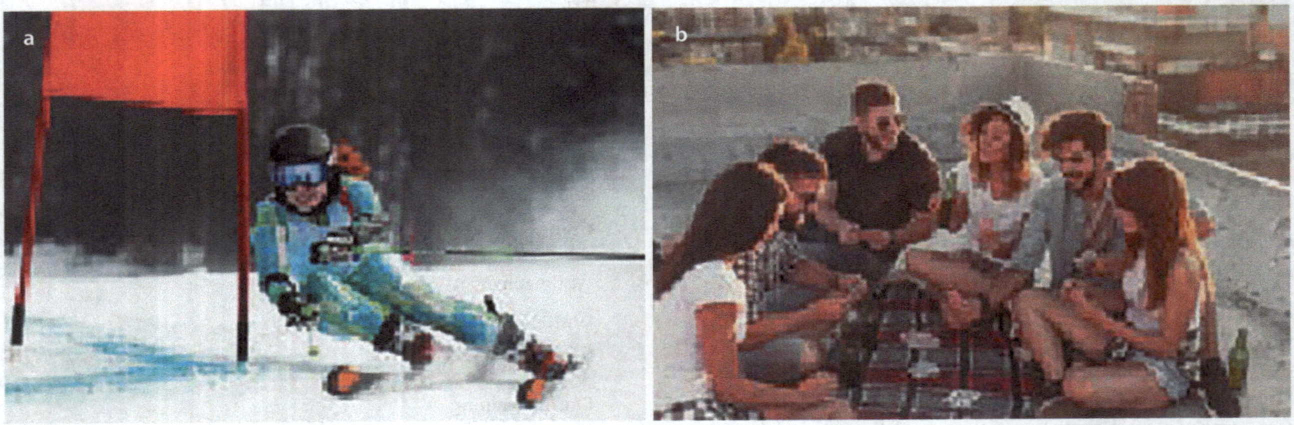

Fig. 13.12 **a, b** Trait-relevant vs. irrelevant situation (**a:** © technotr/Getty Images/iStock; **b:** © vladans/Getty Images/iStock)

13

Exemplary Studies

Trait Relevance in Pressure Situations

Within the research on the prediction of performance under pressure through personality traits, Geukes et al. (2012, 2013a, 2013b) investigated whether the type of pressure situation influences performance prediction through traits (see also Geukes et al. (2017b)). Therefore, two comparisons were made: of low-pressure and high-pressure situations and, within high-pressure situations, of "private" pressure situations, in which money could be won and the importance of the performance was stressed, and "public" pressure situations, in which participants were video-taped, competed against each other, and were observed by up to 2000 spectators.

Regarding the personality traits private self-consciousness (the tendency to introspect and direct attention inward) and narcissism (the tendency to regard oneself as grandiose and to seek the deserved admiration), it was assumed that private self-consciousness would only be relevant in the private pressure situation, whereas narcissism would only be relevant in the public one.

In the studies, trait expressions were assessed, and participants then attempted seven-meter penalty throws in European handball under simulated low- and high-pressure conditions. One-half of the sample was assigned to the private pressure condition and the other half to the public one. In each condition, all athletes threw eight times at a target attached to the handball goal. The aim was to hit the central target hole.

Findings showed (a) that, as expected, none of the assessed personality traits was capable of predicting low-pressure performance (no trait activation) and (b) that the personality traits contributed to performance prediction in different high-pressure situations (trait activation): private self-consciousness negatively predicted performance in the private pressure condition, and narcissism positively predicted performance in the public pressure condition (Geukes et al., 2013a).

13.3.1.3 Situation-Specific Person Effects

A third form of person-situation interaction effects are situation-specific person effects. These effects are present when the prediction of states through personality traits is successful in situations (i.e., significant correlation in each situation), but their associations are differently strong depending on the situation. Situation-specific person effects can go so far that a trait predicts a state positively in one situation but negatively in another.

This possibility is the difference between situation-specific person effects and moderating effects of a situation's strength or trait relevance. Within the latter two, we only find—due to great situation strength or trait irrelevance—differences in a state in one of the considered situations. Accordingly, the state prediction through personality traits is only successful in one but not in both situations.

Let us consider motivation (ranging from *intrinsic*, internally motivated, to *extrinsic*, motivated by rewards) as an example and consider performances of individuals in training and competitive situations (◘ Fig. 13.13). A situation-specific person effect is present when motivation differently predicts performance in both situations.

In this example, extrinsic motivation negatively predicts performance in the training situation. In contrast to highly intrinsically motivated individuals, extrinsically motivated individuals do not see a good reason to make an effort (e.g., no reward) and therefore show rather poor performances. In the competitive situation, extrinsic motivation positively predicts performance. Highly extrinsically motivated individuals, compared to intrinsically motivated individuals, see good reason to make an effort because of the prospect of a reward (e.g., approval, recognition, success, positive press, team nomination) and achieve good performances (◘ Fig. 13.14).

In sport psychology, interaction effects have been found indicating that extraversion and performance are

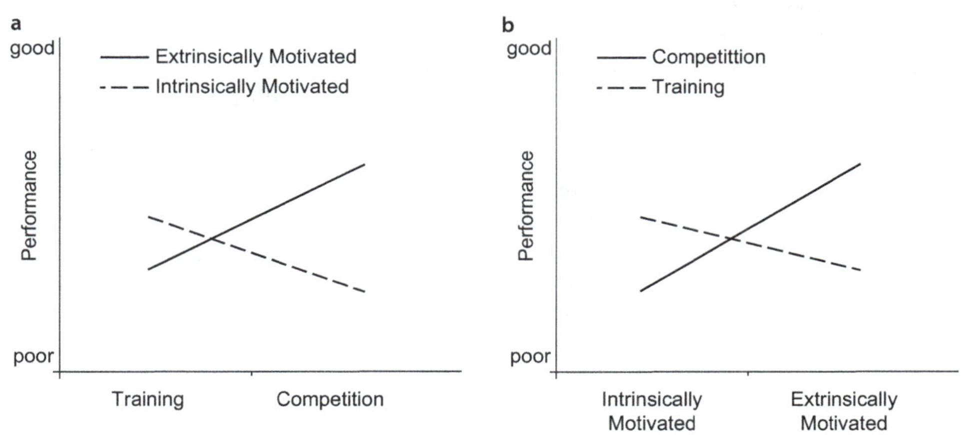

◘ **Fig. 13.13** Extrinsic vs. intrinsic motivation and performance in training and competition presented in two ways

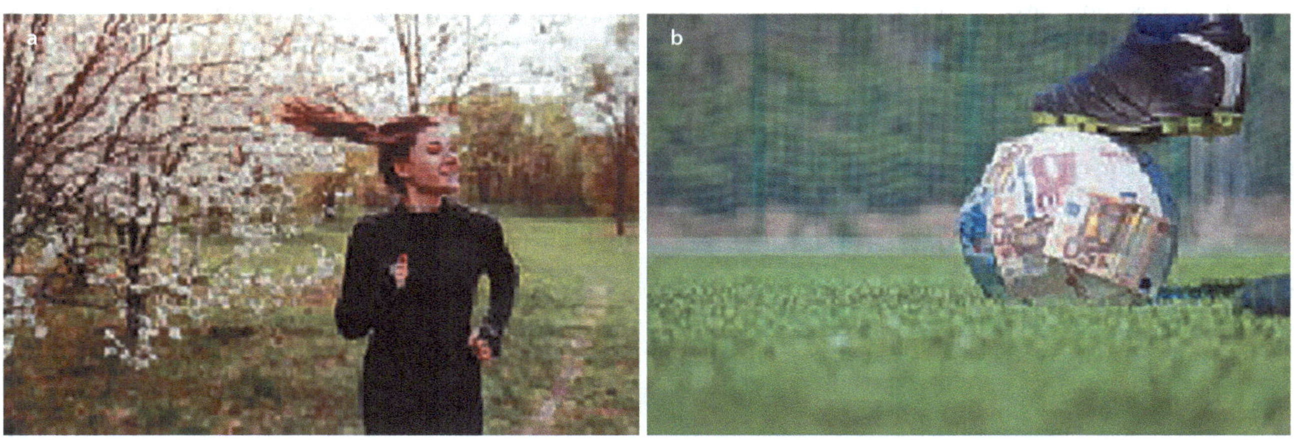

◘ **Fig. 13.14** **a**, **b** Intrinsic vs extrinsic motivation

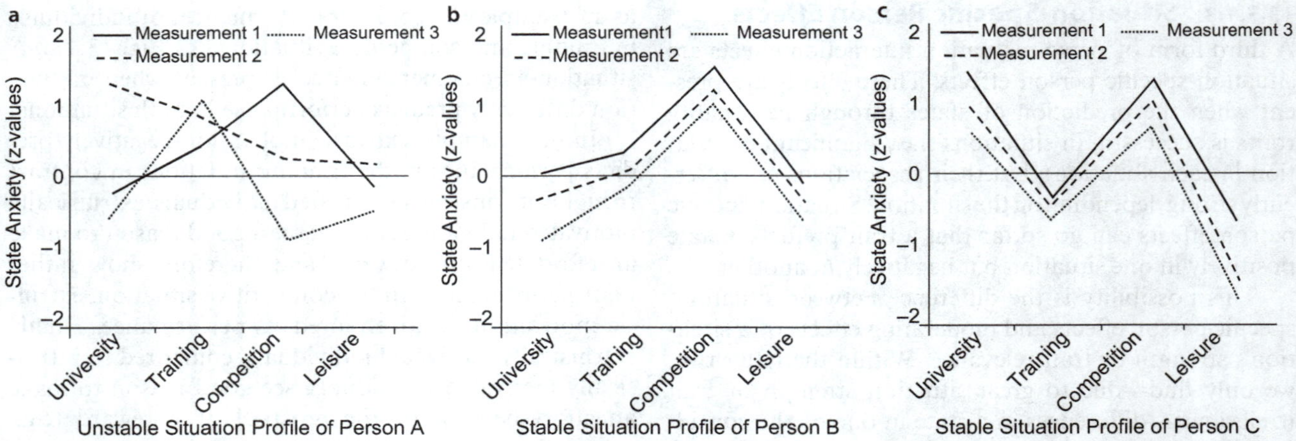

Fig. 13.15 Situation profiles

associated depending on whether or not spectators are present and whether (or not) the situation is anger provoking. When spectators are present (vs. when they are not), extraverts seem to exhibit comparatively better performances (Graydon & Murphy, 1995). Also in anger-provoking (vs. not anger-provoking) situations, extraverts seem to exhibit comparatively better performances (Woodman et al., 2009).

The three forms of the person-situation interaction effects are not always present. Oftentimes, only person effects and situation effects are present. When, however, interaction effects are present, they clearly speak against high relative trans-situational consistency. This becomes particularly evident when we consider the rank orders of individuals as in the example mentioned above. To find such an interaction effect, individuals with high values on extrinsic motivation have to be at the bottom end of the rank order in one situation (training) and at the top end in the other (competition). That way, both the absolute raw scores and relative *z*-scores are different, speaking *against* relative trans-situational consistency.

13

Although many have argued otherwise, the absence of trans-situational consistency does not generally speak against the concept of stable personality differences or personality. The absence of trans-situational consistency does not speak against stable and meaningful personality differences when people, across repeated assessments in different situations, respond similarly. In repeated assessments of performance in training and competition, people with higher values on extrinsic motivation should consistently show comparatively poorer performances in training situations but comparatively better performances in competitive situations. This pattern is labeled "stable situation profiles."

13.3.1.4 Stable Situation Profiles: If... Then... Contingencies

Individually unique momentary experiences and behaviors cannot only be regarded in person-situation interaction effects but also in stable individual situation profiles. These profiles describe stable differences between individuals to respond to specific situations with specific experiences and behaviors. Therefore, one needs to consider repeated measurements of states in different situations.

Figure 13.15 illustrates three measurements of state anxiety in different situations (university, training, competition, leisure) for three persons (Persons A, B, and C), respectively.

Within the left part (**a**) of Fig. 13.5, you see the *z*-scores of Person A, who has an unstable situation profile. She shows the highest state anxiety scores in measurement 1 during competition, in measurement 2 at the university, and in measurement 3 during training. Only in leisure situations does she report rather moderate values. This profile is different for Persons B and C in the center (**b**) and right (**c**) part of Fig. 13.15. Both have a stable situation profile; they possess clear if... then... contingencies. If Person B is in a competition situation, then she has above-average anxiety levels. When she is in one of the other three situations, then she has below-average levels of anxiety. Person C also possesses a stable situation profile, her if... then... rules, however, are different than those of Person B. If Person C is at the university or in a competition, then she has above-average anxiety levels. When in the other two situations, she has average (training) or below-average levels of anxiety (leisure).

Reflection

Imagine you are a goalkeeper of a handball team. Together with your team, you face the decisive match you need to win to advance into the next division. Because the opposing team has an outstanding left-hander in the right-back position, your preparation efforts focus on her. You receive four summaries of her typical shooting habits at goal. All four of them are correct (see ◘ Fig. 13.16).

1. Summary:
   - The left-hander throws into all four corners of the goal.
2. Summary:
   - When she has won a one-against-one and throws from close (solid line), she throws at the bottom corners of the goal.
   - When she throws from behind (dashed line), she throws at the top corners of the goal.
3. Summary:
   - When she throws from the outside (right), she throws at the right corners of the goal.
   - When she throws from the inside (left), she throws at the left corners of the goal.
4. Summary:
   - When she has won a one-against-one to the inside and throws from close (solid line), she throws at the bottom-left corner.
   - When she has won a one-against-one to the outside and throws from close (solid line), she throws at the bottom-right corner.
   - When she throws from behind (dashed line) from the inside, she throws at the top-left corner of the goal.
   - When she throws from behind (dashed line) from the outside, she throws at the top-right corner of the goal.

Which summary would help you most as a goalkeeper? Illustrate the different situation profiles resulting from these different summaries. What are the reasons for the differences?

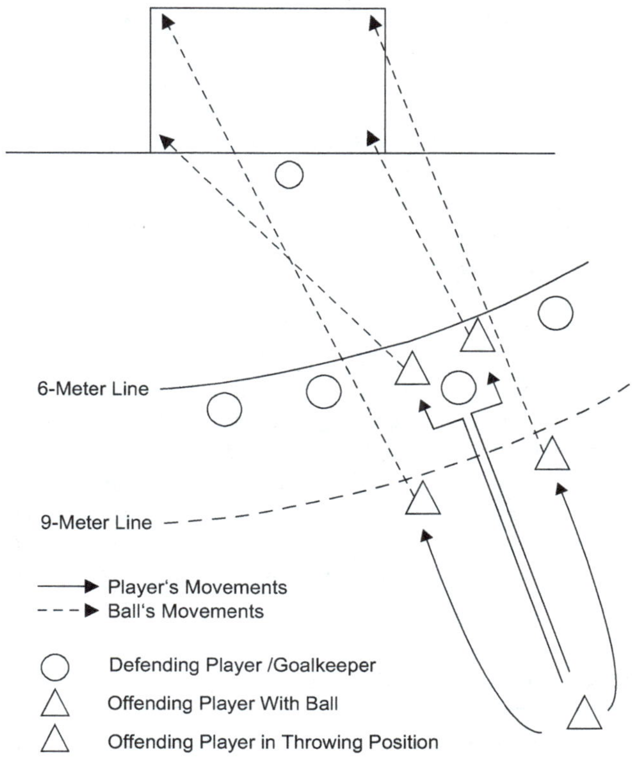

◘ **Fig. 13.16** Stable situation/throw profile of a right-back player in handball

Stable situation profiles, thus, extend the personality concept with the idea that personality does not only describe consistent experiences and behaviors but also stable situation-specific response patterns. Individuals can systematically differ in (a) how (un) stable these individual response patterns are across measurements (Person A vs. B, Person A vs. C) and (b) how different stable response patterns can look and how individuals differ in their if… then… contingencies (Person B vs. C; e.g., Mischel and Shoda (1995)). These situation profiles can, again, be predicted by personality traits.

The concepts of situation-specific person effects and of stable situation profiles share the commonality that their conceptual starting point is low relative trans-situational consistency of states. Both concepts are logically connected. In the case of stable situation profiles, which can be predicted by personality traits, there is a situation-specific person effect across all individuals.

Side Story

The Assessment of Global vs. Situation-Specific Personality Traits

Within the section on the description of personality, we mentioned that we can use global as well as conceptually or situation-specific personality traits to describe personality.

With the aim of better understanding the interplay of persons and situations, the assessment of situation-specific personality traits (e.g., competition anxiety) comes with a major disadvantage, because the assessment of such traits already covers the influence of the situation. The person asked to complete the questionnaire should imagine (only) competitive situations and adjust her responses to her typical experiences and behaviors in such situations. That way, we only receive information about typical responses of a person to the imagined situation. It is possible, however, that this process will identify general person and situation effects as well as person-situation interaction effects (e.g., differences in training and competition) on the basis of situation-specific personality traits.

Of course, there may be applied diagnostic questions in which measuring a person on a situation-specific personality trait is of interest. Thus, in principle, there is nothing wrong with the assessment of such traits. To investigate and better understand the complex interplay of person and situation on a basic level, however, scientific practice should instead measure traits that are *not* specific to situations. Within the group of these nonspecific traits, one can regard global as well as conceptually specific traits. The consideration of conceptually specific traits beyond global traits should at best be empirically justified. Thus, conceptually specific traits should be able to substantially improve the prediction of states through global traits.

13.4 Variability of Personality

13

The focus on single states or on the average of repeatedly assessed states refers to interindividual differences in the *level* of states. This assessment addresses the question of how—in comparison to other individuals—a (average) state (e.g., anxiety) is expressed. When making repeated assessments of states, a second focus may be on differences in fluctuations of individual states and on interindividual differences in *intraindividual variability*. In this case, the question is as follows: How—in comparison to other individuals—does a person fluctuate in a state? For instance, how does a person fluctuate in her anxiety in different situations?

Level and Variability of States

When analyzing states, researchers are typically interested in (at least) two variables: the intraindividual level and the intraindividual variability of states:

1. Regarding the level analysis, the interest is on the average or mean expression of states: On average, how anxious is an individual?
2. Regarding the variability analysis, the interest is on the deviation of the expressions of states: How does a person's anxiety fluctuate across time/situations?

There are persons who always are similarly anxious (or relaxed, low variability), while others, depending on the situation, sometimes show strong, sometimes moderate, and sometimes low anxiety (high variability). Within sports, state variability is not only easy to imagine for anxiety but also, for example, for aggressive behaviors. Imagine we observed players at a soccer match. Some of them may only slightly fluctuate in their aggressiveness, and others may fluctuate considerably. When showing a strong upward fluctuation in aggressiveness, for example, a yellow or even a red card as punishment is likely (◘ Fig. 13.17).

Situation profiles have already shown that individuals report different state values in different situations. Individual density distributions of states further support this finding.

Individual density distributions refer to repeated assessments of a state in a multitude of situations that are plotted within coordinate systems. Each coordinate system summarizes the state reports of one person. On the x-axis, the state scores are plotted and on the y-axis their respective frequency (how often each score occurred). For two persons who reported on their anxiety on respective anxiety items at 50 time points, the density distributions could look like those in ◘ Fig. 13.18.

These distributions can be compared according to many different parameters, for example, the mean, involving information on the level, and the intraindividual standard deviation as an indicator of intraindividual fluctuations. It is evident that Person A in ◘ Fig. 13.18 fluctuates less than Person B. The scores of Person A range between 4 and 5, while the scores of Person B range between 1 and 7.

When investigating level and variability in states, it is important to consider that a very high (or very low) level necessarily goes along with a small standard deviation. There is only one way to achieve a very high (or very low) level, namely, by reporting only many very high (or very low) state values. The moderate range is different. It is possible to achieve a moderate level via many moder-

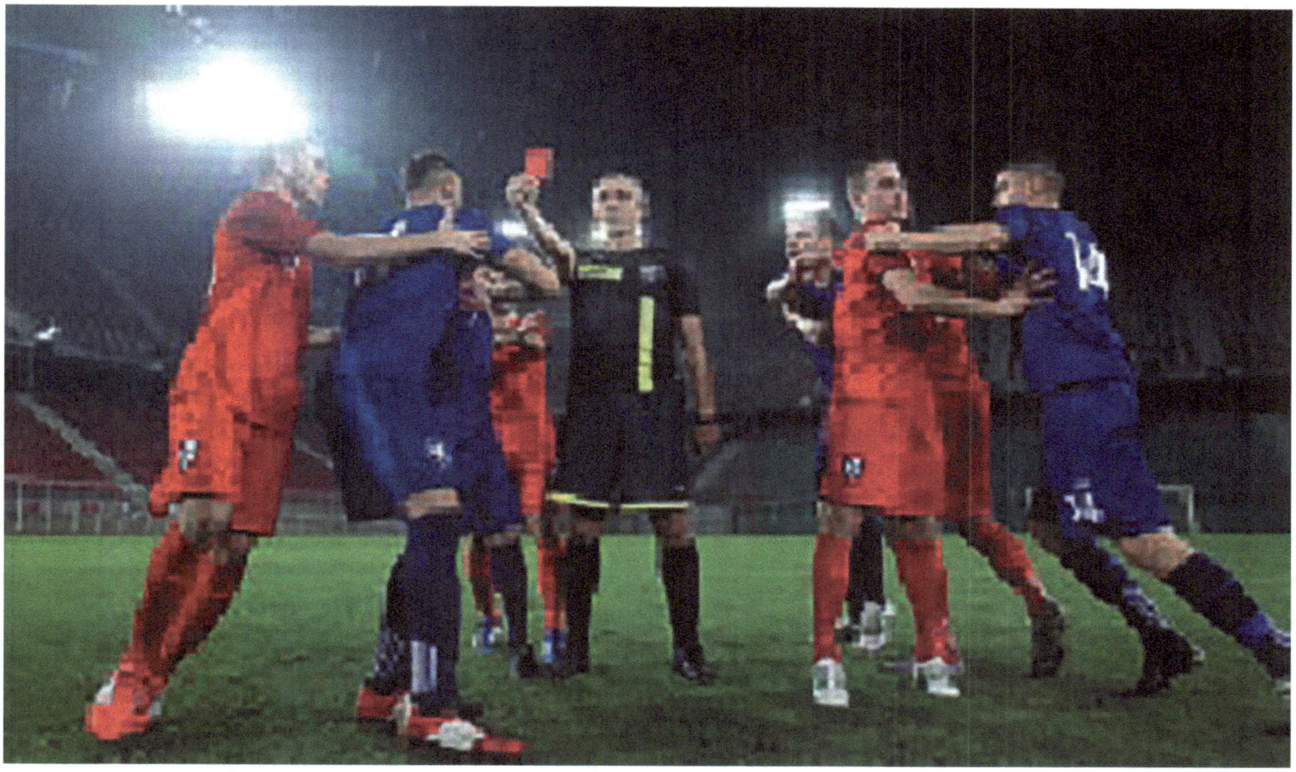

Fig. 13.17 Red card as a consequence of an upward fluctuation in aggressive behavior

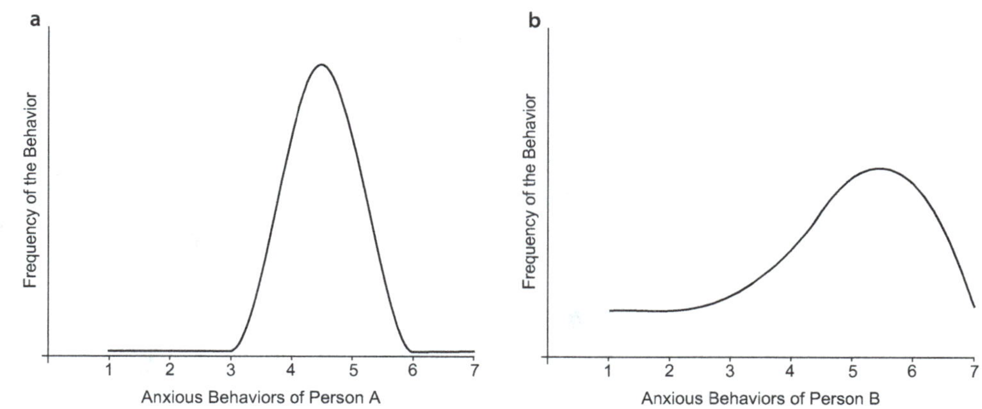

Fig. 13.18 Density distributions of state anxiety in two people

ate values or via a combination of many (very) high and (very) low state values. Thus, the level and variability of states are associated in an inverted U-shaped manner (Fig. 13.19).

Within personality psychology, the interest in inter-individual differences in intraindividual variability is large and has grown within recent years. Similar to personality traits, intraindividual variability characterizes individuals and extends the personality concept by individuals' tendencies to fluctuate in states. To explain differences in state variability, researchers investigate whether these differences can be predicted by personality traits. The most important predictive variable among the Big Five is neuroticism. As Fleeson and Gallagher (2009) have shown in their meta-analysis, the variability in states depends on the expression of this trait ($r = .23$). In addition, they have found that openness (i.e., intellect, $r = .23$) and extraversion ($r = .09$) are significantly positively associated with variability.

The foundation of the calculation of intraindividual variability is the repeated assessment of states. What researchers look for are fluctuations *across time* that individuals experience or show. When having people report on states repeatedly, however, we not only assess

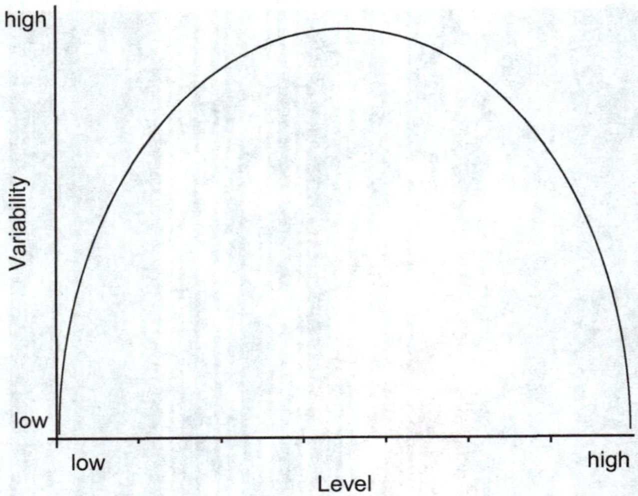

Fig. 13.19 Relationship of level and variability of states

variability across time but also each state assessment in a specific situation. Thus, within intraindividual variability across time, we do not explicitly consider the situations in which a state has been experienced or shown.

13.4.1 Consideration of Situations

In the section on situation effects, it became evident that situations influence momentary experiences and behaviors. They also influence intraindividual variability of states.

Let us consider the upper coordinate system (**a**) in **Fig. 13.20**. Here, the fluctuations in anxiety values of three people in nine different situations are plotted: playing billiards, bowling, singing karaoke, playoff match, regular match, friendly match, birthday coffee and cake, Christmas dinner, and visit with sister.

Fig. 13.20 Interindividual differences in intraindividual variability

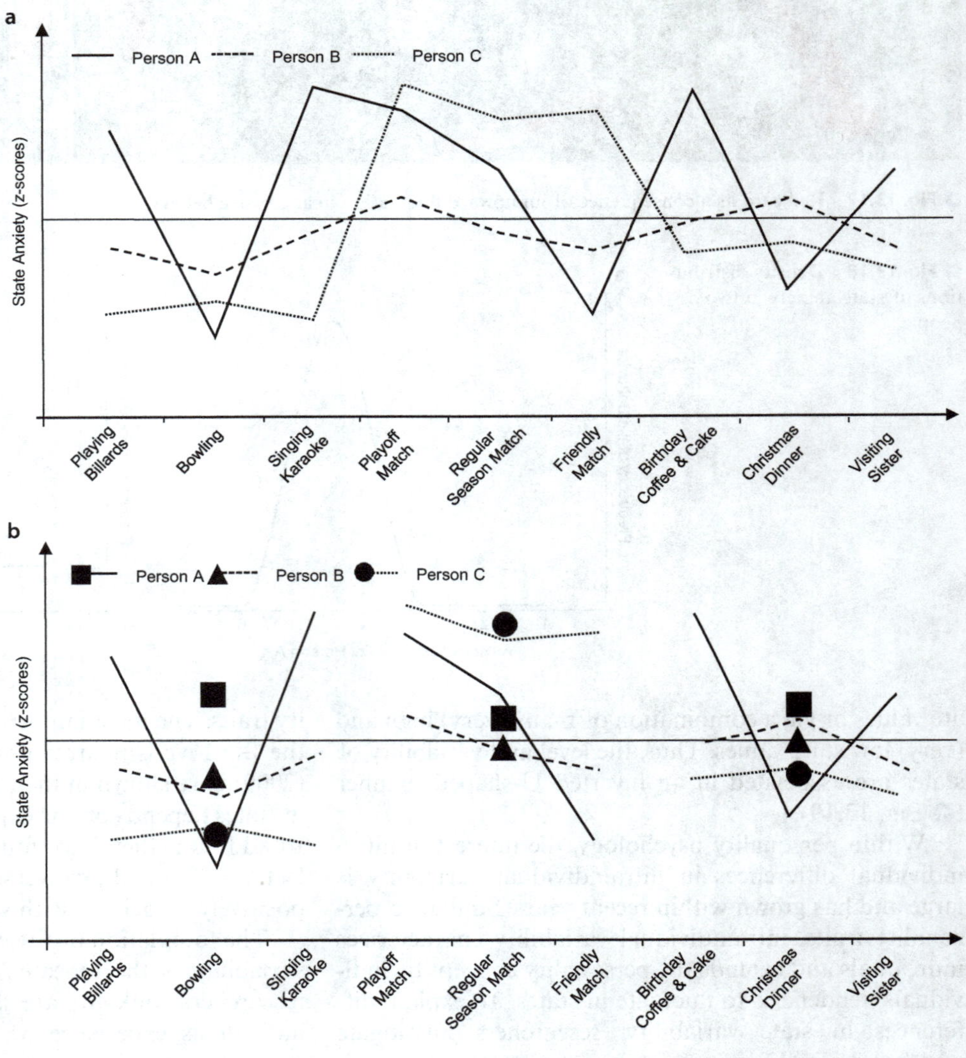

When we ignore the situations, we can see that Person A fluctuates the most and Person B the least. But what conclusion can be drawn when we do consider the situations?

To consider the situations, we group the situations in meaningful categories (contexts) of similar situations: leisure (playing billiards, bowling, singing karaoke), sports (playoff match, regular match, friendly match), and family (birthday coffee and cake, Christmas dinner, visit with sister).

Now, we can separate two types of intraindividual variability: fluctuations within contexts (How much on average does a person fluctuate in her anxiety within leisure, within sports, and within family situations?) and fluctuations across contexts (How much does a person fluctuate across leisure, sports, and family contexts?).

Let us have a look at Person C in the bottom coordinate system (**b**) of ◘ Fig. 13.20. Within each context, this person barely fluctuates (thin dotted lines, the scores are quite similar). Across contexts, however, there are great fluctuations (circles as means). The mean of the state scores in the leisure context is low, high in the sport context, and moderate in the family context. For Person A, the pattern is different: fluctuations within each context are high (thin solid lines); the fluctuation of means across contexts, however, is low (squares as means). Person B does not show great fluctuations within (thin dashed lines) nor across contexts (triangles as means).

The statistical translation is analogous: For the estimation of fluctuations within contexts, one calculates the fluctuations (i.e., the intraindividual standard deviation) for each context and then their average. For the estimation of fluctuations across contexts, one calculates the mean for each context and then the fluctuation (i.e., the intraindividual standard deviation) across these means.

The idea to separate these two types of variability stems from the assumption that a person's state fluctuations may be systematic and justified on the one hand as well as unsystematic and unjustified on the other. Fluctuations within contexts represent unsystematic, unjustified variability (also labeled as *fragility*), because individuals fluctuate even though the situations are similar. Fluctuations across contexts represent systematic, justified variability (also labeled as *flexibility*), because persons are in different contexts with different demands, so that different state means could point to successful adjustment.

Based on the findings of Fleeson and Gallagher (2009), one could conceptually expect that fluctuations within contexts are positively associated with neuroticism and that fluctuations across contexts are positively associated with openness and extraversion. These expectations were empirically supported in a recent study (Geukes et al., 2017b).

13.4.2 Situation Profiles and Interaction Effects

Fluctuations within contexts and across contexts are logically associated with differences in the stability of situation profiles and person-situation interactions.

To describe situation profiles, three measurements of states in different situations (contexts) are graphed in ◘ Fig. 13.21. Accordingly, the variability of Persons A, B, and C (see ◘ Fig. 13.21) can also be plotted as individual situation profiles.

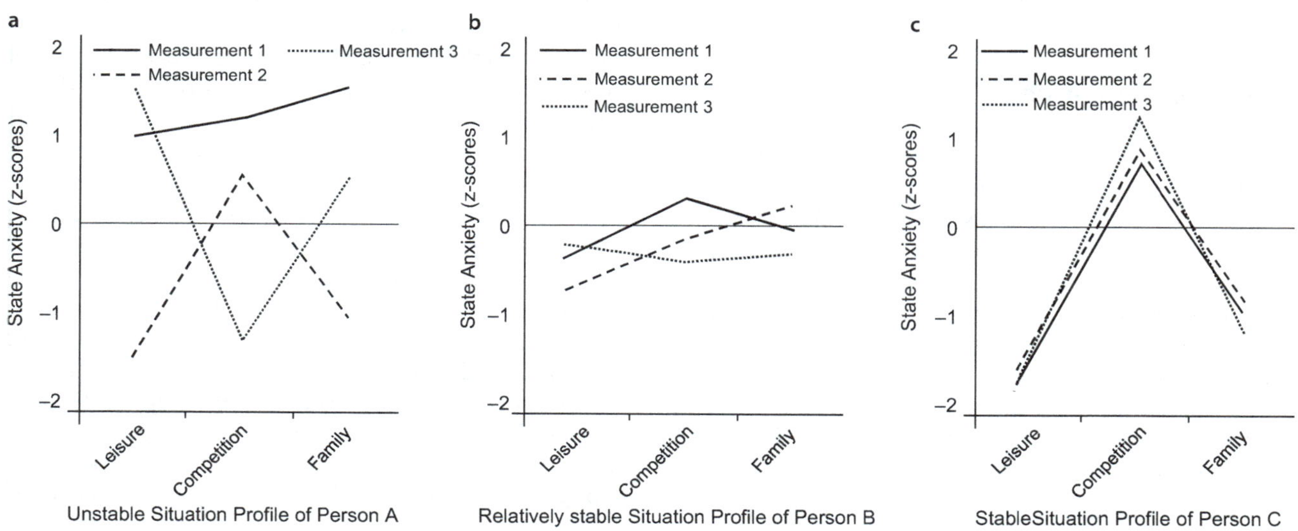

◘ **Fig. 13.21** Situation profiles of Persons **a**, **b** and **c**

For this purpose, we summarized the anxiety scores for playing billiards, competing in a playoff match, and having birthday coffee and cake as assessment 1; bowling, competing in a regular season match, and having Christmas dinner as assessment 2; and singing karaoke, playing in a friendly match, and visiting with one's sister as assessment 3. Transferring the scores of the individuals into the coordinate system of situation profiles, Person A receives an unstable situation profile (**a**), Person B a relatively stable situation profile (**b**), and Person C a stable situation profile (**c**). For Persons B and C, the three assessments for each context are similar (assessment 1 vs. assessment 2 vs. assessment 3); the fluctuations within situations (contexts) are small. The different average z-scores across situations (contexts) highlight that the fluctuations across contexts (leisure vs. competition vs. family) are quite high for Person C but are considerably lower for Person B. Person A, who has an unstable situation profile, shows great fluctuations within situations (contexts), but the fluctuations across situations (contexts) are comparatively small.

Finding great fluctuations across situations (contexts) simultaneously indicates that stable situation profiles as well as person-situation interactions can be found.

13.5 Challenges and Implications

13

The concepts and findings regarding the influences of the person, the situation, and their interplay for momentary experiences and behaviors simultaneously indicate important challenges and implications in sport psychological research and practice. Although we mainly have referred to the performance context in this chapter, the concepts are analogously valid for the health context.

13.5.1 For Research

Within research, the aim is to better understand athletes and their momentary experiences and behaviors. As this chapter comprehensively illustrated, for this purpose, we need to consider the person, the situation, and their interaction.

Therefore, this consideration should inform study designs in psychological research, especially in pure basic research. Only when person variables as well as situation variables are repeatedly assessed, and, moreover, states are repeatedly assessed in similar and dissimilar situations in longitudinal designs, can simultaneous and independent person and situation effects as well effects of their complex interplay be identified.

Particularly, the study of situation characteristics promises new insights for gaining a deeper understanding of their effects on psychological states. What characteristics of a pressure situation produce pressure (cf. Mesagno et al., 2011)? The spectators? One's reputation being at stake? The promised prize money? The anticipated or actual evaluation? This knowledge will inform categorical as well as dimensional approaches to the situation assessment so that we can realize a more goal-directed and therefore meaningful situation assessment in the near future. Person, situation, and their interaction will better explain interindividual and intraindividual differences in states and can be used as a scientifically sound foundation for applied selection and intervention decisions.

To further increase the complexity, for many of these associations (i.e., person, situation, and their interaction effects), the type of the executed task will play an additional important, potentially moderating, role. Optimally, research regarding performance should consider differences in motor tasks and systematically vary these differences to estimate and understand their influence.

13.5.2 For Practical Applications

For sport psychological practice, the complex associations of person, situation, and their interaction for states will play an important role for the selection and the development of individuals as well as for the selection and modification of situations.

Regarding the personality of athletes, the complexity of the various associations speaks against a hasty and global evaluation. Even though a normative (i.e., a generally favorable) personality profile exists, it is still unclear which effects go along with this profile (a) in a specific situation (momentary experience, behavior, or performance) and (b) in the long term (personality development, life satisfaction, well-being, career success). For example, a high score on narcissism can be facilitative under pressure or when getting to know new people, but when dealing with failure or developing long-term friendships, it is commonly found not to be helpful (e.g., Back et al. (2010); Back et al. (2013); Geukes et al. (2013a, 2013b); Leckelt et al. (2015)).

Ultimately, the aim is to establish an optimal match between the person (ability, personality) and the situation (demands, conditions). In the best case, a person—through her abilities and personality—is capable of meeting the situational requirements. If she is not, there are (within the limitations set by the type of sport, competition mode, personal and financial resources, etc.) different opportunities for creating this match. Matches can be made via (a) the selection or placement of individuals (e.g., talent diagnostics, scouting, team composition), (b) the development of individuals (e.g., via training, intervention, and sport psychological counseling), (c) the selection of situations (e.g., via choice of competitions, training methods, and opponents), or (d) the modification of situations (e.g., through habituation and standardization).

Of course, no coach, sport psychologist, or official will change the competition mode to increase the match of a person with a situation. The knowledge about the complex associations, however, might help to successfully target the abovementioned options to improve the match. For Beth, for example, it might be helpful if her success-oriented parents refrained from accompanying her to competitions. Their absence would considerably lower her anxiety, and in the meantime, she could work with a sport psychologist to loosen the close connection of the presence of her parents with her state anxiety.

But who would we select for a decisive 11-meter penalty shot? Aisha, Beth, or Céline? Given their identical shooting accuracy (ability), we would probably go for Céline because she is less anxious than Aisha and Beth.

Learning Control Questions

Basic:

1. How are states, personality, and situation defined and how can they be measured?
2. What are person effects? Provide an example of a strong person effect in sports.
3. What are situation effects? Provide an example of a strong situation effect in sports.
4. How are person and situation effects associated with trans-situational consistency?
5. Which conclusions can be drawn from the person-situation/consistency debate for the prediction of states through the person and the situation?

Advanced:

6. Which two general characteristics of a situation influence the predictive ability of personality for states?
7. What are situation-specific person effects? Provide an example for a situation-specific person effect in sports.
8. How are person-situation interaction effects associated with trans-situational consistency?
9. What are individual density distributions of states? Name two parameters that can be used to compare interindividual differences in intraindividual density distributions of states.

Experts:

10. What types of state variabilities could one differentiate?
11. How are these types of variability associated with (un)stable situation profiles?
12. What tips would you give sport psychological researchers? How should studies optimally be designed?
13. What tips would you give to applied practitioners—(1) for the selection and development of athletes and (2) for the selection and creation of situations?

References

Aidman, E., & Schofield, G. (2004). Personality and individual differences in sport. In T. Morris & J. Summers (Eds.), *Sport psychology: Theory, applications and issues* (pp. 22–47). Wiley.

Allen, M. S., Greenlees, I., & Jones, M. V. (2011). An investigation of the five-factor model of personality and coping behavior in sport. *Journal of Sports Sciences, 29*, 841–850.

Allport, G. W. (1927). Concepts of trait and personality. *Psychological Bulletin, 24*, 284–293.

Allport, G. W. (1937). *Personality: A psychological interpretation*. Holt.

Allport, G. W., & Odbert, H. S. (1936). Trait-names: A psycholexical study. *Psychological Monographs, 47*(1), i.

Asendorpf, J. B. (2003). Head-to-head comparison of the predictive validity of personality types and dimensions. *European Journal of Personality, 17*, 327–346.

Asendorpf, J. B. (2011). *Persönlichkeitspsychologie für Bachelor* (2nd ed.). Springer.

Asendorpf, J. B., Borkenau, P., Ostendorf, F., & van Aken, M. A. G. (2001). Carving personality description at its joints: Confirmation of three replicable personality prototypes for both children and adults. *European Journal of Personality, 15*, 169–198.

Back, M. D., Küfner, A. C. P., Dufner, M., Gerlach, T. M., Rauthmann, J. F., & Denissen, J. J. A. (2013). Narcissistic admiration and rivalry: Disentangling the bright and dark sides of narcissism. *Journal of Personality and Social Psychology, 105*, 1013–1037.

Back, M. D., Schmukle, S. C., & Egloff, B. (2010). Why are narcissists so charming at first sight? Decoding the narcissism-popularity link at zero acquaintance. *Journal of Personality and Social Psychology, 98*, 132–145.

Baumeister, R. F. (1984). Choking under pressure: Self-consciousness and paradoxical effects of incentives on skillful performance. *Journal of Personality and Social Psychology, 46*, 610–620.

Baumeister, R. F., & Showers, C. J. (1986). A review of paradoxical performance effects: Choking under pressure in sports and mental tests. *European Journal of Social Psychology, 16*, 361–383.

Baumeister, R. F., & Steinhilber, A. (1984). Paradoxical effects of supportive audiences on performance under pressure: The home field disadvantage in sports championships. *Journal of Personality and Social Psychology, 47*, 85–93.

Bond, C. F., & Titus, L. J. (1983). Social facilitation: A meta-analysis of 241 studies. *Psychological Bulletin, 94*, 265–292.

Cameron, J. E., Cameron, J. M., Dithurbide, L., & Lalonde, R. N. (2012). Personality traits and stereotypes associated with ice hockey positions. *Journal of Sport Behavior, 35*, 109–124.

Castanier, C., Le Scanff, C., & Woodman, T. (2010). Who takes risks in high-risk sports? A typological personality approach. *Research Quarterly for Exercise and Sport, 81*, 478–485.

Costa, P. T., & McCrae, R. R. (1989). *NEO five-factor inventory (NEO-FFI)*. Psychological Assessment Resources.

Costa, P. T., & McCrae, R. R. (1992). *Revised NEO Personality Inventory (NEO-PIR) and NEO Five Factor Inventory (NEO-FFI) professional manual*. Psychological Assessment Resources.

Darley, J. M., & Batson, C. D. (1973). "From Jerusalem to Jericho": A study of situational and dispositional variables in helping behavior. *Journal of Personality and Social Psychology, 27*, 100–108.

Darley, J. M., & Latané, B. (1968). Bystander intervention in emergencies: Diffusion of responsibility. *Journal of Personality and Social Psychology, 8*, 77–383.

Diener, E., Larsen, R. J., & Emmons, R. A. (1984). Person× Situation interactions: Choice of situations and congruence response models. *Journal of Personality and Social Psychology, 47*, 580–592.

Eagleton, J. R., McKelvie, S. J., & De Man, A. (2007). Extraversion and neuroticism in team sport participants, individual sport participants, and non-participants. *Perceptual and Motor Skills, 105*, 265–275.

Egloff, B., & Jan Gruhn, A. (1996). Personality and endurance sports. *Personality and Individual Differences, 21*, 223–229.

Festinger, L., & Carlsmith, J. M. (1959). Cognitive consequences of forced compliance. *The Journal of Abnormal and Social Psychology, 58*, 203–210.

Fleeson, W., & Gallagher, P. (2009). The implications of Big Five standing for the distribution of trait manifestation in behavior: Fifteen experience-sampling studies and a meta-analysis. *Journal of Personality and Social Psychology, 97*, 1097–1114.

Funder, D. C. (2015). *The personality puzzle: Seventh international student edition*. Norton.

Geukes, K., Mesagno, C., Hanrahan, S. J., & Kellmann, M. (2013a). Activation of self-focus and self-presentation traits under private, mixed, and public pressure. *Journal of Sport & Exercise Psychology, 35*, 50–59.

Geukes, K., Mesagno, C., Hanrahan, S. J., & Kellmann, M. (2013b). Performing under pressure in private: Activation of self-focus traits. *International Journal of Sport and Exercise Psychology, 11*, 11–23.

Geukes, K., Mesagno, C., Hanrahan, S. J., & Kellmann, M. (2012). Testing an interactionist perspective on the relationship between personality and performance under public pressure. *Psychology of Sport and Exercise, 13*, 243–250.

Geukes, K., Nestler, S., Hutteman, R., Küfner, A. C. P., & Back, M. D. (2017b). Trait personality and state variability: Predicting individual differences in within- and cross-context fluctuations in affect, self-evaluations, and behavior in everyday life. *Journal of Research in Personality, 69*, 124–138.

Gosling, S. D., Rentfrow, P. J., & Swann, W. B. (2003). A very brief measure of the Big-Five personality domains. *Journal of Research in Personality, 37*, 504–528.

Graydon, J., & Murphy, T. (1995). The effects of personality on social facilitation whilst performing a sports related task. *Personality and Individual Differences, 19*, 265–267.

Jamieson, J. P. (2010). The home field advantage in athletics: A meta-analysis. *Journal of Applied Social Psychology, 40*, 1819–1848.

Johnson, R. W., & Morgan, W. P. (1981). Personality characteristics of college athletes in different sports. *Scandinavian Journal of Sports Science, 3*, 41–49.

Kirkcaldy, B. D. (1982a). Personality profiles at various levels of athletic participation. *Personality and Individual Differences, 3*, 321–326.

Kirkcaldy, B. D. (1982b). Personality and sex differences related to positions in team sports. *International Journal of Sport Psychology, 13*, 141–153.

Lackie, W. L. (1962). Personality characteristics of certain groups of intercollegiate athletes. *Research Quarterly, 33*, 566–573.

Leckelt, M., Küfner, A. C. P., Nestler, S., & Back, M. D. (2015). Behavioral processes underlying the decline of narcissists' popularity over time. *Journal of Personality and Social Psychology, 109*, 856–871.

Leikas, S., Lönnqvist, J. E., & Verkasalo, M. (2012). Persons, situations, and behaviors: Consistency and variability of different behaviors in four interpersonal situations. *Journal of Personality and Social Psychology, 103*, 1007–1022.

Lewin, K. (1936). *Principles of topological psychology*. McGraw-Hill.

Lucas, R. E., & Diener, E. (2001). Understanding extraverts' enjoyment of social situations: The importance of pleasantness. *Journal of Personality and Social Psychology, 81*(2), 343–356.

McCrae, R. R., & Costa, P. T. (1987). Validation of the five-factor model of personality across instruments and observers. *Journal of Personality and Social Psychology, 52*, 81–90.

McCrae, R. R., & Costa, P. T. (1989). Reinterpreting the Myers-Briggs Type Indicator from the perspective of the five-factor model of personality. *Journal of Personality, 57*, 17–40.

Mesagno, C., Geukes, K., & Larkin, P. (2015). Choking under pressure: A review of current debates, literature, and interventions. In S. D. Mellalieu & S. Hanton (Eds.), *Contemporary advances in sport psychology: A review* (pp. 148–174). Routledge.

Mesagno, C., Harvey, J. T., & Janelle, C. M. (2011). Self-presentational origins of choking: Evidence from separate pressure manipulations. *Journal of Sport & Exercise Psychology, 33*, 441–459.

Milgram, S. (1975). *Obedience to authority*. Harper/Colophon.

Mischel, W. (1968). *Personality and assessment*. Wiley.

Mischel, W., & Shoda, Y. (1995). A cognitive-affective system theory of personality: Reconceptualizing situations, dispositions, dynamics, and invariance in personality structure. *Psychological Review, 102*, 246–268.

Morgan, W. P. (1980). The trait psychology controversy. *Research Quarterly for Exercise and Sport, 51*, 50–76.

O'Sullivan, D. M., Zuckerman, M., & Kraft, M. (1998). Personality characteristics of male and female participants in team sports. *Personality and Individual Differences, 25*, 119–128.

Otten, M. (2009). Choking vs. clutch performance: A study of sport performance under pressure. *Journal of Sport & Exercise Psychology, 31*, 583–601.

Pittenger, D. J. (2004). The limitations of extracting typologies from trait measures of personality. *Personality and Individual Differences, 37*, 779–787.

Rauthmann, J. F., Gallardo-Pujol, D., Guillaume, E. M., Todd, E., Nave, C. S., Sherman, R. A., et al. (2014). The situational eight DIAMONDS: A taxonomy of major dimensions of situation characteristics. *Journal of Personality and Social Psychology, 107*, 677–718.

Rauthmann, J. F., & Sherman, R. A. (2016). Measuring the Situational Eight DIAMONDS characteristics of situations: An optimization of the RSQ-8 to the S8*. *European Journal of Psychological Assessment, 32*, 155–164.

Richard, F. D., Bond, C. F., Jr., & Stokes-Zoota, J. J. (2003). One hundred years of social psychology quantitatively described. *Review of General Psychology, 7*, 331–363.

Rhea, D. J., & Martin, S. (2010). Personality trait differences of traditional sport athletes, bullriders, and other alternative sport athletes. *International Journal of Sports Science and Coaching, 5*, 75–85.

Rhodes, R. E., & Smith, N. E. (2006). Personality correlates of physical activity: A review and meta-analysis. *British Journal of Sports Medicine, 40*, 958–965.

Rogulj, N., Nazor, M., Srhoj, V., & Božin, D. (2006). Differences between competitively efficient and less efficient junior handball players according to their personality traits. *Kinesiology, 38*, 158–163.

Soto, C. J., & John, O. P. (2017a). Short and extra-short form of the Big Five Inventory-2: The BFI-2-S and BFI-2-XS. *Journal of Research in Personality, 68*, 69–81.

Soto, C. J., & John, O. P. (2017b). The next Big Five Inventory (BFI-2): Developing and assessing a hierarchical model with 15 facets to enhance bandwidth, fidelity, and predictive power. *Journal of Personality and Social Psychology, 113*, 117–143.

Strauss, B. (2002). Social facilitation in motor tasks: A review of research and theory. *Psychology of Sport and Exercise, 3*, 237–256.

Ten Berge, M. A., & De Raad, B. (2002). The structure of situations from a personality perspective. *European Journal of Personality, 16*, 81–102.

Tett, R. P., & Guterman, H. A. (2000). Situation trait relevance, trait expression, and cross-situational consistency: Testing a principle of trait activation. *Journal of Research in Personality, 34*, 397–423.

Tok, S. (2011). The big five personality traits and risky sport participation. *Social Behavior and Personality, 39*, 1105–1112.

Williams, L. R., & Parkin, W. A. (1980). Personality factor profiles of three hockey groups. *International Journal of Sport Psychology, 11*, 113–120.

Woodman, T., Davis, P. A., Hardy, L., Callow, N., Glasscock, I., & Yuill-Proctor, J. (2009). Emotions and sport performance: An exploration of happiness, hope, and anger. *Journal of Sport and Exercise Psychology, 31*, 169–188.

Woodman, T., & Hardy, L. (2003). The relative impact of cognitive anxiety and self-confidence upon sport performance: A meta-analysis. *Journal of Sports Sciences, 21*, 443–457.

Wright, E. F., Jackson, W., Christie, S. D., McGuire, G. R., & Wright, R. D. (1991). The home-course disadvantage in golf championships: Further evidence for the undermining effect of supportive audiences on performance under pressure. *Journal of Sport Behavior, 14*, 51–61.

Recommended Readings

Allen, M. S., Greenlees, I., & Jones, M. (2013). Personality in sport: A comprehensive review. *International Review of Sport and Exercise Psychology, 6*, 184–208.

Funder, D. C. (2015). *The Personality Puzzle: Seventh international student edition*. WW Norton & Company.

Kenrick, D. T., & Funder, D. C. (1988). Profiting from controversy: Lessons from the person-situation debate. *American Psychologist, 43*, 23–34.

Personality Development Through Sport

Achim Conzelmann, Claudio R. Nigg and Mirko Schmidt

Contents

J. Schüler et al. (eds.), *Sport and Exercise Psychology*, https://doi.org/10.1007/978-3-031-03921-8_14

Learning Objectives

Basic:

- Being able to name the pedagogical postulates regarding the effects of sport on personality development.
- Being able to specify and delineate the terminology of sport and personality.

Advanced:

- Being able to trace the historical development of personality research in sport science and its essential theoretical and methodological steps.
- Being able to reflect the state of the debate on the question of self-concept development through sport.

Expert:

- Being able to embed the question of personality development through sport in the current developmental theory discussion.

14.1 Introduction

Long before sport psychology began to deal with questions of the relationship between sport and personality, there were, in the traditional theory of physical education, indications in the sense of pedagogical postulates which suggested "what contribution physical activity can make to the formation of a mature personality" (Neumann, 1957, p. 2). Historically, assumptions regarding the positive influence of gymnastics and physical education on character or personality formation go back much further and can already be found in Plato (427–347 BC); Aristotle (384–324 BC); the eighteenth/nineteenth century, for example, in Rousseau, GutsMuths, Jahn, and Coubertin; and around the middle of the twentieth century, for example, in Diem, Spranger, and Nohl (e.g., Grupe and Krüger (1997); Kurz (1973)). The phase of pedagogical postulates on the positive effects of sport on personality development continues to this day. The Swiss philosopher and pedagogue Johann Georg Sulzer stated that

> Physical activity has a non-negligible influence on the soul. It makes the children hard, hearty, patient, steadfast, brave, and, when properly practiced, it imprints something noble on the mind. (Sulzer, 1748, pp. 221–222)

In view of these attributions of meaning, it seems logical that the personality-building effect of sport has been used as an essential justification for the legitimation of school sport. Thus, for example, in the Memorandum on school sport jointly adopted by the German Society of Sport Science, the German Sports Teachers' Association, and the German Olympic Sports Confederation in September 2009, the pedagogical mission of school sport was described as follows: "Basically (...) it is about the double task of both opening up the culture of sport and movement and personality development" (Deutscher Olympischer Sportbund, 2009, p. 5). The series of comparable justifications in position papers on school sport could be extended almost indefinitely at an international level. In short, the positive influence on the personality development of children and young people is seen as a key argument for the legitimacy of physical education in school. Therefore, it is not surprising that, even in the curricula of various countries, school types, and grade levels, the reference to the personality-building significance of school sport is included (► Side Story: International Examples of Pedagogical Postulates for Personality Development Through Physical Education).

14

Side Story

International Examples of Pedagogical Postulates for Personality Development Through Physical Education

Requirements for the subject physical education for schools of general education, secondary schools (Germany): "Physical education helps to develop empathy and promotes the ability to question one's own convictions and world view. It supports pupils in enduring uncertainty and acquiring self-confidence" (Ministry of Education and Vocational Training of the State of Schleswig-Holstein, 2015, p. 10).

Elementary school curriculum, part 7, educational and teaching tasks, as well as teaching material and didactic principles of the mandatory subjects of primary school and upper school, Primary School-Movement and Sport (Austria): "Physical education contributes to improve movement security from a physical and psychological point of view. Furthermore, it contributes significantly to the acquisition of social competences and promotes, in particular, the holistic personality development of the child" (Federal Ministry of Education, 2012, p. 24).

New South Wales Primary School curriculum (Australia): "Personal development, health and physical education is one of the six key learning areas in the NSW primary curriculum. This syllabus makes a unique contribution to the total school curriculum in that it is directly concerned with supporting the development of the student as a whole person" (NSW Board of Studies, 2014, p. 5).

SHAPE America's National Standards and Grade-Level Outcomes for K-12 Physical Education (USA): "**Standard 4:** The physically literate individual exhibits responsible personal and social behavior that respects self and others" (National Standards for K-12 Physical Education, 2013).

Although sport psychology has been trying for more than half a century to prove the positive effects of sport on personality, the empirical evidence is still inconsistent (shown below). But what are the reasons for the so far insufficient empirical evidence for the personality-building effects of sport? Could it be that—contrary to popular opinion—sport cannot influence personality at all? Or are these proclaimed (unidirectional) effects difficult to prove due to the complexity of sport interventions and the complexity of the human personality? Are there at best theoretical and methodological deficits in previous studies that can be held responsible for the lack of proof?

In order to clarify these questions, at first, this contribution is oriented toward the term "personality," which is to be approached from a personality psychology perspective. This perspective is adopted because (a) the construct personality is a genuine object of personality psychology, (b) it has been given a detailed concept specification and operationalization, and (c) specific methodological guidelines for studies on personality development have been developed. It is also important to clarify what is meant by the term "sport" and which directionality is of interest in the relationship between sport and personality. As can be seen from the chapter title, some aspects of personality development is to be stimulated by sport: in other words, it is about the socialization hypothesis of the sport science-related personality research (► Sect. 14.2).

► Section 14.3 describes the historical development of personality research in sport science over the last 60 years with a special focus on theoretical and methodological developments. Among other things, in order to analyze the effects of sport on personality development, personality constructs that are changeable are preferred, because they can be modified in the medium term by exogenous influences.

This demand for plasticity is fulfilled in particular by the personality construct "self-concept," which is why studies on self-concept development through sport have dominated over the last two decades and have proven to be fruitful in answering the question of personality development through sport. The current status of the discussion on self-concept development through sport is presented in ► Sect. 14.4.

The topic "personality development through sport" is a subfield of human development. In ► Sect. 14.5, the topic personality development through sport is therefore discussed from the perspective of current developmental theories (► Side Story: … mens sana in corpore sano?).

Side Story

… Mens Sana in Corpore Sano?

When it comes to personality-shaping effects of sport, reference is often made to a quotation from the Roman satirist Juvenal (first and second centuries), according to which, a healthy mind only resides in a healthy body. However, since this quotation is usually only given in its shortened form, the resulting statement completely misses the criticism of the Roman citizens of this period that was originally formulated by Juvenal. According to Juvenal, his fellow Roman citizens would have turned to the gods with all kinds of prayers for more money or recognition. Upon which, he formulated the following sentence in his satires (X, 356): "Orandum est ut sit mens sana in corpore sano." Translated, this means, "one should pray that in a healthy body a healthy mind dwells." So, if the quotation is reproduced in its full length, it does not mean that only a healthy body can contain a healthy mind. Conversely, the abbreviated interpretation of the phrase would even imply that no healthy spirit can dwell in a sick and weak body.

14.2 The Research Topic "Sport and Personality Development"

In order to specify the research area, the terms "sport" and "personality/personality development," which are familiar to us in everyday language and at the same time relatively vague, need to be defined more precisely and which causal relationships are of interest in the question of personality development through sport need to be clarified.

14.2.1 The Concept of "Personality"

Personality research in sport science examines the construct of personality in close connection with personality psychology and differential psychology, which are interested in systematic variations in the experience and behavior of a person and in systematic differences between persons (groups) and their causes (Pawlik, 1996). Differences in individual personality traits between persons or groups of persons are referred to as differential psychology. In contrast, personality psychology deals with the development of a holistic personality. This chapter focuses on the perspective of personality psychology for two reasons: firstly, it deals with developmental issues (personality development), and secondly, an isolated consideration of the multitude of different personality traits (e.g., development of achievement motivation, intelligence, creativity, fear) would go beyond the scope of this chapter. Therefore, the following deals with the development of a holistic personality in connection with sport activities.

Personality psychology encompasses a multitude of theoretical approaches in which personality is defined in a specific way. In the sense of a common denominator, Herrmann (1991) has presented a minimum consensus-based definition. He understands personality as "a behavioral correlate that is unique to each person, relatively stable and that lasts over time" (p. 29). Behavioral correlate means that our personality influences our behavior. Knowledge of the personality structure, which varies from person to person, allows us to make reasonable behavioral predictions over different situations and with a certain stability over time. However, situational stability should always be understood relatively (in the sense of a tendency). Time stability is also to be seen relatively. What is meant by this is that our personality does not change permanently but remains stable over the short to medium term. However, it can also change over a longer period of time. The potential plasticity of the personality is a prerequisite for a meaningful examination of the extent to which personality development can be influenced by sport.

In psychology, different personality constructs are discussed (e.g., Asendorpf and Neyer (2012)). Among them, personality traits and self-related cognitions were and are of particular interest for personality research in sport science.

? At least four classes of personality constructs are distinguished in psychology (e.g., Asendorpf and Neyer (2012); Krampen (2002); Schneewind (2001)):

- Genetic constitution and physical appearance
- General temperament and personality traits:
  (a) Traits (e.g., Big Five, ► Table 13.4)
  (b) Emotions/states (e.g., fear, anger, moods)
- Performance characteristics:
  (a) Cognitive performance characteristics (e.g., intelligence, creativity, attention, concentration)
  (b) Physical-motor performance characteristics (conditional and coordinative abilities, motor skills)
- Self- and environment-related cognitions:
  (a) Self-related cognitions (e.g., self- and body concept, self-esteem)
  (b) Action characteristics (e.g., motivational constructs, coping styles, action beliefs)
  (c) Appraisal dispositions (e.g., attributions, attitude, values)

14.2.1.1 Trait Concepts

In the trait paradigm (► Chap. 13), "personality" is understood as the organized totality of traits that we can assign to a person (Stemmler et al., 2010). Traits are personality characteristics that are relatively stable over time and allow reasonably accurate predictions of experience and behavior for different situations and longer periods of time (in contrast to the more unstable emotions/states). One goal of this research area is to describe human personality by a manageable number of (independent) personality dimensions. The dimensioning determined by factor analysis led from Cattell's 16 personality factors (1946) via Eysenck's two- or three-dimensional solutions (extraversion, neuroticism, and less clearly psychoticism; Eysenck and Eysenck (1969)) to the Big Five models, which have been favored for more than two decades and are empirically well established, describing the human personality on the basis of five (relatively independent) personality dimensions (e.g., Costa Jr. and McCrae (1992); ► Table 13.4).

14.2.1.2 Self-Concept Approaches

Within the class of cognitive personality characteristics, various concepts have been developed that can be differentiated into self-related cognitions, action characteristics, and appraisal dispositions (e.g., Krampen and Greve (2008)). The approaches that are most frequently taken up in sport science are self-concept approaches (► Sect. 14.4), which are particularly suitable for questions of personality development due to the plasticity of self-concept. The self-concept describes the totality of perception and knowledge about one's own person, that is, the knowledge about one's own abilities, personal characteristics and feelings. An approach often used in sport science is Shavelson's "self-concept model" (Shavelson et al., 1976; ◘ Fig. 14.1).

The model describes the human self-concept as multidimensional and hierarchically structured. At the highest level, a general self-concept is assumed, which includes general expectations and subjective convictions of being able to overcome upcoming problems with one's own competencies (self-esteem). The general self-concept can be divided into an academic and a nonacademic self-concept. These two dimensions can be divided into further subdimensions, which, in turn, can be divided into more specific facets. The degree of universality and stability of the dimensions/facets increases from the base to the top of the pyramid. The self-concept components at the lower levels are thus more exposed to fluctuations and changes than the general self-concept,

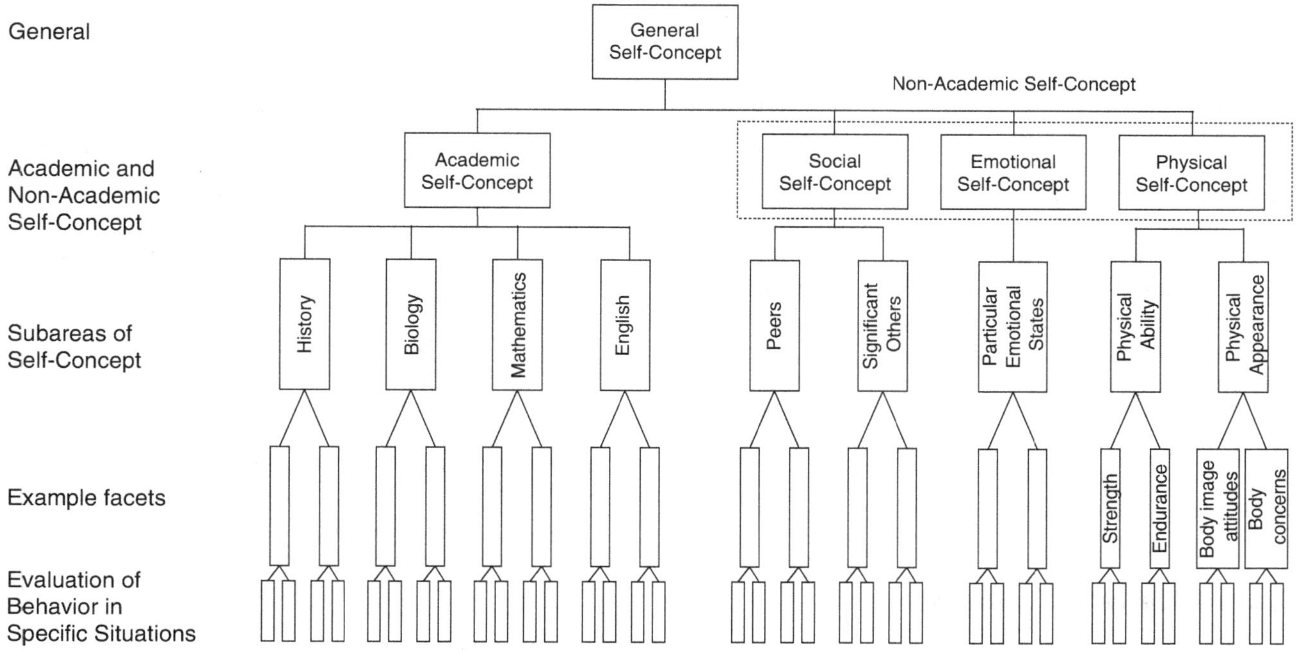

Fig. 14.1 Self-concept model based on Shavelson et al. (1976)

which is considered to be more resistant to change, because the general self-concept is fed from different sources (the subdimensions), which usually do not change simultaneously.

If, for example, a student wins an athletic competition, this should have a positive effect on the physical self-concept, while the academic self-concept, for example, should not be affected by this competition. If the physical self-concept increases and the other self-concept facets remain constant, the general self-concept is, in turn, likely to change only slightly.

The self-concept is also capable of development. Thus, on the one hand, a differentiation of the individual subdimensions and facets becomes apparent. On the other hand, the number of subdimensions increases in the course of childhood to adolescence.

14.2.2 The Term "Sport"

If one asks about the effect of sport on personality, a central question is what is meant by the term "sport"? Sport is an extremely diverse social phenomenon (e.g., Cachay (1990); Digel (1990)). In everyday language, very different activities can be categorized as "sport" (e.g., Willimczik (2001)). In addition, the term is used by different groups of people and institutions, in different cultures, and at different (historical) times with different meanings (Heinemann, 1998), so it is not surprising that there is no uniform definition of this term. Especially from a psychological point of view, it is "problematic to speak of sport because sport (...) is such a complex and inhomogeneous phenomenon (...) that it is challenging to specify consistent conditions and required structures" (Singer, 2004, p. 298). Therefore, for statements on the effects of sport on personality, precise assumptions regarding which personality traits are required in sport or which are influenced by sport are necessary (Conzelmann, 2009). For this reason, theses on the relationship between sport and personality must always include information on which sport activity is meant, in which form, and which effects are expected to arise from precisely this sport activity.

14.2.3 The Sport and Personality (Development) Relationship

A possible (descriptive) connection between sport and personality, for example, in the form of a personality difference between active and inactive persons, offers various potential causal interpretations. In sport science, the socialization and selection hypothesis has been the main topic of discussion so far. While the socialization hypothesis assumes that the variable "sport" has an effect on the variable "personality" (e.g., school sport promotes personality), the selection hypothesis assumes that sport is the criterion and personality the predictor variable (e.g., extroverted people tend to choose team sports). In addition to these two assumptions, which postulate a specific operating direction, a third assumption, the so-called interaction hypothesis, emerged in the course of the nature-nurture debate and through the further development of developmental psychology approaches (▶ Sect. 14.5). The interaction hypothesis assumes a dynamic interaction between sport and personality, that is, an alternating influence of selection and socialization processes over time (▶ Chap. 13). According to this hypothesis, certain personality characteristics favor the choice of a particular sport activity (selection). The regular practice of this sport activity, in turn, changes the personality (socialization), which can lead to an intensification of this sport activity or even to new "choices" (selection) (Conzelmann, 2001, 2009).

14.3 Historical Development

The beginning of systematic scientific research on the topic "sport and personality" in the German-speaking area started around the middle of the 1950s. Since that time, sport psychological personality research has gone through various stages (Conzelmann, 2001, 2009; ◘ Table 14.1).

Following a pre-empirical phase, the mid-1950s saw the beginning of a phase of intensive research activities on questions of the relationship between sport and personality, during which sport science research was primarily oriented toward trait concepts. After that the trait-oriented research on sport and personality had reached a dead-end in the mid-1980s, research activities came at first to a virtual standstill and then, only gradually, experienced a new start and reorientation toward cognitive approaches, developmental approaches, and intervention studies.

◘ **Table 14.1** Stages of sport psychological personality research (Conzelmann, 2009)

Period	Brief characterization	
Until the mid-1950s	**Pre-empirical phase:** Pedagogical postulates on the (positive) relationship between sport and personality	
Mid-1950s to late 1970s	**Phase of empirical individual studies:** "Heyday" of sport personality research in sport science	*Trait*-phase
Mid-1970s to mid-1980s	**Phase of methodologically oriented secondary analyses:** Critical interpretations of inconsistent research findings	
Mid-1980s to mid-1990s	**Phase of relative standstill**	Post-*trait*-phase
From the beginning of the 1990s	**Phase of gradual reorientation:** Cognitivism and dynamic interactionism	

14.3.1 Trait Phase

The monograph by Neumann (1957) marked the beginning of the "heyday of personality research in sport science" in the German-speaking area (Singer, 2004, p. 299). In the 1960s and 1970s, a large number of studies were conducted. The majority of these were studies in which a group of athletes (rarely female athletes) was compared with another group of athletes or with nonathletes with the aim of describing interindividual personality differences, often with the implicit aim of identifying positive effects of sport activities on personality development. However, the findings were not very consistent, and hardly any connections between sport and personality could be detected (Side Story: On the Heterogeneity of Classical Personality Studies in German Language Sport Science).

On the Heterogeneity of Classical Personality Studies in German Language Sport Science

To illustrate the heterogeneity of approaches and findings, three classical studies can be outlined: Neumann (1957) had "student nonathletes," "general athletes," and "training athletes" examined by experts in various sport situations with regard to Lersch's personality dimensions (1938, 1964), and based on his results, he drew a positive picture of the "athlete personality" which differed from that of normal people and which he described with terms such as "high vitality," "strong self-confidence," "elevated basic mood," "self-discipline," and "joy of performance" (1957, pp. 198–199). Steinbach (1968) examined top athletes in various sports. Based on his theoretical approach, the typology of psychopathological personalities according to Schneider (1950), he selected appropriate methods ("Rorschach test," "Minnesota Multiphasic Personality Inventory," constitution-typological procedures) and, in contrast to Neumann, found an (pathologically assessed) "abnormal personality structure" in over 60% of cases. Gabler (1981), on the other hand, concluded that the personality structure of the top swimmers he examined was within the normal range compared to a control group. Following Cattell (1946, 1973), he defined personality as a sum of 16 factors that are collected with the "16 PF (Personality Factor) Questionnaire." Similar to the already mentioned Big Five, the 16 PF describes personality by means of personality dimensions, which result from a content-wise and statistically meaningful summary of characteristic attributions.

The heterogeneity of the findings led to methodologically oriented secondary analyses. It was found that the inconsistent findings were not only due to inconsistent procedures and an ambiguous subject area but also to theoretical-methodological deficiencies. Criticism was leveled at, among other things, the lack of analysis of personality psychology-relevant characteristics in the field of sport, the excessively one-sided orientation toward traits, the lack of theory-based hypothesis generation, the cross-sectional design that is inadequate for causal interpretations, and the unsatisfactory control of social desirability bias or self-representation bias. The secondary analyses also called for more attention to the person-situation interactionism, the need of qualitatively oriented individual case studies, and the use of longitudinal designs (Conzelmann, 2001; Singer, 2004).

? With regard to the question of personality development through sport, three points of criticism are of particular importance from today's perspective (Conzelmann & Müller, 2005; Conzelmann et al., 2011):

1. The orientation toward traits (relatively stable over time and thus resistant to change) (e.g., Costa Jr. and McCrae (1997)) and the orientation toward static personality concepts, which do not consider adequately the dynamic aspect of personality (the possibility to change it)
2. The widespread lack of longitudinal studies and, in particular, the lack of intervention studies that allow differences between athletically active and inactive persons to be interpreted causally in terms of the socialization hypothesis.
3. The conceptual and methodological disregard for the developmental perspective

These theoretical and methodological deficits are likely to have been the major reason why empirical evidence of the supposed positive effects of sport on personality development failed, for a long time, to be convincingly demonstrated. As late as the turn of the century, Singer (2004) concluded that general statements on whether or not sport (in general) shapes the personality in a positive sense are impossible. "It will only be possible to say that sport—depending on its staging and form—can have both a negative and a positive socialization effect on certain groups of test persons, and that these sport-specific socialization impulses will only be effective at the level of general values and behavioral dispositions under very special circumstances" (Singer, 2004, p. 334).

14.3.2 Post-trait Phase

The critical discussion of the 1970s/1980s led to a paralysis of research activities. The number of studies that explicitly dealt with the topic of "sport and personality" decreased significantly in the 1980s in the German-speaking countries.

In the early 1980s, a "fairly bleak picture of personality area, with researchers abandoning the ship in great numbers also became apparent in Anglo-American countries. Even a cursory review of the sport literature reveals that sport personality studies dwindled drastically in the late 1970s and the early 1980s" (Fisher, 1984, p. 79). For the English-speaking world, however, one cannot speak of a "phase of relative standstill."

? In a study based on content analysis, Vealey (1989) was able to show that some promising paths were taken to overcome the "dead-end balance":

1. There was a paradigm shift from static trait concepts to interactionist concepts that allow a more precise approach to understand the complex relationship between the individual, sport environment, and sport behavior.
2. An increasing differentiation into structural and dynamic issues also came into notice, although intervention studies still were rare.
3. Although the methodological approaches still showed weaknesses (correlation studies, unclear operationalizations, unsatisfactory sample selection), the number of intervention studies had increased, and multivariate evaluation strategies (i.e., involving a large number of variables) have largely replaced the univariate ones (focused on individual personality variables).

However, when looking at the Anglo-American-speaking area, it should not be overlooked that the focus of personality research in sport science was primarily on questions that dealt with the influence of personality traits on sport commitment or sport performance (selection hypothesis). The question of the influence of sport on personality, that is, testing the socialization hypothesis, has been largely overlooked (cf. review articles of Allen et al., 2013; Allen & Laborde, 2014; Auweele et al., 1993; Tenenbaum & Bar-Eli, 1995; Vealey, 1992, 2002; Weinberg & Gould, 2003).

The study by Stephan et al. (2014) is, in this context, a more recent exception, which focuses explicitly on the influence of sport on personality development (in the second half of life). Despite two large-scale longitudinal studies, the authors come to a comparatively vague conclusion: "These findings suggest that physical activity may help preserve personality stability and prevent maladaptive personality changes across adulthood and old age" (2014, p. 1). The reasons for the ambiguous results are probably due to the same methodological deficits already noted above. Because of the correlative design of the study, the collection and differentiation of the independent variable sport are insufficient (retrospective self-report on the frequency of participation in "vigorous [e.g., running or lifting heavy objects] and moderate leisure physical activity [e.g., slow or light swimming, brisk walking]"; 2014, p. 2), and a static personality concept was used (Big Five).

In German-speaking countries, it was only since the early 1990s that papers dealing with the topic of "sport and personality" have reemerged. A response to the criticism leveled at the studies published between the 1950s and 1970s has been given in two ways: on the one hand, by increasing the orientation toward cognitive approaches (► Sect. 14.4), and on the other hand, by the adoption of a developmental perspective (► Sect. 14.5).

14.4 Studies on Self-Concept Development Through Sport

The shift away from traits that last for a relatively long time and the preoccupation with cognitive approaches have led to somewhat more consistent findings in the processing of the socialization hypothesis of sport science-related personality research (Conzelmann & Müller, 2005). There are several reasons why this new orientation focuses on the self-concept in particular. On the one hand, a person's self-concept is ascribed a behavior-regulating function in many areas of life (Roebers, 2007). For example, it depends on the self-concept of one's own abilities which goals a person sets for him or herself or to which areas of life he or she devotes time (Schütz & Sellin, 2003). Educational and career decisions, the choice of leisure activities, and interest in a specific sport are also functions of self-concept. For this reason, the formation of a differentiated and realistic, yet positively colored, self-concept is regarded as one of the central developmental tasks and as the basis for healthy personality development (Hurrelmann, 2006). On the other hand, due to the relatively high plasticity (i.e., malleability) of cognitive personality characteristics, it can be assumed that a person's self-concept can be more easily influenced by sport-related interventions than long-term stable traits (e.g., the Big Five already mentioned). But what exactly is the self-concept and how can it be specifically influenced by sport activities?

14.4.1 Self-Concept

The exploration of self-concept has a long tradition in psychology, beginning with the fundamental work of William James at the end of the nineteenth century. In his works, he distinguished between two components of the self: the self as subject ("I") and the self as object ("Me"). While for James (1890) the "I" represents the actor of one's own actions and knowledge, the "Me" represents the object of self-observation. Through this distinction, the self becomes simultaneously subject and object. The "I" recognizes the "Me," so to speak, which makes the self the object of its own cognition. This dichotomy makes it clear that the self is not a passive system that can be accumulated with knowledge but it actively influences and shapes the way we deal with our environment (Hattie, 1992). The self as an object (Me), which can be described as a simple enumeration of items that belong to itself, has been referred to as "self-concept" by subsequent research efforts.

> **Self-Concept**
>
> Self-concept is a person's perception of him or herself. This perception is formed through one's experience with and interpretations of one's environment and is influenced especially by reinforcements, evaluations of significant others, and one's attributions for one's own behavior (Shavelson et al., 1976).

Self-concept approaches describe a person's self-concept as a multidimensional and hierarchically structured construct in which self-related information gained from experience are stored in an area-specific manner. The hierarchical structure of the "self-concept model" of Shavelson et al. (1976), for example, suggests that subdimensions of the self-concept can be influenced more directly by experiences and evaluations than the hierarchically higher general self-concept (◘ Fig. 14.1). But why is a controlled sequence of sport and physical activities integrated into the perception of the self and under what conditions can the higher level of self-esteem be positively influenced?

Sonstroem and Morgan (1989) and, in extension, Sonstroem et al. (1994) describe the relevance of sport-related physical experiences for influencing the physical self-concept in the "Exercise and Self-Esteem Model" (EXSEM). In the sense of a bottom-up process, sport and movement activities contribute to area-specific physical self-efficacy experiences. They lead to the perception of one's own athletic competence, which in turn directly—and meditated via physical acceptance—should lead to positive self-esteem (◘ Fig. 14.2).

Sonstroem and Morgan (1989) developed EXSEM on the basis of the hierarchical "self-concept model" of Shavelson et al. (1976) and the "self-efficacy theory" of Bandura (1977). The use of the term "self-esteem" instead of the general self-concept by Shavelson et al. (1976) illustrates the strong influence of humanistic psy-

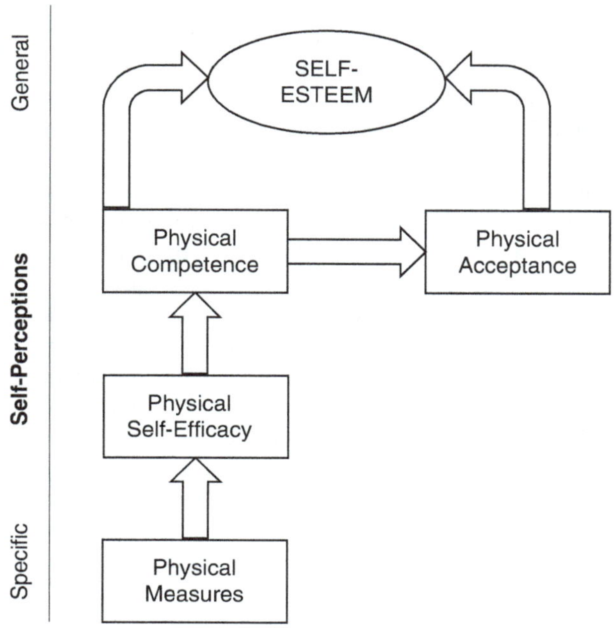

Fig. 14.2 "Exercise and Self-Esteem Model" (based on Sonstroem and Morgan (1989))

chology and its idea of self-realization on the authors. Accordingly, EXSEM focuses on the mechanism of action, how sport and exercise programs can positively influence self-esteem. Although isolated studies have been able to confirm parts of this postulated mechanism (Alfermann & Stoll, 2000; Baldwin & Courneya, 1997; Elavsky, 2010), systematic validation studies on both EXSEM and the expanded model are still pending (Schmidt et al., 2015). Nevertheless, this model does show a possible mechanism of action that can be used to explain possible effects of sport on the self-concept. In order to be able to design targeted interventions, it is not only necessary to have empirical evidence that something works, but one should also understand *why* and *how* something works.

14.4.2 Sport-Related Self-Concept Interventions

Taking into account the hierarchical self-concept structure (e.g., Nigg et al. (2001)) and the mechanism of action presented in EXSEM, it makes little sense to try to promote changes in global, hierarchically higher dimensions through sport-related interventions. This conclusion drawn from theoretical considerations is also supported by empirical studies. O'Mara et al. (2006), for example, show in their meta-analysis of 200 self-concept interventions that particularly the interventions conducted on the subjects who did not strive for changes at the level of the general self-concept, but at the level of dimensions, subdimensions, or facets, tended to have greater effects. In addition, the specificity of the self-concept interventions seems to represent a further condition for success: Interventions that tried to address individual facets by means of tailor-made content achieved the greatest effects (Cohens $d = 0.76$), while those without a clear reference to a particular facet had only small effect sizes (Cohens $d = 0.14$). The more the content corresponds to the facets to be addressed, the more likely it is that the facets will change. An intervention in mathematics teaching will therefore have an effect on the mathematical rather than the physical self-concept. A similar picture emerges for sport-related interventions. While in the meta-analysis by Fox (2000), only half of all studies examined could demonstrate positive effects on the global level of self-esteem, positive effects could be demonstrated for 78% of the study examining area-specific (sport- and body-related) self-concept facets or dimensions.

Not all populations benefit equally from physical activity: children and adolescents are likely to benefit more than adults. Moreover, people with low self-esteem are more easily positively influenced by sport than those with high self-esteem (Alfermann & Stoll, 2000; Whitehead & Corbin, 1997). The findings of Spence et al. (2005) largely confirm these results and highlight, in addition, that the intervention program and the change in fitness induced with the intervention may act as moderating factors. For example, endurance and strength interventions show higher effects than skill-related interventions, and the effects on the self-concept are greater when the intervention actually increases physical fitness. The fact that systematic training is preferable to any sport intervention to achieve such changes is also confirmed by the results of a more recent meta-analysis (Spruit et al., 2016).

In addition to the content of the sport intervention, the setting in which an intervention is carried out also plays a decisive role, as the meta-analysis of Liu et al. (2015) shows. The analysis of 25 randomized and 13 nonrandomized intervention studies showed that sport-related interventions conducted in the school setting had greater effects on self-concept and general self-esteem than those conducted in leisure sports. One possible explanation for the higher effectiveness of sport-related interventions in the school setting can be seen in the fact that they are carried out by pedagogically trained personnel who do not only focus on content but also considered didactic-methodological aspects (▶ Study Box: Bern Intervention Study on School Sport).

Bern Intervention Study on School Sport (BISS)

The importance of the didactic-methodological design of sport-related interventions was also demonstrated in the "Bern Intervention Study on School Sport" (BISS) (Conzelmann et al., 2011). From the background of a dynamic-interactionist perspective, BISS systematically examined the influence of school sport-related interventions on the self-concept development of pupils aged between 11 and 12 years old. The study focused on the principles of competence experience, reflection, and individualization.

Seventeen middle school classes ($M_{age} = 11.91$, $SD = 0.55$ years) underwent two treatment phases of 10 weeks, each during one school year in a quasi-experimental longitudinal study. These treatment phases were developed on a theoretical basis and are characterized by specific sport activities and specific forms of staging. Before and after each intervention part of the three modules "play," "risk," and "performance," different aspects of the social, emotional, and physical self-concept were assessed. For example, an attempt was made to address the social self-concept with the help of specifically staged cooperation games and game development series. As a comparison group, six middle school classes were included in the study, which conducted normal curriculum-oriented physical education classes without specific requirements in terms of (personality-building) learning goals and lesson design.

The findings show that specific facets of pupils' self-concept are positively influenced by specifically designed personality-building physical education. In this context, the targeted orientation of the teaching lessons toward the self-concept facets to be addressed is of central importance. Physical education does not have a positive effect on the child's self-concept per se but only if certain didactic-methodological principles are applied during the lessons.

Sport Practice

How do you give feedback that promotes self-concept?

In the sport context, there are many occasions when a coach wants to give feedback to an athlete or a teacher wants to give feedback to a student. If the focus is not only on the pure improvement of motor skills but also on the promotion of a positive realistic self-concept, Fengler (2009) recommends that the person giving feedback should be guided by the following criteria:

Criteria for self-concept promoting feedback:

1. Immediate and situational
2. Concrete, clear, and precise
3. Behavioral or task-related
4. Descriptive and not interpretive
5. Regularly
6. Honest but fair

Feedback in case of successful task performance: attribute successful achievements to talent and effort (e.g., "You mastered this exercise without any problems because you are extremely courageous and prepared for the exercise very well with your classmates"). In ▸ Chap. 7 (Motivation), for example, the concept of causal attribution (Weiner, 1985) is explained in more detail.

Feedback in case of failed task performance: attribute unsuccessful performance to lack of effort (or at best external circumstances) and not to unchangeable characteristics such as movement ability, height, etc. (e.g., "You would not have slipped off the barrel, if you had used your arms for balance"; ▸ Chap. 6).

14

14.4.3 Veridicality

In the previous remarks, it was assumed that it was clear what was meant by a positive self-concept. And without further clarification of the term "positive," one would probably assume that a positive influence on the self-concept means an increase of the self-concept. It is questionable, however, whether sport-related self-concept interventions should only intend to influence the level of self-concept without making any reference to the actual performance of the study participants. Or formulated as a concrete question: Is it functional to have a high sport-related self-concept if one is in reality a miserable athlete? Could, in addition to the level of the self-concept, the congruency with reality represent a target perspective?

Recommendations from different lines of research regarding the reality relatedness of the self-concept are inconsistent. They range from a self-perception that is as realistic as possible as a "basic condition for healthy personality development" (Hurrelmann, 2006) to a "positive-realistic self-concept" (Sygusch, 2008) and the demand for the highest possible self-concept (Lintunen,

1999; Stiller & Alfermann, 2007). In view of this diversity, it is surprising that most intervention studies found to date in physical education aim at increasing the self-concept of pupils (e.g., Annesi (2007); Calfas and Cooper (1996); Goni and Zulaika (2000); Lloyd and Fox (1992); Magnaguagno et al. (2016); Marsh and Peart (1988); Rubeli et al. (2020)) and disregard veridicality.

Veridicality

Veridicality refers to the degree to which the self-perceptions of one's own abilities and performance correspond to reality (Helmke, 1992, p. 197).

To conclude on the basis of cross-sectional studies that people with a high self-concept perform better than those with a low one and that, therefore, high self-concepts are functional seems problematic, since it is quite possible that people have high self-concepts only because they also possess high abilities in the corresponding domain. In this case, the self-concept would be high, but at the same time, it corresponds to reality. Thus, in addition to the functionality of a high self-concept, the functionality of the veridicality of the self-concept should also be discussed (Schmidt & Conzelmann, 2011).

Bandura (1994) already recognized that situational factors play an important role in answering the question of functionality. He identifies individual situations in which an illusionary overestimation of oneself can be extremely dangerous. If, for example, someone has set himself the goal of crossing a lake by swimming and thereby overestimates his aerobic capacity, this can have just as devastating consequences as overestimating one's cycling abilities in road traffic. Cycling accidents are among the most common causes of serious childhood injuries, according to a study by Rivara (1985): a misjudgment of their own abilities is very often involved. Plumert (1995) was able to show in a study with children aged between 6 and 8 years old that an overestimation of one's own physical abilities is related to the number and to the severity of everyday injuries. Thus, the more children overestimate themselves, the greater the risk of injury. Gender-specific evaluations showed that this effect was stronger among boys than among girls. Since results of further studies by this same working group point in the same direction (Plumert et al., 2004; Plumert & Schwebel, 1997; Schwebel & Bounds, 2003), the authors warn against overestimating one's own abilities, especially during physical or sport activities. However, they also stress that these results should in no way lead to the proclamation that an underestimation is a functional state. Even if underestimating one's own physical abilities can protect children from accidents, Schwebel and Plumert (1999) anticipate negative consequences for the group of underestimators, similar to Bandura (1994)—because those who underestimate themselves miss opportunities to prove their abilities and learn new things. However, appropriate physical and psychological development, especially in childhood and adolescence, involves trying out new things and "growing" from them (Bjorklund & Green, 1992). While overestimation in dangerous situations can increase the risk of accidents, their functionality as a motor for development in non-hazardous or supervised situations is certainly conceded. Thus, without considering the specific situation, a meaningful determination of functionality seems hardly possible.

After their theoretical analysis and review of empirical studies, Schmidt and Conzelmann (2011) conclude that an underestimation of one's own abilities inhibits performance-related behavior as a result of an unproductive persistence (McFarlin et al., 1984) or an inadequate choice of tasks (Harter, 1998). Severe overestimation, on the other hand, can lead to an increased risk of accidents (Schwebel & Plumert, 1999) and is often accompanied by high narcissism values (Bushman & Baumeister, 1998), which can be particularly dysfunctional in social interactions. According to these explanations, a realistic self-assessment or even a moderate overestimation of one's own abilities should be the ideal target perspective. Self-concept interventions should therefore aim at a "positive-realistic self-concept" (Sygusch, 2008, p. 143). While the self-concept of overestimators should be reduced to a more realistic level, underestimators are more likely to benefit from instructional stagings that attempt to increase their self-concept.

Individual-Importance Hypothesis

The individual-importance hypothesis states that "the contribution of a specific domain to global self-concept may be larger when its perceived importance is greater and, conversely, the contribution of a specific domain to global self-concept may be smaller when its perceived importance is of lesser value. In essence, the importance of a specific domain of self-concept may have a critical role in the development of global self-concept." (Hardy & Moriarty, 2006, p. 378).

The view of a multidimensional and hierarchically structured self-concept implies that there must be certain compensation possibilities for an individual within this system. Differential psychologically oriented self-concept research tries to address this by considering not only the individual dimensions but also the personal relevance, significance, or importance of the respective dimensions. Thomas (1989) speaks of "centrality" in this context and means the "extent of the self-reference of processes and attributes" (p. 22). This extent is understood as a continuum ranging from a particularly high or strong to a low or no self-reference. These considerations originate from a hypothesis that was already formulated more than 100 years ago: the individual-importance hypothesis (James, 1890). According to this hypothesis, self-concept dimensions to which an individual attaches greater importance influence general self-esteem or general self-concept to a greater extent than less relevant self-concept dimensions (Hardy & Moriarty, 2006). For example, research in personality psychology (Marsh, 2008), developmental psychology (Harter, 2012), or sport science (Rubeli et al., 2019) assumes that physical self-concept is a central self-concept, especially for children and adolescents, and thus plays a particularly important role in the development of general self-concept. Thus, if a child attaches a high degree of importance to physical performance but produces poor results in sport activities, this will have a negative effect on his or her general self-concept. On the other hand, a child whose general self-concept mainly builds on the child's guitar playing skills will be less negatively influenced by the poor sport activity results. Although the individual-importance hypothesis is constantly being discussed in the general and sport psychological literature (Marsh & Scalas, 2018), empirical support for the hypothesis is surprisingly elusive (Lindwall et al., 2011; Rubeli et al., 2019; Scalas et al., 2013, 2014).

14

> In summary, it can be said that sport can positively influence specific facets of the self-concept. However, the weak to moderate effects must not lead to the assumption that sport would per se contribute to a positive influence on self-concept. Depending on the way it is staged, different effects on the self-concept can be expected, which suggest that sport pedagogically oriented interventions should take into account the content and methodology of their design. For example, a teaching unit dedicated to learning the backflip can either focus on the social-cooperative aspects of helping and securing (social self-concept) or address the fear that the execution of this movement can trigger (emotional self-concept). Moreover, in addition to a general psychological perspective, a differential perspective is always advisable, since it cannot be assumed that one specific sport activity has the same effect on all individuals (Schmidt et al., 2013).

14.5 Theoretical Considerations on the Topic of Personality Development Through Sport

The findings reported in the previous chapter show that, under certain conditions, specific characteristics of the personality can be (positively) influenced. Nevertheless, it remains unclear how these changes come about. Which theoretical approaches can be used to explain personality changes? Which approaches describe and explain personality development?

From a structural viewpoint, the question of personality development through sport involves assumptions about changes in the dependent variable personality (P) resulting from the influence of the independent variable sport (S). Conceptual specifications on different levels are necessary to problematize $P = f(S)$ hypotheses (▣ Fig. 14.3). First, it is necessary to clarify what is meant by the descriptive construct personality (this is usually defined by personality theories); second, the explicative construct sport has to be specified; and third, it has to be clarified which theories can be used to describe and explain personality changes between two measurement points (▶ Sect. 14.2). If one also takes a developmental perspective, which is interested in changes over longer periods of time (life span development), the question of suitable theories of personality development arises.

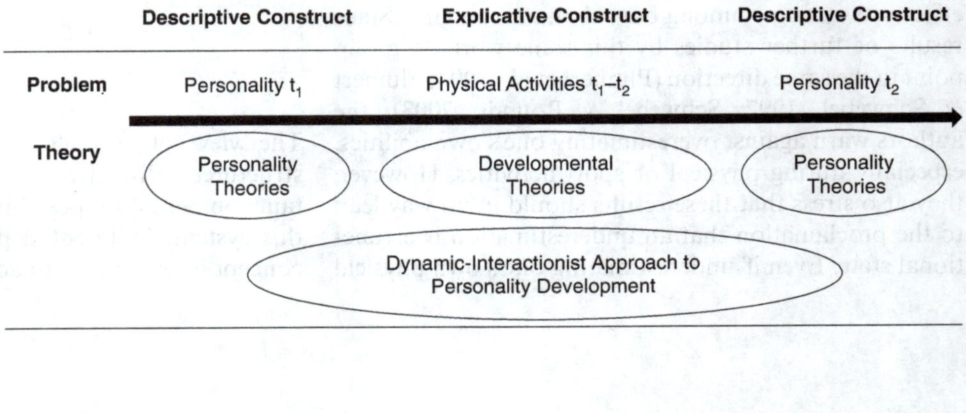

▣ Fig. 14.3 The structure of $P = f(S)$ hypotheses

Personality theories are suitable in different ways for conceptualizing personality changes. Theories that focus on the structure of personality (e.g., trait concepts) usually exclude process-related aspects of personality (see Krampen and Greve (2008), within sport science: Conzelmann (2009)). For questions of personality development, on the other hand, theoretical approaches that address the process character of personality and thus personality development seem appropriate. In the context of the current discussion, dynamic-interactionist approaches to personality development are highly recommended (Overton & Molenar, 2015).

Magnusson (1990) summarizes the basic assumptions of the dynamic-interactionist approach to human functioning and development as follows: "(1) An individual develops and functions as a total, integrated organism; current functioning and development do not take place in single aspects per se, in isolation from the totality. (2) An individual develops and functions in a dynamic, continuous and reciprocal process of interaction with his or her environment. (3) The characteristic way in which an individual develops and functions, in interaction with the environment, depends on and influences the continuous reciprocal process of interaction among subsystems of mental and biological facts" (p. 196; see also Lerner (2002); Magnusson and Stattin (2006)).

? For dynamic-interactionist approaches, the following are key basic assumptions of the field's research (e.g., Magnusson (2001); ► Fig. 13.4):

(a) The current behavior is the result of a continuous process of multidirectional interaction between the individual and the situation in which the individual finds himself/herself.
(b) In this interaction process, the individual has an active (acting) role.
(c) At the personal level, cognitive and motivational factors are major determinants of behavior.
(d) At the situational level, the psychological significance of a situation is the main determinant of behavior.

Human development is thus understood as a reciprocal process of interaction that takes place on three levels (e.g., Magnusson (1990); Magnusson and Stattin (2006); ◘ Fig. 14.4): intraorganismic interactions, extraorganismic interactions, and person-environment interactions.

Dynamic-interactionist approaches are particularly suitable for dealing with questions of personality development, because they establish a connection between personality and developmental psychology by simultaneously observing the functionality related to current behavior and the change in this functionality in ontogenesis, thus doing justice to the dynamic character of personality development.

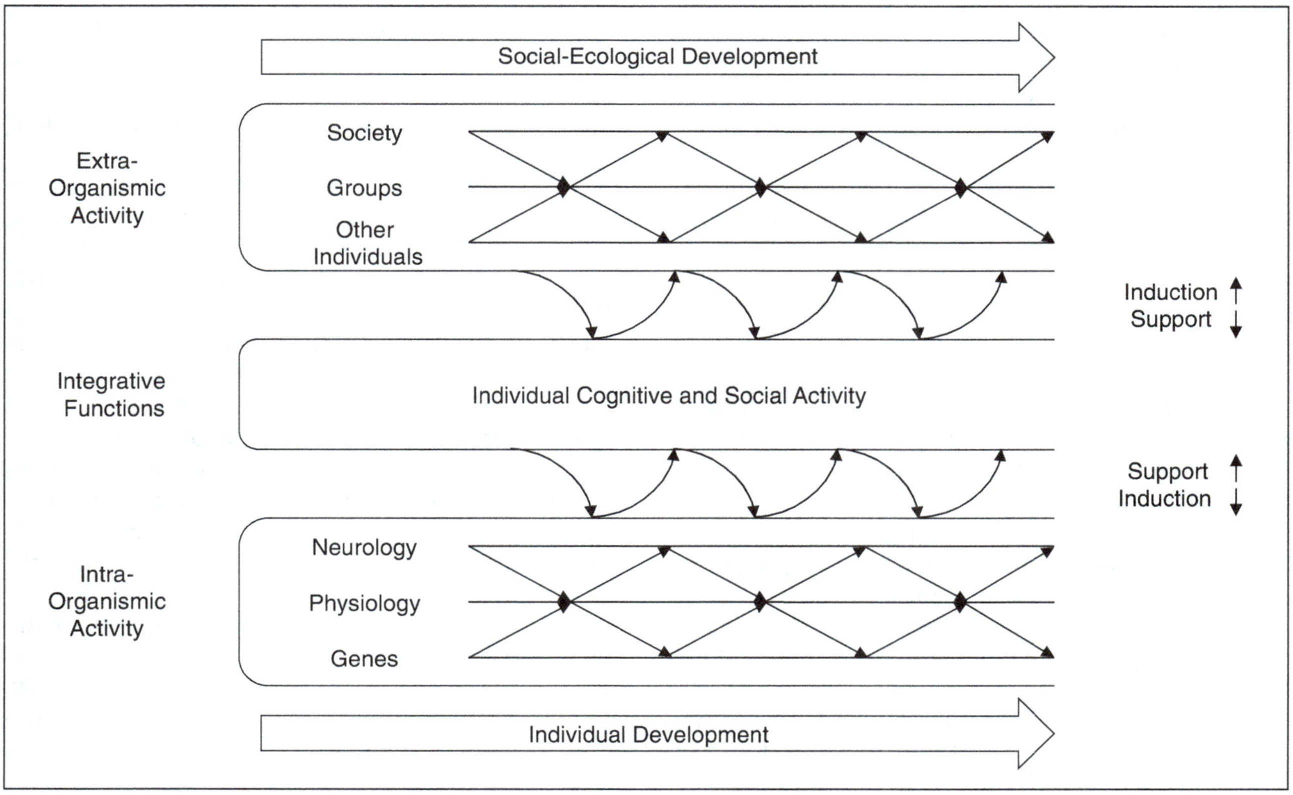

◘ **Fig. 14.4** The model of holistic dynamic interaction (based on Gariépy (1996), p. 88; published by Conzelmann et al. (2013), p. 326)

The dynamic-interactionist view of personality development has implications for the hypotheses discussed in ► Sect. 14.2 regarding the relationship between sport and personality. On the one hand, applied sport science is interested in being able to empirically investigate the effect of sport on personality development and, in the best case, to confirm it. This is because, in many cases, the socialization hypothesis is an important argument for the legitimization for the state support of sport (e.g., for the legitimization of school sport or the financial support of club sport). On the other hand, clear evidence for a unidirectional effect of sport on personality development is not to be expected, since there is a constant interaction between the person and the environment. Socialization and selection effects therefore constantly alternate.

In the "assumption of an action-mediated interaction between biological potential and environmental conditions" (Baur, 1989, p. 84), the role of the (intentional) individual as a shaper of his or her own development (Brandtstädter, 1998, 2001; Lerner & Busch-Rossnagel, 1981) is emphasized (cf. ◘ Fig. 14.4, in which the actions of the individual are characterized by the term "individual cognitive and social activity"). For sure, environmental influences are important for human development. However, an analysis of environmental influences cannot be carried out without taking into account the personality system, which changes and varies between individuals in the course of ontogenesis. Without considering the individual personality and the individual stage of development of the athlete, it is not possible to accurately examine whether and how, for example, competitive sport activities affect personality.

It is therefore not a question of how much influence sport activities have on a more or less passive individual but rather a question of the proportional relation between personal effects (e.g., through the choice of certain sport activities) and environmental effects (e.g., effects of a sport setting that the person has chosen). It should be noted that "culture, action and development are so closely intertwined, both conceptually and functionally, that an adequate theoretical version of one area is hardly possible without reference to the other" (Brandtstädter, 2001, p. 28).

The dynamic-interactionist approach recommends to view human development from a systemic perspective (e.g., Lerner (2002); Magnusson and Cairns (1996); Overton (2015); Shoda and Mischel (2000)). Dynamic systems not only have the property of increasing stability and thus of becoming increasingly less changeable over the course of a lifetime, but they also have the property of nonlinearity (e.g., Petermann and Rudinger (2002); Witherington (2015)). This, in turn, suggests—with reference to the topic of sport and personality development—that it is not necessary to look for causal connections. In other words, the question of whether sport influences personality or whether personality is responsible for a person's choice of a particular sport is not meaningful in the context of a person's development. Only if it were possible to develop less complex partial theories (which do not involve reciprocal interactions) for partial questions of sport scientific personality research, the search for cause-and-effect sequences would be meaningful (this is partly the case with the intervention studies described in ► Sect. 14.4). As long as the holistic personality is considered in its course of development, as it is the case in the dynamic interactionism, the search for linear processes makes no sense.

For a comprehensive understanding of personality development, the dynamic-interactionist approach is a suitable framework concept, but due to its complexity, it is hardly accessible to empirical testing, since intra- and extraorganismic change processes and their complex interaction over time must be recorded synchronously. In this respect, it is not surprising that a methodology that does justice to the interactive model in its entirety is not yet available (Hurrelmann, 2006, p. 91; Magnusson & Cairns, 1996, p. 20 f).

An important methodological consequence of dynamic interactionism is that it is not sufficient to take an exclusively variable-oriented approach, which means to consider only some individual characteristics of a person and make interindividual comparisons for these characteristics. Ideally, this approach should be supplemented by person-oriented strategies in which the individual person is the central (intraindividual) unit of investigation (Von Eye & Spiel, 2010).

The person-oriented approach has been used in sport-scientific personality research, for example, in the longitudinal study on self-concept development in adolescence by Müller and colleagues (Müller et al., 2012, 2013). From the authors' point of view, the person-oriented approach offers the possibility of a holistic perspective by considering other contexts such as school, family, or peers in addition to the developmental context of sport. In this way, the contribution of sport as one of several developmental contexts that interact in a complex way with other contexts can be presented in a more differentiated way in the process of self-concept development in the future. The studies show that the unsatisfactory findings in variable-oriented studies on self-concept development through sport (e.g., Alfermann et al. (2003); Burrmann (2004); Heim (2002)) are not exclusively due to the lack of personality-building effects of sport activities but rather to the insufficient consideration of other development contexts (Müller et al., 2013).

Learning Control Questions

Basic:

1. What pedagogical postulates are there addressing the effect of sport activities on personality development?
2. How can the construct "personality" be defined from a psychological point of view?
3. Which classes of personality constructs (areas of personality) can be distinguished?

Advanced:

4. Why does it not make sense from a theoretical perspective to talk about the effects of sport on personality?
5. Why are self-concept studies more promising than trait studies for investigating possible effects of sport on personality development?
6. How do the socialization and selection hypothesis differ? What role does the interaction hypothesis play in this context?
7. How can the different stages of sport psychological personality research be characterized? What differences in historical development can be seen in the Anglo-American- compared to the German-speaking area?
8. How can the positive influence of sport and exercise programs on self-esteem be explained according to the "Exercise and Self-Esteem Model" (Sonstroem & Morgan, 1989)?

Expert:

9. Why is it important that self-concept interventions are not basically aimed at increasing self-concept but rather at forming a "positive-realistic self-concept"?
10. What are the basic assumptions of dynamic-interactionist developmental concepts? What are the consequences of a dynamic-interactionist perspective for addressing the question of personality development through sport?

References

Alfermann, D., Stiller, J., & Würth, S. (2003). Das physische Selbstkonzept bei sportlich aktiven Jugendlichen in Abhängigkeit von sportlicher Leistungsentwicklung und Geschlecht. *Zeitschrift für Entwicklungspsychologie und Pädagogische Psychologie, 35*, 135–143. https://doi.org/10.1026//0049-8637.35.3.135

Alfermann, D., & Stoll, O. (2000). Effects of physical exercise on self-concept and well-being. *International Journal of Sport Psychology, 30*, 47–65.

Allen, M. S., Greenlees, I., & Jones, M. (2013). Personality in sport: A comprehensive review. *International Review of Sport and Exercise Psychology, 6*(1), 184–208. https://doi.org/10.1080/1750984X.2013.769614

Allen, M. S., & Laborde, S. (2014). The role of personality in sport and physical activity. *Current Directions in Psychological Science, 23*(6), 460–465. https://doi.org/10.1177/0963721414550705

Annesi, J. J. (2007). Relations of age with changes in self-efficacy and physical self-concept in preadolescents participating in a physical activity intervention during afterschool care. *Perceptual and Motor Skills, 105*, 221–226. https://doi.org/10.2466/PMS.105.1.221-226

Asendorpf, J. B., & Neyer, F. (2012). *Psychologie der Persönlichkeit (5. vollständig überarbeitete Aufl.)*. Springer.

Auweele, Y. V., De Cuyper, B., Van Mele, V., & Rzewnicki, R. (1993). Elite performance and personality: From description and prediction to diagnosis and intervention. In R. N. Singer & L. Tennant (Eds.), *Handbook of research on sport psychology* (pp. 257–289). McMillan.

Baldwin, M. K., & Courneya, K. S. (1997). Exercise and self-esteem in breast cancer survivors: An application of the exercise and self-esteem model. *Journal of Sport & Exercise Psychology, 19*(4), 347–358. https://doi.org/10.1123/jsep.19.4.347

Bandura, A. (1977). *Social learning theory*. Prentice-Hall.

Bandura, A. (1994). Self-efficacy. In V. S. Ramachaudran (Ed.), *Encyclopedia of human behavior* (Vol. 4, pp. 71–81). Academic Press.

Baur, J. (1989). *Körper- und Bewegungskarrieren*. Hofmann.

Bjorklund, D. F., & Green, B. L. (1992). The adaptive nature of cognitive immaturity. *American Psychologist, 47*, 46–54.

Brandtstädter, J. (1998). Action perspectives on human development. In R. M. Lerner (Ed.), *Handbook of child psychology: Volume 1 Theoretical models of human development* (pp. 807–863). Wiley.

Brandtstädter, J. (2001). *Entwicklung, Intentionalität, Handeln*. Kohlhammer.

Burrmann, U. (2004). Effekte des Sporttreibens auf die Entwicklung des Selbstkonzepts Jugendlicher. *Zeitschrift für Sportpsychologie, 11*, 71–82. https://doi.org/10.1026/1612-5010.11.2.71

Bushman, B., & Baumeister, R. F. (1998). Threatened egotism, narcissism, self-esteem, and direct and displaced aggression: Does self-love or self-hate lead to violence? *Journal of Personality and Social Psychology, 75*, 219–229. https://doi.org/10.1037/0022-3514.75.1.219

Cachay, K. (1990). Versportlichung der Gesellschaft und Entsportung des Sports—Systemtheoretische Anmerkungen zu einem gesellschaftlichen Phänomen. In H. Gabler & U. Göhner (Eds.), *Für einen besseren Sport-Themen, Entwicklungen und Perspektiven aus Sport und Sportwissenschaft* (pp. 97–113). Hofmann.

Calfas, K. & Cooper, D. (1996). Effect of a 5 week exercise training program on self-worth among adolescent girls. A randomised controlled study. Medicine and Science in Sports and Exercise, 28, 135.

Cattell, R. B. (1946). *The description and measurement of personality*. World Book.

Cattell, R. B. (1973). *Die empirische Erforschung der Persönlichkeit*. Beltz.

Conzelmann, A. (2001). *Sport und Persönlichkeitsentwicklung: Möglichkeiten und Grenzen von Lebenslaufanalysen*. Hofmann.

Conzelmann, A. (2009). Differentielle Sportpsychologie—Sport und Persönlichkeit. In W. Schlicht & B. Strauß (Hrsg.), Enzyklopädie der Psychologie: Themenbereich D Praxisgebiete, Serie V Sportpsychologie, Band 1 Grundlagen der Sportpsychologie (S. 375-439). : Hogrefe.

Conzelmann, A., Schmidt, M., & Valkanover, S. (2011). *Persönlichkeitsentwicklung durch Schulsport. Theorie, Empirie und Praxisbausteine der Berner Interventionsstudie Schulsport (BISS)*. Huber.

Conzelmann, A., Hänsel, F., & Höner, O. (2013). Individuum und Handeln—Sportpsychologie. In A. Güllich & M. Krüger (Eds.), *Das Lehrbuch für das Sportstudium (Reihe Bachelor)* (pp. 271–337). Springer.

Conzelmann, A., & Müller, M. (2005). Sport und Selbstkonzeptentwicklung—Ein Situationsbericht aus entwicklungstheoretischer Perspektive. *Sportpsychologie, 12*, 108–118. https://doi.org/10.1026/1612-5010.12.4.108

Costa, P. T., Jr., & McCrae, R. R. (1992). *Revised NEO Personality Inventory and NEO Five Factor Inventory professional manual*. Psychological Assessment Resources.

Costa, P. T., Jr., & McCrae, R. R. (1997). Longitudinal stability of adult development. In R. Hogan, J. Johnson, & S. Briggs (Eds.), *Handbook of personality psychology* (pp. 269–290). Academic Press.

Deutscher Olympischer Sportbund. (2009). *Memorandum zum Schulsport*. DOSB.

Digel, H. (1990). Die Versportlichung unserer Kultur und deren Folgen für den Sport—Ein Beitrag zur Uneigentlichkeit des Sports. In H. Gabler & U. Göhner (Eds.), *Für einen besseren Sport-Themen, Entwicklungen und Perspektiven aus Sport und Sportwissenschaft* (pp. 73–96). Hofmann.

Elavsky, S. (2010). Longitudinal examination of the exercise and self-esteem model in middle-aged women. *Journal of Sport & Exercise Psychology, 32*(6), 862–880. https://doi.org/10.1123/jsep.32.6.862

Eysenck, H. J., & Eysenck, S. B. G. (1969). *Personality structure and measurement*. Routledge.

Federal Ministry of Education (Bundesministerium für Bildung). (2012). Lehrplan der Volksschule, Siebenter Teil, Bildungs- und Lehraufgaben sowie Lehrstoff und didaktische Grundsätze der Pflichtgegenstände der Grundschule und der Volksschuloberstufe, Grundschule—Bewegung und Sport. Eigenverlag.

Fengler, J. (2009). *Feedback geben. Strategien und Übungen* (4. Aufl.). : Beltz.

Fisher, A. C. (1984). New directions in sport personality research. In J. M. Silva & R. S. Weinberg (Eds.), *Psychological foundations of sport* (pp. 70–80). Human Kinetics.

Fox, K. R. (2000). Self-esteem, Self-perceptions and Exercise. *International Journal of Sport Psychology, 31*, 228–241.

Gabler, H. (1981). *Leistungsmotivation im Hochleistungssport* (3. Aufl.). : Hofmann.

Gariépy, J.-L. (1996). The question of continuity and change in development. In R. B. Cairns, G. H. Elder, & E. J. Costello (Eds.), *Developmental science* (pp. 78–96). University Press.

Goni, A., & Zulaika, L. (2000). Relationships between physical education classes and the enhancement of fifth grade pupils' self-concept. *Perceptual and Motor Skills, 91*, 246–250. https://doi.org/10.2466/PMS.91.5.246-250

Grupe, O., & Krüger, M. (1997). *Einführung in die Sportpädagogik*. Hofmann.

Hardy, L., & Moriarty, T. (2006). Shaping self-concept: The elusive importance effect. *Journal of Personality, 74*(2), 377–401. https://doi.org/10.1111/j.1467-6494.2005.00379.x

Harter, S. (1998). The development of self-representations. In N. Eisenberg (Ed.), *Handbook of child psychology* (Social, emotional and personality development) (Vol. 3, 5th ed., pp. 553–617). Wiley.

Harter, S. (2012). *The construction of the self. Developmental and sociocultural foundations* (2nd ed.). Guilford Press.

Hattie, J. A. (1992). *Self-concept*. Lawrence Erlbaum.

Heim, R. (2002). *Jugendliche Sozialisation und Selbstkonzeptentwicklung im Hochleistungssport* (2. Aufl.). : Meyer & Meyer.

Heinemann, K. (1998). *Einführung in die Soziologie des Sports* (4. Aufl.). : Hofmann.

Helmke, A. (1992). *Selbstvertrauen und schulische Leistungen*. Hogrefe.

Herrmann, T. (1991). *Lehrbuch der empirischen Persönlichkeitsforschung* (6. Aufl.). : Hogrefe.

Hurrelmann, K. (2006). *Einführung in die Sozialisationstheorie* (9. Aufl.). : Beltz.

James, W. (1890). *The principles of psychology*. Holt.

Krampen, G. (2002). Persönlichkeits- und Selbstkonzeptentwicklung. In R. Oerter & L. Montada (Hrsg.), *Entwicklungspsychologie* (5. Aufl., S. 675-710). : Beltz.

Krampen, G. & Greve, W. (2008). Persönlichkeits- und Selbstkonzeptentwicklung über die Lebensspanne. In R. Oerter & L. Montada (Hrsg.), *Entwicklungspsychologie* (6. Aufl., S. 652-686). : Beltz.

Kurz, D. (1973). Gymnastische Erziehung bei Platon und Aristoteles. In H. Lenk, S. Moser, & E. Beyer (Eds.), *Philosophie des Sports* (pp. 163–184). Schorndorf.

Lersch, P. (1938). *Aufbau der Person* (1. Aufl.). : Barth.

Lersch, P. (1964). *Aufbau der Person* (9. Aufl.). : Barth.

Lerner, R. M. (2002). *Concepts and theories of human development* (3rd ed.). Erlbaum.

Lerner, R. M., & Busch-Rossnagel, N. A. (Eds.). (1981). *Individuals as producers of their development*. Academic Press.

Lindwall, M., Asci, F. H., Palmeira, A., Fox, K. R., & Hagger, M. S. (2011). The importance of importance in the physical self. support for the theoretically appealing but empirically elusive model of James. *Journal of Personality, 79*(2), 303–334.

Lintunen, T. (1999). Development of self-perceptions during the school years. In Y. V. Auweele, F. Bakker, S. Biddle, M. Durand, & R. Seiler (Eds.), *Psychology for physical educators* (pp. 115–134). Human Kinetics.

Liu, M., Wu, L., & Ming, Q. (2015). How does physical activity intervention improve self-esteem and self-concept in children and adolescents? Evidence from a meta-analysis. *PLoS One, 10*(8), e0134804. https://doi.org/10.1371/journal.pone.0134804

Lloyd, J., & Fox, K. R. (1992). Achievement goals and motivation to exercise in adolescent girls. A preliminary investigation study. *British Journal of Physical Education Research Supplement, 11*, 12–16.

Magnaguagno, L., Schmidt, M., Valkanover, S., Sygusch, R., & Conzelmann, A. (2016). Programm- und Outputevaluation einer Intervention zur Förderung des sozialen Selbstkonzepts im Sportunterricht. *Zeitschrift für Sportpsychologie, 23*(2), 56–65. https://doi.org/10.1026/1612-5010/a000163

Magnusson, D. (1990). Personality development from an interactional perspective. In L. A. Pervin (Ed.), *Handbook of personality: Theory and research* (pp. 193–222). Guilford.

Magnusson, D. (2001). Interactionism and personality. In N. J. Smelser & P. Baltes (Eds.), *International encyclopedia of the social & behavioral sciences, Band 11* (pp. 7691–7695). Elsevier.

Magnusson, D., & Cairns, R. B. (1996). Developmental science: Toward a unified framework. In R. B. Cairns, G. H. Elder, & E. J. Costello (Eds.), *Developmental science* (pp. 7–30). University Press.

Magnusson, D., & Stattin, H. (2006). The person in context: A Holistic-interactionistic approach. In R. M. Lerner (Ed.), *Handbook of child psychology: Vol. 1. Theoretical models of human development* (6th ed., pp. 400–464). Wiley.

Marsh, H. W. (2008). The elusive importance effect: More failure for the Jamesian perspective on the importance of importance in shaping self-esteem. *Journal of Personality, 76*(5), 1081–1122. https://doi.org/10.1111/j.1467-6494.2008.00514.x

Marsh, H. W., & Peart, N. (1988). Competitive and cooperative physical fitness training programs for girls: Effects on physical fitness and on multidimensional self-concepts. *Journal of Sport*

14

and Exercise Psychology, 10, 390–407. https://doi.org/10.1123/jsep.10.4.390
Marsh, H. W., & Scalas, L. F. (2018). Individually weighted-average models: Testing a taxonomic SEM approach across different multidimensional/global constructs because the weights "don't make no nevermind". *Structural Equation Modeling: A Multidisciplinary Journal, 25*(1), 137–159. https://doi.org/10.1080/10705511.2017.1370377
McFarlin, D. B., Baumeister, R. F., & Blascovich, J. (1984). On knowing when to quit: Task failure, self-esteem, advice, and non-productive persistence. *Journal of Personality, 52*, 138–155. https://doi.org/10.1111/j.1467-6494.1984.tb00349.x
Ministry of Education and Vocational Training of the State of Schleswig-Holstein (Ministerium für Schule und Berufsbildung des Landes Schleswig-Holstein). (2015). *Fachanforderungen Sport für die allgemein bildenden Schulen, Sekundarstufe I & II*. Schmidt & Klaunig.
Müller, M., Schmidt, M., & Conzelmann, A. (2012). Sport und Selbstkonzeptentwicklung—Musteranalysen als methodische Implikation personorientierter Ansätze. *Spectrum der Sportwissenschaften, 24*, 17–40.
Müller, M., Schmidt, M., Zibung, M., & Conzelmann, A. (2013). Muster, Entwicklungstypen und Persönlichkeit—Zur Rolle des Sports für das Selbstkonzept Heranwachsender. *Zeitschrift Sportpsychologie, 20*, 150–162. https://doi.org/10.1026/1612-5010/a000107
National Standards for K-12 Physical Education. (2013). SHAPE America-Society of Health and Physical Educators, Reston, VA. Retrieved from www.shapeamerica.org.
Neumann, O. (1957). *Sport und Persönlichkeit*. Barth.
Nigg, C. R., Norman, G. J., Rossi, J. S., & Benisovich, S. V. (2001). Examining the Structure of Physical Self-Description Using an American University Sample. *Research Quarterly for Exercise and Sport, 72*(1), 78–83. https://doi.org/10.1080/02701367.2001.10608936
NSW Board of Studies. (2014). Personal Development, Health and Physical Education K-6 Syllabus. Sydney: Board of Studies NSW. Retrieved August 17, 2020, from https://educationstandards.nsw.edu.au/wps/wcm/connect/f63e7d9d-fa2a-471b-bf3c-d5b362fddb00/k6_pdhpe_syl.pdf?MOD=AJPERES&CVID
O'Mara, A. J., Marsh, H. W., Craven, R. G., & Debus, R. (2006). Do self-concept interventions make a difference? A synergistic blend of construct validation and meta-analysis. *Educational Psychologist, 41*(3), 181–206. https://doi.org/10.1207/s15326985ep4103_4
Overton, W. F. (2015). Process, relations, and relational-developmental-systems. In I. W. F. Overton & P. C. M. Molenar (Eds.), *Handbook of child psychology and developmental science. Volume 1: Theory and method* (7th ed., pp. 9–62). Wiley.
Overton, W. F., & Molenar, P. C. M. (2015). *Handbook of child psychology and developmental science. Volume 1: Theory and Method* (7th ed.). Wiley.
Pawlik, K. (1996). Differentielle Psychologie und Persönlichkeitsforschung: Grundbegriffe, Fragestellungen, Systematik. In K. Pawlik (Ed.), *Grundlagen und Methoden der Differentiellen Psychologie* (pp. 3–30). Hogrefe.
Petermann, F. & Rudinger, G. (2002). Quantitative und qualitative Methoden der Entwicklungspsychologie. In R. Oerter & L. Montada (Hrsg.), *Entwicklungspsychologie* (5. Aufl., S. 999-1028). : Beltz.
Plumert, J. M. (1995). Relations between children's overestimation of their physical abilities and accident proneness. *Developmental Psychology, 31*, 866–876.
Plumert, J. M., Kearney, J. K., & Cremer, J. F. (2004). Children's perception of gap avoidances: Bicycling across traffic-filled intersections in an immersive virtual environment. *Child Development, 75*, 1243–1253.
Plumert, J. M., & Schwebel, D. C. (1997). Social and temperamental influences on children's overestimation of their physical abilities: Links to accidental injuries. *Journal of Experimental Child Psychology, 67*, 317–337.
Rivara, F. P. (1985). Traumatic deaths of children in the United States: Currently available prevention strategies. *Pediatrics, 75*, 456–462.
Roebers, C. M. (2007). Entwicklung des Selbstkonzeptes. In M. Hasselhorn & W. Schneider (Eds.), *Handbuch der Entwicklungspsychologie* (pp. 381–391). Hogrefe.
Rubeli, B., Oswald, E., Conzelmann, A., & Schmidt, M. (2019). Predicting global self-esteem in early adolescence: The importance of individual and gender-specific importance of perceived sports competence. *Sport, Exercise, and Performance Psychology, 9*(4), 519–531. https://doi.org/10.1037/spy0000196
Rubeli, B., Oswald, E., Conzelmann, A., Schmid, J., Valkanover, S., & Schmidt, M. (2020). Promoting schoolchildren's self-esteem in physical education: Testing the effectiveness of a five-month teacher training. *Physical Education and Sport Pedagogy, 25*(4), 346–360. https://doi.org/10.1080/17408989.2020.1712348
Scalas, L. F., Marsh, H. W., Nagengast, B., & Morin, A. J. (2013). Latent-Variable Approaches to the Jamesian Model of Importance-Weighted Averages. *Personality and Social Psychology Bulletin, 39*(1), 100–114.
Scalas, L. F., Morin, A. J. S., Marsh, H. W., & Nagengast, B. (2014). Importance models of the physical self: Improved methodology supports a normative-cultural importance model, but not the individual importance model. *European Journal of Social Psychology, 44*, 154–174.
Schmidt, M., Blum, M., Valkanover, S., & Conzelmann, A. (2015). Motor ability and self-esteem: The mediating role of physical self-concept and perceived social acceptance. *Psychology of Sport & Exercise, 17*, 15–23. https://doi.org/10.1016/j.psychsport.2014.11.006
Schmidt, M., & Conzelmann, A. (2011). Selbstkonzeptförderung im Sportunterricht. Eine psychologische Betrachtung einer pädagogischen Zielperspektive. *Sportwissenschaft, 41*, 190–201. https://doi.org/10.1007/s12662-011-0195-7
Schmidt, M., Valkanover, S., Roebers, C. M., & Conzelmann, A. (2013). Promoting a functional physical self-concept in physical education: Evaluation of a 10-week intervention. *European Physical Education Review, 19*(2), 232–255. https://doi.org/10.1177/1356336X13486057
Schneewind, K. A. (2001). Persönlichkeit. In G. Wenninger (Ed.), *Lexikon der Psychologie* (pp. 237–240). Spektrum.
Schneider, K. (1950). *Klinische Psychopathologie*. Thieme.
Schwebel, D. C., & Bounds, M. L. (2003). The role of parents and temperament on children's estimation of physical ability: Links to unintentional injury prevention. *Journal of Pediatric Psychology, 28*, 505–516.
Schwebel, D. C., & Plumert, J. M. (1999). Longitudinal and concurrent relations among temperament, ability estimation, and injury proneness. *Child Development, 70*, 700–712. https://doi.org/10.1111/1467-8624.00050
Schütz, A., & Sellin, I. (2003). Selbst und Informationsverarbeitung. *Zeitschrift für Differentielle und Diagnostische Psychologie, 24*, 151–161.
Shavelson, R. J., Hubner, J. J., & Stanton, G. C. (1976). Self-concept: Validation of construct interpretations. *Review of Educational Research, 46*, 407–441. https://doi.org/10.3102/00346543046003407

Shoda, Y., & Mischel, W. (2000). Reconciling contextualism with the core assumptions of personality psychology. *European Journal of Personality, 14*, 407–428. https://doi.org/10.1002/1099--0984(200009/10)14:53.0.CO;2-3

Singer, R. (2004). Sport und Persönlichkeit. In H. Gabler, J. R. Nitsch & R. Singer (Hrsg.), *Einführung in die Sportpsychologie. Teil 1 Grundthemen* (3. Aufl., S. 289-336). : Hofmann.

Sonstroem, R. J., Harlow, L. L., & Josephs, L. (1994). Exercise and self-esteem. Validity of model expansion and exercise associations. *Journal of Sport & Exercise Psychology, 16*(1), 29–42. https://doi.org/10.1123/jsep.16.1.29

Sonstroem, R. J., & Morgan, W. P. (1989). Exercise and self-esteem. Rationale and model. *Medicine and Science in Sports and Exercise, 21*, 329–337. https://doi.org/10.1249/00005768-198906000-00018

Spence, J. C., McGannon, K. R., & Poon, P. (2005). The effect of exercise on global self-esteem: A quantitative review. *Journal of Sport and Exercise Psychology, 27*, 311–334. https://doi.org/10.1123/jsep.27.3.311

Spruit, A., Assink, M., van Vugt, E., van der Put, C., & Stams, G. J. (2016). The effects of physical activity interventions on psychosocial outcomes in adolescents: A meta-analytic review. *Clinical Psychology Review, 45*, 56–71. https://doi.org/10.1016/j.cpr.2016.03.006

Stephan, Y., Sutin, A. R., & Terracciano, A. (2014). Physical activity and personality development across adulthood and old age: Evidence from two longitudinal studies. *Journal of Research in Personality, 49*, 1–7. https://doi.org/10.1016/j.jrp.2013.12.003

Steinbach, M. (1968). *Pathocharakterologische Motivation sportlicher Höchstleistungen bei mehrdimensionaler Betrachtung maßgeblicher Bedingungen*. Manuskript, Universität Mainz.

Stemmler, G., Hagemann, D., Amelang, M. & Bartussek, D. (2010). *Differentielle Psychologie und Persönlichkeitsforschung* (7. Aufl.). : Kohlhammer.

Stiller, J., & Alfermann, D. (2007). Promotion of a healthy self-concept. In J. Liukkonen, Y. V. Auweele, B. Vereijken, D. Alfermann, & Y. Theodorakis (Eds.), *Psychology for physical educators. Student in focus* (Vol. 2, pp. 123–140). Human Kinetics.

Sulzer, J. G. (1748). *Versuch von der Erziehung und Unterweisung der Kinder*. Orell.

Sygusch, R. (2008). Selbstkonzeptförderung im Jugendsport—Zufall oder zielgerichtet? In A. Conzelmann & F. Hänsel (Eds.), *Sport und Selbstkonzept. Struktur, Dynamik und Entwicklung* (pp. 140–156). Hofmann.

Tenenbaum, G., & Bar-Eli, M. (1995). Personality and intellectual capabilities in sport psychology. In D. H. Saklofske & M. Zeidner (Eds.), *International Handbook of Personality and Intelligence* (pp. 687–710). Plenum.

Thomas, M. (1989). *Zentralität und Selbstkonzept*. Huber.

Vealey, R. S. (1989). Sport personology: A paradigmatic and methodological analysis. *Journal of Sport and Exercise Psychology, 11*, 216–235. https://doi.org/10.1123/jsep.11.2.216

Vealey, R. S. (1992). Personality and sport: A comprehensive view. In T. S. Horn (Ed.), *Advances in sport psychology* (pp. 25–59). Human Kinetics.

Vealey, R. S. (2002). Personality and sport behavior. In T. S. Horn (Ed.), *Advances in sport psychology* (2nd ed., pp. 43–82). Human Kinetics.

Von Eye, A., & Spiel, C. (2010). Conducting person-oriented research. *Zeitschrift für Psychologie – Journal of Psychology, 218*(3), 151–154. https://doi.org/10.1027/0044-3409/a000024

Weinberg, R. S., & Gould, D. (2003). *Foundations of sport and exercise psychology* (3rd ed.). Human Kinetics.

Weiner, B. (1985). An attributional theory of achievement motivation and emotion. *Psychological Review, 92*(4), 548–573.

Whitehead, J. R., & Corbin, C. (1997). Self-esteem in children and youth. The role of sport and physical education. In K. R. Fox (Ed.), *The physical self: From motivation to well-being* (pp. 175–203). Human Kinetics.

Willimczik, K. (2001). Sportwissenschaft interdisziplinär—Ein wissenschaftstheoretischer Dialog. In *Band 1 Geschichte, Struktur und Gegenstand der Sportwissenschaft*. Czwalina.

Witherington, D. C. (2015). Dynamic systems in developmental science. In W. F. Overton & P. C. M. Molenar (Eds.), *Handbook of child psychology and developmental science. Volume 1: Theory and Method* (7th ed., pp. 63–112). Wiley.

Physical Activity Across the Life Span: Personality, Physical Activity, and Sedentary Behavior

Ines Pfeffer and Ryan E. Rhodes

Contents

J. Schüler et al. (eds.), *Sport and Exercise Psychology*, https://doi.org/10.1007/978-3-031-03921-8_15

Learning Objectives

Basic:

- Describing the prevalence of physical activity and sedentary behavior for different age groups
- Justifying of personality as a determinant of various physical activity behaviors and a sedentary lifestyle

Advanced:

- Explaining the associations between personality, health behavior, and health
- Outlining evidence for personality-based interventions for physical activity
- Discussing motivational approaches that explain the relationship between personality and physical activity behavior

Experts:

- Outlining a heuristic model of personality, physical activity, sedentary behavior, and health across the life span

15.1 Introduction

Regular physical activity is a protective factor for physical and mental health (Powell et al., 2011; Rhodes et al., 2017). Physical inactivity is the fourth largest risk factor for the development of cardiovascular diseases and is associated with an increased risk for diseases of civilization such as obesity, diabetes mellitus type 2, and breast or colon cancer (World Health Organization, 2010; on the effects of physical activity on various facets of health see ► Chaps. 26 and 27). Furthermore, a sedentary lifestyle seems to be an additional serious risk factor for the development of diseases, regardless of how physically active an individual is (Biswas et al., 2015; Ekelund et al., 2019; Sutin et al., 2016). Therefore, a physically active lifestyle as well as the reduction of the time spent sedentary during the day can be defined as an important public health goal. A sound knowledge of the influencing factors of both types of health behavior is relevant for developing theory-guided and effective prevention and health promotion programs.

15

Research has increasingly focused on the role of personality traits for health and health behavior such as physical activity and sedentary behaviors (Bogg & Roberts, 2013). Physical activity and sedentary behavior are therefore discussed as possible mediators (mechanisms) between personality and health (Wilson & Dishman, 2015). In ◘ Fig. 15.1, the mediating effect of health behavior (Z) for the relationship between personality (X) and health (Y) is displayed.

Mediator Variable

A mediator variable (Z) is a third variable, which is assumed to explain the relationship (effect) between a variable (X) and a variable (Y).

In this chapter (as shown in ◘ Fig. 15.1), relevant terms and different concepts of physical activity and sedentary behavior are introduced (► Sect. 15.2), and the patterns of physical activity and sedentary behavior are described for different age groups (► Sect. 15.3). Based on the Big Five personality dimensions, findings about the relationship of personality traits (► Chap. 13) with health (► Sect. 15.4.1; ◘ Fig. 15.1, arrow 1; Chapman et al., 2011) and health behavior (physical activity or sedentary behavior; ► Sect. 15.4.2; ◘ Fig. 15.1, arrow 2) are discussed. The association between physical activity and (mental) health (◘ Fig. 15.1, arrow 3) is addressed in detail in ► Chaps. 26 and 27 of this book. The mediating effect of physical activity behavior as a mechanism of the relationship between personality and health will be highlighted (► Sect. 15.4.3). Explanations for the association between personality and physical activity behavior are focused on (► Sect. 15.5), and approaches for interventions are discussed (► Sect. 15.6).

◘ **Fig. 15.1** Health behavior as mediator between personality and health

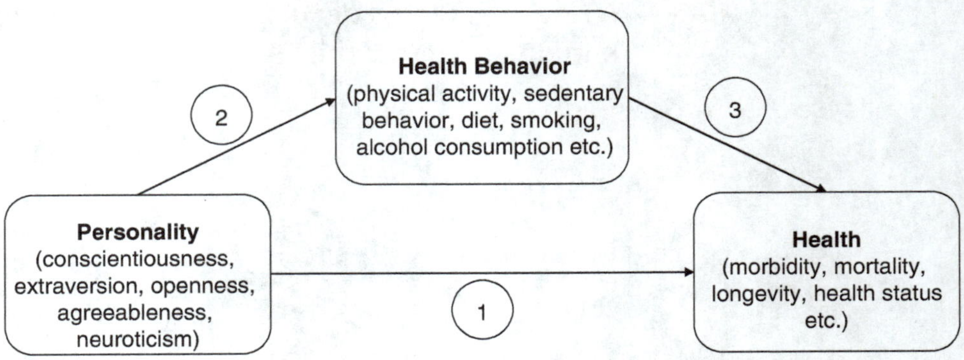

Summarizing the chapter, a heuristic model is presented (► Sect. 15.7) that might be directive to derive hypotheses for future research about personality, health behavior, and health across the life span. Finally, practical implications are discussed (► Sect. 15.8).

15.2 Key Concepts and Terminology

In the context of exercise and health, various terms and concepts are used in the literature which first need to be clarified. In particular, the terms physical activity, sport, exercise, physical inactivity, and sedentary behavior have to be introduced.

Physical Activity

Physical activity is the general term for any bodily action that is produced by the skeletal muscles and significantly increases the basal metabolic rate. It is an umbrella term for different human behaviors and includes sport activities, exercises, as well as everyday physical activities such as gardening, domestic work, or trips that are made by foot (walking) or by bicycle (Bouchard & Sheppard, 1994). There is a positive correlation between physical activity and physical fitness (Biddle & Mutrie, 2007). A person is considered to be physically active if he or she meets the current recommendations for health-promoting physical activity of almost daily for at least 30 min (150 min/week) with moderate-to-vigorous intensity (≥3 MET (metabolic equivalent of task); see ► Methods Box: Metabolic Equivalent).

Sports

Sports is historically and culturally defined subcategory of physical activity that is associated with high performance, competition, record, and adherence to specific rules. These activities are performed with the aim to use and improve physical abilities and skills. This comprises participation in typical sports such as gymnastics, athletics, tennis, football, volleyball, and judo, which are often practiced with high intensities (≥6 MET).

Exercise

Exercise is a subcategory of physical activity, which is planned, structured, and repeatedly performed for the purpose of conditioning and increasing as well as maintaining physical fitness and health. Aspects of sports are partly adopted without necessarily taking the characteristics of sport such as competition or specific rules into account.

Physical Inactivity

Individuals are described as physically inactive if they fail to follow the recommendations for health-promoting physical activity because they are either physically active less often (< 600 MET minutes per week with moderate-to-vigorous intensity) or with lower intensities (1.6–2.9 METs).

Sedentary Behavior

Sedentary behavior is a behavior in which an awake person is sitting, reclining, or lying and has low energy expenditure (1–≤ 1.5 METs; Bames et al., 2012). This includes behavior such as watching television, playing computer games, driving, reading, or working at a computer.

In this chapter, the term physical activity is used as a higher-order term. Specific terms (sport or exercise) are used where a distinction is necessary. With regard to the dose-response relationship, that is, the question of how much physical activity should be performed to reach an optimal health benefit, the WHO (2010) has published global evidence-based recommendations for health-promoting physical activities for different populations (e.g., age groups) based on a review of the literature. The recommendations are valid for the prevention of cardiovascular diseases (e.g., coronary heart disease, stroke, high blood pressure), metabolic diseases (e.g., obesity and diabetes mellitus type 2), diseases of the postural and locomotor system (e.g., osteoporosis, arthrosis), mental illnesses (e.g., depression), and cancer (e.g., breast and colon cancer) or the prevention of falls in older age.

WHO Recommendations on Physical Activity

WHO recommendations for children and adolescents aged 5–17 years include physical activities such as play, sports, transportation (e.g., bicycling or walking), physical education, and leisure activities. Children and adolescents should be physically active for at least 60 min a day with moderate-to-vigorous intensity. Activities lasting more than 1 h provide additional health benefits. These activities should predominantly include aerobic endurance activities improving cardiovascular health. Unstructured physical activities strengthening resistance of muscles and bones (e.g., sprinting, climbing, use of playground equipment) should be additionally performed on 3 days a week. Several shorter periods of activity (e.g., of 15 min each) can be accumulated over the day (e.g., 4 × 15 min a day = 60 min).

Adults aged 18–64 years should be physically active for at least 150 min per week at moderate intensity (3–5.9 METs, or on the rating of perceived exertion scale (RPE scale; Borg, 1982) from 0 to 10 relative to an individuals' capacity at a value of 5–6; sweating and breathing harder) or at least 75 min with vigorous intensity (≥ 6 METs, or on the rating of perceived exertion scale relative to an individuals' capacity from

0 to 10 at a value of 7–8; sweating heavily and breathing much harder) or a combination of moderate and vigorous physical activities. By increasing the physical activity level to 300 min per week (or 150 min with vigorous intensity), the effects on health can be further increased. Twice a week physical activities strengthening the large muscle groups and bones should be performed. Activity bouts should last at least 10 min at a time.

The WHO recommendations for people of 65 years and older are comparable with those for young- and middle-aged adults. Additional aims for this target group are to counteract age-related cognitive decline and to prevent falls in older people with impaired mobility balance skills that should be trained three or more days a week. If these recommendations can no longer be achieved due to illnesses and/or age-related health restrictions, older people should be as physically active as possible and to an extent that corresponds with their abilities and health status.

Physically inactive people fail to achieve the abovementioned physical activity recommendations, because they are either physically active less often or with lower intensities (Bucksch & Schlicht, 2014). Previously, a physically inactive lifestyle was put on a level with a sedentary lifestyle. However, studies have shown that sedentary behavior patterns must be seen as an independent risk factor additionally contributing in explaining overall mortality (mortality) and chronic illnesses beyond the physical activity level (Allen et al., 2017; Ekelund et al., 2019). Sedentary behaviors are defined as a group of waking behaviors while in a sitting, reclining, or lying posture, which are associated with an energy expenditure of less than 1.5 METs (Bames et al., 2012). The daily time spent with sedentary behaviors is associated with various chronic diseases and health conditions (e.g., overweight and obesity, depressive symptoms, diabetes mellitus, cardiovascular diseases), regardless of the physical activity level of an individual. Due to our modern lifestyle, sedentary behaviors can be seen as a widespread risk factor. However, based on the current knowledge, a specification of the dose-response relationship between sedentary behavior patterns and health outcomes is not yet defined, although Canada has recently put this at maximum of 8 h based on an extensive review of all available literature (Ross et al., 2020). It is recommended to reduce the sedentary time during work and during leisure time and transportation and to interrupt sedentary behaviors as often as possible by standing and/or physical activity.

The metabolic equivalent (MET) of a task can be used to further define and compare the intensities of physical activities. Sedentary behavior is indicated with a metabolic equivalent of 1–1.5 METs. Physical activities with low intensity are classified between 1.6 and 2.9 METs. For moderate physical activities, 3–5.9 METs are given and for high-intensity activities ≥6 METs (Fig. 15.2; ► Methods Box: Metabolic Equivalent).

Metabolic Equivalent

The metabolic equivalent (MET) of task describes the metabolic rate of a person in relation to the resting rate (sitting quietly) in relation to his/her body weight. One MET corresponds to a calorie consumption of 1 kcal per kilogram body weight per hour. METs thus indicate the calorie consumption of physical activities as a multiple of the basal metabolic rate and are used to compare the energy expenditure of different physical activities (Fig. 15.2). A compendium of various physical activities and their metabolic equivalent was provided by Ainsworth's research group (Ainsworth et al., 2011, 1993, 2000). MET minutes describe the minutes accumulated with increased energy expenditure and thus specify the accumulated physical activity MET minutes per week.

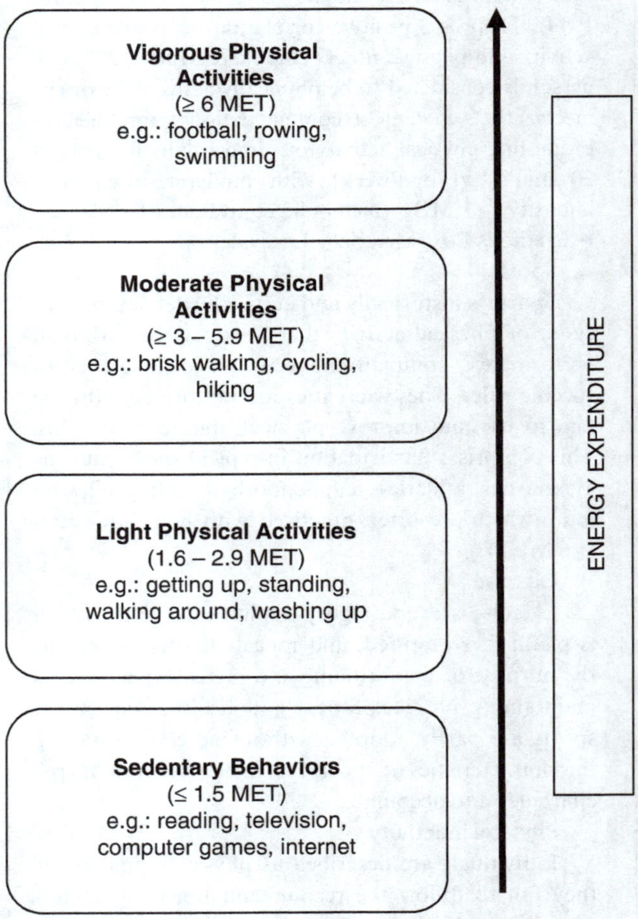

Fig. 15.2 Physical activity, sedentary behavior, and energy expenditure. (Based on Bucksch & Schlicht, 2014, p. 16)

15.3 Prevalence of Physical Activity, Inactivity, and Sedentary Behavior

In 2012, the World Health Organization provided a review with data from 122 countries representing 89% of the world's population, which was updated in 2016 and 2018/2020 (Guthold et al., 2018, 2020; Hallal et al., 2012; Sallis et al., 2016). Data from about two-thirds of countries worldwide enabled a comparative assessment of physical activity behavior (Hallal et al., 2012). Physical activity prevalence for the adult population was mainly based on the IPAQ (International Physical Activity Questionnaire; Craig et al., 2003) and the GPAQ (Global Physical Activity Questionnaire; Bull et al., 2009), two well-established and widely used subjective measures of physical activity behavior.

Childhood and Adolescence

In the study of 2012, 80% of 13–15-year-olds do not do 60 min of moderate-to-vigorous physical activity per day. Girls are less active than boys. Estimates were much higher than were those reported in adults (Hallal et al., 2012). The proportion of adolescents not achieving 60 min per day was equal to or greater than 80% in 56 (53%) of 105 countries in boys and 100 (95%) of 105 countries for girls. In 2016 (Sallis et al., 2016), estimates were available for adolescents aged 11–17 years from 120 countries, with data mainly from the Global School-based Student Health Survey (GSHS) and the Health Behaviour in School-aged Children (HBSC) Study. Consistent with 2012, inactivity prevalence continued to be extremely high, with a global average of 78% for boys and 84% for girls. In the vast majority of countries (115 of 120 countries with data), more than a quarter of adolescents did not reach the recommended level of activity (Fig. 15.3). Global prevalence of physical inactivity was about 80% for adolescents (Guthold et al., 2020; Sallis et al., 2016). According to country income group, no clear pattern was observed (Guthold et al., 2020).

The HBSC data from 40 countries in Europe and North America revealed that about two-thirds of the boys (66%) and girls (68%) aged 13–15 years spent 2 h or more per day in front of the television (Hallal et al., 2012). In 2016, the sedentary time spent was not examined. Guthold et al. (2010) reported that in more than half of the 34 studied countries of the WHO regions, more than a third of students spent 3 h or more per day doing sedentary activities during their leisure time. Another study revealed that nearly half (47%) of US children exceed ≥2 h/day of time in sedentary behavior (Sisson et al., 2009). The systematic review by Arundell et al. (2016) found that on average, children spent between 41% and 51% of the after-school period in sedentary time, while adolescents spent 57% of the after-school period with sitting. TV viewing and other screen-based behaviors make up to 26% of this period, while non-screen-based sedentary behaviors (e.g., social sedentary behaviors, motorized transport, homework, and reading) comprise 54% of the after-school period. Therefore, the after-school period holds great potential for interventions that aim to reduce sedentary time.

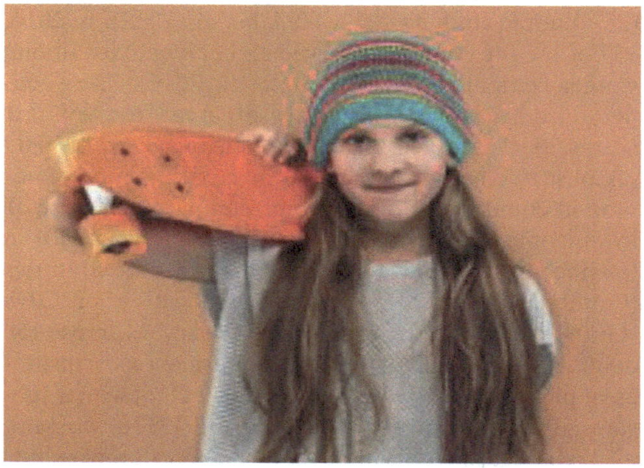

Fig. 15.3 Physical activity in childhood is very important

> Only a small percentage of children and adolescents achieve the WHO recommended level of health-promoting physical activity of at least 60 min per day. In addition, a large proportion of children and adolescents spend too much sedentary time on television or other media consumption during their leisure time.

Young- and Middle-Aged Adults

With regard to vigorous-intensity physical activity, 31% of adults report to be active on three or more days per week, with large differences between WHO regions. For example, 38% of individuals in Africa report such activity, 25% in North America, 25% in Europe, and 43% in Southeast Asia. In all age groups, men are more likely to reach the recommendation in vigorous-intensity physical activity than women (Hallal et al., 2012).

Worldwide, 31% of adults are physically inactive and do not reach the WHO recommendation of moderate-to-vigorous physical activity. For example, 43% of people in North America, 28% in Africa, 35% in Europe, and 17% in Southeast Asia are not sufficiently active to gain health benefits. Between 2012 and 2016, estimated global prevalence of inactivity among adult populations worldwide decreased from 31% to 23% (Hallal et al., 2012; Sallis et al., 2016). However, this reduction can be primarily explained by changes in the definition of sufficient physical activity rather than a real decrease in inactivity. Women were more inactive (34%) than men

(28%) in the study in 2012 (Hallal et al., 2012). In 2016, 137 of the 146 countries showed higher inactivity among women compared to men (Sallis et al., 2016). These gender differences were especially observed for younger adults. Physical inactivity increased with age in all WHO regions. Furthermore, physical inactivity is more common in countries of high income compared to those of low income (Hallal et al., 2012). Prevalence was 16% in low-income countries and 37% in high-income countries (Guthold et al., 2018). In the publication of 2018 (Guthold et al., 2018), data from 358 surveys across 168 countries were included. Global prevalence of insufficient physical activity was calculated at 28%, with a substantial sex difference (23% in men and 32% in women).

With regard to sitting time, the proportion of adults spending four or more hours per day sitting is 42%. The value varied greatly between WHO regions: 38% of individuals sit for four or more hours per day in Africa, 55% in North America, 64% in Europe, and 24% in Southeast Asia. For adults aged 15–59 years, the proportion spending 4 h or more per day sitting does not vary substantially. No sex differences were observed (Hallal et al., 2012). Data from the Eurobarometer across 32 European countries resulted in an average reported weekday sitting time of 309 min/day (SD 184 min/day; Bennie et al., 2013).

> Worldwide, only about 72% of the adult population is physically active according to WHO recommendations. Men achieve the WHO recommendations significantly more often than women. The time spent sitting also decreases with increasing age.

Older Adults (60 Years and Older)

Participation in vigorous physical activity strongly decreases from ages 60 years and older. Adults aged 60 years and older from Southeast Asia are much more active than are individuals of the same age from all other WHO regions and actually more active than are young adults (aged 15–29 years) from North America or Europe (Hallal et al., 2012). In the study of 2016, older age groups continue to be at higher risk for inactivity, with the oldest age category (80 years or older) showing more than double the prevalence (55%) of the youngest (19%; 18–29 years) (Sallis et al., 2016).

The percentage of people spending >4 h per day sitting is highest in the age group of 60 years and older (Hallal et al., 2012). Almost 60% of older adults reported sitting for more than 4 h per day (Harvey et al., 2013). With regard to the type of sedentary behavior, 65% sit in front of a screen for more than 3 h daily, and over 55% report watching more than 2 h of TV. However, based on objective data, it was found that 67% of the older population were sedentary for more than 8.5 h per day (Stamatakis et al., 2012).

> The percentage of people who do not achieve the WHO recommendations of health-promoting physical activity increases continuously in later adulthood, with an essential decline in vigorous physical activities. Furthermore, the sedentary time also increases in older age compared to young- and middle-aged adults.

Conclusion

The available epidemiological data on physical activity and sedentary behavior are predominantly based on cross-sectional data and self-report measures (i.e., questionnaire), while the instruments used varied across countries. Therefore, it has to be considered that the age differences might not represent real age effects but could merely reflect cohort effects. Cohorts are groups of persons born in the same period. Cohort effects are therefore differences between persons of different cohorts, which are based on different environmental or social influences. Large-scale longitudinal studies have been lacking to date. Furthermore, more population-based studies using direct measures of physical activity behavior (e.g., accelerometers), which may provide more reliable and valid ways to assess the frequency, duration, and intensity of physical activity behavior, are needed (Hallal et al., 2012). Nevertheless, the current data prove the necessity of promoting a physically active lifestyle and reducing sedentary behaviors in all age groups and across most countries in the world. In order to develop theory-guided programs for physical activity promotion, a broad knowledge of relevant factors influencing a physically active lifestyle is necessary. In recent years, there has been increasing evidence, particularly on the basis of the Big Five personality dimensions (► Chap. 13), that health and physical activity behavior are related to personality traits.

15.4 Personality, Health, and Physical Activity

Psychological factors play an important role in the development of various diseases and particularly of widespread lifestyle diseases. To clarify which factors contribute to increased morbidity and premature mortality is of particular interest. The question of *who* gets sick and *why* has received much attention in psychological research. Which psychological characteristics make people susceptible to diseases? And which mechanisms might explain these relationships? The answers on these research questions can help to develop effective disease prevention and health promotion programs and to identify individuals at risk timely, who can then benefit from appropriate programs. Central psychological factors that are investigated in this context are personality traits and health behaviors.

Personality traits are defined as relatively stable, gradually developed personal characteristics that influence a person's thinking, feeling, will, and behavior across a wide range of contexts and situations. They can also be understood as phenotypic dimensions of interindividual differences that reflect both genetic and environmental influences (▶ Chap. 13). The Big Five personality dimensions *openness*, *conscientiousness*, *extraversion*, *agreeableness*, and *neuroticism* have been a fruitful conception of personality for research in the last decades (▶ Chaps. 13 and 14). These personality dimensions were shown to be related to different health parameters, and some longitudinal studies even revealed a relevant association between personality and morbidity, mortality or longevity (Chapman et al., 2011; Jokela et al., 2013).

? Which dimensions and *facets* (examples) does the five-factor model of personality comprise?
- Openness: *creative*, *flexible*, *cultivated*, *open-minded*, and *curious*
- Conscientiousness: *diligent*, *dutiful*, *systematic*, *focused*, *reliable*, *careful*, and *ambitious*
- Extraversion: *sociable*, *active*, *cordial*, *sensation seeking*, *determined*, and *cheerful*
- Agreeableness: *trusting*, *sincere*, *altruistic*, *modest*, *sensitive*, and *cooperative*
- Neuroticism: *anxious*, *irritable*, *pessimistic inhibited*, *impulsive*, and *vulnerable*

15.4.1 Personality and Health

In this section, empirical findings about the relationship between personality and health are reviewed (◘ Fig. 15.1, arrow 1). Studies have shown that conscientiousness is associated with lower blood pressure, fewer diabetes cases, and a reduced number of strokes (Goodwin & Friedman, 2006). And even in cases of pre-existing disease, conscientiousness can have a positive influence on life expectancy (Christensen & Moran, 2001). This could be due to a better disease management of conscientious compared to less conscientious people. Conscientiousness is defined as a relatively stable tendency to being orderly, dutiful, and achievement/goal striving as well as to control impulses and to plan and to be able to postpone rewards.

The meta-analysis (▶ Methods Box: Systematic Review and Meta-analysis) by Jokela et al. (2013) was the first to summarize the relationship between the Big Five personality dimensions and all-cause mortality across seven large-scale prospective cohort studies with a total of 76,000 individuals. All-cause mortality quantifies the mortality from all causes of death taken together. Conscientiousness proved to be a consistent correlate of all-cause mortality. With regard to the degree of conscientiousness, the lowest third (tercile) of the sample showed a 37% higher mortality risk than persons in the middle and upper tercile. The strength of the association between conscientiousness and longevity is comparable with the association between socioeconomic status or IQ and longevity (Chapman et al., 2011). No consistent effects were observed for the other four personality traits.

Systematic Review
A systematic review is a type of scientific article based on a clear review question in which systematic methods are used to identify and critically evaluate as well as summarize findings in order to provide a complete, exhaustive, transparent, and replicable summary of current evidence.

Meta-analysis
A meta-analysis is a statistical procedure based on a systematic review in which the results of the included studies are summarized quantitatively to provide the overall effect size across all included studies (Kunz et al., 2009).

Due to the increasing evidence, Bogg and Roberts (2013) emphasize conscientiousness as an important epidemiological factor. A possible explanation for the missing or less consistent links between the other Big Five personality dimensions and mortality or longevity could be that the dimensions consist of different facets, each of which may be associated with mortality and longevity to different degrees and in different directions. More differentiated analyses, based on subordinate facets of the Big Five personality dimensions, could provide a deeper insight.

› Conscientiousness has been shown to be a consistent factor explaining health status, all-cause mortality, and longevity. Conscientiousness should therefore be considered as an epidemiological factor in both public health and medical research (Bogg & Roberts, 2013).

15.4.2 Personality, Physical Activity, and Sedentary Behavior

Various studies investigated the associations between the Big Five personality dimensions and physical activity, physical inactivity, or sedentary behavior (Fig. 15.1, arrow 2).

15.4.2.1 Personality and Physical Activity

A meta-analysis on the topic of personality and physical activity, which summarized 33 studies (Rhodes & Smith, 2006), found positive correlations between conscientiousness and extraversion and physical activity behavior as well as a negative correlation for neuroticism. No correlations were found for the dimensions agreeableness and openness. However, the findings were very heterogeneous across the studies. Robust moderator analyses on sample characteristics such as age and gender or characteristics of the study (e.g., study design or type of physical activity measure) could not be conducted due to the small number of effects included in the analyses. Only six of the included studies had a prospective design with an interval of at least 1 year, nine studies were based on a prospective design of a few days up to 28 weeks between the points of measurement, and 18 studies were based on a cross-sectional design only (Background Information: Correlation Coefficient r).

> **Correlation Coefficient *r***
> The correlation coefficient r reflects the relationship between two variables and indicates the extent to which the expression of a variable X corresponds to the value of a variable Y. Correlation coefficients indicate how strongly an empirical relationship is pronounced. In case of a positive correlation, the following applies: The higher/lower the value of variable A, the higher/lower the value of variable B. In case of a negative correlation, the higher/lower variable A is pronounced, the lower/higher variable B is pronounced. By convention, Cohen (1988) describes a correlation coefficient of $r = 0.10$ as small, $r = 0.30$ as medium, and $r = 0.50$ as large.

15

Wilson and Dishman (2015) extended the meta-analysis of Rhodes and Smith (2006) and included 64 studies with a total of 88,4000 subjects in their meta-analysis. Comparable positive effects were shown for extraversion ($r = 0.11$) and conscientiousness ($r = 0.10$) and very small effects for openness ($r = 0.03$) and neuroticism ($r = -0.07$). No significant correlation was found for the dimension agreeableness. A further meta-analysis (Sutin et al., 2016), which summarized results from a total of 16 large-scale national surveys, concluded that all Big Five personality dimensions are related to the physical activity level: small effects for extraversion ($\beta = 0.11$), conscientiousness ($\beta = 0.10$), and openness ($\beta = 0.09$) and very small relations for neuroticism ($\beta = -0.07$) and agreeableness ($\beta = 0.04$). The beta coefficient is the standardized regression weight and indicates the relative contribution of an independent variable (predictor) to the prediction of a dependent variable (criterion). The interpretation is similar to that of the correlation coefficient.

The observed correlations between physical activity and personality can be classified as small but appear plausible and are in line with the results of general personality research in other contexts. How can these correlations be explained? In contrast to introversion, extraversion is accompanied by the search for strong sensory stimulation and social contacts (Eysenck et al., 1982). Both can be realized in the context of physical activity. Therefore, extraverted persons may seek for physical activity contexts more often than introverted persons. Conscientious people are characterized as disciplined, dutiful, and thoughtful. They may become more involved in health behaviors such as physical activity (Bogg & Roberts, 2004, 2013), as they are considered to be useful and socially desirable. Conscientious people also have better abilities to self-regulate, which could lead to a more successful adoption and maintenance of physical activity (Rhodes et al., 2002). Furthermore, the physical activity context is suitable for satisfying the need for experiencing competence, which is distinct in conscientious individuals (Ingledew et al., 2004). People with higher values in openness to new experiences are usually receptive to new ideas and opportunities to gather new experiences and are, therefore, often inclined to try out new behaviors. The physical activity context, due to the high number of different sports and types of exercises, offers many opportunities to try out new things and gain a wide variety of experiences. It therefore seems obvious that people with high levels of openness tend to engage in different sports and forms of exercise and are therefore more physically active than less open people (Wilson & Dishman, 2015). Persons with high values in the variable neuroticism show increased anxiety and emotional instability. In addition, neuroticism is associated with an increased sensitivity to intense stimuli and a tendency to negative affect (Wilson & Dishman, 2015). These characteristics could potentially undermine participation in physical activity and sport, especially if increased exertion and physiological arousal during these activities are experienced as negative.

> Extraversion and conscientiousness are positively associated with physical activity behavior. Effects for openness, neuroticism, and agreeableness are inconsistent and/or very small.

Personality and Specific Physical Activity Behavior

Physical activity is a collection of movement behavior with different skill requirements and energy expenditure costs (Ainsworth et al., 2011; Pate et al., 1995), so any exploration of personality traits and physical activity may benefit from a more refined examination of specific behaviors. Further, personality would conceivably be more strongly linked to certain physical activity behaviors than others. As an example, Rhodes and Smith (2006) found that extraversion was positively associated with aerobic activity, while neuroticism was negatively associated with this aerobic activity. In an even more focused appraisal, Howard et al. (1987) showed that extraverts were more likely to engage in swimming, aerobic conditioning, dancing, and tennis than introverts. By contrast, introverts were more likely to engage in gardening and various forms of home improvement as physical activities of choice. Howard and colleagues showed no associations between personality and walking, jogging, golf, and cycling, suggesting that these types of activities were equally prevalent regardless of extraversion or neuroticism. This same finding was replicated by Rhodes et al. (2007) by showing no relationship with neuroticism, extraversion, or conscientiousness and walking. Taken together, the results support more robust relationships between personality and specific physical activity behaviors that require more extreme energy requirements, competitiveness, and skill, which was also supported in a recent meta-analysis (Wilson & Dishman, 2015).

In line with this theorizing, considerable research has explored higher-risk physical activities (i.e., also known as high-risk sports and adventure activities) and personality. A recent review of 39 studies on the topic showed that high-risk participants scored higher on sensation seeking, extraversion, and impulsivity compared to comparison groups who did not participate in these activities (McEwan et al., 2019). By contrast, the contrast groups were found to have higher neuroticism, while there was no association in high-risk sports for agreeableness, conscientiousness, or openness.

Sensation seeking in particular has been studied extensively with high-risk sports and activities. One of the earliest examinations in this area was skydiving, where Hymbaugh and Garrett (1974) reported higher levels of sensation seeking scores for skydivers compared to a normative control group. Skydivers were even shown to score higher on sensation seeking compared to pathological gamblers (Myrseth et al., 2012). Sensation seeking involves a willingness to take physical risks for the attainment of novel, varied, and intense sensations/experiences (Zuckerman 1994) so high-risk sports do seem like a natural behavioral outlet for this trait.

The positive relationship between extraversion and participation in a range of high-risk sports, is likely an extension of the relationship between extraversion and general higher-intensity physical activities (Rhodes & Smith, 2006; Wilson & Dishman, 2015). Extraversion tends to be manifested through energetic behaviors (McEwan et al., 2019). Individuals with lower levels of neuroticism seem more likely to participate in high-risk sports, which also may be an extension of the general physical activity research. Neuroticism is characterized by feelings of worry, fear, or anxiety (Costa & McCrae, 1995), so it seems plausible that individuals who are inclined toward neuroticism would be less likely to participate in high-risk activities. Finally, it is interesting that the McEwan et al.'s review did not show a relationship between high-risk sports and conscientiousness and agreeableness. While it may be tempting to label high-risk sport participants as reckless and disagreeable, the evidence suggests that these traits are not congruent with high-risk sports. High-risk sport participants are no more reckless, nonconformist, or angry compared to individuals who do not partake in such activities.

> Personality has been associated with some physical activities more than others. Extraversion, for example, is associated with physical activities that require extreme energy requirements, competitiveness, and skill. High-risk physical activities, such as skydiving, are also more often performed by extraverts (particularly those who are sensation seekers) and avoided by those who are higher in neuroticism.

Personality traits also seem to be associated with exercise addiction, a further risk behavior. For example, Andreassen et al. (2013) found that exercise addiction was positively associated with neuroticism (β = 0.18), extraversion (β = 0.27), and conscientiousness (β = 0.29) and negatively with agreeableness (β = –0.15). Personality explained about 14% in the variance of exercise addiction. Another study found positive relationships for extraversion (β = 0.19) and neuroticism (β = 0.17) with exercise dependence and a negative association between agreeableness and exercise dependence symptoms (β = –0.19; Hausenblas & Giacobbi, 2004).

The positive association between neuroticism and exercise dependence might be explained by the general vulnerability of neurotic individuals to develop psychopathology (Winter & Kuiper, 1997). Exercise dependence may also be a result of a maladaptive coping strategy for the concerns about their own appearance or health of neurotic individuals (Hausenblas & Giacobbi, 2004). For extraversion, it can be assumed that extraverted people seek out stimulation (Eysenck, 1963) and are typically energetic and active, which may make them vulnerable for excessive exercising and exercise dependence (Hausenblas & Giacobbi, 2004; Hill et al., 2000). The positive association between conscientiousness and exercise dependence might be due to high self-control, planning abilities, and weak temptations in conscientious individuals, which may support excessive exercise behavior. Furthermore, exercise dependence can be seen as a positive addiction, which is characterized by producing feelings of self-efficacy (Glasser, 1976), which is particularly appreciated by conscientious individuals. With regard to agreeableness, an explanation might be that people with exercise dependence often come into conflict with others (e.g., friends, partner, family) due to their excessive behavior (Weinstein & Lejoyeux, 2010). This would be contrary to being likeable, pleasant, and emphasizing harmony in relationships with others, which is highly important for agreeable individuals (Graziano & Tobin, 2009). High scores on agreeableness may protect the development of exercise dependence, due to the intention to avoid interpersonal conflicts.

15.4.2.2 Personality and Sedentary Behavior

Sedentary behavior impairs health and has to be seen as a discrete risk behavior independent of an individual's physical activity level. Knowledge about the personality factors that determine a sedentary lifestyle is increasing. A meta-analysis by Allen et al. (2017) revealed very small positive correlation between neuroticism and sedentary behavior ($r = 0.08$; high emotional lability is associated with increased sitting) and a negative correlation between conscientiousness and sedentary behavior ($r = -0.08$; high conscientiousness is associated with less pronounced sedentary behavior) across 23 cross-sectional studies and 3 prospective longitudinal studies. Differentiating between the three sedentary behaviors of playing electronic games, general use of the Internet, and the use of social media, a more differentiated picture emerged: a positive correlation between extraversion and the use of social media, but not computer gaming, was observed. Neuroticism was also associated with the use of social media, but not with the general use of the Internet. Furthermore, age moderated the relationship between personality and sedentary behavior. In participants of 35 years and older, a negative correlation between openness for new experiences and sedentary behavior was found, whereas this correlation was not observed for persons aged 24 years and younger. With regard to agreeableness, a significant and negative correlation was found among those under 35 years of age, but not for those over 35 years of age. The meta-analysis by Sutin et al. (2016) showed similar findings. In five of the included studies, sedentary behavior was examined. Again, higher values in neuroticism were associated with a more pronounced sedentary lifestyle and higher values in conscientiousness with a lower degree of sedentary behaviors.

> Sedentary behavior is positively linked to the personality dimension of neuroticism and negatively to conscientiousness. Since sedentary behavior subsumes a multitude of different behaviors driven by diverse motives, a more differentiated view seems to be valuable.

Overall, the Big Five personality dimensions show correlations with physical activity behavior and sedentary behavior. According to Cohen (1988), the correlations can be classified as small, but the finding has been reliable across several meta-analyses across many years, even as the research literature has grown. However, a cause-and-effect relationship of personality on physical activity behavior can hardly be derived from these results, since the study designs are predominantly cross-sectional, which only allows conclusions about a general relationship but not about a specific direction of influence between these variables. Longitudinal studies assessing personality at a first point of measurement and health behaviors several years later are still rare. Certainly, longitudinal studies are also observational studies and therefore of limited use in proving causality. However, the direction of the relationship could be tested, for example, within a longitudinal cross-lagged panel design in which personality and health behavior are observed in parallel over several points of measurement and the mutual predictive power of the variables (in the sense of a causal effect) is then tested in both directions (► Methods Box: Study Designs). The unidirectional view of personality on health behavior ignores the fact that physical activity or sedentary behavior might also affect personality itself.

Study Designs

Observational studies (e.g., cross-sectional and longitudinal studies) are nonexperimental study designs that can be conducted to investigate a relationship between two variables. A cause-and-effect relationship between these two variables can only be examined to a limited extent. Causal conclusions can merely be drawn from longitudinal research through specific statistical analysis methods (cross-lagged panel design).

In randomized controlled trials (RCTs; experimental study with randomized allocation of the subjects to test and control group), the independent variable (here: personality) is manipulated, and the effect of this manipulation is examined on the dependent variable (here: health behavior or health) in comparison to a control group without or a placebo manipulation. With this approach, researchers aim to document that the treatment "causes" the dependent variable/outcome. This study design is most eligible ("gold standard") to establish causal conclusions (cause-and-effect relationships).

15.4.3 Health Behavior as a Mediator Between Personality and Health

A possible explanation for the relationship between personality and health (total mortality) is provided by health behavior. Many illnesses and damages to health are fostered by an individual's behavior. This is particularly true for so-called diseases of civilization such as high blood pressure, heart attack, stroke, overweight, diabetes mellitus type 2, back pain, osteoporosis, and arthrosis. Health behavior influences health through various psychological and physiological mechanisms. There is ample evidence that the personality is associated with a variety of health behaviors including physical activity and sedentary behavior (► Sect. 15.4.2). Thus, health behavior can be assumed to be a mechanism explaining the association between personality and health (health status, morbidity, mortality, or longevity; ◘ Fig. 15.1).

▪ Physical Activity as a Mediator Between Personality and Health

The abovementioned studies and meta-analyses confirm the relationships between personality and health (mortality) as well as between personality and health behavior. However, they only examined the single paths, but not the assumed mediating effect of health behavior. Only few studies have aimed to examine the mediating role of physical activity behavior for the personality-health relationship. In a cohort study over two waves of personality, health behavior and brain health a cohort of people born in 1936 were investigated (Booth et al., 2014). The aim was to determine correlations between personality and different indicators of brain health (e.g., loss of brain tissue), which were determined by imaging techniques, and to examine the mediating effect of a number of health behaviors (e.g., physical activity, smoking, diet, BMI) based on a large sample. Physical activity was shown to be the most consistent and significant mechanism between personality and brain health.

A study by Armon (2014) investigated the extent to which personality is related to the concentration of serum lipids such as cholesterol (HDL (high-density lipoprotein), LDL (low-density lipoprotein)) and triglycerides and if this association can be explained by physical activity behavior (Excursus: Serum Lipids). The results of the prospective longitudinal study over two points of measurement at an interval of 2.5 years showed interesting relationships. The concentration of HDL could be prospectively predicted by the personality dimensions neuroticism (negative), extraversion (negative), conscientiousness (positive), and openness (positive), and 24% of the variance in HDL could be explained. However, these effects almost completely disappeared when smoking, body weight, and physical activity were controlled for as potential mediators (Armon, 2014). The personality dimension openness remained the only significant predictor. Physical activity behavior at the first point of measurement predicted HDL significantly. Furthermore, physical activity behavior (positive) and the body weight (negative) assessed at the second point of measurement were significantly related to HDL. A total of 32% of the variance in HDL could be explained by the predictors involved.

Side Story

Serum Lipids

Serum lipids such as LDL (low-density lipoprotein) cholesterol and triglycerides can be pathologically elevated by an unhealthy lifestyle (e.g., unhealthy diet, physical inactivity, sedentary lifestyle, obesity) and, for example, promote deposits in the arteries, which can promote the development of cardiovascular disease. Elevated levels of LDL and triglycerides should therefore be avoided.

HDL (high-density lipoprotein) cholesterol, on the other hand, is a protective factor and promotes the transport of excessive cholesterol from the tissue (e.g., deposits in the blood vessels) to the liver, where it is broken down and excreted. High levels of HDL in blood serum are therefore desirable.

LDL cholesterol was not predicted by any of the personality dimensions, but physical activity behavior was a significant negative predictor of LDL and thus a protective factor. Body weight (second point of measurement) was also positively associated with LDL cholesterol. However, only 9% of the variance in LDL could be explained. The author interprets the missing associations between personality and LDL by the fact that LDL levels are often adjusted by medication and that the influence of lifestyle could therefore only be examined to a limited extent. This also explains why the LDL cholesterol did not show any association with personality traits.

The concentration of triglycerides was prospectively predicted by the personality dimensions of extraversion (positive), conscientiousness (negative), and openness (negative). Thus, 7% of the variance in triglycerides could be explained. These relationships were reduced in accordance with the mediation hypothesis when health behavior was included in the model. The physical activity level was a negative predictor of the triglyceride levels, which suggests a protective effect. A total of 16% of the variance in triglycerides could be explained with this model. The findings of Armon (2014) affirm the mediating effect of health behavior between personality and health by physiological mechanisms (such as the concentration of serum lipids; Fig. 15.1).

The Role of Health Behavior for the Personality-Health Association

The study by Hampson et al. (2007) is one of the few studies that examined correlations between personality, health behavior, and health in a prospective longitudinal study design from childhood to middle adulthood (N = 1054). In this research, correlations between personality, health behavior (smoking, diet, and physical activity), and subjectively assessed health status were examined. Personality was assessed by the teachers in the first, second, fifth, or sixth grade in childhood. The educational level and health behavior and the subjective health status were surveyed in the same sample about 30–40 years later at the ages of 41–50 years. It was assumed that the educational level and health behavior can explain the effect of personality on health status. A direct and significant correlation between extraversion and physical activity behavior was found. Physical activity and dietary behavior were the strongest positive predictors of the perceived health status, and smoking behavior also showed a significant correlation with this variable. The level of education was predicted by conscientiousness and to a lesser extent by agreeableness. However, contrary to expectations and previous findings, the level of education showed a negative correlation with physical activity behavior. Conscientiousness and educational level were directly related to subjective health. Emotional stability (neuroticism) showed no significant correlation with the examined variables. The findings suggest that the personality dimension of extraversion has a positive influence on the perceived health status via physical activity behavior (Hampson et al., 2007).

Overall, the findings support the assumed mediator effect of physical activity, although the effect sizes are often to be classified as low. However, since there is a multitude of different health behaviors that are influenced by different personality dimensions, even small effects in a specific behavior can be considered to be relevant.

> Physical activity behavior can partially explain the effect of personality on health. Even if personality was assessed in early childhood, this effect can be observed up to middle adulthood.

15.5 Explanations for the Personality-Physical Activity Relationship

The evidence of personality influencing physical activity behavior has increased in recent years. But how can the association between personality and physical activity be explained (Fig. 15.1, arrow 2)? Personality models such as the five-factor model can describe interindividual differences in behavior, but they do not explain the underlying mechanisms by which personality influences certain behaviors. One explanation attempt is based on motivational processes that are determined by personality dimensions.

Smith and Spiro (2002) postulate social-cognitive middle units (Mischel & Shoda, 1995, 2000) as mediating mechanisms between personality and behavior, based on an approach by Mischel and Shoda (1995) and McAdams (1995). These middle units comprise, for example, **mental representations** (e.g., self- and relationship schematics), **motivational processes** (e.g., goals and expectations), **affective processes** (e.g., feelings and physiological reactions), **competencies** (e.g., strategies and social skills), and **self-regulation** (e.g., self-evaluation and delayed reward). These constructs are codetermined by personality and influence, for example, health behavior. These examples illustrate the manifold mechanisms that can intervene between personality and health behavior.

Middle Units

Social-cognitive middle units are mechanistic representations of the influences of personality on health behavior and describe how personality can influence health. Social-cognitive middle units are predictors of health behavior and health and illustrate the broadness of the influence of personality on psychophysiological processes and thus on health and disease (Smith & Spiro, 2002).

Ingledew and Markland (2008) also assume that the relationship between personality and physical activity behavior is based on motivational processes and that participation motives and behavioral regulation might explain this association (◘ Fig. 15.4). Participation motives are an individual's goals that cause him or her to participate in certain types of behavior (e.g., physical activity). They can be defined as classifications of outcomes or states that an individual approaches or avoids (Austin & Vancouver, 1996). Participation motives motivate people to increase and maintain a physically active lifestyle and are determined by personality traits (► Self-Reflection: Participation Motives of Physical Activity).

Personality traits can activate participation motives, which can subsequently be satisfied by appropriate behaviors. It is also assumed that personality traits influence the life goals of individuals, which causes them to select and form suitable social contexts. Ingledew and Markland (2008) further assume that the participation motives also influence the regulation of behavior. The "self-determination theory" (Deci & Ryan, 1985, 2000) distinguishes between external, introjected, identified, integrated, and intrinsic behavioral regulations (► Chap. 8: Organismic Integration Theory). If the cause or the control of one's behavior lies within the person himself or herself (e.g., "I go jogging because I enjoy it"), the person has an intrinsic regulation, which is the prototype of autonomous regulation. If an individual has an external behavioral regulation, the cause or control of the behavior lies outside of the person (e.g., "I go jogging because my doctor advised me to do so"). The external and the introjected regulation belongs to the externally determined, controlled forms of regulation, while the identified and integrated regulations are also extrinsic but are more strongly assigned to the self-determined forms of behavioral regulation. In a first study, Ingledew et al. (2004) have shown that personality is related to the behavioral regulation of physical activity. For members of a sport club who were in the maintenance phase of physical activity behavior, neuroticism proved to be a positive correlate of an introjected regulation and extraversion a positive correlate of an identified and intrinsic regulation, openness was negatively associated with external regulation, and a higher degree of conscientiousness was associated with a lower external and a higher intrinsic motivation. Thus, it can be assumed that neuroticism is rather associated with an externally controlled external form of regulation, whereas extraversion, conscientiousness, and openness correspond to a lower externally controlled and more self-determined (intrinsic) regulation of physical activity.

Participation Motives of Physical Activity

Participation motives, defined as individual goal content, are classifications of behavioral outcomes or states that an individual approaches or avoids (Austin & Vancouver, 1996). Participation motives of physical activity behavior are multifaceted and can be assessed, for example, with the "Exercise Motivations Inventory" Version 2 (EMI-2) by Markland and Ingledew (1997). The questionnaire consists of 51 items that describe possible reasons for being physically active.

The items are introduced with the words "Personally, I exercise (or might exercise), ..." and are answered on a six-point scale ranging from 0, "not at all true for me," to 5, "very true for me." You may respond to the following questions in order to find out about your own motive to participate in physical activity:

The 51 items split up to the following 14 subscales (item example in parentheses):

1. Stress management (e.g., "... to help manage stress")
2. Revitalization (e.g., "... to recharge my batteries")

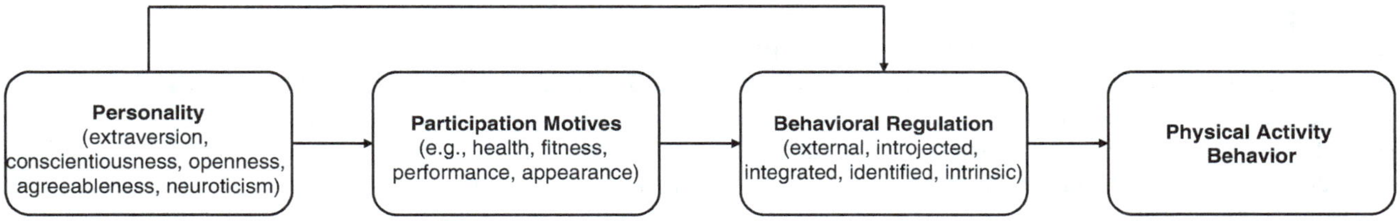

◘ **Fig. 15.4** Motivational model of personality and physical activity behavior. (Based on Ingledew & Markland, 2008)

3. Enjoyment (e.g., "… because I feel at my best while exercising")
4. Challenge (e.g., "… to give me personal challenges to face")
5. Social recognition (e.g., "… to show my worth to others")
6. Affiliation (e.g., "… to spend time with friends")
7. Competition (e.g., "… because I like trying to win in physical activities")
8. Health pressure (e.g., "… because my doctor advised me to exercise")
9. Ill-health avoidance (e.g., "… to avoid heart disease")
10. Positive health (e.g., "… to have a healthy body")
11. Weight management (e.g., "… to stay slim")
12. Appearance (e.g., "… to have a good body")
13. Strength and endurance (e.g., "… to build up my strength")
14. Nimbleness (e.g., "… to maintain flexibility")

Personality, Participation Motives, Behavioral Regulation, and Physical Activity

Ingledew and Markland (2008) assume that an individuals' participation motives might mediate the effect of personality on behavioral regulation and behavioral regulation in turn mediates the effect of participation motives on physical activity behavior (Fig. 15.4). These assumptions were tested in an empirical cross-sectional study in which the participation motives were assessed with the EMI-2 ("Exercise Motivations Inventory Version 2"; Markland & Ingledew, 1997). The subscales of the EMI-2 were submitted to a main component analysis and thus combined into three superordinate components: health/fitness, appearance/body weight, and social motives. Personality was assessed via the "NEO Five-Factor Inventory" (Costa & McCrae, 1992) and behavioral regulation with the Behavioral Regulation in Exercise Questionnaire-2 (BREQ-2; Markland & Tobin, 2004). The results based on the mediator model outlined in Fig. 15.4 revealed at least partially support for the expected mediator effects and the assumed mechanisms. The participation motive appearance/body weight mediated the effect of the personality dimension neuroticism on an external and introjected and thus rather externally determined behavioral regulation. The participation motive health/fitness mediated between openness and an identified (i.e., rather self-determined) regulation, which in turn was positively associated with physical activity behavior. Furthermore, the external regulation mediated the association between appearance/body weight and physical activity behavior as well as between conscientiousness and physical activity. The participation motive appearance/body weight was linked to the personality dimension neuroticism and an external behavioral regulation and was negatively related to physical activity behavior. From an applied perspective, it can be concluded that physical activity instructors should pay attention to promoting an intrinsic motivation, which is particularly relevant for people with high levels of neuroticism, and a pronounced physical activity participation motive of appearance and weight management. Overall, the results confirm the assumption that the relationship between personality and physical activity can be explained by underlying motivational processes and that participation motives as well as behavioral regulation can explain this association.

15

It should be noted, however, that these relationships can change over the life course. This is because personality and participation motives, preferences, and physical activity behavior are subject to change over the course of a lifetime. For example, the health motive becomes more important with increasing age, while the motive competition tends to decrease over the life course. Moreover, participating in physical activities can also change personality traits (▶ Chap. 14). Therefore, the relationship between personality and physical activity may be dependent on the social context (e.g., whether physical activity is carried out alone and self-organized or within a fixed group and an instructor) and should be considered as a bidirectional relationship.

Participation motives and behavioral regulation are motivational mechanisms that explain the relationship between personality and physical activity behavior. Neuroticism is particularly linked to the motives appearance and weight management and a more external behavioral regulation, which has a negative effect on physical activity behavior. In contrast, openness is associated with the participation motives of health and fitness and an identified behavioral regulation, which leads to higher physical activity levels.

15.6 Personality Traits in the Context of Social-Cognitive Models

In the last decades, a number of social-cognitive theories were proposed that try to explain health behavior and behavior change (▶ Chap. 25). In addition to the "social-cognitive learning theory" (Bandura, 1986), the "transtheoretical model of behavioral change" (Prochaska & DiClemente, 1983), or the "health action process approach" (Schwarzer, 1992), the "theory of planned behavior" (Ajzen, 1985, 1991) is a widely used framework for predicting physical activity behavior.

15.6.1 Theory of Planned Behavior

The "theory of planned behavior" (Ajzen, 1985, 1991) assumes that the intention (e.g., the goal to be regularly physically active) is the most important determinant of physical activity behavior (Fishbein & Ajzen, 1975). Intentions are influenced by attitudes and subjective norms. While attitudes are the positive or negative evaluation of the behavior in question (cognitive and affective), subjective norms are more socially determined and reflect the perceived social pressure to take up a physically active lifestyle. A person develops an intention if he or she either evaluates a continuous physical activity behavior as positive and/or if he or she is convinced that relevant persons from his or her environment believe that they should this behavior (◘ Fig. 15.5).

The model also describes which factors are involved in the formation of attitudes and subjective norms (Ajzen, 1991). Attitudes are determined on the one hand by behavioral expectations, that is, the expected consequences of the behavior, and on the other hand by evaluation of these consequences (desirability). The subjective norms are a function of the normative expectations of relevant persons (their opinion on whether the person should show a certain behavior or not) and the individual willingness to agree to these norms (the motivation of a person to do what other people expect of him or her).

In order to be able to predict behavior that cannot be completely controlled by the person and that is partly dependent on the availability of internal or external resources, Ajzen (1985) extended his model by a further construct: perceived behavioral control (◘ Fig. 15.5). It describes the individual's assessment of how easy or difficult it will be to perform the behavior under consideration. Perceived behavioral control is determined by the belief in one's own resources and abilities and is formed by the reflection of experiences and the anticipation of obstacles and barriers related to physical activity. If the perceived behavioral control is high, the probability of being physically active is also higher. In this way, the "theory of planned behavior" also considers real or perceived barriers that might prevent the execution of a behavior. Thus, intention is not only a function of attitude and subjective norm but is additionally determined by perceived behavioral control. Furthermore, perceived behavioral control has a direct effect on the behavior itself.

> In the "theory of planned behavior" attitudes, subjective norms and the perceived behavioral control predict the intention to perform a behavior (intention to act). The intention and the perceived behavioral control are predictors of the behavior (e.g., physical activity behavior), while intention is the strongest and most proximal predictor.

Social-cognitive constructs such as attitudes, subjective norms, perceived behavioral control, and intention play an important role in explaining and predicting physical activity behavior (McEachan et al., 2011). By including personality dimensions, a more comprehensive understanding of physical activity behavior could be achieved. In particular, two facets of the Big Five personality dimensions, namely, diligence (a facet of the dimension conscientiousness) and activity (a facet of the dimension extraversion), have proven to be particularly relevant for physical activity behavior (Bogg, 2008; Hoyt et al., 2009; Rhodes et al., 2005; Vo & Bogg, 2015). People who show high values on the activity facet are characterized as busy and engaged, as "always on the go." With regard to physical activity behavior, this facet has direct effects on attitude toward the behavior and perceived behavioral control (Rhodes & Courneya, 2003; Vo & Bogg, 2015), which in turn pre-

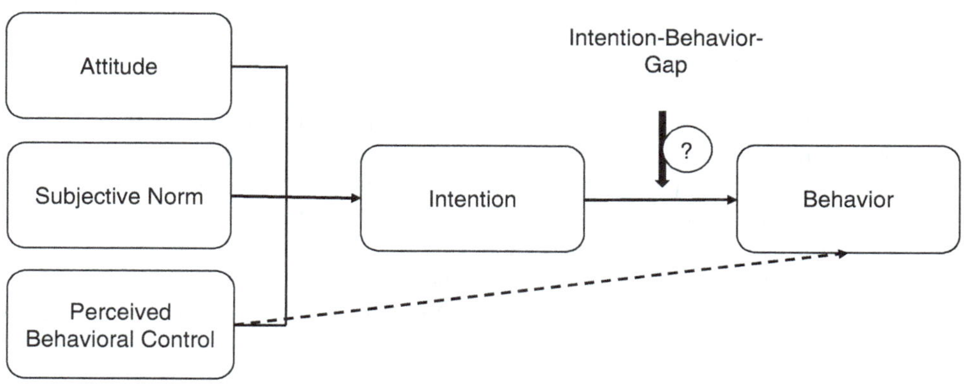

◘ **Fig. 15.5** The theory of planned behavior and the intention-behavior gap dict intention (indirect effects on intention) but also show direct effects on intention (Hoyt et al., 2009). People who score high on the facet diligence are described as hardworking, persistent, ambitious, imaginative, and confident. Hardworking people exhibit higher perceived behavioral control, subjective norms and more positive attitudes toward physical activity behavior, and a closer intention-behavior relationship than less hardworking people (Rhodes & Courneya, 2003; Vo & Bogg, 2015).

15.6.2 Personality Dimensions as Moderators Within the Theory of Planned Behavior

In addition to the observed direct and indirect effects of personality on the social-cognitive constructs of the "theory of planned behavior," personality was tested as a moderator variable. These studies investigated to what extent the strength of the relationship between the social-cognitive constructs varies according to the characteristics of the different Big Five personality dimensions. It is quite plausible to assume that the strength of the association between the social-cognitive constructs (e.g., attitude and intention or subjective norm and intention) is modified by personality traits.

Moderator Variable
A moderator variable is a third variable (C) that changes the relationship between a variable (X) and a variable (Y). The relationship between the variable (X) and the variable (Y) is different depending on the characteristic of (C). Researcher, which model personality (C) is a moderator variable, assume, for example, that the relationship between attitude (X) and intention (Y) is changed by the value in the personality dimension extraversion (C).

15

? Social-cognitive variables (middle units; ◘ Fig. 15.6) might act as mediators between personality and health behavior. However, why is it useful to investigate the Big Five personality dimensions also as moderators within the framework of the "theory of planned behavior" (Yap & Lee, 2013)?

1. Studies have shown that the Big Five personality dimensions are related to physical activity behavior (► Sect. 15.4.2.1).
2. Ajzen (1991) assumes that some people build their behavioral intentions based on attitudes and others more on subjective norms. This theoretical assumption implies the presence of moderating variables, and personality dimensions might be respective factors.
3. The moderating role of personality has been rarely examined, although initial studies have provided evidence of a moderating effect.

Rhodes et al. (2002) investigated the Big Five personality dimensions as moderators of the relationships between social cognitions and physical activity intention. The authors found a moderating effect of conscientiousness on the attitude-intention relationship. Attitude was a stronger predictor of intention for less conscientious compared to more conscientious persons. That is, people with lower values in conscientiousness hold a stronger affective attitude-intention relationship. In addition, the relationship between subjective norms and intention is moderated by the personality dimension neuroticism. People with higher values of neuroticism show a stronger association between subjective norm and intention than people with lower values of neuroticism. People with higher levels of neuroticism have a vulnerable and inhibited personality and that is why they may be more inclined to give in to social pressure, while people with lower levels of neuroticism, for example, are less concerned and may therefore be less likely to be guided by social expectations to manage their concerns. Furthermore, the relationship between subjective norms and intention is moderated by the dimension of extraversion. Extraverted people show a lower correlation between subjective norms and intention than introverted individuals. Extraverts are more sociable, optimistic, and assertive and therefore possibly less susceptible to social expectations and social pressure than introverts.

The study by Yap and Lee (2013) also found moderating effects of personality in the context of the "theory of planned behavior." In contrast to the study by Rhodes et al. (2002), conscientiousness and neuroticism moderated the relationship between perceived behavioral control and intention. The association between behavioral control and intention is stronger for more conscientious and less neurotic people. Conscientious people seem to feel more in control about the behavior and thus are more motivated to be physically active. People low in conscientiousness may lack in goal striving and self-discipline and are therefore less motivated to be physically active. Due to their disposition toward negativity, highly neurotic people might be less motivated because they lack the perception of opportunities to become physically active. Furthermore, extraversion moderated the attitude-intention relationship. The association between affective attitude and intention was stronger for extraverted compared to less extraverted people. Physical activity intention seems to be affected by feelings (e.g., enjoyment, pleasure) particularly in extraverted individuals. Extrovert people prefer higher levels of arousal and hence seek out for stimulation, which they can find in the physical activity context. This might be a reason why their motivation to participate in physical activities is more driven by affect (i.e., affective attitude; Rhodes et al., 2002; Yap & Lee, 2013).

From an applied perspective, physical activity instructors should foster positive affective attitudes toward physical activity behavior, notably among people with lower levels of conscientiousness and extraversion. Furthermore, it can be assumed that interventions on sustaining normative beliefs might be effective particularly for people with lower values in extraversion and higher values in neuroticism (Rhodes et al., 2002). Interventions promoting perceived behavioral control might be important for people with low conscientiousness and high neuroticism, as they might lack goal striving, self-discipline, and the perception of opportunities due to overestimation of obstacles and barriers to become physically active.

Particularly, the facets diligence and activity are highly relevant for explaining physical activity behavior and have an independent effect on attitude, subjective norm, perceived behavioral control, and intention. The dimensions conscientiousness, neuroticism, and extraversion moderate the associations between the social-cognitive constructs of the "theory of planned behavior." However, the findings are heterogeneous with respect to the relationships to be moderated and their direction.

15.6.2.1 Intention-Behavior Gap

The fact that many people intend to engage in regular physical activity but do not act accordingly describes the phenomenon of the intention-behavior gap (▶ Chap. 10; Volition in Sport). In the "theory of planned behavior," the intention to perform a behavior is the strongest predictor of that behavior, and it is assumed that a strong intention (i.e., high motivation) will translate into behavior. However, meta-analyses (Rhodes & de Bruijn, 2013) show that the variance of physical activity behavior can only partially be explained by intentions and that a large proportion of the variance in behavior remains unexplained. Including personality in the model could help to explain which people are particularly successful in translating their intention into action and which might be less successful. Thus, the relationship between intention and behavior should be further specified (◘ Fig. 15.5; Background Information: intention-behavior gap).

Side Story

Intention-Behavior Gap

Intention has been shown to be the most significant predictor of physical activity behavior in social-cognitive models of health behavior (e.g., "theory of planned behavior"). Meta-analyses have shown, however, that only 20–30% of the behavioral variance can be explained by intention (Hagger et al., 2002; McEachan et al., 2011). A recent review shows that only about half of the people who have formed an intention actually show the behavior (Rhodes & de Bruijn, 2013; Sheeran & Webb, 2016). This discrepancy between intention and behavior is widely known as the intention-behavior gap (Orbell & Sheeran, 1998). This phenomenon shows that many people have difficulties to translate their intention into action. This insight led to the question which additional factors are relevant between intention and behavior. The concept of **implementation intentions** (i.e., planning; Gollwitzer, 1999) is currently the most extensively examined approach known to bridge the intention-behavior gap (▶ Chap. 25). Once a person has formed the intention to be physically active on a regular basis, the next step should be to develop detailed action plans that define **when**, **how**, **where**, **how long**, **how often**, and **with whom** which physical activities should be carried out. Linking a specific situation to a concrete behavior facilitates the implementation of intentions (Hagger & Luszczynska, 2014). In addition to planning, personality may also play an important role in whether the intention to engage in physical activity behavior is successfully translated into action or not.

In their systematic review, Rhodes and Dickau (2013) investigated different personality dimensions as moderator variables of the intention-behavior gap. Conscientiousness proved to be a consistent moderator of the intention-behavior relationship. Higher values on the scale of conscientiousness were associated with a closer relationship between intention and behavior (i.e., a smaller intention-behavior gap). More conscientious people are more successful in translating their intention into actual behavior compared to less conscientious people. Conscientious people generally tend to have greater self-discipline and better self-regulation and to fulfill social expectations, which may explain the moderating effect. They are better able to put their intentions into practice. On a practical level, this means that people with low values in the dimension of conscientiousness, who are considered rather unorganized and undisciplined, could benefit from planning interventions in the sense of implementation intentions (Gollwitzer, 1999). They are guided to develop precise action and coping plans (▶ Chaps. 10 and 25; by specifying, for example, when, where, how long, how often, and with whom which physical activities could be performed (Rhodes & Dickau, 2013). Furthermore, extraversion has been identified as a moderator of the intention-behavior relationship in three out of five of the included studies. Individuals with higher values in the variable extraversion showed a closer relationship between intention and behavior. The authors explain this effect with the general tendency of extraverts to seek out situations in which they can be active, together with other people, and in which they experience stimulation. These tendencies can be realized and satisfied in the physical activity context. No effects have been found for the personality dimensions of openness, agreeableness, and neuroticism.

> The personality dimensions of conscientiousness and extraversion modify the relationship between intention and behavior. The more conscientious and extraverted people are, the better they succeed in translating their physical activity intention into actual behavior. The results are more consistent for conscientiousness compared to extraversion.

15.7 Physical Activity Interventions Using Personality Traits

Given the importance of shifting population to physical activity, a move from descriptive to predictive research in personality to its role in physical activity promotion would be helpful. Unlike social-cognitive or social environmental variables, an association between personality and physical activity represents a potentially challenging obstacle and not a target for change. Rather, personality traits resemble other intractable correlates of physical activity such as age, disability, or gender. Thus, health promoters need to consider responsive interventions for personality types (Rhodes & Boudreau, 2017). Personality assessments may help clinicians and public health professionals recommend activities with features that have been reported to appeal to people according to their personality. As an example, extraverts like being active with others and open individuals prefer unsupervised, outdoor activities (Courneya & Hellsten, 1998), so one might recommend joining an unsupervised, socially supported (i.e., recruit a walking buddy), outdoor walking program to an open, extraverted person, compared to someone who is less extraverted. Personality may also interact with recruitment materials and might moderate intervention strategies to impact intervention effectiveness and subsequent physical activity. Finally, personality might predict which people are likely to maintain physical activity following an initial intervention, and those who may be at risk for dropout or poor maintenance, which is an essential information for practitioners.

Despite the appeal of personality and physical activity intervention, there remains very limited research on this approach at present (Rhodes & Wilson, 2020). One potential pathway that personality-matched interventions may be able to promote physical activity is via planning interventions among less conscientious individuals. Conscientiousness represents organization and achievement striving and thus has been shown to moderate the planning to physical activity link (Lippke et al., 2018). Thus, Rhodes and Matheson (2008) examined whether a planning intervention among low conscientiousness individuals could help improve physical activity over a control group. The effects were null, but they may have been from an ineffective intervention as most of the participants reported that they did not even complete the planning worksheet. By contrast, Why and colleagues (Why et al., 2010) examined the effects of a walking intervention and found that messages were more effective in increasing walking behavior among conscientious individuals than their less conscientious counterparts. The results underscore that personality traits may need targeting to help less conscientious individuals (Smith et al., 2017).

More recently, a series of studies have explored how extraversion and/or neuroticism may interact with the success of physical activity interventions. Lepri and colleagues (Lepri et al., 2016) showed some evidence that extraverts and those higher on neuroticism increased physical activity under a social comparison strategy but not using peer pressure. Kahlin et al. (2016) found no evidence that personality moderated the success of a school-based intervention among inactive female adolescents. By contrast, Zaitsu et al. (2015) showed evidence that older adults who were more neurotic and introverted than their counterparts were advantaged by participating in an exergame intervention, yet the intervention had no relationship with conscientiousness. These mixed results show that a continuation of this research is needed, to ascertain the utility of personality-matched intervention.

> Understanding personality traits may help clinicians and health professionals recommend physical activity programs that match individual preferences and capabilities. Personality may also interact with recruitment materials and impact intervention effectiveness. Despite the appeal of personality and physical activity intervention, at present, very limited research exists on this approach. Furthermore, the current evidence has shown mixed results in terms of whether personality can determine the success of an interven-

tion. A continuation of this type of research is needed to decide on whether it is important to use personality-matched intervention for physical activity.

15.8 A Heuristic Model of Personality, Physical Activity Behavior, and Health Across the Life Span

A physically active lifestyle has positive effects on physical and mental health. There is increasing evidence that extensively engaging in sedentary behaviors is an independent risk factor for diseases. Nevertheless, many people are not sufficiently physically active and spend too much time with sedentary behavior. Interventions aimed at promoting a physically active lifestyle or reducing sedentary behavior are yet insufficiently successful. Personality as an influencing factor and moderator of intervention effects has hardly been investigated to date (Wilson & Dishman, 2015). Physical activities should be maintained throughout the entire life span to optimally influence health. Knowledge about the underlying mechanisms of the relationship between personality and health (behavior) can help to develop more effective interventions for specific target groups (e.g., for people low in conscientiousness or extraversion).

Figure 15.6 outlines a heuristic model that can be useful for specifying further research questions and hypotheses on personality and health, taking physical activity and sedentary behavior and different psychophysiological mechanisms as mediators into account. Smith and Spiro (2002) recommend that these associations should be examined from a life span perspective, since the influence of personality on health status, mortality, and longevity is mediated by behavioral patterns that often have beneficial or harmful effects on health only in the long run. Civilization diseases such as cardiovascular diseases, diabetes mellitus type 2, and cancer generally develop slowly and over a longer period of time (Hampson & Friedman, 2008; Smith & Spiro, 2002). The life span perspective is not a specific theory but rather a specific view of development and change in the life course.

According to this model, the health status of an individual is determined by environmental or contextual factors as well as individual factors, which are interrelated as a person-environment interaction (Adler & Matthews, 1994). Since social contexts and social interactions change during the life course, a research perspective across the life span is necessary. It is known that social contexts (e.g., socioeconomic status, educational level, occupation) play an important role for health and illness. Social stressors, which, for example, arise from social interactions with important attachment figures (e.g., family, friends, colleagues, peer group), and social roles (e.g., mother, father, employee) can trigger neuroendocrine reactions and lead to a cardiovascular stress response (e.g., increased heart rate, increased blood pressure). Neuroendocrine cardiovascular stress reactions such as the continuous activation of the sympathetic nervous system (Caspi & Roberts, 2001) can lead to health problems (e.g., cardiovascular diseases, increased susceptibility to infections), particularly if they occur frequently and over a longer period of time. A lack of social support can further increase this stress. Likewise, personality (e.g., people become more conscientious with increasing age) or the health status can

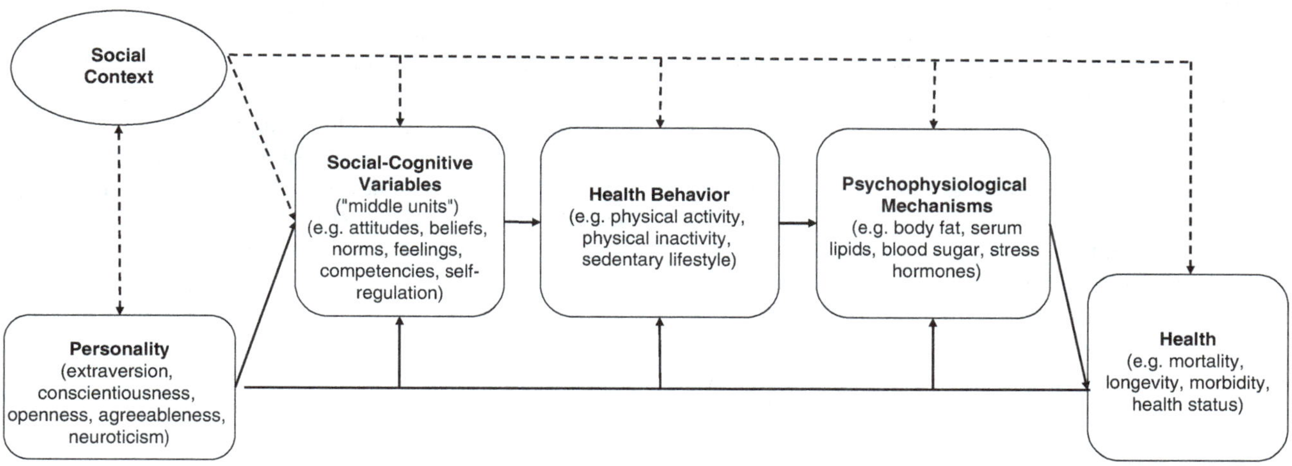

Fig. 15.6 Heuristic model of personality, health behavior (e.g., physical activity, sedentary behavior), and health across the life span. (Based on Smith & Spiro, 2002)

change over the life course. It is conceivable that stress is exacerbated by personality traits. Conscientious people might be more likely to have the ability to avoid or cope successfully with stressful situations, while people with high levels of neuroticism may be more likely to be drawn into stress situations (Letter, 2012). Personality is also related to different health behaviors, which can be assumed to be mediators between personality and health. Physical activity, for example, can mitigate the consequences of stress and act as a stress buffer. On the other hand, stress can have a negative influence on health behavior and, for example, discourage physical activity, as it can be perceived as an additional stressor in difficult life situations (Stults-Kolehmainen & Sinha, 2014; ► Chap. 27).

The influences of personality and social context on health and illness are unlikely to be one-dimensional. In a study by Jaconelli et al. (2013), it was shown that neuroticism was negatively associated with physical functioning in people between 60 and 91 years with a low and medium level of education, but not with a high level of education. A high level of education mitigates and even eliminates the negative association between neuroticism and physical functioning. This finding points to the interaction of personality traits with social context factors. A person in a job with low qualifications, long and changing working hours (shift work), is very likely to be exposed to stress and one-sided physical strain. This can reduce the time and energy for health-conscious behavior such as physical activity during leisure time. In addition, the social environment of these individuals (e.g., friends, colleagues) may also have a low level of education and an unfavorable health behavior (social norms), which further increases this effect, since physical activity (or sports) is associated with socioeconomic status and can lead to reduced physical functioning (in old age). The personality of this person (e.g., high levels of neuroticism, low levels of conscientiousness) can then further promote health impairments together with the educational level and the social environment (Jaconelli et al., 2013).

Studies that investigate the relationships between contextual characteristics, personality, health behavior, and health in prospective designs, over longer periods of time and in different populations from different social contexts, can provide further insight into these complex relationships. These effects should be investigated in different phases or stages of life (e.g., childhood, adolescence, middle adulthood, old age, vocational training, starting a family, retirement) and their transitions as well as under consideration of specific aspects of these phases or stages. A consistent attention of the Big Five personality dimensions and their facets is useful, since the mediators of the personality-mortality relationship are strongly dependent on the respective personality dimension, the health behavior taken into account, and the health outcome measured (Chapman et al., 2011).

Side Story

Become More Conscientious and Live Healthier and Lon ger?

Taking the Big Five personality dimensions into account, it can be specified which interventions aimed at promoting a physically active lifestyle or reducing sedentary behaviors work well or less well for whom (i.e., for people with high or low expression of a certain personality trait). Interventions can thus be specifically tailored to the characteristics of different personality dimensions and facets. Conscientiousness has so far emerged as a highly consistent factor of health behavior and health (Bogg & Roberts, 2013; Kern & Friedman, 2008). Becoming more conscientious could therefore be a convincing way to live healthier and longer. The question of the extent to which personality dimensions such as conscientiousness can be changed through targeted interventions and training has not yet been satisfactorily answered (Bogg & Roberts, 2013). Nevertheless, the results of therapy studies suggest that personality traits can be changed, even if these changes were not usually the primary goal of therapy. Randomized controlled intervention studies examining if the personality dimension of conscientiousness is modifiable are therefore needed. In addition, long-term efficacy studies have to challenge if the changes in one personality dimension are reflected in changes of health behavior (e.g., physical activity or sedentary behavior patterns) and thus have a positive influence on health.

What Can We Do to Strengthen Conscientiousness?

Even if personality cannot be changed easily: the Harvard Health Letter (Hammerness & Moore, 2012), which distributes health information to the general population, provides simple tips on how individuals can possibly become more conscientious and therefore healthier:

- Focus on specific areas: Becoming more conscientious in general is a major task. Therefore, focus on specific areas such as being on time or cleaning up your desk. With specific changes, you will probably be more successful.
- Make plans and work on them daily: Making and keeping a daily schedule supports organization and self-discipline.
- Use memory aids: Use reminders on your smartphone or computer to enhance the likelihood that your plans are realized successfully.

- Be social: There is a social component to conscientiousness. Being in contact with other people promotes conscientious behavior such as being on time or expressing gratitude.

Although it has been shown that personality traits can be changed through intervention, there are hardly any studies to date that have had the primary goal of changing conscientiousness (and not just underlying facets; Bogg & Roberts, 2013).

Learning Control Questions

Basic:

1. Define and characterize the constructs sport, exercise, physical activity, physical inactivity, and sedentary behaviors.
2. Describe the WHO recommendations on health-promoting physical activity for different age groups.
3. Describe the physical activity patterns of population for children and adolescents, young- and middle-aged adults, as well as persons of older age.

Advanced:

4. What do you understand by middle units in the context of the personality-health relationship, and what do they try to explain?
5. What personality traits describe high-risk physical activities like skydiving?
6. Which mechanisms can be assumed between personality and physical activity behavior, and which empirical findings can be cited?
7. Describe the "theory of planned behavior," and explain to what extent the Big Five personality dimensions can further specify the model.
8. What personality traits predict the intention-behavior gap in physical activity?

Experts:

9. Why and how should personality traits be taken into account in promoting a physically active lifestyle? Give concrete examples.
10. Which of the Big Five personality dimensions proves to be the most consistent influencing factor on health and health behavior, and how can that be explained?
11. Describe a heuristic model of the relationship between personality and health, and pay particular attention to physical activity behavior.

References

Adler, N., & Matthews, K. (1994). Health psychology: Why do some people get sick and some stay well? *Annual Review of Psychology, 45*(1), 229.

Ainsworth, B. E., Haskell, W. L., Herrmann, S. D., Meckes, N., Bassett, D. R., Jr., Tudor-Locke, C., et al. (2011). 2011 compendium of physical activities: A second update of codes and MET values. *Medicine and Science in Sports and Exercise, 43*(8), 1575–1581. https://doi.org/10.1249/MSS.0b013e31821ece12

Ainsworth, B. E., Haskell, W. L., Leon, A. S., Jacobs, D. R., Jr., Montoye, H. J., Sallis, J. F., & Paffenbarger, R. S., Jr. (1993). Compendium of physical activities: Classification of energy costs of human physical activities. *Medicine and Science in Sports and Exercise, 25*(1), 71–80.

Ainsworth, B. E., Haskell, W. L., Whitt, M. C., Irwin, M. L., Swartz, A. M., Strath, S. J., et al. (2000). Compendium of physical activities: An update of activity codes and MET intensities. *Medicine and Science in Sports and Exercise, 32*(9 Suppl), S498–S504.

Ajzen, I. (1985). From intentions to actions: A theory of planned behavior. In J. Kuhl & J. Beckmann (Eds.), *Action-control: From cognition to behavior* (pp. 11–39). Springer.

Ajzen, I. (1991). The theory of planned behavior. *Organizational Behavior and Human Decision Processes, 50*(2), 179–211. https://doi.org/10.1016/0749-5978(91)90020-T

Allen, M. S., Walter, E. E., & McDermott, M. S. (2017). Personality and sedentary behavior: A systematic review and meta-analysis. *Health Psychology, 36*(3), 255–263. https://doi.org/10.1037/hea0000429

Andreassen, C. S., Griffiths, M. D., Gjertsen, S. R., Krossbakken, E., Kvam, S., & Pallesen, S. (2013). The relationships between behavioral addictions and the five-factor model of personality. *Journal of Behavioral Addictions, 2*(2), 90–99.

Armon, G. (2014). Personality and serum lipids: Does lifestyle account for their concurrent and long-term relationships. *European Journal of Personality, 28*(6), 550–559.

Arundell, L., Fletcher, E., Salmon, J., Veitch, J., & Hinkley, T. (2016). A systematic review of the prevalence of sedentary behavior during the after-school period among children aged 5–18 years. *International Journal of Behavioral Nutrition and Physical Activity, 13*(1), 93.

Austin, J. T., & Vancouver, J. B. (1996). Goal constructs in psychology: Structure, process, and content. *Psychological Bulletin, 120*(3), 338–375. https://doi.org/10.1037/0033-2909.120.3.338

Bames, J., Behrens, T. K., Benden, M. E., Biddle, S., Bond, D., Brassard, P., et al. (2012). Letter to the editor: Standardized use of the terms "sedentary" and "sedentary behaviours". *Applied Physiology, Nutrition, and Metabolism, 37*, 540–542.

Bandura, A. (1986). *Social foundations of thought and action: A social cognitive theory*. Prentice Hall.

Bennie, J. A., Chau, J. Y., van der Ploeg, H. P., Stamatakis, E., Do, A., & Bauman, A. (2013). The prevalence and correlates of sitting in European adults-a comparison of 32 Eurobarometer-participating countries. *International Journal of Behavioral Nutrition and Physical Activity, 10*(1), 107.

Biddle, S. J., & Mutrie, N. (2007). *Psychology of physical activity: Determinants, Well-being and interventions*. Routledge.

Biswas, A., Oh, P., Faulkner, G., Bajaj, R., Silver, M., Mitchell, M., & Alter, D. (2015). Sedentary time and its association with risk for disease incidence, mortality, and hospitalization in adults: A systematic review and meta-analysis. *Annals of Internal Medicine, 162*(2), 123–132.

Bogg, T. (2008). Conscientiousness, the Transtheoretical model of change, and exercise: A neo-Socioanalytic integration of trait and social-cognitive frameworks in the prediction of behavior. *Journal of Personality, 76*(4), 775–802.

Bogg, T., & Roberts, B. W. (2004). Conscientiousness and health-related behaviors: A meta-analysis of the leading behavioral contributors to mortality. *Psychological Bulletin, 130*(6), 887–919. https://doi.org/10.1037/0033-2909.130.6.887

Bogg, T., & Roberts, B. W. (2013). The case for conscientiousness: Evidence and implications for a personality trait marker of health and longevity. *Annals of Behavioral Medicine, 45*(3), 278–288. https://doi.org/10.1007/s12160-012-9454-6

Booth, T., Mõttus, R., Corley, J., Gow, A. J., Henderson, R. D., Maniega, S. M., et al. (2014). Personality, health, and brain integrity: The Lothian birth cohort study 1936. *Health Psychology, 33*(12), 1477–1486. https://doi.org/10.1037/hea0000012

Borg, G. (1982). Psychophysical bases of perceived exertion. *Medicine & Science in Sports & Exercise, 14*(5), 377–381.

Bouchard, C., & Sheppard, R. (1994). Physical activity, fitness, and health: The model and key concepts. In C. Bouchard, R. J. Shephard, & T. Stephens (Eds.), *Physical activity, fitness, and health* (pp. 77–88). Human Kinetics Books.

Bucksch, J., & Schlicht, W. (2014). Sitzende Lebensweise als ein gesundheitlich riskantes Verhalten. *Deutsche Zeitschrift fur Sportmedizin, 65*(1), 15–21.

Bull, F. C., Maslin, T. S., & Armstrong, T. (2009). Global physical activity questionnaire (GPAQ): Nine country reliability and validity study. *Journal of Physical Activity and Health, 6*(6), 790–804.

Caspi, A., & Roberts, B. W. (2001). Personality development across the life course: The argument for change and continuity. *Psychological Inquiry, 12*(2), 49–66.

Chapman, B. P., Roberts, B., & Duberstein, P. (2011). Personality and longevity: Knowns, unknowns, and implications for public health and personalized medicine. *Journal of Aging Research, 2011*, 759170–759170. https://doi.org/10.4061/2011/759170

Christensen, A. J., & Moran, P. J. (2001). Psychological aspects of end-stage renal disease. In D. W. Johnston, M. Johnston, A. S. Bellack, & M. Hersen (Eds.), Health psychology, Vol. 8. Comprehensive clinical psychology (pp. 321–338). Elsevier. https://doi.org/10.1016/B0080-4270(73)00091-2

Cohen, J. (1988). *Statistical power analysis for the behavioral sciences*. Lawrence Erlbaum Associates.

Courneya, K. S., & Hellsten, L. A. M. (1998). Personality correlates of exercise behavior, motives, barriers and preferences: An application of the five-factor model. *Personality and Individual Differences*, 24(5), 625–633.

Costa, P. T., & McCrae, R. R. (1992). *Revised NEO personality inventory (NEO-PI-R) and NEO five factor inventory (NEO FFI) professional manual*. Psychological Assessment Resources.

Costa, P. T., & McCrae, R. R. (1995). Domains and facets: Hierarchical personality assessment using the revised NEO personality inventory. *Journal of Personality Assessment, 64*, 21–50.

Craig, C. L., Marshall, A. L., Sjöström, M., Bauman, A. E., Booth, M. L., Ainsworth, B. E., et al. (2003). International physical activity questionnaire: 12-country reliability and validity. *Medicine & Science in Sports & Exercise, 35*(8), 1381–1395.

Deci, E. L., & Ryan, R. M. (1985). *Intrinsic motivation & self-determination in human behavior*. Plenum Press.

Deci, E. L., & Ryan, R. M. (2000). The 'what' and 'why' of goal pursuits: Human needs and the self-determination of behavior. *Psychological Inquiry, 11*(4), 227.

Ekelund, U., Brown, W. J., Steene-Johannessen, J., Fagerland, M. W., Owen, N., Powell, K. E., et al. (2019). Do the associations of sedentary behaviour with cardiovascular disease mortality and cancer mortality differ by physical activity level? A systematic review and harmonised meta-analysis of data from 850060 participants. *British Journal of Sports Medicine, 53*(14), 886–894.

Eysenck, H. J. (1963). Biological basis of personality. *Nature, 199*(4898), 1031–1034.

Eysenck, H. J., Nias, D. K. B., & Cox, D. N. (1982). Sport and personality. *Advances in Behaviour Research and Therapy, 4*(1), 1–56.

Fishbein, M., & Ajzen, I. (1975). *Belief, attitude, intention, and behavior: An introduction to theory and research*. Addison-Wesley.

Glasser, W. (1976). *Positive addiction*. Harper & Row.

Gollwitzer, P. M. (1999). Implementation intentions: Strong effects of simple plans. *American Psychologist, 54*(7), 493–503. https://doi.org/10.1037/0003-066X.54.7.493

Goodwin, R. D., & Friedman, H. S. (2006). Health status and the five-factor personality traits in a nationally representative sample. *Journal of Health Psychology, 11*(5), 643–654.

Graziano, W. G., & Tobin, R. M. (2009). Agreeableness. In M. R. Leary & R. H. Hoyle (Eds.), *Handbook of individual differences in social behavior* (pp. 46–61). Guilford Press.

Guthold, R., Cowan, M. J., Autenrieth, C. S., Kann, L., & Riley, L. M. (2010). Physical activity and sedentary behavior among schoolchildren: A 34-country comparison. *The Journal of Pediatrics, 157*(1), 43–49.e41.

Guthold, R., Stevens, G. A., Riley, L. M., & Bull, F. C. (2018). Worldwide trends in insufficient physical activity from 2001 to 2016: A pooled analysis of 358 population-based surveys with 1·9 million participants. *The Lancet Global Health, 6*(10), e1077–e1086.

Guthold, R., Stevens, G. A., Riley, L. M., & Bull, F. C. (2020). Global trends in insufficient physical activity among adolescents: A pooled analysis of 298 population-based surveys with 16 million participants. *The Lancet Child and Adolescent Health, 4*(1), 23–35.

Hagger, M. S., Chatzisarantis, N. L. D., & Biddle, S. J. H. (2002). A meta-analytic review of the theories of reasoned action and planned behavior in physical activity: Predictive validity and the contribution of additional variables. *Journal of Sport & Exercise Psychology, 24*(1), 3–32. https://doi.org/10.1123/jsep.24.1.3

Hagger, M. S., & Luszczynska, A. (2014). Implementation intention and action planning interventions in health contexts: State of the research and proposals for the way forward. *Applied Psychology. Health and Well-Being, 6*(1), 1–47. https://doi.org/10.1111/aphw.12017

Hallal, P. C., Andersen, L. B., Bull, F. C., Guthold, R., Haskell, W., Ekelund, U., & Lancet Physical Activity Series Working Group. (2012). Global physical activity levels: Surveillance progress, pitfalls, and prospects. *Lancet, 380*(9838), 247–257.

Hammerness, P., & Moore, M. (2012). *Organize your mind, organize your life: Train your brain to get more done in less time*. Harlequin.

Hampson, S. E., & Friedman, H. S. (2008). Personality and health: A lifespan perspective. In O. P. John, R. W. Robins, L. A. Pervin, O. P. John, R. W. Robins, & L. A. Pervin (Eds.), *Handbook of personality: Theory and research* (3rd ed., pp. 770–794). Guilford Press.

Hampson, S. E., Goldberg, L. R., Vogt, T. M., & Dubanoski, J. P. (2007). Mechanisms by which childhood personality traits influence adult health status: Educational attainment and healthy behaviors. *Health Psychology, 26*(1), 121–125.

Harvey, J. A., Chastin, S. F., & Skelton, D. A. (2013). Prevalence of sedentary behavior in older adults: A systematic review. *International Journal of Environmental Research and Public Health, 10*(12), 6645–6661.

Hausenblas, H. A., & Giacobbi, P. R. (2004). Relationship between exercise dependence symptoms and personality. *Personality and Individual Differences, 36*(6), 1265–1273.

Hill, S. Y., Shen, S., Lowers, L., & Locke, J. (2000). Factors predicting the onset of adolescent drinking in families at high risk for developing alcoholism. *Biological Psychiatry, 48*(4), 265–275.

Howard, J. H., Cunningham, D. A., & Rechnitzer, P. A. (1987). Personality and fitness decline in middle-aged men. *International Journal of Sport Psychology, 18*, 100–111.

Hoyt, A. L., Rhodes, R. E., Hausenblas, H. A., & Giacobbi, P. R. (2009). Integrating five-factor model facet-level traits with the theory of planned behavior and exercise. *Psychology of Sport and Exercise, 10*(5), 565–572. https://doi.org/10.1016/j.psychsport.2009.02.008

Hymbaugh, K., & Garrett, N. D. J. (1974). Sensation seeking among skydivers. *Perceptual and Motor Skills, 38*, 118.

Ingledew, D. K., & Markland, D. (2008). The role of motives in exercise participation. *Psychology & Health, 23*(7), 807–828.

Ingledew, D. K., Markland, D., & Sheppard, K. E. (2004). Personality and self-determination of exercise behaviour. *Personality and Individual Differences, 36*(8), 1921–1932. https://doi.org/10.1016/j.paid.2003.08.021

Jaconelli, A., Stephan, Y., Canada, B., & Chapman, B. P. (2013). Personality and physical functioning among older adults: The moderating role of education. *The Journals of Gerontology. Series B, Psychological Sciences and Social Sciences, 68*(4), 553–557.

Jokela, M., Batty, G. D., Nyberg, S. T., Virtanen, M., Nabi, H., Singh-Manoux, A., & Kivimäki, M. (2013). Personality and all-cause mortality: Individual-participant meta-analysis of 3,947 deaths in 76,150 adults. *American Journal of Epidemiology, 178*(6), 667–675.

Kahlin, Y., Werner, S., Edman, G., Raustorp, A., & Alricsson, M. (2016). Physical self-esteem and personality traits in Swedish physically inactive female high school students: An intervention study. *International Journal of Adolescent Medicine and Health, 28*, 363–372.

Kern, M. L., & Friedman, H. S. (2008). Do conscientious individuals live longer? A quantitative review. *Health Psychology, 27*(5), 505–512.

Kunz, R., Khan, K. S., Kleijnen, J., & Antes, G. (2009). *Systematische Übersichtsarbeiten und Meta-Analysen: Einführung in Instrumente der evidenzbasierten Medizin für Ärzte, klinische Forscher und Experten im Gesundheitswesen*. Huber.

Lepri, B., Staiano, J., Shmueli, E., Pianesi, F., & Pentland, A. (2016). The role of personality in shaping social networks and mediating behavioral change. *User-Model User Adaptation Interface, 26*, 143–175.

Letter, H. H. (2012). *Raising your conscientiousness* [Press release]. http://search.ebscohost.com/login.aspx?direct=true&db=ccm&AN=104565316&site=ehost-live.

Lippke, S., Pomp, S., & Fleig, L. (2018). Rehabilitants' conscientiousness as a moderator of the intention–planning-behavior chain. *Rehabilitation Psychology, 63*, 460–467.

Markland, D., & Ingledew, D. K. (1997). The measurement of exercise motives: Factorial validity and invariance across gender of a revised exercise motivations inventory. *British Journal of Health Psychology, 2*, 361–376. https://doi.org/10.1111/j.2044-8287.1997.tb00549.x

Markland, D., & Tobin, V. (2004). A modification to the behavioural regulation in exercise questionnaire to include an assessment of amotivation. *Journal of Sport & Exercise Psychology, 26*(2), 191–196.

McAdams, D. P. (1995). What do we know when we know a person? *Journal of Personality, 63*(3), 365–396. https://doi.org/10.1111/j.1467-6494.1995.tb00500.x

McEachan, R. R. C., Conner, M., Taylor, N. J., & Lawton, R. J. (2011). Prospective prediction of health-related behaviours with the theory of planned behaviour: A meta-analysis. *Health Psychology Review, 5*(2), 97–144.

McEwan, D., Boudreau, P., Curran, T., & Rhodes, R. E. (2019). Personality traits of high-risk sport participants: A meta-analysis. *Journal of Research in Personality, 79*, 83–93.

Mischel, W., & Shoda, Y. (1995). A cognitive-affective system theory of personality: Reconceptualizing situations, dispositions, dynamics, and invariance in personality structure. *Psychological Review, 102*(2), 246–268. https://doi.org/10.1037/0033--295X.102.2.246

Mischel, W., & Shoda, Y. (2000). A cognitive-affective system theory of personality: Reconceptualizing situations, dispositions, dynamics, and invariance in personality structure. In E. T. Higgins, A. W. Kruglanski, E. T. Higgins, & A. W. Kruglanski (Eds.), *Motivational science: Social and personality perspectives* (pp. 150–176). Psychology Press.

Myrseth, H., Tverå, R., Hagatun, S., & Lindgren, C. (2012). A comparison of impulsivity and sensation seeking in pathological gamblers and skydivers. *Scandinavian Journal of Psychology, 53*, 340–346.

Orbell, S., & Sheeran, P. (1998). 'Inclined abstainers': A problem for predicting health-related behaviour. *British Journal of Social Psychology, 37*(2), 151–165. https://doi.org/10.1111/j.2044-8309.1998.tb01162.x

Pate, R. R., Pratt, M., Blair, S., Haskell, W. L., Macera, C. A., & Bouchard, C. (1995). Physical activity and public health: A recommendation from the centers of disease control and prevention and the American College of Sports Medicine. *Journal of the American Medical Association, 273*, 402–407.

Powell, K. E., Paluch, A. E., & Blair, S. N. (2011). Physical activity for health: What kind? How much? How intense? On top of what? *Annual Review of Public Health, 32*, 349–365. https://doi.org/10.1146/annurev-publhealth-031210-101151

Prochaska, J. O., & DiClemente, C. C. (1983). Stages and processes of self-change of smoking: Toward an integrative model of change. *Journal of Consulting and Clinical Psychology, 51*(3), 390–395. https://doi.org/10.1037/0022-006X.51.3.390

Rhodes, R. E., & Boudreau, P. (2017). *Physical activity and personality traits*. Oxford Press.

Rhodes, R. E., & Courneya, K. S. (2003). Relationships between personality, an extended theory of planned behaviour model and exercise behaviour. *British Journal of Health Psychology, 8*(1), 19–36. https://doi.org/10.1348/135910703762879183

Rhodes, R. E., Courneya, K. S., Blanchard, C. M., & Plotnikoff, R. C. (2007). Prediction of leisure-time walking: An integration of social cognitive, perceived environmental, and personality factors. *International Journal of Behavioral Nutrition and Physical Activity, 4*, 51.

Rhodes, R. E., Courneya, K. S., & Hayduk, L. A. (2002). Does personality moderate the theory of planned behavior in the exercise domain? *Journal of Sport & Exercise Psychology, 24*(2), 120–132.

Rhodes, R. E., Courneya, K. S., & Jones, L. W. (2005). The theory of planned behavior and lower-order personality traits: Interaction effects in the exercise domain. *Personality and Individual Differences, 38*(2), 251–265. https://doi.org/10.1016/j.paid.2004.04.005

Rhodes, R. E., & de Bruijn, G.-J. (2013). How big is the physical activity intention-behaviour gap? A meta-analysis using the action control framework. *British Journal of Health Psychology, 18*(2), 296–309. https://doi.org/10.1111/bjhp.12032

Rhodes, R. E., & Dickau, L. (2013). Moderators of the intention-behaviour relationship in the physical activity domain: A systematic review. *British Journal of Sports Medicine, 47*(4), 215–225. https://doi.org/10.1136/bjsports-2011-090411

Rhodes, R. E., Janssen, I., Bredin, S. S., Warburton, D. E., & Bauman, A. (2017). Physical activity: Health impact, prevalence, correlates and interventions. *Psychology & Health, 32*(8), 942–975.

Rhodes, R. E., & Matheson, D. H. (2008). Does personality moderate the effect of implementation intentions on physical activity? *Annals of Behavioral Medicine, 35*, S209.

Rhodes, R. E., & Smith, N. E. I. (2006). Personality correlates of physical activity: A review and meta-analysis. *British Journal of Sports Medicine, 40*, 958–965.

Rhodes, R. E., & Wilson, K. E. (2020). Personality and physical activity. In D. Hackfort & R. J. Schinke (Eds.), *The Routledge international encyclopedia of sport and exercise psychology* (pp. 413–425). Taylor and Francis.

Ross, R., Chaput, J., Giangregorio, L., Janssen, I., Saunders, T. J., Kho, M. E., et al. (2020). Canadian 24-hour movement guidelines for adults aged 18–64 years and adults aged 65 years or older: An integration of physical activity, sedentary behaviour, and sleep. *Applied Physiology, Nutrition, and Metabolism, 45*(10 Suppl. 2), S165–S179.

Sallis, J. F., Bull, F., Guthold, R., Heath, G. W., Inoue, S., Kelly, P., et al. (2016). Progress in physical activity over the Olympic quadrennium. *The Lancet, 388*(10051), 1325–1336.

Schwarzer, R. (1992). Self-efficacy in the adoption and maintenance of health behaviors: Theoretical approaches and a new model. In R. Schwarzer (Ed.), *Self-efficacy: Thought control of action* (pp. 217–243). Hemisphere Publishing Corp.

Sheeran, P., & Webb, T. L. (2016). The intention–behavior gap. *Social and Personality Psychology Compass, 10*(9), 503–518. https://doi.org/10.1111/spc3.12265

Sisson, S. B., Church, T. S., Martin, C. K., Tudor-Locke, C., Smith, S. R., Bouchard, C., et al. (2009). Profiles of sedentary behavior in children and adolescents: The US National Health and nutrition examination survey, 2001–2006. *International Journal of Pediatric Obesity, 4*(4), 353–359.

Smith, G., Williams, L., O'Donnell, C., & McKechnie, J. (2017). The influence of social-cognitive constructs and personality traits on physical activity in healthy adults. *International Journal of Sport and Exercise Psychology, 15*, 540–555.

Smith, T. W., & Spiro, A. (2002). Personality, health, and aging: Prolegomenon for the next generation. *Journal of Research in Personality, 36*(4), 363–394.

Stamatakis, E., Hamer, M., Tilling, K., & Lawlor, D. A. (2012). Sedentary time in relation to cardio-metabolic risk factors: Differential associations for self-report vs accelerometry in working age adults. *International Journal of Epidemiology, 41*(5), 1328–1337.

Stults-Kolehmainen, M. A., & Sinha, R. (2014). The effects of stress on physical activity and exercise. *Sports Medicine, 44*(1), 81–121.

Sutin, A. R., Stephan, Y., Luchetti, M., Artese, A., Oshio, A., & Terracciano, A. (2016). The five-factor model of personality and physical inactivity: A meta-analysis of 16 samples. *Journal of Research in Personality, 63*, 22–28. https://doi.org/10.1016/j.jrp.2016.05.001

Vo, P. T., & Bogg, T. (2015). Testing theory of planned behavior and neo-socioanalytic theory models of trait activity, industriousness, exercise social cognitions, exercise intentions, and physical activity in a representative U.S. sample. *Frontiers in Psychology, 6*, 1114.

Weinstein, A., & Lejoyeux, M. (2010). Internet addiction or excessive internet use. *The American Journal of Drug and Alcohol Abuse, 36*(5), 277–283.

Why, Y. P., Huang, R. Z., & Sandhu, P. K. (2010). Affective messages increase leisure walking only among conscientious individuals. *Personality and Individual Differences, 48*, 752–756.

Wilson, K. E., & Dishman, R. K. (2015). Personality and physical activity: A systematic review and meta-analysis. *Personality and Individual Differences, 72*, 230–242.

Winter, K. A., & Kuiper, N. A. (1997). Individual differences in the experience of emotions. *Clinical Psychology Review, 17*(7), 791–821.

World Health Organization. (2010). *Global recommendations on physical activity for health*. http://search.ebscohost.com/login.aspx?direct=true&db=mdc&AN=26180873&site=ehost-live.

Yap, S. F., & Lee, C. K. C. (2013). Does personality matter in exercise participation? *Journal of Consumer Behaviour, 12*(5), 401–411. https://doi.org/10.1002/cb.1442

Zaitsu, K., Nishimura, Y., Matsuguma, H., & Higuchi, S. (2015). Association between extraversion and exercise performance among elderly persons receiving a videogame intervention. *Games for Health Journal, 4*, 375–380.

Zuckerman, M. (1994). Behavioral expressions and biosocial bases of sensation seeking. Cambridge university press.

Social Processes

Contents

Group Performance

Jeannine Ohlert, Christian Zepp and Mark Eys

Contents

J. Schüler et al. (eds.), *Sport and Exercise Psychology*, https://doi.org/10.1007/978-3-031-03921-8_16

Learning Objectives

Basic:
- Knowledge of the definition of a group
- Ability to describe different types of groups
- Understand the development of groups and the phases that play a role in a sport context
- Ability to explain under which conditions people perform better in groups than individually and vice versa
- Ability to explain those phenomena theoretically

Advanced:
- Knowledge of how to prevent a loss of performance in sport teams
- Understand the reasons why a team consisting of individually less competent players is sometimes able to defeat a team consisting of individual players with higher competencies
- Ability to explain which intra-team processes are significantly involved in determining the performance of a team

Experts:
- Knowledge of how intra-team processes can be measured and diagnosed
- Understand how to find weaknesses in one's own team

16.1 Introduction

"TEAM = Together, Everyone, Achieves, More", or "The chain is only as strong as its weakest link"?

People complete all kinds of tasks in groups or teams, whether in small departments in a business, in assignment groups for academic study, or in team sports. In athletics, the type of sport determines whether competitions are held in a team or individually. In addition, for typical individual sports (e.g., athletics or judo), the question arises to what extent group processes play a role within training or during competition and how they affect the performance of all group members.

16

Due to the participation of many people with different personalities, as well as the social processes that occur, the scientific investigation of groups is very complex. In the context of business, many case studies show that organizing employees in small groups can have positive (but also negative) effects on the cohesion, leadership, interaction, employee satisfaction, and productivity of the company (Forsyth, 2014). However, the efficiency and thus the performance of groups cannot be described solely by productivity as an output. In fact, Hackman (2002) described three key points that should be considered in order to realistically assess group performance. The first (and probably the most important) point is the **productivity** of a group, since in most cases, the group was formed and assembled for the very reason of achieving certain goals and practical results. Therefore, productivity describes and records the direct performance of the group. Furthermore, Hackman identified two indirect performance outputs of the group: **growth** of the group and the **individual development** of the group members. A truly successful team becomes stronger over time and can master greater challenges and more difficult tasks in the future (Forsyth, 2014). Nevertheless, there are situations in which the group inhibits the individual development of its members or prevents individual members from feeling comfortable. As a consequence, the affected members may feel frustrated and disillusioned and may even leave the group. As a result, the costs for achieving the group's goals increase (Hackman, 2002).

The current chapter focuses on groups in sport. In some cases, the research in sport is inconclusive to make clear statements, and therefore, studies from other areas (e.g., organizational psychology) are included. After giving a definition of groups and teams, theoretical approaches of **group research** are presented, followed by a description of phenomena that contribute to reducing or increasing performance in groups. Finally, various social processes that affect group performance are discussed.

16.2 What Accounts for a Group?

When dealing with group performance, it is important to first understand the point at which a gathering of people can be considered a group. Does a volleyball team differ from a choir, a school class, the audience in a stadium, or people who train together in a fitness studio with regard to their performance-relevant conditions?

16.2.1 Definition of a Group

Colloquially, the term group or "team" is used in various contexts. For example, when several people happen to be standing in front of the Cathedral of Cologne looking at it at the same time, we describe them as a group. However, in order to deal with groups and group processes scientifically, a more precise definition of the term "group" is important. In the past, scientists used various criteria to define a group (e.g., degree of interdependence, social influence, common social identity; DeLamater, 1974). However, there is still no final consensus among scientists on how to define a group specifically. Including the developmental "life" of a group in a definition would require the consideration of countless criteria and factors, which would in consequence be too detailed for proper use. Nevertheless, it is important to deal with the most important **criteria** that describe a group. Johnson and Johnson (2009) were able to identify a total of seven **characteristics** that are often mentioned in scientific definitions of a group: (1) a group consists of at least two persons who also consider themselves as members of that group, (2) the group members interact with each other directly, (3) the interaction of the group members is structured by roles and group norms, (4) the group members are dependent on each other, (5) the group members influence each other, (6) the group members come together to achieve a goal, and (7) the group members are motivated to be part of the group to satisfy a need. When applying these seven characteristics to the example above, it becomes evident that a gathering of people in front of the Cathedral of Cologne cannot be considered as a group in the scientific sense. Even if they interact with each other, they likely neither perceive themselves as members of the "cathedral viewer group" nor are their interactions structured by specific roles or group norms. In this case, the scientific term for this collection of people would be a **crowd**, in which social processes are different from those in a group. Similarly, spectators in a stadium are not considered a group in the scientific sense, because even if they were all assigned to the group of fans of a particular club, their interaction is not structured and many of the group members are not dependent on each other (unless they belong to a fan club).

Group

A **group** is defined as two or more people in direct interaction with each other, who are aware of their positive interdependence in achieving their goals, who are aware of their membership in the group, and who consciously perceive the other persons belonging to the group.

It should be noted that researchers do not necessarily have consensus regarding the definition of a group. Some definitions presume that a group must consist of at least three people (Moreland & Levine, 2012). Researchers justify this criterion by stating that dyads (a group of two people) are more simply structured and organized than groups consisting of three or more people. For instance, dyads can be formed and dispersed more quickly. A beach volleyball team that has to disperse as soon as one member is injured is a good example of a dyad's organizational structure. The healthy members cannot compete in tournaments on their own; therefore, a completely new team with a new partner must be formed (at least temporarily). Alternatively, the original team does not exist at all for the duration of the injury. However, in larger groups, there are always substitute members who could step in for the injured person in order to retain the group (e.g., an indoor volleyball team). Some researchers also argue that important group processes and phenomena such as the influence of a majority or coalition formation may not occur in dyads (Moreland & Levine, 2012). Therefore, the dyad is usually understood as a special case of a group.

It is also interesting that some researchers distinguish between groups and **teams** (Johnson & Johnson, 2009). They explicitly emphasize the added value of a team by referring to a common goal and a joint effort of the team members to achieve a team outcome (in addition to individual goals and outcomes). Consequently, a hockey team would be considered more reflective of a team relative to members of a track-and-field training group. However, both examples are groups when referring to the common definition.

16.2.2 Different Types of Groups and Group Tasks

The examples mentioned above show that groups can be very diverse. They differ in a broad range of characteristics, such as the goals of their members (e.g., church community vs. voluntary fire department), the size of the group (e.g., beach volleyball team vs. students of a school), the duration of the group (e.g., study group at the university vs. LGBTQ+ activist group), and the degree of organization (e.g., emergency medical team vs. fan club). Nevertheless, it can be assumed that comparable social processes occur in all of these groups, influencing the behavior of the group members.

A frequently used distinction of groups in sport refers to the specific task a group wants to or should manage. Based on the original categorization proposed by Steiner (1972), there are four different types of tasks that are relevant in sport.

Group Tasks

- **Additive/compensatory**: The performances of all group members are summed up independently from each other. For additive tasks, the sum is used as a criterion (e.g., ski jumping in a team). For compensatory tasks, the total sum is then divided by the number of group members to achieve an average value (which occurs in sports only when the grading of judges is calculated).
- **Disjunctive**: The group members act co-actively to enable their strongest group member to perform at their best. Only the performance of the strongest team member is taken as the result (e.g., teams in cycling races promoting their captain).

- **Conjunctive (not dividable)**: The group members interact with each other; all group members have (almost) the same task (e.g., rowing eight). The result is a joint group performance that cannot be traced back to the performance of the individuals and is limited by the worst group member.
- **Conjunctive (dividable)**: The group members interact with each other, but there are different tasks for the individual members (e.g., handball). The result is a joint group performance that cannot be traced back completely to the performance of individuals.

16.3 Theoretical Approaches to Groups and Group Performance

In order to understand how group performance develops, and which factors are influencing performance, it is helpful to initially consider which theoretical aspects are potentially important. In business, a distinction is made between models dealing with the temporal development and change of groups, theories of group roles, input-process-output models, and other theoretical approaches (e.g., four-factor theory of innovation, team reflexivity; cf. Van Dick & West, 2013). For sport teams, two different models have been used to help explain group performance.

16.3.1 Model of Small Group Development

Often used to describe the sequential development of small groups, the **Phase Model of Team Development** (Tuckman, 1965; Tuckman & Jensen, 1977) considers the temporal development and change of groups. Tuckman assumed that there are five different temporal phases in the development of a small group on its way to peak performance: *Forming*, *Storming*, *Norming*, *Performing*, and *Adjourning*. The *Forming* phase occurs immediately after the formation of a group. In this phase, the group members make first *contact* and try to discover accepted behaviors as well as the boundaries of the group. All members are dependent on each other regarding their behavior and rules are formed or reinforced. In the second phase, *Storming*, individuals try to find their place in the group hierarchy. Conflicts often occur among the group members. The subsequent phase, *Norming*, is characterized by group members focusing on group cohesion and the shared tasks of the group. Group members develop shared norms and values that should help them to be successful and enter an unwritten contract with the mutual acceptance of these norms. After successfully completing this phase (and typically occurring throughout the previous phases), the group *Performs*; all roles within the group become clarified, a hierarchy is established, and a considerable level of group cohesion is achieved. In this phase, the group attempts to achieve its best performance through cooperation. Once the group goal has been achieved, the task is completed (e.g., the season is over), and the *Adjourning* phase ensues, in which the group disperses.

Originally, Tuckman's model mainly referred to groups in therapy and health, but the application of this model is also useful as a starting point for thinking about group development in sport. A sport example shows that characteristics of Tuckman's model are experienced by teams (Applied Sport Psychology: Practical Application of Tuckman's Phase Model). However, the duration of the different phases depends on many aspects (e.g., the personalities involved, the club culture, the coaches, or the integration of sport psychologists). Therefore, a criticism regarding the model focuses on the linear and inflexible sequence. In reality, groups are dynamic for many reasons across their life span. For example, a central group member may drop out (e.g., injury) or a new member joins. In addition, groups that exist for a longer period of time (i.e., sport teams) do not strictly complete the *Adjourning* phase (e.g., veteran players return the following season). Conversely, there are national teams who have a different composition of players almost every time they meet. As such, the developmental stages of sport teams do not follow consistent or linear paths, though Tuckman's model offers a starting point from which to discuss the life span of a group.

> **Applied Sport Psychology**
>
> **Practical Application of Tuckman's Phase Model**
>
> To illustrate the phase model of Tuckman, the development of the German women's national handball team can be used as an example. Several years ago, the team gathered together during the preparation for the World Championships. After the first training camp, the core team for the first preparatory phase was formed (*Forming* phase). After a short period of time, the *Storming* phase took place, in which one key player attracted particular attention because repeated conflicts occurred between her and other players. These conflicts escalated to such an extent that the national coach finally removed her from the team and continued the preparation without this key player. However, within the games, the team suffered from not being able to draw on her talents. Hence, the national coach got together with the team's sport psychologist and the team council, and they decided that the player should be reintegrated. Still, very strict rules were enforced for the entire team, which the player had to agree to in order to be

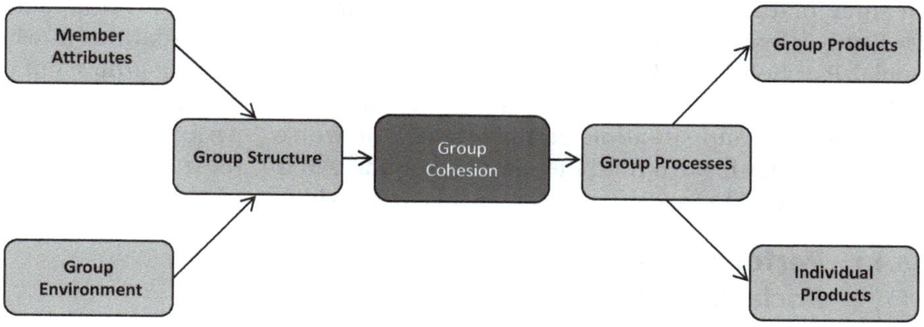

■ **Fig. 16.1** A conceptual framework for the study of sport teams by Eys, Evans, and Benson (2020b, p. 17). Used with permission from the FiT Publishing, West Virginia University

allowed to compete in the World Cup (*Norming* process). Since the World Cup participation was very important to her, she adhered to the rules and followed them like everyone else, which allowed the team to perform at a higher level at the World Cup.

16.3.2 A Conceptual Framework for the Study of Sport Teams

The **conceptual framework for the study of sport teams** (Carron & Eys, 2012; Carron & Hausenblas, 1998; Eys et al., 2020b) is an input-throughput-output model regarding the functionalities of groups. *Inputs* include, for example, the characteristics of the individual group members or the environment in which the group has to perform. These inputs influence the *structure* (e.g., roles), *processes* (e.g., communication), and *emergent states* (e.g., cohesion) of the group, which then influence the *outputs* in the third step. *Outputs* are the final products or results of the group, such as group performance or member satisfaction.

The model broadly highlights two *input* factors. One factor contains the characteristics of the group members (e.g., gender, age, skills, needs, and motivation). The other factor comprises the environment and conditions of the sport group (e.g., group size, motivational climate of the group, spectators, and media coverage). These *input* factors will affect the structure of the sport group. This refers to aspects such as the leadership structure and hierarchy within the group and member roles. Also affected will be key processes like communication and coordinative actions, as well as broader conceptions of the group itself (i.e., emergent states) in terms of its cohesion and collective efficacy. Ultimately, these throughputs will contribute to *outputs*, which are divided into individual and group products. Examples for possible individual products are the individual performance of the athletes, their satisfaction within the team, and the general well-being of the athletes. Group products primarily describe the objective group performance (■ Fig. 16.1).

16.4 Performance Gains and Losses in Groups

Reflection

How would you react? Imagine the following group situations, and consider whether and how your personal motivation of performing at your best would change compared to an individual situation:

- You are having a tug-of-war and know that you are the strongest person in your team.
- You are supposed to clear out an apartment together with eight other people.
- You discuss in your volleyball team that everyone takes turns in washing jerseys on a voluntary basis after the games. There will be no documentation of who completed the task at any point.
- You carry a football goal/net with five other team members, and you are the smallest and weakest person in the group.
- You play a tennis doubles match with a partner who is performing a little bit better than you are.
- You are brainstorming in a group, and you are well versed in the topic. However, there is another expert on the topic in the group.
- You are in a rowing eight, and you know that the individual effort of each person is recorded by sensors.

In the following chapter, you will learn about the reactions of most other people and about the reasons for individual behavior within a group.

In some of the first social-psychological experiments (▶ Study Box: The Ringelmann Effect: The First Social-Psychological Experiment; see related works ▶ Chap. 17), researchers wanted to explore whether people in a group situation perform better or worse than when they have to fulfil the same task alone. After more than a 100 years of research in this area (which is still not completed by far), the answer is both! There are situations in which people perform best when they are in a group, but conversely, there are also situations where the group situation leads to a decrease in the performance of the individuals. In the next section, these two opposing phenomena will be examined.

16.4.1 Performance Losses in Groups: Social Loafing

Study Box

The Ringelmann Effect: The First Social-Psychological Experiment

Research on social loafing has its origin in the experiments of the French agricultural engineer Max Ringelmann. Between 1882 and 1887, he conducted experiments on pulling and pushing to find out how loads can be moved most effectively by people and animals. He carried out the experiments in groups of 7 or 14 people as well as individually. In his publication from Ringelmann, 1913, Ringelmann reported (see Kravitz and Martin, 1986) that only 63–84% of the individual strength potential was achieved in the group situations. However, since he was not really interested in these results—as an agricultural engineer, he was more intrigued by the effectiveness of his tug-of-war method in comparison to other methods—he did not further investigate these results and did not calculate whether the differences he found were statistically significant. Therefore, the experiment itself did not attract scientific attention at first. However, a small table did, which could be found in the text with the note "Supplementary findings on this topic." In that table, results were presented comparing the work performance of one person versus groups of two to eight people, but without further explanation about the origin of the data and their context. A German researcher named Moede used these data in Moede, 1927 and reported the loss of performance under the name "Ringelmann effect." It was not until the 1970s that research on social loafing was finally continued, referring back to Moede and Ringelmann.

The most interesting aspect about this story is that Ringelmann was long regarded as a German psychologist (and a student of Moede) and that only the data of his supplemental table was passed on. Therefore, it was suspected that the experiment was carried out only in the twentieth century. Finally, Kravitz and Martin found the original document, published the correct experiment in 1986, and clarified that the experiments had already taken place much earlier, thus before the experiments on social facilitation (▶ Chap. 17). However, despite this clarification, many textbooks still contain incorrect information about Ringelmann and his experiments and which study was the first social-psychological experiment.

Important: In contrast to social loafing, the Ringelmann effect merely refers to the fact that the performance of a group is worse than the sum of the performance of the individual group members. The reason for this decrease in performance can simply be a **coordination problem** between the group members—a reason that Ringelmann also gave in his article.

16

A loss of performance in a group means that an individual reduces his or her performance in the group situation compared to the individual situation. A typical example of this would be a rower, who produces less individual power in a quadruple scull boat compared to a single scull boat. It could be argued that the reduced power is explained by the fact that single scull rowers must concentrate only on themselves, whereas in the quadruple scull boat, the rowers need to also focus on the coordination with the others in their boat. Thus, they cannot use the maximum force. As a result, researchers try to separate **the coordination losses** from **the motivation losses** (i.e., the physical from the psychological processes). This was shown for the first time by Ingham et al. who investigated a blindfolded tug-of-war in their experiment (Ingham et al., 1974). The subjects thought that they were performing the tug-of-war in groups of different sizes, but in fact, they were pulling the tug-of-war alone while the persons behind them were not using any power ("pseudo groups"). Losses of coordination could be ruled out in this manner, but the performance of the participants in the pseudo group situation still decreased significantly compared to the individual situation. Thus, Ingham et al. had created an experimental paradigm that significantly accelerated research in this area. Latané et al. (1979) were able to replicate the effect in an experiment with clapping and shouting in an individual situation as well as in pseudo groups and subsequently named the phenomenon *social loafing*.

Social Loafing

Social loafing describes a reduction of a person's motivation and effort in a collective situation compared to a co-active or individual situation.

As stated in the definition, a distinction is made between collective and **co-active situations in groups**. A co-active situation describes a kind of group work with clearly divided and identifiable tasks and achievements for each individual person, whereas in a collective situation, a clear assignment within the group performance to single individuals is not possible. A typical example of a co-active situation is a 100-meter relay team in swimming: The group performance is the total time of all swimmers together, but also each individual swimmer's performance is identifiable because all individual times are announced after the end of the race. If this was handled differently and only a total time was recorded, it would be a **collective performance situation**, such that the personal contribution of each swimmer would not be identifiable. According to the definition, it can be assumed that slower times (i.e., social loafing) would occur in such a collective situation. Williams et al. (1989) were able to support this proposition in an experiment with college swimmers.

Factors That Influence Social Loafing

In each case, the situation with more social loafing is mentioned.

Characteristics of the task:

- Collective task
- No evaluation of personal performance
- Perceived redundancy of personal contributions
- Very easy task

Characteristics of the group and the situation:

- Large group
- Low importance of the group for the person
- Low identification with the team (▶ Sect. 16.5.5)
- Low group cohesion (▶ Sect. 16.5.6)
- Role ambiguity (▶ Sect. 16.5.3)
- Poor quality of interaction with the team leader
- Perceived unfairness (injustice) in coaches' decisions

Personal characteristics:

- Male
- Member of Western culture
- Individualistic attitude (vs. collectivistic attitude)
- Ego orientation (vs. task orientation, ▶ Sect. 16.5.1)
- Narcissism

Overall, a high degree of **identifiability** of one's own performance (personally and/or through others) enhances the motivation to make an effort, while a low degree of identifiability reduces motivation and thus one's own performance (especially for individuals with individualistic characteristics, ▶ Sect. 16.4.3).

Most studies on social loafing contain either basic experiments or are economic studies (for a summary, see Ohlert, 2009). However, several studies on social loafing have also been conducted in the sport setting. In addition to the study with swimming relay teams previously mentioned (Williams et al., 1989), social loafing has been demonstrated in sprint relay situations as long as the individual running times were not announced (Huddleston et al., 1985; Swain, 1996). Social loafing under **training conditions** (i.e., not in competition) has been reliably demonstrated; in addition to the studies already mentioned, it was shown in swimmers (Everett et al., 1992; Miles & Greenberg, 1993) and female rowers (Anshel, 1995).

The quality of the opponent also appears to influence social loafing behaviors. Heuzé and Brunel (2003) examined competitive sport students performing a dart competition in dyads. However, the researchers manipulated the participants' expectations of winning by reporting the alleged scores achieved by the opposing dyad beforehand, which were either realistically achievable or much higher than the dyad's own performance. They were able to show that the effort in the collective situation only decreased when the participants believed they did not have a good chance to beat their opponents. No social loafing was detected in the situation with a realistically achievable score. Unfortunately, what happens when the opponents are considered to be much weaker than the own team was not investigated.

Furthermore, sport-related research has demonstrated that prior information about the existence of social loafing does not prevent the effect. The sprint relay study by Huddleston et al. (1985), as well as a replication with bicycle ergometers (Nilsen et al., 2014), revealed that social loafing occurred when the participants had been explicitly informed about the phenomenon beforehand. Thus, social loafing seems to be an **unconscious process**, at least to some extent.

In several studies, Ohlert (Ohlert, 2009; Ohlert & Kleinert, 2013) investigated an extension of social loafing to the preparation phase of a group task: the *pre-loafing effect*. For example, male participants prepared less conscientiously for a group tug-of-war situation in comparison with an individual tug-of-war situation (Ohlert, 2009). A replication of the study based on a hand strength task demonstrated a less thorough preparation in the group situation, especially for the female participants (Ohlert & Kleinert, 2013). This experiment revealed almost no connection between preloafing and social loafing. This means that participants engaged in social loafing either during preparation *or* in the actual performance situation; thus, it was not the same persons who engaged in preloafing and social loafing. Finally, the effect of *preloafing* can be seen in sport settings through debilitative preparation related to general health behavior (alcohol consumption, smoking, nutrition, and sleeping behavior) in competitive team athletes compared to individual athletes (Ohlert, 2009).

The swimming relay study by Williams and colleagues is also illuminating with regard to the fact that social loafing could be demonstrated in the context of a competitive situation with "real" relay teams. However, this only occurred if the individual times could not be identified—a condition that rarely exists in swimming competitions. Hardy and Latané (1988) found a similar effect in cheerleaders even during an induced competition: cheerleaders performed worse in the collective situation compared to a co-active situation. Hence, a **competitive situation** does not completely prevent social loafing. It should still be noted that the effects occurred during field experiments in artificial competitive situations. Social loafing has yet to be investigated during a real competition, in which athletes are exposed to completely different pressures than in a laboratory. The reason behind this is the fact that in a real sporting competition, the performance of the individual is either always accessible (e.g., in relays) or not at all (e.g., in rowing). A situation in which athletes believe that their individual performance is not identifiable, but other people still have knowledge about it, does not exist in regular sporting competitions.

Since social loafing can apparently still occur during competitions, researchers have tested alternative methods for recording social loafing in more recent studies. For example, Høigaard and Ingvaldsen (2006) tried to operationalize the **effort** of floorball players by monitoring the heart rate and creating an index of objective performance via different game parameters. However, they discovered no differences between situations with low and high identifiability. Especially in ball games, it is subject to discussion as to whether objective parameters such as heart rate, running distance, or shots on goal can reflect the actual performance of a player, because tactical expectations of a coach for a player of a certain position do not necessarily involve maximum effort for certain criteria (e.g., number of shots).

Another attempt to assess social loafing in sports is the measurement of **perceived loafing** in teammates (de Backer et al., 2015; Høigaard & Ingvaldsen, 2006), although the extent to which perceived loafing is related to (objective) social loafing has yet to be confirmed. In other recent studies, social loafing is partly investigated on the basis of **self-reports** (self-reported social loafing); participants are asked to indicate whether they do their best or whether they let themselves down (de Backer et al., 2015; Høigaard et al., 2010). There are some difficulties regarding this type of questioning because of the high likeliness of social desirability bias and the fact that unconscious parts of social loafing cannot be detected in this manner.

Overall, social loafing can be characterized as quite stable under certain circumstances that are characteristic of team sport. Since performance will never be completely objective, especially in ball games, social loafing may always be a threat (during both training and competitions as well as preparation and warm-up phases; ► Study Box: How to Prevent Social Loafing in Sports?).

Applied Sport Psychology

How to Prevent Social Loafing in Sport?

Unfortunately, there is no evidence of applied intervention programs to reduce social loafing (neither in sport nor in other relevant areas). However, based on the factors found to influence social loafing, some methods can be derived that should prevent or at least reduce social loafing in sport teams (see also Hardy, 1990):

- Increase the **identifiability of individual** performance wherever possible. It is important for the athletes to have the feeling that their individual performance is noticed. A possible implementation could be via individual meetings or breaking down group tasks into individual parts for each person (if possible).
- Establish **individual goals** for all athletes, which are reviewed and adjusted regularly. This increases the identification with the goals, and the athletes more likely feel that their performance is noticed.
- Try to increase the **personal importance** of the task for the athletes. The higher the relevance of the task and the intrinsic motivation, the less social loafing will occur.
- Increase **identification with the team** (► Sect. 16.5.5) and **group cohesion** (► Sect. 16.5.6) through team building exercises (► Chap. 22). With higher value of the group for a person, social loafing will be reduced.
- At least in training, try to work in **small groups** more often to increase the visibility of the individuals.
- Clarify the tasks and **role expectations in the team** for all athletes individually (Sect. 16.5.3). Commu-

nicate and justify decisions, and try to establish the **same rules** for all and follow them consistently.
- Work with your athletes in **a task-oriented** manner (▶ Sect. 16.5.1).
- Keep an eye on people with a high level of **ego orientation** and a high drive for prestige (narcissism). Intervene consistently if you have the feeling that individuals are slowing down at the expense of others.

Study Box

The Turning Point in Games

A research question in the field of group performance has to do with momentum shifts. A well-known example in recent years is the 2017 Super Bowl (American football). As described by Sobleski (2017), "After leading by 25 points with 18 minutes left to play, Atlanta allowed the biggest comeback in Super Bowl history, as the Patriots roared back with 31 unanswered points to emerge with a 34–28 overtime victory. An inevitable argument occurs after a slim margin decides any major contest: Did the winner earn the victory, or did the loser give it away?" (para. 2–3).

Assuming the latter in this case, researchers refer to such a situation as a **collective collapse** (Apitzsch, 2006; Wergin et al., 2018). Boss and Kleinert (2015) assume that the collective collapse is preceded by an automatic **social contagion,** which ultimately causes the "collapse" of the team. Social contagion can refer to emotions as well as attitudes and behavior and, according to theory, occurs unconsciously as well as without intentional control of this contagion by the initiating person. Moll et al. (Moll et al., 2010) were able to support this phenomenon for positive situations by finding a correlation between the reaction of a successful penalty kicker and the probability that the following team member will also score: if the successful player showed obvious pride and dominance in his reaction, the probability of the subsequent kicker to score increased as well. Within preliminary studies, Boss and Kleinert (2015) tried to investigate the existence of social contagion in negative situations. They conducted two experiments with dyads and discovered a reduction of the **quality of the relationship** with a partner when the partner's performance drops. Furthermore, there was a tendency for the individuals to decrease their own performance. Further studies need to research whether and how social contagion is actually responsible for a collective collapse.

16.4.2 Performance Gains in Groups

There are also conditions in which a group is actually more than the sum of its parts, because individuals increase their performance when they are part of a group. In this context, an important phenomenon is the effect of social facilitation, which is discussed elsewhere in this book (▶ Chap. 17). Additionally, there is the so-called Köhler effect and the phenomenon of social compensation.

16.4.2.1 The Köhler Effect

Initial investigations into the **Köhler effect** can be traced back to a similar timeframe as the Ringelmann effect. The Köhler effect is named after the German industrial psychologist Otto Köhler, who published his first experiments on performance gains in group situations in 1926 and 1927 (Köhler, 1926, 1927).

Köhler Effect

The **Köhler effect** describes the increase in motivation and effort of the weakest member of a group in a collective performance situation compared to an individual task.

In his original experiments, Köhler (Köhler, 1926) conducted studies on endurance performance in weightlifting in dyads compared to individuals. He used a conjunctive task by having both male subjects of a **dyad** pull a bar, which was connected to an 82 kg weight by a rope. The kind of construction used in the experiment only enabled a successful lift of the weight when both test persons were exerting sufficient force. The task was to lift the weight up to a certain point and to release it again as often as possible. The total distance lifted was measured and compared to the individual distances of each subject when lifting a 41 kg weight under the same conditions. The researcher discovered that for dyads with (almost) equally strong members, social loafing occurred and that the overall performance was lower than the average of the individual performances. The same held true for dyads where the **difference in performance** was quite large in the individual tests. However, for those dyads with one member slightly (between 20% and 35%) weaker than the other, an increase in group performance of up to 25% could be found compared to the individual performances. Köhler did not investigate, however, whether the effect occurred due to an increase in performance of the weaker or the stronger person. In another experiment investigating groups of three people, he was able to replicate the effect, but less pronounced than before.

Researchers started to investigate the effect again in the 1990s. A series of experiments trying to replicate the original experiments of Köhler were successful. Hence, Stroebe et al. (1996) were able to detect the "Köhler effect" when there was a moderate difference in performances between the two members of a dyad. Furthermore, they were able to prove that the performance gain was almost solely due to an increased effort in the weaker person. In their meta-analysis, Weber and Hertel (2007) finally demonstrated a medium size of the effect as well as enabling conditions. Specifically, it occurs within conjunctive tasks (► Sect. 16.2.2), when information on the performance of the partner is constantly available and when a physical task needs to be completed.

Overall, very little research on the Köhler effect is documented (the meta-analysis by Weber and Hertel found only 17 studies, three of which were unpublished). In addition, there is limited practical application with regard to performance-oriented sport. The double boats in rowing and canoe racing might be a relevant example for the Köhler effect, since these are conjunctive tasks in dyads. However, scientific studies do not exist in this area of application. Also, the Köhler effect during conjunctive, but dividable, tasks (e.g., beach volleyball, dancing, or figure skating pairs) has not yet been examined (Digression: The Köhler Effect in Exergames).

Side Story

Digression: The Köhler Effect in Exergames

A line of research deals with the application of the Köhler effect in so-called **exergames**, which are special computer games that involve active movement. Feltz and Kerr were able to demonstrate that a Köhler effect occurs in exergames when playing with a human partner via Skype (Kerr et al., 2013) and also when playing with a **virtual partner** who is moderately superior in performance (Feltz et al., 2011). The effect is not as strong in virtual partners compared to real partners (Feltz et al., 2014) but can be shown quite well for both strength endurance and aerobic endurance tasks (Irwin et al., 2012). Over a longer period of time (several sessions), the Köhler effect is particularly stable when the challenge consists of two tasks and the real person feels superior to the virtual partner at least in one of the tasks (Kerr et al., 2013) or when the more dominant virtual partner shows signs of fatigue and weakness (Max et al., 2016). However, the latter effect could only be discovered for male subjects. Overall, this research represents an exciting area in which social-psychological processes in physical activity are linked with virtual reality. However, whether the effects can also be transferred to performance-oriented e-sports has not yet been examined.

16.4.2.2 Social Compensation

Social Compensation

Social compensation refers to the effect that individuals in collective situations increase their effort to compensate for the expected lack of performance of other group members.

In contrast to the Köhler effect, social compensation focuses on the person in a group who is, from their own point of view, the best performer. Williams and Karau (1991) initially demonstrated that, in dyads of **heterogeneous abilities,** the stronger person tries to compensate for the weaker person's lack of ability during performance situations. Within their three experiments, the researchers found social compensation, as opposed to social loafing, under the conditions that the participants both (a) cared about the task and (b) judged their partner to be unreliable, reluctant, or lacking ability regarding the respective task. In particular, this effect was found in collective situations (i.e., when the performance of the individuals was not visible). To date, the effect could only be demonstrated for dyads. Obviously, social compensation serves to avoid poor group performance in a task that is important for the person. Moreover, the effect only occurs when performing with a **stranger**, but not with friends (Karau & Williams, 1997). Interestingly, this is also a condition where social loafing would be expected. Since competitive sports rarely creates situations in which the performance *of a stranger* who is showing apathy or little ability has to be compensated, it can be assumed that the effect will only rarely occur or not at all. In the area of **physical activity**, the phenomenon could be used in analogy to the considerations about the Köhler effect. However, no studies have yet been conducted in this area. Still, the effect was robustly shown in experiments (e.g., Hart et al., 2001; Hüffmeier et al., 2013a; Todd et al., 2006) but seems to occur only under these particular conditions.

16.4.3 Theoretical Explanations for Performance Losses and Gains in Groups

Reflection

Now that you have been introduced to situations and conditions under which motivation in groups (and thus personal performance) increases or decreases—what do you think is the reason for these fluctuations of group performance? Which theories and mechanisms would you use to explain social loafing, the Köhler effect, and social compensation?

Various research projects have already been able to demonstrate triggering conditions for social loafing and social compensation. Nevertheless, a theoretical explanation of why and when these phenomena occur is also very important and helpful for researchers as well as practitioners. Several explanations and models already exist, especially in the area of motivation losses.

16.4.3.1 Theoretical Explanations of Performance Losses

One of the earlier theoretical approaches explaining social loafing is **social impact theory** (Latané, 1981), which is described in detail elsewhere in this book (► Chap. 17). It would be assumed that the attention—and therefore the social impact—of an observing or controlling person (e.g., experimenter, coach) will be distributed over several persons in a group situation. Thus, the impact on one person is smaller than in an individual situation. A similar explanation was developed in the **drive theory approach** (Jackson & Williams, 1985), which assumes that the presence of others, as well as their focus of attention, increases one's own level of arousal. However, if the attention is distributed over several individuals (as in a group situation), the arousal will be shared and therefore reduced. In an experiment consisting of easy and difficult tasks, social loafing was present for easy tasks due to the reduced arousal, whereas the performance for difficult tasks increased in collective situations (Jackson & Williams, 1985). The increased arousal caused by the difficult task compensated for the reduced arousal induced by the presence of others.

Other researchers (e.g., Harkins, 1987; Harkins and Szymanski, 1989) considered the reduced **possibility to evaluate** individual performance as a trigger for social loafing. In a collective situation, the evaluation of individual performance is not possible; therefore, individuals cannot be held responsible for poor performance. Similarly, outstanding performance cannot be recognized either. The authors were able to verify their assumptions, demonstrating that social loafing disappears as soon as individual performance is made recognizable and quantifiable for all participants of a collective situation.

The **dispensability of one's own contributions** (Kerr & Bruun, 1983) is another potential reason for individual performance loss and reflects decreased motivation if members perceive their own contribution to a group performance as unnecessary or redundant. As soon as people feel that their individual contributions make little difference to the overall performance of the group, their motivation and thus their performance decrease. In particular, this should be true for disjunctive group tasks (Sect. 16.2.2).

As a final example, **social identity theory** (► Sect. 16.5.4) has been proposed to explain social loafing (Van Dick et al., 2009). This theory proposes that social loafing disappears, and the motivation to perform may increase, when the respective group is significant for the social identity of the members. This would likely be the case for many athletes who are members of sport teams. In contrast, in situations where groups have only been formed for an experiment, for example, there would be minimal identification with the group and stronger potential for social loafing to occur.

The theoretical approaches discussed above contribute to the understanding of social loafing, but none of these theories is able to explain the phenomenon completely. Nevertheless, they function as a foundation for implementing specific intervention programs for social loafing. For example, an intervention based on the theory of social identity would attempt to increase the positive valence of a group for the respective persons in order to increase their motivation and willingness to perform.

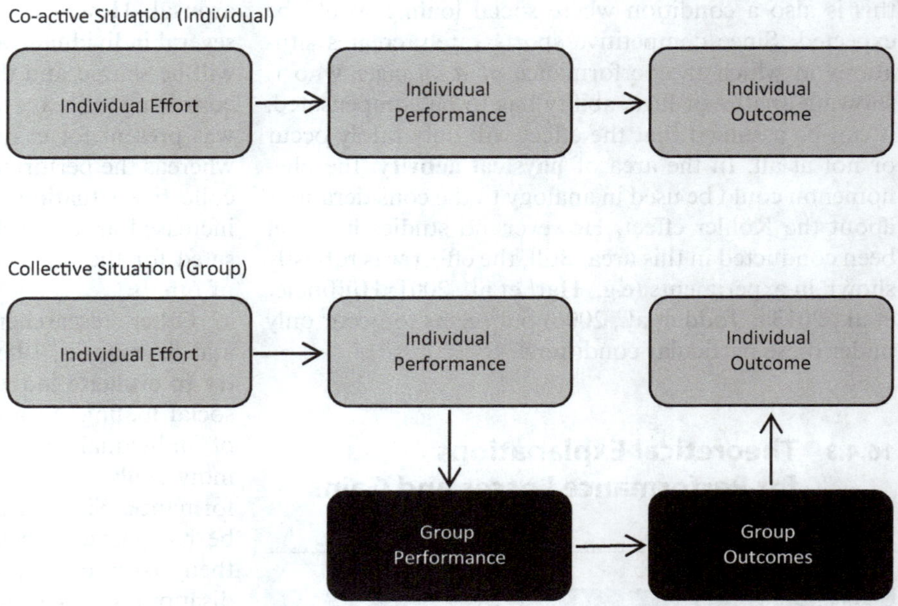

Fig. 16.2 The "collective effort model" (CEM) by Karau and Williams (1993)

16.4.3.2 Theoretical Explanations of Performance Gains in Groups

The Köhler effect is usually explained by two processes: On one hand, it is assumed that the slightly weaker persons make a **social comparison** and notes their inferiority with regard to the task to be performed. This promotes goal setting for their individual contribution to the task to match or outperform the superior person (competition within the group). On the other hand, in contrast to social loafing, the **indispensability of one's own contribution** to the dyad seems to play a role as well. Specifically, conjunctive tasks produce this effect, since the group performance is determined by the weakest group member.

In the area of social compensation, it was initially assumed that a person compensates in order to accomplish something: If they achieve a good group result, the person knows that they are primarily responsible for the good performance, because the partner was clearly weaker (and possibly lacked willingness). In the case of a poor group result, the person who performed worse can always be held responsible (Williams & Karau, 1991). However, more recent studies have applied the "collective effort model" as a foundation, as it provides a more comprehensive model for group performance.

16.4.3.3 The "Collective Effort Model": Integration of Theoretical Approaches

The **collective effort model** (CEM) was developed by Karau and Williams (1993) in order to unite existing models at that time, which were mostly limited to a few unique situations. Their aim was to create a comprehensive model than can explain motivation gains and losses in groups.

Figure 16.2 shows the basic components of the CEM. Based on expectancy-value theories (Heckhausen, 1977; Vroom, 1964; ▶ Chap. 6), the CEM assumes that people are fundamentally hedonistic and will therefore always try to derive the **maximum benefit** from their actions. Accordingly, a person is only motivated if he/she has the expectation that the individual effort is (a) crucial for achieving a valued result and (b) will lead to a result that is valuable to him or her personally. Both the expectation of goal attainment and the value of the result must be greater than zero, because the expectancy-value theory assumes that the person's motivational strength can be calculated by multiplying the expectation by the value of the result. As a consequence, in a situation in which either the expectation to achieve the result or the value of the result for a person equals zero, a person will exhibit a lack of motivation. Within the CEM, this applies equally for individual, co-active, and collective situations. In the co-active and individual situations, however, the performing person knows that their personal effort is crucial for performance, as well as the value that the performance result has for them. If thesis assessments are positive, the person is usually motivated. In contrast, in a collective situation, the **instrumentality** of the individual performance is not immediately evident. As such, the increased complexity of interrelations for the group task reduces the clarity of the instrumentality of one's own actions. This leads to a situation in which it is harder for a person to assess whether their efforts will help in achieving the desired result as well as whether the group results will ultimately lead to a personally valuable individual outcome. According to the model, individual motivation decreases as soon as these connections assumed in the model are not clear to the person.

In their meta-analysis, Karau and Williams (1993) were able to show support for their model. In subsequent years, the model was tested and supported repeatedly by other researchers, particularly by those in the area of social loafing (e.g., Feuchter and Funke, 2004; Hart et al., 2004). Furthermore, the model is also able to explain social compensation and the Köhler effects (Karau et al., 2000) and thus creates a foundation for targeted interventions in order to increase individual motivation.

Criticism regarding this model mainly concerns the fact that the CEM is a purely **cognitive model**. However, the authors emphasized that people in group situations do not necessarily process all factors systematically and consciously. On the contrary, the model assumes that people usually **process** familiar situations **automatically**, meaning that a kind of script is activated in order to keep the cognitive load in a situation as low as possible. Support for this cognitive approach was provided by Thompson and Thornton (2007), who investigated social loafing in children aged 3–5 years. They demonstrated that those children who were able to discern other people's perspectives (i.e., engage in perspective-taking), indicative of a higher level of cognitive development, demonstrated social loafing tendencies. The (mostly younger) children who were not yet able to demonstrate these perspective-taking abilities worked just as intensively during the collective condition as during the co-active one. Additionally, it could be assumed that older children had also gained more group experiences than the younger ones and, hence, may have tended to the automatic processing of group situations (i.e., to social loafing).

Overall, the CEM is the theoretical model that can help explain performance losses and gains in groups comprehensively and can also accompany other theoretical approaches (e.g., Social Identity Theory; ► Sect. 16.5.4). Therefore, the CEM is now considered an important model for explaining individual performance motivation in groups. It provides a pathway to explain why people reduce their performance in groups under some conditions, increase it in other situations, or perform in a similar way independent of the setting (► Study Box: Performance Gains in Relay Swimmers).

Study Box

Performance Gains in Relay Swimmers

Hüffmeier and colleagues investigated a special case of performance gains in relay swimming within three studies (Hüffmeier et al., 2012; Hüffmeier & Hertel, 2011; Hüffmeier et al., 2013b). In the first study (Hüffmeier & Hertel, 2011), they evaluated the swimming times of all individual swimmers in the freestyle relay semifinal at the Olympic Games in 2008 and compared these times with the performances of the individual competitions. The authors' assumption was that swimmers with a later position within the relay team would perform better in team situations, because they have to assume that a potential weak performance cannot be compensated anymore (compared to the swimmers in the lead positions). Their results confirmed the assumption, because those swimmers in the leading positions did not swim faster than their individual competitions but those in the later positions did.

In the second study (Hüffmeier et al., 2012), the authors expanded their sample size in order to test additional effects. They analyzed data from the finals of all international competitions (Olympic Games, World Championships, and European Championships) between 1996 and 2010. All swimmers who had reached both the individual and relay finals were included in the sample ($N = 199$). In addition to the position within the relay team, the team's probability to win the contest (high vs. low) was also included in the analyses. The results revealed that the effect of performance gains from the first study could be replicated for the later positions in the relay, but only for those relay teams who had a high probability of winning. For relay teams with a low probability of winning, the relay times were at the same level as the individual times.

Within their third study (Hüffmeier et al., 2013b), the authors made a comparison between freestyle relay teams and medley relay teams (i.e., teams of four athletes, but every athlete has to perform in another style of swimming). They assumed that the effect would not occur in a medley relay team because the swimmers could not estimate their probability of winning from the current position in the race (time differences for a specific distance vary greatly across swimming styles). For this purpose, they evaluated the freestyle and medley relay results of the Olympic Games from 1996 to 2008 and found exactly the expected effect.

Based on the CEM (Sect. 16.4.3.3), the authors explained the results of all three studies as a reflection of a strong connection between individual performance and group performance (i.e., when their own performance is considered **indispensable** and can no longer be compensated). Additionally, a connection between group performance and the group result must be perceived (i.e., a realistic chance to win a medal). This phenomenon only occurred when the relay team was performing well and only for freestyle relays and not the medley.

16.5 Group-Related Phenomena Affecting Group Performance

As already described through the Conceptual Framework for Research on Sport Teams, several **group-related phenomena** have an influence on the performance of a team (see also Kleinert et al., 2012; Ohlert & Zepp, 2016). These include, but are not limited to, (1) motivational climate, (2) leadership structure within the team, (3) role perceptions within a team (► Chap. 22) (4) identity of the team, (5) identification with the team, (6) group cohesion, (7) collective efficacy, (8) team trust, and (9) communication (► Chap. 18). It is important to consider that these factors do not independently influence the functionality of a team and consequently its performance. Rather, there are many reciprocal relationships among the variables (Digression: The "Too-Much-Talent Effect").

Side Story

Digression: The "Too-Much-Talent Effect"

Swaab and colleagues (Swaab et al., 2014) investigated the importance of the ideal composition of a sport team via a phenomenon termed the **too-much-talent effect**. This effect means that the overall performance of a group declines as soon as too many people with very high abilities are gathered in the group. According to the authors, a lot of energy is devoted to striving **for dominance** when the hierarchy for the best performers is not clear. This energy is then diverted from the group's performance. In order to gain advantages in the hierarchy, group members might not support, or even obstruct, each other under some circumstances. The authors were able to demonstrate the effect for the qualifier games of the FIFA World Cup in 2010 and 2014. Teams with many players from top clubs won less often than they should have based on the talent in their team. The same could be shown for the US National Basketball Association. Interestingly, however, the effect does not occur in sports where less interaction among the group members is needed. In the American Major League Baseball, a linear effect of talent on team performance was found—teams with the best players also achieved the best results. Apparently, due to a reduced need for interaction, the players cannot hinder each other in their actions. Incidentally, the authors assume that the effect is also **dependent on testosterone** and should therefore be stronger in men's teams than in women's; however, there is still no scientific evidence for this suggestion.

16.5.1 Motivational Climate

16

The concept of motivational climate is based on **achievement goal theory** (Ames, 1992). This theory states that every person has a certain goal orientation when it comes to achieving performance. It distinguishes between task orientation and ego orientation. In **task orientation**, the performance goal is self-referenced (e.g., to further develop oneself), whereas in **ego orientation**, comparison to others is crucial, so the performance goal is externally focused. These goal orientations are held in varying degrees by everybody but can also be influenced by the prevailing motivational climate in a group (Duda & Balaguer, 2007). The **motivational climate** in a group can be created by group members and their goal orientations (i.e., peer-created motivational climate), but above all by the group leader (e.g., the coach or teacher). Therefore, the goal orientation of the coach mainly determines the motivational climate within a sport group (coach-created motivational climate). Depending on the situation, the motivational climate can be either ego-oriented and/or task-oriented (Duda & Balaguer, 2007).

Motivational Climate

A **task-oriented climate** (in some studies also called *mastery climate*) is characterized by an environment that stresses effort, skill development, and cooperative learning, such that all athletes are perceived and treated as equally as possible. In an **ego-oriented climate**, mistakes are punished, athletes are treated differently depending on their performance level, and rivalry within the team is encouraged.

Research on the **coach-created motivational climate** shows that a task-oriented climate is positively associated with (among others) higher self-esteem among the athletes, a better moral understanding by athletes, and higher perceived social support from the coach. Conversely, a high ego-oriented climate is associated with higher competitive anxiety, dropouts, and conflicts within the sport team (for a summary, see Duda and Balaguer, 2007). When examining group performance, positive correlations to a task-oriented climate are detected both for the subjective assessment of performance by the athletes and for objective group performance (Balaguer et al., 2002; Hodge et al., 2014). A practical intervention concept for developing a task-oriented climate in school classes and sport groups is called the **TARGET model** (for an overview, see Woolfolk, 2019; Digression: Empowering Climate).

Side Story

Digression: Empowering Climate

An **empowering climate** is a current development within motivational climate research, which also considers components of "self-determination theory" (SDT; Deci & Ryan, 2000). SDT assumes that every person has three basic psychological needs: the need for competence, autonomy, and relatedness. The better these **basic needs** are satisfied in a certain situation, the higher the probability of the person's intrinsic motivation. In sport, the situation and thus the satisfaction of basic needs can be influenced by the coach. In this sense, **autonomy-supportive** coaches consider the wishes of their athletes, involve them in decisions, and try to understand their perspectives. By contrast, **controlling** (and not autonomy-supportive) coaches behave in an intimidating and restrictive way and put pressure on the athletes. Coaches who value the need for relatedness behave in a socially supportive manner by showing that they value each individual athlete, both as an athlete and as a human being. In addition, they create a structure that is characterized by an unambiguous description of expectations as well as by clear, timely, and informative feedback.

If these SDT-based constructs are combined with the two factors of the motivational climate, two overarching dimensions can be formed (Duda & Appleton, 2016). First, an **empowering climate** consists of a focus on task orientation, autonomy support, social support, and structure. Second, ego orientation and control are assigned to the **disempowering climate**. Initial studies on an *empowering* climate show that it is associated with positive effects such as greater satisfaction, fewer dropouts, and better performance, while a *disempowering* climate is accompanied by negative feelings, burnout, and reduced self-esteem (for a summary, see Duda and Appleton, 2016). Based on the conceptual considerations and the "TARGET model of motivational climate," an intervention tool for teachers and coaches was developed (Duda, 2013).

16.5.2 Leadership Structure Within the Team

In addition to leadership by coaches, there is usually a **leadership structure** within a group with roles and status for each person (▶ Chap. 22). This leadership structure is based on various formal and informal leaders (Fransen et al., 2014b; Loughead et al., 2006). Although formal leaders in sport are often determined or chosen by the coach or the team, informal leadership develops over time through intra-team interactions. Within a team, there are four different types of informal leaders: (1) the **task-oriented leader**, who takes responsibility for the goals and tactical behavior of the team; (2) the **motivational leader**, who motivates the other players and supports them to do their best; (3) the **social leader**, who takes care of the harmony within the team and the positive relationships among players; and (4) the **external leader**, who facilitates contact with the coach, the club, the media, and other people outside the team (Fransen et al., 2014a; Fransen et al., 2014b). These leadership functions may be the responsibility of one person but are usually spread over several people in a group. The quality of the overall leadership within a team influences its efficacy and helps to achieve common goals (Fransen et al., 2014b; Glenn & Horn, 1993). Furthermore, the development of informal leaders has a positive correlation with individual and team performance (Zhang et al., 2012).

16.5.3 Role Ambiguity

Role Ambiguity

Role ambiguity refers to a lack of understanding by a group member regarding the expectations for his/her role responsibilities.

Role ambiguity represents one of several cognitions individuals hold about their group responsibilities (e.g., role commitment, role satisfaction), though role ambiguity to date has been a major focus of research efforts. In their role ambiguity conceptual model, Beauchamp et al. (2002) described four areas that are important to consider with respect to understanding one's role in a sport team. The first area deals with the general scope of **responsibility** that a player must understand within a team. The second area relates to understanding the **behavioral patterns** that are necessary to successfully complete the responsibilities assigned to a person. The third area consists of the understanding of the **evaluation** of the role performance. The fourth and last area deals with the degree of knowledge one has regarding the consequences of failing to successfully perform the assigned role and responsibilities (for further information on the subject of roles, see ► Chap. 22). Relating this role ambiguity to group performance, research shows that role ambiguity has negative consequences for individual group members as well as the whole group and also limits the performance of groups (Cunningham & Eys, 2007). Although there is no direct empirical evidence for a connection between team performance and other aspects of team roles, it is generally accepted that role perceptions and behaviors are important for group processes, emergent states, and team performance (Kleinert et al., 2012). In particular, this holds true for the communication within the group (Cunningham & Eys, 2007) and group cohesion (Eys et al., 2005; Digression: Group Socialization).

Side Story

Digression: Group Socialization

The **model of group socialization** by Moreland and Levine (1982) explains how individuals in groups establish their respective roles. The theory distinguishes between five different kinds of role classes: prospective group member, new group member, full group member, marginal group member, and former group member. Prior to joining a group (**prospective group member**), the person tries to be informed about the group's past, opportunities the group offers for further development, possible success of the group, and other important aspects. This includes considering what role the person might fulfill within the group in the future. At the same time, the group tries to recruit new members in order to improve in certain areas (e.g., technique, tactics, leadership). Therefore, the group will offer potential roles and responsibilities to interesting prospective group members (see Kramer (1998)). If a person decides to join the group, his or her willingness to work for the interests and the performance of the group increases (**new group member**). At the same time, the socialization of the new group member toward becoming a **full group member** begins. From the point of view of the existing full group members, a new group member has no experience, which means that the person cannot be trusted completely until the group norms and the individual role have been accepted. The more that individuals establish themselves in the group and develop to a full member, the more their commitment and willingness to perform increase. However, if he or she becomes a **marginal group member** because of a change in the situation, their behaviors, or certain characteristics and/or abilities, the commitment and willingness to perform decrease. This group member may subsequently become a **former group member** when they decide to leave the group (or they are dismissed). As a consequence, only a full group member can truly contribute to the success of the group (Forsyth, 2014). To apply this phenomenon to practical situations, this means that marginal group members have to be integrated into the group at an early stage in order to prevent a decline in the performance of the individual and the group. The assignment of specific tasks, appraisal for positive behavior and personal success, and/or social integration in activities outside the actual group context might be helpful for this issue.

Researchers have started to examine the concept of socialization tactics within sport groups (Benson et al., 2016). Benson and Eys (2017) identified three primary tactics that facilitate newcomer adjustment within teams. First, serial tactics occur when veteran athletes share information and advice with newcomers who help them understand task responsibilities and needs. Second, social inclusionary tactics are shared group experiences that focus on the development of interpersonal relationships among members. Finally, coach-initiated role communication tactics directly address the responsibilities of incoming members and have an explicit task focus with consequences for individual and group performance. Their initial work demonstrated theoretically supported links between socialization tactics and newcomers' perceptions of commitment to teammates and coaches, as well as group cohesion (Benson & Eys, 2017), serving to illustrate the importance of this variable during the early group development stage.

16.5.4 Social Identity

Social Identity

Social identity is a part of an individual's self-concept that derives from the knowledge about his/her membership in a social group (or groups), coupled with the value and emotional meaning of that membership.

By developing **social identity theory** (SIT), Tajfel and Turner (1979, 1986) explained that the individual self-concept is not only defined by characteristics that distinguish a person from others but also by memberships to different social groups and the social aspects associated with them. Accordingly, this theory is very important for various aspects of behavior in sports (Rees et al., 2015). In essence, SIT assumes that people desire to give a positive impression in front of others, but also for themselves, in order to maintain a positive self-concept. For this purpose, the person makes comparisons between groups within the same social context that consequently lead to distinctions between one's own group (**ingroup**) and comparable other groups (**outgroup**). In order to appear positively, the ingroup is attributed with positive characteristics, while comparable outgroups (subjectively speaking) tend to be assessed less positively.

The social categories that form the basis for social identity are based on **prototypical attributes** of all team members and refer to norms, values, rules, perceptions, feelings, behaviors, or goals (Turner et al., 1987; Zepp et al., 2013). Although SIT assumes that the **team identity** shared by the majority of members has a positive influence on team performance and results, only a few studies can directly demonstrate this correlation (Murrell & Gaertner, 1992). Nevertheless, it is assumed that if team members do not behave in accordance with the norms, this can lead to destructive conflicts within the team, which in turn have an impact on its efficacy and performance (LaVoi, 2007). Furthermore, a positive correlation with leadership behavior within a team has been shown (de Cremer et al., 2010). However, in order to achieve optimal performance within a team, it is not only necessary that the team possesses a positive social identity. It is also crucial that team members differ on individual personal characteristics and that in addition to a social identity, different personal identities exist inside the team (see Baumeister et al., 2016; Zepp & Kleinert, 2015; Digression: Social Identity in Practice).

Side Story

Digression: Social Identity in Practice

FC Bayern Munich dominated the men's soccer Bundesliga in Germany between the 2012/2013 and 2021/2022 seasons, in some seasons very clearly. The players in other clubs of the league often worked on strategies to defeat FC Bayern Munich's team during this period. How did the players and club managers of the other teams manage to give their best in every training session and every match, despite the prospect of not having a realistic chance of achieving a comparable level of performance in the foreseeable future? One explanation for this is social identity. What can be observed repeatedly is the clear separation of one's own club and FC Bayern Munich's team. The team members of the other clubs have perceived and developed characteristics and attributes of their own team (ingroup) while assuming that the players of Bayern (outgroup) do not have these characteristics. For example, players from other clubs would say "We have more amazing fans," "We stick together even if we don't win the championship," "We have a lower match load," or "We have more fun in training." With the help of these attributes, the players of the other clubs can distinguish themselves from FC Bayern Munich and maintain a positive identity and, thus, a **positive self-concept**, despite perhaps lower success in sports.

16.5.5 Identification with the Team

Identification

Identification describes the positive emotional, cognitive, and affective evaluation of the relationship between the self and the own group (*ingroup*; Brown et al., 1986; Henry et al., 1999).

The identification process of a person with a sport team is always connected with (1) the identification of the group as a team, (2) the differentiation from other teams (of the same sport), (3) the personal identification as a team member, and (4) the personal meaning of belonging to this team. Cognitive, affective, and evaluative processes are responsible for identification with a team (Postmes et al., 2013; Tajfel, 1978). **Cognitive processes of identification** refer to the perception of the identity of a team and to the personal and rational comparison of this identity with one's personal identity. **Affective processes of identification** describe the emotional connection that a person has with a particular team. The **evaluative processes of identification** deal with the relevance of belonging to a particular team (Brown et al., 1986; Henry et al., 1999; Tajfel & Turner, 1979). Obviously, social identity and identification consist of cognitive and emotional aspects. The difference between the two is that whereas we are likely to possess a certain social identity due to our formal membership to a group, we might not necessarily give any importance to that particular identity (i.e., we do not identify with the respective group or category). One example for such a case would be a basketball player who has been traded to a new club where he necessarily needs to adopt the social identity of that team. However, he might not see the team as part of who he personally is (cognitive identification), does not enjoy being together with fellow team members (affective identification), or does not consider it important for him personally to be part of this specific team with their specific social identity.

Team members who identify strongly with their team show a greater willingness to make an effort and to perform well than team members whose identification with the team is less pronounced (Fielding & Hogg, 2000). Baumeister et al. (2016) assume that groups can perform best when, initially, an identification with the team and the willingness to make an effort are developed, followed by the development or assignment of distinct (i.e., clearly defined) identities and roles for the individual group members. The authors were also able to show that identification with a group motivates the individual group members to show more commitment and to accept existing norms and values of the group.

16

16.5.6 Group Cohesion

Group cohesion is an important construct in Eys et al.' (2020a) Conceptual Framework for Research on Sport Teams (► Sect. 16.3.2). As the definition shows, group cohesion is more than just liking each other within a group.

Group Cohesion

Group cohesion is a dynamic emergent state, which is "reflected in the tendency for a group to stick together and remain united in the pursuit of its instrumental objectives and/or for the satisfaction of member affective needs" (Carron et al., 1998, p. 213).

Characteristics of Group Cohesion (Carron et al., 1985)

- **Group cohesion is multidimensional:** There is not "one" overall dimension of group cohesion, but it consists of several factors.
- **Group cohesion is dynamic**: Group cohesion changes constantly depending on current events within and around the team.
- **Group cohesion is instrumental**: All groups have a sense of purpose, even if that purpose is a social one (e.g., to meet and have fun together). Therefore, group cohesion deals with the achievement of mutual goals.
- **Group cohesion is related to emotions**: Group cohesion is also about liking and respecting each other. The individual group members always develop relationships with each other.

In sport, group cohesion is generally described based on the concept of Carron et al. (1985), which particularly emphasizes the **multidimensional nature of cohesion**. This approach distinguishes between an individual level of group membership and the level of the whole group. For example, it could be possible that a female basketball player perceives a high level of group cohesion in her team; however, she herself may not feel too integrated into the group.

In addition, group cohesion can be considered from task- and social-related perspectives. The task-related perspective refers to the specific goals of the group. For example, in a sport situation, the goal of an ice hockey team could be to get promoted at the end of the season. The social perspective relates to relationships among the group members. Therefore, it is possible that the members of a water polo team do not actually get along very well; hence, the social cohesion would be rather low. However, since everyone's goal is the championship title, the task-related cohesion may be very high.

When combining the two levels and perspectives, the four-dimension concept of group cohesion emerges. It contains an individual-, task-related factor (*attraction to the group-task*, ATG-T), an individual-, social-related factor (*attraction to the group-social*, ATG-S), a group- and task-related factor (*group integration-task*, GI-T), and a group- and social-related factor (*group integration-social*, GI-S).

Furthermore, research found evidence for the influence of various aspects on group cohesion with important situational, personal, leadership, and team factors (for a summary, see Carron and Eys (2012); ◘ Table 16.1).

In addition to the fact that group cohesion is related to many performance-related aspects of group structure

Table 16.1 Factors that correlate with group cohesion

Situational factors	Contracts of the individual players
	Cultural/normative pressure
	Level of performance
	Physical/functional proximity of the group
	Permeability of the group (openness to nonmembers)
	Group size
Personal factors	Similarity in demographic aspects
	Gender
	Shared perceptions
	Attribution of responsibility for wins/losses
	Anxiety/depression
	Satisfaction
	Personal sacrifices for the group
	Attendance
	Social loafing
Leadership factors	Leadership behavior of the coach
	Decision style of the coach
	Coach-athlete relationship
Group factors	Perception of status
	Role behavior
	Group norms
	Collective efficacy
	Motivational climate/conflicts

and group processes, numerous studies investigated the direct relationship between group cohesion and group performance. The results are quite clear: a meta-analysis of 46 studies by Carron et al. (2002) reveals that group performance and group cohesion are correlated, both for the social and task dimensions. Thus, higher social cohesion and task cohesion are related to better group performance. A more recent meta-analysis by Castaño et al. (2013) concluded the same phenomenon for groups outside sport. Moreover, the effect is reciprocal, such that higher group cohesion leads to higher performance but conversely better group performance also increases group cohesion (Carron et al., 2002). Furthermore, the relationship between group cohesion and performance appears to be stronger in women's teams than in men's teams, although the reasons for this finding are not yet clear (Eys et al., 2015). The cohesion-performance link is also relevant for co-acting and individual sport contexts (Carron et al., 2002; Ohlert, 2012; Digression: Group Cohesion in Other Areas of Sport).

Despite the clear meta-analytic results, the benefits of group cohesion are repeatedly discussed in sport science and sport practice. There are still challenges with respect to the operationalization of group performance, the adaptation of questionnaires to different sport contexts, and a lack of consensus regarding the underlying theoretical definition/conceptualization across contexts (Ohlert et al., 2015). Additionally, there are discussions regarding how to collate individual responses to represent a group-oriented construct (e.g., using of average values of individuals, using the consistency of the results within a team; Drescher et al., 2012; Digression: Case Study: Unexpected Positive Performance at the European Football Championship Due to Positive Group Processes?)

Digression

Case Study: Unexpected Positive Performance at the European Soccer Championship Due to Positive Group Processes?

At the men's European Soccer Championship in France 2016, two teams, Iceland and Wales, reached the quarterfinals unexpectedly (Wales even reached the semifinals). Experts had predicted that both teams would be eliminated in the qualifying round (Iceland in one group with the Netherlands, among others). Furthermore, after the group phase, they made it through the round of 16 before they were finally defeated in the quarterfinals and semifinals, respectively. Obviously, something had developed in those teams who made them stronger than expected, according to their position in the world ranking. Additionally, statistics analyzed during the championship emphasized this low world ranking: Iceland had the lowest rate of ball possession (36%) and the second worst rate of passing accuracy (75%). Wales' stats demonstrated average performance at best. In contrast, in terms of blocked balls and saves, both teams showed the highest performance. Hence, what is the reason for the unexpected success of these teams? Unfortunately, this cannot be answered scientifically unless a retrospective survey will be conducted with the players of all teams involved. Alternatively, an observation system that would allow for the objective assessment of group cohesion within a team would be very helpful, but this does not exist at the moment. Further, the development of a reliable and valid observational tool is very challenging to create. Ultimately, only speculation and personal assumptions suggest that the increased performance was caused by a high level of **identification with their team and their nation** as well as a high level of **group cohesion** without personal fights for dominance between individual star players (see above Digression: The "Too-Much-Talent Effect"). Because of this feeling of solidarity and common identity, it is possible that they ran more for each other, helped each other more often than players of other teams, and made more sacrifices for each other (unfortunately, there are no statistics for this). Processes such as social comparisons or the perception of the indispensability of one's own performance may also have played a role (▶ Sect. 16.4.3.2). If this could be scientifically proven, it would be the perfect example of the effect of group processes on one's own performance. Or perhaps, it was just caused by superior tactics of the coach and the optimal implementation by the team.

Generally speaking, having high cohesion in a team is viewed as a positive characteristic. However, there may also be negative effects of having too much group cohesion. For example, groups who have high levels of cohesion show an increased level of alcohol consumption (Ohlert & Kleinert, 2014), as well as increased **self-handicapping** and an increased tendency to "overlook" social loafing in their teammates (Carron & Eys, 2012). In addition, increased group cohesion leads to higher conformity to group norms than in less cohesive groups (Prapavessis & Carron, 1997). This effect may explain why group cohesion can also have negative consequences: If negative behaviors exist in a group due to certain group norms, they are further emphasized by a high degree of group cohesion. Thus, group cohesion can also be seen as reinforcing factor for other group processes (both positive and negative).

Side Story

Digression: Group Cohesion in Other Areas of Sport

In addition to competitive sports, **recreational sports and physical activity** represent an important field of research in the area of group cohesion. The consideration of task cohesion is very interesting in this area, since the shared goal is likely not as focused on winning, table positions/standings, or the like. In this context, individual and group goals are more heterogeneous and can range from the acquisition of skills to weight loss, to the improvement of endurance performance, etc. High group cohesion can therefore be characterized by the fact that the group members have very similar **individual goals** and support each other in achieving them. In addition, it should be noted that the term *performance* can be used in the context of recreational sports; however, it may be less relevant in connection with physical activity. For these reasons, it makes sense to look at other positive consequences of group cohesion in physical activity, such as how often and regularly the group members participate in the offered classes, how often they **drop out** of courses, or how positive their attitude is toward exercise.

Overall, studies demonstrated that group cohesion in physical activity groups is positively correlated with attendance, positive attitudes, and (less) dropout (Burke et al., 2008). Thus, group members benefit from liking the others in their group and pursuing similar goals.

There are also initial approaches in the consideration of group cohesion in specific fields of activity, for example, in **physical education in schools** (Kleinknecht et al., 2014), in **rehabilitation sports** (Fraser & Spink, 2002), in individual sports (Evans et al., 2012), or in **children's and youth sport** (Eys et al., 2009), but there are still not enough studies available to make reliable statements. Although the results on group cohesion in typical team sports and physical activity environments can be considered as informative, there is still a significant need for further research in these specific fields.

16.5.7 Collective Efficacy

The construct of collective efficacy describes a group's belief about having the skills to successfully organize and execute actions and behaviors within the group, which are necessary to achieve a particular group goal (Bandura, 1997), even when obstacles and difficulties arise (Feltz & Lirgg, 2001). In addition, alternative definitions have been developed in the scientific literature that pay particular attention to the interactive aspect of collective efficacy within groups.

Collective Efficacy

Collective efficacy is defined most comprehensively as a "group's shared belief in its conjoint capability to organize and execute the courses of action required to produce given levels of attainment" (Bandura, 1997, p. 477).

The degree of collective efficacy within a group influences how individual members of a team, as well as the team as a whole, behave, how much **effort** they put into achieving the goals, and how persistent the team is in pursuing its goals (Bandura, 1997). As a consequence, teams with high collective efficacy choose more **challenging goals** (Silver & Bufanio, 1996), apply more effort, and are more persistent in trying to achieve their goals even under difficult conditions (Greenlees et al., 1999). Many studies and meta-analyses referring to different kinds of sports have empirically demonstrated a positive relationship between the degree of a team's collective efficacy and its performance (Gully et al., 2002; Petitta et al., 2015). Some studies even seem to indicate that collective efficacy is more important to the performance of a team than the individual strengths of the team members (e.g., Fransen et al., 2012).

16.5.8 Team Trust

Trust

Trust describes the intention to make oneself vulnerable to another person, based on positive expectations of that person's actions and behavior.

In recent literature, a distinction has been established between trust, trustworthiness, and the propensity to trust others (for a comprehensive description, see Colquitt et al., 2007). **Trustworthiness** refers to the abilities, care, and integrity of the person whom someone wants to or has to trust. The **propensity to trust** others describes a general willingness to rely on others. On a higher level, **trust** is the conscious decision to be vulnerable to others, in the positive assumption that this person has the skills and qualities to successfully master a situation and not take advantage of one's own weakness. Behavior that can have a negative effect on trust within a group includes noncompliance with rules, a (unjustified) change in norms and values, shirking responsibility, breaking promises, lying, stealing ideas, or passing on confidential information (Franz, 2012). These behaviors influence the group members' trust in the group's hierarchy or leadership structure. Other negative behaviors that affect trust in another person include publicly criticizing others, accusing others unfairly or falsely for negative events, and insulting group members or the whole group. If trust within a group has been damaged, group members may react in different ways, which in the worst case can affect the efficacy of the group and consequently group performance (Franz, 2012). A lack of trust can have several negative outcomes that range in severity from smaller consequences (e.g., doing nothing, fantasizing about possible revenge) to more influential outcomes (e.g., social withdrawal of individual group members; Bies and Tripp, 1996).

Once trust within a group is damaged in any way, it must be rebuilt to restore the group's full functionality. Basic strategies for rebuilding trust are openness, honesty, behaving ethically, appreciation of commitment, communication with others, and consistent and moral actions (Whipple, 2009). Both the efficacy of a team and the communication that is necessary for interaction between group members are based on trust between members (Breuer et al., 2016; Yukelson, 1993).

16.6 Diagnostics of Performance-Relevant Group Processes

In order to carry out targeted sport psychology interventions with groups to improve various group processes, it is necessary to determine the current state of the group. It is immensely important to use valid and reliable instruments, otherwise the results are not meaningful and subsequent interventions cannot achieve targeted effects (Kleinert et al., 2012).

16.6.1 Overview of Available Instruments

▫ Table 16.2 shows an overview of the available **diagnostic tools** in the area of group processes which have support for their reliability and validity.

Table 16.2 Overview of available diagnostic tools for group processes

Construct/instrument	Context	Authors
Motivational climate		
Peer motivational climate in youth sport questionnaire (PeerMCYSQ)	Elite sports Leisure sports Physical activity	Ntoumanis and Vazou (2005)
Perceived motivational climate in sport Questionnaire-2 (PMCSQ-2)	Elite sports Leisure sports Physical activity	Newton et al. (2000)
Observational system for motivational climate (with the BEST software)	Elite sports Leisure sports Physical activity	Morgan et al. (2005)
Empowering and disempowering motivational climate questionnaire-coach (EDMCQ-C)	Elite sports Leisure sports Physical activity	Appleton et al. (2016)
Multidimensional motivational climate observation system (MMCOS)	Elite sports Leisure sports Physical activity	Smith et al. (2015)
Role perceptions		
Role ambiguity scale (RAS)	Team sports	Beauchamp et al. (2002)
Role commitment scale for sport	Team sports	Eys et al. (2020a)
Social identity		
Questionnaire for the perception of prototypes within a team (PWT)	Elite sports Leisure sports Physical activity	Zepp et al. (2013)
Identification with a group		
Scale for the identification with a group (SIG)	Elite sports Leisure sports Physical activity	Zepp and Kleinert (2015)
Group cohesion		
Group environment questionnaire (GEQ)	Elite sports	Carron et al. (1985) and Ohlert et al. (2015)
Physical activity group environment questionnaire (PAGEQ)	Leisure sports Physical activity	Estabrooks and Carron (2000)
Youth sport environment questionnaire (YSEQ)	Adolescents from 12 years of age	Eys et al. (2009)
Child sport cohesion questionnaire	Children 9–12 years of age	Martin et al. (2012)
Collective efficacy		
Collective efficacy questionnaire in sports (CEQS)	Elite sports	Short et al. (2005)
Trust		
VIST-scale	Elite sports	Hertel (2002)

16.6.2 Diagnosing the Needs of the Team

Based on the Conceptual Framework for Research on Sport Teams (▶ Sect. 16.3.2), attempts have been made to provide some guidance toward team interventions in terms of what to focus on when developing the group. Bruner et al. (2020) created a brief 11-item questionnaire (i.e., Team Environment AssessMent) to quickly assess team members' perceptions of the state of the group environment, structure, and processes. The goal is to identify those aspects that need specific attention rather than providing a broad teambuilding intervention. In their work with an elite hockey team, the initial responses to the questionnaire identified role acceptance and leadership as targets. This knowledge helped direct intervention activities, and post-intervention responses to the same survey suggested some success in modifying the athletes' perceptions of these variables in a positive manner.

As a second example, Ohlert and Zepp developed a theoretically based **team diagnostic process** for assessing performance-relevant group processes in sport teams, called the "momentum TEAMdiagnostik" (Ohlert & Zepp, 2016). In order to obtain an overview of the sociopsychological state of a group as holistically and comprehensively as possible, the "TEAMdiagnostik" uses various methods during training and competition situations, including questionnaires, interviews with players, as well as systematic observations. ◘ Table 16.3 provides an overview of the methods used in the "TEAMdiagnostik" to assess the different sociopsychological processes or constructs.

◘ **Table 16.3** Overview of the methods used in "TEAMdiagnostik" (based on Ohlert and Zepp (2016))

Construct	Online questionnaire	Observation	Interview
Motivational climate		X	X
Leadership structure	X		X
Communication		X	X
Collective efficacy	X		
Group cohesion	X	X	X
Team trust	X		
Identification	X		
Perceived roles	X		X
Identity	X		

Team diagnosis is divided into four phases: (1) initial interview and **analysis of needs**, (2) diagnostics, (3) analyses, and (4) feedback of results. During the initial interview, the content-related focus and organizational aspects of the team diagnostics are discussed. This process starts about 10 days prior to being present at a practice or competition with the dissemination of an online questionnaire to the coach and the players. After 10 days, the second step includes videotaping a training and competition session and capturing the statements of the coach with a lapel microphone. In order to keep the reactivity of the group members as low as possible, the research team behaves as unobtrusively as possible. Individual interviews are conducted with a total of six group members (e.g., formal leader, one or two informal leaders, three to four randomly selected additional group members) in order to obtain the most comprehensive impression of the social processes within the team. After the measurement sessions, the questionnaire data, the video and audio recordings, and the interviews, all responses are evaluated, analyzed, and prepared in terms of content and graphics. The written report contains information about the **resources and potential** of the group, which the coach can utilize and integrate with the team. About 2 weeks after the diagnostics are presented, personal feedback of the results takes place. In this personal conversation, the sport psychology consultant presents the diagnostic results to the coaches, followed by a discussion about available resources and intervention approaches. In order to ensure the quality and **sustainability** of the diagnostics, the coach is contacted approximately 1 month after the personal conversation to discuss the development and possible changes in the group or to clarify any questions about the results. Experience shows that individual intervention approaches can be derived for each group based on the results (Ohlert & Zepp, 2016).

Learning Control Questions

Basic:

1. How can a "real group" be distinguished from a collection of people?
2. What distinguishes a disjunctive group task from an additive group task?
3. How should a coach of a team act according to Tuckman's "Phase Model of Team Development" in the *Storming* phase?

Advanced:

4. What are some general group processes according to the conceptual framework for the study of sport groups by Carron et al.?

5. How does social loafing differ from the Ringelmann effect?
6. Which theoretical model can be applied to explain the Köhler effect?
7. What are the differences between motivational climate and *empowering* climate?

Experts:

8. Which nine factors and processes within a team are relevant for team performance?
9. How do members of a weaker sport team maintain a positive team identity?
10. Which four factors are part of group cohesion?

References

Ames, C. A. (1992). Achievement goals, motivational climate, and motivational processes. In G. C. Roberts (Ed.), *Motivation in sport and exercise* (pp. 161–176). Human Kinetics.

Anshel, M. H. (1995). Examining social loafing among elite female rowers as a function of task duration and mood. *Journal of Sport Behavior, 18*(1), 39–49.

Apitzsch, E. (2006). Collective collapse in team sports: A theoretical approach. In F. Boen, B. de Cuyper, & J. Opdenacker (Eds.), *Current research topics in exercise and sport psychology in Europe* (pp. 35–46). LannooCampus Publishers.

Appleton, P. R., Ntoumanis, N., Quested, E., Viladrich, C., & Duda, J. L. (2016). Initial validation of the coach-created Empowering and Disempowering Motivational Climate Questionnaire (EDMCQ-C). *Psychology of Sport and Exercise, 22*, 53–65. https://doi.org/10.1016/j.psychsport.2015.05.008

Balaguer, I., Duda, J. L., Atienza, F. L., & Mayo, C. (2002). Situational and dispositional goals as predictors of perceptions on individual and team improvement, satisfaction and coach ratings among elite female handball teams. *Psychology of Sport and Exercise, 3*, 293–308.

Bandura, A. (1997). *Self-efficacy. The exercise of control*. Freeman.

Baumeister, R. F., Ainsworth, S. E., & Vohs, K. D. (2016). Are groups more or less than the sum of their members? The moderating role of individual identification. *Behavioral and Brain Sciences, 39*, e137. https://doi.org/10.1017/S0140525X15000618

Beauchamp, M. R., Bray, S. R., Eys, M. A., & Carron, A. V. (2002). Role ambiguity, role efficacy, and role performance: Multidimensional and mediational relationships within interdependent sport teams. *Group Dynamics: Theory, Research, and Practice, 6*(3), 229–242. https://doi.org/10.1037//1089-2699.6.3.229

Benson, A., & Eys, M. (2017). Understanding the consequences of newcomer integration processes: The Sport Team Socialization Tactics Questionnaire. *Journal of Sport & Exercise Psychology, 39*, 13–28. https://doi.org/10.1123/jsep.2016-0182

Benson, A. J., Evans, B., & Eys, M. A. (2016). Organizational socialization in team sport environments. *Scandinavian Journal of Medicine and Science in Sports, 26*, 463–473. https://doi.org/10.1111/sms.12460

Bies, R., & Tripp, T. M. (1996). Beyond trust: "Getting even" and the need for revenge. In R. D. Kramer & T. R. Tyler (Eds.), *Trust in organizations: Frontiers of theory and research* (pp. 246–260). Sage Publications.

Boss, M., & Kleinert, J. (2015). Explaining social contagion in sport applying Heider's balance theory: First experimental results. *Psychology of Sport and Exercise, 16*(3), 160–169. https://doi.org/10.1016/j.psychsport.2014.10.006

Breuer, C., Hüffmeier, J., & Hertel, G. (2016). Does trust matter more in virtual teams? A meta-analysis of trust and team effectiveness considering virtuality and documentation as moderators. *Journal of Applied Psychology, 101*(8), 1151–1177.

Brown, R., Condor, S., Matthews, A., Wage, G., & Williams, J. (1986). Explaining intergroup differentiation in an industrial organization. *Journal of Occupational Psychology, 59*, 273–286. https://doi.org/10.1111/j.2044-8325.1986.tb00230.x

Bruner, M. W., Eys, M., Carreau, J. M., McLaren, C., & Van Woezik, R. (2020). Utilizing the Team Environment AssessMent (TEAM) to enhance team building in sport. *The Sport Psychologist, 34*, 62–70. https://doi.org/10.1123/tsp.2018-0174

Burke, S. M., Carron, A. V., & Shapcott, K. M. (2008). Cohesion in exercise groups: An overview. *International Review of Sport and Exercise Psychology, 1*(2), 107–123. https://doi.org/10.1080/17509840802227065

Carron, A. V., Brawley, L. R., & Widmeyer, W. N. (1998). The measurement of cohesiveness in sport groups. In J. L. Duda (Ed.), *Advancements in sport and exercise psychology measurement* (pp. 213–226). Fitness Information Technology.

Carron, A. V., Colman, M. M., Wheeler, J., & Stevens, D. (2002). Cohesion and performance in sport. A meta analysis. *Journal of Sport and Exercise Psychology, 24*, 168–188.

Carron, A. V., & Eys, M. A. (2012). *Group dynamics in sport* (4th ed.). Fitness Information Technology.

Carron, A. V., & Hausenblas, H. A. (Eds.). (1998). *Group dynamics in sport* (2nd ed.). Fitness Information Technology.

Carron, A. V., Widmeyer, W. N., & Brawley, L. R. (1985). The development of an instrument to assess cohesion in sport teams: The Group Environment Questionnaire. *Journal of Sport Psychology, 7*, 244–266. https://doi.org/10.1177/104649640003100105

Castaño, N., Watts, T., & Tekleab, A. G. (2013). A reexamination of the cohesion–performance relationship meta-analyses. A comprehensive approach. *Group Dynamics: Theory, Research, and Practice, 17*(4), 207–231. https://doi.org/10.1037/a0034142

Colquitt, J. A., Scott, B. A., & LePine, J. A. (2007). Trust, trustworthiness, and trust propensity: A meta-analytic test of their unique relationships with risk taking and job performance. *Journal of Applied Psychology, 92*(4), 909–927. https://doi.org/10.1037/0021-9010.92.4.909

Cunningham, I., & Eys, M. A. (2007). Role ambiguity and intra-team communication in interdependent sport teams. *Journal of Applied Social Psychology, 37*(10), 2220–2237.

de Backer, M., Boen, F., de Cuyper, B., Høigaard, R., & Vande Broek, G. (2015). A team fares well with a fair coach: Predictors of social loafing in interactive female sport teams. *Scandinavian Journal of Medicine and Science in Sports, 25*, 897–912. https://doi.org/10.1111/sms.12303

de Cremer, D., van Dijke, M., & Mayer, D. M. (2010). Cooperating when "you" and "I" are treated fairly: The moderating role of leader prototypicality. *Journal of Applied Psychology, 95*(6), 1121–1133. https://doi.org/10.1037/a0020419

Deci, E. L., & Ryan, R. M. (2000). The "what" and "why" of goal pursuits. Human needs and the self-determination of behavior. *Psychological Inquiry, 11*(4), 227–268. https://doi.org/10.1207/S15327965PLI1104_01

DeLamater, J. (1974). A definition of "group". *Small Group Research, 5*(1), 30–44. https://doi.org/10.1177/104649647400500103

Drescher, S., Burlingame, G. M., & Fuhriman, A. (2012). Cohesion: An Odyssey in empirical understanding. *Small Group Research, 43*(6), 662–689. https://doi.org/10.1177/1046496412468073

16

Duda, J. L. (2013). The conceptual and empirical foundations of empowering coaching™: Setting the stage for the PAPA project. *International Journal of Sport and Exercise Psychology, 11*(4), 311–318. https://doi.org/10.1080/1612197X.2013.839414
Duda, J. L., & Appleton, P. R. (2016). Empowering and disempowering coaching climates: Conceptualization, measurement issues, and intervention implications. In M. Raab, P. Wylleman, R. Seiler, A.-M. Elbe, & A. Hatzigeorgiadis (Eds.), *Sport and exercise psychology research* (pp. 373–388). Elsevier.
Duda, J. L., & Balaguer, I. (2007). Coach-created motivational climate. In S. Jowett & D. Lavallee (Eds.), *Social psychology in sport* (pp. 117–130). Human Kinetics.
Estabrooks, P. A., & Carron, A. V. (2000). The Physical Activity Group Environment Questionnaire. An instrument for the assessment of cohesion in exercise classes. *Group Dynamics: Theory, Research, and Practice, 4*, 230–243. https://doi.org/10.1037/1089-2699.4.3.230
Evans, M. B., Eys, M. A., & Bruner, M. W. (2012). Seeing the "we" in "me" sports: The need to consider individual sport team environments. *Canadian Psychology/Psychologie Canadienne, 53*(4), 301–308. https://doi.org/10.1037/a0030202
Everett, J. J., Smith, R. E., & Williams, K. D. (1992). Effects of team cohesion and identifiability on social loafing in relay swimming performance. *International Journal of Sport Psychology, 23*(4), 311–324.
Eys, M., Beauchamp, M. R., Godfrey, M., Dawson, K., Loughead, T. M., & Schinke, R. J. (2020a). Role commitment and acceptance in a sport context. *Journal of Sport & Exercise Psychology, 42*, 89–101. https://doi.org/10.1123/jsep.2019-0057
Eys, M. A., Carron, A. V., Beauchamp, M. R., & Bray, S. R. (2005). Athletes' perceptions of the sources of role ambiguity. *Small Group Research, 36*(4), 383–403. https://doi.org/10.1177/1046496404268533
Eys, M. A., Evans, M. B., & Benson, A. (2020b). *Group dynamics in sport* (5th ed.). Fitness Information Technology.
Eys, M. A., Loughead, T. M., Bray, S. R., & Carron, A. V. (2009). Development of a cohesion questionnaire for youth: The youth sport environment questionnaire. *Journal of Sport & Exercise Psychology, 31*, 390–408.
Eys, M. A., Ohlert, J., Evans, B., Wolf, S. A., Martin, L., VanBussel, M., et al. (2015). Cohesion and performance for female and male sport teams. *The Sport Psychologist, 29*(2), 97–109. https://doi.org/10.1123/tsp.2014-0027
Feltz, D. L., Forlenza, S. T., Winn, B., & Kerr, N. L. (2014). Cyber buddy is better than no buddy: A test of the Köhler motivation effect in exergames. *Games for Health, 3*(2), 98–105.
Feltz, D. L., Kerr, N. L., & Irwin, B. C. (2011). Buddy up: The Köhler effect applied to health games. *Journal of Sport & Exercise Psychology, 33*, 506–526.
Feltz, D. L., & Lirgg, C. D. (2001). Self-efficacy beliefs of athletes, teams, and coaches. In R. N. Singer, H. A. Hausenblas, & C. M. Janelle (Eds.), *Handbook of sport psychology* (2nd ed., pp. 340–361). Wiley.
Feuchter, A., & Funke, J. (2004). Positive Effekte sozialen Faulenzens beim Lösen komplexer Probleme [positive effects of social loafing when solving complex problems]. *Kölner Zeitschrift für Soziologie und Sozialpsychologie, 56*(2), 304–325.
Fielding, K. S., & Hogg, M. A. (2000). Working hard to achieve self-defining group goals: A social identity analysis. *Zeitschrift für Sozialpsychologie, 31*(4), 191–203. https://doi.org/10.1024//0044-3514.31.4.191
Forsyth, D. R. (2014). *Group dynamics* (6th ed.). Wadsworth Cengage Learning.
Fransen, K., Coffee, P., Vanbeselaere, N., Slater, M., de Cuyper, B., & Boen, F. (2014a). The impact of athlete leaders on team members' team outcome confidence: A test of mediation by team identification and collective efficacy. *The Sport Psychologist, 28*(4), 347–360. https://doi.org/10.1123/tsp.2013-0141
Fransen, K., Vanbeselaere, N., de Cuyper, B., Vande Broek, G., & Boen, F. (2014b). The myth of the team captain as principal leader: Extending the athlete leadership classification within sport teams. *Journal of Sports Sciences, 32*(14), 1389–1397. https://doi.org/10.1080/02640414.2014.891291
Fransen, K., Vanbeselaere, N., Exadaktylos, V., Vande Broek, G., de Cuyper, B., Berckmans, D., et al. (2012). "Yes, we can!": Perceptions of collective efficacy sources in volleyball. *Journal of Sports Sciences, 30*, 641–649. https://doi.org/10.1080/02640414.2011.653579
Franz, T. M. (2012). *Group dynamics and team interventions. Understanding and improving team performance*. Blackwell.
Fraser, S. N., & Spink, K. S. (2002). Examining the role of social support and group cohesion in exercise compliance. *Journal of Behavioral Medicine, 25*(3), 233–249.
Glenn, S. D., & Horn, T. S. (1993). Psychological and personal predictors of leadership behavior in female soccer athletes. *Journal of Applied Sport Psychology, 5*(1), 17–34. https://doi.org/10.1080/10413209308411302
Greenlees, I. A., Graydon, J. K., & Maynard, I. (1999). The impact of collective efficacy beliefs on effort and persistence in a group task. *Journal of Sports Sciences, 17*, 151–158.
Gully, S. M., Incalcaterra, K. A., Joshi, A., & Beubien, J. M. (2002). A meta-analysis of team-efficacy, potency, and performance: Interdependence and level of analysis as moderators of observed relationships. *Journal of Applied Psychology, 87*, 819–832.
Hackman, J. R. (2002). *Leading teams: Setting the stage for greater performances*. Harvard Business School Press.
Hardy, C. J. (1990). Social loafing. Motivational losses in collective performance. *International Journal of Sport Psychology, 21*, 305–327.
Hardy, C. J., & Latané, B. (1988). Social loafing in cheerleaders: Effect of team membership and competition. *Journal of Sport & Exercise Psychology, 10*, 109–114.
Harkins, S. (1987). Social loafing and social facilitation. *Journal of Experimental Social Psychology, 23*, 1–18. https://doi.org/10.1016/0022-1031(87)90022-9
Harkins, S., & Szymanski, K. (1989). Social loafing and group evaluation. *Journal of Personality and Social Psychology, 56*, 934–941. https://doi.org/10.1037/0022-3514.56.6.934
Hart, J. W., Bridgett, D. J., & Karau, S. J. (2001). Coworker ability and effort as determinants of individual effort on a collective task. *Group Dynamics: Theory, Research, and Practice, 5*(3), 181–190.
Hart, J. W., Karau, S. J., Stasson, M. F., & Kerr, N. A. (2004). Achievement motivation, expected coworker performance, and collective task motivation: Working hard or hardly working? *Journal of Applied Social Psychology, 34*(5), 984–1000.
Heckhausen, H. (1977). Achievement motivation and its constructs. A cognitive model. *Motivation and Emotion, 1*, 283–329.
Henry, K. B., Arrow, H., & Carini, B. (1999). A tripartite model of group identification: Theory and measurement. *Small Group Research, 30*, 558–581. https://doi.org/10.1177/104649649903000504
Hertel, G. (2002). Management virtueller teams auf der basis sozialpsychologischer Theorien. Das VIST-Modell. [Management of virtual teams based on social psychological theories. The VIST model]. In F. H. Witte (Ed.), *Sozialpsychologie wirtschaftlicher Prozesse* (pp. 172–202). Pabst.
Heuzé, J.-P., & Brunel, P. C. (2003). Social loafing in a competitive context. *International Journal of Sport and Exercise Psychology, 1*(3), 246–263.
Hodge, K., Henry, G., & Smith, W. (2014). A case study of excellence in elite sport. Motivational climate in a world champion team.

The Sport Psychologist, 28(1), 60–74. https://doi.org/10.1123/tsp.2013-0037

Høigaard, R., Fuglestad, S., Peters, D. M., de Cuyper, B., de Backer, M., & Boen, F. (2010). Role satisfaction mediates the relation between role ambiguity and social loafing among elite women handball players. *Journal of Applied Sport Psychology, 22*(4), 408–419. https://doi.org/10.1080/10413200.2010.495326

Høigaard, R., & Ingvaldsen, R. P. (2006). Social loafing in interactive groups. The effects of identifiability on effort and individual performance in floorball. *Athletic Insight, 8*(2), 52–63.

Huddleston, S., Doody, S. G., & Ruder, M. K. (1985). The effect of prior knowledge of the social loafing phenomenon on performance in a group. *International Journal of Sport Psychology, 16*, 176–182.

Hüffmeier, J., Dietrich, H., & Hertel, G. (2013a). Effort intentions in teams: Effects of task type and teammate performance. *Small Group Research, 44*(1), 62–88.

Hüffmeier, J., & Hertel, G. (2011). When the whole is more than the sum of its parts. Group motivation gains in the wild. *Journal of Experimental Social Psychology, 47*(2), 455–459. https://doi.org/10.1016/j.jesp.2010.12.004

Hüffmeier, J., Kanthak, J., & Hertel, G. (2013b). Specificity of partner feedback as moderator of group motivation gains in Olympic swimmers. *Group Processes & Intergroup Relations, 16*(4), 516–525. https://doi.org/10.1177/1368430212460894

Hüffmeier, J., Krumm, S., Kanthak, J., & Hertel, G. (2012). Don't let the group down: Facets of instrumentality moderate the motivating effects of groups in a field experiment. *European Journal of Social Psychology, 42*, 533–538.

Ingham, A. G., Levinger, G., Graves, J., & Peckham, V. (1974). The Ringelmann effect. Studies of group size and group performance. *Journal of Experimental Social Psychology, 10*, 371–384.

Irwin, B. C., Scorniaenchi, J., Kerr, N. L., Eisenmann, J. C., & Feltz, D. L. (2012). Aerobic exercise is promoted when individual performance affects the group: A test of the Kohler motivation gain effect. *Annals of Behavioral Medicine: A Publication of the Society of Behavioral Medicine, 44*(2), 151–159. https://doi.org/10.1007/s12160-012-9367-4

Jackson, J. M., & Williams, K. D. (1985). Social loafing on difficult tasks. Working collectively can improve performance. *Journal of Personality and Social Psychology, 49*, 937–942. https://doi.org/10.1037/0022-3514.49.4.937

Johnson, D. W., & Johnson, F. P. (2009). *Joining together: Group theory and group skills* (10th ed.). Pearson.

Karau, S. J., Markus, M. J., & Williams, K. D. (2000). On the elusive search for motivation gains in groups. Insights from the collective effort model. *Zeitschrift für Sozialpsychologie, 31*(4), 179–190.

Karau, S. J., & Williams, K. D. (1993). Social loafing. A meta-analytic review and theoretical integration. *Journal of Personality and Social Psychology, 65*(4), 681–706.

Karau, S. J., & Williams, K. D. (1997). The effects of group cohesiveness on social loafing and social compensation. *Group Dynamics: Theory, Research, and Practice, 1*(2), 156–168. https://doi.org/10.1037/1089-2699.1.2.156

Kerr, N. L., & Bruun, S. (1983). The dispensability of member effort and group motivation losses: Free rider effects. *Journal of Personality and Social Psychology, 44*, 78–94. https://doi.org/10.1037/0022-3514.44.1.78

Kerr, N. L., Forlenza, S. T., Irwin, B. C., & Feltz, D. L. (2013). '… been down so long …': Perpetual vs. intermittent inferiority and the Köhler group motivation gain in exercise groups. *Group Dynamics: Theory, Research, and Practice, 17*(2), 67–80.

Kleinert, J., Ohlert, J., Carron, A. V., Eys, M. A., Feltz, D. L., Harwood, C., et al. (2012). Group dynamics in sport. An overview and recommendations on diagnostic and intervention. *The Sport Psychologist, 26*, 412–434.

Kleinknecht, C., Kleinert, J., & Ohlert, J. (2014). Erfassung von „Kohäsion im Team von Freizeit- und Gesundheitssportgruppen" (KIT-FG) [Measuring group cohesion in recreational and health sport (KIT-FG]. Zeitschrift für Gesundheitspsychologie, 22(2), 68–78.

Köhler, O. (1926). Kraftleistungen bei Einzel- und Gruppenarbeit [Power performance in individual and group tasks]. *Industrielle Psychotechnik, 3*, 274–282.

Köhler, O. (1927). Über den Gruppenwirkungsgrad der menschlichen Körperarbeit und die Bedingung optimaler Kollektivkraftreaktion [On group efficiency of physical human work and the conditions of optimal collective power reactions]. *Industrielle Psychotechnik, 4*, 209–226.

Kramer, R. M. (1998). Paranoid cognition in social systems: Thinking and acting in the shadow of doubt. *Personality and Social Psychology Review, 2*, 251–275.

Kravitz, D. A., & Martin, B. (1986). Ringelmann rediscovered: The original article. *Journal of Personality and Social Psychology, 50*(5), 936–941.

Latané, B. (1981). The psychology of social impact. *American Psychologist, 36*, 343–356. https://doi.org/10.1037/0003-066X.36.4.343

Latané, B., Williams, K. D., & Harkins, S. (1979). Many hands make light the work: The causes and consequences of social loafing. *Journal of Personality and Social Psychology, 37*(6), 822–832. https://doi.org/10.1037/0022-3514.37.6.822

LaVoi, N. M. (2007). Interpersonal communication and conflict in the coach-athlete relationship. In S. Jowett & D. Lavallee (Eds.), *Social psychology in sport* (pp. 29–40). Human Kinetics.

Loughead, T. M., Hardy, J., & Eys, M. A. (2006). The nature of athlete leadership. *Journal of Sport Behaviour, 29*, 142–158.

Martin, L. J., Carron, A. V., Eys, M. A., & Loughead, T. (2012). Development of a cohesion questionnaire for children's sport teams. *Group Dynamics: Theory, Research, and Practice, 16*, 68–79. https://doi.org/10.1037/a0024691

Max, E. J., Samendinger, S., Winn, B., Kerr, N. L., Pfeiffer, K. A., & Feltz, D. L. (2016). Enhancing aerobic exercise with a novel virtual exercise buddy based on the Kohler effect. *Games for Health Journal, 5*(4), 252–257. https://doi.org/10.1089/g4h.2016.0018

Miles, J. A., & Greenberg, J. (1993). Using punishment threats to attenuate social loafing effects among swimmers. *Organizational Behavior and Human Decision Processes, 56*(2), 246–265.

Moede, W. (1927). Die Richtlinien der Leistungs-Psychologie [Benchmarks for performance psychology]. *Industrielle Psychotechnik, 4*, 193–207.

Moll, T., Jordet, G., & Pepping, G.-J. (2010). Emotional contagion in soccer penalty shootouts: Celebration of individual success is associated with ultimate team success. *Journal of Sports Sciences, 28*(9), 983–992.

Moreland, R. L., & Levine, J. M. (1982). Socialization in small groups: Temporal changes in individual-group relations. *Advances in Experimental Social Psychology, 15*, 137–192.

Moreland, R. L., & Levine, J. M. (2012). A history of small group research. In A. W. Kruglanski & W. Stroebe (Eds.), *Handbook of the history of social psychology* (pp. 383–405). Taylor & Francis.

Morgan, K., Sproule, J., Weigand, D., & Carpenter, P. J. (2005). A computer-based observational assessment of the teaching behaviours that influence motivational climate in physical education. *Physical Education & Sport Pedagogy, 10*(1), 83–105.

Murrell, A. J., & Gaertner, S. L. (1992). Cohesion and sport team effectiveness. The benefit of a common group identity. *Journal of Sport & Social Issues, 16*(1), 1–14. https://doi.org/10.1177/019372359201600101

16

Newton, M. L., Duda, J. L., & Yin, Z. (2000). Examination of the psychometric properties of the Perceived Motivational Climate in Sport Questionnaire-2 in a sample of female athletes. *Journal of Sports Sciences, 18*(4), 275–290.
Nilsen, T., Haugen, T., Reinboth, M., Peters, D. M., & Høigaard, R. (2014). Explicit prior knowledge of social loafing does not reduce social loafing in subsequent team cycle trial performance. *Kinesiologia Slovenica, 20*(2), 17–25.
Ntoumanis, N., & Vazou, S. (2005). Peer motivational climate in youth sport. Measurement development and validation. *Journal of Sport & Exercise Psychology, 27*(4), 432–455.
Ohlert, J. (2009). *Teamleistung. Social loafing in der Vorbereitung auf eine Gruppenaufgabe [Team performance. Social loafing during preparation for a group task]*. Kovač.
Ohlert, J. (2012). Kohäsionsfragebogen für Individual- und Teamsport—Leistungssport (KIT-L)—A German-language instrument for measuring group cohesion in individual and team sports. *International Journal of Sport and Exercise Psychology, 10*(1), 39–51. https://doi.org/10.1080/1612197X.2012.645129
Ohlert, J., & Kleinert, J. (2013). Social loafing during preparation for performance situations. The preloafing effect. *Social Psychology, 44*, 231–237. https://doi.org/10.1027/1864-9335/a000107
Ohlert, J., & Kleinert, J. (2014). Sozialer Kontext und antizipierter Alkoholkonsum bei Leistungssportlern [Social context and anticipated alcohol consumption in elite athletes]. *SUCHT, 60*(2), 73–83.
Ohlert, J., Kleinknecht, C., & Kleinert, J. (2015). Group cohesion reworded—Measuring group cohesion feelings in sport. *Sportwissenschaft, 45*(3), 116–126. https://doi.org/10.1007/s12662-015-0364-1
Ohlert, J., & Zepp, C. (2016). Theory based team diagnostics and interventions. In M. Raab, P. Wylleman, R. Seiler, A.-M. Elbe, & A. Hatzigeorgiadis (Eds.), *Sport and exercise psychology research* (pp. 347–370). Elsevier.
Petitta, L., Jiang, L., & Palange, M. (2015). The differential mediating roles of task, relations, and emotions collective efficacy on the link between dominance and performance. A multilevel study in sport teams. *Group Dynamics: Theory, Research, and Practice, 19*(3), 181–199. https://doi.org/10.1037/gdn0000031
Postmes, T., Haslam, S. A., & Jans, L. (2013). A single-item measure of social identification: Reliability, validity, and utility. *British Journal of Social Psychology, 52*(4), 597–617. https://doi.org/10.1111/bjso.12006
Prapavessis, H., & Carron, A. V. (1997). Sacrifice, cohesion, and conformity to norms in sport teams. *Group Dynamics: Theory, Research, and Practice, 1*(3), 231–240. https://doi.org/10.1037/1089-2699.1.3.231
Rees, T., Alexander Haslam, S., Coffee, P., & Lavallee, D. (2015). A social identity approach to sport psychology: Principles, practice, and prospects. *Sports Medicine, 45*(8), 1083–1096. https://doi.org/10.1007/s40279-015-0345-4
Ringelmann, M. (1913). Recherches Sur les moteurs animes: Travail de l'homme [Research on living machines: Work of human]. *Annales de l'Institut National Agronomique, 12*(1), 1–40.
Short, S. E., Sullivan, P. J., & Feltz, D. L. (2005). Development and preliminary validation of the collective efficacy questionnaire for sports. *Measurement in Physical Education and Exercise Science, 9*(3), 181–202.
Silver, W. S., & Bufanio, K. M. (1996). The impact of group efficacy and group goals on group task performance. *Small Group Research, 27*, 347–359.
Smith, N., Tessier, D., Tzioumakis, Y., Quested, E., Appleton, P., Sarrazin, P., et al. (2015). Development and validation of the multidimensional motivational climate observation system. *Journal of Sport & Exercise Psychology, 37*(1), 4–22. https://doi.org/10.1123/jsep.2014-0059
Sobleski, B. (2017, February 6). *How did the Atlanta falcons blow super bowl LI?* Bleacher Report. https://bleacherreport.com/articles/2691400-how-did-the-atlanta-falcons-blow-super-bowl-xli
Steiner, I. D. (1972). *Group processes and productivity*. Academic Press.
Stroebe, W., Diehl, M., & Abakoumkin, G. (1996). Social compensation and the Koehler effect. Toward a theoretical explanation of motivation gains in group productivity. In E. H. Witte & J. H. Davis (Eds.), *Understanding group behavior. Small group processes and interpersonal relations* (pp. 37–65). Lawrence Erlbaum; Lawrence Erlbaum Associates.
Swaab, R. I., Schaerer, M., Anicich, E. M., Ronay, R., & Galinsky, A. D. (2014). The too-much-talent effect. Team interdependence determines when more talent is too much or not enough. *Psychological Science, 25*(8), 1581–1591.
Swain, A. (1996). Social loafing and identifiability: The mediating role of achievement goal orientations. *Research Quarterly for Exercise and Sport, 67*(3), 337–344.
Tajfel, H. (1978). Social categorization, social identity and social comparison. In H. Tajfel (Ed.), *Differentiation between social groups* (pp. 61–76). Academic Press.
Tajfel, H., & Turner, J. C. (1979). An integrative theory of intergroup conflict. In W. G. Austin & S. Worchel (Eds.), *The social psychology of intergroup relations* (2nd ed., pp. 33–47). Brooks/Cole.
Tajfel, H., & Turner, J. C. (1986). The social identity theory of intergroup behavior. In S. Worchel & W. G. Austin (Eds.), *Psychology of intergroup relations* (2nd ed., pp. 7–24). Nelson-Hall.
Thompson, B., & Thornton, B. (2007). Exploring mental-state reasoning as a social-cognitive mechanism for social loafing in children. *The Journal of Social Psychology, 147*(2), 159–174.
Todd, A. R., Seok, D.-H., Kerr, N. L., & Messé, L. A. (2006). Social compensation: Fact or social-comparison artifact? *Group Processes & Intergroup Relations, 9*(3), 431–442.
Tuckman, B. W. (1965). Developmental sequences in small groups. *Psychological Bulletin, 63*, 348–399.
Tuckman, B. W., & Jensen, M. A. C. (1977). Stages of small-group development revisited. *Group & Organization Management, 2*(4), 419–427. https://doi.org/10.1177/105960117700200404
Turner, J. C., Hogg, M. A., Oakes, P. J., Reicher, S. D., & Wetherell, M. S. (Eds.). (1987). *Rediscovering the social group. A self-categorization theory*. Blackwell.
Van Dick, R., Stellmacher, J., Wagner, U., Lemmer, G., & Tissington, P. A. (2009). Group membership salience and task performance. *Journal of Managerial Psychology, 24*(7), 609–626. https://doi.org/10.1108/02683940910989011
Van Dick, R., & West, M. A. (2013). *Teamwork, Teamdiagnose, Teamentwicklung [Teamwork, team diagnosis, team development]* (2nd ed.). Hogrefe.
Vroom, V. H. (1964). *Work and motivation*. Wiley.
Weber, B., & Hertel, G. (2007). Motivation gains of inferior group members: A meta-analytical review. *Journal of Personality and Social Psychology, 93*(6), 973–993. https://doi.org/10.1037/0022-3514.93.6.973
Wergin, V. V., Zimanyi, Z., Mesagno, C., & Beckmann, J. (2018). When suddenly nothing works anymore within a team - causes of collective sport team collapse. *Frontiers in Psychology, 9*, 2115. https://doi.org/10.3389/fpsyg.2018.02115
Whipple, R. (2009). Reinforcing candor: It builds trust and transparency. *Leadership Excellence, 26*(6), 17.
Williams, K. D., & Karau, S. J. (1991). Social loafing and social compensation. The effects of expectations of co-worker performance. *Journal of Personality and Social Psychology, 61*(4), 570–581.

Williams, K. D., Nida, S. A., Baca, L. D., & Latané, B. (1989). Social loafing and swimming. Effects of identifiability on individual and relay performance of intercollegiate swimmers. *Basic and Applied Social Psychology, 10*, 73–81.

Woolfolk, A. (2019). *Educational Psychology* (14th ed.). Pearson Studium.

Yukelson, D. P. (1993). Communicating effectively. In J. Williams (Ed.), *Applied sport psychology: Personal growth to peak performance* (pp. 122–136). Mayfield Publishing.

Zepp, C., & Kleinert, J. (2015). Symmetric and complementary fit based on prototypical attributes of soccer teams. *Group Processes & Intergroup Relations, 18*(4), 557–572. https://doi.org/10.1177/1368430214556701

Zepp, C., Kleinert, J., & Liebscher, A. (2013). Inhalte und Strukturen prototypischer Merkmale in Fußballmannschaften [contents and structure of prototypical attributes in soccer teams]. *Sportwissenschaft, 43*(4), 283–290. https://doi.org/10.1007/s12662-013-0305-9

Zhang, Z., Wladman, D. A., & Wang, Z. (2012). A multilevel investigation of leader-member exchange, informal leader emergence, and individual and team performance. *Personnel Psychology, 65*(1), 49–78.

Social Influence of Sport Spectators

Bernd Strauss, Kathrin Staufenbiel, Edda van Meurs and Clare MacMahon

Contents

J. Schüler et al. (eds.), *Sport and Exercise Psychology*, https://doi.org/10.1007/978-3-031-03921-8_17

Learning Objectives

Basic:
- To define social influence and how it can be related to sport
- To describe various forms of social influence

Advanced:
- To outline and compare the main theories and models that explain social influence
- To present the key seminal studies on social influence

Experts:
- To elucidate how spectators may be a significant factor in causing the home advantage

17.1 Introduction

Social influence has been summarized as the change in one's beliefs, behavior, or attitudes due to external pressure that may be real or imagined (Cialdini, 2001).

In this chapter, we focus on the question of how (sports-relevant) behavior and athletic performances are influenced by others, especially passive observers (see ► Sect. 17.3) and active sport spectators (see ► Sect. 17.4).

You have probably already experienced giving a presentation in front of a group of people. Were you influenced by the presence of your audience? Was your performance better, worse, or unaffected compared to the rehearsal session when you practiced alone? Is your performance influenced differently when the audience listens attentively as opposed to when they are noisily not paying attention? How does this presence of others impact performances and behaviors in motor tasks and in the context of sports? In sports, social influence has already been investigated extensively (cf. Epting et al., 2011; Strauss, 2002b). A particular interest within social influence research is the home advantage in team sports (Allen & Jones, 2014; Carron et al., 2005). Research in this field is concerned with understanding whether the performance of the home team is better due to more of *their* fans being in the stadium.

17

17.2 Forms of Social Influence of Spectators

The most basic differentiation of social influence is the one between a "directly evident" and "not directly evident" influence (see Strauss & MacMahon, 2014).

A *directly evident influence* is experienced when it is obvious and directly observable and there is no doubt that one or more spectators had an impact on the performance or behavior of the athletes. This may occur in the form of a spectator running onto the field to stop play or competition or in an attempt to hurt or kill a player. A terrible example of the latter is the on-court assault of famous tennis player Monica Seles in 1993 by a fanatic spectator.

A *not directly evident influence* is harder to account for and thus needs to be explained and embedded in psychological or sociological theory. This may mean that it is doubtful that the influence even exists at all. Moreover, the underlying explanation for the influence is not directly evident, is probabilistic in nature, and has theoretical and empirical support. In this chapter, we give an overview of this *not directly evident influence*.

To continue to generally discuss spectator influences, we can go back to 1935, when Dashiell published a list of potential types of not directly evident influences exerted by people on performers. Dashiell's list (see ◘ Table 17.1) is useful to derive ideas for potential areas to study in this field.

This collection of possible types of influencers distinguishes first between the involvement with the actor (e.g., "passive audience," "competitors," "co-actors," "cooperating or interacting"). Secondly, it highlights further characteristics of the other persons (e.g., "size and status of the audience"), and thirdly, it describes specific behaviors (e.g., "giving ratings," "passing on information", "volume"). According to Dashiell's classification (Dashiell, 1935), a "passive audience" occurs when others are merely present, i.e., when others are only observing the actor and do not interact, support, or discourage them. In the context of sports, various types of influencers may be present: sport spectators, who may either be observing the sporting performance passively (mere presence) or engage in directly influencing behaviors like reinforcement, razzing, and encouragement (Landers & McCullagh, 1976). Spectators may come in small num-

◘ **Table 17.1** Types of influencers by Dashiell (1935), cf. Guerin (1993)

(1) A passive audience
(2) A co-worker not in competition with the performer
(3) A contestant
(4) An evaluator making comments on the work
(5) A cooperator, dedicated to the same goal
(6) An information controller
(7) A prestigious or large audience

bers to practice sessions, or in tens of thousands, e.g., to the Soccer World Cup final (large and prestigious audiences; Dashiell, 1935). In either situation, the spectators are commonly separated from the athletes, do not actively participate in the performance, and thus do not interact with the athlete. Spectators' social relationship with the actor of interest may vary from being fans who have never met the athlete to relatives who are close to the athlete. The relationship between a performer and the audience was also found to impact the performance (Cox, 1966).

On the other hand, an athlete might be influenced by the co-actors and competitors present. Allport (1924) discriminated between effects resulting from the presence of a co-actor or rival in competitive situations. The diverging influences are most likely due to the confounding role of competitive motivation in the presence of a competitor (Aiello et al., 1979). Co-actors are a borderline case in terms of their classification as spectators: they perform the same activity (in principle) at the same time as the actors (Zajonc, 1965), e.g., rowers or sprinters. They can be in competition with the actor or not (e.g., chess players in a tournament, who play simultaneously but not against each other). Co-actors and competitors are often more limited in number in comparison to spectators, and in many cases show similar personal characteristics (gender, age).

Coaches and referees are an integral social part of sports. They can be considered interactors that convey important information about the qualitative or quantitative evaluation of the performance. Rather than spectators who pass on general information to the actors (e.g., information about the end of the match, "cheering" as information for a home competition), coaches, judges, and referees provide information about the performance result (e.g., "you were offside when you received that pass") or the quality of the performance (e.g., "lower and upper leg were at an angle of 90 degrees"). They have other reasons for observing and are therefore not sports spectators in the strict sense of the word.

Starting with the seminal work of Kelman (1958), there have been various attempts to develop general models of social influence to explain the circumstances under which performance, beliefs, and attitudes change (for an overview, see Flake et al., 2017). A prominent example was formulated by Latané (1981), who proposed a *general theory of social influence*. It is kept "general" because this theory should refer to all facets of social influence and not to specific social processes.

The basic idea by Latané (1981) is that of a social force field in which there are sources of influence and one or more goals of influence. Different forces (the sources of influence) act on one or more goals, which, according to Latané (1981), can be divided into three aspects: "strength," "immediacy," and "number." "Strength (S)" can be described as the frequency, significance, power, or intensity of the source of influence and is for example operationalized through the status of the source (e.g., whether the audience includes experts, friends, fans, opponents, etc.), the behavior of the sources of influence (e.g., supportive, unsupportive), or the predictable relationship to the target (e.g., emotional ties between the athlete and the audience). "Immediacy (I)" is the temporal and spatial immediacy of the source of influence and refers, e.g., to the observable, the immediate presence of an audience in a stadium, as well as the not immediate presence of a media audience. "Number (N)" indicates the absolute number of persons present who may act as a source of influence in a specific case.

According to Latané (1981), the social force, "social impact (SI)," is a multiplicative function of these characteristics: strength (S), immediacy (I), and number (N). The multiplicative relationship signals that if one of the three aspects of a source of influence is eliminated, social influence does not occur. It is also interesting to note that Latané (1981) formulated another principle regarding the influence of the number of spectators, which he called the psychosocial law of the marginal impact (Latané, 1981, p. 349): The more spectators are present, the smaller the influence of each additional spectator. This is particularly interesting in the context of the presence of others (for more information, see ► Sect. 17.4).

17.3 Social Facilitation: Social Influence of Passive Spectators

In Burnham (1910), Burnham published the first scoping review that synthesized a number of studies on the presence of other performers (as co-actors or in competition). In this article, reference was made to the article "The Dynamogenic Factors in Pacemaking and Competition" by Norman Triplett (1898), a pioneering study that is included in any textbook on social and sports psychology (for a critical discussion related to the interpretation of the results, see Martin, 2020; Stroebe, 2012).

Study Box

Triplett (1898) looked at the influence of co-acting persons who are in competition with the performing person. First, in an archival study, he reported that cyclists with pacers (riders setting the cycling pace) were about 25% faster than those without pacers. Triplett (1898) discussed several explanations, e.g., the encouragement, the social comparison between competitors, and their reciprocal distraction. He argued that the physical presence of a competitor leads to an "idea" of one's own movement and thus releases one's own energy ("dynamogenic explanation", p. 531).

Secondly, he conducted an experiment in which his subjects (school children) had to turn a crank as quickly as possible on a "competition machine", either while performing simultaneously with someone standing directly beside them or while alone. Surprisingly, while some subjects' performance improved as expected, others showed a performance decline or even remained unaffected by the presence of the competitor. The latter was explained by Triplett (1898) as a potential overstimulation.

Burnham (1905, 1910) also reported some early academic and pedagogical-psychological studies conducted in Germany (e.g., by Mayer, 1904; Meumann, 1904), which did not investigate the effects of the presence of others in a competitive context (like Triplett, 1898), but in a co-acting setting. E.g., Meumann (1904) found that children's performance was always poorer in the alone condition in comparison to conditions where others were co-acting with them. He assumed that the pupils would be distracted by the presence of spectators but would show increased performance through increased effort. On the other hand, Burnham (1910) argued that this difference occurred mainly due to rivalries and the intention to impress, rather than distractions (cf. Guerin, 1993).

During the following decade, a few other seminal studies on the presence of others were conducted (e.g., Moede, 1920; Moore, 1917). In 1913, Moede (a former student of Wilhelm Wundt, a German psychologist, who established the first experimental psychological laboratory in Leipzig in 1879, and who is widely considered as one of the founders of experimental psychology, see, e.g., Danziger, 2000) conducted a series of experimental studies in Germany with pupils and students who had to complete various tasks (e.g., measures of strength, concentration, and memory) alone or in the presence of others ("just watching" as well as under conditions of co-acting with and without competition). The German report "Experimentelle Massenpsychologie" ("Experimental Crowd Psychology"), which strongly influenced the history of psychology and in particular social psychology, could only be published in 1920 due to the First World War.

In his experiments, Moede determined that on average, performance increased when others were present, but that the variation of performances compared to the alone condition decreased. Moede (1920) explained the increases in performance with, among other reasons, people's ambition and striving for satisfaction. Interestingly enough, he was already indirectly referring to the conditional aspects of strength tasks (and their energetically determined nature).

> It was not until 1924 that the term *social facilitation* was coined by Floyd Allport. Allport published an English textbook that had a considerable influence on social psychological research. Here, he laid the foundation for experimental social psychology. He gave two explanations for the findings described when the presence of others was investigated: firstly, the rivalry between the actor and the co-actors, and secondly *social facilitation*, "… which consists of an increase in response merely from the sight or sound of others making the same movement" (Allport, 1924, p. 262).

Allport (1920, 1924), in his numerous experiments, used, e.g., association tasks, among others. His subjects were asked to solve the tasks under alone conditions as well as under conditions with an audience (four or five persons, no competition). This spectator condition was different compared to studies such as Triplett (1898), in which conditions were competitive and thus spectator influence and competition were combined. With this distinction, Allport hoped to use the conditions of cooperation to investigate the "real" influence of spectators. It turned out that under the conditions of co-action, the quantitative performance with regard to the associative tasks was increased. More ideas were also identified in the production of critical arguments. Contradictory to these findings, Meumann (1904) and Burnham (1910) found that creative tasks that involved active problem-solving were inhibited rather than facilitated in the classroom, where co-actors are present.

This newly identified field of social facilitation was soon picked up by various disciplines: similar experiments were conducted with nonhuman animals (e.g., monkeys, ants, finches, cockroaches, rats, turtles, sunfish; for an overview of the anthology, see Zajonc, 1969) as well as with human subjects (e.g., pupils, students, workers). The majority of these studies compared performances in cognitive (or motor) tasks in the presence

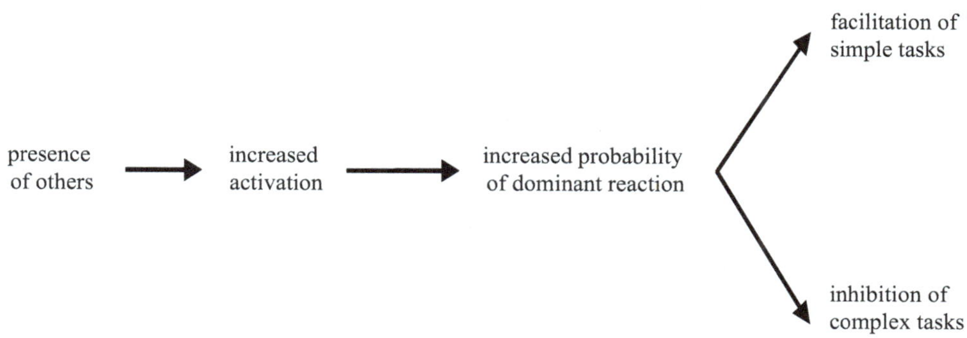

Fig. 17.1 Social facilitation and social inhibition (adapted from Zajonc, 1965)

of spectators or co-actors to performances alone (the usual control group).

After four decades of numerous empirical studies with human as well as animal subjects, which were carried out without a sound theoretical framework (for a detailed overview, see Guerin, 1993; Strauss, 2002a), both performance improvements and deteriorations were observed in the presence of spectators or co-actors, yet it was not until 1965 that a satisfactory theoretical framework to explain the contradictory results from human and animal experiments was provided with the groundbreaking work by Robert B. Zajonc (1965).

Zajonc (1965) developed an integrated activation theory model to explain the partly contradictory research results. Zajonc (1965) distinguished between two types of tasks: well-learned, i.e., easy tasks, and novel, i.e., complex tasks. He put forward the hypothesis that well-learned, easy routine tasks are more likely to be positively affected by the presence of others (*social facilitation*), while complex, novel tasks are more likely to be negatively affected (*social inhibition*). To support his argument, Zajonc referred to the *drive theory* (Hull, 1943; Spence, 1956), according to which the presence of others from the same species leads to an innate increase in arousal and a willingness to respond to the actions of others.

Figure 17.1 shows how, according to Zajonc (1965), the presence of others leads to either social facilitation or inhibition. According to this, arousal tends to lead to an increased probability of reactions that have priority in a person's behavioral repertoire, so-called dominant reactions, which are considered easy behaviors. On the other hand, social presence inhibits non-dominant reactions, i.e., novel and complex behaviors.

Another activation-based model places particular emphasis on the evaluation apprehension of people who perform a task in the presence of others (Cottrell et al., 1968). Here, arousal through the presence of others is not attributed to an innate drive, but to the learned expectation and concern of being evaluated by others. Experimental studies show that this evaluation could play an important role when performing a task in the presence of others (Maxwell et al., 2008; Worringham & Messick, 1983). These results also follow the expectations arising from the *social impact theory* described above (Latané, 1981). For example, the assumption of being evaluated leads to better performance among people with high self-efficacy expectations (expectations of their own ability) than the assumption of not being evaluated (Sanna, 1992). A subsequent meta-analysis by Uziel (2007) found that subjects with high levels of extraversion and self-esteem (positive orientation) experienced performance increments, while subjects with high levels of neuroticism and low self-esteem (negative orientation) performed significantly worse in both simple and complex tasks.

Other explanatory models following these first two approaches focus on attentional processes (see Strauss, 2002a), which are disturbed by the mere or active presence of others. In these models, it is assumed that the presence of an audience impairs the optimal alignment of the actor's attention to the task to be performed. This can lead to conflicts of attention. Here, two directions can be distinguished: Firstly, there may be a conflict between the attention paid to a social stimulus—such as the audience, the co-actor, or the experimenter (see Brown & Harkins, 2020)—and non-social stimuli—such as noise—and the task ("distraction"). On the other hand, there can be an attentional conflict between the self and the task ("self-attention").

Several theoretical advances revolve around this concept of cognitive overload and an exhaustion of the attentional capacity (overload hypothesis, Baron, 1986; capacity model, Manstead & Semin, 1980; distraction-conflict hypothesis, Sanders et al., 1978, Fig. 17.2). To avoid task failure, a "priority ranking" of the conflicting stimuli is created (Boggs & Simon, 1968), which narrows the attentional range and taxes the cognitive capacity. Their hypothesis states that new, complex tasks with high attentional demands are impaired, whereas well-learned tasks that require less attention are not impaired or even facilitated in this context.

The biopsychosocial model by Blascovich and Tomaka (1996) and Blascovich et al. (1999) integrates theoretical frameworks in the domain of human behav-

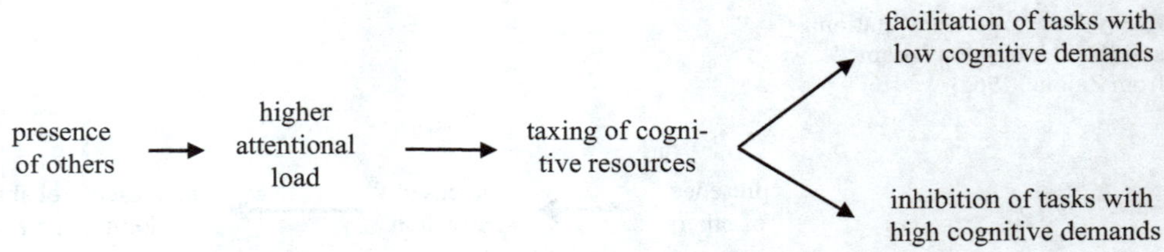

Fig. 17.2 Visualization of the capacity model (Manstead & Semin, 1980)

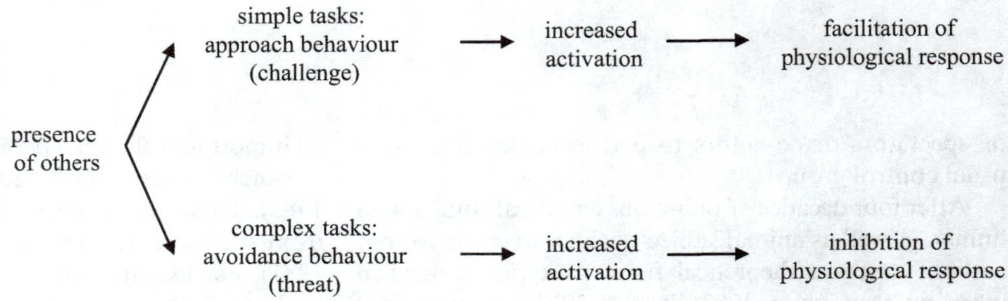

Fig. 17.3 Visualization of the biopsychosocial model in the context of social facilitation

ior and emphasizes the social, information-processing processes of the actor. In addition to physiological (e.g., arousal) and cognitive processes (e.g., attention, cognitive assessment), their model addresses emotional processes (e.g., positive or negative feelings). If a situation is perceived as relevant and important to the goal, the person's own resources and possible actions are evaluated in order to cope with it. This evaluation can be innate or learned, unconscious or conscious. If one's resources are considered sufficient, the situation is perceived as a challenge, and if insufficient, it is perceived as a threat (Fig. 17.3). This ultimately influences behavior and performance in this situation. According to Blascovich et al. (1999), the mere or active presence of others increases the importance of a situation and thus the probability of perceiving it as a challenge or threat. Derived from this, the presence of others in simple, well-learned tasks is more likely to lead to the situation being perceived as challenging and to better performance than when the task is performed alone. On the other hand, during complex or new tasks, the presence of others will cause the actor to perceive the situation as a threat and should therefore lead to decreased performance.

17

The proposal of these theoretical explanations led to a significant increase in the number of studies investigating social facilitation and social inhibition. This growth was especially noticeable for research into social influence on motor performances (see van Meurs et al., 2022, p. 26).

By 1983, the quantity of empirical evidence allowed for the estimation of the overall magnitude and direction of the social facilitation effect: in a meta-analysis, Bond and Titus (1983) quantified the magnitude of the social facilitation effect due to the presence of others on human performance. They included 241 studies, in which the participants primarily worked on cognitive tasks. The overall influence of the presence of others was very small, and the authors concluded that only 0.3–3% of the variance in performance parameters can be explained by social influence. The task's difficulty (simple vs. complex) and its requirements (speed vs. accuracy requirements) moderated the influence of others' presence on task performance. Yet, it has to be noted that the quality of the experiments was mostly low due to low internal validity and the potentially confounding presence of the experimenter (Guerin, 1993).

In the context of sports, social facilitation due to the mere presence of spectators was investigated in numerous studies (see Strauss, 2002a). Very few studies used distinct motor tasks. Rather, this research employed cognitive tasks with fine motor coordination skill demands: e.g., pursuit rotor task (Martens, 1969a, 1969b, 1969c; Wankel, 1977) or a finger labyrinth task (e.g., Miyamoto, 1979; Rajecki et al., 1977). Other gross motor tasks involved balancing (e.g., Landers, 1975; Lau et al., 2019; Murray, 1982), running, and measures of strength (e.g., Feltz et al., 2011; Martens & Landers, 1969; Moede, 1920; Sheridan et al., 2019). In a comprehensive narrative review, Strauss (2002a) distinguished between studies on the spectators' influence during predominantly condition-based tasks (performance highly dependent on energetic potentials, e.g., strength, endurance, speed), during predominantly coordination-based tasks (performance highly dependent on information-processing skills, e.g., fine motor skills), and during tasks that require a mixture of both condition and coordination. Overall, however, the empirical results do not support one theory. Strauss (2002a) found that the presence of others positively affected condition-based, also called energy-based/effort-based, tasks (*general drive hypothesis*, Zajonc, 1965) and negatively affected coordination-based, also called skill-based, tasks due to higher cognitive demands (*overload hypothesis*, Manstead & Semin, 1980): during tasks with high condition demands, the presence of others tends to result in an increase in performance; in tasks with high coordination demands, the presence of others tends to lead to a decrease in performance. This is especially true if the task is not yet well learned. If the task requires both condition and coordination, no difference in performance is to be expected when others are present (Strauss, 2002a). A recent and comprehensive systematic review and meta-analysis considering 100 years of experimental research of the existing empirical evidence (van Meurs et al., 2022) indicates a similar trend in line with the findings by Bond and Titus (1983) and Strauss (2002a): condition-based tasks mostly reliant on speed appear to be facilitated (e.g., Feltz et al., 2011; Worringham & Messick, 1983), while coordination-based tasks performed under time and precision pressure show inconsistent results (e.g., Lau et al., 2019; Miyamoto, 1979). Effect sizes for tasks with coordination demands are smaller and show more variability. Van Meurs et al. (2022) conclude that the findings in the context of motor performances support both the drive and the overload hypothesis as expected.

Nonetheless, Strauss' narrative review (2002a) as well as van Meurs et al.'s (2022) review and meta-analysis suggest that theoretical models on the influence of spectators in relation to a precise taxonomy of sporting performance still need to be developed. In general, the social influence of the passive or co-active presence of others during sporting performance—as well as during cognitive tasks (Bond & Titus, 1983)—seems to be rather small. Yet, several questions remain unanswered to this day: is social facilitation driven by activation or attention? What is the role of the experimenter in empirical studies? How does virtual presence affect cognitive and even motor performance? This latter question has received particular attention in the last decade. In the *social impact theory* (Latané, 1981), a virtual presence is represented by the immediacy aspect. Several studies have made first advances to study whether a social influence occurs in digital virtual realities without the physical presence of others (Feltz et al., 2011; Murray et al., 2016; Snyder et al., 2012). College students were able to hold a plank position (fitness exercise) longer when co-planking with another subject via Skype in comparison to planking alone (Feltz et al., 2011). Female subjects performed better on a rowing ergometer if they were presented not only with a virtual reality environment, but also with a virtual teammate with whom they cooperated (Murray et al., 2016). New empirical and theoretical insights into the social influence of others are expected in using digitalization and the development of ever-improving virtual reality (VR) environments. The research should be mindful of the difference between virtual and real-world situations, however, and avoid simple generalization of results from one to the other.

Study Box

Murray et al. (2016) developed a study design to test the use of virtual reality during exergaming. More specifically, they wanted to know how a virtual environment might affect both performance and subjective evaluation measures as well as the additive effect of a virtual co-actor. To do so, they had $N = 60$ female subjects ($M = 20.20$ years old) row in either of the three conditions:

No virtual reality (NVR): no virtual-reality environment was presented during the rowing exercise.

Individual virtual reality (IVR): participants saw a virtual-reality environment; however, no teammate was present, and no mention was made of it.

Co-actor virtual reality (CVR): participants saw a third-person virtual-reality environment with another boat rowing next to them. They were told that they were rowing simultaneously with another subject (which was a cover story and "confirmed" via a telephone call with a confederate).

In the CVR condition, participants were told that the team score would be derived from the shortest distance rowed in 9 min. Meanwhile, the teammate's performance was manipulated in such a way that the second boat was 40% faster than the baseline performance by the subject.

While the CVR group covered a significantly greater distance than the IVR group and thereby had a higher heart rate, this difference was not associated with the other performance measures (power and strokes per minute). Moreover, the subjective self-reports of felt arousal, positive feelings, affect and enjoyment during the exercise, perceived exertion, and intrinsic motivation did not differ between the two groups, indicating that these psychological measures did not account for the increase in performance in the presence of a teammate. The authors suggest that the teammate's performance may have been used as a benchmark or that a more representative pacing strategy was employed.

While this experiment does add to the objective quantification that another person's presence (physical or virtual, see also Blascovich & McCall, 2013; Feltz et al., 2011, 2014) may positively affect performance outcomes, it does not yet clarify the psychosocial or attentional processes at the heart of this effect.

17.4 Home Advantage and Disadvantage: Social Influence of Active Spectators

Spectators in a sports-relevant context are usually not merely present or co-acting, but also behave, sometimes consciously, and may exert social influence, e.g., to support the actors during their performances. Additionally, they may have a negative influence, e.g., by behaving dismissively, which prevents actors from performing optimally. These behaviors include visual (e.g., waving flags, distracting clothing) as well as auditory characteristics (e.g., noise, shouting, singing). As long ago as 216 BC, the writer Polybius reported that a fistfight at the Panhellenic Games in Olympia between Cleitomachus and Aristonikus (see Guttmann, 1986) was significantly influenced by the audience's shouts. These other behaviors that spectators can engage in determine the "strength" aspect in the *social impact theory* by Latané (1981) or, with regard to the "immediacy" aspect, the direct or indirect presence of spectators (e.g., spectators may be in the stadium, but also on the internet or in front of the TV). The influence of digitalization on the "number" (N) aspect has increased massively in the last few years, as can be seen in the TV ratings and the online streaming services, next to the physically present number of spectators in the stadium.

Laird (1923) carried out what was likely the first experimental investigation of the influence of the hostile behavior of spectators in a sports-relevant context. He examined the influence of a mocking ("*razzing*") audience on various motor skills. "*Razzing*" represents an attempt to discourage the athlete and can be understood as a negative feedback. In Laird's (1923) experiment, the test subjects had to complete several tests in the presence of calm and friendly spectators at first, followed by the same tests, this time performed in front of scoffing spectators. It turned out that, especially in coordination tests, performance dropped significantly when the subjects had to perform in front of razzing spectators.

17

However, it cannot be assumed that non-supportive behavior always leads to a decrease in performance (and supportive behavior to an increase), as a study by Kozar (1973) showed. He had his subjects learn a balancing task either alone or in front of a supportive or a non-supportive audience. The learning progress across multiple trials did not depend on the behavior of the audience.

Other coordination-based skills that have received research attention were closed motor skills from different sports. Epting et al. (2011) examined individual actions in basketball (free throw), baseball (pitching), and golf (hitting a golf ball) in an experimental study design (with the three observer conditions cheering, jeering, and silence). The free-throw performances remained unaffected by the experimental manipulation, while baseball players were negatively influenced by the jeering and golfers performed significantly worse both in the cheering and jeering conditions. Hence, the influence appears to be dependent on the type of sport; however, it remains unclear why these differences exist.

For predominantly condition- (or energy-/effort-) based tasks (requiring the consumption of oxygen, e.g., endurance, speed, power tasks), it is often assumed that encouragement of an active spectator leads to an increase in effort and motivation and finally to an increase in performance, resp. to an decrease in the case of discouragement of an active spectator (see, e.g., Strauss & MacMahon, 2014; Wallace et al., 2005). However, there are only a few controlled experiments testing this assumption. Recently, Edwards et al. (2018) showed that a verbally encouraging spectator leads to relevant performance increments in an endurance task (20 min on an ergometer) and a speed task (a sprint cycling test with two 30-s bouts) when compared to a control condition with a passive spectator. Otte et al. (2021) experimentally tested the effect of noise on passes (passing times and accuracy) of soccer players in a standardized technical training environment called "Footbonaut". The players were faster (passing times) in the (0) baseline condition (constant light signals and beep sound signals, 75dB) in comparison to the condition in which (1) no auditory information was available, as well as in comparison to (2) the negative auditory-cue condition (e.g., loud crowd booing presented through speakers, 85 dB), but not in comparison to (3) the positive auditory-cue condition (loud crowd singing, also presented through speakers, 85dB). Passing accuracy was not affected by the noise conditions.

The direct or indirect social influence of active sports spectators has been studied in the context of home advantage, where the outcome of a competition on a group level but also individual level in so-called home and away situations (e.g., winning and losing statistics at home, won yards in football) is investigated. From here on, we will focus on large audiences as categorized by Dashiell (1935).

Side Story

In an article in the New York Times on 9 January 1972, the renowned sports columnist Leonard Koppett was probably one of the first observers to introduce a definition of home field advantage in a sports context: "Being at home increases your chance of winning." In the sports science literature, home advantage is described as the increased probability of successfully completing a sporting competition under "home" conditions (one's "own" sports stadium, one's "own" bobsleigh run, etc.; see examples in Carron et al., 2005; Courneya & Carron, 1992).

A home advantage in individual sports has rarely been documented to date, and if so, the effect was found to be relatively small (see, e.g., the concerned chapters in Gómez-Ruano et al., 2021; Jones, 2013). In a recent study, the opposite—a home disadvantage—was found for biathlon shooting performances across tournaments from 2001 to 2017: athletes from the top quartile of the ranking missed significantly more shots when performing in their home country as opposed to when performing abroad (Harb-Wu & Krumer, 2019). However, after a review of the available literature, Jones (2013) concludes that a home advantage in individual sports can only be identified (and if so, only at a very low level) if the result is mediated by a subjective component, e.g., because refereeing judgements are included.

Unlike in individual sports, it has been shown consistently that a home advantage exists in team sports (for a comprehensive overview, see the edition by Gómez-Ruano et al., 2021). Many comparing overviews show a lot of variation in the size of the home advantage (see, e.g., Carron et al., 2005; Courneya & Carron, 1992; Jamieson, 2010; Pollard et al., 2017; Staufenbiel et al., 2015; Strauss & MacMahon, 2014): interestingly, the magnitude of the home advantage differs as a function of the type of sport. In reviewing the existing evidence, the home advantage was strongest in soccer and weakest in baseball and cricket (e.g., Jamieson, 2010; Jones, 2018). Moreover, a number of archival studies show that home advantage in soccer and other sports varies between countries (e.g., Pollard et al., 2017; Pollard & Gómez, 2014b; Riedl et al., 2014) as well as between men and women (Pollard et al., 2017; Pollard & Gómez, 2014a). In male team sports leagues, the home advantage is usually higher than in female leagues. For soccer in particular (but also in other team sports), it was found that home advantage has declined in recent decades, in some cases significantly (Palacios-Huerta, 2004; Peeters & van Ours, 2020; Pollard & Pollard, 2005; Riedl et al., 2014).

A key question in the understanding of home advantage revolves around the underlying mechanisms. The most frequently investigated reasons so far are the influence of spectators as well as that of referees (see, e.g., Pollard & Armatas, 2017). However, travel factors, (competition/tournament) rules, familiarity with the venue, tactics/strategies of coaches, and physiological and psychological variables are also taken into account. These potential influencing factors can also be found in the seminal additive framework model developed by Carron et al. (2005).

When athletes, coaches, referees, or fans themselves are interviewed, they report that they perceive spectators to be the most important factor for the home advantage (Anderson et al., 2012; Fothergill et al., 2014). Fothergill et al. (2014) interviewed professional soccer players and coaches and asked for their views on home advantage. Overall, the respondents assumed that fans have an influence on the players. For example, one soccer player explained that it is very important for players to have the fans' support: "[…] of course for a player the big thing is to have the fans behind you […] the best thing when you play at home is the fans" (Fothergill et al., 2014, p. 323). The influence of the spectators is therefore often considered to be the decisive factor for the home advantage, e.g., when a loud audience supporting the home team or local athletes is assumed, or even when spectators are present in large numbers. This is frequently called the thesis of social support (Strauss, 2002b).

The "classic" assumption is that higher spectator numbers (or the measures derived from them) are advantageous for the home team and disadvantageous for the away team. Schwartz and Barsky (1977) argue that a large number of spectators would indicate higher social support for the home team from "their" home audience and at the same time create social rejection for the away team. In line with this thinking is the idea that a larger number of spectators would result in a higher degree of partiality, which is expressed in the form of different public behavioral characteristics such as cheering and booing. This is used to forecast increases in performance for the home team and decreases in performance for the away team.

Various studies (e.g., Peeters & van Ours, 2020; Pollard & Armatas, 2017; Strauss & Bierschwale, 2008; Strauss & Höfer, 2001) examining a large number of games have shown that the number of spectators significantly correlates with the result, but only slightly at best, i.e., a weak effect. It is consistent e.g., with the results reported by Leite and Pollard (2018), who, in a worldwide analysis of 47 countries, found that the home advantage in the second soccer division is almost always higher than that in the first division. As a rule, however, the average number of spectators in the first division is higher than that in the second division. Moreover, some studies have shown that there is a relevant home advantage in youth soccer (e.g., Staufenbiel et al., 2018) and in amateur soccer leagues (e.g., Wunderlich et al., 2021), although the number of spectators is usually very small in these games (often only 50–200 spectators, if spectators are present at all).

The few studies on games behind closed doors before the COVID-19 pandemic (see the Side Story for studies focussing on the absence of spectators during the COVID-19 pandemic) that have been published in peer-reviewed journals before the pandemic started, commonly report a very small N (and are thus fraught with high uncertainty). Generally, they show no change in home advantage when no spectators are present; for example, in a small archival study of Italian soccer, Van de Ven (2011) examined 20 games behind closed doors (due to restrictions on clubs where there had been previous spectator riots). Moore and Brylinsky (1993) similarly observed 11 basketball games in the North American college league, which were played without spectators due to a measles epidemic. When compared to matches played by the same teams in the presence of spectators, there were no significant differences in various performance measures (e.g., number of points, free-throw rate). However, these studies are limited by the small number of matches that can be considered as matches without spectators, and by the fact that the home advantage statistics in a league vary considerably from season to season (see, e.g., Peeters & van Ours, 2020; Pollard & Pollard, 2005; Riedl et al., 2014). Several thousand matches are necessary to identify substantial trends and correlations. This necessity is probably caused by the random variability in team success that is particularly high in soccer, averaging 80% in one game, as physicist Heuer (2020) has calculated for the German Premier League in soccer. Consequently, this means that only 20% of the total variance (on average) is left for substantial possible cause to explain differences in the home advantage.

Side Story

In 2020, the number of games behind closed doors across many countries and sports increased substantially. As a result of the COVID-19 pandemic, from May 2020 onwards, soccer matches in the professional leagues throughout Europe and worldwide were played without (with the German soccer league being the first to declare this) or very few spectators until the end of the 19/20 season in July/August 2020, and again in some parts in the season 20/21. The number of publications analyzing the now available data on the absence of spectators increased quickly (for an overview, see Benz & Lopez, 2021), conducted by various research groups (cf. international comparisons: Benz & Lopez, 2021; Bilalić et al., 2021; Bryson et al., 2021; McCarrick et al., 2021; Wunderlich et al., 2021), but often only analyzing one or a few soccer leagues (e.g., Tilp & Thaller, 2020 for the German Premier soccer league). These differ considerably not only in the direction of the results but also regarding the number of leagues included, the number of matches that were considered, the characteristics of the matches chosen for comparison, as well as the methodologies and performance indicators. Although this special situation in the stadium appears to be similar to previous games held behind closed doors, there are a few disparities that may distort the results if not considered. The additional hygiene protocols and regular tests for COVID-19 in combination with a tightened match schedule and hardly any preparation are assumed to affect the players' performance. Additionally, the change of rules, allowing five substitutions rather than three, has considerable potential to alter the individual demands of the game. Notwithstanding these limitations, the large international comparison studies like Bryson et al. (2021) are the most informative. This study examined all matches from 23 professional soccer leagues in 17 countries and compared the matches without spectators during the pandemic to those with spectators before the COVID-19 pandemic (a total of $N = 6481$ matches). Bryson et al. (2021) showed that, across all leagues, the average results (i.e., goal differences or points) of the games behind closed doors do not differ, while in other studies that compared leagues, they only differ slightly from the pre-COVID games (see e.g., the studies by Benz & Lopez, 2021; Bilalić et al., 2021; Bryson et al., 2021; McCarrick et al., 2021; Wunderlich et al., 2021, which identify overall a—mostly small—reduction of the home wins, but the home advantage still exists in games played behind closed doors, e.g. McCarrick et al. (2021) found a small reduction of won home games from 43% to 41%), but there are changes in the number of yellow cards awarded. "We find that the absence of a partisan home crowd has no effect on the final match scoreline, but it does result in a reduction of one-third of a yellow card for away teams relative to home teams" (Bryson et al., 2021, p. 4). With respect to refereeing decisions, a similar pattern of results has also been reported, e.g., by McCarrick, Bilalić, Neave, and Wolfson (2021), who investigated the COVID-19-related changes and their effect on a number of measures for 15 European leagues. These measures included the outcome, as well as the dominance of a team (measured by the number of corners, shots, and shots on target) and the refereeing decisions (fouls, yellow and red cards). Bilalić, Gula, and Vaci (2021) used parts of the same archival data (12 European leagues), supplemented by a few other (control) variables, and tested successfully a so-called joint Home Advantage Mediated (HAM) model, which includes direct and indirect paths, using a joint Bayesian mixed effects model. Here, the dominance of a team – now called team performance – and refereeing decisions are used as mediating predictors for the games' outcome (points and goals, see also McCarrick et al., 2021, who called this team performance).

Similar to so many other studies investigating spectator influences and various home advantage outcomes (e.g., goals, points, see above), the variance between the several leagues is considerable. On the one hand, there was an increase in the home advantage observed in Italy and Portugal, while on the other hand, a considerable decrease was found in Greece or the Premier League in Germany (see Tilp & Thaller, 2020), but not the second and third divisions in Germany (see Fischer & Haucap, 2021).

Home advantage has also been investigated in other sports, however, not as exhaustively as soccer, and still presenting a lot of variance. This variation between different sports does not allow the conclusion that a large crowd is mainly responsible for the home advantage. For the COVID-19 season 19/20, Higgs and Stavness (2021) found a reduction of home wins in the NHL and the NBA, which were finished in a bubble, excluding spectators and limiting all games to the same location, but no change in the NFL and the World Series Baseball league. For the following season 20/21, in which some games were played without and some with spectators (often limited in size), Szabo (2022) found a reduction in the home wins in the NFL (American Football) and in the NBA (basketball), but not in the NHL (hockey). Fazackerley et al. (2022) investigated individual performance statistics of players in the professional Australian National Rugby League (NRL) and did not find any substantial differences in effort-based (e.g., running distance) or skill-based performance measures (e.g., decoys) for the same players in games with and without a large audience. They concluded that "the findings suggest that NRL players' performance appears unlikely to be affected by the presence or absence of a crowd" (Fazackerley et al., 2022, p. 1).

An additional emphasis on the explanation of home advantage is the capacity utilization of a stadium (spectator density; cf. e.g., Agnew & Carron, 1994). It is often argued that a higher spectator density (actual number of spectators present divided by the number of seats) is responsible for the home advantage, e.g., because it is more likely to create an intense, uproarious atmosphere which leads to a special home advantage. Nevertheless, the empirical evidence does not support this hypothesis: Strauss and Bierschwale (2008) found a correlation of spectator density and matches won of almost $r = 0$ for the German handball league. Pollard (1986) and Pollard and Armatas (2017) also did not find a correlation between home advantage and spectator density.

Overall, there is little to no correlation between the number of spectators or spectator density and home advantage. The theory of social support—according to which more spectators provide more social support and therefore may positively affect the home team's performance—cannot be supported by the results at present, even if ongoing evaluations regarding COVID-19 pandemic-related spectator-less conditions are still emerging, which may warrant a reassessment. If one follows the *social impact theory* by Latané (1981), a linear relationship between crowd density or number of spectators and home advantage is not expected according to his "psychosocial law of the marginal impact": he argued that the influence of each additional spectator decreases. The usual studies on number and density, however, use linear correlations, so that for conceptual reasons (Latané, 1981) as well as for statistical reasons, no relevant association can be expected.

In light of these findings, it could be argued that social support is not expressed in terms of number or density, but only in terms of concrete supportive or opposing behavior, and that this must be investigated consistently. If, however, we do not look at anecdotes and self-reports like Polybius (see above), but at the studies that examine the influence of specific spectator behavior (cheering, jeering, aggressive behavior) on athletic performance or behavior in a competitive situation, we find that the number of studies is negligible for cheering (Epting et al., 2011; Salminen, 1993; Strauss, 2002b), jeering (Epting et al., 2011; Greer, 1983), and aggressive behavior (Thirer & Rampey, 1979). On the other hand, although the number of fouls is influenced by spectator behavior, among other things, performance is not. This was demonstrated by Greer (1983): In a study with American basketball teams, he examined the influence of spectator protest ("spectator booing") on the number of fouls, turnovers, and baskets. When booing occurred for at least 15 seconds in a game, the five minutes following were called the "booing interval." Booing usually was a reaction to refereeing decisions against the home team or the actions of the away team. It was found that neither home nor visiting teams benefited significantly from the booing with regard to shot success and turnovers, but there were changes in the number of fouls: more fouls were called against the visiting teams than the home teams. Meanwhile, the number of fouls decreased for the home teams in the "booing interval." Yet again, this study (as well as the basketball study by Epting et al., 2011) did not show an effect of booing on sporting performance.

Following the methodological idea of Greer (1983), Strauss (2002b) conducted a study examining the effect of cheering on American Football performance by analyzing the sporting performance of a team in several games and the behavior of parts of the audience. He found no evidence that supportive spectator behavior such as cheering during the time before the action has an influence on subsequent performances. Salminen (1993) also found no effects caused by spectator behaviors in various sports. These few studies that examine the specific behavior of viewers may show either no or little or at best highly specific influences (see Epting et al., 2011).

So far, the question of the *direct* influence of spectators on sporting performance has been considered. Since in all team sports referees are in control of the event, it is also conceivable that the spectators influence the referee, which in turn would have an impact on the development and outcome of the game. The question of this *indirect* social influence of spectators on athletes mediated by distorted refereeing decisions is examined particularly in the context of "noise from spectators and refereeing decisions" (e.g., MacMahon & Strauss, 2014). It is assumed, for example, that referees receive cues (e.g., increased noise) from the audience, especially in ambiguous situations, that indicate a foul. The subsequent decisions would then favor the home team.

17

The classic experiments of Nevill et al. (1999, 2002) show that judges take into account the information from the spectators (here: noise) in their decision-making process. Soccer referees, coaches, and players were shown soccer matches with and without sound. The participants attributed more fouls to the visiting team (in comparison to the away team) when they watched the recordings with sound. The decisions made when watching the situations with sound also mirrored the actual referee's decision in the game. Unkelbach and Memmert (2010) were able to replicate this experiment, however, using a significantly improved methodology. In the first—experimental—part of their investigation, Unkelbach and Memmert (2010) found that referees awarded more yellow cards under the influence of noise. Additionally, they conducted an archival analysis, which confirmed that away teams were awarded significantly more yellow cards than home teams. This difference correlates significantly with spectator density, indicating that spectators act as an additional source of information for referees. They also found that the difference in the yellow cards given to home and away teams correlated significantly with the difference in goals (their measure of home advantage) but explained only a small proportion of the variance (approx. 1%), suggesting that referees can explain only a small part of the home advantage at best.

This difference in the number of fouls may indeed affect the match outcome. Lehman and Reifman (1987) report in an older archival study that top players in the Los Angeles Lakers (a team in the North American professional basketball league NBA) were awarded fewer fouls in home games than in away games in 1984 and 1985. This corresponds to the observation by Nevill et al. (1996) that about two-thirds of penalties in soccer are awarded to the home team (see also Boyko et al., 2007). Additionally, two-thirds of the yellow/red cards are given to the away team, which in turn can lead to a home advantage, among other things, because of the numbers advantage this creates when players are dismissed (red card; Pollard & Armatas, 2017). Interestingly, when analyzing games in the European Rugby Cup, Dawson et al. (2020) found that the number of yellow cards awarded to away teams increased after implementing the Television Match Official (TMO). The authors speculated that before the TMO, the on-field referees tried to avoid favoring the home team, whereas this consideration was then absent for the TMO.

Nonetheless, the interpretation of the entirety of empirical data regarding the allocation of fouls and cards remains vague. It is unclear what the driving mechanisms are behind the results found by, e.g., Bryson et al. (2021), McCarrick et al. (2021), or Bilalić et al. (2021) regarding yellow or red cards in games behind closed doors. One explanation lies in the lack of stimuli from the spectators, but the correlation could also be attributed to athletes and their change in tactics due to the lack of noise (see, e.g., the recent experiment on passing times and accuracy in soccer by Otte et al., 2020, or the arguments made by Benz & Lopez, 2021). On the one hand, the referee could be influenced by the spectators; on the other hand, however, the "away athletes" could also appear to be more aggressive and the referee's decision would thus be a necessary and logical, undistorted consequence to ensure game control and management (Raab et al., 2020). So far, in our opinion, no attempt has been made to consider the conflicting demands of possible audience influence on player behavior and the referee's decision outside cross-sectional archival studies (e.g., Bilalić et al., 2021). A field experimental study or longitudinal design to separate the effects in this process is needed.

It should be noted that although distorted refereeing decisions can occur in numerous decision-making situations, often studies in controlled experiments (for an overview, see e.g., MacMahon & Strauss, 2014; Raab et al., 2019), no significant impact of such specific decisions on home advantage has been found. An archival study that statistically investigated the question of whether an existing referee bias (here the so-called injury bias in soccer) actually leads to greater home advantage—measured in points or goals—was conducted by Riedl et al. (2015). It is a well-established finding, first shown by Sutter and Kocher (2004), that referees in the German Premier League award more extra time after the 90th minute if the home team is behind by one goal, as opposed to if the home team is up by one goal. Riedl et al. (2015) were able to confirm this, indicating that, on average, the injury time was 18 seconds longer. Beyond this effect, Riedl and colleagues were the first to statistically test whether this also translated into more goals or points and thus would result in a home advantage. This was not the case. The study shows that the existence of the referee bias does not explain the home advantage. It is therefore doubtful that referees contribute significantly to home advantage (e.g., because the effects are too small or occur only rarely).

All in all, for now, it can be said that there is little empirical support that the home advantage results from social support through spectators and is directly or indirectly mediated by referees. On the contrary, the theory of social support can be countered by the theory of social pressure exerted by spectators in some situations (Strauss, 2002b; Wallace et al., 2005).

The research and empirical evidence of "choking under pressure" are particularly relevant, both theoretically and methodologically, in the area of motor learning (see, e.g., in addition to numerous other studies, Marchant et al., 2014). As a consequence, multiple sport psychological intervention techniques have been developed that prevent choking (for a systematic review, see Gröpel & Mesagno, 2019). Sian Beilock has presented numerous influential publications on "choking under pressure" and the correlation with neural activities (see, e.g., the popular science book "Choke"; Beilock, 2011). At this point, we will only refer to some of the investigations concerning this wide field of research. A critical in-depth discussion of different theoretical choking approaches has been provided by Gray (2020).

> Baumeister (1984) defines choking under pressure as a deterioration in performance under pressure, although the person is essentially motivated to perform optimally.

Factors that can exert pressure on a person ("pressure variables") are, for example, competition and its conditions, presence of spectators, size of the reward, and expectation of negative consequences. Positive and negative public expectations are also considered "pressure variables" (Baumeister et al., 1985; Baumeister & Steinhilber, 1984).

The seminal study on "choking under pressure", was carried out by Baumeister and Steinhilber (1984). They claim that the anticipation of success in situations in which the athlete could achieve a new, desired social identity, can lead to performance decrements. They argue that the prospect of becoming a master, e.g., increases self-awareness. This means that an internal focus on one's own body and behavior is adopted. Numerous experimental studies on coordination- and condition-based tasks have shown that this internal focus tends to decrease performance compared to an external focus (e.g., greater muscular tension, more oxygen consumption; cf. e.g., Chua et al., 2021; Wulf, 2013).

Study Box

To provide evidence that increased self-awareness during important matches leads to a decrease in performance, Baumeister and Steinhilber (1984) used the results of the World Series finals from 1924 to 1982 (baseball) and the finals and semifinals of the NBA from 1967 to 1982 (basketball). In both leagues, the winner is determined according to a "best of seven" tournament, i.e., the winner of the final or semifinal must have won four matches. Baumeister and Steinhilber (1984) argued that the home disadvantage should occur particularly in the seventh or last game, when pressure is at its highest. Games 1–4 in the basketball and games 1 and 2 in the baseball analysis were chosen as benchmarks for comparison. As expected, in games 1–4, a home advantage was found and linked to the fact that the outcome did not hinge on these games. However, the last three games (games 5, 6, or 7) were won more often by the away team, as predicted.

According to Baumeister and Steinhilber (1984), the probability of negative performance changes in decisive matches increases for the home team relative to the increased self-awareness. In the following decades, an intense controversy developed. Baumeister and Steinhilber (1984) were criticized in particular for the suggestion that increased self-awareness hinders performance. Heaton and Sigall (1989) reinterpreted Baumeister and Steinhilber's (1984) results, stating that it is not the possible attainment of a positive identity that triggers the home disadvantage, but the athletes' fear of attaining a negative identity or the fear of failure.

Schlenker et al. (1995) repeated the analysis of Baumeister and Steinhilber (1984), with one difference: the period of analysis now extended to 1993. For this period, it was now difficult to prove a home disadvantage in decisive games. From this, they deduced the inadequacy of the statement by Baumeister and Steinhilber (1984). A controversial discussion developed about the correct interpretation. However, it must be stated that when more games are included in the analysis, the effect found by Baumeister and Steinhilber (1984) in basketball levels out or disappears. This was reported by Tauer et al. (2009) in a comprehensive analysis of 50 years of NBA play-offs, where a choking effect was no longer found.

Following the debate in the 1990s, Butler and Baumeister (1998) published a study in which they once again provided evidence for the negative influence of supportive spectators, this time on performance in difficult tasks. In their first experiment, the subjects were asked to solve mental arithmetic tasks either in front of a friend (condition 1) or in front of a stranger (condition 2). The people watching were not visible to the participants and could not make their presence known. It turned out that the worst performances occurred in front of a friendly audience. Butler and Baumeister (1998) were also able to show in two additional experiments that a supposedly supportive audience led to a decrease in performance when working on difficult tasks. This effect did not occur with easy tasks. An interesting side note from the experiments by Butler and Baumeister (1998) is that the actors in front of this audience felt more comfortable and less stressed and preferred to work under this condition. They did not notice that their personal performance scores decreased.

17

Law et al. (2003) also showed in an experiment with table tennis players, who had to learn a table tennis shot, that a supportive audience that increases internal focus (see above, e.g., Chua et al., 2021) has a deteriorating effect if the shot has been learned explicitly.

Wallace et al. (2005) transferred the arguments taken from the Butler and Baumeister (1998) experiments to the real-world situation in a home- and away-related competitive scenario with a supportive audience. They found that choking can occur more frequently for home teams in mostly skill-based tasks (like penalties in soccer, or free throws in basketball). The performances in effort-related tasks (e.g., running time of players) should benefit from the home supportive situation. This argument is very similar to the conclusion that Strauss (2002a) already presented in his narrative review about social facilitation effects of observers (merely present or co-active) on motor tasks (see ► Sect. 17.3).

There is some empirical support for Wallace et al.'s (2005) transfer from Butler and Baumeister (1998). For example, Dohmen (2008) found in an archival study with data from the German Premier soccer league (1963–2004) that the away team was more successful in scoring a penalty (73.59%) than the home teams (75.83%). In a recent detailed analysis of NBA basketball games, Böheim et al. (2019) showed that a large crowd is associated with lower free-throw efficiency for players on the home team (but only in the first half). Some of the results therefore suggest a decrease in performance, in contrast to theories of social support. McEwan (2019) investigated 100 years of NHL (hockey) archives and found that away teams in comparison to home teams have an advantage for winning the play-off series if it comes to an overtime situation. McEwan and Hofmann (2021) argue in an overview that choking is not an overall phenomenon that can easily be found in archival data, but that the effect exists for specific situations.

One of these specific situations is dart throwing, which can be classified as a coordination/skill-based task. For the successful execution of a throw, concentration and focus are necessary. Outside the home advantage-related research, Greve et al. (2022) investigated the effects of an actively present audience, of no spectators, and of a simulated audience (due to the COVID-19 pandemic) on the performances of top-class dart throwers in all archived high-level competitions from 2018 to 2021. The real presence of spectators was the condition with the worst performances in comparison with the two others.

What about comparing skill- and effort-based tasks? Heinrich et al. (2021) analyzed all archived competition outcomes of world-class biathletes before COVID-19 and during COVID-19 (without an audience) and showed that the skiing times (the conditioning-based part of their overall performances) were better in front of an active large audience and that the shooting performances (the coordination-based part) improved during COVID-19, i.e., when crowds were not present. This pattern of results confirms the assumption of Strauss (2002a) and Wallace et al. (2005). However, the pattern only holds for male biathletes, not for females, where the observed pattern was the opposite (skiing times did not improve, shooting performance did) and counters previous assumptions.

Looking at some of the results of the "choking under pressure" research following Baumeister and Steinhilber's (1984) approach on decisive and crucial games, it can also be argued that a larger number of spectators than usual tend to have a (small) performance-decreasing effect on the home team and would lead to more home losses. Strauss and Höfer (2001) argued that a larger number of spectators or higher spectator density than usual could be associated with greater importance of the game. The number of spectators, audience density, corresponding spectator behavior, or other measures would thus function as indicators for the importance of a performance, which would lead to greater social pressure for the home team. They found a small tendency of an increase of home losses in the German Premier soccer league (1963–1998) with a greater number of spectators than usual (using the numbers from the previous season as the teams' standard level). Interestingly, Fischer and Haucap (2021) made a similar argument—but in the opposite direction—to explain the decrease of home wins for some German soccer teams in the three professional leagues during the COVID-19 season (2019/2020) in closed-door games. They found that teams that usually enjoy a very large home audience suffer the most, with a drop in the number of home-field wins in games behind closed doors. For teams with a traditionally smaller or moderate crowd size (measured pre-COVID restrictions), there was no relevant decrease in the home advantage. Discussing the findings by Strauss and Höfer (2001) and Fischer and Haucap (2021) together, one can speculate that relevant deviations from the previously experienced standard level of spectators (the "usual") could lead to more social pressure, and hence, the likelihood of choking under pressure increases. Summarizing this, some of the described results suggest a decrease in performance, in contrast to the theories of social support.

Overall, there has been—and still is—a lack of robust empirical evidence that spectators are directly (or even indirectly via, e.g., referees) strongly involved in the home advantage (beyond what we have introduced in the beginning of this chapter as directly evident influence).

Of course, future studies can change and challenge the lack of empirical evidence. Indeed, with ongoing COVID-19 pandemic changes, limited spectator attendance, a comparison to "normal" and subsequent increases of spectators, fewer or no restrictions, and improved methodologies within the area (like specific statistical multilevel approaches), the understanding of audience effects may improve. Some archival studies investigating the home advantage situation during COVID-19 games behind closed doors claimed to find a (strong) direct (or in a few cases also indirect) spectator effect, while others suggest the opposite. These contrasting positions are not surprising due to the large random effects and variance in home advantage outcomes. In addition, it is not only the number of spectators that changed dramatically during the pandemic, but also other aspects like hygiene protocols, match rules, and match preparation times. For an overall assessment and conclusion on the impact of spectators on the home advantage, it is also necessary to consider not only archival and correlational COVID-19 studies, but also, and moreover, the whole literature, theories, and methodological (from correlational to experimental) approaches and thousands of studies, starting with Schwarz and Barsky (1977).

Taking the current evidence, spectators are not considered to be the main causal factor for the home advantage, as is the case in the models of Courneya and Carron (1992) and Carron et al. (2005). They should not be considered as the main underlying force for home advantage, but rather as a situational condition that is cognitively evaluated by athletes. It therefore seems appropriate to investigate the effects of a potential social influence through spectators on the athletes themselves, their information processing, even the tactical behavior of the coaches (Staufenbiel et al., 2015), or the learning processes for home and away games (Staufenbiel et al., 2018).

17.5 Final Remarks

Whether merely present or actively behaving, spectators have an impact on sporting performance—if certain conditions are met. The social influence of spectators seems to depend more on the cognitive assessment of the situation by the actors, as suggested, e.g., by the biopsychosocial theory of Blascovich et al. (1999) or Wallace et al. (2005), rather than on direct external influence and related factors (such as number, density, specific behavior). This concept illustrates the importance of investigating the information processing of athletes and coaches. These evaluations can be investigated using experimental research designs in both social facilitation and home advantage research.

The psychological (and physiological) correlates such as athletes' (or also coaches') expectations (e.g., self-efficacy, self-fulfilling prophecy, learning processes, cf. Allen & Jones, 2014; Bray et al., 2002; Staufenbiel et al., 2015, 2018) and thus their ability to efficiently process information likely play a key role in the reasons for home advantage, and this is where ongoing investigations should focus.

Learning Control Questions

Basic:

- Define social influence in general and apply this definition to the sports context.
- What are Dashiell's (1935) seven types of influence of other people on actors? To what extent are these seven types of influence also relevant to the sports context?
- What sources of influence does Latané (1981) describe?

Advanced:

- Describe the most famous study on the influence of others by Triplett (1898).
- Compare activation theory models and models of attention processes to explain social influence.
- Describe the theory of Zajonc (1965). To what extent is this model supported by research results from sport?
- What is the result of the meta-analysis by Bond and Titus (1983)?

Experts:

- Which research findings support the hypothesis that athletes are influenced by spectators at home games, and which dismiss the hypothesis?
- To what extent do spectators have an influence on referees?
- What is meant by *choking under pressure*? Put this in the context of research on social influence.

References

Agnew, G. A., & Carron, A. V. (1994). Crowd effects and the home advantage. *International Journal of Sport Psychology, 25*(1), 53–62.

Aiello, J. R., Nicosia, G., & Thompson, D. (1979). Physiological, social, and behavioral consequences of crowding on children and adolescents. *Child Development, 50*(1), 195–202.

Allen, M. S., & Jones, M. V. (2014). The "Home Advantage" in Athletic competitions. *Current Directions in Psychological Science, 23*(1), 48–54.

Allport, F. H. (1920). The influence of the group upon association and thought. *Journal of Experimental Psychology, 3*(3), 159–182. https://doi.org/10.1037/h0067891

Allport, F. H. (1924). Response to social stimulation in the group. In *Social psychology* (1st ed., pp. 260–291). Erlbaum.

Anderson, M., Wolfson, S., Neave, N., & Moss, M. (2012). Perspectives on the home advantage: A comparison of football players, fans and referees. *Psychology of Sport and Exercise, 13*(3), 311–316. https://doi.org/10.1016/j.psychsport.2011.11.012

Baron, R. S. (1986). Distraction-conflict theory: Progress and problems. *Advances in Experimental Social Psychology, 19*(C), 1–40. https://doi.org/10.1016/S0065-2601(08)60211-7

Baumeister, R. F. (1984). Choking under pressure: Self-consciousness and paradoxical effects of incentives on skillful performance. *Journal of Personality and Social Psychology, 46*(3), 610–620. https://doi.org/10.1037/0022-3514.46.3.610

Baumeister, R. F., Hamilton, J. C., & Tice, D. M. (1985). Public versus private expectancy of success. Confidence booster or performance pressure? *Journal of Personality and Social Psychology, 48*(6), 1447–1457. https://doi.org/10.1037/0022-3514.48.6.1447

Baumeister, R. F., & Steinhilber, A. (1984). Paradoxical effects of supportive audiences on performance under pressure: The home field disadvantage in sports championships. *Journal of Personality and Social Psychology, 47*(1), 85–93. https://doi.org/10.1037/0022-3514.47.1.85

Beilock, S. (2011). *Choke*. Free Press.

Benz, L. S., & Lopez, M. J. (2021). Estimating the change in soccer's home advantage during the Covid-19 pandemic using bivariate Poisson regression. *AStA Advances in Statistical Analysis*. https://doi.org/10.1007/s10182-021-00413-9

Bilalić, M., Gula, B., & Vaci, N. (2021). Home advantage mediated (HAM) by referee bias and team performance during covid. *Scientific Reports, 11*(1), 21558. https://doi.org/10.1038/s41598-021-00784-8

Blascovich, J., & McCall, C. (2013). Social influence in virtual environments. In K. E. Dill (Ed.), *Oxford library of psychology. The Oxford handbook of media psychology* (pp. 305–315). Oxford University Press.

Blascovich, J., Mendes, W. B., Hunter, S. B., & Salomon, K. (1999). Social 'facilitation' as challenge and threat. *Journal of Personality and Social Psychology, 77*(1), 68–77. https://doi.org/10.1037/0022-3514.77.1.68

Blascovich, J., & Tomaka, J. (1996). The biopsychosocial model of arousal regulation. In M. P. Zanna (Ed.), *Advances in experimental social psychology* (Vol. 28, pp. 1–52). Academic Press, Inc.

Boggs, D. H., & Simon, J. R. (1968). Differential effect of noise on tasks of varying complexity. *Journal of Applied Psychology, 52*(2), 148–153. https://doi.org/10.1037/h0025496

Böheim, R., Grübl, D., & Lackner, M. (2019). Choking under pressure—Evidence of the causal effect of audience size on performance. *Journal of Economic Behavior and Organization, 168*, 76–93. https://doi.org/10.1016/j.jebo.2019.10.001

Bond, C. F., & Titus, L. J. (1983). Social facilitation: A meta-analysis of 241 studies. *Psychological Bulletin, 94*(2), 265–292. https://doi.org/10.1037/0033-2909.94.2.265

Boyko, R. H., Boyko, A. R., & Boyko, M. G. (2007). Referee bias contributes to home advantage in English Premiership football. *Journal of Sports Sciences, 25*(11), 1185–1194. https://doi.org/10.1080/02640410601038576

Bray, S. R., Jones, M. V., & Owen, S. (2002). The influence of competition location on athletes' psychological states. *Journal of Sport Behavior, 25*(3), 231–242.

Brown, A. J., & Harkins, S. G. (2020). Social facilitation and social loafing: Opposite sides of the same coin. In S. J. Karau (Ed.), *Individual motivation within groups* (pp. 297–330). Academic Press.

Bryson, A., Dolton, P., Reade, J. J., Schreyer, D., & Singleton, C. (2021). Causal effects of an absent crowd on performances and refereeing decisions during Covid-19. *Economics Letters, 198*, 109664. https://doi.org/10.1016/j.econlet.2020.109664

Burnham, W. H. (1905). The hygiene of home study. *The Pedagogical Seminary, 12*(2), 213–230. https://doi.org/10.1080/08919402.1905.10532755

Burnham, W. H. (1910). The group as a stimulus to mental activity. *Science, 31*(803), 761–767.

Butler, J. L., & Baumeister, R. F. (1998). The trouble with friendly faces: Skilled performance with a supportive audience. *Journal of Personality and Social Psychology, 75*(5), 1213–1230.

Carron, A. V., Loughhead, T. M., & Bray, S. R. (2005). The home advantage in sport competitions: Courneya and Carron's (1992)

17

conceptual framework a decade later. *Journal of Sports Sciences, 23*(4), 395–407. https://doi.org/10.1080/02640410400021542
Chua, L.-K., Jimenez-Diaz, J., Lewthwaite, R., Kim, T., & Wulf, G. (2021). Superiority of external attentional focus for motor performance and learning: Systematic reviews and meta-analyses. *Psychological Bulletin, 147*(6), 618–645. https://doi.org/10.1037/bul0000335
Cialdini, R. B. (2001). *Influence: Science and practice* (4th ed.). Harper Collins.
Cottrell, N. B., Wack, D. L., Sekerak, G. J., & Rittle, R. H. (1968). Social facilitation of dominant responses by the presence of an audience and the mere presence of others. *Journal of Personality and Social Psychology, 9*(3), 245–250. https://doi.org/10.1037/h0025902
Courneya, K. S., & Carron, A. V. (1992). The home advantage in sport competitions: A literature review. *Journal of Sport & Exercise Psychology, 14*(1), 13–27.
Cox, F. N. (1966). Some effects of test anxiety and presence or absence of other persons on boys' performance on a repetitive motor task. *Journal of Experimental Child Psychology, 3*(1), 100–112. https://doi.org/10.1016/0022-0965(66)90065-8
Danziger, K. (2000). Making social psychology experimental: A conceptual history, 1920–1970. *Journal of the History of the Behavioral Sciences, 36*(4), 329–347. https://doi.org/10.1002/1520-6696(200023)36:4
Dashiell, J. F. (1935). Experimental studies of the influence of social situations on the behavior of individual human adults. In E. Murchinson (Ed.), A handbook of social psychology (pp. 1097–1158). Clark University Press.
Dawson, P., Massey, P., & Downward, P. (2020). Television match officials, referees, and home advantage: Evidence from the European Rugby Cup. *Sport Management Review, 23*(3), 443–454. https://doi.org/10.1016/j.smr.2019.04.002
Dohmen, T. J. (2008). Do professionals choke under pressure? *Journal of Economic Behavior & Organization, 65*(3), 636–653. https://doi.org/10.1016/j.jebo.2005.12.004
Edwards, A. M., Dutton-Challis, L., Cottrell, D., Guy, J. H., & Hettinga, F. J. (2018). Impact of active and passive social facilitation on self-paced endurance and sprint exercise: Encouragement augments performance and motivation to exercise. *BMJ Open Sport & Exercise Medicine, 4*(1), e000368. https://doi.org/10.1136/bmjsem-2018-000368
Epting, L. K., Riggs, K. N., Knowles, J. D., & Hanky, J. J. (2011). Cheers vs. Jeers: Effects of audience feedback on individual athletic performance. North. *American Journal of Psychology, 13*(2), 299–312.
Fazackerley, L. A., Gorman, A. D., Minett, G. M., Caia, J., & Kelly, V. G. (2022). The influence of absent crowds on National Rugby League match player statistics and running metrics. *Psychology of Sport & Exercise, 60*, 102163. https://doi.org/10.1016/j.psychsport.2022.102163
Feltz, D. L., Forlenza, S. T., Winn, B., & Kerr, N. L. (2014). Cyber Buddy is better than no buddy: A test of the Köhler motivation effect in exergames. *Games for Health Journal, 3*(2), 98–105. https://doi.org/10.1089/g4h.2013.0088
Feltz, D. L., Kerr, N. L., & Irwin, B. C. (2011). Buddy up: The Köhler effect applied to health games. *Journal of Sport and Exercise Psychology, 33*(4), 506–526. https://doi.org/10.1123/jsep.33.4.506
Fischer, K., & Haucap, J. (2021). Does crowd support drive the home advantage in professional football? Evidence from German ghost games during the COVID-19 pandemic. *Journal of Sports Economics, 22*(8), 982–1008. https://doi.org/10.1177/15270025211026552
Flake, J. K., Pek, J., & Hehman, E. (2017). Construct validation in social and personality research. *Social Psychological and Personality Science, 8*(4), 370–378. https://doi.org/10.1177/1948550617693063
Fothergill, M., Wolfson, S., & Little, L. (2014). A qualitative analysis of perceptions of venue: Do professional soccer players and managers concur with the conceptual home advantage framework? *International Journal of Sport and Exercise Psychology, 12*(4), 316–332. https://doi.org/10.1080/1612197X.2014.932826
Gómez-Ruano, M. A., Pollard, R., & Lago-Peñas, C. (2021). *Home advantage in sport: Causes and the effect on performance*. Routledge.
Gray, R. (2020). Attentional theories of choking under pressure revisited. In G. Tenenbaum & R. C. Eklund (Eds.), Handbook of sport psychology (pp. 595–610). John Wiley & Sons, . doi: https://doi.org/10.1002/9781119568124.ch28
Greer, D. L. (1983). Spectator booing and the home advantage: A study of social influence in the basketball arena. *Social Psychology Quarterly, 46*(3), 252–261.
Greve, J., van Meurs, E., & Strauss, B. (2022). "…and the crowd goes wild!" – Performance in elite darts players, the presence of crowds and the simulation of a crowd during the COVID-19 pandemic. *Journal of Sport & Exercise Psychology, 44*, S81.
Gröpel, P., & Mesagno, C. (2019). Choking interventions in sports: A systematic review. *International Review of Sport and Exercise Psychology, 12*(1), 176–201. https://doi.org/10.1080/1750984X.2017.1408134
Guerin, B. (1993). *Social facilitation*. Cambridge University Press.
Guttmann, A. (1986). *Sports spectators* (1st ed.). Columbia University Press.
Harb-Wu, K., & Krumer, A. (2019). Choking under pressure in front of a supportive audience: Evidence from professional biathlon. *Journal of Economic Behavior and Organization, 166*, 246–262. https://doi.org/10.1016/j.jebo.2019.09.001
Heaton, A. W., & Sigall, H. (1989). The 'Championship Choke' revisited: the role of fear of acquiring a negative identity1. *Journal of Applied Social Psychology, 19*(12), 1019–1033. https://doi.org/10.1111/j.1559-1816.1989.tb01236.x
Heinrich, A., Müller, F., Stoll, O., & Cañal-Bruland, R. (2021). Selection bias in social facilitation theory? Audience effects on elite biathletes' performance are gender-specific. *Psychology of Sport and Exercise, 55*, 101943. https://doi.org/10.1016/j.psychsport.2021.101943
Heuer, A. (2020). *From identification of random contributions to determination of the optimum forecast of a soccer match*. https://doi.org/10.48550/arXiv.2003.09352
Higgs, N., & Staveness, I. (2021). Bayesian analysis of home advantage in north american professional sports before and during COVID-19. *Scientific Reports, 11*(1). https://doi.org/10.1038/s41598-021-93533-w
Hull, C. L. (1943). *Principles of behavior* (1st ed.). Appleton-Century-Crofts.
Jamieson, J. P. (2010). The home field advantage in athletics: A meta-analysis. *Journal of Applied Social Psychology, 40*(7), 1819–1848.
Jones, M. B. (2013). The home advantage in individual sports: An augmented review. *Psychology of Sport and Exercise, 14*(3), 397–404. https://doi.org/10.1016/J.PSYCHSPORT.2013.01.002
Jones, M. B. (2018). Differences in home advantage between sports. *Psychology of Sport & Exercise, 34*, 61–69. https://doi.org/10.1016/j.psychsport.2017.07.012
Kelman, H. C. (1958). Compliance, identification, and internalization: Three processes of attitude change. *Journal of Conflict Resolution, 2*(1), 51–60.
Kozar, B. (1973). The effects of a supportive and nonsupportive audience upon learning a gross motor skill. *International Journal of Sport Psychology, 4*(1), 11–30.

Laird, D. A. (1923). Changes in motor control and individual variation under the influence of 'Razzing'. *Journal of Experimental Psychology, 6*(3), 236–246. https://doi.org/10.1037/h0072891

Landers, D. (1975). Observational learning of a motor skill: Temporal spacing of demonstrations and audience presence. *Journal of Motor Behavior, 7*(4), 281–287. https://doi.org/10.1080/00222895.1975.10735047

Landers, D., & McCullagh, P. D. (1976). Social facilitation of motor performance. *Exercise and Sport Sciences Reviews, 4*(1), 125–162. https://doi.org/10.1249/00003677-197600040-00006

Latané, B. (1981). The psychology of social impact. *American Psychologist, 36*(4), 343–356. https://doi.org/10.1037/0003-066X.36.4.343

Lau, A., Schwarz, J., & Stoll, O. (2019). Influence of social facilitation on learning development using a Wii Balanceboard (TM). *German Journal of Exercise and Sport Research, 49*(1), 97–102.

Law, J., Masters, R., Bray, S. R., Eves, F., & Bardswell, I. (2003). Motor performance as a function of audience affability and metaknowledge. *Journal of Sport and Exercise Psychology, 25*(4), 484–500. https://doi.org/10.1123/jsep.25.4.484

Lehman, D. R., & Reifman, A. (1987). Spectator influence on basketball officiating. *Journal of Social Psychology, 127*(6), 673–675.

Leite, W., & Pollard, R. (2018). International comparison of differences in home advantage between level 1 and level 2 of domestic football leagues. *German Journal of Exercise and Sport Research, 48*(2), 271–277. https://doi.org/10.1007/s12662-018-0507-2

MacMahon, C., & Strauss, B. (2014). The psychology of decision making in sports officials. In A. G. Papaioanno & D. Hackfort (Eds.), *Routledge companion to sport and exercise psychology* (1st ed., pp. 223–235). Routledge.

Manstead, A. S. R., & Semin, G. R. (1980). Social facilitation effects: Mere enhancement of dominant responses? *British Journal of Social and Clinical Psychology, 19*(2), 119–135. https://doi.org/10.1111/j.2044-8260.1980.tb00937.x

Marchant, D., Maher, R., & Wang, J. (2014). Perspectives on choking in sport. In A. G. Papaioanno & D. Hackfort (Eds.), *Routledge companion to sport and exercise psychology* (pp. 446–459). Routledge.

Martens, R. (1969a). Effect on performance of learning a complex motor task in the presence of spectators. *Research Quarterly of the American Association for Health, Physical Education and Recreation, 40*(2), 317–323. https://doi.org/10.1080/10671188.1969.10614830

Martens, R. (1969b). Palmar sweating and the presence of an audience. *Journal of Experimental Social Psychology, 5*(3), 371–374. https://doi.org/10.1016/0022-1031(69)90061-4

17

Martens, R. (1969c). Effect of an audience on learning and performance of a complex motor skill. *Journal of Personality and Social Psychology, 12*(3), 252–260. https://doi.org/10.1037/h0027710

Martens, R., & Landers, D. (1969). Coaction effects on a muscular endurance task. *Research Quarterly of the American Association for Health, Physical Education and Recreation, 40*(4), 733–737. https://doi.org/10.1080/10671188.1969.10614911

Martin, J. J. (2020). What triplett didn't find and what Lewin never said first. *Kinesiology Review, 9*(2), 89–91. https://doi.org/10.1123/kr.2020-0006

Maxwell, J. P., Masters, R., & Poolton, J. M. (2008). Self-consciousness, perceived evaluation and performance of a continuous motor task. *International Journal of Sport Psychology, 39*(3), 179–191.

Mayer, A. (1904). Über Einzel- und Gesamtleistung des Schulkindes. In *Sammlungen von Abhandlungen zur Psychologischen Pädagogik I, Band 4*. Heft.

McCarrick, D., Bilalic, M., Neave, N., & Wolfson, S. (2021). Home advantage during the COVID-19 pandemic: Analyses of European football leagues. *Psychology of Sport & Exercise, 56*, 102013. https://doi.org/10.1016/j.psychsport.2021.102013

McEwan, D. (2019). A home advantage? Examining 100 years of team success in National Hockey League playoff overtime games. *Psychology of Sport & Exercise, 43*, 195–199. https://doi.org/10.1016/j.psychsport.2019.02.010

McEwan, D., & Hofmann, M. D. (2021). Does a home disadvantage ever exist? In M. A. Gómez-Ruano, R. Pollard, & C. Lago-Peñas (Eds.), *Home advantage in sport* (1st ed., pp. 131–143). Routledge. doi: https://doi.org/10.4324/9781003081456-15

Meumann, E. (1904). *Haus- und Schularbeit*. Barth.

Miyamoto, M. (1979). Social Facilitation in Finger Maze Learning. *Japanese Psychological Research, 21*(2), 94–98. https://doi.org/10.4992/psycholres1954.21.94

Moede, W. (1920). *Experimentelle Massenpsychologie: Beiträge zur Experimentalpsychologie der Gruppe*. Hirzel.

Moore, H. (1917). Laboratory tests of anger, fear and sex interest. *The American Journal of Psychology, 28*(3), 396. https://doi.org/10.2307/1413610

Moore, J. C., & Brylinsky, J. A. (1993). Spectator effect on team performance in college basketball. *Journal of Sport Behavior, 16*(2), 77–84.

Murray, E., Neumann, D. L., Moffitt, R. L., & Thomas, P. R. (2016). The effects of the presence of others during a rowing exercise in a virtual reality environment. *Psychology of Sport and Exercise, 22*, 328–336. https://doi.org/10.1016/j.psychsport.2015.09.007

Murray, J. F. (1982). Construction of a stabilometer capable of indicating the variability of non-level performance. *Perceptual and Motor Skills, 55*, 1211–1215. https://doi.org/10.2466/pms.1982.55.3f.1211

Nevill, A. M., Balmer, N., & Williams, M. (1999). Crowd influence on decisions in association football. *Lancet, 353*(9162), 1416. https://doi.org/10.1016/S0140-6736(99)01299-4

Nevill, A. M., Balmer, N., & Williams, M. (2002). The influence of crowd noise and experience upon refereeing decisions in football. *Psychology of Sport and Exercise, 3*(4), 261–272. https://doi.org/10.1016/S1469-0292(01)00033-4

Nevill, A. M., Newell, S. M., & Gale, S. (1996). Factors associated with home advantage in english and Scottish soccer matches. *Journal of Sports Sciences, 14*(2), 181–186. https://doi.org/10.1080/02640419608727700

Otte, F. W., Millar, S.-K., & Klatt, S. (2020). What do you hear? The effect of stadium noise on football players' passing performances. *European Journal of Sport Science, 21*(7), 1035–1044. https://doi.org/10.1080/17461391.2020.1809714

Otte, F. W., Millar, S. K., & Klatt, S. (2021). What do you hear? The effect of stadium noise on football players' passing performances. *European journal of sport science, 21*(7), 1035–1044. https://doi.org/10.1080/17461391.2020.1809714

Palacios-Huerta, I. (2004). Structural changes during a century of the world's most popular sport. *Statistical Methods and Applications, 13*(2), 241–258. https://doi.org/10.1007/s10260-004-0093-3

Peeters, T., & van Ours, J. (2020). Seasonal home advantage in English professional football; 1973–2018. *SSRN Electronic Journal*. https://doi.org/10.2139/ssrn.3603228

Pollard, R. (1986). Home advantage in soccer: A retrospective analysis. *Journal of Sports Sciences, 4*(3), 237–248. https://doi.org/10.1080/02640418608732122

Pollard, R., & Armatas, V. (2017). Factors affecting home advantage in football World Cup qualification. *International Journal of Performance Analysis in Sport, 17*(1–2), 121–135. https://doi.org/10.1080/24748668.2017.1304031

Pollard, R., & Gómez, M. A. (2014a). Comparison of home advantage in men's and women's football leagues in Europe. *European*

Journal of Sport Science, 14(Suppl. 1), 77–83. https://doi.org/10.1080/17461391.2011.651490

Pollard, R., & Gómez, M. A. (2014b). Components of home advantage in 157 national soccer leagues worldwide. *International Journal of Sport and Exercise Psychology, 12*(3), 218–233. https://doi.org/10.1080/1612197X.2014.888245

Pollard, R., & Pollard, G. (2005). Long-term trends in home advantage in professional team sports in North America and England (1876–2003). *Journal of Sports Sciences, 23*(4), 337–350. https://doi.org/10.1080/02640410400021559

Pollard, R., Prieto, J., & Gómez, M. Á. (2017). Global differences in home advantage by country, sport and sex. *International Journal of Performance Analysis in Sport, 17*(4), 586–599. https://doi.org/10.1080/24748668.2017.1372164

Raab, M., Avugos, S., Bar-Eli, M., & MacMahon, C. (2020). The referee's challenge: A threshold process model for decision making in sport games. *International Review of Sport and Exercise Psychology, 1–21*. https://doi.org/10.1080/1750984X.2020.1783696

Raab, M., Bar-Eli, M., Plessner, H., & Araújo, D. (2019). The past, present and future of research on judgment and decision making in sport. *Psychology of Sport & Exercise, 42*, 25–32. https://doi.org/10.1016/j.psychsport.2018.10.004

Rajecki, D. W., Ickes, W., Corcoran, C., & Lenerz, K. (1977). Social facilitation of human performance: Mere presence effects. *Journal of Social Psychology, 102*(2), 297–310. https://doi.org/10.1080/00224545.1977.9713277

Riedl, D., Staufenbiel, K., Strauss, B., & Heuer, A. (2014). The global home advantage in Soccer: Status, developments and causes. *J Exerc Mov Sport, 12*, 218–233. Available since February 17, 2022, at PsyArXiv. https://doi.org/10.31234/osf.io/zaujy

Riedl, D., Strauss, B., Heuer, A., & Rubner, O. (2015). Finale furioso: Referee-biased injury times and their effects on home advantage in football. *Journal of Sports Sciences, 33*(4), 327–336. https://doi.org/10.1080/02640414.2014.944558

Salminen, S. (1993). The effect of the audience on the home advantage. *Perceptual and Motor Skills, 76*(Suppl. 3), 1123–1128. https://doi.org/10.2466/pms.1993.76.3c.1123

Sanders, G. S., Baron, R. S., & Moore, D. L. (1978). Distraction and social comparison as mediators of social facilitation effects. *Journal of Experimental Social Psychology, 14*(3), 291–303. https://doi.org/10.1016/0022-1031(78)90017-3

Sanna, L. J. (1992). Self-Efficacy Theory: Implications for social facilitation and social loafing. *Journal of Personality and Social Psychology, 62*(5), 774–786. https://doi.org/10.1037/0022-3514.62.5.774

Schlenker, B. R., Phillips, S. T., Boniecki, K. A., & Schlenker, D. R. (1995). Where is the home choke? *Journal of Personality and Social Psychology, 68*(4), 649–652. https://doi.org/10.1037/0022-3514.68.4.649

Schwartz, B., & Barsky, S. F. (1977). The home advantage. *Social Forces, 55*(3), 641–661.

Sheridan, A., Marchant, D. C., Williams, E. L., Jones, H. S., Hewitt, P. A., & Sparks, A. (2019). Presence of spotters improves bench press performance: A deception study. *Journal of Strength and Conditioning Research, 33*(7), 1755–1761.

Snyder, A. L., Anderson-Hanley, C., & Arciero, P. J. (2012). Virtual and live social facilitation while exergaming: Competitiveness moderates exercise intensity. *Journal of Sport and Exercise Psychology, 34*(2), 252–259.

Spence, K. W. (1956). *Behavior theory and conditioning*. Yale University Press.

Staufenbiel, K., Lobinger, B., & Strauss, B. (2015). Home advantage in soccer—A matter of expectations, goal setting and tactical decisions of coaches? *Journal of Sports Sciences, 33*(18), 1932–1941. https://doi.org/10.1080/02640414.2015.1018929

Staufenbiel, K., Riedl, D., & Strauss, B. (2018). Learning to be advantaged: The development of home advantage in high-level youth soccer. *International Journal of Sport and Exercise Psychology, 16*(1), 36–50. https://doi.org/10.1080/1612197X.2016.1142463

Strauss, B. (2002a). Social facilitation in motor tasks: A review of research and theory. *Psychology of Sport and Exercise, 3*(3), 237–256. https://doi.org/10.1016/S1469-0292(01)00019-X

Strauss, B. (2002b). The impact of supportive spectator behavior on performance in team sports. *International Journal of Sport Psychology, 33*(4), 372–390.

Strauss, B., & Bierschwale, J. (2008). Zuschauer und der Heimvorteil in der Handballbundesliga. *Zeitschrift Für Sportpsychologie, 15*(3), 96–101. https://doi.org/10.1026/1612-5010.15.3.96

Strauss, B., & Höfer, E. (2001). Spectators and the home advantage in team sports. In A. Papaioammou, M. Goudas, & Y. Theodorakis (Eds.), Proceedings of the 10th world congress of sport psychology (Vol. 4, pp. 210–212). Christodoulidi Publications.

Strauss, B., & MacMahon, C. (2014). Audience influences on athlete performances. In A. G. Papaioanno & D. Hackfort (Eds.), *Routledge companion to sport and exercise psychology* (1st ed. pp. 213–222). Routledge.

Stroebe, W. (2012). The truth about triplett (1898), but nobody seems to care. *Perspectives on Psychological Science, 7*(1), 54–57. https://doi.org/10.1177/1745691611427306

Sutter, M., & Kocher, M. G. (2004). Favoritism of agents—The case of referees' home bias. *Journal of Economic Psychology, 25*(4), 461–469. https://doi.org/10.1016/S0167-4870(03)00013-8

Szabó, D. Z. (2022). The impact of differing audience sizes on referees and team performance from a North American perspective. *Psychology of Sport & Exercise, 60*, 102162. https://doi.org/10.1016/j.psychsport.2022.102162

Tauer, J. M., Guenther, C. L., & Rozek, C. (2009). Is there a home choke in decisive playoff basketball games? *Journal of Applied Sport Psychology, 21*(2), 148–162.

Thirer, J., & Rampey, M. S. (1979). Effects of abusive spectators' behavior on performance of home and visiting intercollegiate basketball teams. *Perceptual and Motor Skills, 48*(Suppl. 3), 1047–1053. https://doi.org/10.2466/pms.1979.48.3c.1047

Tilp, M., & Thaller, S. (2020). Covid-19 has turned home advantage into home disadvantage in the German Soccer Bundesliga. *Frontiers in Sports and Active Living, 2*. https://doi.org/10.3389/fspor.2020.593499

Triplett, N. (1898). The dynamogenic factors in pacemaking and competition. *The American Journal of Psychology, 9*(4), 507–533.

Unkelbach, C., & Memmert, D. (2010). Crowd noise as a cue in referee decisions contributes to the home advantage. *Journal of Sport and Exercise Psychology, 32*(4), 483–498. https://doi.org/10.1123/jsep.32.4.483

Uziel, L. (2007). Individual differences in the social facilitation effect: A review and meta-analysis. *Journal of Research in Personality, 41*(3), 579–601. https://doi.org/10.1016/j.jrp.2006.06.008

Van de Ven, N. (2011). Supporters are not necessary for the home advantage: Evidence from same-stadium Derbies and games without an audience. *Journal of Applied Social Psychology, 41*(12), 2785–2792. https://doi.org/10.1111/j.1559-1816.2011.00865.x

van Meurs, E., Greve, J., & Strauss, B. (2022). Moving in the presence of others—A systematic review and meta-analysis. *International Review of Sport and Psychology*, 1–12. https://doi.org/10.1080/1750984X.2022.2111663

Wallace, H. M., Baumeister, R. F., & Vohs, K. D. (2005). Audience support and choking under pressure: A home disadvantage? *Journal of Sports Sciences, 23*(4), 429–438. https://doi.org/10.1080/02640410400021666

Wankel, L. M. (1977). Audience size and trait anxiety effects upon state anxiety and motor performance. *Research Quarterly of the*

American Alliance for Health, Physical Education and Recreation, 48(1), 181–186. https://doi.org/10.1080/10671315.1977.10762168

Worringham, C. J., & Messick, D. M. (1983). Social facilitation of running: An unobtrusive study. *Journal of Social Psychology, 121*(1), 23–29. https://doi.org/10.1080/00224545.1983.9924462

Wulf, G. (2013). Attentional focus and motor learning: A review of 15 years. *International Review of Sport and Exercise Psychology, 6*(1), 77–104. https://doi.org/10.1080/1750984X.2012.723728

Wunderlich, F., Weigelt, M., Rein, R., & Memmert, D. (2021). How does spectator presence affect football? Home advantage remains in European top-class football matches played without spectators during the COVID-19 pandemic. *PLoS ONE, 16*(3), e0248590. https://doi.org/10.1371/journal.pone.0248590

Zajonc, R. B. (1965). Social facilitation. *Science, 149*, 142–146.

Zajonc, R. B. (1969). *Animal social psychology: A reader of experimental studies*. Wiley.

Interaction and Communication

Andreas Lau and Henning Plessner

Contents

J. Schüler et al. (eds.), *Sport and Exercise Psychology*, https://doi.org/10.1007/978-3-031-03921-8_18

Learning Objectives

Basic:
- To comprehend basic theories for understanding people as social beings
- To define and differentiate interaction and communication as types of social actions

Advanced:
- To demonstrate interaction and communication as social processes
- To discuss task-based and social interactions in sport

Experts:
- To know how to apply principles and examples of effective communication in sport

18.1 Introduction

Humans are social beings. Our ability to live in community with others gave our ancestors an evolutionary advantage. The human abilities of thinking and speaking could not have developed if prehistoric man had not lived in organizational structures in which interaction and communication were vital. The interaction and communication required in these organizational structures also served as a significant source for individual development and the effectiveness of social action. These process-like, inter-individual occurrences are inseparably interwoven. Social interaction, however, is considered to be the broader concept of the two, because it encompasses every type of interrelated behavior of persons, while communication primarily represents the process of information exchange between the actors. In this chapter, the nature of interaction and communication will be discussed fundamentally in order to highlight applied aspects of sport afterward.

18.2 Social Interaction

The term "interaction" is used in many ways. In science, it is applied by various disciplines to define events that are borne by the mutual influence of things, persons, or institutions. Physics, for example, covers interactions between elementary particles, pharmacy is concerned with pharmaceutical interactions that need to be considered, and biology examines the mutual influence of organisms and substances within an ecosystem. Computer science understands the design of interactive user interfaces as a type of human-computer interaction (i.e., an interrelationship between man and machine) for which there are numerous other examples in technology and economics. In sociology, the term interaction is also applied to the cooperation of organizations and institutions. In psychology, interaction stands for a "related action of two or more persons" (Bierhoff & Jonas, 2011, p. 132) and is understood as a *social interaction* as opposed to the types described above. Other defining **characteristics of social interactions** include:

1. Reachability/presence of at least two or more actors
2. Possibility of direct or indirect contact
3. Time-relatedness and influencing the actors through action and reaction
4. Unity of conscious and unconscious influence on or by the other actor
5. Differentiation into task- and relationship-related aspects of social interaction
6. Communication as a mediator of social interactions
7. Influence of the interaction results on the quality of the relationship between the interaction partners and their social environment

Social Interaction

Social interaction refers to the mutual influence as well as the interrelated (interdependent) actions and behavior of at least two actors.

The course of social interactions is largely determined by social cognitions, motives, and emotions of the interacting persons. To this end, the participants bring their own goals, expectations, experiences, and competences into the interaction, but those of the other person are also perceived and interpreted. The success of a social interaction can be measured by the extent to which participants succeed in setting or achieving their own or common goals and expectations (▶ Chap. 22). Since social interactions are part of the essence of interpersonal relationships, it is not surprising that social science theories and models for these relationships emerged very early on and have been continuously developed further. The most fundamental of these are presented in the next section.

18.2.1 Social Exchange Theories

G. H. Mead (1863–1931) provided an early social behaviorist approach termed "symbolic interactionism" that is one of the main directions of the so-called Interpretative Program. This perspective involves the assumption that social reality arises from the changing, interrelated, and interpretive actions of individuals. In this behaviorist tradition, Mead characterizes humans, as distinct from animals, as symbol-using creatures that have gained further forms of interaction through the use of language (verbal gestures) as well as through meaningful vocal (sounds) and nonvocal gestures (facial expressions), which he describes as significant symbols. This language-mediated interaction between the actors is determined by two decisive characteristics: (a) the ability to perceive oneself and (b) the ability to anticipate behavior. In his thesis of the "Generalized Other," Mead postulates that a person is fundamentally able to change his or her perspective when interacting. In addition, people are able to assess their own behavior from the perspective (seeing themselves through the eyes of the other) and, at the same time, to predict (anticipate) the behavior of the other actor (e.g., their emotional reaction), i.e., to put themselves in other's shoes (adoption of perspective). Accordingly, the identity of an individual (self) is constituted by the subjective assumptions about oneself (I) and the social self (me), in which the expectations of important reference persons or groups are reflected. The **concept of the "Generalized Other"** is seen as an important interface between the individual and the social perspective of a person, since it emphasizes their special feature of being able to orient their behavior toward others on the basis of processes of interpretation and to be capable of communication, cooperation, and self-reflection. This practical **intersubjectivity** thus establishes the social essence of man (Mead, 1934; Treibel, 2000).

H. Blumer (1900–1987), a pupil of Mead, formulated three additional premises that form the foundation of this approach (Blumer, 1969):

1. People behave toward things (objects, other people) on the basis of the meanings they have for them.
2. The meanings of such things derive from the social interaction one enters into with them.
3. These meanings are used and adapted by people for their interaction with others as a result of an interpretative process.

Thus, for the actors involved, their social interaction is in particular an interpretation process (Treibel, 2000, p. 118).

G. C. Homans (1910–1989) is regarded as one of the founders of behavioral theory in sociology, who, like Mead, was guided by the basic assumptions of behaviorism and explains human social behavior as an exchange process. His basic thesis states: A universal principle of social action is based on the fact that every actor strives to achieve the maximization of the expected extent of rewards and a minimization of punishment. In other words, people exchange material and immaterial goods (e.g., affection, recognition, prestige) in their interactions with the aim of increasing their personal benefit or maximizing their profit. Homans' theses are based on the human image of *homo economicus,* which assumes that humans are fully informed about possible options for power and exchange, foresee their consequences, and make rational decisions on this basis. Accordingly, the behavior of individuals is cost-conscious and maximizes benefits. In addition, the own benefit of an interaction is always measured by the success or failure of the other actors. Seen in this light, social exchange explains the forms of interaction cooperation and competition (▶ Sect. 18.2.2; Cook & Rice, 2003; Treibel, 2000).

Rusbult's (1983) "investment model" was a valuable further development based on "theory of social exchange" principles alongside the "equity theory" (Walster et al., 1973) and the "interdependence theory" (Kelley & Thibaut, 1978). Above all, it introduced **commitment** as the central predictor of satisfaction with social interaction (▶ Chap. 22).

In summary and in addition, it can be stated that social exchange: a) focuses on the mutual interdependence of the interaction partners; b) includes forms of reward deferral; c) also includes intangible goods such as feelings, social recognition, and status changes in the sense of costs and benefits; and d) does not have to correspond to a zero-sum game (benefit of A corresponds to the costs of B), but longer-term interactions can, in their overall assessment, create a win-win situation for both actors (Cook & Rice, 2003).

On the basis of these theoretical approaches, numerous applied topics and fields of research have developed, especially in the field of social psychology. Examples for these are the topics of power, conformity, social influence, and leadership (▶ Chaps. 5, 16, and 17). In corresponding interaction analyses, as already suggested by Bales (1976), a distinction is made between task-related and social interactions and usually a dyadic- or group-related interaction situation is taken as a basis. The diversity of social interactions in sport will be discussed in the next section.

18.2.2 Social Interaction in Sport

The forms of social interaction in sport are as diverse as sport itself. Even the recreational athlete who laces up his running shoes and is initially alone on his running route is in most cases acting in a social context, for example, because social motives encourage him to run regularly (e.g., recognition by his partner), because he may hope to see or be seen by a like-minded person or walker, or because he changes (adjusts) his running pace when he sees a runner in front of or behind him on his route. Both the imagined and the actual presence of others has a social influence on one's own behavior and experience in sport (▶ Chap. 16) and can be interpreted as social interaction in a broader sense. The example of the recreational runner also illustrates that the task and social aspects of interaction are closely interwoven and are only considered separately from each other formally or for methodological reasons. As soon as the runner decides to join another runner in order to continue running together, both runners have to coordinate their running pace, the running distance, and, if necessary, the running breaks. If a runner takes part in a race, his run becomes an immediate and obvious part of social interactions, namely, a mutual influence of all involved actors (e.g., runner, audience). A distinction can be made between **direct social interaction** (e.g., running with a pacemaker or partner) and **indirect interaction** (e.g., initial pace of the runner crowd or audience applause). This means that the occurrence and extent of social interactions and their effects on people's behavior and experience are largely determined by the **situational context** in which people engage in sport.

In the following, only those situations in sport will be considered in which two or more actors interact in an intended, direct, and interrelated way. Such interactions usually take place in sporting activities and behavior during training and competition. Constitutive elements in the development of interactions and the evaluation of the quality of interaction (e.g., appropriateness, proportionality, effectiveness, success) between athletes are the objectives and tasks that need to be achieved as well as the real conditions which normatively determine the actors' scope for action and decision-making. This means that, as in everyday life, typical social interaction in sport is often determined by the fact that a person has to choose between contrary alternatives of action. It is irrelevant whether the interactions are task- or relationship-oriented, as the following three examples show.

Case Studies

A handball player can make more selfish decisions when in possession of the ball, by trying to solve the situation with an action of her own (e.g., breakthrough to the goal, attempt to score a goal). Or in principle she plays in a team-oriented manner and only throws on goal herself if there is no (tactically) better alternative (e.g., pass to the free player).

A fair playing defender of a football team meets a very unfairly acting opponent in a betting game. However, his fairness is damaging to his team, as the opponent's striker has already used a dive to take a free kick that led to a goal.

It is customary for the men's team to meet up in the clubhouse for a cozy get-together after the final training on Friday. But some players are already married and would much rather spend time with their spouse instead of fulfilling this social obligation.The examples show that the respective actors are in fact in a tight spot when it comes to deciding on their further course of action, as their own interests are in conflict with the interests of others. In social psychology, this interaction situation corresponds to the classic prisoner dilemma (Excursus: Classical Prisoner's Dilemma), which is similar to the problem of social exchange (▶ Sect. 18.2.1). Social interaction is thus about the recurring decision to help each other (cooperation) or to refuse help (competition). The **social dilemma** is created above all by the fact that, initially independent of the behavior of the other person, uncooperative behavior (egoistic, unfair, uncompanionable; see examples), on the one hand, always pays off for the individual actor (e.g., egoistic play leads to more own goals). On the other hand, group effectiveness and the group climate suffer all the more the more members of the group behave competitively. This means that the individual benefit can only be maximized at the expense of the team and also depends on what the other players decide to do in the situation (Mosler & Brucks, 2006; ▶ Side Story: Classical Prisoner's Dilemma).

Side Story

Classical Prisoner's Dilemma

The prisoner's dilemma is a metaphor for the general problem of the social dilemma into which two people can be drawn under certain circumstances. It originates from the following story: Two criminals accused of bank robbery are being questioned by the prosecution simultaneously but independently. In the absence of evidence, the prosecutor makes the following offer to both defendants: A confession of the crime leads to a shortened imprisonment, while the accomplice receives the full sentence, as long as he or she does not confess. If both confess independently, both receive the same, only slightly reduced sentence. If both don't confess and remain silent, they will be sentenced to 1 year of imprisonment because of weak circumstantial evidence. These options inevitably make both prisoners fall into a trust dilemma, as they cannot know for sure how their partner will react to this offer. Silence is the best option, but only if both can rely on the other person and know that the other one does not break his or her silence and confesses to the bank robbery in favor of both of them receiving a greatly reduced sentence (Rapoport & Chammah, 1965).

Fig. 18.1 Interdependent decisions of two athletes based on the prisoner's dilemma model (Lau, 2005)

	Player B: teamwork, fair, social	Player B: selfish, unfair, antisocial
Player A: teamwork, fair, social	+ / +	− − / + +
Player A: selfish, unfair, antisocial	+ + / − −	− / −

In relation to the above examples, the following results: Each of the players has to decide between team-oriented (see handball player), fair (see football defender), or comradely (see team member) behavior or the opposite. A decision that is beneficial to all concerned is always the "team beneficial" (or fair, social) one, while a "self-centered" decision is of no benefit to either side. However, a maximum **benefit** (+ +) or **disadvantage** (− −) results when one actor chooses to be selfish and the other actor chooses to act cooperatively (Fig. 18.1).

Of course, it is not enough to simply explain the nature of the social dilemma. Rather, it is necessary to describe and discuss situational and personal conditions as well as rules of conduct which help the persons involved to solve this inner conflict. In his "Theory of Cooperation and Competition and Beyond," Deutsch (2011) scientifically examines the conditions for the occurrence of cooperative or competing behavior of conflict parties and demands that the mutual influence of the motives and objectives of all parties involved has to be analyzed. A negative correlation has to be expected if the success of one party goes hand in hand with the loss of the other (*win-lose orientation*). A positive tendency is to be expected if the implementation of one's own goals makes the success of both parties possible (*win-win orientation*). Consequently, a distinction is made between constructive and destructive processes in the resolution of conflict situations. It can be shown that cooperative behavior of both parties implies constructive solutions rather than competitive behavior. Cooperative relations between the conflict parties are characterized by numerous positive features such as effective communication, an open and friendly attitude, and the mutual willingness to strengthen the other party. Competing relationships in turn result precisely from contrary features (summarized in Deutsch, 2011).

> Without binding agreements or the orientation toward known preferences and experiences with regard to the decision-making behavior of the actors, a social dilemma is rationally hardly solvable.

Sport Practice

The following experiences and measures should be communicated in order to optimize social interactions and avoid social dilemmas between the participants (Lau & Plessner, 2016):

Creating trust

The confidence that the partner makes reliable decisions that can be derived from his/her fundamental attitudes and motives provides a solid basis for decision-making. Both actors should assure each other of their trust and communicate changes in their basic values in a timely manner. A person who operates distrustfully in a social dilemma is more likely to rely on competition than on cooperation, while more familiarity generates stronger willingness to cooperate.

Communicating reliability

Personal motives, attitudes, and values should be conveyed to the participants through appropriate self-management. A person who is obviously led by fixed and clearly recognizable premises in behavior makes it easier for the partner to anticipate the decision options in the current interaction. Jumpy, emotional, and mood-guided behavior as well as constantly changing, or inappropriate, strategies of action increase the risk of not being reliably assessed by the partner.

Promoting communication

Open, regular, and targeted communication between the actors (e.g., between group members) can help avoid interpretation problems and clear up misunderstandings. This can counteract judging others with a focus on pursuing self-interest and promote a willingness to realize common interests.

Considering time perspectives
Especially in repeated interactions (e.g., in-season training), social dilemmas may occur frequently. From the short-term perspective, in which each decision choice is valid only in this situation, the decision to compete seems to promise more success. If one looks rather at the long-term perspective (e.g., at the end of the season), in which there is a final accounting of all social dilemma solutions, then the early attention to mutual cooperation proves to be more valuable.

Accepting standards
One of the most effective measures for solving social dilemmas, especially within groups, is the establishment of common behavioral standards and decision rules. Within this, social norms represent a behavioral regulator and promote conformity processes in the group (► Chap. 16). A universal and cross-cultural norm for interpersonal behavior is the rule of reciprocity. Through defensive or reactive behavior, where the first step is expected from the interaction partner, both joint cooperation and competition are possible as captured in vernacular phrases such as "What goes around comes around!" or "Tit for tat." The so-called tit-for-tat strategy promotes active cooperation right at the beginning of the interaction. This strategy basically contains two rules (Mosler & Brucks, 2006):

1. First, offer your cooperation and present yourself as friendly and open.
2. Then, all of your further decisions are in accordance to the response of your partner. If he cooperates, the strategy will determine this for the next interactions, if not, competition will follow.

These rules of conduct presented so far have been designed for the classic prisoner dilemma (i.e., as solution strategies for two actors). However, in general and especially in sports, there is a need for explanatory approaches involving several actors. Here we speak of the **N-person prisoner's dilemma,** which is characterized by two premises (Dawes, 1980):

1. The individual benefits from the competitive choice more than cooperation.
2. However, all individuals benefit if all parties involved rely on cooperation.

As with the classic social dilemma, cooperation in principle is given a long-term advantage. Nevertheless, the overall situation must be regarded as more diffuse, and the occurrence of defensive behavior patterns on the part of individuals, as well as social loafing and free-riding cannot be ruled out (► Chap. 17).

The "All-or-Nobody Treaty" is to be seen here as a solution example that can be used in groups. With this contract, which can be concluded formally or informally, a norm is created that focuses primarily on equal treatment and justice. In principle, the aim is to establish cooperation as the goal of majority decision-making in open communication. The agreed rules of conduct are then—without ifs and buts—binding for all.

In summary, it can be said that the actors in social interactions often have to decide between cooperative or competitive behavior. The choice of one's own behavior is guided by the principles of social exchange (individual benefit maximization). Inner conflicts (social dilemmas) arise primarily from the uncertainty of the behavior of the other person. The choice of the optimal behavior is made more difficult by the number of participants, by misinterpretation of behavior due to lack of experience and trust in the other person, and by communication disorders (► Sect. 18.3). Even though the development of social norms can support the development of action strategies, it is not possible to fully control and predict social interaction processes (Bierhoff & Jonas, 2011; Mosler & Brucks, 2006).

Further research results on the effects of social interactions in sport are available in connection with group processes (► Chap. 17), spectator behavior (► Chap. 16) parental influence (Knight et al., 2016), and leadership behavior in and by groups (► Chap. 17). However, as the interaction between the coach and his/her athlete is of central importance in all sports (LaVoi, 2007), it will be discussed in more detail below. While the emphasis in ► Sect. 18.2.3 is on the social relationships between coach and athlete, the communication requirements are discussed in ► Sect. 18.4.

18.2.3 Coach-Athlete Interaction

The coach as the leader is responsible for the implementation of a planned, systematic, and age-appropriate training process. It is often the coach's responsibility to take over the competition control (coaching) for the athlete. The promotion of athletic performance is primarily to be evaluated as task-related interaction, which is reflected above all in the coach's leadership behavior. The "multidimensional model of leadership in sport" by Chelladurai (2007) predicts athlete performance and satisfaction as a consequence of the interaction of personal and situational characteristics and the resulting leadership behavior of the coach (◘ Fig. 18.2). It will be explained in more detail here, as it explicitly focuses on the coach-athlete interaction (◘ Fig. 18.3).

First of all, three input factors must be characterized. Thus, each situation in the sports context has some specific characteristics which may differ with regard to the objective, the methodological-didactical requirements, and the material-technical conditions. The situational conditions determine above all the **behavior required** (in this situation), if there are only a few appropriate alternatives for action. The more action alternatives appear to be useful for the solution of a group task, the more likely it is that the **behavior preferred** by the group members can be incorporated into the leadership decision in this situation. The preferred behavior is, of course, primarily determined by the preferences, experiences, and expectations of the athletes, whereas the required behavior of the coach is determined by the current performance and development level of the athletes. As a third influencing factor, the model considers the personality traits of the leader (i.e., the behavioral options available to him/her to shape the leadership task). Ideally, the leader should be familiar with several leadership styles, which he/she can credibly and successfully implement behaviorally. Openness and flexibility of the leader are especially important when he/she has to adapt **current leadership behavior** to the overall situation. The model makes it clear that the coach should include personal assessments and perceptions of required and preferred behavior in the decision on current leadership behavior. This way, the model plausibly explains that being too one-sided in leadership behavior orientation toward the required *or* preferred behavior can result in a long-run loss of performance or satisfaction among athletes. Rather, the leader must be able to use his or her leadership skills to achieve the necessary balance between the required and preferred leadership behavior (congruence) and thus to achieve optimal results with their actual leadership behavior (Chelladurai, 2007; ▶ Study Box: Coach Behavior, Satisfaction, and Performance).

	Helpful/caring	
Prizewinning	Effective and successful	Ineffectiv and successful
	Effective and unsuccessful	Ineffectiv and unsuccessful

◘ **Fig. 18.3** The "2×2 model of coach-athlete interaction" (modified after Jowett & Poczwardowski, 2007)

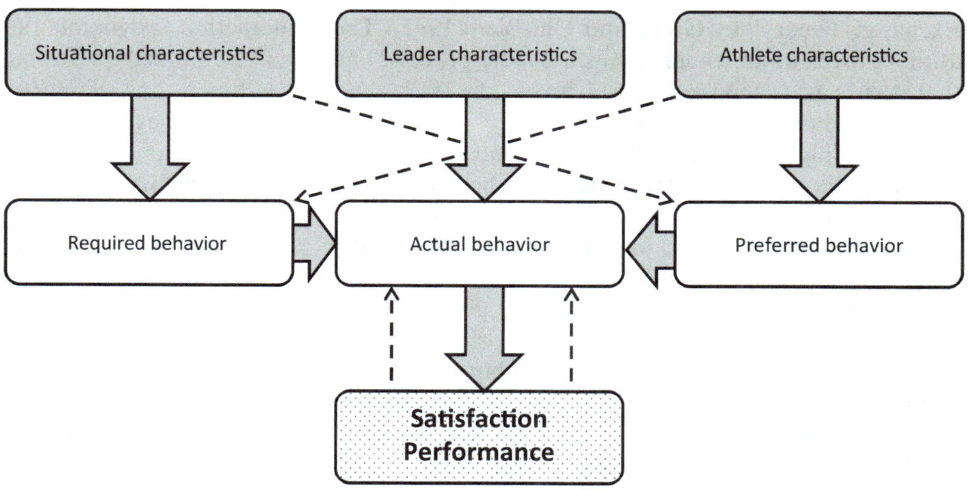

◘ **Fig. 18.2** The "multidimensional model of guidance in sports" (modified according to Chelladurai, 2007, with kind permission of John Wiley and Sons)

Study Box

Coach Behavior, Satisfaction, and Performance

Based on the "multidimensional model" (Fig. 18.2), Pfeffer et al. (2004) examined differences and correlations between the subjective perception of the coach-athlete interaction, performance development, and satisfaction in individual and team sports. The results uncovered differences between the individual and team sports: While the longitudinal development of performance among young people from the individual sports were associated *above* all with a high degree of subjectively perceived instructions and a task-oriented training climate, in team sports, it was obviously more closely linked to the level of perceived social support. But the current level of performance was not related to the evaluation of the coach-athlete interaction. The more pronounced the instructive behavior of the coach, the more satisfied the athletes were with the training.

In a cross-sectional analysis, Pfeffer and Gallitschke (2008) examined female soccer players and female and male coaches in competitive football and could show that gender is a coach personality trait (Fig. 18.2) which also has an influence on the evaluation of the coach-athlete interaction. Male coaches were evaluated as more socially supportive, more rewarding, and more democratically valued in leadership by the players than their female colleagues. As a cause for this surprising result, the authors assume that the dominant-male context of football leads female coaches to try and use their behavior more in line with that of their male colleagues, while conversely, male coaches of women's football learn how to adapt their behavior to their presumed expectation preferences of the women. Obviously, gender-specific role models and expectations, at least for women's football, exert considerable influence on assessments of coach-athlete interactions.

In a nutshell, Alfermann (Alfermann, 2010) summarizes the previous findings by saying that a) the results are rather inconsistent, b) the connection between satisfaction and actual (current) leadership behavior is greatest when this also corresponds to the coach behavior perceived by the athletes, and c) the influences of leadership behavior on performance or performance development are not very clear.

Classic behavioral leadership concepts focus on the interaction between the leader and the person being led, but expect a universally equal positive effect on all group members. Later on, different **sociopsychological leadership concepts** have been developed to at least complement these approaches, such as the "Leader-Member Exchange Theory" by Green and Uhl-Bien (1995). The authors focus upon leadership as a dyadic process; one that occurs as a social exchange between the leader and each individual group member.

It is mainly thanks to Sophia Jowett and her research team that the emotional-social quality of the relationship between coach and athlete has become a more important topic in sport psychology. Jowett (2007) fundamentally assumes that the coach-athlete interaction is characterized by interdependence and a common goal and that its quality is reflected in the athlete's performance development and success (success vs. failure) but also in athlete personality development and maturity (effective vs. ineffective) (Fig. 18.3). Furthermore, the perceived satisfaction with the relationship between coach and athlete is determined by the combination of athletic success or aspired performance progress and effective, age-appropriate personality development. The (temporary) absence of success in sport may be less of a threat to the **coach-athlete relationship** than a negative assessment on a social level, where the coach and/or athlete feel that the relationship is more likely to be detrimental to their personal development and becomes a socio-emotional burden. If performance and relationship development remain ineffective for a longer period of time, a breakdown in the cooperation between coach and athlete seems inevitable (Jowett & Poczwardowski, 2007).

The quality of the relationship in a coach-athlete interaction is dynamic rather than stable. According to the "3C model" by Jowett (2007) it can be divided into the dimensions *closeness* (proximity, affection), *commitment* (obligation, bin- dung), and *complementarity* (cooperation) and operationalized in them. With the help of the "Coach-Athlete Relationship Questionnaire (CART-Q)" by Jowett and Ntoumanis (2004), the coach and his athlete or his athletes estimate the measure of these three relationship components, first from their own and then from the presumed perspective of the other. Further analysis of the relationship can also be used to check the agreement (co-orientation, congruence) between the perceived relationship quality of the coach and the athlete(s), which represents a significant extension of the original model to the "3 + 1 C model". Although the psychometric quality of the CART-Q has been questioned (Alfermann, 2010), this differentiated, multidimensional assessment of relationship quality seems to be very relevant in practice, as it makes clear, to coaches in particular, the importance of the affective relationship component for successful, satisfactory, and lasting social interaction.

18.3 Basics Principles of Communication

Every social interaction also generates communication. Even in the case of short-term and casual social contacts (e.g., when two athletes meet at the entrance to the stadium), an act of communication takes place, provided that one follows Paul Watzlawick's thesis that one cannot not communicate (Watzlawick et al., 1967). In social psychological theory formation, the two terms are, however, distinguished in that **communication** primarily focuses on the exchange of information and the establishment of common understanding. **Interaction**, on the other hand, includes all processes that take place between individuals, groups, and institutions. Communication can take place verbally and nonverbally and leads to the exchange of information (synonym: messages) via the communicant's own empathy, perception, thinking, remembering, and feeling. For the description and analysis of an act of communication, the following components must be assessed: Who (sender) says what (message, information, action) to whom (receiver) with what (sign, symbol, language) via which medium (channel) with what purpose (intention, awareness) and with what effect (reaction of the receiver) (Traut-Mattausch & Frey, 2006)?

Most of the basic psychological communication models follow technical transmitter-receiver models (◘ Fig. 18.4), not only in terms of their content but also conceptually. The starting point of a human act of communication is the intention of a person (transmitter) to transmit information to a target person (receiver). The transmitter selects an available and suitable channel for information transmission. While radio technicians are concerned with the choice of frequency range, the choice between acoustic, optical, and tactile sensory channels, or a combination of these, is of primary importance from a psychological point of view and is influenced by the accessibility of the receiver and, if necessary, by environmental influences (e.g., ambient noise, distance). Further distinctions between **forms of communication** are:

- Direct (face-to-face) or indirect communication (both communicators cannot see each other and are only in contact with each other through technical means)
- Acoustic communication: vocal (not linguistic bound sounds, e.g., whistling) or verbal (speaking)
- Verbal communication: oral or written use of language
- Nonverbal communication: arbitrary gestures, facial expressions, eye and body contact (e.g., clapping), body poses and activity (e.g., jumping around) or involuntary physiological reactions (e.g., perspiration, blushing), posture and body activation (e.g., trembling, yawning)
- Interpersonal communication (e.g., dialogue or group discussion) or mass communication (indirect, one-sided dissemination of information by one person to a large number of recipients such as occurs in brochures, posters, reports)

The information is thus encoded (synonymously: coded, encrypted) by the transmitter depending on the available channel and then transmitted. The receiver

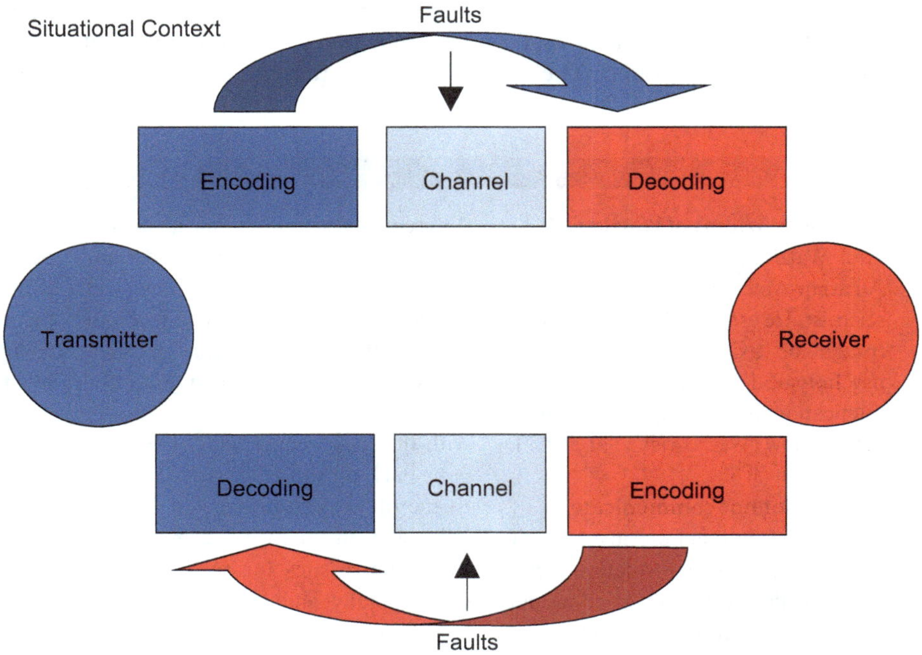

◘ **Fig. 18.4** General transmitter-receiver model (modified according to Traut-Mattausch & Frey, 2006)

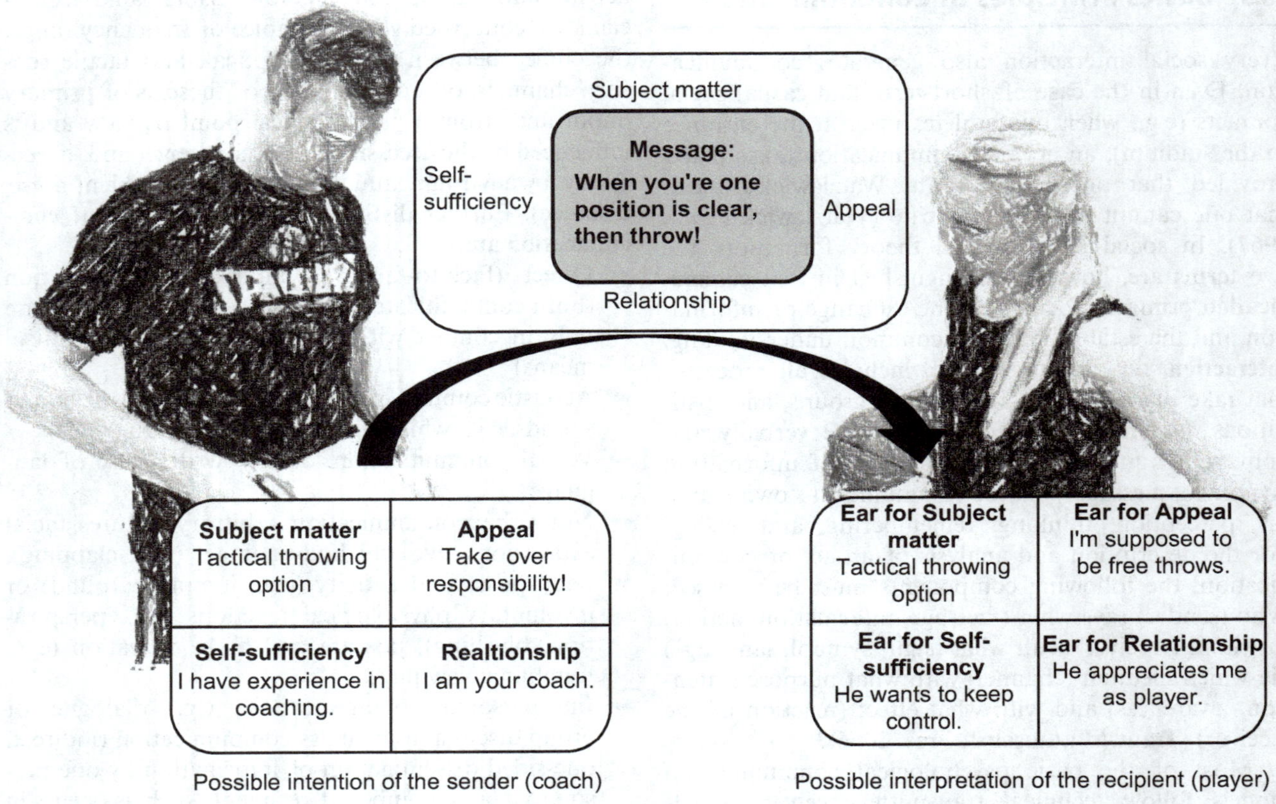

Fig. 18.5 Four sides of a message (modified according to Schulz von Thun, 2008)

uses his sensory organs to perceive the message and must decode (decrypt) it. This means that the receiver interprets the content of the message and tries to understand it. Whereas in technical models the act of communication is considered complete with this, in **psychologically determined models** a second phase of communication is added. The receiver becomes the sender of a reaction (feedback) to the received message and lets the first sender become the receiver. This feedback becomes a significant element of the act of communication, because it is the indicator for the success or failure or the end or continuation of the act of communication (Fig. 18.5; ► Side Story: Pragmatic Axioms of Watzlawick).

18

Side Story

Pragmatic Axioms of Watzlawick

Paul Watzlawick (1921–2007) was an Austrian-American communication scientist. He established five basic rules (pragmatic axioms) which point to psychological aspects in human communication and are explained in more detail below (Watzlawick et al., 1967).

One cannot not communicate

Any social interaction involves the transmission of information, even if no explicit intention to communicate exists. Even if two athletes from different backgrounds meet during competition preparation and do not communicate via words, they will still tell each other how they feel and evaluate the situation. Behaviors such as looking down, keeping a great distance, not greeting someone, dealing with the sports equipment or turning your back on the other person signal to the other person that you are not interested in intensive communication. The reasons for such behavior can be many and varied (e.g., insecurity in the encounter, bad mood, or the focus on the upcoming competition). Friendly, questioning eye contact, approach, and attention, on the other hand, at least convey the willingness to communicate with the other person.

Every communication has a content and a relationship level

The content aspect corresponds to the information content, that is, it describes the factual information that the sender wants to transmit to the receiver. However, even the most factual information is influenced by the existing relationship between sender and receiver and is often implicitly included. The intended request of the coach to an athlete to show more effort (factual content), will be discussed in their formulation and verbalization (voice) in a more trusting and mutually respectful manner in a controlled coach-athlete relationship (e.g., "Come on, you can do it!") than in a relationship in which the coach generally does not trust the athlete and has doubts about his willingness to make the effort (e.g., "Finally pull yourself together!"). This is particularly problematic when the necessary communication of factual information is burdened by conflicts of interest between the actors.

Communication is symmetrical or complementary

This axiom also refers to the meaning of the relationship and status characteristics for communication. A basic distinction must be made between *symmetrical* and *complementary* communication. In a symmetrical communication both actors perceive themselves as like-minded, on the same level (status), with equal rights and equipped with the same information and resources (e.g., knowledge, skills, competences). A conversation between two coaches, team members, or friends would typically implicate symmetrical communication. Communication is complementary when there are clear differences in status between the actors. Here, for example, the coach talks to the athlete, the teacher to students, the team captain with a teammate, or the stadium security guard with a spectator. In particular, positions of leadership and power generate or demand complementary communication. In German, the transition from the "formal you" ("Sie") to the "informal you" ("du") can show a (desired) change of the communication basis. This example also makes clear that transition from formal to informal might be indicative of a transition from complementary to symmetrical communication between individuals.

Communication is always cause and effect

This axiom refers mainly to the typical case of uninterrupted communication between two actors, referring to what has been said before, between two actors, e.g., a dispute. This type of communication takes place in a circle, without beginning or end. Subjectively, each actor determines his or her own course of communication structure, which does not have to match the subjective reflection of the sequence of events of the other actor. It is therefore normal that, especially in problematic communication between two actors, subjectively different records of when the quarrel began and who provoked it exist. Although cause and effect can hardly be separated, everyone insists on their version of the events and their sequence, which usually worsens the problem instead of solving it. An example: Player A is known to be impulsive and easily irritable. Player B likes to provoke with his behavior and appearance. Both repeatedly get into heated debates and small fights, but nobody wants to give in. At the coach's request what their disagreements were actually about, A says: "B provoked me" and B claims: "A overreacted." Everyone subjectively interprets the communication that has taken place in their own favor only as a response (effect) to the other's behavior (cause).

Human communication makes use of analogical and digital modalities

In general, several available channels are used simultaneously for the transmission of information in human communication. Two types of modalities (analogical and digital) are used to encode a message for the receiver. The analogical part includes the chosen language, the used terms, and the choice of words. If both actors use the same verbalization and have the same vocabulary, there is nothing that prevents successful analogical communication. A problem arises, however, when both actors do not speak the same language. When that occurs, the message of the transmitter does not have an analogical equivalent in the receiver's language. This can cause by not only actual language and speech barriers but also by differences between the transmitter and the receiver in age, experience, and motivation. Digital modalities include all forms of information transmission by means of nonverbal communication. The spoken word and its meaning are always combined with nonverbal signals from the transmitter when there is face-to-face contact. In line with nonconceptually coded (digital) signals (e.g., facial expressions, voice coloring, volume, posture, and gestures), the transmitter encrypts subjective significance, emotions, and intention into the message being communicated the recipient. However, nonverbal signals can also be expressed unconsciously (i.e., out of the sender's intentional control). The abundance of possible emotions and subjective states as well as the very individual possibilities and competences to express them make it difficult to communicate clearly interpretable digital signals to the other person. Another problem is the incongruence of analog and digital signals. This is the case when what is being said is combined with ambiguous nonverbal signals or when it is not possible for the recipient to interpret both modalities appropriately. Thus, an athlete may reasonably doubt the coach's intent to reward him or her, if the coach makes the remark "You did a great job!" with an unimpressed voice and a grim look on his face.

The German psychologist and communication scientist Friedemann Schulz von Thun followed the axioms of communication but extended the dual view of the second axiom (content and relationship aspect) by a more differentiated consideration of the relationship aspect. He developed the "four-sides model" (Schulz von Thun, 2008), which describes the sending (with four mouths) and receiving (with four ears) of messages but also explains possible communication disturbances (◘ Fig. 18.5).

The "four-sides model" explicitly refers to the verbal-bound communication and points out that each spoken message can contain three additional messages to the recipient in addition to the actual factual content. The self-revelation contains personal details of the sender, which should convey something about him- or herself (e.g., current state of mind, status). The appeal encodes the sender's expectations of the recipient (i.e., what the recipient is to be induced to do by the statement). The relationship hint should convey to the recipient what the sender receives from the recipient (sympathy vs. antipathy) and in which relationship mode he or she sees him- or herself (e.g., friend vs. opponent).

All four messages can resonate with each message, even if the broadcaster deliberately highlights one side and/or the other. The square symbolizes that all four sides of a message are of equal importance. In any case, the message sender must be aware of the fact that the recipient can also hear and interpret the message with "four ears" (◘ Fig. 18.5). Whether and which side of the message particularly penetrates the recipient's consciousness depends above all on his or her subjective assessment of the situation (environment) and the person (sender), on his or her own experiences, competencies, and expectations, as well as on his or her current state of mind.

This model is well suited for the diagnosis of communication disturbances on the transmitter side, but also for tracing them back to an overly one-sided interpretation of messages by the receiver. Factual content, for example, can drift into the background if the recipient is, figuratively speaking, lying in wait with the "relationship ear" due to expectations and subjective assessment of the situation. An overestimation of self-development and relationship content of the message can result. Of course, the receiver's subsequent emotional feedback may also irritate the transmitter, because he or she actually only tried to give a factual instruction.

18

People who have known each other for a long time often think they know exactly what the other person means. In communication, however, **misunderstandings** or **disturbances** occur much more often than one might think and even among people who know each other very well. The German Sociologist Niklas Luhmann (1997) even assumes that communication is extremely susceptible to disruptions and that the unlikelihood of successful communication outweighs the probability of misunderstanding because the intentions of what is meant and what is understood are often not congruent. In order to recognize communication disturbances, to become clear about "hidden" bottlenecks and to uncover faulty communication patterns, it can be helpful—also proactive—to communicate on communication. This form is called metacommunication. It clarifies in which way a communication takes place.

Communication is not simply and exchange of information. Through evaluation and interpretation processes, it can lead to mutual social influence. Consequently, numerous research and application fields have used communication analyses to scientifically clarify aspects of the formation and change of attitudes and prejudices, the optimization of counselling interviews, and the conduct of discussions in groups (▶ Chap. 22).

The following section describes and analyses aspects of the coach-athlete communication in more detail.

18.4 Communication in Competitive Sports

The coach is of central importance for the athlete. He or she is responsible for the training and competition control and should lead his or her athletes to maximum performance and competition victories. With all his or her competences, experience and empathy, he or she has to influence the athlete in such a way that he or she is willing and able to exploit his or her performance potential in training and competition or to even exceed it. In competitive sports, the performance shown by the athlete is always evaluated as a product of this social interaction between coach and athlete. However, communication is the only way for the coach to influence the performance of his athlete. The successful work of the coach therefore depends to a large extent on the communication between him or her and his or her athlete (LaVoi, 2007; Yukelson, 2021). The conditions (context) in competitive sport, in which communication is possible, are very complex and challenging. For example, the following aggravating conditions for training should be mentioned:

- Frequency and long-term nature of training
- Inevitability and often contractual obligations of cooperation
- Age and gender differences between coach and athlete
- Double bond problems (e.g., a parent is also the coach)

The following sources of interference are often found in competition:

- Spectator volume
- Prohibition to speak
- Long distance (e.g., in a stadium)
- Lack of eye contact
- Danger of being overheard by the athletic opponent

Borggrefe and Cachay (2013, 2015, 2016) see the real challenge in **coach-athlete relationship** in successful communication. Based on their theoretical model of coach-athlete communication in top-class sport, they, above all, use qualitative methods (e.g., interviews, behavioral observation) to generate insights into communication requirements, problems and solution strategies in training and competition. Overall, they have been able to analyze empirical material from 26 coaches and 135 athletes from six different individual and team sports. They identified overarching requirements for coach-athlete communication, which are presented below.

18.4.1 Securing Understanding

Communication should not be seen by the coach as a simple transmission process where he or she just has to put desired information (message) into the athlete's head and expect the athlete to translate it into behavior. Rather, it must be a matter of functionally coordinating: (1) Information selection ("What do I want to tell the athlete?/What do I want to achieve with him or her?"), (2) communication behavior ("What is the best channel (verbal and/or nonverbal modality) through which I can best reach the athlete?"), and (3) understanding ("How can I ensure that the athlete has received the message consistently?").

The coach and the athlete must speak a **common language** in order for them to understand each other. In addition to language comprehension problems, which can arise from special features concerning age, gender, culture, and environment (e.g., when supervising foreign athletes), the use of technical language (e.g., technical, tactical terms) must be precisely agreed upon. The repertoire of sports- or team-specific hand signals, gestures, as well as signal and correction words for task-related communication is large and requires very precise coordination between the actors in order to avoid misinterpretations. Ultimately, it is the coach's responsibility to closely observe the follow-up communication and the behavior of his athlete (reflexive communication) in order to immediately notice any misunderstandings that occur and to avoid misinterpretations through a renewed and/or modified communication sequence.

18.4.2 Control Strategies

Even if the communication between coach and athlete is secured, another central problem is the control of the athlete's behavior. It is not automatically possible to count on the athlete's agreement with the message received from the coach. In other words, athletes can accept (identify with) control attempts by their coach, only comply (show compliance), or reject them (communicate "no"). The likelihood that the athlete will do what the coach appeals to increases by creating a communicative context that causes the athletes to meaningfully control themselves. That means the coach should be able to communicate in a way that it appears to the athlete as meaningful cooperation if he or she behaves accordingly. This control strategy has a greater effect if power, morality, sympathy, trust, or truth are included, which are currently important for the coach-athlete relationship and therefore make it easier for the athlete to orientate his or her own behavior toward the intention of the coach.

18.4.3 Conflict Regulation

Frequently, a conflict begins if a communication is followed by a communicated "no" as an answer. According to Messmer (2003), such a conflict can be divided into a conflict of facts, a conflict of relationships, and a conflict of power. All too often it is not understood that conflicts do not necessarily have to mean something negative per se but can also have a functional benefit in coach-athlete communication, for example, when creative solutions to the communicated problem arise from the joint resolution of the conflict. Once the form of conflict has been prioritized (power and relationship problems must be clarified before factual conflicts), the **principle of respectful communication** is considered necessary in conflict regulation, alongside **meta-communicative approaches**. This is based on the fact that both communicators, in their perception and mindfulness, communicate the view of the other (e.g., "I can understand your opinion, but …"). At the same time, it is important that the right to speak is distributed symmetrically and that both actors meet each other respectfully and politely (e.g., being able to listen, let them finish). Ultimately, the following applies to conflict parties not only to pursue enforcement intentions but also to always signal willingness to communicate and find solutions.

18.4.4 Moral Communication

Every message sent contains an appeal to the receiver (▶ Sect. 18.3). Appeals from coaches often remind their athletes of honor, attitude, courage, will, passion, effort, and so on, in order to influence their behavior, especially in critical situations. Basically, moral communication relates behavior to the norms and values specific to the social context (e.g., "one must never give up in competition"). Those who do not adhere run the risk of disappointing the moral expectations of not only the coach but their entire social environment. The danger here is that such moral expectations are often only polarized in "this is good/this is bad" schemes, which "outlaw" not just the behavior but the person as a whole where "ostracization" can follow failure or "glorification" in case of success. Above all, **moral expectation deceptions** and **blame assignments** by the coach quickly lead to emotionally charged states in the athlete (e.g., shame, anger). The well-intentioned moralizing communication by the coach can even lead to the opposite behavior (e.g., escalation of conflict, protest, aggression, withdrawal). This can happen, for example, through a too strong person-relatedness and emotionality in the athlete's reflection. It is, therefore, necessary to formulate criticism, blame, or even sanctions in coach-athlete communication in such a way that they are not interpreted by the athlete as a deliberate personal violation or discreditation.

18.4.5 Participation

Participation is the active and goal-oriented **inclusion** of the athlete in the coach-athlete communication. It is important on at least three accounts. Firstly, it should be emphasized that the athlete can only contribute to communication understanding if he or she is willing and able to provide the coach with feedback in his or her follow-up communication that can be interpreted meaningfully, so that the coach can see what effect his or her communication has had on the athlete. Secondly, the athlete's participation facilitates the coach's steering efforts if he or she succeeds in the communicative discourse in reading the athlete's opinion in the decision-making process (e.g., for certain strategic-tactical behavioral options) or at least gives the athlete the feeling that he or she is involved. Jointly agreed decisions create a deeper identification of the athlete with the subject matter. Thirdly, it can be assumed that a culture of participation encourages the athlete to contradict critically and to communicate problems that may not be apparent from the coach's point of view even in situations that are difficult and confusing for him or her and the coach (e.g., during a competition). In these cases, the coach may deviate from the intentions communicated beforehand and accepts changes in the athlete's behavior.

Also, in sports, the dialogue remains the most important form of communication. Based on the basic communication model (◘ Fig. 18.5), most authors distinguish between communication rules for the transmitter, the receiver, and a functional feedback. The most important recommendations are summarized below (Lau & Plessner, 2016).

18.4.6 Recommendations for the Transmitter

- **Openness:** Open yourself up and communicate what is going on inside of you.
  - Wrong: You have lost the game once again
  - Right: I am disappointed that it was not enough to win, but you gave everything.
- **"I"-Use:** Talk about your own thoughts and feelings. Use "I"-sentences instead of "you"-sentences.
  - Wrong: You screwed up big time again.
  - Right: I wish you would have tried harder.
- **Concreteness:** Address concrete situations or behavior and avoid generalizations (e.g., "always," "never") or judgmental insinuations (e.g., "typical of you," "You are incapable."). Separate your statements from your feelings and thoughts.
  - Wrong: You are simply incapable of implementing the tactic.
  - Right: I think it would have been better if you had acted tactically differently in this game situation.
- **Relevance of the topic:** Make sure to only communicate such contents that are relevant to the current topic and make it clearer to your partner what it is all about. Avoid unnecessary trivialities and embellishments.
  - Wrong: Maybe you got up on the wrong side of the bed or slept badly, and it's really none of my business, but…
  - Right: I have the impression that you were not concentrating during training today.
- **Authenticity:** Stay true to yourself by being truthful and credible, instead of pretending to be someone else or adapting to the opinion or attitude of the interlocutor.
  - Wrong: If you think it might have been A's fault, then it must be so.
  - Right: I think that you both—A and you—are not entirely innocent in this situation.

18

- **Congruence:** Support your statements with the same directed nonverbal signals. Body posture, facial expressions, and gestures should support your position clearly and recognizably for the interviewer.
  - Wrong: Coach praises A and looks at the ground.
  - Right: Coach praises A and looks friendly and openly into his or her eyes.

18.4.7 Recommendations for Recipients and Feedback Providers

- **Receptive listening**: Show your partner that you are listening to him or her and that you are interested in his or her statements by means of supporting gestures, eye contact, or consenting interjections. Encourage him or her to continue if he or she falters or signals uncertainty about whether to continue.
- **Summarizing**: If possible, describe the transmitter's main messages in your own words to show that you understand him or her. If you find this difficult, use the transmitter's choice of words. Word-for-word repetition helps you understand the transmitter and may reveal misunderstandings.
- **Asking openly**: To obtain a better understanding of the statements from the interlocutor, ask him or her open questions (e.g., "How did you feel about it?", "Was there a reason for it?"). A question will save you unnecessary or incorrect interpretations and will show the transmitter your interest in getting involved in the chosen topic.
- **Praising:** Praise the transmitter for open and understandable statements (e.g., "I now see where the problem lies because you addressed it so clearly and openly.").
- **Feedback on triggered feelings:** In conversations that trigger strong feelings of anger, insecurity, or joy, and when it is not possible for you to react to the speaker with understanding, you should avoid feedback on content for the time being. In such situations, it is better to directly reflect the feelings triggered by the message (e.g., "I am completely surprised…", "I am disappointed that…", "I'm happy with your offer and don't know what to say.").
- **Do not launch a counterattack:** If criticism is directed at you, you should react calmly and not immediately "push back" by defending or justifying your statement. In the case of serious accusations, you can also ask for time to consider and thus defuse emotionally charged situations and avoid escalations. You can take your time to put your thoughts in order and react afterward. Try to figure out the intention of the verbal attack as there mostly are comprehensible motives (e.g., fear, anger, frustration).
- **Positive and useful aspects first**: Every message contains useful and positive aspects which should be considered in the feedback first. In this way, you signal to the interlocutor that you acknowledge his or her efforts to establish a constructive dialogue.
- **Criticizing behavior:** Feedback should not be used to harm another person (e.g., insults, generalizations, general suspicion) but should only refer to the effects of their behavior.
- **Asking meaningful and open questions:** Instead of a hasty interpretation and inappropriate reaction, a meaningful question can be used as feedback to either gain clarity about what has been heard or to give the partner the opportunity to formulate his intended message more clearly by asking him to repeat his response.
- **Respecting the other person's point of view:** Everyone has their own values and attitudes. You should not judge others, because the individuality and self-determination of each person is a great asset of our culture. A conversation with a person who has a different point of view can be very enriching, as long as you respect the other opinion, don't immediately oppose it, and consciously consider it. Differences of opinion on minor issues are certainly more acceptable than on matters of principle. Here, argumentation must be possible and respected by both sides in order to reach a consensus. In doing so, you should always remain self-contained and not pretend to be someone else.
- **Do not lecture**: Avoid making lecturing comments. Try to find out what is behind the statements and which causes justify the behavior of the other person. Inspire your interlocutor to a consensus and not to confrontation and hostility. If you approach someone with a request, it is much more likely that they will meet you halfway if you express it in a friendly manner instead of backing them up with accusations or criticism.

In any case, a thorough preparation of important conversations is recommended to increase the probability of effective and successful communication. To expand your knowledge on the topic of communication it is worth taking a look at the following:

- Clampitt, P. G. (2016). *Communicating for managerial effectiveness* (sixth ed.). Sage Publications.
- Schulz von Thun, F. (2008). *Six tools for clear communication -The Hamburg approach in English language.* Schulz von Thun Institut.

Learning Control Questions

Basic:

1. How can the terms "interaction" and "communication" be defined and what are the differences between them?
2. How does human communication work and why are disturbances inevitable?

Advanced:

3. What are the four sides of a message according to Schulz von Thun (2008)?
4. What do the 3Cs of Jowett (2007) mean and what are they supposed to promote?

Experts:

5. Which rules apply to the transmitter and which to the recipient of a message if they want to successfully communicate with each other?

References

Alfermann, D. (2010). Trainer- und Trainerinnenverhalten [Coach behavior]. In O. Stoll, I. Pfeffer, & D. Alfermann (Eds.), *Lehrbuch Sportpsychologie [Text book sport psychology]* (pp. 149–172). Huber.

Bales, R. F. (1976). *Interaction process analysis. A model for the study of small groups*. University of Chicago Press.

Bierhoff, H.-W., & Jonas, E. (2011). Soziale Interaktion [Social interaction]. In D. Frey & H.-W. Bierhoff (Eds.), *Sozialpsychologie—Interaktion und Gruppe [Social psychology—Interaction and groups]* (pp. 131–159). Hogrefe.

Blumer, H. (1969). *Symbolic interactionism: Perspective and method*. Prentice-Hall.

Borggrefe, C., & Cachay, K. (2013). Communicative challenges of coaches in elite-level sports. System theoretical reflections on successful coaching strategies. *European Journal for Sport and Society, 10*(1), 7–29.

Borggrefe, C., & Cachay, K. (2015). *Kommunikation als Herausforderung [Communication as a challenge]*. Hofmann.

Borggrefe, C., & Cachay, K. (2016). 'You've got to go where it hurts'. Forms, functions and effects of moral communication in elite sport. *Sport in Society, 19*(7), 990–1019.

Chelladurai, P. (2007). Leadership in sports. In G. Tenenbaum & R. C. Eklund (Eds.), *Handbook of psychology* (3rd ed., pp. 113–135). Wiley.

Cook, K. S., & Rice, E. (2003). Social exchange theory. In J. Delamater (Ed.), *Handbook of social psychology* (pp. 53–76). Kluwer.

Dawes, R. M. (1980). Social dilemmas. *Annual Review of Psychology, 31*, 169–193.

Deutsch, M. (2011). A theory of co-operation and competition and beyond. In P. Van Lange, A. Kruglanski, & E. T. Higgins (Eds.), *Handbook of theories of social psychology* (Vol. 2, pp. 275–294). Sage Publications.

Green, G. B., & Uhl-Bien, M. (1995). Development of leader-member exchange (LMX) theory of leadership over 25 years: Applying a multi-level multi-domain perspective. *The Leadership Quarterly, 6*, 219–247.

Jowett, S. (2007). Interdependence analysis and the 3+1 Cs in the coach-athlete relationship. In S. Jowett & D. Lavallee (Eds.), *Social psychology in sport* (pp. 15–27). Human Kinetics.

Jowett, S., & Ntoumanis, N. (2004). The coach-athlete relationship questionnaire (CART-Q): Development and initial validation. *Scandinavian Journal of Medicine and Science in Sports, 14*, 245–257.

Jowett, S., & Poczwardowski, A. (2007). Understanding the coach-athlete relationship. In S. Jowett & D. Lavallee (Eds.), *Social psychology in sport* (pp. 3–14). Human Kinetics.

Kelley, H. H., & Thibaut, J. W. (1978). *Interpersonal relations: A theory of interdependence*. Wiley-Interscience.

Knight, C. J., Dorsch, T. E., Osai, K. V., Haderlie, K. L., & Sellars, P. A. (2016). Influences on parental involvement in youth sport. *Sport Exercise and Performance Psychology, 5*, 161–178.

Lau, A. (2005). *Die kollektive Leistung in den Sportspielen—Eine interdisziplinäre Analyse* [The collective performance in sports games—An interdisciplinary analysis] [Unpublished Habilitation thesis]. Martin-Luther-Universität Halle-Wittenberg.

Lau, A., & Plessner, H. (2016). *Sozialpsychologie und Sport. Ein Lehrbuch in 12 Lektionen [Social psychology and sport. A textbook in 12 lessons]*. Meyer & Meyer.

LaVoi, N. M. (2007). Interpersonal communication and conflict in the coach-athlete relationship. In S. Jowett & D. Lavallee (Eds.), *Social psychology in sport* (pp. 29–40). Human Kinetics.

Luhmann, N. (1997). *Die Gesellschaft der Gesellschaft [The society of the society]*. Suhrkamp.

Mead, G. H. (1934). *Mind, self and society. From the standpoint of a social behaviorist*. University of Chicago Press.

Messmer, H. (2003). *Der soziale Konflikt. Kommunikative Emergenz und systemtheoretische Reproduktion [Social conflict. Communicative emergence and systems-theoretical reproduction]*. Lucius & Lucius.

Mosler, H.-J., & Brucks, W. M. (2006). Kooperation und Wettbewerb in sozialen Dilemmas [cooperation and competition in social dilemmas]. In H.-W. Bierhoff & D. Frey (Eds.), Handbuch der Sozialpsychologie und Kommunikationspsychologie [*Handbook of social psychology and communication psychology*] (pp. 676–683). Hogrefe.

Pfeffer, I., & Gallitschke, M. (2008). Trainerinnen und Trainer im Frauenfußball aus Sicht der Athletinnen [Coaches in women's soccer from the point of view of the athletes]. *Zeitschrift für Sportpsychologie*, 15, 88–95.

Pfeffer, I., Würth, S., & Alfermann, D. (2004). Die subjektive Wahrnehmung der Trainer-Athlet-Interaktion in Individualsportarten und Mannschaftsspielen [Subjective perceptions of coach-athlete interaction in individual sports and team games]. *Zeitschrift für Sportpsychologie*, 11, 24–32.

Rapoport, A., & Chammah, A. M. (1965). *Prisoner's dilemma: A study in conflict and cooperation*. University of Michigan Press.

Rusbult, C. E. (1983). A longitudinal test of the investment models: The impact on job satisfaction, job commitment, and turnover of variations in rewards, costs, alternatives, and investments. *Journal of Applied Psychology, 68*, 429–438.

Schulz von Thun, F. (2008). *Six tools for clear communication -the Hamburg approach in English language*. Schulz von Thun Institut.

Traut-Mattausch, E., & Frey, D. (2006). Kommunikationsmodelle [models of communication]. In H.-W. Bierhoff & D. Frey (Eds.), *Handbuch der Sozialpsychologie und Kommunikationspsychologie [Handbook of social psychology and communication psychology]* (pp. 536–544). Hogrefe.

Treibel, A. (2000). *Einführung in soziologische Theorien der Gegenwart [Introduction to contemporary sociological theories*]. Leske + Budrich.

Walster, E., Berscheid, E., & Walster, G. W. (1973). New directions in equity research. *Journal of Personal and Social Psychology, 25*, 151–176.

Watzlawick, P., Bavelas, J. B., & Jackson, D. D. (1967). *Pragmatics of human communication: Study of interactional patterns, pathologies and paradoxes*. Norton.

Yukelson, D. P. (2021). Communicating effectively. In J. M. Williams & V. Krane (Eds.), *Applied sport psychology* (8th ed., pp. 139–156). McGraw Hill.

The Self in Sport and Exercise

Robert C. Eklund, Catherine M. Sabiston, and Ulrich Kühnen

Contents

J. Schüler et al. (eds.), *Sport and Exercise Psychology*, https://doi.org/10.1007/978-3-031-03921-8_19

Learning Objectives

After examining this chapter, readers should:

Basic:

- Have acquired knowledge on definitions and conceptual differences among constructs employed in sport and exercise psychology research such as self-concept, self-esteem, physical self-concept, and self-efficacy
- Be able to explain differences between unidimensional, multidimensional, and hierarchical conceptualizations of the self
- Be able to describe and differentiate self-conscious emotions and experiences in sport and exercise settings

Advanced:

- Understand the conceptual organization of self-constructs varying in stability across hierarchical models of the self
- Understand that individuals' sense of self develops in their cultural context and hence is informed and shaped by knowledge and beliefs specific to their culture
- Be able to provide examples of self-presentation in physical activity involvement and describe underlying processes implicated in their manifestation

Experts:

- Be able to identify and critique the differences between the skill development and self-enhancement hypotheses relative to the hierarchical model of self-concept
- Understand how cultural differences across individualist and collectivist societies tend to result in, respectively, independent and an interdependent self-construals and their consequences for self-related judgments in the domain of sport

19.1 Introduction

"No topic is more interesting to people than people. For most people, moreover, the most interesting person is the self" (Baumeister, 1999, p. 1). According to Baumeister (1999), there are three core functions of selfhood: First, there is reflexive consciousness—our ability to think about ourselves. Second, the self has an executive function. It allows us to become agents and make conscious choices for our actions. And finally, the self is a member of groups and relationships and enables people to relate to others, thus becoming interpersonal beings. All three functions are crucial and salient in sport and exercise contexts (Sabiston et al., 2019). Much of the research on the self has centered on developing an understanding of the content and structure of the self-system. Furthermore, the core interest in understanding the self is to examine whether sport and exercise participation enhances individuals' self-perceptions and/or whether different self-perceptions influence participation behaviors. In the current chapter, prevalent "self" constructs and conceptual perspectives studied in sport and exercise contexts are described under the headings of self-esteem and self-concept, self-presentation, and self-conscious emotions, with the final section of the chapter being focused on the self as a self-construal which varies as a function of the cultural context in which one has been developmentally situated.

Core Functions of Selfhood

The three core functions of selfhood include:

- Reflexive consciousness which provides the ability to think about ourselves
- Executive function which affords the agency to make conscious choices in our actions
- Interpersonal function which involves the ability to recognize the self as a member of groups and relationships enabling people to relate to others as interpersonal beings (Baumeister, 1999)

19.2 Self-Esteem and Self-Concept

Self-esteem has commonly been studied as the way an individual thinks about his or her own value or worth as a person (i.e., self-worth), whereas self-concept is broadly defined as an individual's self-description of what she or he believes to be true about the self based on his/her experiences and interpretations of their environment (Shavelson et al., 1976). In this way, the self-esteem construct takes into account how people *feel* about their sense of self, while the self-concept construct is more focused on how individuals *describe* themselves. Both constructs are inherently interrelated as a consequence and also very broad in nature. Self-esteem is regarded to be an individual's overall self-assessment or self-evaluation of the worthiness of one's overall self-description. The stability of these self-assessments has been a matter of interest from a self-determination theory perspective with true self-esteem (intrapsychic feelings of personal worth and autonomy) being regarded as featuring greater stability and contingent self-esteem being regarded as less stable and contingent on interpersonal outcomes and achievements (Deci & Ryan, 1995). Of interest to sport and exercise psychology, contingent self-esteem is grounded in the approval of others, social comparison, and/or the outcome of events (i.e., fluctuations in an individual's self-esteem resulting from success or failure). Specifically, an athlete may self-evaluate with high worth when accomplishing goals in sport engagement (e.g., scoring a goal in a critical game) and low worth when self-perceiving failure in sport engagement (e.g., having a bad soccer game).

Self-Esteem and Self-Concept

- *Self-concept* is the individual's self-description of what is believed to be true about the self, based on his/her experiences and interpretations of interactions with the environment.
- *Self-esteem* is a construct that is focused on an individual's overall self-assessment, or self-evaluation, of the worthiness of what is held to be true about the self.

Self-efficacy is another self-construct that is often confused with self-esteem and self-concept, but self-efficacy is a very narrow self-construct that is focused upon an individual's beliefs of his or her capabilities to organize and execute actions needed to produce specific outcomes at a given time in a given context (Bandura, 1997). In this way, self-efficacy is not a reflective of a holistic evaluative description of the self in any way. In this chapter, we focus on self-esteem and self-concept instead. For further reading in self-efficacy, please refer to ► Chap. 25.

19.2.1 Multidimensional and Hierarchical Self Structure

In a very general sense, self-perceptions can be defined as the way people think about themselves including reference to their traits, beliefs, roles, identities, and descriptions (Leary & Tangney, 2003). Self-perception fosters reflexive consciousness and thinking that is important for individuals' interpretations of their social, physical, and emotional circumstances and in the regulation of their behaviors. An individual's sense of self is also shaped in interactions with the world and others and involves processes such as self-comparison (e.g., comparing actions and behaviors with current personal standards or across time), social comparison (e.g., comparing actions and behaviors to those of significant or relevant others), and evaluations from significant others such as positive and negative feedback from peers, family, coaches, trainers, and teachers (Harter, 2012; Stets & Burke, 2003). These processes are theorized to lead to the development of a multidimensional self-concept, with the physical self-concept being an area of self-concept differentiation that tends to be integral to overall self-esteem.

Early models of the self were primarily unidimensional (e.g., one self-concept representing the entirety of the person's roles, responsibilities, beliefs, and feelings; see Fox, 1997); however, prominent work by self-concept theorists including Coopersmith (1967) and Fitts (1965) demonstrated that the self is multidimensional in nature (see ◘ Fig. 19.1). This multidimensional conceptualization of the self was comprised of a number of domain-specific self-concepts that have roots in areas such as work and employment (i.e., employment self), morality (i.e., moral self), social connections and relationships (i.e., social or relational self), education and pedagogy (i.e., academic self), and physical functioning and appearance (i.e., physical self). Nowadays, most researchers agree that the self is multidimensional (Hattie & Fletcher, 2005; Marsh & Craven, 2006). In sport and exercise psychology research, the physical self has been the prominent focus.

The physical self-concept can motivate, limit, or prevent sport and exercise behaviors and is also a factor impacting sport and exercise experiences while studied also as an outcome associated with sport and exercise behaviors (Fox, 1997). The physical self-concept is generally rooted in perceptions on what the body can do (i.e., perceived competencies in function and fitness) and

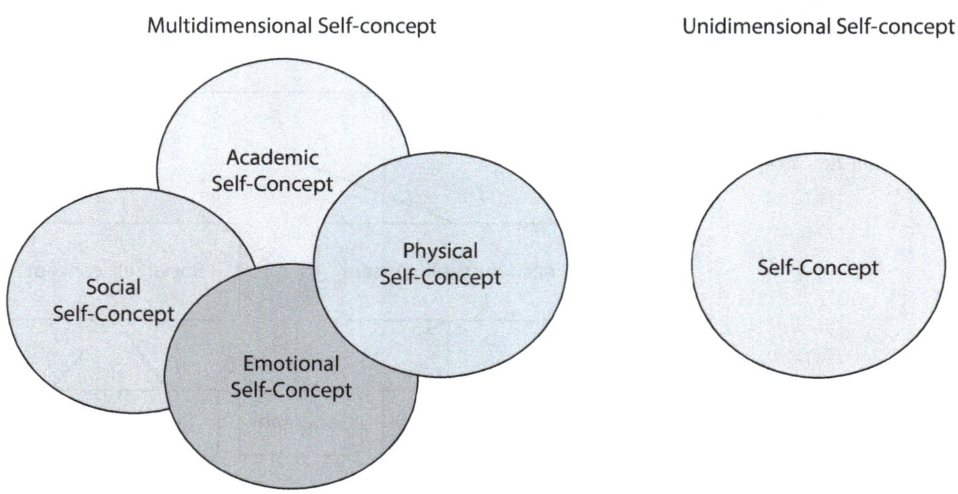

◘ **Fig. 19.1** Schematic representation of multidimensional vs. unidimensional conceptualizations of self-concept

what the body looks like (i.e., appearance and weight competency perceptions). Intuitively, sport and exercise participation may offer greater opportunities for changes in the physical self-perceptions tied to functional perceptions compared to appearance and weight perceptions. Also, physical self-perceptions specific to strength and endurance (i.e., functional self-perceptions) may protect from detrimental physical self-perceptions of appearance and weight (Vani et al., 2021). Specifically, all physical self-perceptions intersect and interact in a complex way that requires more research attention.

The multi-dimensionality of the self has long been argued to have a hierarchical structure (Sonstroem, 1976). Global self-esteem/self-concept has been conceptualized as the apex construct of the self-perception hierarchy (see ◘ Fig. 19.2) that is situated over multiple domain-specific self-concepts (e.g., social, academic, physical). Each of these domain-specific self-concepts are then defined by subdomain competency self-perceptions. Of most relevance to sport and exercise psychology, the physical self-concept is defined by general competency self-perceptions that are broadly related to what the body can do (e.g., sport competence, endurance, strength) and what the body looks like (e.g., body fat, appearance). These physical self-perceptions are considered subdomain levels, which are further differentiated and specified into facet level competencies (e.g., sport competence in basketball) and sub-facet level competencies relating to specific self-perceptions of skills (e.g., a layup or free throw).

Even though self-concept as a hierarchical organization of self-beliefs makes intuitive sense, it is not a conceptualization that has achieved full consensus (Hattie & Fletcher, 2005; Kowalski et al., 2003). Researchers arguing for a hierarchical structure have suggested that global self-constructs (i.e., those residing at the top of the model such as self-esteem) are more stable (or trait-like) than self-constructs further down in the hierarchy. One can reasonably expect that situational constructs, such as perceptions of basketball layup skill at any given contextual moment (i.e., skill specific self-efficacy) would be subsumed under, and less stable than, broader sport competence self-perceptions such as one's overall capability as a basketball player (Shavelson et al., 1976).

Sport scientists have considered bottom-up and top-down alternatives to causal flow across these general hierarchical perspectives of the self. A bottom-up causal flow example might be engagement in training behaviors (e.g., throwing and catching a baseball) that causally enhances self-efficacies related to the specific skill being trained (e.g., "I can confidently throw and catch a baseball in game situations") which might enhance more general sport competence self-perceptions (e.g., "I am good in sport"), physical self-worth perceptions (e.g., "I am physically good"), and ultimately global self-esteem (e.g., "I am a good person"). A top-down causal flow, which is essentially the flip of the bottom-up effects, would involve global self-worth perceptions having self-consistency effects on, in turn, physical self-worth perceptions and perceptions of physical competencies that results in specific beliefs about behavioral capabilities and behaviors themselves that are consistent with the individual's global sense of self overtime. Horizontal effects are also possible across time wherein specific self-perceptions and self-concepts are most affected by previous levels on those same self-perceptions at the same level of the hierarchy. For example, baseball throwing continues to enhance baseball throwing distance and speed over time but may also transfer to Frisbee throwing or basketball passing—ultimately enhancing these self-perceptions.

19

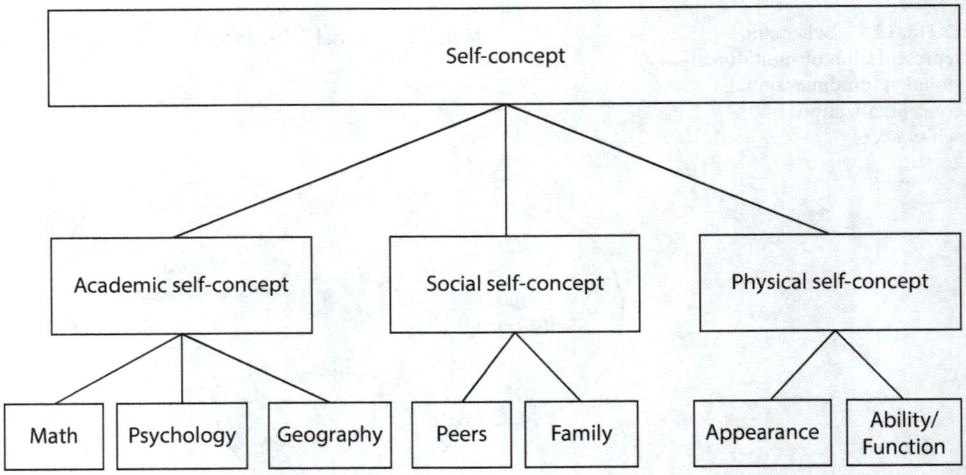

◘ **Fig. 19.2** The hierarchical model of self-concept. Adapted from: Shavelson, R., Hubner, J., & Stanton, G. (1976). Self-concept: Validation of construct interpretations. *Review of Educational Research*, *46*, 407–441

19.2.2 Linking Sport and Exercise Participation and Self-Esteem

The bottom-up and top-down approaches offer frameworks for understanding the association between sport and exercise participation and constructs related to the self.

Sport and exercise, physical self-perceptions, and self-esteem: The skill development hypothesis. The exercise and self-esteem model (EXSEM; Sonstroem & Morgan, 1989) is an example of a bottom-up approach whereby sport and exercise participation is proposed to influence global self-esteem by affecting contextual aspects of the self (see ◘ Fig. 19.3). Within the EXSEM, sport and exercise behavior is proposed to change physical outcomes (e.g., muscular strength, aerobic conditioning), which then enhances related perceptions of physical self-efficacy, and self-perceptions on physical competence (e.g., competences in sport, physical conditioning, strength, and physical appearance as postulated by Fox, 1997). Increases in these self-perceptions (i.e., the specific efficacies involved and the more general beliefs about physical competencies) are then expected to result in a sense of greater physical self-worth and ultimately a greater sense of self-esteem (Sonstroem, 1997; Sonstroem et al., 1994). Of importance to understanding the EXSEM tenets, self-efficacy relates to judgments of particular skills, or abilities, in a specific situation (e.g., successfully making a free-throw shot in basketball in the particular moment) whereas perceptions of competence are more general judgments (e.g., perception that one has, overall, good basketball skills). Physical competence perceptions are directly related to physical self-concept and self-esteem but are also proposed to have an effect through physical acceptance (i.e., the extent to which an individual accepts his/her physical strengths and weaknesses or satisfaction). In this way, physical competence and physical self-acceptance are both amenable to change through sport and exercise and both alter global sense of self.

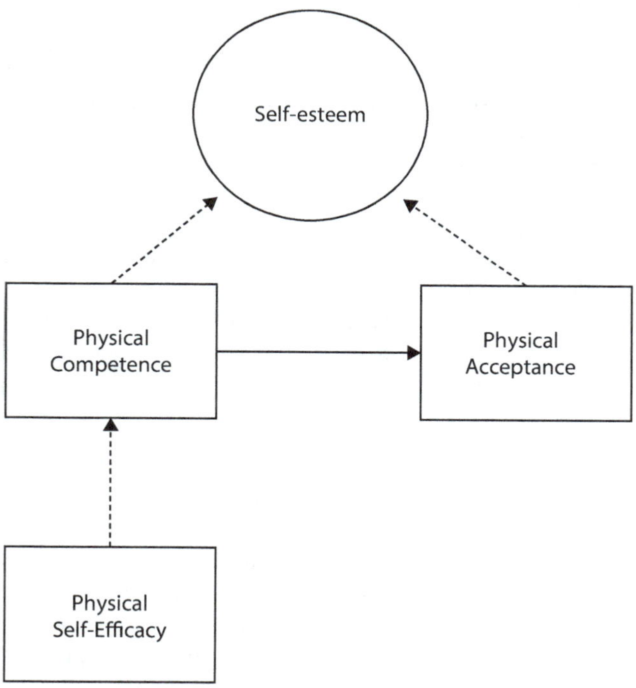

◘ **Fig. 19.3** Depiction of the general relationships in the exercise and self-esteem model (EXSEM; Sonstroem & Morgan, 1989)

Support for the general tenets of the EXSEM has been demonstrated in samples ranging from children and adolescents to older adults (e.g., Barber et al., 2001; Elavsky, 2010; Elavsky & McAuley, 2007; Findlay & Bowker, 2009; Fredricks & Eccles, 2006; Slutzky & Simpkins, 2009; Welk & Eklund, 2005). Overall, there is general support for the bottom-up perspective that is characteristic of the EXSEM. Engagement in sport and exercise has been shown to effect change in participants' contextual self-perceptions, which in turn result in changes at the higher levels of the self-perceptual system. In investigations directly testing EXSEM contentions, the observed effects of sport and exercise participation on self-esteem have been consistently in the small to moderate. Interestingly enough, there is some evidence that self-efficacy and changes in sport and exercise outcomes (e.g., fitness) co-occur temporally rather than sequentially or hierarchically (Babic et al., 2014; Dishman et al., 2006; McAuley et al., 2000, 2005). Finally, the role of the physical acceptance construct in understanding the EXSEM relationships is underdeveloped. Researchers are encouraged to focus on establishing support for the hierarchical bottom-up links specified in the EXSEM.

Self-perceptions to sport and exercise participation: The self-enhancement hypothesis. The top-down effect suggests that more global aspects of the self (i.e., at the apex of the self-hierarchy) influence more specific self-perceptions that then, in turn, influence behavioral engagement and participation in sport and exercise. Drawing on a top-down model perspective, individuals are highly motivated to engage in tasks and behaviors in which they can demonstrate their abilities and in which they feel capable of achievement (e.g., Harter, 2012). For example, a person who reports high self-esteem and high perceptions of competence in the sport domain would be likely to seek out opportunities, and likely more challenging ones, for participation in such activities. It is a hypothesis that makes a great deal of sense, but most of the supporting evidence has been cross-sectional which precludes an understanding of the direction of causal effects (Babic et al., 2014; Bauman et al., 2012). Some more convincing descriptive longitudinal support exists too (e.g., Lemoyne et al., 2015; Lindwall et al., 2014), but it is fair to wonder about how strong the supporting evidence might be (see ► Study Box: How Strong is the Support for the Self-Enhancement Hypothesis?).

How Strong is the Support for the Self-Enhancement Hypothesis?

Lindwall et al. (2014) found some support for the self-enhancement hypothesis in supplementary longitudinal growth curve analyses of data obtained at three time points, each separated by a year, from 705 Canadian female students from Saskatoon Saskatchewan starting in Grade 9 (aged 14–15 years) and continuing for 2 successive years. They obtained data on global self-esteem, physical self-perceptions physical activity using questionnaires:

- **Global self-esteem/worth** was assessed using a five-item self-report questionnaire recommended for use with adolescents (Harter, 1988). Participants are first asked to decide which kind of teenagers he or she is most like, those on the left or those on the right in each statement ("Often unhappy/happy with self" "Like/don't like the way they're leading their lives"). Then they decide whether the description on the side he/she chose is "Really True for Me" or "Sort of True for Me."
- **The physical self-perceptions profile** (Fox & Corbin, 1989) consists of five sub-scales representing the perceptions of physical self-worth, sport (sport competence), body (body attractiveness), condition (physical conditioning and exercise), and strength (physical strength and muscular development).As in Harter's (1988) questionnaire, the items consist of a matched pair of statements (e.g., "Some people feel that they are not very good when it comes to sports" vs. "Others feel that they are really good at just about every sport"). Respondents indicate which description is more like them and whether the selected description is "Really True for Me" or "Sort of True for Me."
- The physical activity questionnaire for adolescents (PAQ-A; Kowalski et al., 1997) is an 8-item self-report assessing 7-day participation in various types of physical activity including activity during physical education, lunch break, after school, during evenings, and weekends (5-point scale, with "1" indicating low and "5" a high level of PA).

Their secondary exploration of associations of change in self-esteem, the various physical self-perceptions, and self-reported physical activity provided evidence consistent with the self-enhancement hypothesis. They observed that girls higher in self-esteem were more likely to engage in physical activity but observed no skill development hypothesis evidence indicating greater participation in physical activity enhanced girls' self-esteem.

Similarly, Lemoyne et al. (2015) recruited a sample of 418 Canadian college students to examine reciprocal relationships across two time points separated by 3 months between multiple types of physical activity (exercise, sport participation, and weight training measured with questions from the Kohl et al., 1988, aerobic longitudinal cooper study questionnaire) and a French translation of Fox and Corbin's physical self-perception measures of endurance, sport competence, strength, and bodily attractiveness (Ninot et al., 2001). Consistent with the self-enhancement hypothesis, higher perceptions of competence in a given dimension (e.g., sports competence) were associated with higher participation in that corresponding physical activity behavior (e.g., playing sports) with weaker associations were observed across domains (e.g., between perceived sports competence and the behavior of lifting weights). So, in short, tantalizing bits of evidence are available supporting this hypothesis but, overall, the evidentiary base is weak and limited.

19.2.3 In Summary

There is longitudinal evidence, albeit limited and somewhat more ambiguous, to support for both top-down and bottom-up causal influence. Elavsky (2010), for example, tested the competing models with a sample of middle-aged women and exercise engagement and found support for both directional effects. Wagnsson et al. (2014) also found support for both the skill development and self-enhancement models in a sample of school-aged children. Overall, the evidence paints an ambiguous picture, so more research is needed to test competing approaches using longitudinal and experimental designs in individuals across the lifespan to advance understanding in the area. It is, nonetheless, evident that an individual's sense of self shapes, and is shaped by, involvement in sport and exercise activity as described earlier in this section.

Although our self-perceptions and sense of self inform our behavioral engagements, it is also true that our behavioral enactments and engagements serve to communicate *to others* who we are and what we are like. These self-presentational processes play an important role in interaction in life broadly, so it should not be surprising that self-presentational aspects of engagements in sport and exercise settings, as discussed in the coming section, are also implicated in the social and personal definition and construction of the self.

19.3 Self-Presentation

Self-presentation was originally defined by Baumeister (1982) as "the use of behavior to communicate some information about oneself to others" (p. 3). Leary and Kowalski (1990) extended the definition and described self-presentation as the "process by which individuals attempt to control the impressions others form of them" (p. 34). In this way, self-presentation generally involves selectively presenting one's characteristics to create the desired impression and also selectively omitting characteristics to avoid creating an undesired impression (Leary, 1992; Schlenker & Leary, 1982). Self-presentation is a deliberate, goal-directed process whereby individuals engage in to convey desired images in order to influence how others perceive and treat them (Leary & Kowalski, 1990; Schlenker & Leary, 1982). Although this description includes the possibility of deceptive self-presentations, evidence indicates that most self-presentations are almost exclusively and narrowly confined to what individuals believe to be true about themselves. People do tend to want to be perceived in the best light possible—but relative to who they actually perceive themselves to be. The self-presentational costs of going beyond what is perceived to be true (i.e., making false presentations of the self) are understood to be nontrivial by most individuals.

It is fair to say that self-presentation permeates human behavior, and engagements in sport, exercise, and recreational physical activity are not exempt from that generalization (Leary, 1992). Individuals across the lifespan are motivated to participate in sport, exercise, and physical activity for self-presentational reasons (Conroy et al., 2000; Howle et al., 2015; Leary, 1992) and to employ self-presentational strategies in those engagements (Conroy et al., 2000; Crawford & Eklund, 1994; Eklund & Crawford, 1994)—while also accruing self-presentational benefits (or suffering self-presentational detriments) in the process (Howle & Eklund, 2013; Martin Ginis, Latimer, & Jung, 2003; Renfrew et al., 2017). The importance of self-presentation in shaping physical activity involvement and outcomes is widely acknowledged in sport and exercise psychology (Dimmock et al., 2020; Eklund & Howle, 2017; Hausenblas et al., 2004; Howle et al., 2015; Martin Ginis et al., 2007; Martin Ginis & Mack, 2012).

Side Story

What Do You Remember Most About Junior High School Physical Education?

What do you remember most about Junior High School physical education? Some remember it as a joyous experience involving an amalgam of opportunities relating to the development of knowledge, the display of physical capabilities, and energetic motoric engagement in sport, exercise, or physical activity with peers at the same grade level. Others' memories are focused differently, and sometimes not because of a dislike of the material covered in physical education but instead because of the obligatory trials of the locker room (Eklund & Bianco, 2000). Adolescence is an incredibly complex developmental phase of life that involves biological maturation, including readily observable changes in physicality as well as the less visible cognitive and psychosocial developments. New social roles and responsibilities are adopted, often in social contexts novel to prior experience, that are coupled with urges to start test old boundaries of independence. Entry into a world of seeking approval and acceptance from new relationship partners is underway, and it is one where peer comparison and peer evaluation have become very influential sources of information about the nature and worthiness of the self. The locker room can present particularly daunting self-presentational trials as a consequence, with the memories of physical education for some being dominated by the self-presentational perils of the mandatory changes of attire into gym clothing and/or the shower room afterward. Or sometimes those memories are dominated by encounters with teachers or coaches who regarded the young person's struggles to maintain a sense of dignity in physical self-presentation as displays of defiance or insolence instead of self-protective reluctance. Those memories of physical education can boil down to regularly scheduled encounters with being caught between a rock (disciplinary action) and a hard place (the perceived self-presentational tyranny of the locker room). What experiences do you remember most about junior high school physical education? Are they positive, negative, or some mix of both? And to what extent did self-presentational processes shape your recollection of those experiences?

Unfortunately, Tetlock and Manstead's (1985) complaint about the absence of formally defined theory of self-presentation (also known as impression management) remains as salient for researchers today as it was more than three decades ago. Sport and exercise psychology researchers have forged ahead in conducting interesting and useful self-presentational research anyway by relying upon various conceptual models and frameworks to organize and categorize self-presentational processes of interest. Leary and Kowalski's (1990) two-component model of impression management is probably the most widely referenced model in sport and exercise psychology but Howle et al.'s (2015a) recent 2 × 2 model of self-presentational motives in physical activity in particular is progressively garnering more attention. These models are addressed subsequently.

Leary and Kowalski's (1990) two component model is focused upon two types of self-presentation processes (i.e., impression motivation, impression construction). The *impression motivation* component of the model is focused upon the extent to which individuals experience an interest in managing others' impressions about them within a particular social encounter (see ► Key Points: Factors Giving Rise to Impression Motivation). Individuals tend to experience heightened impression motivation in a situation when they perceive that others' impressions of them in that situation have implications for their goals in terms of material or social outcomes, self-esteem maintenance, and/or identity development. *Impression construction* processes relate to the choices and strategies implicated in the crafting of desired images and/or in avoiding undesired images (see ► Key Points: Factors Determining Content and Actions Taken in the Impression Construction Process). The distinction between impression motivation and impression construction is important because the former deals with the motivation behind making an impression while the latter deals with the content and extent to which actions are taken to make that impression. If someone is motivated to manage the impressions formed by others, Leary and Kowalski posit that his/her choices about desired impressions and how to pursue their creation (i.e., impression construction) are determined by five factors (i.e., the self-presenter's self-concept, desired and undesired identity images, present role-related norms and standards of behavior, values of the self-presentational target, and the individual's current and potential social image).

Factors Giving Rise to *Impression Motivation*

From Leary and Kowalski's (1990) perspective, impression motivation is elevated when self-presenters:

- Believe that how they are perceived by others in the situation has goal-relevant implications in terms of material or social outcomes, maintenance of self-esteem, and/or identity development
- Place a high value on the goal
- Perceive that a discrepancy exists between their desired image and the image that others in the situation currently hold of them

Factors Determining Content and Actions Taken in the *Impression Construction* Process

When someone is motivated to manage the impressions formed by others, Leary and Kowalski (1990) posit that his/her choices about desired impressions and how to pursue their creation (i.e., impression construction) are determined by five factors including:

- The self-presenter's self-concept
- The self-presenter's desired and undesired identity images
- Present role-related norms and standards of behavior
- The values of the self-presentational target
- The self-presenter's beliefs about his/her current and potential social image (◘ Fig. 19.4)

It has been argued for several decades that self-presentational imperatives can be implicated in individuals' engagement sport and exercise activity (e.g., Conroy et al., 2000; Crawford & Eklund, 1994; Eklund & Crawford, 1994; Leary, 1992; Martin Ginis et al., 2007; Sadalla et al., 1988), and Leary and Kowalski's

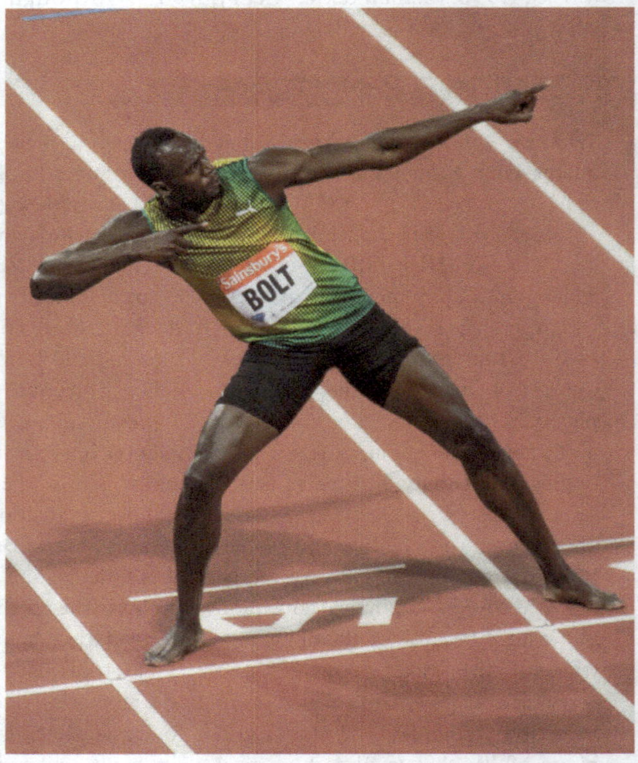

◘ **Fig. 19.4** Check the factors giving rise to Impression Motivation (see ► Key Points). Do they apply to Usain Bolt?

(1990) two component model has provided a useful conceptual framework for interpretation of extant findings and the advancement of research in the area. Sadalla et al. (1988), for example, had previously observed commonly held stereotypes among American university students about personality characteristics and social identities of participants in different sport activities (i.e., bowling, skiing, golf, tennis, motocross). They argued, albeit without supporting data, that the self-presentational implications emanating from the students' awareness of sport stereotypes likely served to shape the impression motivation preferences in sport and physical activity relative to the pursuit of the desired social identities as well as the avoidance of undesired social identities. Evidence has been subsequently presented of positive associations between college students' impression motivation and self-reported number of days per week of exercise as well as their impression construction and the percentage of time spent exercising (Conroy et al., 2000). In contrast, Gammage et al. (2004) found that low-frequency exercisers (i.e., exercised once or twice per week) and high-frequency exercisers (i.e., exercised three or more times per week) did not differ significantly on their reported levels of impression motivation. They did not, however, examine impression construction in their study which may indicate the importance of studying both impression motivation and impression construction to understand the influence of self-presentational processes in physical activity settings.

Indications of why the consideration of both impression motivation and impression construction is available across studies. In the Conroy et al. (2000) study, negative associations were observed in simple correlations between physical self-presentation confidence and the impression motivation and impression construction constructs. In the Gammage et al. (2004) study, low-frequency and high-frequency exercisers did not differ significantly on their reported levels of impression motivation, but high-frequency exercisers reported stronger perceptions in their ability to convey the desired impression and placed more importance on portraying the desired impression than females who exercise less frequently. Woodgate et al.'s (2003) examination of self-presentation efficacy (or confidence) as a moderator of the relationship between social physique anxiety (a construct with motivating/demotivating self-presentational properties) and physical activity behavior was revealing on that account. Specifically, women high in self-presentation efficacy and low social physique anxiety (to be discussed further in the next section) were more likely to exercise than women who were low in both social physique anxiety and self-presentation efficacy. Based on these findings, it may be individuals' levels of self-presentational efficacy or confidence that determines the extent of physical activity engagement or avoidance while also potentially serving to moderate the relationship between self-presentation processes and physical activity behavior. Despite the intriguing possibilities offered by the two-component model, the extent to which to measures developed for sport and exercise settings (i.e., Conroy et al., 2000; Payne et al., 2013) assessed impression motivation beyond an interest in being positively perceived by others (e.g., the avoidance of undesired perceptions—which, incidentally, is not the same as lacking interest in being positively perceived) was limited.

Howle et al.'s (2015) recent introduction of the 2 × 2 framework of self-presentation motives in physical activity contexts, as well as an associated measurement tool (Howle et al., 2015b), has addressed some limitations of understanding self-presentation processes. Their 2 × 2 framework was a result of configural integration of two well-established and well-supported conceptual distinctions (i.e., approach/avoidance, Elliot, 2008; agency/communion, Bakan, 1966) evident in extant motivational theory. Acquisitive (or approach-oriented) motives have to do with individual orientations toward positive outcomes (i.e., gains in social approval), whereas avoidance-oriented (or protective) motives have to do with individual orientations away from negative outcomes (i.e., losses in social approval). Agentic motives have to do with a focus on task achievement and individual competency whereas communal motives have to do with a focus on interpersonal connections and relationships.

As depicted in ◘ Fig. 19.5, integration of these motives from a self-presentational perspective resulted in the 2 × 2 framework of *acquisitive-agentic*, *acquisitive-communal*, *protective-agentic*, and *protective-communal* self-presentation motives (also see Definition Box).

Self-presentation Motives in Physical Activity in Howle et al.'s (2015a) *2 × 2 Framework include:*

1. *Acquisitive-agentic motive* which relates to the desire to gain social approval from others in terms of their perceptions of one's physical qualities and task ability
2. *Acquisitive-communal motive* which relates to the desire to gain social approval from others in terms of their perceptions of one's interpersonal qualities
3. *Protective-agentic motive* which relates to the desire to avoid social disapproval (or losses of social approval) from others in terms of their perceptions of one's physical qualities and task ability
4. *Protective-communal motive* which relates to the desire to avoid social disapproval (or losses of social approval) from others in terms of their perceptions of one's interpersonal qualities

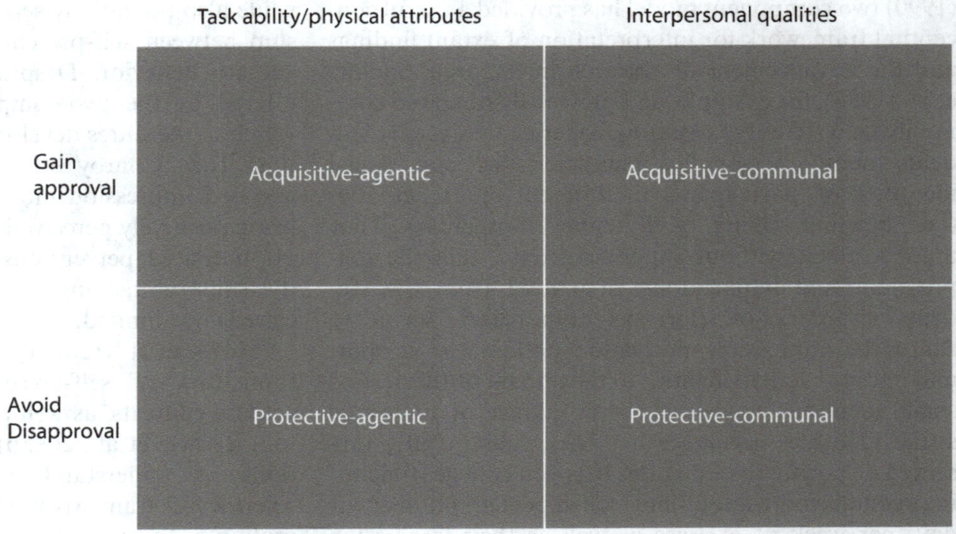

Fig. 19.5 2 × 2 Self-presentation motive framework. Note: vertical axis represents the approach (acquisitive) and avoidance (protective) dimension and the horizontal axis represents the agentic and communal dimension. From: Eklund, R. C., & Howle, T. (2017). Self-presentation and communication in physical activity settings. In B. Jackson & J. Dimmock (Eds.), *Communication and Persuasion in Sport, Exercise, and Physical Activity* (pp. 250–265). Milton Park, UK: Routledge/Psychology Press

Consistent with their respective theoretical underpinnings, Howle et al. (2015a) posited that acquisitive motives would energize engagement within physical activity tasks (i.e., acquisitive agency) and an affiliative approach to interpersonal interactions (i.e., acquisitive communion) while protective motives would result in a more reluctant style of participation or even task withdrawal (i.e., protective agency) and more hesitant interpersonal interaction (i.e., protective communion). Communal motives were thought to have particular potential relevance for understanding interpersonal processes in physical activity settings.

Evidence has also started to accumulate from research grounded in the 2 × 2 model that supports the theorizing by Howle et al. (2015). In a sport setting, Australian undergraduate students' scores on the acquisitive communal self-presentation motive were positively predictive of the favorability of teammate communal evaluations, while protective communal motives and those communal evaluations were negatively associated (Howle et al., 2016). Moreover, acquisitive agentic motive scores were positively related to the coding of task behavior during the game. Howle et al. (2016) found indirect positive effects (via personal task goals) on Australian undergraduate students' persistence on a wall-sit task from their scores on the acquisitive-agentic motive but negative indirect effects from scores on the protective agentic motive. Verma et al. (2019) reported a positive indirect effect (via physical activity identity) from acquisitive agency to physical education class engagement but a negative indirect effect from protective agency.

These previous sections have focused on the way individuals think about and describe themselves as well as communicate information about the self to others. Perceptions and cognitions are important to understanding the self-system. Emotional or affective perspectives are also key to advancing understanding on the way the self-system is associated with experiences and behaviors in sport and exercise.

19.4 Self-Conscious Emotions

Self-conscious emotions involve a self-evaluative process, wherein individuals' emotions are impacted through their thought processes and evaluations of themselves. Self-reflective processes are also vital to the experience of self-conscious emotions (Tangney & Tracy, 2012). Furthermore, the self-conscious emotions can be distinguished by state levels as well as the proneness to experience them. State level refers to an emotion felt in response to a specific event or behavior. For example, an individual who regrets skipping a workout might experience state guilt. In comparison, proneness is an emotional disposition which refers to the likelihood that an individual will experience the emotion. For example, people can vary in the extent to which they are prone to regretting their behavioral choices and hence be prone to the experience of guilt relative to those choices.

19.4.1 Emotions Specific to the Physical Self

Each self-conscious emotion can shape individuals' experiences within sport and exercise, and equally these body-related emotions can be influenced by such behaviors. Specific to body image emotions, the majority of empirical investigations have focused on body-related shame (Castonguay et al., 2014; Pila et al., 2016; Sabiston et al., 2010) and guilt (Calogero & Pina, 2011;

Pila et al., 2016; Sabiston et al., 2010). There is also early evidence indicating the importance of understanding the role of body-related envy (Pila et al., 2014) and body-related embarrassment (Vani et al., 2021) in sport and exercise settings. Body-related pride, the only positively appraised self-conscious emotion, has been explored as an important emotion linked to sport and exercise experiences (Castonguay et al., 2013; Gilchrist & Sabiston, 2018; Mack et al., 2015). Furthermore, social physique anxiety has been studied extensively as a common emotion in the sport and exercise context (Sabiston et al., 2014). While not empirically studied under the umbrella of a self-conscious emotion, social physique anxiety shares common features of self-conscious emotions and is presented here to best understand the main body-related emotions tied to the physical self. See ◘ Fig. 19.6 for a broad depiction of the variety of self-conscious emotions specific to both appearance (i.e., how the body looks) and function (i.e., how the body performs).

Social Physique Anxiety Social physique anxiety is a widely studied, negatively valenced emotion, defined as the anxiety a person experiences as a result of perceived or actual judgments of his or her physical being by others (Hart et al., 1989). Rooted in social anxiety, self-presentation, and physical self-related literature, social physique anxiety is often experienced in social settings that highlight the physique and ability of individuals (Crombie et al., 2011; Sabiston et al., 2014). Given these features, it is not surprising that social physique anxiety is frequently experienced in sport and exercise contexts. This emotion is not often studied under the umbrella of self-conscious emotions, yet the social evaluative, judgment-based, and self-reflective nature of the emotion suggests there is an underlying self-consciousness to the experience of social physique anxiety.

A number of negative outcomes have been linked to experiences of social physique anxiety, including reduced perceptions of competence and enjoyment, symptoms of disordered eating, depression and competitive anxiety, and behavioral avoidance (see Sabiston et al., 2014). Specific to avoidance, individuals who experience social physique anxiety tend to avoid scenarios where their physical body may be on display, such as in sport or exercise contexts (Kowalski et al., 2006). Repeated experiences of social physique anxiety are negatively associated with physical activity in adolescence and adulthood (Sabiston et al., 2014). Therefore, one of the critical outcomes of social physique anxiety is a reduction in sport and exercise participation.

Interpersonal factors are linked to social physique anxiety. Youth who felt accepted and like they belonged in their peer group experienced lower social physique anxiety in physical education class (Cox et al., 2013). However, mothers of adolescents (Sabiston et al., 2007) and teachers and coaches that emphasize appearance (Krane et al., 2001) trigger social physique anxiety. Furthermore, older adolescents and young adults report experiencing greater social physique anxiety around peers compared to parents (Brunet & Sabiston, 2011). From an environmental perspective, social physique anxiety is heightened when individuals exercise in front of a mirror or when they view videos that display physique salient instructors (Martin Ginis et al., 2008; Martin Ginis, Jung, & Gauvin, 2003). Further examples include a desire to become more muscular (Brunet et al., 2010), changing in front of others in locker rooms (Ladwig et al., 2018), and wearing mandatory uniforms in physical education classes (Sabiston et al., 2007) that also elicit greater social physique anxiety. Although specific aspects of sport and exercise may increase social physique anxiety, there is some evidence to show that engaging in sport and exercise may reduce this emotion. For example, Gammage et al. (2016) found that engagement in one resistance exercise class or yoga class can reduce state social physique anxiety, with yoga having a larger effect on this affective state.

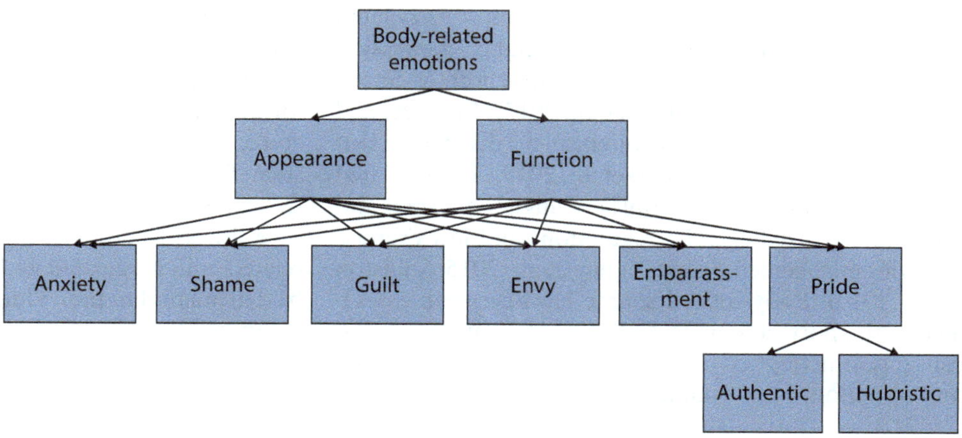

◘ **Fig. 19.6** Schematic representation of body-related self-conscious emotions relative to self-perceptions of appearance and function

As a general summary, social physique anxiety is an emotion that both promotes and prevents sport and exercise behavior across the lifespan. It is a negatively valenced emotion that has some commonalities with experiences of shame and embarrassment emotions.

Body-Related Shame Shame is an emotion individuals' feel when their sense of self includes a self-perceived fundamental flaw; often one believed to be visible to others. Individuals who experience shame often feel worthless and desire to hide and be unseen; they perceive or fear a loss of social status while failing to meet internal standards for oneself (Lewis, 2008). Shame is a strong negative and painful emotion that can often arise as a result of self-perceptions pertinent to body image.

Body-related shame results from causal attributions to the self that are controllable and stable and lead to many poor cognitive and behavioral outcomes (Tracy & Robins, 2004; also consider the commentary in ▶ Chap. 7 on causal attributions). In early work testing these attributions with body-related emotions, Crocker et al. (2014) reported that body-related shame was predicted by controllability and globality attributions, but not stability. Other common predictors of body-related shame are proposed to be similar to those outlined for social physique anxiety (e.g., environmental considerations that heighten awareness on the body, such as mirrors, social comparisons, and evaluative contexts; as well as social factors such as the presence of others who may judge one's appearance and function). Furthermore, physical self-discrepancies (Brunet et al., 2012; Morin et al., 2015; Woodman & Hemmings, 2008), objectification (Fredrickson & Harrison, 2005; Slater & Tiggemann, 2011), and body surveillance (Calogero & Pina, 2011) are all additional proposed predictors of body-related shame. In a recent study of over 500 adolescent girl athletes, body surveillance (which is a heightened attention on the body)was a unique significant predictor of the experience of body-related shame and related to changes in body-related shame over a 3-year period (Sabiston et al., 2020).

There are many psychosocial outcomes associated with body-related shame, including higher depression symptoms and worse self-esteem (Bessenoff & Snow, 2006; Brunet et al., 2019; Pila et al., 2015). Body-related shame may also lead to avoidance or disengagement from sport and exercise (Pearl et al., 2015). Body-related shame can also result in reports of higher external and lower internalized exercise regulations and low exercise behavior engagement (Castonguay et al., 2015; Sabiston et al., 2010). Body-related shame has also been associated with sport outcomes. For example, among adolescent girl athletes, body-related shame about appearance and function were significantly negatively associated with sport enjoyment and commitment and positively associated with competitive sport anxiety, over 3 years (Pila et al., 2020). These associations were consistent at the within-person and between-person levels—suggesting that girls with higher body-related shame compared to other athletes reported poorer sport experiences, as well as when their body-related shame was higher than usual the emotion was associated with these sport experiences.

The most important take-away message about shame is that it is an intense negatively valanced emotion that often leads to behavioral avoidance and poor outcomes in sport and exercise settings. Feelings of shame are also often accompanied by experiences of guilt, although guilt is not as an intense emotion. It may lead to behavioral engagement as well as avoidance (Tangney & Tracy, 2012).

Body-Related guilt Body-related guilt is a negative affective experience that is evoked when an individual's physical appearance and/or function are not aligned with personal or societal standards. This misalignment appears to motivate reparatory behavior rather than aversive avoidance as occurs with the experience of shame. Guilt is often tied to attributions about one's behavior. Because of this, body-related guilt can sometimes be perceived as an adaptive emotion as it can facilitate reparative behaviors such as exercise with subsequent adaptive consequences (Gino & Pierce, 2009).

Contrary to the general premise that guilt is elicited by specific and unstable attributions (Tracy & Robins, 2004), body-related guilt has been shown to be predicated on stable and global attributions (Crocker et al., 2014). Lower perceptions of physical self-concept were also associated with higher reports of body-related guilt. Body surveillance has also been identified as a key predictor of body-related guilt (Sabiston et al., 2020). Furthermore, women are more likely to experience body-related guilt compared to men, and individuals of higher weight status (Pila et al., 2016) may also report greater body-related guilt. As such, gender and weight status may be key distinguishing factors in the experience of body-related guilt.

Body-related guilt leads to higher reports of exercise for men and women (Castonguay et al., 2015; Sabiston et al., 2010). It is important to note that this guilt may stem from maladaptive behaviors such as overeating (Mond & Calogero, 2009) or monitoring one's behavior on a fitness tracker (Ledger & McCaffrey, 2014). Body-related guilt associated with appearance is more likely to be detrimental to individuals physical and mental health compared to guilt associated with fitness or function of the body (Calogero & Pina, 2011; Castonguay et al., 2014, 2016). In sport, body-related guilt was associated with poorer sport experiences among girl athletes, including lower reports of enjoyment and commitment and higher competitive anxiety over 3 years (Pila et al., 2020). Of note, function-based emotions were stronger predictors of the sport experiences and remained significant in models when appearance-based emotions were also included. Furthermore, it is likely that adolescent boys may also report body-related guilt that may influence sport experiences. Research efforts are needed to test the body-related emotions and sport and exercise outcomes in boys.

Body-related guilt is a negative emotion specific to behavior and may lead to reparative actions such as engagement in sport and exercise. Nonetheless, guilt can also be harmful to performance outcomes and it is important to focus on ways to help athletes reduce or manage feelings of guilt.

Body-Related Envy Body-related envy is experienced when individuals desire the possessions or characteristics possessed by others. It is typical for body-related envy to be categorized as either benign or malicious (Pila et al., 2014). The more benign form of envy is associated with feelings of inferiority as well as admiration of body-related attributes of the other, albeit without negative feelings toward that individual. In contrast, the more malicious form of envy is typically associated with feelings of hostility and ill-will. Malicious envy is more maladaptive than benign envy because the experience of malicious envy often involves perceptions of an injustice accompanied with feelings of resentment and hostility. Individuals who experience malicious envy often do not acknowledge these feelings and sometimes are not consciously aware of the envious feelings. Researchers typically focus on more malicious forms of envy due to its maladaptive consequences and sometimes severe implications such as attempts to thwart other's success and/or the experience of enjoyment in others' failures.

The experience of malicious forms of envy tends to be associated with maladaptive forms of behavior, such as a lack of sustained exercise behaviors or avoidance. On the other hand, individuals who experience benign envy are often inspired or motivated to improve aspects of their self that are the target of the comparison and this improvement may involve engagement in sport and exercise (Pila et al., 2014). Qualitative findings of sport experiences suggest these feelings of benign and malicious body-related envy may be distinguishable and may be linked to sport drop among girl athletes (Vani et al., 2021). Nonetheless, there has been little emphasis on body-related envy in general, or the specific subtypes of envy, in sport and exercise research to date.

Body-Related Embarrassment Body-related embarrassment is a negatively valenced self-conscious emotion that is experienced following an individual's perception of a public violation of social standards regarding physical appearance or function (i.e., dressing inappropriately, receiving negative comments about one's body weight or shape, accidentally exposing body parts in the change room). This body-related emotion most often occurs in social contexts in the presence of others, although they can occur, albeit to a lesser degree, in anticipation of public exposure (Vani et al., 2020). Body-related embarrassment is actually considered the most social of the self-conscious emotions (Robbins & Parlavecchio, 2006) (◘ Fig. 19.7).

Body-related embarrassment is often described similarly to shame, and some measures of body-related shame and guilt use items of embarrassment (e.g., "the appearance of my body is embarrassing for me in front of others"; Conradt et al., 2007). Yet, embarrassment is distinct from shame and guilt. Body-related embarrassment is not linked to an inferior global self (shame) and occurs in public, contrasting with guilt and shame emotions that can occur

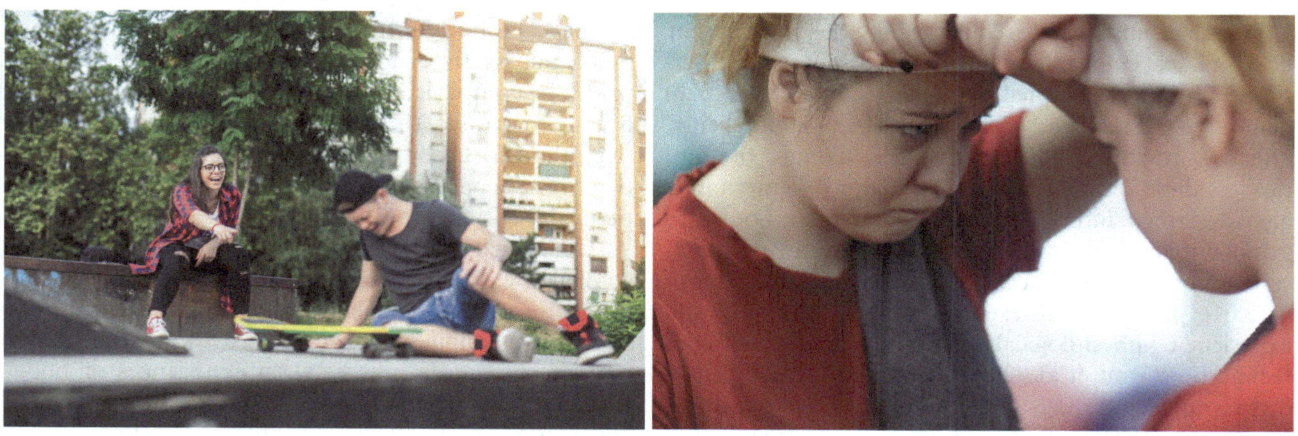

◘ **Fig. 19.7** What negatively valenced self-conscious emotions are at work here?

publicly and privately (Beer & Keltner, 2004; Vani et al., 2020). Body-related embarrassment occurs in response to social convention violations whereas social physique anxiety is elicited from a fear of negative evaluation. Further, body-related embarrassment is more transient when compared to body-related shame, guilt, and social physique anxiety (Beer & Keltner, 2004; Tangney et al., 1996).

In sport and exercise contexts, empirical investigations of body-related embarrassment are limited. Global embarrassment (i.e., embarrassment not contextualized to the body) is often reported in sport and exercise contexts and frequently acts as a barrier to activity engagement (Lascar et al., 2014; McHugh et al., 2008; More et al., 2019; Sabiston et al., 2007; Toft & Uhrenfeldt, 2015). Contextualized to the body, a narrative study among older adolescents and young adults suggested that about half of the participants described experiencing body-related embarrassment in sport and exercise contexts (e.g., sports, gym; Vani et al., 2020). These contexts included both aesthetic (e.g., swimming) and non-aesthetic (e.g., soccer) activities, suggesting that body-related embarrassment is not only experienced in sport and exercise settings that emphasize public displays of the body but is also reported in non-aesthetic contexts. In these ways, antecedents for experiencing body-related embarrassment in sport and exercise settings include fearing appearance evaluation (e.g., public weighing and body fat assessments in gym class), body talk and weight commentary (e.g., being teased for body weight in gym class), sport-related mistakes (e.g., missing a catch in football), accidents occurring in public (e.g., falling on the ice during hockey), and upward body comparisons (e.g., perceiving others as more muscular in the gym; Vani et al., 2020). These experiences have been reported by men and women in a variety of sport and exercise settings, and it's likely because there is tremendous opportunity for experiencing body-related embarrassment while participating in sport and exercise.

There is limited research describing the outcomes of body-related embarrassment in sport and exercise settings. Within the limited research, Vani et al. (2020) demonstrated that body-related embarrassment elicited affective, cognitive, and behavioral outcomes. In addition to these outcomes, adolescents and young adults also described hiding or covering up their bodies to avoid public displays of the body, withdrawing themselves from physical activity altogether, feeling motivated to participate in exercise or to lose weight, and experiencing physiological reactions such as blushing or feeling hot (Vani et al., 2020). Using avoidance behaviors to manage feelings of body-related embarrassment may impact future sport and exercise experiences and participation (Cash et al., 2005). Furthermore, body related-embarrassing experiences that motivate exercise are likely rooted in external motivation and therefore may only motivate short-term change and can be harmful to physical and mental health (Assor et al., 2009; Ingledew & Markland, 2008). Therefore, the outcomes of body-related embarrassment may lead to negative consequences for sport and exercise experiences and behavior.

Overall, body-related embarrassment is a unique experience to feelings of shame, guilt, and social physique anxiety. The emotion is fleeting, which means it may not last a long time, but researchers have to study the rumination and specific attention on the body-related embarrassment that extends beyond the quick experience of the emotion.

Body-Related Pride Body-related pride is a positive self-conscious emotion that individuals can feel about their fitness or appearance (Gilchrist, Pila, et al., 2018; Tracy & Robins, 2004). Pride can facilitate and sustain motivation that is often required when engaging in adaptive behaviors such as sport and exercise.

Pride can be experienced pertaining to body-related appearance or function and also as a state or disposition. Also, there may be hubristic and authentic facets of pride (Castonguay et al., 2013; Tracy & Robins, 2004). Hubristic pride is derived from perceptions of superiority through downward comparisons between oneself and others. In contrast, individuals feel authentic pride from the satisfaction and achievement through their own effort and hard work. It is the individuals' explanations for why they present with certain body-related function and appearance characteristics (i.e., their attributions) that are believed to elicit the different facets of pride. Feelings of hubristic pride are derived from attributions that are relatively uncontrollable and stable across time. For example, individuals who believe they are in good shape because they have "good genes" (something which people do not have a lot of control over and is unlikely to change much across time) are more likely to feel hubristic pride. In comparison, individuals who attribute their fitness to causes that are controllable and unstable (e.g., the effort they put in at the gym or at sport practice over the past few months) are likely to feel authentic pride.

Compared to generalized experiences of pride as studied by Tracy and Robins (2007), body-related authentic and hubristic pride may be more conceptually similar. Castonguay et al. (2014, 2016) noted a similar pattern of relationships between experiences of body-related authentic and hubristic pride. Similarly, high correlations ($r \geq 0.70$) have been reported between body-related hubristic and authentic pride among girl athletes (Pila et al., 2020; Sabiston et al., 2020). Furthermore, there is some evidence that the measurement of hubristic pride has met limited success, leading some to question its existence as a distinct facet of pride (Holbrook et al., 2014). These trends need to be further explored in the context of body-relate pride, especially since the two facets of body-related pride have been measured with scales developed to overcome challenges associated with the measurement of hubristic pride (Castonguay et al., 2014, 2016).

Feelings of pride arise when an individual evaluates the actual self (i.e., how he/she currently appears) as congruent with the ideal self (i.e., how he/she would ideally like to appear). Greater congruence between actual and ideal self-perceptions of fitness (function) has been associated with greater anticipated authentic pride among young adults (Gilchrist, Sabiston, & Kowalski, 2018). Greater congruence between actual weight and ideal weight has been associated with greater authentic pride among adult females (Castonguay et al., 2012). In another study, the congruence between actual and ideal perceptions of muscularity and thinness was significantly associated with hubristic and authentic pride in male adults (Mackowiak et al., 2019). As such, congruence in actual and ideal self-perceptions of weight, function, muscularity, and thinness contributes to feelings of body-related pride.

Pride is associated with favorable health-related behaviors. Specifically, Gilchrist and colleagues (2018) found that both hubristic and authentic pride in one's fitness were positively associated with higher levels of moderate-to-vigorous physical activity (MVPA). Appearance-related hubristic and authentic pride, however, were not related to MVPA, indicating that pride pertinent to fitness and function might be a stronger predictor of physical activity than pride pertinent to appearance (Gilchrist, Pila, et al., 2018). Mack et al. (2015) also found a positive association between both functional facets of both authentic and hubristic pride and engagement in MVPA. These results suggest that experiences of body-related hubristic and authentic pride about function are associated with engagement in physical activity. Pila et al. (2020) found similar associations between body-related authentic and hubristic pride and positive sport experiences over time among girl athletes. Body-related pride focused on fitness was a stronger predictor of sport enjoyment and commitment compared to appearance pride emotions, and these associations held over time. Based on this research, the beneficial effects of promoting feelings of body-related fitness pride need to be integrated into sport and exercise programming, with a limited focus on one's appearance.

19.4.2 Anticipated and Experienced Emotions

All body-related self-conscious emotions have been studied in the context of body appearance and fitness/function. As can be seen, the emotions are both positive and negative in valence and can also be studied as state and trait/proneness. Body-related emotions can also be described as experienced/felt (i.e., in the moment emotion) or anticipated (i.e., a future experience of the emotion); however, there is very little work exploring anticipated emotions.

Anticipated emotions have been studied predominantly framed around negative emotions. For example, Gilchrist et al. (2020) found a negative association between physical self-concept and anticipated body-related shame among young adult women but not men. Physical self-concept was not associated with anticipated body-related guilt, although men reported anticipating more guilt compared to women. These findings demonstrate potential uniqueness among the anticipation of shame and guilt emotions. When linked to behavior, anticipated emotions have been mostly studied with psychological and behavioral indices of eating disorders (e.g., body size misperception, caloric consumption; fear of weight gain). For example, Troop's program of research has articulated the important and unique distinction between experienced and anticipated body shame with relevance to disordered eating (Troop, 2016; Troop & Redshaw, 2012). In this work, even if an individual does not currently experience shame about their weight, self-regulation and behavioral modification may occur to avoid the onset of shame in the future. Drawing on this work, the anticipation of negative emotions may also be motivational or discouraging for exercise or sport participation (Gilchrist, Conroy, & Sabiston, 2017; Gilchrist & Sabiston, 2018; Gilchrist, Sabiston, et al., 2018; Gilchrist et al., 2020). Furthermore, the association between anticipated authentic and hubristic pride and engagement in moderate-to-vigorous physical activity (MVPA) has been reported among young adults (Gilchrist & Sabiston, 2018). In this study, intentions to be physically active significantly *mediated* the association between anticipated authentic and hubristic pride and MVPA. These recent findings focused on anticipated positive emotions suggest that targeting anticipated hedonic outcomes of MVPA may be valuable in interventions targeting exercise participation.

Although much more work is needed, early evidence suggests that understanding distinctions between experienced and anticipated emotions, and association to behavioral outcomes, may be valuable to sport and exercise.

19.5 A Cultural Perspective on the Self

The self develops as individuals grow-up in and actively navigate through various social contexts and attune themselves to these by asking questions such as "Who am I?" "What should I be doing?" and "How do I relate to others?" These contexts vary in complexity, from the specific current situation to society as a whole. Individual behavior within these various contexts is informed by (frequently implicit) knowledge and beliefs about what is appropriate and morally justified, and what it means "to be a good person." Markus and Kitayama (1991, 2010) have linked cultural differences between individualist and collectivist societies to two ways of construing identity or two different self-construals: An independent and an interdependent way of understanding the self (see ◘ Fig. 19.8).

Within the independent perspective, as explained by Markus and Kitayama (1991, 2010), the self is primarily defined by characteristics that distinguish the person from others, like traits, attitudes, or abilities. The interdependent self, however, incorporates elements of the social world, such as close and stable relationships, contexts for behavior, important roles, and group memberships. While presumably all people everywhere *can* think about the self in either way, research has identified systematic inter- and intra-individual variations in the emphasis that individuals place on independence or interdependence, respectively.

Within the independent construal that is prevalent in many Western individualist societies, the self is seen as clearly separate from others (Markus & Kitayama, 1991, 2010). Although these other people vary in how close they are to the self, the distinction between the self and others is always pronounced. Coinciding with this distinction is the fact that attachment to one's in-groups is comparatively loose. While group-based social identities (such as one's sport team) can be salient in a given context, it, generally speaking, is the internal repertoire of autonomous features ("I am particularly good at…") of the self that is subjectively seen as most self-defining. People with independent self-construal tend to have many social identities, each of which does not figure very prominently in one's sense of the self—social identities between which the person can flexibly switch. A further important aspect of independent self-definitions is the fact that they are acquired by aggregating the self-descriptive features across the various contexts one encounters and are hence abstract and context-free in nature. For example, if one defines the self as being "honest" (an independent concept), it is implied that one frankly tells the truth in most if not all contexts wherever that is possible. In this view, one's personal degree of honesty is a feature of the self and less so of the context one happens to be in.

The interdependent self-construal (see right-hand panel of ◘ Fig. 19.8) is prevalent in many Eastern collectivist cultures (e.g., East Asia) and stresses the exact opposite. According to this view, the self is fundamentally connected and inseparably linked to others. Interdependent self-aspects include one's relationships to others (e.g., "I am a caring partner"). It is not possible to think about the self in interdependent terms, while not at the very same moment thinking about relevant others. Put differently, the mental representation of the self and close others overlap. Coinciding with this view is the fact that group-based social identities are subjectively highly important. One cannot exist in interdepen-

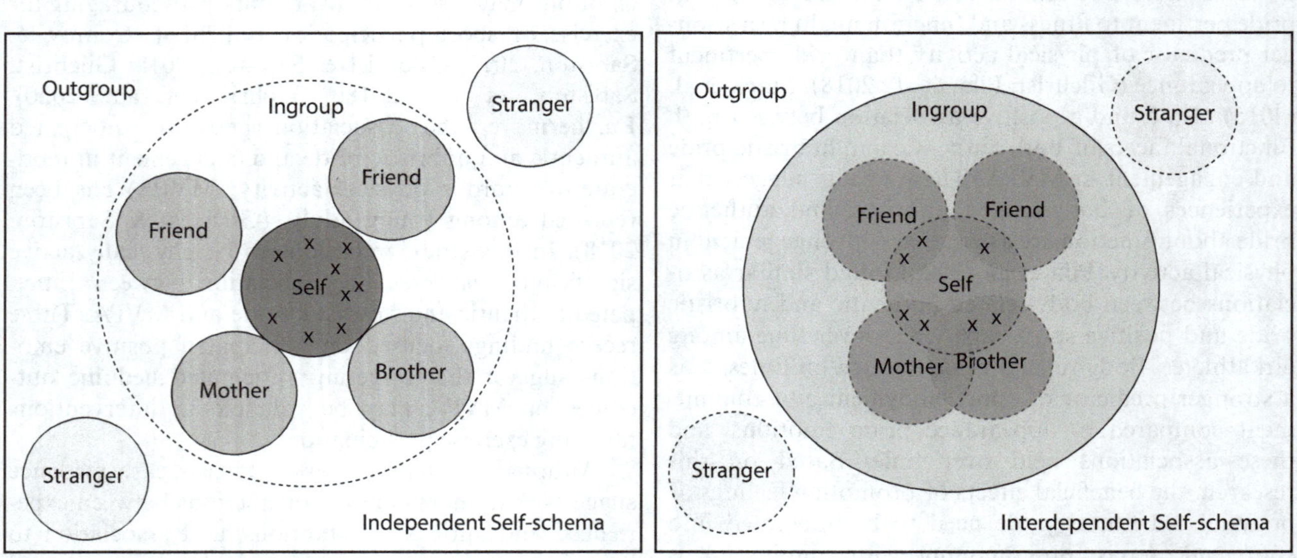

◘ **Fig. 19.8** The independent (left) and interdependent (right) construal of the self (from Markus & Kitayama, 2010). Adapted from Markus, H. R., & Kitayama, S. (2010). Cultures and selves: A cycle of mutual constitution. *Perspectives on Psychological Science, 5*, 420–430

dence with others while being disconnected from them. Therefore, social group membership tends to be highly selective but also strongly binding and long lasting. Furthermore, because the self is defined by relationships to others who are encountered in specific social contexts only, interdependent self-aspects are more concrete and context-related (e.g., Rhee et al., 1995). To use the abovementioned example once more: The interdependent self-definition "I am a caring partner" implies that one is a caring person in the context of one's marriage; it does however not imply that one is caring about all others in general.

Markus and Kitayama (1991, 2010) argued that the very nature of the self-construal has important consequences for thinking, feeling, and action. This contention is in line with the three basic functions of the self as identified by Baumeister (1999) referred to previously. The self not only enables self-reflection but also executive function that provides free consciousness and allows for agency in life. Finally, the self regulates social relationships thus making us interpersonal beings. The degree of independence/interdependence of self-construal influences and shapes the responses of an individual with regard to all three basic functions of the self. Markus and Kitayama (1991) reviewed a broad range of cultural differences in cognition, emotion, and motivation, and argued that they all can be parsimoniously explained by invoking cultural differences in self-construal. The same holds true for some of the sport and exercise phenomena discussed in this chapter so far.

To give an example, recall the earlier discussed skill development hypothesis of the hierarchical conceptualization of the self, wherein sport and exercise involvement is postulated to enhance perceptions of self-efficacy and ultimately increase self-esteem. Both self-esteem and self-efficacy are partly influenced by a person's cultural background. Many studies converge in showing that East Asians tend to report lower levels of self-esteem than Westerners. In reviewing research in the area, Heine et al. (1999) have reported that more than 93% of European-Canadians endorsed items on self-esteem inventories about their value as individuals above the scale theoretical midpoint, and only roughly 55% of Japanese did so. Interestingly, Heine et al. (1999) argue that these differences are not simply a function of moderacy response sets, nor cultural differences in socially desirable responding. They instead point to culture and note that Western cultures emphasize the pursuit of personal goals and an attendant sense of the self as efficacious and in control to a much greater degree than East Asian cultures. Interpretation of these response differences by taking the independence-interdependence cultural distinctions, therefore, has relevance. Within the independent cultural framework, the pursuit of personal goals is justified and even appreciated. Culturally speaking, people are motivated to self-enhance; that is, they have a desire to see the self positively. By contrast the interdependent cultural framework highlights responsiveness to the needs and expectations of social others and a resulting sense of the self that is harmoniously connected to others. Sticking out (even in positive direction) may threaten relational harmony and hence the sense of interdependence with others.

Findings indicating that Asians report lower levels of self-esteem do not inherently imply that they feel less positivity toward the self, but rather that the "goodness" of their self-evaluations comes from a different sociocultural perspective; one that, at least in part, also involves features or characteristics outside of the self (as understood in Western Cultural terms) such as social relational embeddedness of the self, interpersonal harmony, and so on. Whether or not these findings hold for athletes in these cultures remains unclear but finding the right balance between true self-confidence as an inner feeling of capability on the one hand and the avoidance of cockiness on the other hand can be assumed to be a crucial issue for many high achievers in sports. What is regarded as the "right" balance can almost certainly be assumed to vary between cultures.

Consistent with this analysis, a growing body of literature on self-serving motivations across cultures has demonstrated that Americans are much more likely than Asians to seek and confirm a positive view of self. Specifically, Kitayama et al. (1995) have reported cross-cultural differences in self-serving or self-enhancing motivations relative to causal attributions for success (i.e., attributing one's successes to internal forces such as personal talent or ambition) and failure (i.e., attributing one's failures to external forces such as tough luck or unfair treatment by others). Note, however, that these authors (like many others) did not look specifically at attributions for *sport* performance. Typical examples in sport could include readily accepting credit for win as a matter of having had the right attitude (e.g., "We always believed in ourselves") and complaining about a referee's decision being biased and unfair if about to lose a match (thereby attributing the potential failure to an external factor) as depicted in the picture of the Juventus Turin players in blue appealing to the referee about a call that they perceive to be "unjust" (◘ Fig. 19.9).

Based on the findings that self-serving biases are often stronger among individualist than collectivist culture members, one might therefore expect similar tendencies when athletes from different cultures explain their performance. The evidence is somewhat mixed but a recent meta-analysis by Allen et al. (2020) on the strength of self-serving attribution biases particularly in the competitive domain of organized sport showed that

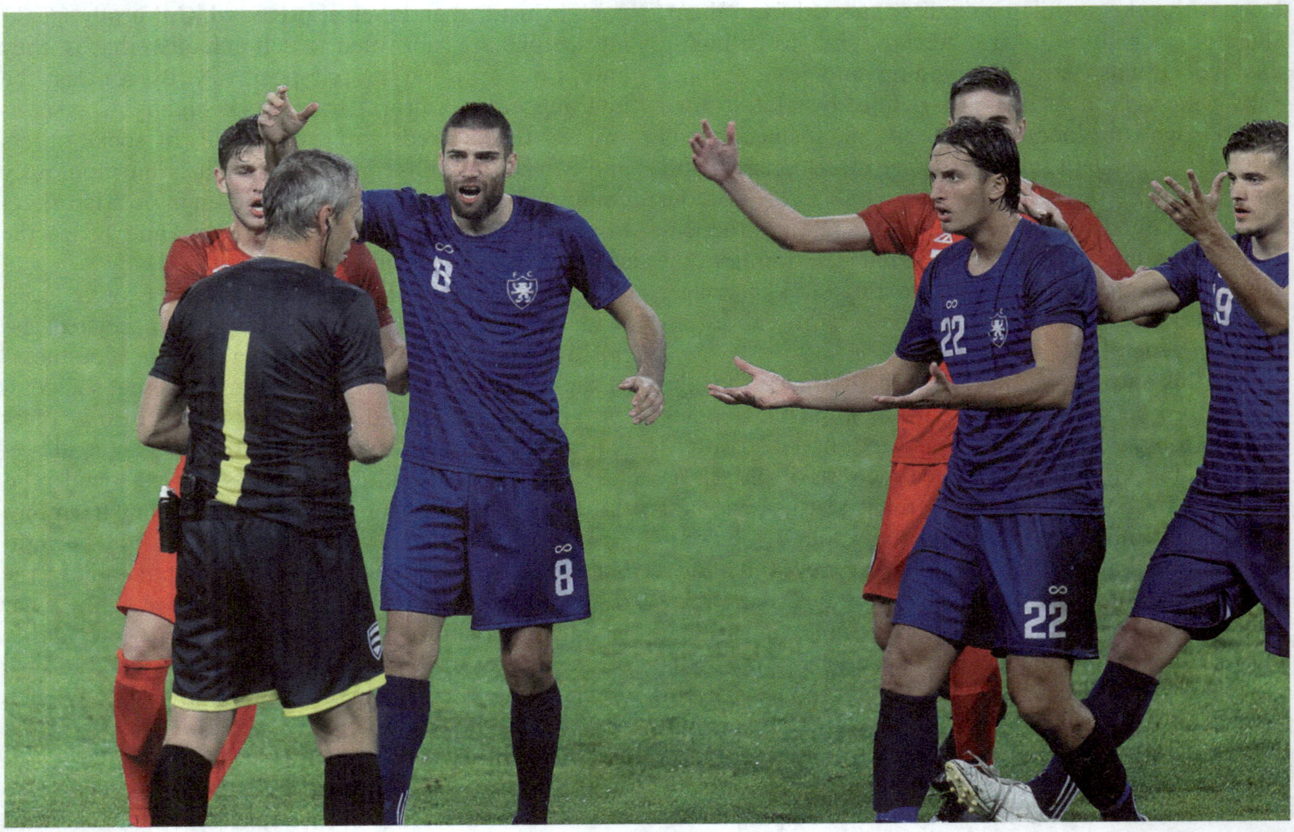

Fig. 19.9 Is the Referee's Call Perceived to be Fair or "Unjust" by the Players in Blue?

sport performers do have a tendency to a) attribute personal success internally and failure externally, b) attribute team success to factors within the team and failure to factors outside the team, and c) claim more personal responsibility for team success and less personal responsibility for team failure. Importantly, these tendencies were more pronounced among athletes from North America—arguably the most individualist world region—than among athletes from less individualist European countries.

Cultural differences in attributional self-enhancement tendencies in newspaper reports about outcomes in international sport events have also been reported. Lee et al. (1996) analyzed newspaper reports about soccer matches from the US and from Hong Kong and found that the US reporters included many more dispositional attributions for the success of the teams (e.g., the team's quality and ambition), whereas Hong Kong newspapers attributed the same events more strongly to situational circumstances (e.g., mere luck). Other studies, however, suggest strong self-serving biases may exist even in collectivist cultures. For example, contrary to the prediction that would follow from Lee and colleagues' findings, Aldrige and Islam (2012) found that self-serving biases in attributions for success and failure by Olympic athletes in the reporting of both Japanese and Australian newspapers. This inconsistency calls for further investigation.

Furthermore, Heine and Hamamurra (2007) conducted a meta-analysis on cultural differences in various indicators of self-enhancement, including the tendency to see the self as better than average, and the tendency to recall information about personal successes better than about personal failures. Westerners overall showed strong tendencies for self-enhancement, whereas East Asians did not (see ▶ Study Box: Cultural Differences in Child Rearing). Overall, evidence clearly suggests that individuals with an independent construal of the self are more likely to self-enhance and to strive for positive self-esteem than individuals with an interdependent construal of the self. This is not to say that a positive self-view is not important to East Asians. Another way of maintaining a positive sense of the self is through the concept of "face" which can be defined as the amount of social value granted by others when living up to the standards associated with one's position (e.g., Ho, 1976).

Cultural Differences in Child Rearing

Cultural differences in attributional self-enhancement have been identified in child rearing practices and educational beliefs in interviews with parents from the USA and Taiwan. Miller et al. (1997), for example, reported that the stories told by European-American parents to their children more often pertained to the past success of the child than was the case for Taiwanese parents who, by comparison, told more stories about past transgressions of the child. Regarding the role of self-esteem in education, US parents tended to see self-esteem as a positive quality that enhances a child's development (and therefore should be cultivated), while Taiwanese parents were much more critical and believed that too much self-esteem might lead to frustration for a child when things go wrong.

Many studies show that "losing face" yields much stronger emotional consequences for East Asians than for Westerners. One implication of the concept of face is that it is more easily lost than gained. Given this fact, it seems a plausible strategy to cautiously avoid acting in a way that might lead to the disapproval by others. This line of thought leads to an intriguing prediction: Different kinds of performance feedback in sport and exercise settings might motivate people with independent vs. interdependent self-construal. For independent people, positive (success) feedback might be more motivating than negative (failure) feedback, because positive feedback induces pride and as a consequence increases self-esteem, not so, however, for interdependent people. For them negative feedback might be more motivating, because it signals potential disapproval by others which one should anxiously avoid by trying harder. More abstractly speaking, while self-enhancement motivation might be stronger in independent cultures, self-improvement motivation (i.e., attempts to seek out potential weaknesses and to correct them) might be more motivating in East Asian contexts. In fact, many studies confirm this prediction. For instance, Oishi and Diener (2003) gave people with European American or Asian backgrounds the choice of playing either basketball or darts. While European Americans chose the activity they were good at, Asian Americans did not. Similarly, when given alleged positive or negative feedback on a performance test, Canadian participants subsequently persisted longer on the task after positive than negative feedback, while the exact opposite was found for Japanese (Heine et al., 2001).

Another important implication of the distinction between the independent and interdependent construal of the self pertains to intrinsic motivation and how it can be fostered. Abundant studies, mainly in Western cultures, converge in showing that one of the most important predictors of intrinsic motivation is freedom of choice: We are motivated to try harder in tasks that are self-chosen than on tasks that are given to us by others (e.g., Deci & Ryan, 1985) (see also ► Chap. 8 about self-determination theory and intrinsic motivation). Again, this finding may rest on the independent construal of the self where agency is regarded as a feature of the individual and disjoint from others (Markus & Kitayama, 2003). Within this model of agency, actions are chosen freely and according to one's preferences with the goal to affirm the independent self. Not so, however, among people with interdependent self-views. They regard agency as conjoint in the sense that actions are responsive to perceived social expectations. Fulfilling the expectations of important others affirms the interdependence with them.

In line with this reasoning, Iyengar and Lepper (1999) conducted a study with children with either individualist (USA) or collectivist (India) cultural background who were supposed to work on a number of puzzles. In one condition, the children were able to choose which puzzles to work on themselves, while in a second condition the same puzzles were administered to the children by the experimenter. Replicating previous findings, children from both cultural backgrounds persisted longer on the puzzles when they had freely chosen to work on them. In a third condition; however, children were informed that the puzzles had actually been chosen by a close other (i.e., their mother). For kids with American background, persistence in this condition was comparable to the experimenter-choice condition. In other words, for these children, the crucial difference in intrinsic motivation existed between puzzles they had chosen for themselves versus not (irrespective of the relationship with the other person choosing for them). Children with Asian background, however, persisted the strongest on puzzles that they presumed to have been chosen by their mother. In other words, these kids regarded the assignment from the perspective of conjoint agency implicated in the interdependence cultural construal of social expectations wherein the fulfillment of the expectations of important others affirms interdependence and prevents social disappointment. These cultural differences may also appear in sport and exercise settings. Hudson et al. (2010), for example, reported differences in constraints to engaging in downhill skiing among non-skiing Anglo-Canadian (independent) and Chinese-Canadian (interdependent) participants. Anglo-Canadians reported being primarily constrained by structural fac-

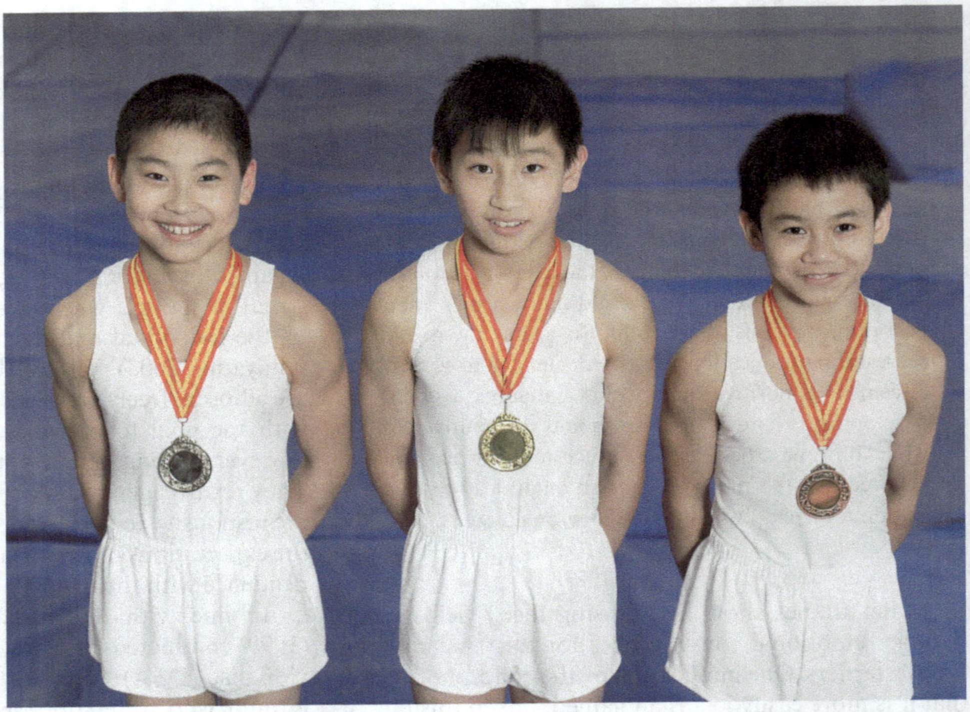

Fig. 19.10 Expressing and feeling pride as self-conscious emotion that is formed by culture

tors (e.g., time, money), whereas Chinese-Canadians reported being more constrained by the lack of friends to ski with, or by parental barriers, supporting the contention that they highly value conformation to social expectations.

The nature of the self in terms of independence or interdependence has also been shown to have consequences for self-conscious emotions. Research by Kitayama et al. (2006) assessed the frequency and intensity of different types of emotions in US and Japanese participants. Socially disengaging emotions—such as pride, anger, or irritation—were found to be more frequent and intense in European American than in Japanese participants. This finding is consistent with the European American emphasis on autonomy and independence. In line with the East Asian emphasis on relatedness and interdependence, however, Kitayama et al. found socially engaging emotions—such as close feelings, shame, guilt, or indebtedness—to be more frequent and intense in Japanese than in European American participants. Applying these findings to the domain of sport, one would predict that Asian gold medalists exhibit less pride in the Olympic Games than Western athletes, a hypothesis that has been tested in several studies. Van Osch et al. (2015), for example, found exactly this pattern—at least relative to outperforming an in-group member: Chinese gold medalists outperforming another Chinese showed lower levels of pride than Americans outperforming a fellow American (Fig. 19.10).

When outperforming an out-group member, however, this difference was negligible. It seems plausible that these differences may also affect body-related emotions (i.e., shame, pride, or guilt), a speculation that for the time being, however, awaits investigation.

19.6 Summary and Concluding Remarks

To summarize, in this chapter, we have discussed the role of the self in sport and exercising, and we have focused on such important concepts as self-concept and self-esteem, self-presentation (including self-enhancement), and self-conscious emotions. In all these areas, cultural differences in the construal of the self in terms of independence or interdependence are likely to be relevant, because, as Markus and Kitayama (1991) suggested, whenever a cognitive, motivational, or emotion process implicates the self, the degree of independence or interdependence is likely to shape the outcome.

19

Learning Control Questions

Basic:

1. How do the constructs of self-concept, self-esteem, physical self-concept, and self-efficacy differ conceptually?
2. What are the differences between unidimensional, multidimensional, and hierarchical conceptualizations of the self?
3. What is self-presentation and when are self-presentational imperatives most likely to be salient for individuals?
4. How are self-conscious emotions linked to individuals' self-concept/self-esteem?

Advanced:

5. With regard to the hierarchical model of self-esteem, what are the key differences between, and implications of, the skill development and self-enhancement hypotheses?
6. Are there meaningful differences between the two prominent models of self-presentation? Why or why not?
7. How might the various body-related self-conscious emotions be elicited in sport and exercise settings?

Experts:

8. What prominent self-presentation motives can be manifest in sport and exercise settings and how might they shape behavioral enactments in those settings?
9. When elicited in sport and exercise settings, what are key differentiating features among/between the body-related self-conscious emotions of (a) anxiety, guilt, shame, and embarrassment, (b) authentic and hubristic pride, and (c) benign and malicious envy?
10. How might individuals' self-construals differ across societies with individualist and collectivist cultures, and what are potential manifestations of these self-construal differences in sport and exercise settings?

References

Aldrige, L. J., & Islam, M. R. (2012). Cultural differences in athlete attributions for success and failure: The sports pages revisited. *International Journal of Psychology, 47*, 67–75.

Allen, M. S., Robson, D. A., Martin, L. J., & Laborde, S. (2020). Systematic review and meta-analysis of self-serving attribution biases in the competitive context of organized sport. *Personality and Social Psychology Bulletin, 46*, 1027–1043.

Assor, A., Vansteenkiste, M., & Kaplan, A. (2009). Identified versus introjected approach and introjected avoidance motivations in school and in sports: The limited benefits of self-worth strivings. *Journal of Educational Psychology, 101*, 482–497.

Babic, M. J., Morgan, P. J., Plotnikoff, R. C., Lonsdale, C., White, R. L., & Lubans, D. R. (2014). Physical activity and physical self-concept in youth: Systematic review and meta-analysis. *Sports Medicine, 44*, 1589–1601.

Bakan, D. (1966). *The duality of human existence: Isolation and communion in Western man*. Beacon.

Bandura, A. (1997). *Self-efficacy: The exercise of control*. Freeman.

Barber, B. L., Eccles, J. S., & Stone, M. R. (2001). Whatever happened to the jock, the brain, and the princess? Young adult pathways linked to adolescent activity involvement and social identity. *Journal of Adolescent Research, 16*, 429–455.

Bauman, A. E., Reis, R. S., Sallis, J. F., Wells, J. C., Loos, R. J. F., & Martin, B. W. (2012). Correlates of physical activity: Why are some people physically active and others not? *Lancet, 380*, 258–271.

Baumeister, R. F. (1982). A self-presentational view of social phenomena. *Psychological Bulletin, 91*, 3–26.

Baumeister, R. F. (Ed.). (1999). *The self in social psychology*. Psychology Press (Taylor & Francis).

Beer, J. S., & Keltner, D. (2004). What is unique about self-conscious emotions? *Psychological Inquiry, 15*, 126–170.

Bessenoff, G. R., & Snow, D. (2006). Absorbing society's influence: Body image self-discrepancy and internalized shame. *Sex Roles, 54*, 727–731.

Brunet, J., Pila, E., Solomon-Krakus, S., Sabiston, C. M., & O'Loughlin, J. (2019). Self-esteem moderates the associations between body-related self-conscious emotions and depressive symptoms. *Journal of Health Psychology, 24*, 833–843.

Brunet, J., Sabiston, C., Castonguay, A., Ferguson, L., & Bessette, N. (2012). The association between physical self-discrepancies and women's physical activity: The mediating role of motivation. *Journal of Sport and Exercise Psychology, 34*, 102–123.

Brunet, J., & Sabiston, C. M. (2011). In the company we keep: Social physique anxiety levels differ around parents and peers. *Journal of Health Psychology, 16*(1), 42–49.

Brunet, J., Sabiston, C. M., Dorsch, K. D., & McCreary, D. R. (2010). Exploring a model linking social physique anxiety, drive for muscularity, drive for thinness and self-esteem among adolescent boys and girls. *Body Image, 7*, 137–142.

Calogero, R. M., & Pina, A. (2011). Body guilt: Preliminary evidence for a further subjective experience of self-objectification. *Psychology of Women Quarterly, 35*(3), 428–440.

Cash, T. F., Santos, M. T., & Williams, E. F. (2005). Coping with body-image threats and challenges: Validation of the body image coping strategies inventory. *Journal of Psychosomatic Research, 58*, 190–199.

Castonguay, A. L., Brunet, J., Ferguson, L., & Sabiston, C.M. (2012). Weight-related actual and ideal self-states, discrepancies, and shame, guilt, and pride: Examining associations within the process model of self-conscious emotions. Body Image, 9(4), 488–494. https://doi.org/10.1016/j.bodyim.2012.07.003.

Castonguay, A. L., Gilchrist, J. D., Mack, D. E., & Sabiston, C. M. (2013). Body-related pride in young adults: An exploration of the triggers, contexts, outcomes and attributions. *Body Image, 10*, 335–343.

Castonguay, A. L., Pila, E., Wrosch, C., & Sabiston, C. M. (2015). Body-related self-conscious emotions relate to physical activity motivation and behavior in men. *American Journal of Men's Health, 9*, 209–221.

Castonguay, A. L., Sabiston, C. M., Crocker, P. R. E., & Mack, D. E. (2014). Development and validation of the body and appearance self-conscious emotions scale (BASES). *Body Image, 11*(2), 126–136.

Castonguay, A. L., Sabiston, C. M., Kowalski, K. C., & Wilson, P. M. (2016). Introducing an instrument to measure body and fitness-related self-conscious emotions: The BSE-FIT. *Psychology of Sport and Exercise, 23*, 1–12.

Conradt, M., Dierk, J.-M., Schlumberger, P., Rauh, E., Hevebrand, J., & Rief, W. (2007). Development of the weight- and body-related shame and guilt scale (WEB-SG) in a non-clinical sample of obese subjects. *Journal of Personality Assessment, 88*, 317–327.

Conroy, D. E., Motl, R. W., & Hall, E. G. (2000). Progress toward construct validation of the self-presentation in exercise questionnaire (SPEQ). *Journal of Sport & Exercise Psychology, 22*, 21–38.

Coopersmith, S. (1967). *The antecedents of self-esteem*. W. H. Freeman and Company.

Cox, A. E., Ullrich-French, S., & Sabiston, C. M. (2013). Using motivation regulations in a person-centered approach to examine the link between social physique anxiety in physical education and physical activity-related outcomes in adolescents. *Psychology of Sport and Exercise, 14*, 461–467.

Crawford, S., & Eklund, R. C. (1994). Social physique anxiety, reasons for exercise, and attitudes toward exercise settings. *Journal of Sport & Exercise Psychology, 16*, 70–82.

Crocker, P. R. E., Brune, S. M., Kowalski, K. C., Mack, D. E., Wilson, P. M., & Sabiston, C. M. (2014). Body-related state shame and guilt in women: Do causal attributions mediate the influence of physical self-concept and shame and guilt proneness. *Body Image, 11*, 19–26.

Crombie, P.-A., Brunet, J., & Sabiston, C. M. (2011). Stop staring! Proposed strategies to reduce students' body-related concerns in physical education. *Journal of Physical Education Recreation and Dance, 82*, 39–43.

Deci, E. L., & Ryan, R. M. (1985). *Intrinsic motivation and self-determination in human behaviour*. Plenum.

Deci, E. L., & Ryan, R. M. (1995). Human autonomy: The basis for true self-esteem. In M. H. Kernis (Ed.), *Plenum series in social/clinical psychology. Efficacy, agency, and self-esteem* (pp. 31–49). Plenum.

Dimmock, J. A., Howle, T. C., & Jackson, B. (2020). Self-presentation in sport and exercise. In G. Tenenbaum & R. C. Eklund (Eds.), *Handbook of sport psychology* (4th ed.). Wiley.

Dishman, R. K., Hales, D. P., Pfeiffer, K. A., Felton, G. A., Saunders, R., Ward, D. S., et al. (2006). Physical self-concept and self-esteem mediate cross-sectional relations of physical activity and sport participation with depression symptoms among adolescent girls. *Health Psychology, 25*, 396–407.

Eklund, R. C., & Bianco, T. (2000). Social physique anxiety and physical activity among adolescents. *Reclaiming Children and Youth, 9*, 139–142.

Eklund, R. C., & Crawford, S. (1994). Active women, social physique anxiety, and exercise. *Journal of Sport & Exercise Psychology, 16*, 431–448.

Eklund, R. C., & Howle, T. (2017). Self-presentation and communication in physical activity settings. In B. Jackson & J. Dimmock (Eds.), *Communication and persuasion in sport, exercise, and physical activity* (pp. 250–265). Routledge/Psychology Press.

Elavsky, S. (2010). Longitudinal examination of the exercise and self-esteem model in middle-aged women. *Journal of Sport & Exercise Psychology, 32*, 862–880.

Elavsky, S., & McAuley, E. (2007). Physical activity and mental health outcomes during menopause: A randomized controlled trial. *Annals of Behavioral Medicine, 33*, 132–142.

Elliot, A. J. (2008). *Handbook of approach and avoidance motivation*. Taylor & Francis.

Findlay, L. C., & Bowker, A. (2009). The link between competitive sport participation and self-concept in early adolescence: A consideration of gender and sport orientation. *Journal of Youth and Adolescence, 38*, 29–40.

Fitts, W. (1965). *Manual for the Tennessee self-concept scale*. Counselor Recordings and Tests.

Fox, K. R. (1997). *The physical self: From motivation to well-being*. Human Kinetics.

Fox, K. R., & Corbin, C. B. (1989). The physical self-perception profile: Development and preliminary validation. *Journal of Sport and Exercise Psychology, 11*(4), 408–430.

Fredricks, J. A., & Eccles, J. S. (2006). Is extracurricular participation associated with beneficial outcomes? Concurrent and longitudinal relations. *Developmental Psychology, 42*, 698–713.

Fredrickson, B. L., & Harrison, K. (2005). Throwing like a girl: Self-objectification predicts adolescent girls' motor performance. *Journal of Sport & Social Issues, 29*(1), 79–101.

Gammage, K. L., Drouin, B., & Lamarche, L. (2016). Comparing a yoga class with a resistance exercise class: Effects on body satisfaction and social physique anxiety in university women. *Journal of Physical Activity and Health, 13*, 1202–1209.

Gammage, K. L., Hall, C. R., & Martin Ginis, K. A. (2004). Self-presentation in exercise contexts: Differences between high and low frequency exercisers. *Journal of Applied Social Psychology, 34*, 1638–1651.

Gilchrist, J. D., Conroy, D. E., & Sabiston, C. M. (2017). Experienced and anticipated pride and shame as predictors of goal-directed behavior. Journal of Sport and Exercise Psychology, 39(6), 438–442. https://doi.org/10.1123/jsep.2017-0011.

Gilchrist, J.D., Pila, E., Castonguay, A., Sabiston, C.M., & Mack, D.E. (2018). Body pride and physical activity: Differential associations between fitness- and appearance-related pride in young adult Canadians. Body Image, 27, 77–85. https://doi.org/10.1016/j.bodyim.2018.08.010

Gilchrist, J.D., Sabiston, C.M., Conroy, D.E., & Atkinson, M. (2018). Authentic pride regulates runners' trainng progress. Psychology of Sport and Exercise, 38, 10–16. https://doi.org/10.1016/j.psychsport.2018.05.007.

Gilchrist, J. D., & Sabiston, C. M. (2018). Intentions mediate the association between anticipated pride and physical activity in young adults. *Sport Exercise and Performance Psychology, 7*, 308–317.

Gilchrist, J. D., Sabiston, C. M., & Kowalski, K. C. (2018b). Associations between actual and ideal self-perceptions and anticipated pride among young adults. *Journal of Theoretical Social Psychology, 3*, 127–134.

Gilchrist, J. D., Solomon-Krakus, S., Pila, E., Crocker, P., & Sabiston, C. M. (2020). Associations between physical self-concept and anticipated guilt and shame: The moderating role of gender. *Sex Roles, 83*, 763–772.

Gino, F., & Pierce, L. (2009). Dishonesty in the name of equity. *Psychological Science, 20*, 1153–1160.

Hart, E., Leary, M. R., & Rejeski, J. W. (1989). The measurement of social physique anxiety. *Journal of Sport & Exercise Psychology, 11*, 94–104.

Harter, S. (1988). *The self-perception profile for adolescents* [Unpublished manual]. University of Denver.

Harter, S. (2012). *The construction of the self: A developmental perspective*. Guilford.

Hattie, J., & Fletcher, R. (2005). Self-esteem = success/pretensions. In H. W. Marsh, R. G. Craven, & D. McInerney (Eds.), *International advances in self research* (New frontiers for self research) (Vol. 2, pp. 123–152). Information Age Publishers.

Hausenblas, H. A., Brewer, B. W., & Van Raalte, J. L. (2004). Self-presentation and exercise. *Journal of Applied Sport Psychology, 16*, 3–18.

Heine, S., Lehman, D. R., Peng, K., & Kitayama, S. (1999). Is there a universal need for positive self-regard? *Psychological Review, 106*, 766–794.

Heine, S. J., & Hamamurra, T. (2007). In search of East Asian self-enhancement. *Personality and Social Psychology Review, 11*, 4–27.

Heine, S. J., Kitayama, S., Lehman, D. R., Takata, T., Ide, E., Leung, C., & Matsumoto, H. (2001). Divergent consequences of success and failure in Japan and North America: An investigation of self-improving motivations and malleable selves. *Journal of Personality and Social Psychology, 81*, 599–615.

Ho, D. Y. F. (1976). On the concept of face. *American Journal of Sociology, 81*, 867–884.

Holbrook, C., Piazza, J. R., & Fessler, D. M. T. (2014). Further challenges to the "authentic"/"hubristic" model of pride: Conceptual clarifications and new evidence. *Emotion, 14*, 38–42.

Howle, T., & Eklund, R. C. (2013). The effect of induced self-presentation concerns on cognitive appraisal and affect. *Anxiety, Stress, and Coping, 26*, 700–710.

Howle, T. C., Dimmock, J. A., & Jackson, B. (2016a). Relations between self-efficacy beliefs, self-presentation motives, personal task goals, and performance on endurance-based physical activity tasks. *Psychology of Sport and Exercise, 22*, 149–159.

Howle, T. C., Dimmock, J. A., Whipp, P. R., & Jackson, B. (2015a). Moving to self-present: An investigation into proposed antecedents of 2 × 2 self-presentation motives. *Journal of Sport & Exercise Psychology, 37*, 547–558.

Howle, T. C., Dimmock, J. A., Whipp, P. R., & Jackson, B. (2015b). The self-presentation motives for physical activity questionnaire: Instrument development and preliminary construct validity evidence. *Journal of Sport & Exercise Psychology, 37*, 225–243.

Howle, T. C., Jackson, B., Conroy, D. E., & Dimmock, J. A. (2015). Winning friends and influencing people: Self-presentation motives in physical activity settings. *International Review of Sport and Exercise Psychology, 8*, 44–70.

Howle, T. C., Jackson, B., & Dimmock, J. A. (2016b). On the formation of favourable impressions: Associations between self-presentation motives, task behaviour, and others' evaluations of the self in a team-sport setting. *Psychology of Sport and Exercise, 26*, 40–47.

Hudson, S., Hinch, T., Walker, G., & Simpson, B. (2010). Constraints to sport tourism: A cross-cultural analysis. *Journal of Sport & Tourism, 15*, 71–88.

Ingledew, D. K., & Markland, D. (2008). The role of motives in exercise participation. *Psychology and Health, 23*, 807–828.

Iyengar, S. S., & Lepper, M. R. (1999). Rethinking the value of choice: A cultural perspective on intrinsic motivation. *Journal of Personality and Social Psychology, 76*, 349–366.

Kitayama, S., Mesquita, B., & Karasawa, M. (2006). Cultural affordances and emotional experience: Socially engaging and disengaging emotions in Japan and the United States. *Journal of Personality and Social Psychology, 91*, 890–903.

Kitayama, S., Takagi, H., & Matsumoto, H. (1995). Seiko to shippai no kiin: Nihonteki jiko no bunka-shinrigaku [Causal attribution of success and failure: Cultural psychology of Japanese selves]. *Japanese Psychological Review, 38*, 247–280.

Kohl, H. W., Blair, S. N., Paffenbarger, R. S., Macera, C. A., & Kronenfeld, J. J. (1988). A mail survey of physical activity habits as related to measured physical fitness. *American Journal of Epidemiology, 127*(6), 1228–1239.

Kowalski, K. C., Crocker, P. R. E., & Kowalski, N. P. (1997). Convergent validity of the physical activity questionnaire for adolescents. *Pediatric Exercise Science, 9*(4), 342–352.

Kowalski, K. C., Crocker, P. R. E., Kowalski, N. P., Chad, K. E., & Humbert, M. L. (2003). Examining the physical self in adolescent girls over time: Further evidence against the hierarchical model. *Journal of Sport & Exercise Psychology, 25*, 5–18.

Kowalski, K. C., Mack, D. E., Crocker, P. R. E., Niefer, C. B., & Fleming, T. (2006). Coping with social physique anxiety in adolescence. *Journal of Adolescent Health, 39*, 275.e9–275.e16.

Krane, V., Waldron, J., Stiles-Shipley, J., & Michalenok, J. (2001). Relationships among body satisfaction, social physique anxiety, and eating behaviors in female athletes and exercisers. *Journal of Sport Behavior, 24*, 247–264.

Ladwig, M., Vazou, S., & Ekkekakis, P. (2018). "My best memory is when I was done with it": PE memories are associated with adult sedentary behavior. *Translational Journal of the American College of Sports Medicine, 3*, 119–129.

Lascar, N., Kennedy, A., Hancock, B., Jenkins, D., Andrews, R. C., Greenfield, S., & Narendran, P. (2014). Attitudes and barriers to exercise in adults with type 1 diabetes (T1DM) and how best to address them: A qualitative study. *PLoS One, 9*(9), e108019.

Leary, M. R. (1992). Self-presentational processes in exercise and sport. *Journal of Sport & Exercise Psychology, 14*, 339–351.

Leary, M. R., & Kowalski, R. M. (1990). Impression management: A literature review and two-component model. *Psychological Bulletin, 107*, 34–47.

Leary, M. R., & Tangney, J. P. (2003). The self as an organizing construct in the behavioral and social sciences. In M. R. Leary & J. P. Tangney (Eds.), *Handbook of self and identity* (pp. 3–14). Guilford.

Ledger, D., & McCaffrey, D. (2014). *Inside wearables, how the science of human behavior change offers the secret to long-term engagement*. https://medium.com/@endeavourprtnrs/inside-wearable-how-the-science-of-human-behavior-change-offers-the-secret-to-long-term-engagement-a15b3c7d4cf3

Lee, F., Hallahan, M., & Herzog, T. (1996). Explaining real-life events: How culture and domain shape attributions. *Personality and Social Psychology Bulletin, 22*, 732–741.

Lemoyne, J., Valois, P., & Guay, F. (2015). Physical self-concept and participation in physical activity in college students. *Medicine and Science in Sports and Exercise, 47*, 142–150.

Lewis, M. (2008). Self-conscious emotions: Embarrassment, pride, shame, and guilt. In *Handbook of emotions* (3rd ed., pp. 742–756). Guilford.

Lindwall, M., Asci, H., & Crocker, P. (2014). The physical self in motion: Within-person change and associations of change in self-esteem, physical self-concept, and physical activity in adolescent girls. *Journal of Sport & Exercise Psychology, 36*, 551–563.

Mack, D. E., Kouali, D., Gilchrist, J. D., & Sabiston, C. M. (2015). Pride and physical activity: Behavioural regulations as a motivational mechanism? *Psychology and Health, 30*, 1049–1062.

Mackowiak, R., Lucibello, K. M., Gilchrist, J. D., & Sabiston, C. M. (2019). Examination of actual and ideal body-related characteristics and body-related pride in adult males. *American Journal of Men's Health, 13*, 1–8.

Markus, H., & Kitayama, S. (1991). Culture and the self: Implications for cognition, emotion, and motivation. *Psychological Review, 98*, 224–253.

Markus, H. R., & Kitayama, S. (2003). Models of agency: Sociocultural diversity in the construction of action. In V. Murphy-Berman & J. J. Berman (Eds.), *Vol. 49 of the Nebraska symposium on motivation. Cross-cultural differences in perspectives on the self* (pp. 18–74). University of Nebraska Press.

Markus, H. R., & Kitayama, S. (2010). Cultures and selves: A cycle of mutual constitution. *Perspectives on Psychological Science, 5*, 420–430.

Marsh, H. W., & Craven, R. G. (2006). Reciprocal effects of self-concept and performance from a multidimensional perspective: Beyond seductive pleasure and unidimensional perspectives. *Perspectives on Psychological Science, 1*, 133–163.

Martin Ginis, K. A., Jung, M. E., & Gauvin, L. (2003a). Effects of exercising in mirrored environments on sedentary women's feeling states and self-efficacy. *Health Psychology, 22*, 354–361.

Martin Ginis, K. A., Latimer, A. E., & Jung, M. E. (2003b). No pain no gain? Examining the generalizability of the exercise stereotype to moderately active and excessive active targets. *Social Behavior and Personality, 31*, 283–290.

Martin Ginis, K. A., Lindwall, M., & Prapavessis, H. (2007). Who cares what other people think? Self-presentation in exercise and sport. In G. Tenenbaum & R. C. Eklund (Eds.), *Handbook of sport psychology* (3rd ed., pp. 136–157). Wiley.

Martin Ginis, K. A., & Mack, D. (2012). Understanding exercise behavior: A self-presentational perspective. In G. Roberts & G. Treasure (Eds.), *Advances in motivation in sport and exercise* (pp. 327–356). Human Kinetics.

Martin Ginis, K. A., Prapavessis, H., & Haase, A. M. (2008). The effects of physique-salient and physique non-salient exercise videos on women's body image, self-presentational concerns, and exercise motivation. *Body Image, 5*, 164–172.

McAuley, E., Blissmer, B., Katula, J., Duncan, T. E., & Mihalko, S. L. (2000). Physical activity, self-esteem, and self-efficacy relationships in older adults: A randomized controlled trial. *Annals of Behavioral Medicine, 22*, 131–139.

McAuley, E., Elavsky, S., Motl, R. W., Konopack, J. F., Hu, L., & Marquez, D. X. (2005). Physical activity, self-efficacy, and self-esteem: Longitudinal relationships in older adults. *The Journals of Gerontology, 60*, 268–275.

McHugh, T. L. F., Kowalski, K. C., MacK, D. E., Crocker, P. R. E., Junkin, S. E., Lejbak, L. K., & Martin, S. (2008). Young women's experiences of social physique anxiety. *Feminism and Psychology, 18*, 231–252.

Miller, P. J., Wiley, A. R., Fung, H., & Liang, C.-H. (1997). Personal storytelling as a medium of socialization in Chinese and American families. *Child Development, 68*, 557–568.

Mond, J. M., & Calogero, R. M. (2009). Excessive exercise in eating disorder patients and in healthy women. *Australian and New Zealand Journal of Psychiatry, 43*, 227–234.

More, K. R., Phillips, L. A., & Eisenberg Colman, M. H. (2019). Evaluating the potential roles of body dissatisfaction in exercise avoidance. *Body Image, 28*, 110–114.

Morin, A. J. S., Scalas, L. F., & Marsh, H. W. (2015). Tracking the elusive actual-ideal discrepancy model within latent subpopulations. *Journal of Individual Differences, 36*, 65–72.

Ninot, G., Fortes, M., & Delignières, D. (2001). A psychometric tool for the assessment of the dynamics of the physical self. *European Review of Applied Psychology, 51*(3), 205–216.

Oishi, S., & Diener, E. (2003). Culture and well-being: The cycle of action, evaluation, and decision. *Personality and Social Psychology Bulletin, 29*, 939–949.

Payne, S. M., Hudson, J., Akehurst, S., & Ntoumanis, N. (2013). Development and initial validation of the impression motivation in sport questionnaire-team. *Journal of Sport & Exercise Psychology, 35*, 281–298.

Pearl, R. L., Puhl, R. M., & Dovidio, J. F. (2015). Differential effects of weight bias experiences and internalization on exercise among women with overweight and obesity. *Journal of Health Psychology, 20*, 1626–1632.

Pila, E., Brunet, J., Crocker, P. R. E., Kowalski, K. C., & Sabiston, C. M. (2016). Intrapersonal characteristics of body-related guilt, shame, pride, and envy in Canadian adults. *Body Image, 16*, 100–106.

Pila, E., Sabiston, C. M., Brunet, J., Castonguay, A. L., & O'Loughlin, J. (2015). Do body-related shame and guilt mediate the association between weight status and self-esteem? *Journal of Health Psychology, 20*, 659–669.

Pila, E., Sabiston, C. M., Mack, D. E., Wilson, P. M., Brunet, J., Kowalski, K. C., & Crocker, P. R. E. (2020). Fitness and appearance-related self-conscious emotions and sport experiences: A prospective longitudinal investigation among adolescent girls. *Psychology of Sport and Exercise, 47*, 101641.

Pila, E., Stamiris, A., Castonguay, A., & Sabiston, C. M. (2014). Body-related envy: A social comparison perspective in sport and exercise. *Journal of Sport and Exercise Psychology, 36*, 93–106.

Renfrew, J., Howle, T., & Eklund, R. C. (2017). Self-presentation concerns may contribute towards the understanding of athletes' affect when trialling for a new sports team. *Journal of Applied Sport Psychology, 29*, 484–492.

Rhee, E., Uleman, J. S., Lee, H. K., & Roman, R. J. (1995). Spontaneous self-descriptions and ethnic identities in individualistic and collectivistic cultures. *Journal of Personality and Social Psychology, 69*, 142–152.

Robbins, B. D., & Parlavecchio, H. (2006). The unwanted exposure of the self: A phenomenological study of embarrassment. *Humanistic Psychologist, 34*, 321–345.

Sabiston, C. M., Brunet, J., Kowalski, K. C., Wilson, P. M., Mack, D. E., & Crocker, P. R. E. (2010). The role of body-related self-conscious emotions in motivating women's physical activity. *Journal of Sport and Exercise Psychology, 32*, 417–437.

Sabiston, C. M., Gilchrist, J., & Brunet, J. (2019). Self-system and processes. In T. Horn & A. Smith (Eds.), *Advances in sport and exercise psychology*. Human Kinetics.

Sabiston, C. M., Pila, E., Crocker, P. R. E., Mack, D. E., Wilson, P. M., Brunet, J., & Kowalski, K. C. (2020). Changes in body-related self-conscious emotions over time among youth female athletes. *Body Image, 32*, 24–33.

Sabiston, C. M., Pila, E., Pinsonnault-Bilodeau, G., & Cox, A. E. (2014). Social physiqueanxiety experiences in physical activity: A comprehensive synthesis of research studies focused on measurement, theory, and predictors and outcomes. *International Review of Sport and Exercise Psychology, 7*, 158–183.

Sabiston, C. M., Sedgwick, W. A., Crocker, P. R. E., Kowalski, K. C., & Mack, D. E. (2007). Social physique anxiety in adolescence: An exploration of influences, coping strategies, and health behaviors. *Journal of Adolescent Research, 22*, 78–101.

Sadalla, E. K., Linder, D. E., & Jenkins, B. A. (1988). Sport preference: A self-presentational analysis. *Journal of Sport & Exercise Psychology, 10*, 214–222.

Schlenker, B. R., & Leary, M. R. (1982). Social anxiety and self-presentation: A conceptualization and model. *Psychological Bulletin, 92*, 641–669.

Shavelson, R., Hubner, J., & Stanton, G. (1976). Self-concept: Validation of construct interpretations. *Review of Educational Research, 46*, 407–441.

Slater, A., & Tiggemann, M. (2011). Gender differences in adolescent sport participation, teasing, self-objectification and body image concerns. *Journal of Adolescence, 34*(3), 455–463.

Slutzky, C. B., & Simpkins, S. D. (2009). The link between children's sport participation and self-esteem: Exploring the mediating role of sport self-concept. *Psychology of Sport and Exercise, 10*, 381–389.

Sonstroem, R. J. (1976). The validity of self-perceptions regarding physical and athletic ability. *Medicine and Science in Sports, 8*, 126–132.

Sonstroem, R. J. (1997). The physical self-system: A mediator of exercise and self-esteem. In K. R. Fox (Ed.), *The physical self: From motivation to well-being* (pp. 3–26). Human Kinetics.

Sonstroem, R. J., Harlow, L. L., & Josephs, L. (1994). Exercise and self-esteem: Validity of model expansion and exercise associations. *Journal of Sport & Exercise Psychology, 16*, 29–42.

Sonstroem, R. J., & Morgan, W. P. (1989). Exercise and self-esteem: Rationale and model. *Medicine & Science in Sports & Exercise, 21*, 329–337.

Stets, J. E., & Burke, P. J. (2003). A sociological approach to self and identity. In M. Leary & J. Tangney (Eds.), *Handbook of self and identity* (pp. 128–152). Guilford.

Tangney, J. P., Miller, R. S., Flicker, L., & Barlow, D. H. (1996). Are shame, guilt, and embarrassment distinct emotions? *Journal of Personality and Social Psychology, 70*, 1256–1269.

Tangney, J. P., & Tracy, J. L. (2012). Self-conscious emotions. In M. R. Leary & J. P. Tangney (Eds.), *Handbook of self and identity* (pp. 446–478). Guilford.

Tetlock, P. E., & Manstead, A. S. (1985). Impression management versus intrapsychic explanations in social psychology: A useful dichotomy? *Psychological Review, 92*, 59–77.

Toft, B. S., & Uhrenfeldt, L. (2015). The lived experiences of being physically active when morbidly obese: A qualitative systematic review. *International Journal of Qualitative Studies on Health and Well-Being, 10*, 1.

Tracy, J. L., & Robins, R. W. (2004). Putting the self into self-conscious emotions: A theoretical model. *Psychological Inquiry, 15*, 103–125.

Tracy, J. L., & Robins, R. W. (2007). The psychological structure of pride: A tale of two facets. *Journal of Personality and Social Psychology, 92*, 506–525.

Troop, N. A. (2016). The effect of current and anticipated body pride and shame on dietary restraint and caloric intake. *Appetite, 96*, 375–382.

Troop, N. A., & Redshaw, C. (2012). General shame and bodily shame in eating disorders: A 2.5-year longitudinal study. *European Eating Disorders Review, 20*, 373–378.

Van Osch, Y., Zeelenberg, M., & Breugelmans, S. (2015). On the context dependence of emotion displays: Perceptions of gold medalists' expressions of pride. *Cognition and Emotion, 30*, 1332–1343.

Vani, M. F., De Jonge, M., Pila, E., Solomon-Krakus, S., & Sabiston, C. M. (2021). 'Can you move your fat ass off the baseline?' Exploring the sport experiences of adolescent girls with body image concerns. *Qualitative Research in Sport and Exercise, 13*(4), 671–689. https://doi.org/10.1080/2159676X.2020.1771409

Vani, M. F., Pila, E., Willson, E., & Sabiston, C. M. (2020). Body-related embarrassment: The overlooked self-conscious emotion. *Body Image, 32*, 14–23.

Verma, N., Eklund, R. C., Howle, T., Arthur, C., & Gibson, A.-M. (2019). Transformational teaching, self-presentation motives, and identity in adolescent female physical education. *Journal of Sport & Exercise Psychology, 41*, 1–9.

Wagnsson, S., Lindwall, M., & Gustafsson, H. (2014). Participation in organized sport and self-esteem across adolescence: The mediating role of perceived sport competence. *Journal of Sport & Exercise Psychology, 36*, 584–594.

Welk, G., & Eklund, B. (2005). Validation of the children and youth physical self-perception profile for young children. *Psychology of Sport and Exercise, 6*, 51–65.

Woodgate, J., Martin Ginis, K. A., & Sinden, A. R. (2003). Physical activity and social physique anxiety in older women: The moderating effects of self-presentation efficacy. *Journal of Applied Biobehavioral Research, 8*, 116–127.

Woodman, T., & Hemmings, S. (2008). Body image self-discrepancies and affect: Exploring the feared body self. *Self and Identity, 7*, 413–429.

Competitive Sport

Contents

Self-Regulation in Competitive Sports

Jürgen Beckmann, Denise Beckmann-Waldenmayer, and Svenja Anna Wolf

Contents

J. Schüler et al. (eds.), *Sport and Exercise Psychology*, https://doi.org/10.1007/978-3-031-03921-8_20

Learning Objectives

Basic:

- Being able to describe and differentiate between self-regulation theories in sport and exercise
- Being able to distinguish between self-regulation and self-control

Advanced:

- Being able to describe skills and different techniques for self-regulation in sport

Experts:

- Being able to explain the mediating role of positive and negative effects in self-regulation

20.1 The Function of Self-Regulation in Competitive Sports

How does a football player manage to concentrate fully on the penalty kick that decides the world cup in front of 70,000 cheering spectators, and who above all support the opposing team? How can a marathon runner resist the impulse to give up at 35 km when he feels that he is at the end of his tether? Why do some athletes regularly manage to complete their full training schedule without the coach's control, while others fail to do so? The answer to these behavioral phenomena lies in the concept of self-regulation.

Self-regulation refers to providing psychological resources for an activity for which motivation is not or is no longer sufficient to successfully complete the activity (Beckmann, 2001). Most sport psychological interventions are designed to strengthen such self-regulation processes, for example, in the context of emotion management, concentration, motivation, self-confidence, and mental preparation (Mahoney et al., 1987). Furthermore, the training example above shows that individuals differ regarding their self-regulation abilities, which needs to be taken into account when designing psychological interventions. In this chapter, we will give an overview of basic concepts of self-regulation in psychology and specifically in sport psychology.

20

20.2 Definition of Self-Regulation

In a very broad sense, self-regulation refers to the regulation of mental states and functions by individuals (Beckmann, 2001). It begins with the basic assumption that mental processes are flexible and adaptable and that actors can influence these deliberately. However, motivation alone is not sufficient for this. For example, a lack of sufficient motivation could be the problem for not initiating an activity or motivation may wane during a long and arduous period, thus leading to the discontinuation before the goal is achieved. In this respect, self-regulation has its roots in the psychology of will (Kuhl & Beckmann, 1985). Frequently, the terms self-control, action control, will, or volitional processes are used synonymously. We propose that it is useful to differentiate between different types of self-regulation. Specifically, we will distinguish between *self-regulation* and *self-control* as types of self-regulation with different functions and different consequences.

Self-Regulation

Self-regulation refers to the regulation of mental states and functions by individuals. Frequently, the terms self-control, action control, will, or volitional processes are used synonymously

Karoly (1993) defines self-regulation as internal or transactional processes that enable individuals to pursue their goal-oriented actions. This implies the regulation of cognitive processes and affect through intentional or automatic mechanisms and skills. Processes of self-regulation are initiated when internal or external obstacles arise that endanger the efficient realization of an intended action. Therefore, Kuhl (2001) uses *action control* as the general term for self-regulation. In connection with self-regulation or action control, Kuhl also speaks of auxiliary processes that support basic action processes such as attention and motivation if the basic action processes are not sufficient to ensure optimal action.

> Processes of self-regulation are initiated when **internal** or **external obstacles** arise that endanger the efficient realization of an intended action

Baumeister and Vohs (2007) understand self-regulation as the ability of the self to change its own actions. Here, the term "action" is used very broadly, because self-regulation can also consist of changing an emotional state. Self-regulation can also be necessary when different beliefs or self-perceptions do not match, such as "I am a team player" and "It's every man for himself." Perception of this discrepancy results in the unpleasant state of cognitive dissonance, which motivates a reduction of the dissonance (Festinger, 1957). Dissonance reduction can be achieved, for example, by adding cognitive arguments to reconcile the statements, such as "Good individual performance will benefit the team." Hence, dissonance reduction is ultimately a form of self-regulation that supports action stabilization (or action control; Beckmann & Irle, 1985; Harmon-Jones & Harmon-Jones, 2019).

Similarly, emotion regulation, that is, individuals' efforts to influence the quality, intensity, and timing of their emotional experiences and expressions (Gross, 2015) also constitutes a form of self-regulation to reduce the discrepancy between actual and desired emotional states (Friesen et al., 2019). Emotion regulation refers to the individuals' efforts to influence the quality, intensity, and timing of their emotional experiences and expressions. It is a form of self-regulation in the sense that it reduces the discrepancy between actual and desired emotional states.

The prerequisite for self-regulation is that the problem situation is recognized and evaluated in order to decide which resources (skills, competences, strategies) are available to deal with the problem. Positive or negative self-talk (e.g., "I can do it" vs. "it will never work out") influences the perception of resources as well as the efficiency of the selection and the resultant use of resources (Kirschenbaum, 1984; Williams et al., 2000). All of these processes can take place both consciously and unconsciously. According to Karoly (1993), the effectiveness of self-evaluation and resource-selection depends on individuals' mental skills for identifying discrepancies between desired goals and current actions, whereby the initial problem identification is the result of effective self-monitoring.

❓ In total, effective self-regulation presupposes three essential prerequisites (see ◘ Fig. 20.1):

1. The person must have an idea of the target state they try to achieve (e.g., via binding standards or ideals).
2. The person must have access to their own self through which they can organize psychological processes and functions to remove blockades and achieve the desired target states.
3. The person must possess (meta-cognitive and/or meta-motivational) knowledge about resources they can use to cope with critical situations. This knowledge does not necessarily have to be explicit or conscious. In many cases, rather, it is an implicit competence.

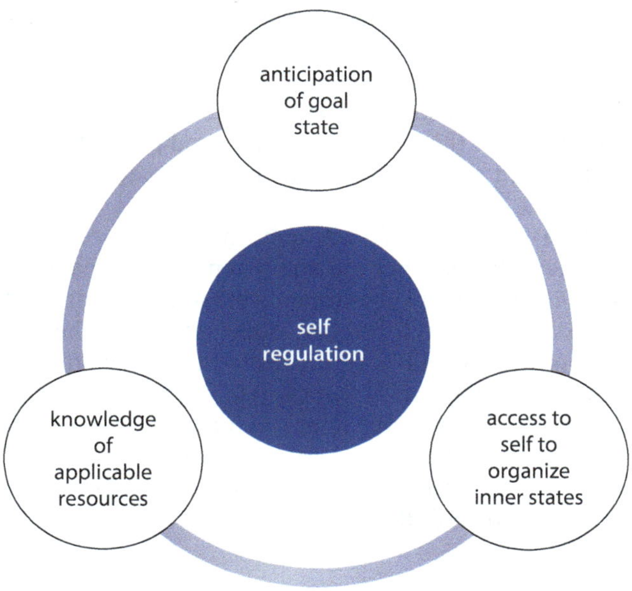

◘ **Fig. 20.1** Components of self-regulation

In summary, self-regulation processes are conscious as well as unconscious auxiliary processes that ensure that goal-oriented activity or performance is maintained even when external or internal obstacles occur and impulses need to be controlled and that action is aligned appropriately with the given situation.

❓ According to Kuhl et al. (2006), there are three basic functions of self-regulation:

1. The maintenance of an action
2. The inhibition of competing action tendencies or the inadequate initiation of an action
3. The removal of execution inhibition if conditions are considered favorable

20.3 Origins of the Psychological Concept of Self-Regulation

The beginning of modern sport psychology in the 1960s and 1970s was dominated by relaxation interventions, which can be considered a very basic form of self-regulation. For this reason, they continue to constitute an integral component of basic sport psychology training (Beckmann & Elbe, 2015).

In psychology, there is a longer tradition of addressing self-regulation as a process of will (cf. Kuhl & Beckmann, 1985). Mischel's (1974, 2014) experiments on delay of gratification, the postponement of rewards, were groundbreaking investigations in the study of self-regulation (see ► Chap. 10). Here, self-regulation serves to suppress the impulse to take immediate, consuming action in the case of an attractive reward (one marshmallow) when a considerably higher reward (two marshmallows) could be obtained if one managed to wait (◘ Fig. 20.2).

Because the higher reward is not immediately available and can only be obtained by not consuming the immediately available one, strategies are required to resist the impulse to take the immediately available smaller reward and manage to wait. Follow-up studies showed that their parents also rated children who dis-

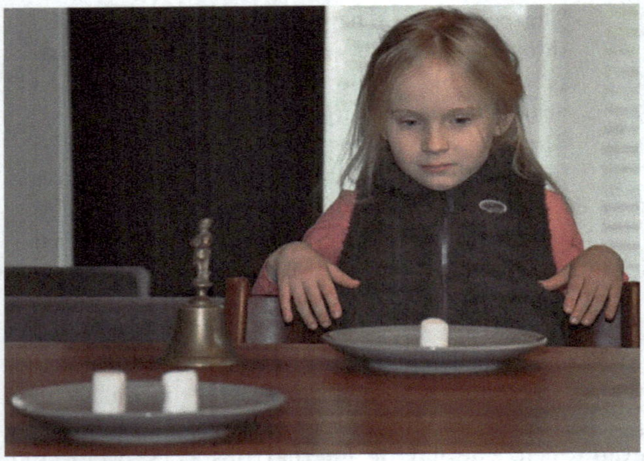

Fig. 20.2 The "Marshmallow Test." Resisting to taking the immediate small reward (one marshmallow) for getting a delayed larger reward (two marshmallows). Note. The figure can be found in the German version of the book. The picture was taken by the authors themselves and is not available to us. The illustration is available to Springer (Heidelberg) as ► Fig. 19.2

played greater stamina in this so-called marshmallow experiment as more socially competent, frustration-tolerant, and successful in school (Shoda et al., 1990). In addition, they had better scores in English and Mathematics on the Scholastic Aptitude Test (SAT). Watts et al. (2018) criticize Mischel's original studies in terms of representativeness and found in their own research only a weak increase in the ability to postpone rewards from the age of 4 to the age of 15. In contrast, other more recent replication studies (e.g., Duckworth et al., 2013) confirm Mischel's (1974) assumptions that the ability to delay gratification refers to the basic ability to control oneself.

Self-Control in Psychological Skill Training

Since the 1960s, behavioral therapists have increasingly included self-control processes in their therapeutic procedures. Cognitive processes are addressed as problem-solving strategies such as "structuring" or "clarifying inconsistencies" that enable individuals to better control and manage their own behavior (or actions; cf., e.g., Kanfer, 1970). Toward the end of the 1970s, models and techniques of behavioral control from clinical psychology increasingly found their way into the developing field of applied sport psychology (e.g., Mahoney & Avener, 1977). These self-control strategies have become the core elements of "mental training" or "psychological skill training."

20.4 Self-Regulation Skills and Techniques

20.4.1 Naïve Self-Regulation Techniques

Self-regulation is very important in everyday life, such as resisting the temptation to eat sweets when you have newly decided to go on a diet. In martial arts, for example, athletes must follow strict diets in order to reach or maintain their fighting weights, although their strenuous training may result in increased hunger. Competitive sports generally require a high degree of such self-discipline, which is a form of self-regulation. This includes the young swimmer who manages to pull herself out of bed every day for swim practice before school, the marathon runner who holds out when his stamina is dwindling, as well as the Alpine skier who starts the high-risk downhill run despite a fear of injury. In many of these cases, athletes employ naïve self-regulation techniques. These are highly personalized techniques for situations in which a challenge or threat is perceived. Everyday self-regulation strategies can be referred to as "naïve" because they are not based on scientific knowledge and therefore their actual effectiveness is not validated. These techniques develop through the person's experience of the situation and subjective assessment of what appears to be helpful in the situation. Naïve self-regulation often also consists of superstitious behavior combined with various rituals (Keinan, 2002). It can be observed that the frequency of the use of naïve self-regulation techniques increases with the pressure to perform and one's own insecurity (Dömötör et al., 2016). Dömötör et al. (2016) state in their literature review that superstitious behavior can certainly contribute to the self-regulation of affect (e.g., reduction of anxiety) and thus to athletic success. However, this may be merely a placebo effect that leads to an increased perception of control and self-confidence in uncertain competitive situations.

A disadvantage of such naïve self-regulation techniques can be that they are not systematically related to factors that actually impair performance. As mentioned above, they may involve superstitious behavior. Therefore, they will not be consistently successful. At some point, the coach's team will lose, even if he wears his lucky sweater. In the long run, naive self-regulation techniques are thus less successful than the formal and structured psychological skills provided by sport psychology (Morris & Bull, 1991).

20.4.2 Self-Regulation and Self-Control: Two Fundamental Modes

As mentioned before, different terms for self-regulation are occasionally used synonymously. The previously given examples show that self-regulation can involve quite different mechanisms and strategies. Kuhl (1994) proposed a fundamental differentiation between self-regulation and self-control in terms of functionality and consequences, including them under a super ordinate concept of volitional strategies or self-management. According to Kuhl, *self-regulation* describes a strengthening of current intention through different individual resources (e.g., beliefs, values, incentives). Conversely, *self-control* captures a defense against disturbances by inhibiting competing impulses.

> *Self-regulation* describes a strengthening of current intention through different individual resources (e.g., beliefs, values, incentives).

> *Self-control* captures a defense against disturbances by inhibiting competing impulses (e.g., suppression of emotional expressions; Gross, 2015).

In line with this distinction, Beckmann (1989) found that individuals use two types of self-regulation processes when they face obstacles that interfere with the realization of an intended action. On the one hand, relatively simple mechanisms such as increased effort in the attempt to concentrate and block out disturbing elements are used to fight the interference. For example, if the motivation to continue is exhausted, marathon runners could tell themselves continuously to "keep going." On the other hand, more elaborate strategies are used, for example, to achieve motivation control. For example, the marathon runners could imagine the positive reactions of people who are important to them after crossing the finish line. Importantly, the simpler mechanism, self-control, is only successful over a limited period of time because it consumes energy resources and may sometimes be inconsistent with individuals' regular preferences (e.g., implicit needs). Rothbart et al. (2000) also speak of "exerted control," referring primarily to executive attention regulation and inhibitory control. This is in essence what Kuhl and Beckmann (1994a) have described as processes involved in self-control. Baumeister et al. (1998) also associated the term "volitional exhaustion" (i.e., volitional depletion or ego depletion) with this type of self-control, neglecting the more sophisticated alternative of self-regulation. In contrast to resource-consuming, strained self-control, self-regulation is a more complex strategy that can be used in the long term without leading to exhaustion (Kuhl & Beckmann, 1994a). In fact, if the marathon runners manage to focus on the subjective incentives of running (i.e., motivation control), they may potentially get into a state of flow. Flow is characterized by the complete absorption in an activity resulting in an effortless nature of the performance (Csikszentmihalyi, 1975).

> **Flow**
>
> Flow is characterized by the complete absorption in an activity resulting in an effortless nature of the performance

The cognitive costs of self-control are especially apparent in the context of emotion regulation. In particular, both reappraisal (i.e., the attempt to change one's cognitive evaluation of a situation, comparable to self-regulation) and expressive suppression (i.e., the attempt to inhibit one's emotion expression, comparable to self-control) are effective strategies to regulate one's emotional response (Gross, 2015). However, in this process, expressive suppression (i.e., self-control) consumes important cognitive capacity that impairs individuals' memory (Gross, 2002; Richards & Gross, 2000), effort (Low et al., 2017), and, specific to a sport context, (cycling and tennis) performance (Monaci & Veronesi, 2019; Wagstaff, 2014). Conversely, reappraisal (i.e., self-regulation) leaves cognitive capacity (i.e., memory) and performance intact (Gross, 2002; Monaci & Veronesi, 2019; Richards & Gross, 2000).

The function of both self-control and self-regulation is to maintain control over actions and to ensure that goals are achieved. The strategies pursue different routes, however, to fulfill this function. Self-control is primarily concerned with inhibiting disturbing mental processes, such as a low self-efficacy or competing action tendencies and the associated disturbing thoughts. Self-regulation, on the other hand, involves coordinating personal subsystems (motivational, affective, cognitive) in such a way that the intended action tendency is strengthened and facilitated (cf. Kuhl, 2001). With regard to self-control, one could also speak of self-discipline or willpower. In the example of the marathon runners who feel they are about to withdraw from the race due to their exhausted motivation, may find themselves repeating the mantra "I must not give up" once a television camera is pointed in their direction. This therefore results in the runners pushing themselves to finish the race successfully. Thus, because there is a constant need for this type of volitional strategy in competitive sports, self-control can be used very effectively. Although extremely useful in the moment, sophisticated self-regulation can actually be considered much more pleasant and in the long run, more beneficial. Here, an attempt is made to influence the motivational basis of the current activity in such a way that the temptation to change actions, for example, to skip swimming training, disappears. In this case, swimmers may look for aspects of the training that they particularly enjoy or they may visualize personally important goals that can only be achieved through consistent practice.

If athletes solely rely on self-control in the long term, negative effects can ensue as they may experience alienation from their preferred intentions (cf. Kuhl & Beckmann, 1994b). Rather than relying and therefore acting on their own interests, they instead are driven by obligation. This leads to a loss of the sense of self-determination and competence that is fundamental to intrinsic motivation (cf. Deci & Ryan, 1985). Various studies suggest that by blocking access to one's own (implicit) self, creative potential is lost. The midfielder in football, for example, is no longer the designer of his team's game (Kazen, Kuhl et al., 2015; Kuhl & Beckmann, 1994a, 1994b). Additionally, a perceived loss of autonomy may also lead to mental health problems (Cresswell & Eklund, 2007).

The same applies to performers' emotion-regulation. If their environment (e.g., sport, organizational, or team norms; Tamminen et al., 2016; Tibbert et al., 2015; Wagstaff et al., 2012) constantly requires them to align their emotions with their prescribed (work) roles (i.e., perform emotional labor; Hochschild, 1983), this can take a toll on performers' mental health. Specifically, if individuals such as coaches (Lee & Chelladurai, 2016) use self-control (i.e., surface acting, e.g., expressive suppression; Grandey & Melloy, 2017) to achieve the desired emotional responses, they feel depleted in their willpower and report more strain, dissatisfaction, and exhaustion (Grandey & Melloy, 2017; Trougakos et al., 2015). Conversely, if coaches draw upon self-regulation (i.e., deep acting, e.g., reappraisal; Grandey & Melloy, 2017), this has no impact on their levels of exhaustion (Lee & Chelladurai, 2016).

While self-control focuses on the inhibition of unwanted activities, self-regulation activates supporting processes (e.g., self-talk, emotions). Neuroscientific research shows that training such executive functions can actually change the architecture of the brain (Kühn et al., 2013). Specifically, these processes of neuronal plasticity are related to mindfulness-based procedures. Kühn et al. (2013) found that different areas of the brain are activated when an emotional response is self-regulated via mindfulness in comparison to when an attempt is made to suppress the specific emotion on command. This approach offers numerous possibilities for (sport) psychological interventions, which we will discuss in more detail below (Sect. 20.6.8; ◘ Fig. 20.3).

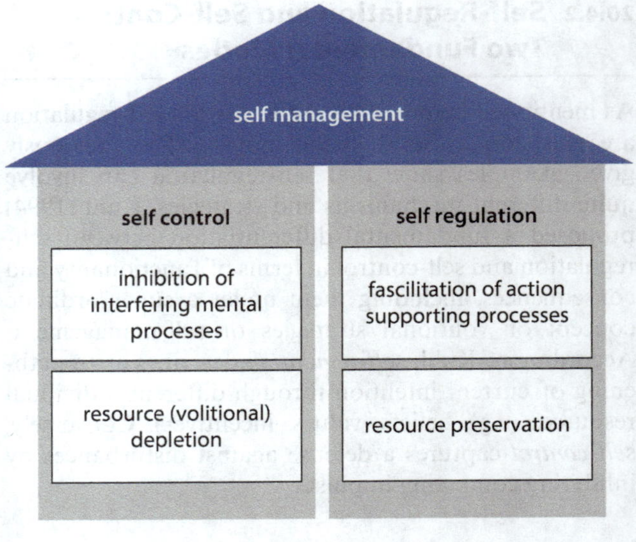

◘ **Fig. 20.3** Types of self-control

20.5 Development of Self-Regulation: How to Develop and Train the Will Muscle

The development of self-regulation is generally regarded as a decisive factor for successful adaptation in childhood and adolescence (cf. Mischel, 2014). But how do self-regulation skills develop? Recent research reveals that the development of self-regulatory skills is not completed in childhood but continues into later stages. Notably, basic forms of self-regulatory competence develop in childhood (King et al., 2013) and become increasingly elaborate during adolescence (Roberts et al., 2001). Corresponding developments both at the behavioral level (Monahan et al., 2009) and the neurobiological level (Luna et al., 2004; King et al., 2013) occur at least into early adulthood (cf. Beckmann et al., 2006).

According to Kuhl and Kraska (1989), rudimentary forms of self-regulation can already be found in early childhood. In Mischel's marshmallow experiments (Mischel, 1974), for example, even 4-year-old children resisted the temptation to eat the marshmallow immediately by occupying themselves with other things or simply **blocking** out the marshmallows by closing their eyes. Conversely, elaborate strategies, such as **incentive con-**

trol, in which motivational incentives are sought, do not develop until adolescence and adulthood, because they are based on the development of meta-motivational knowledge. An important prerequisite for the development of the elaborated strategies is that children and adolescents are given opportunities to master difficult situations. However, it is essential that they deal with the challenges in a self-determined way (Kuhl & Kraska, 1989). By conceptualizing the will as a muscle that needs to be trained, Lindworsky (1923) demanded a practice of the will by independent accomplishments of difficult challenges already.

Development of Self-Regulation Skills in Young Athletes

Beckmann et al. (2006) later confirmed these assumptions of Lindworsky's school of will empirically in a longitudinal study. In this study, athlete and non-athlete students from seventh to twelfth grade were tested annually over 6 years (September 1998 through October 2003) for the development of motivational and volitional parameters. The study revealed that young athletes showed a stronger volitional development than non-athlete students. This is easily understood, considering that young athletes experience many challenges in their sports independently from an early age. Therefore, this places demands on persistence and failure management. Thus, they are not merely training their physical muscles but also their "will muscle."

Beckmann et al.'s study also found that with increasing age, simpler forms of self-regulation (e.g., anxious self-motivation) are replaced by more elaborate ones (e.g., positive self-motivation). The strongest development of elaborate self-regulation was found in young athletes who lived in specialized boarding schools. This effect can be explained by the superior amount of self-determined leisure time of the boarding school athletes. At first sight, it might be surprising that athletes at boarding schools had more self-determined leisure time than athletes living at home. At second glance, it makes sense, however, because self-determined leisure time of young athletes who lived with their parents was consumed almost completely by the necessary traveling between school, sport facilities, and their parental homes.

Finally, advantages in the area of the volitional abilities of young athletes compared to the volitional abilities of regular students partly existed prior to the time of enrollment in the seventh grade. Interestingly, the probability of premature career termination increased when leaders (e.g., coaches, boarding school teachers) did not take into account young athletes' previously well-developed self-regulation skills and restricted the young athletes in the use of their abilities (Elbe et al., 2003). This generated conflicts between self-determined actions and external control, resulting in frustration and reduced motivation ultimately leading to a dropout (Fig. 20.4).

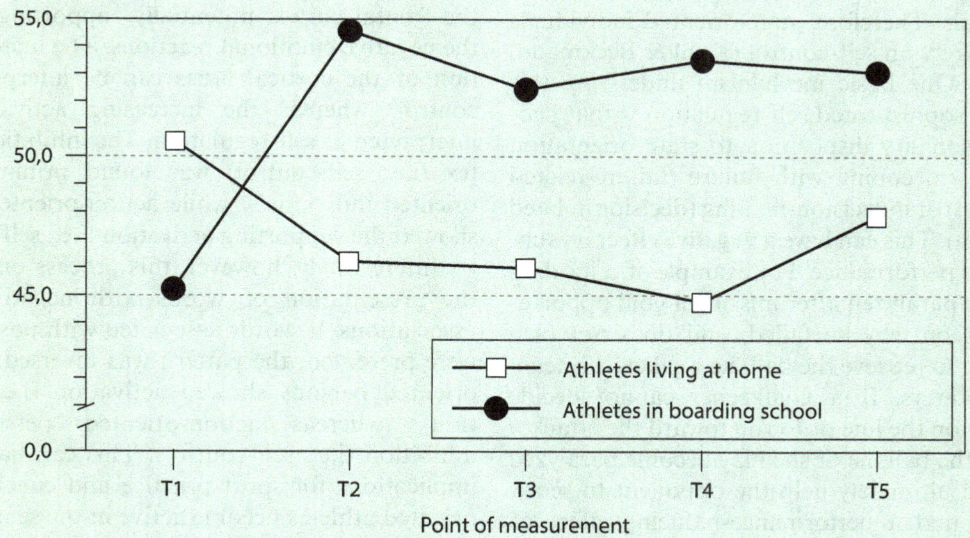

Fig. 20.4 Developmental increase of self-regulation skills in boarding school athletes compared to athletes living at home (Beckmann et al., 2006)

20.5.1 Individual Differences in Self-Regulation

Individual differences in self-regulation are already present in early childhood. For example, differences in temperament, which have a great impact on impulse control, are found to be partly genetic and thus available at a young age (Auerbach et al., 2001). Furthermore, correlates of individual differences can also be found at the neural level. Specifically, the orbitofrontal cortex (OFC), referred to as the "Executive Brain" (Goldberg, 2009) seems to play a crucial role in self and emotion regulation. Petrovic et al. (2015) found a correlation between the volume of the OFC and the ability to regulate emotions. Furthermore, a reduced volume of this brain area was also found in patients with borderline personality disorder and antisocial personality disorder. In addition, Dolcos et al. (2015) discovered that adults with a larger OFC were less anxious and more optimistic. Finally, research has shown that the central modulation is related to the personality trait of action and state orientation (▶ Chap. 10).

In general, connections between personality traits and athletic performance are described as very weak (Conzelmann, 2001). However, in the area of self-regulation there are numerous findings demonstrating that the disposition to action versus state orientation affects self-regulation and thereby athletic performance. It can be said that action-oriented individuals can use self-regulation strategies very efficiently, whereas sophisticated self-regulation is generally impaired in state-oriented individuals. Therefore, state-oriented individuals mostly need to rely on self-control (Kuhl & Beckmann, 1994a, 1994b). One basic mechanism underlying this impairment of sophisticated self-regulation is that people with a personality disposition to state orientation have difficulties in coping with failure (failure-related state orientation) or indecision-making (decision-related state orientation). This can have a negative effect on subsequent athletic performance. For example, if a football player becomes paralyzed after missing a goal opportunity, ruminates on why he failed, and does not turn around and run to retrieve the ball, he weakens his team in defensive powers. If a goalkeeper cannot decide whether to stay on the line or to run toward the attacker who possesses the ball, he or she may become paralyzed in inaction and ultimately help the opponent to score. Kuhl (1981) found a performance-reducing effect of such "learned helplessness" caused by a series of failures on a subsequent cognitive task-performance in the case of individuals with high state rather than high action orientation. In a study by Strang et al. (1987), sport students first received a series of failure experiences (failure training) before they performed a complex motor task. The number of errors on this task was four times as high for state-oriented participants compared to action-oriented participants.

> Action orientation as a personality variable refers to the disposition to deliberately but not necessarily consciously focus attention on factors that support the execution of the action.

> State orientation is associated with an increased shift of attention to situational factors and mental persevering (rumination), which impairs the intuitive execution of the action.

The different effects of the dispositions for action or state orientation are particularly evident in pressure situations, such as athletic competitions. State-oriented individuals show chronic negative affect or a lack of positive affect and tend to ruminate excessively over failures or decision alternatives. Consequently, the self-regulation capacity of state-oriented people is reduced. Conversely, action-oriented people show a high efficiency in self-regulation. This is illustrated in a study by Kuhl et al. (1994), in which two different reactions to the presentation of words associated with negative emotions were found in the EEG. One was an increasing inhibition of cortical areas emanating from the frontal cortex. The other reaction to the same words consisted of increasing activation of cortical areas starting from the frontal cortex, potentially supporting coping with the negative emotional reactions. The increasing inhibition of the cortical areas can be interpreted as self-control, whereas the increasing activation can be interpreted as self-regulation. The inhibition of the cortex (i.e., self-control) was found primarily in state-oriented individuals, while action-oriented individuals showed the supporting activation (i.e., self-regulation).

Interestingly, however, this process only applied to the presentation of words with negative emotional associations. If words associated with positive emotion were presented, the pattern was reversed. Then, state-oriented persons showed activation (i.e., self-regulation), whereas action-oriented persons showed inhibition (i.e., self-control). This can have important implications for sport practice and coaching: Action-oriented athletes become active in the sense of self-regulation when the situation is rather stressful or even aversive. In contrast, if the situation is less demanding and rather positive, the self-regulation mode is not activated in action-oriented persons (cf. Antoni & Beckmann, 1989). State-oriented athletes can also use the resource-activating self-regulation mode, but only in a situation that is positive or relaxed. In some areas, the disposition to state orientation can have advantages. Because state-oriented individuals consider more variants of a current action than those who are action-oriented, they should also have more problem-solving options. Indeed, Beckmann and Trux (1991) found that state-oriented playmakers had an advantage over action-oriented playmakers. At least in this study, playmakers in higher divisions (first and second Bundesliga) in basketball and volleyball were in the majority state- rather than action-oriented.

Action-Oriented Athletes

- Show stable performance in high-pressure situations (e.g., under time pressure, under fatigue, after failure) and in competitions
- Risk more and take on responsibility in sports
- Can be found in executing positions in sport games such as the striker in soccer or the center in basketball

State-Oriented Athletes

- Constantly perform at a high level in practice but tend to show performance decreases in competitions and high-pressure situations
- Are sensitive to and need coaches' and teammates' support and precise instructions, yet implement these instructions and follow tactical routes accurately
- Excel in maximum strength sports such as 100 m sprint
- Can be found in organizing/playmaking positions in sport games such as the midfielder in soccer or the point guard in basketball

The perception of state orientation can be analyzed differently dependent on the individual's current situation. Kuhl (1994), for example, assumes that state orientation is associated with a rather rigid and context-insensitive acceptance of rules imposed by others. In this respect, coaches will favor state-oriented athletes as they have the need to consistently comply with instructions as well as follow the given tactical routes (Beckmann & Trux, 1991). However, state-oriented athletes will only succeed in doing so as long as their tendency to ponder, for example, over a failed action, does not interfere with their plans. Sahre (1991) was able to show that in critical game situations (e.g., a close score toward the end of a game) action-oriented players are more likely to control their nerves and thus take advantage of scoring opportunities than state-oriented players.State-oriented players obviously need as concrete and precise instructions as possible from the coach, whereas such instructions can conflict with the flexible self-regulation potential action-oriented players may possess. The latter can even benefit from pressure situations, which in turn may be more likely to cause problems in state-oriented athletes. This was confirmed in a study by Heckhausen and Strang (1988). A record instruction (i.e., trying to beat the high score) in a basketball task resulted in increased effort for both action and state-oriented players, but resulted in enhanced scoring for action-oriented athletes only. State-oriented players ran faster under the record construction than in normal conditions, but did not score more baskets. In contrast, action-oriented players also increased the number of baskets while simultaneously increasing running speed (cf. Sahre, 1991). The reason for this seems to be that action-oriented players know how to regulate the utilization of their available resources more effectively than state-oriented players and only put in as much effort as is beneficial to performance. Such an effective regulation of effort is not feasible for state-oriented players. Accordingly, under the record-breaking instruction their resources were quickly exhausted. Building on these findings, Häger et al. (2015) found a connection between the disposition to action versus state orientation and the chronic self-regulatory focus of a person (Higgins, 1997). According to Higgins' Regulatory Focus Theory, goals with a promotion focus (focus is on hope and fulfillment) are distinguished from goals with a prevention focus (focus is on duty and security). Häger et al. discovered that failure-related state orientation in basketball players related to a chronic prevention focus. In contrast, action-oriented players tended to have a high promotion focus. According to regulatory focus theory, this should be associated with a better focus on achieving personally important goals or personally important ideas.

20.6 Applied Perspectives: Mental Skills Training

In a qualitative study by Heiss (2012), elite athletes reported which volitional strategies (self-regulation strategies) they use for self-management. The most frequent strategies mentioned were environmental control (prevention), mental programming and routines to switch off thinking, positive self-talk (self-motivation), and relaxation. The athletes were found to have used both naive self-regulation strategies as well as strategies taught through mental skills training. In the following, we will give an overview of basic contents of mental skills used for self-regulation in sports (for detailed practical information on mental skills training, see, e.g., Beckmann & Elbe, 2015). First, we will address forms of

Fig. 20.5 Overview of sport psychological basic and skills trainings

Basic Training		
Relaxation	• Breathing • Progressive Muscle Relaxation • Autogenic Training	Increasing Complexity
Skills Training		
Motivational Skills	Goal Setting	Specific, hard but realistic goals
	Positive/Negative Self Motivation	e.g. focus on positive incentives
Volitional Skills	Attention Regulation	Focus on execution-relevant information
	Emotion Control	Make use of supportive emotions
	Self-Efficacy	Positive beliefs regarding own competencies
	Self-Talk Regulation	Positive, supportive inner dialogue
Embodiment Skills	Dynamic Handgrip	Dynamic clenching of left hand to generate relaxation
	Posture Control	Upright posture, “Gait of the matadors”

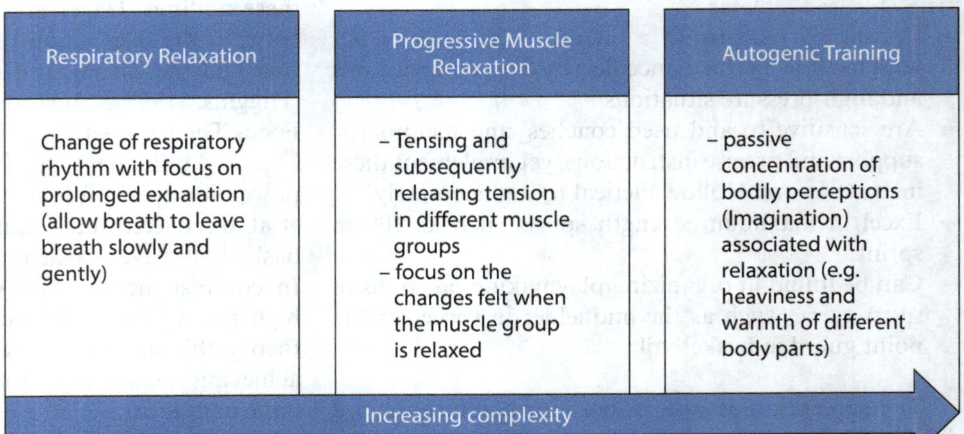

Fig. 20.6 Forms of relaxation training

self-regulation that regulate basic organismic functions comprehensively. These include activation regulation and maintenance of a stress-recovery balance. Subsequently, we will address more specific skills that belong to the standard repertoire of psychological skills training such as goal-setting, imagery, and self-talk (Fig. 20.5).

20.6.1 Activation Regulation: The Individual Zone of Optimal Functioning

A very basic form of self-regulation is **activation regulation**. Because it is a very basic and overarching skill, Beckmann and Elbe (2015) also speak of basic training. For quite some time, the assumption of an inverted U-curve regarding the relationship of arousal or activation and performance, with medium activation as optimal for performance (Yerkes & Dodson, 1908) prevailed. However, modern approaches have become more differentiated. A current orientation is provided by Hanin's (2000) so-called IZOF model. According to this model of an “individual optimal zone of functioning” (IZOF), each athlete has an optimal level of activation for a specific task (see also ► Chap. 11). With regard to the influence of IZOF, various studies have shown that successful athletes reported activation levels prior to competition that were significantly closer to their IZOF than less successful athletes (Raglin & Hanin, 2000). In order to enable athletes to reach their individual optimal zone, classical relaxation methods such as **respiratory relaxation, progressive muscle relaxation,** and **autogenic training** have proven particularly helpful (Kellmann et al., 2018; Fig. 20.6).

These methods can also be used to modulate the cognitive and emotional components of one's state such as worry. For example, when disturbing thoughts are triggered by anxiety (see ▶ Chap. 12), overly analytical focusing on technical elements can be reduced or eliminated. Furthermore, in competitions, respiratory relaxation appears to be particularly successful. It relieves tension and thereby reduces straining thoughts (worries) instantaneously without diminishing the necessary competition tension. Outside of competitions, progressive muscle relaxation and autogenic training in particular can lead to more serenity and less anxiety in the end. However, the latter methods reduce the competition tension necessary for optimal functioning and should therefore not be used immediately before the start of a competition.

20.6.2 Stress-Recovery Balance: Getting Physical and Psychological Rest

An important area for maintaining a high level of performance in sports over a longer period of time and avoiding overtraining and burnout is a balance of experienced stress and recovery. The recovery-stress questionnaire (RESTQ, Kallus & Kellmann, 2016) can be used to assess and monitor athletes' recovery-stress balance. It has also been used in numerous studies and applied settings (see Kellmann & Beckmann, 2018).

Self-Reflection

The REST-Q (Kallus & Kellmann, 2016) is used to monitor athletes' recovery-stress balance over time. How recovered or stressed are you at the moment? Use the following example items from the REST-Q to visualize your personal recovery-stress levels.

In the past 3 days…	1-never	2	3	4	5	6	7-always
1 general stress. …I felt down							
2 emotional stress. … I was in a bad mood							
3 social stress. … I was angry with someone							
4 conflicts/ pressure. … I felt under pressure							
5 fatigue. … I was overtired							
6 lack of energy. … I was unable to concentrate well							
7 physical complaints. … I felt uncomfortable							
8 success. … I finished important tasks							
9 social recovery. … I had a good time with my friends							
10 physical recovery. … I felt at ease							
11 general Well-being. … I was in a good mood							
12 sleep quality. … I had a satisfying sleep							
13 disturbed breaks. … too much was demanded of me during the breaks							
14 emotional Exhaution. … I felt that I wanted to quit my sport							
15 injury. My performance drained me physically							
16 being in shape. … I was in a good condition physically							
17 personal accomplishments. … I dealt very effectively with my teammates' problems							

In the past 3 days...	1-never	2	3	4	5	6	7-always
18 self-efficacy. … I was convinced that I had trained well							
19 self-regulation. … I prepared myself mentally for performance							

If athletes do not manage to terminate preoccupation with athletic activities, which is often the case after failure, this lack of deactivation generates continued stress and can also impair or disrupt a subsequent recovery through continued brooding (Eccles & Kazmier, 2019). Recently, the importance of post-actionable self-regulation to deactivate thinking about this action has been applied to the area of recovery (Beckmann, 2002). It has been shown that the dispositions of both action and state orientation as well as volitional skills have an influence on recovery. State-oriented people, who generally show impaired self-regulation, particularly in processing failure, were found to have a less favorable recovery-stress balance than action-oriented people This means that their stress level remains relatively high over a longer period of time, while their recovery is comparatively low (Beckmann & Kellmann, 2004).

Strategies that help to focus attention on the here and now such as the concept of mindfulness, which will be addressed later, have proven to be helpful to cease ruminations and obstructive evaluations. For example, the "54,321 exercise" (Dolan, 1991) could lead to a thought-stop at this point. In this method, athletes first fixate on a spot in the environment and then name five things they see, five things they hear, and five things they feel. In the next step, they name four things, then three, and so on. If athletes also have an idea of which thoughts are personally most helpful for them, they can further combine such post-actionable deactivation exercises with a new orientation toward positive thoughts.

20.6.3 Goal Setting as Self-Regulation: A Motivational Technique

From our perspective, goal setting is a volitional or self-regulation technique to increase motivation. Hence, not surprisingly, the concept of goal setting is practiced more or less systematically in almost all sports (Weinberg, 1992). In fact, setting difficult, specific goals can improve athletic performance. Specifically, in a review of 201 studies in different performance areas with more than 40,000 participants, Locke and Latham (1990) found that 91% of success was related to setting difficult, specific goals. A nice example of the effect of setting a specific goal can be seen in the field of physiotherapy. When patients with movement restrictions in the shoulder and elbow joints are told, "close your eyes and lift your arm as high as possible…, higher…, even higher," they reach considerably lower than when they follow the specific request "please grab that book up there from the shelf." When setting goals as a self-regulation measure, it is of further crucial importance that these goals are accepted and consequently internalized by athletes (Erez & Zidon, 1984).

Research shows that many athletes set at least two types of goals for themselves, namely, outcome goals and process goals (Jones & Hanton, 1996). However, if outcome goals relate only to performance results and consequences, they may in turn lead to increased anxiety levels (Burton, 1989) and may even result in withdrawal from a competition (Roberts, 1986). In contrast, as a study by Kingston and Hardy (1997) illustrated, golfers who used process-oriented goals ("Where do I play the ball") were able to concentrate better and control negative thoughts more efficiently than golfers who used outcome-oriented goals. Additionally, a third type of goal is performance goals. Performance goals are objectives that an athlete expects to achieve within a set period of time. Higher-level, long-term performance goals (i.e., career goals) are very important for stabilizing motivation, especially under difficult conditions. After an injury, it can be important to focus attention on long-term performance goals to maintain motivation during the sometimes-lengthy rehabilitation process. In competition, on the other hand, performance can be stabilized primarily by attention-directing process goals (Orlick & Partington, 1988).

Athletes should be made aware that different goals can be used at different times—depending on individual progress and needs (Hardy, 1996). According to available research findings, a multiple-objective strategy with an even balance between outcome, performance, and process goals seems to lead to the best performance (Filby et al., 1999). Another area of importance is the repeated evaluation of goals and, if necessary, the adaption to change them. This ensures that the process of goal setting as a self-regulation technique in the sense of maintaining or increasing motivation functions sustainably.

Key Points

An even balance between different types of goals benefits athletic performance (see also ► Chap. 7)

Outcome Goals
Outcome goals describe what outcome is aspired to (e.g., the ranking in a competition)

Process Goals
Process goals define specific aspects of the executions of an action in sports, and they are concerned with strategies or skills performed in a certain sport situation (e.g., a calm breath during swimming).

Performance Goals
Performance goals describe individual performance parameters and focus on self-related standards of excellence (e.g., improve the number of successful passes compared to the previous game).

20.6.4 Imagination and Imagination Training: Programming Successful Performance

In the study by Heiss (2012) cited above, the self-regulation strategy (self-management) athletes mentioned most frequently was imagery or imagination training. In imagery, a certain action or movement is mentally practiced to improve or stabilize a certain athletic skill. "For this purpose, an internal representation of the action is activated and the execution of this action—as optimally as possible—is repeated and mentally simulated in a selected context. This mental simulation takes place without any observable physical activity (Schack, 2006, p. 255). Among other uses, imagery can be employed in sports in which training runs are limited due to the given conditions (e.g., bobsleigh, luge, and skeleton). Additionally, this method can be used to prepare for performance immediately before a competition, such as mentally skiing through a slalom course in one's own imagination before the start.

Imagination is a comprehensive form of mental programming in which a reality is created with all of the senses without the actual stimuli being present (MacIntyre et al., 2013). Imagination goes beyond mere imagery because it involves as many senses as possible and is not limited to the retrieval of a pictorial or linguistic image of the execution of the motor skill. Therefore, as an idea of the feeling of an optimally realized movement (athletic skill), it can in many cases be completely independent of verbal representations, because the focus is on the physical perceptions associated with the performance. Imagination thus strengthens the pattern of optimal movement execution in the brain and includes regulation of activation, the strengthening of self-efficacy. It can also support the healing process after sport injuries.

Orlick and Partington (1988) report that 99% of the top athletes they studied use imagery. Overall, top athletes make more use of imagery than less successful athletes (Hall et al., 1991). High-performance and competitive athletes use imagination more frequently, more purposefully and with greater focus, and consider this method to be more relevant and significant than recreational athletes (Nordin et al., 2006). These athletes also incorporate more varied forms of imagination in their practice.

20.6.5 Routines: Helping to Prepare and Focus

In the study by Heiss (2012), athletes also mentioned routines as important self-regulation strategies. A routine is referred to as a process that proceeds in approximately the same way every time it is executed (Beckmann & Elbe, 2015). According to the general understanding of the term, having a routine means that you can confidently carry out a task without having to think about its execution. If an individual acts routinely, the possibility of falling out of rhythm and thus becoming disturbed or preoccupied by other thoughts is less likely to occur.

Routine
A routine is a structured process that proceeds in approximately the same way every time it is executed. A routine in sports includes psychological skills that are functional for the solution of a task at hand (cf. Schack et al., 2005).

In contrast to rituals, which can be considered naïve self-regulation strategies, routines are well organized but still allow flexibility (Schack et al., 2005). The most important difference between rituals and routines is that routines include psychological or self-regulation skills that are functional for solving the task at hand, for example, because they eliminate disturbing thoughts and instead build up concentration. Rituals, on the other hand, are rather ceremonial and may contain superstitious elements. The function of routines is to stabilize action through self-regulation skills. They create a "deliberate microcosm that can be controlled" (Schack et al., 2005, p. 145). The objective of routines is to optimize the preparation of athletic performance or, in the case of a post-performance routine, to terminate an action that has been executed. Routines combine several of the aforementioned self-regulation skills such as respiratory relaxation and imagery in a fixed, functional order. Using a routine helps athletes to prepare for performance or terminate mental occupation with a finished activity. It is very important that a routine consist of a meaningful or functional sequence of self-regulation skills in a relatively fixed time sequence, leaving no room for disturbing thoughts or worries.

Because athletes' needs in the preparation for performance are highly individual, the development of their own personal routines is essential. The better they understand their needs and the functions of their routine, the more likely their needs are to be met and the effectiveness of their routine is increased (cf. Schack et al., 2005, p. 138). Numerous studies confirm this theory (Cohn, 1990; Mesagno et al., 2008). For example, Crews and Boutcher (1986) found that experienced and successful female golfers had much more elaborate pre-shot routines than inexperienced golfers and in turn, applied them much more consistently.

Studies in various sports such as diving (Highlen & Bennett, 1983), golf (Cohn et al., 1990), tennis (Moore, 1986), gymnastics (Mahoney & Avener, 1977), and volleyball (Schack, 1997) show that the best performance effects are achieved with routines that include both cognitive elements (e.g., attention focusing, slogans) and physical elements (e.g., breathing, trial movement). Another important aspect of self-regulation can be found in the so-called post-performance routines. These routines are carried out after the completion of an athletic activity (e.g., after a golf shot or after firing a shot in sport shooting) and thus involve a conscious termination of the activity. Especially for state-oriented athletes, post-performance routines can be essential for maintaining or regaining good performance in the further progress of the competition (Beckmann & Elbe, 2015).

> Routines help stabilize sport performance:
> - If they include a functional set of relaxation techniques and are organized in a fixed time sequence, leaving no room for disturbance
> - If they are highly individual
> - If they involve cognitive (e.g., attention focusing) and physical elements (e.g., breathing)
> - Because they benefit the preparation of a performance
> - Because they help terminate conscious occupation with an athletic performance after completion

20

20.6.6 Embodiment: How the Body Affects the Mind

In addition to the physical elements of breathing and trial movements, routines can also include specific embodiment techniques. Human information processing takes place in a constant interaction between the body, its sensorimotor state, and its mental representation, a process, which is called "embodiment" (Koch, 2011; see also ► Chap. 6 in this book). Mental states affect physical states such as facial expressions, posture, and body tension, and vice versa, bodily states affect mental states. For example, dejection after failure is frequently manifested in a bent back and drooping shoulders. At the same time, however, the state of the body also has a reverse effect on information processing, motivation, and, in particular, how one feels. For example, if the muscles that are necessary for laughing are activated, this leads to a better mood even without any positive event (Strack et al., 1988).

Because physical states can be influenced deliberately, a self-regulation of psychological processes such as affect can be achieved through changes in posture and other bodily expressions. Instead of letting their shoulders sag, athletes can deliberately show a proudly swollen chest despite failure; instead of letting the corners of their mouths fall, they can paste on a smile. This increases the chances that their motivational and emotional states will improve accordingly. In addition, such expressive changes activate brain structures that access representations of one's own strengths, thus enhancing self-confidence and self-efficacy. In addition, the athletes do not disclose potential weaknesses to their opponents but demonstrate self-confidence and strength. Another advantage of embodiment techniques as self-regulation strategies is that they do not rely on verbal instructions and can therefore be easily and quickly realized.

For example, a very simple embodiment technique that can be effortlessly incorporated into routines is the squeezing of a ball with the left hand. Dynamic left-hand clenching was found to lead to a relaxation effect in the brain, effectively eliminating thoughts that interfere with a smooth execution of a motor skill (Cross-Villasana et al., 2015). A number of studies in various sports have shown that this can prevent choking under pressure, for instance, during penalty shootouts (Beckmann et al., 2013) and tennis serves (Beckmann et al., 2021).

20.6.7 Self-Talk Regulation: Optimizing the Inner Dialogue

The self-regulation strategies outlined above attempt to switch off conscious thinking especially task-irrelevant, disturbing thoughts or focus thinking on task-promoting aspects. However, another option is to maintain conscious thinking or the "inner dialogue," yet regulate it to be more adaptive. Often, athletes lose a competition when their inner dialogue has turned negative. In the sense of Gallwey (1976), the inner "voice of doubt" with its negative messages gains the upper hand here. Statements such as, "I can't play long passes today,"

"Today is not my day," or "My serve simply won't come today" characterize the soliloquy in this case. This is often accompanied by an inner dialogue marked by helplessness: "I don't know what's going on either," "Why am I so bad?" After such statements, one can hardly expect to return to a good level of performance. Various research studies have illustrated that such negative self-talk is associated with mediocre athletic performance (van Raalte et al., 1994) and that athletic performance can be improved by practicing self-talk regulation (Hatzigeorgiadis et al., 2009). Self-talk can be used successfully to increase effort (Rushall, 1984), direct attention to relevant stimuli (Beckmann-Waldenmayer & Aeply, 2012; Schmid & Peper, 1993),, induce a change of mood (Hardy & Fazey, 1990), reduce competition anxiety (Hatzigeorgiadis et al., 2009), and support rehabilitation after a sport injury (Levleva & Orlick, 1991).

Self-talk helps:
- Increase effort
- Direct attention to relevant stimuli
- Change your mood
- Rehabilitation after sport injury

Hardy (2006) also distinguishes between motivational and instructive self-talk. Motivational self-talk (e.g., "Let's go! Let's go now!") should be used for activation regulation. Instructional soliloquies (e.g., "Exact and snappy!" when aiming in biathlon) are suitable for fine motor tasks where the execution of movements, timing, and accuracy play a decisive role. Furthermore, the effectiveness of self-talk can be enhanced by the addition of imagination (Cumming et al., 2006).

Accordingly, the optimization of the inner dialogue is an important goal of psychological skills training. To improve their self-talk, athletes first need to determine which self-statements are detrimental and which are beneficial for them. The initial step is generally to become aware of disturbing and performance-inhibiting thoughts. In a second step, these thoughts are then reformulated or reframed in order to positively support performance. These self-statements must be systematically practiced and thus integrated into the athletic training (Table 20.1).

A very effective method to better understand and optimize self-talk is to set up an "inner team" (Schulz von Thun, 1998). This metaphor addresses the different, partly contradictory trains of thoughts that can run through our heads when trying to make a decision. It aims to identify as many inner voices as possible in order to be able to use them in a helpful and functional way. Athletes should first give names to their inner voices or team members (e.g., the coach, the self-confident, the fearful, the defiant, or references to people that have a certain significance to them; e.g., Messi) and write down a characteristic sentence or statement for each voice. Afterward, the respective benefit of each voice's contribution is assessed (e.g., helps me in my further development, promotes social contacts). This intervention allows the athletes to assume a meta-perspective regarding their inner dialogue and to ultimately change and enhance this with the help of preexisting self-statements (e.g., other more helpful voices). Furthermore, experience has shown that most athletes are rather surprised to discover the "negative" voices do indeed have functional or beneficial aspects dependent on their specific amount or "volume." The superior "I" of the athlete assumes either a passive observer role or the mediating role between the different members of the inner team in this inner dialogue. It can thus consciously control positive change. Through this, athletes can develop the confidence that they have control over their own thoughts and thus are able to use them beneficially for themselves.

Table 20.1 Example for the optimization of inner dialogues

Negative self-talk	Rephrased positive self-talk alternative
My heart is beating out of my chest—I am so incredibly nervous!	I can clearly feel my activation—Now I am ready to go!
If I make a mistake, I have failed!	If I make a mistake, I will learn from it!
Only if I win today, I can be satisfied.	If I do my best today, I will be satisfied.

20.6.8 Mindfulness Training: An Alternative Avenue to Strengthen Self-Regulation

Previous research has shown that a dispositional state orientation can be shifted toward action orientation through behavioral therapy measures (Hartung & Schulte, 1994). For example, Altfeld et al. (2017) found that mental training in basketball can increase players' action orientation. As mentioned, Lindworsky (1923) compared the will (volition) with a muscle that needs to be trained, and sport seems to provide favorable conditions for such training. Young athletes experience many failures and through their experience, learn how to master difficult situations time and time again. As the findings of a longitudinal study with adolescent athletes show, this seems to contribute to the strengthening of volitional abilities (Beckmann et al., 2006).

The development and use of more elaborate self-regulation strategies requires access to one's own resources. Every person has highly individual resources to cope with or master problem situations (Langosch, 2015). While purely behavioral therapeutic interventions primarily aim to teach individual's concrete self-control strategies, other therapeutic methods focus on helping clients to discover and develop their own coping resources. Although such a procedure promises long-term success, it first requires access to one's own implicit self (Kuhl, 2001). Mindfulness-based methods can help to facilitate this access.

There are numerous definitions of the concept of mindfulness in the psychological literature. For this chapter, we refer to a frequently cited definition by Kabat-Zinn (1982). He understands mindfulness as a specific form of attention that is intentional and nonjudgmental and refers to the current moment of experience (the here and now). Accordingly, current external and internal processes such as thoughts, feelings, and body perceptions are perceived attentively without further evaluation. Mindfulness-based interventions have been implemented and evaluated in psychotherapy since the 1970s (see Ospina et al., 2007). Although there were some methodological shortcomings in the evaluation studies, the effectiveness of mindfulness-based interventions on emotion regulation via fMRI has since been demonstrated in initial studies (Creswell et al., 2007; Way et al., 2010).

Mindfulness

Mindfulness is a specific form of attention that is intentional and nonjudgmental and refers to the current moment of experience (e.g., thoughts, feelings, body perceptions) without further evaluation.

In accordance with the construct of mindfulness, (sports) psychological interventions aim to enable athletes to stay in the here and now with their thoughts, rather than remain fixated on a previous mistake or failure that would lead to concern in the future. Through the intervention, they learn to detach themselves consciously from disturbing thoughts in order to focus on the current situation. Furthermore, as described above (▶ Sect. 20.6.2), athletes also learn to approach feelings and body perceptions mindfully. For example, sport shooters who act attentively after a miss would perceive that they experience feelings of anger and rage, but would not identify with these negative feelings—they *have* the feelings, but they are not controlled *by* their feelings. The shooters can manage not to succumb to the negative feelings, for instance, by practicing wide mindful attention and observing that, positive feelings (e.g., pride that they qualified for this competition, hope to place the next shots well) are also present at the same time. An important part of this mindful attitude is not to evaluate these feelings, but only to perceive them. Therefore, having such feelings would not be labeled as "good" or "bad," but rather acknowledged for being present, and able to change again in the following moments. This way, athletes have an opportunity to distance themselves from the negative feelings and "let them go." Additionally, a helpful technique for athletes would be, for example, to first pause consciously for a moment—perhaps with a long exhalation. Then, they would direct their attention to all the stimuli perceived by their senses (i.e., what can they see, hear, smell, feel, taste?). Perhaps, athletes could also observe how the thoughts pass by—how thoughts come and go again—only to gradually refocus on the task at hand. Mindfulness techniques are thus recommended as thought stopping techniques, as relaxation techniques in the sense of (short) meditation, as impulse control for emotion regulation, or as a part of sport psychological routines. As previously mentioned, various studies have shown that mindfulness can help to stabilize and improve athletic performance (Bühlmayer et al., 2017).

Mindfulness techniques are recommended as:
- Thought-stopping techniques
- Relaxation techniques (e.g., meditation)
- Impulse control techniques for emotion regulation
- Part of sport psychological routines

20.6.9 Music as a Self-Regulation Strategy: Marching to Your Own Rhythm

Music has long been used by athletes for self-regulation. More recently, Karageorghis (2017) has included music as a means of self-regulation based on systematic research on the effect of music on athletic performance. He distinguishes three different forms of intervention: synchronous, asynchronous, and preparatory interventions. In synchronous interventions, the rhythmic aspects of music are used to regulate movement patterns. For example, a three-fourth beat can structure a golf swing. The synchronous aspect can also be used to regulate energy in endurance sports, thereby increasing efficiency. In asynchronous interventions, there is no conscious synchronization. The music rather plays in the background and shows positive effects in terms of reduced perceived exhaustion and increased joy in the activity. Finally, music can be used to prepare for a performance, for example, to activate or relax and to posi-

20

tively influence the mood of athletes or teams before a competition. In general, according to Karageorghis (2017), fast, loud music has a stimulating effect and can be used for a so-called "psyching-up." Quiet, slow music, on the other hand, has a calming effect.

20.6.10 Emotion Regulation: Prevention Is Better Than Cure

As this chapter shows, influencing emotions and mood is a central theme of self-regulation. According to Gross' (1998) process model of emotion regulation (see also ▶ Chaps. 11 and 12), individuals can draw upon both antecedent- and response-focused strategies to attain their desired responses. Research has shown, however, that response-focused strategies (e.g., expressive suppression; Gross' (1998) detract self-control resources from the primary task and hence reduce performance (Monaci & Veronesi, 2019; Wagstaff, 2014). Thus, from a self-regulation and cognitive resource perspective, athletes, coaches, and other performers should rather employ antecedent-focused strategies (e.g., reappraisal; Gross, 1998). In other words, as the British Association of Sport and Exercise Sciences put it in their Expert Statement on emotion regulation in sport (Lane et al., 2012), "where dysfunctional emotions in sport are concerned, prevention might be better than cure" (p. 1192).

Side Story

On September 12, 2021, Novak Djokovic had the chance to win the US Open and with this be the first male player to complete a tennis grand slam (i.e., win all four major tournaments of the season) in 52 years. Djokovic, who to that date had been ranked the world's number one for 337 consecutive weeks and not lost a single three-set match the entire season, however, lost to Daniil Medvedev in three straight sets. Remarkably, toward the end of the match, when it started to become clear that Medvedev was going to win, Djokovic suddenly burst into tears as a response to the audience's audible and continued support and could not stop crying, even while playing his final set. He was "overcome with emotion" a number of media outlets titled and indeed, it seemed as if Djokovic had not enough self-control left to contain his emotional response that likely had built up over the course of the pressurized match and maybe the whole tournament. Of course, we do not know how Djokivic had played, had he not be tasked with controlling his emotions, if he would indeed have been able to devote these self-control resources to his match play instead. Yet, it seems clear how pressurized and emotionally taxing competitive sports can be and how much self-control and regulation they require before the performers indeed "spill over."

Nonetheless, attaining an optimal emotional state is crucial, also for performers' self-regulation. Kuhl (2001) postulates in his theory of personality-system interactions (PSI theory) that positive affect activates intuitive action control, while negative affect activates discrepancy-sensitive object recognition. This means that with positive effect, initiative is shown and action is taken, while with negative affect the person becomes cautious and reactions are controlled by the situation. The own potential (e.g., creative ideas) is not used. Particularly the presence of positive affect and the absence of negative affect seem to have a significant performance-supporting effect, even if negative emotions can occasionally trigger a reactance effect ("Now more than ever!"; Kuhl, 2001). Many coaches still seem to rely on giving their players a "good talking to" after a bad first half and thereby creating negative team affect (Staw et al., 2019; van Kleef et al., 2019). According to Kuhl (2001), however, this blocks many functions that would be required in the game, such as creativity and initiative. Consequently, teams of coaches displaying (excessive) anger at halftime performed worse rather than better in the second half of the match (Staw et al., 2019; van Kleef et al., 2019), likely because they experienced more anger themselves (van Kleef et al., 2019). Conversely, research has shown that positive effect, or the extent to which a person feels enthusiastic, active, and lively, promotes flexible and creative thinking (Isen et al., 1987). Indeed, teams whose coaches displayed happiness instead of anger performed better, likely because they experienced greater happiness themselves (van Kleef et al., 2019). It would therefore be desirable for the coach to aim for the reduction of negative affect and the induction of positive affect during the halftime break.

Key Points

According to Kuhl (2001), affect can powerfully influence sport performance:

Positive Affect

- Helps taking initiative and action
- Makes people more enthusiastic and lively and promotes flexible and creative thinking
- Leads to activation of intuitive action control

Negative Affect
- Makes athletes cautious and actions controlled by the situation
- Leads to activation of discrepancy-sensitive object recognition

Positive Affect can be increased by self-regulation (emotion regulation):
- Coaches' speeches
- The design of a workout and prosocial actions (e.g., by teammates)
- Feedback and positive reinforcement (e.g., by coaches and teammates)
- Humor

Coaches' efforts in these situations can described as extrinsic (Gross, 2015) or interpersonal emotion regulation (Niven et al., 2009). Coaches can influence their athletes' emotions not only via speeches (Evans et al., 2018) but via a variety of strategies including the design of a workout, distraction, and positive reinforcement (Braun & Tamminen, 2020). Teammates, too, can influence each other's emotions strategically, for example, via positive and technical feedback, cueing, or prosocial actions (Palmateer & Tamminen, 2018; Tamminen & Crocker, 2013; Wolf et al., 2018). With this, teammates and coaches could be great resources to athletes because athletes can "outsource" their emotion regulation and dedicate their self-regulation capacities to the primary performance task.

In this context, humor could be a particularly beneficial strategy, both as players' self-regulation against the influence of a negative coach or teammate as well as an interpersonal emotion regulation strategy to induce positive affect and enable players' full potential. This is supported in a study by Burke et al. (1995) who found positive correlations between humorous behaviors of the coach and positive evaluations by his athletes. In addition, teammates frequently use humor to regulate each other's emotions (Palmateer & Tamminen, 2018; Tamminen & Crocker, 2013) or cope with stressors together (Leprince et al., 2019).

20.7 Concluding Remarks

20

The explanations in this chapter illustrate the many different forms of self-regulation used in sport, specifically in competitive sports, and their ability to support and stabilize athletic performance. This has been well-proven empirically in numerous studies (e.g., Weinberg & Comar, 1994). Not only competition performance but also training and regeneration are supported by self-regulation. It is important to distinguish between self-control and self-regulation as different self-regulation strategies, because there are differences in functionality and resource consumption. For sport psychologists in applied settings, as well as coaches, knowledge of this and the related individual differences in self-regulation is important. As the knowledge about the neurophysiological basis of self-regulation increases, neurofeedback training maybe a promising avenue to increase athletes' competence in self-regulation in the future (Mirifar et al., 2017).

Learning Control Questions

Basic:
1. What is the difference between self-regulation and self-control?
2. What's the marshmallow test?
3. What's the difference between state orientation and action orientation?

Advanced:

4. Can you name some forms of relaxation trainings?
5. Can you define what a routine is and how it can help to prepare and focus?
6. Explain how self-talk can help self-regulation.

Experts:

7. How does emotion regulation relate to self-regulation and self-control?
8. What would be the best way to regulate emotions from a self-regulation perspective?
9. Why use mindfulness procedures? And how?

References

Altfeld, S., Langenkamp, H., Beckmann, J., & Kellmann, M. (2017). Evaluation of psychological orientated basketball exercises in team practice to improve self-regulation. *International Journal of Sports Science and Coaching, 12*, 725–736.

Antoni, C., & Beckmann, J. (1989). An action control conceptualization of goal setting and feedback effects. In U. E. Kleinbeck, H. H. Quast, H. Thierry, & H. Häcker (Eds.), *Work motivation* (pp. 41–52). Erlbaum.

Auerbach, J. G., Ebstein, R., Kahana, M., & Levine, J. (2001). The association of the dopamine D4 receptor gene (DRD4) and the serotonin transporter promoter gene (5-HTTLPR) with temperament in 12-month-old infants. *Journal of Child Psychology and Psychiatry, 42*, 777–783.

Baumeister, R. F., Bratslavsky, E., Muraven, M., & Tice, D. M. (1998). Ego depletion: Is the active self a limited resource? *Journal of Personality and Social Psychology, 74*, 1252–1265.

Baumeister, R. F., & Vohs, K. D. (2007). Self-regulation, ego depletion, and motivation. *Social and Personality Psychology Compass, 1*, 115–128. https://doi.org/10.1111/j.1751-9004.2007.00001.x

Beckmann, J. (1989). Erhöhte Leistung nach unzureichender Motivationskontrolle. *Zeitschrift für Experimentelle und Angewandte Psychologie, 36*, 1–15.

Beckmann, J. (2001). Self-regulation of athletic performance. In N. J. Smelser & P. B. Baltes (Eds.), *International encyclopedia of the social and behavioral sciences* (pp. 14947–14952). Elsevier.

Beckmann, J. (2002). Interaction of volition and recovery. In M. Kellmann (Ed.), *Enhancing recovery: Preventing underperformance in athletes* (pp. 269–282). Human Kinetics.

Beckmann, J., & Elbe, A. (2011). *Praxis der Sportpsychologie in Wettkampf- und Leistungssport* (2nd ed.). Spitta-Verlag.

Beckmann, J., & Elbe, A. (2015). *Sport psychological interventions in competitive sports*. Cambridge Scholars Publishing.

Beckmann, J., Elbe, A.-M., Szymanski, B., & Ehrlenspiel, F. (2006). *Chancen und Risiken vom Leben im Verbundsystem von Schule und Leistungssport—Psychologische, soziologische und sportliche Leistungsaspekte*. Sport und Buch Strauß.

Beckmann, J., Fimpel, L., & Wergin, V. V. (2021). Preventing a loss of accuracy of the tennis serve under pressure. *PLoS ONE, 16*(7), e0255060. https://doi.org/10.1371/journal.pone.0255060

Beckmann, J., Gröpel, P., & Ehrlenspiel, F. (2013). Preventing motor skill failure through hemisphere-specific priming: Cases from choking under pressure. *Journal of Experimental Psychology: General, 142*, 679–691.

Beckmann, J., & Irle, M. (1985). Dissonance and action control. In J. Kuhl & J. Beckmann (Eds.), *Action control: From cognition to behavior* (pp. 129–150). Springer.

Beckmann, J., & Kellmann, M. (2004). Self-regulation and recovery: Approaching an understanding of the process of recovery from stress. *Psychological Reports, 95*, 1135–1153.

Beckmann, J., & Trux, J. (1991). Wen lasse ich wo spielen? Persönlichkeitseigenschaften und die Eignung für bestimmte Positionen in Sportspielmannschaften. *Sportpsychologie, 5*, 18–21.

Beckmann-Waldenmayer, D., & Aeply, J.-E. (2012). Sportschießen Pistole—Das kennt doch jeder, oder doch nicht?! In D. Beckmann-Waldenmayer & J. Beckmann (Eds.), *Handbuch sportpsychologischer Praxis* (pp. 177–187). Spitta.

Braun, C., & Tamminen, K. A. (2020). Coaches' interpersonal emotion regulation and the coach-athlete relationship. *Movement and Sports Sciences—Science et Motricite, 105*(3), 37–51. https://doi.org/10.1051/sm/2019011

Bühlmayer, L., Birrer, D., Röthlin, P., Faude, O., & Donat, L. (2017). Effects of mindfulness practice on performance-relevant parameters and performance outcomes in sports: A metaanalytic review. *Sports Medicine, 47*(11), 2309–2321.

Burke, K. L., Peterson, D., & Nix, C. L. (1995). The effects of the coaches' use of humor on female volleyball players' evaluation of their coaches. *Journal of Sport Behavior, 18*, 83–90.

Burton, D. (1989). Winning isn't everything: Examining the impact of performance goals on collegiate swimmers' cognitions and performance. *The Sport Psychologist, 3*, 105–132.

Cohn, P. J. (1990). Pre-performance routines in sport: Theoretical support and practical applications. *The Sport Psychologist, 4*, 301–312.

Cohn, P. J., Rotella, R. J., & Lloyd, J. W. (1990). Effects of a cognitive-behavioral intervention on the preshot routine and performance in golf. *The Sport Psychologist, 4*, 33–47.

Conzelmann, A. (2001). *Sport und Persönlichkeitsentwicklung*. Hofmann.

Cresswell, S. L., & Eklund, R. C. (2007). Athlete burnout: A longitudinal qualitative study. *The Sport Psychologist, 21*(1), 1–20.

Creswell, J. D., Way, B. M., Eisenberger, N. I., & Lieberman, M. D. (2007). Neural correlates of dispositional mindfulness during affect labeling. *Psychosomatic Medicine, 69*, 560–565.

Crews, D., & Boutcher, S. H. (1986). An exploratory observational behaviour analysis of professional female golfers during tournament play. *Journal of Sport Behavior, 9*, 51–58.

Cross-Villasana, F., Gröpel, P., Doppelmayr, M., & Beckmann, J. (2015). Unilateral left-hand contractions produce widespread depression of cortical activity after their execution. *PLoS One, 10*(12), e0145867. https://doi.org/10.1371/journal.pone.0145867

Csikszentmihalyi, M. (1975). *Beyond boredom and anxiety*. Jossey-Bass Publishers.

Cumming, J., Nordin, S. M., Horton, R., & Reynolds, S. (2006). Examining the direction of imagery and self-talk on dart-throwing performance and self-efficacy. *The Sport Psychologist, 20*, 257–274.

Deci, E. L., & Ryan, R. M. (1985). *Intrinsic motivation and self-determination in human behavior*. Springer Science & Business Media.

Dolan, Y. (1991). *Resolving sexual abuse: Solution-focused therapy and Ericksonian hypnosis for adult survivors*. W.W. Norton.

Dolcos, S., Hu, Y., Iordan, A. D., Moore, M., & Dolcos, F. (2015). Optimism and the brain: Trait optimism mediates the protective role of the orbitofrontal cortex gray matter volume against anxiety. *Social Cognitive and Affective Neuroscience, 11*, 263–271. https://doi.org/10.1093/scan/nsv106

Dömötör, Z., Ruíz-Barquín, R., & Szabo, A. (2016). Superstitious behavior in sport: A literature review. *Scandinavian Journal of Psychology, 57*, 368–382. https://doi.org/10.1111/sjop.12301

Duckworth, A. L., Tsukayama, E., & Kirby, T. A. (2013). Is it really self-control? Examining the predictive power of the delay of gratification task. *Personality and Social Psychology Bulletin, 39*, 843–855. https://doi.org/10.1177/0146167213482589

Eccles, D. W., & Kazmier, A. W. (2019). The psychology of rest in athletes: An empirical study and initial model. *Psychology of Sport and Exercise, 44*, 90–98.

Elbe, A.-M., Beckmann, J., & Szymanski, B. (2003). Das Dropout Phänomen an Eliteschulen des Sports—ein Problem der Selbstregulation? *Leistungssport, 33*, 46–49.

Erez, M., & Zidon, I. (1984). Effects of goal acceptance on the relationship of goal difficulty to performance. *Journal of Applied Psychology, 69*, 69–78.

Evans, A. L., Turner, M. J., Pickering, R., & Powditch, R. (2018). The effects of rational and irrational coach team talks on the cognitive appraisal and achievement goal orientation of varsity football athletes. *International Journal of Sports Science and Coaching, 13*, 431–438. https://doi.org/10.1177/1747954118771183

Festinger, L. (1957). *A theory of cognitive dissonance*. Stanford University Press.

Filby, W. C., Maynard, I. W., & Graydon, J. K. (1999). The effect of multiple-goal strategies on performance outcomes in training and competition. *Journal of Applied Sport Psychology, 11*, 230–246.

Friesen, A., Stanley, D., Devonport, T., & Lane, A. M. (2019). Regulating own and teammates' emotions prior to competition. *Movement and Sports Sciences—Science et Motricite, 105*(3), 5–15. https://doi.org/10.1051/sm/2019014

Gallwey, T. (1976). *Inner tennis: Playing the game*. Random House.

Goldberg, E. (2009). *The new executive brain*. Oxford University Press.

Grandey, A. A., & Melloy, R. C. (2017). The state of the heart: Emotional labor as emotion regulation reviewed and revised. *Journal of Occupational Health Psychology, 22*, 407–422. https://doi.org/10.1037/ocp0000067

Gross, J. J. (1998). The emerging field of emotion regulation: An integrative review. *Review of General Psychology, 2*, 271–299. https://doi.org/10.1037/1089-2680.2.3.271

Gross, J. J. (2002). Emotion regulation: Affective, cognitive, and social consequences. *Psychophysiology, 39*, 281–291. https://doi.org/10.1017/s0048577201393198

Gross, J. J. (2015). Emotion regulation: Current status and future prospects. *Psychological Inquiry, 26*, 1–26. https://doi.org/10.1080/1047840X.2014.940781
Häger, J., Schlapkohl, N., & Raab, M. (2015). Lassen sich Leistungsunterschiede im Basketballfreiwurf durch die Regulatory Focus Theorie und die Handlungskontrolltheorie erklären? *Zeitschrift für Sportpsychologie, 21*, 149–160. https://doi.org/10.1026/1612-5010/a000128
Hall, C. R., Rogers, W. M., & Buckolz, E. (1991). The effect of an imagery training program on imagery ability, imagery use and figure skating performance. *Journal of Applied Sport Psychology, 3*, 109–125.
Hanin, Y. L. (2000). Individual zones of optimal functioning (IZOF) model: Emotion-performance relationships in sport. In Y. L. Hanin (Ed.), *Emotions in sport* (pp. 65–89). Human Kinetics.
Hardy, J. (2006). Speaking clearly: A critical review of the self-talk literature. *Psychology of Sport and Exercise, 7*, 81–97.
Hardy, L. (1996). Testing the predictions of the cusp catastrophe model of anxiety and performance. *Sport Psychologist, 10*, 140–156.
Hardy, L., & Fazey, J. (1990). *Mental rehearsal: A guide for sports performance*. National Coaching Foundation.
Harmon-Jones, E., & Harmon-Jones, C. (2019). Understanding the motivation underlying dissonance effects: The action-based model. In E. Harmon-Jones (Ed.), *Cognitive dissonance: Reexamining a pivotal theory in psychology* (pp. 63–89). American Psychological Association. https://doi.org/10.1037/0000135-004
Hartung, J., & Schulte, D. (1994). Action- and state-orientations during therapy of phobic disorders. In J. Kuhl & J. Beckmann (Eds.), *Volition and personality: Action versus state orientation* (pp. 217–232). Hogrefe & Huber.
Hatzigeorgiadis, A., Zourbanos, N., Mpoumpaki, S., & Theodorakis, Y. (2009). Mechanisms underlying the *self-talk*-performance relationship: The effects of motivational self-talk on self-confidence and anxiety. *Psychology of Sport and Exercise, 10*, 186–192.
Heckhausen, H., & Strang, H. (1988). Efficiency under record performance demands: Exertion control - an individual difference variable? *Journal of Personality and Social Psychology, 55*, 489–498.
Heiss, C. (2012). *How do elite athletes lead themselves? Transferring a revised concept of self-leadership to sport psychology* [Dissertation]. Technische Universität München.
Higgins, E. T. (1997). Beyond pleasure and pain. *American Psychologist, 52*, 1280–1300. https://doi.org/10.1037/0003-066X.52.12.1280
Highlen, P. S., & Bennett, B. B. (1983). Elite divers and wrestlers: A comparison between open- and closed-skill athletes. *Journal of Sport Psychology, 5*, 390–409.
Hochschild, A. R. (1983). *The managed heart*. University of California Press.
Isen, A. M., Daubman, K. A., & Nowicki, G. P. (1987). Positive affect facilitates creative problem solving. *Journal of Personality and Social Psychology, 52*, 1122–1131.
Jones, G., & Hanton, S. (1996). Interpretation of competitive anxiety symptoms and goal attainment expectancies. *Journal of Sport and Exercise Psychology, 18*, 144–157.
Kabat-Zinn, J. (1982). An outpatient program in behavioral medicine for chronic pain patients based on the practice of mindfulness meditation: Theoretical considerations and preliminary results. *General Hospital Psychiatry, 4*, 33–47.
Kallus, W., & Kellmann, M. (Eds.). (2016). *RESTQ. The recovery-stress-questionnaires*. Pearson.
Kanfer, F. (1970). Self-regulation: Research, issues, and speculations. In C. Neuringer & J. Michaels (Eds.), *Behavior modification in clinical psychology* (pp. 178–220). Appleton-Century-Crofts.
Karageorghis, C. I. (2017). *Applying music in exercise and sport*. Human Kinetics.
Karoly, P. (1993). Mechanisms of self-regulation: A systems view. *Annual Review of Psychology, 44*, 23–52.
Keinan, G. (2002). The effects of stress and desire for control on superstitious behavior. *Personality and Social Psychology Bulletin, 28*(1), 102–108.
Kellmann, M., & Beckmann, J. (Eds.). (2018). *Sport, recovery, and performance*. Routledge.
Kellmann, M., Pelka, M., & Beckmann, J. (2018). Psychological relaxation techniques to enhance recovery in sports. In J. Kellmann & J. Beckmann (Eds.), *Sport, recovery, and performance* (pp. 247–259). Routledge.
King, K. M., Lengua, L. J., & Monahan, K. C. (2013). Individual differences in the development of self-regulation during pre-adolescence: connections to context and adjustment. *Journal of Abnormal Child Psychology, 41*(1), 57–69.
Kingston, K., & Hardy, L. (1997). Effects of different types of goals on processes that support performance. *The Sport Psychologist, 11*, 277–293.
Kirschenbaum, D. S. (1984). Self-regulation and sport psychology: Nurturing an emerging symbiosis. *Journal of Sport Psychology, 6*, 159–183.
Koch, S. (2011). *Embodiment. Der Einfluss von Eigenbewegung auf Affekt, Einstellung und Kognition. Experimentelle Grundlagen und klinische Anwendungen*. Logos.
Kuhl, J. (1981). Motivational and functional helplessness: The moderating effect of state versus action orientation. *Journal of Personality and Social Psychology, 40*, 155–170.
Kuhl, J. (1994). Motivation and volition. In G. d'Ydevalle, P. Bertelson, & P. Eelen (Eds.), *Current advances in psychological science: An international perspective* (pp. 311–340). Erlbaum.
Kuhl, J. (2001). *Motivation und Persönlichkeit*. Hogrefe.
Kuhl, J., & Beckmann, J. (1985). Historical perspectives in the study of action control. In J. Kuhl & J. Beckmann (Eds.), *Action control. From cognition to behaviour* (pp. 89–100). Springer.
Kuhl, J., & Beckmann, J. (Eds.). (1994a). *Volition and personality: Action and state orientation*. Hogrefe & Huber.
Kuhl, J., & Beckmann, J. (1994b). Alienation. Ignoring one's preferences. In J. Kuhl, J. Beckmann, & J. (Eds.), *Volition and personality: Action and state orientation* (pp. 375–390). Seattle.
Kuhl, J., Kazén, M., & Koole, S. L. (2006). Putting self-regulation theory into practice: A user's manual. *Applied Psychology. An International Review, 55*, 408–418.
Kuhl, J., Koole, S. L., & Quirin, M. (2015). Being someone: The integrated self as a neuropsychological system. *Social and Personality Psychology Compass, 9*, 115–132. https://doi.org/10.1111/spc3.12162
Kuhl, J., & Kraska, K. (1989). Self-regulation and metamotivation: Computational mechanisms, development and assessment. In R. Kaufer, P. L. Ackerman, & R. Cudeck (Eds.), *Abilities, motivation, and methodology: The Minnesota symposium on learning and individual differences* (pp. 343–374). Lawrence Erlbaum Associates.
Kuhl, J., Schapkin, S., & Gusew, A. (1994). *A theory of volitional inhibition and an empirical test: Individual differences in the topography of ERP patterns for action- versus state-oriented processing of emotional words* [Unveröffentlichtes Manuskript]. Universität Osnabrück.
Kühn, S., Haggard, P., & Brass, M. (2013). Differences between endogenous and exogenous emotion inhibition in the human brain. *Brain Structure and Function, 219*, 1129–1138. https://doi.org/10.1007/s00429-013-0556-0
Lane, A. M., Beedie, C. J., Jones, M. V., Uphill, M., & Devonport, T. J. (2012). The BASES expert statement on emotion regulation in sport. *Journal of Sports Sciences, 30*(11), 1189–1195.

Langosch, A. (2015). *Ressourcenorientierte Beratung und Therapie*. Reinhardt.
Lee, Y. H., & Chelladurai, P. (2016). Affectivity, emotional labor, emotional exhaustion, and emotional intelligence in coaching. *Journal of Applied Sport Psychology, 28*, 170–184.
Leprince, C., D'Arripe-Longueville, F., Chanal, J., & Doron, J. (2019). Development and preliminary validation of the communal coping strategies inventory for competitive team sports. *Psychology of Sport and Exercise, 45*(August), 101569. https://doi.org/10.1016/j.psychsport.2019.101569
Levleva, L., & Orlick, T. (1991). Mental links to enhanced healing: An exploratory study. *The Sports Psychologist, 5*, 25–40.
Lindworsky, J. (1923). *Der Wille: Seine Erscheinung und seine Beherrschung* (3rd ed.). Barth.
Locke, E. L., & Latham, G. P. (1990). *A theory of goal setting and task performance*. Prentice Hall.
Low, R. S. T., Overall, N. C., Hammond, M. D., & Girme, Y. U. (2017). Emotional suppression during personal goal pursuit strivings and achievement. *Emotion, 17*(2), 208–223. https://doi.org/10.1037/emo0000218
Luna, B., Garver, K. E., Urban, T. A., Lazar, N. A., & Sweeney, J. A. (2004). Maturation of cognitive processes from late childhood to adulthood. *Child Development, 75*, 1357–1372.
MacIntyre, T. E., Moran, A., Collett, C., & Guillot, A. (2013). An emerging paradigm: A strength-based approach to exploring mental imagery. *Frontiers in Human Neuroscience, 7*, 104. https://doi.org/10.3389/fnhum.2013.00104
Mahoney, M., Gabriel, T., & Perkins, T. S. (1987). Psychological skills and exceptional athletic performance. *The Sport Psychologist, 1*, 181–199.
Mahoney, M. J., & Avener, M. (1977). Psychology of the elite athletes: An exploration study. *Cognitive Therapy and Research, 1*, 135–141.
Mesagno, C., Marchant, D., & Morris, T. (2008). A pre-performance routine to alleviate choking in "choking-susceptible" athletes. *The Sport Psychologist, 22*, 439–457. https://doi.org/10.1123/tsp.22.4.439
Mirifar, A., Beckmann, J., & Ehrlenspiel, F. (2017). Neurofeedback as supplementary training for optimizing athletes' performance: A systematic review with implications for future research. *Neuroscience & Biobehavioral Reviews, 75*, 419–432.
Mischel, W. (1974). Processes in delay of gratification. In L. Berkowitz (Ed.), *Advances in experimental social psychology* (Vol. 7, pp. 249–292). Academic Press.
Mischel, W. (2014). *The marshmallow test. Mastering self-control*. Little Brown.
Monaci, M. G., & Veronesi, F. (2019). Getting angry when playing tennis: Gender differences and impact on performance. *Journal of Clinical Sport Psychology, 13*, 116–133.
Monahan, K. C., Steinberg, L., Cauffman, E., & Mulvey, E. P. (2009). Trajectories of antisocial behavior and psychosocial maturity from adolescence to young adulthood. *Developmental Psychology, 45*, 1654–1668.
Moore, W. E. (1986). *Covert-overt service routines: The effects of a service routine training programme on elite tennis players* [Doctoral dissertation]. University of Virginia, Charlottesville, VA.
Morris, T., & Bull, S. J. (1991). *Mental training in sport: An overview* (BASS monograph (3). British Association of Sports Sciences). National Coaching Foundation.
Niven, K., Totterdell, P., & Holman, D. (2009). A classification of controlled interpersonal affect regulation strategies. *Emotion, 9*, 498–509. https://doi.org/10.1037/a0015962
Nordin, S. M., Cumming, J., Vincent, J., & McGrory, S. (2006). Mental practice or spontaneous play? Examining which types of imagery constitute deliberate practice in sport. *Journal of Applied Sport Psychology, 18*, 345–362.
Orlick, T., & Partington, J. (1988). Mental links to excellence. *The Sport Psychologist, 2*, 105–130.
Ospina, M. B., Bond, K., Karkhaneh, M., Tjosvold, L., Vandermeer, B., Liang, Y., Bialy, L., Hooton, N., Buscemi, N., Dryden, D. M., & Klassen, T. P. (2007). Meditation practices for health: State of the research. *Evidence Report/Technology Assessment (Full Report), 155*, 1–263.
Palmateer, T., & Tamminen, K. (2018). A case study of interpersonal emotion regulation within a varsity volleyball team. *Journal of Applied Sport Psychology, 30*, 321–340. https://doi.org/10.1080/10413200.2017.1367335
Petrovic, P., Ekman, C.-J., Klahr, J., Tigerström, L., Rydén, G., Johansson, A. G. M., Sellgren, C., Golkar, A., Olsson, A., Öhman, A., Ingvar, M., & Landén, M. (2015). Significant gray matter changes in a region of the orbitofrontal cortex in healthy participants predicts emotional dysregulation. *Social Cognitive and Affective Neuroscience, 11*, 1041–1049.
Raglin, J., & Hanin, Y. (2000). Competitive anxiety and athletic performance. In Y. Hanin (Ed.), *Emotions in sport* (pp. 93–112). Human Kinetics.
Richards, J. M., & Gross, J. J. (2000). Emotion regulation and memory: The cognitive costs of keeping one's cool. *Journal of Personality and Social Psychology, 79*(3), 410–424. https://doi.org/10.1037/0022-3514.79.3.410
Roberts, B. W., Caspi, A., & Moffitt, T. E. (2001). The kids are alright: Growth and stability in personality development from adolescence to adulthood. *Journal of Personality and Social Psychology, 81*(4), 670–683.
Roberts, G. C. (1986). The growing child and the perception of competitive stress in sport. In G. Gleeson (Ed.), *The growing child in competitive sport* (pp. 130–144). Hodder & Stoughton.
Rothbart, M. K., Ahadi, S. A., & Evans, D. E. (2000). Temperament and personality: Origins and outcomes. *Journal of Personality and Social Psychology, 78*, 122–135.
Rushall, B. S. (1984). The content of competitive thinking. In W. F. Straub & J. M. Williams (Eds.), *Cognitive sport psychology* (pp. 51–62). Sport Science Associates.
Sahre, E. (1991). Wer behält die Nerven, wenn es darauf ankommt? Zum Einfluss von Handlungs- und Lageorientierung auf die Spielleistung im Basketball unter psychischer Belastung und physischer Beanspruchung. *Sportpsychologie, 5*, 11–15.
Schack, T. (1997). *Ängstliche Schüler im Sport—Interventionsverfahren zur Entwicklung der Handlungskontrolle*. Hofmann.
Schack, T. (2006). Mentales training. In M. Tietjens & B. Strauss (Eds.), *Handbuch Sportpsychologie* (pp. 254–261). Hofmann.
Schack, T., Whitmarsh, B., Pike, R., & Redden, C. (2005). Routines. In J. Taylor & G. Wilson (Eds.), *Applying sport psychology* (pp. 137–150). Human Kinetics.
Schmid, A., & Peper, E. (1993). Training strategies for concentration. In J. M. Williams (Ed.), *Applied sport psychology: Personal growth to peak performance* (2nd ed., pp. 262–273). Mayfield.
Schulz von Thun, F. (1998). *Miteinander reden 3 – Das "innere Team" und situationsgerechte Kommunikation. Kommunikation, Person, Situation*. Rowohlt.
Shoda, Y., Mischel, W., & Peake, P. K. (1990). Predicting adolescent cognitive and social competence from preschool delay of gratification: Identifying diagnostic conditions. *Developmental Psychology, 26*, 978–986.
Staw, B. M., DeCelles, K. A., & de Goey, P. (2019). Leadership in the locker room: How the intensity of leaders' unpleasant affective displays shapes team performance. *Journal of Applied Psychology, 104*(12), 1547–1557.

Strack, F., Martin, L., & Stepper, S. (1988). Inhibiting and facilitating conditions of the human smile: A nonobtrusive test of the facial feedback hypothesis. *Journal of Personality and Social Psychology, 54*, 768–777.

Strang, H., Wegner, M., & Schwarze, S. (1987). Die Bewältigung von Misserfolgserfahrungen. *Sportpsychologie, 1*, 22–25.

Tamminen, K. A., & Crocker, P. R. E. (2013). "I control my own emotions for the sake of the team": Emotional self-regulation and interpersonal emotion regulation among female high-performance curlers. *Psychology of Sport and Exercise, 14*, 737–747. https://doi.org/10.1016/j.psychsport.2013.05.002

Tamminen, K. A., Palmateer, T. M., Denton, M., Sabiston, C., Crocker, P., Eys, M., & Smith, B. (2016). Exploring emotions as social phenomena among Canadian varsity athletes. *Psychology of Sport and Exercise, 27*, 28–38. https://doi.org/10.1016/j.psychsport.2016.07.010

Tibbert, S. J., Andersen, M. B., & Morris, T. (2015). What a difference a "mentally toughening" year makes: The acculturation of a rookie. *Psychology of Sport and Exercise, 17*, 68–78. https://doi.org/10.1016/j.psychsport.2014.10.007

Trougakos, J. P., Beal, D. J., Cheng, B. H., Hideg, I., & Zweig, D. (2015). Too drained to help: A resource depletion perspective on daily interpersonal citizenship behaviors. *Journal of Applied Psychology, 100*, 227–236. https://doi.org/10.1037/a0038082

van Kleef, G. A., Cheshin, A., Koning, L. F., & Wolf, S. A. (2019). Emotional games: How coaches' emotional expressions shape players' emotions, inferences, and team performance. *Psychology of Sport and Exercise, 41*, 1–11. https://doi.org/10.1016/j.psychsport.2018.11.004

van Raalte, J. L., Brewer, B. W., Rivera, P. M., & Petitpas, A. J. (1994). The relationship between observable self-talk and competitive junior tennis players' match performances. *Journal of Sport and Exercise Psychology, 16*, 400–415.

Wagstaff, C. R. D. (2014). Emotion regulation and sport performance. *Journal of Sport & Exercise Psychology, 36*, 401–412.

Wagstaff, C. R. D., Fletcher, D., & Hanton, S. (2012). Exploring emotion abilities and regulation strategies in sport organizations. *Sport Exercise and Performance Psychology, 1*, 268–282. https://doi.org/10.1037/a0028814

Watts, T. W., Duncan, G. J., & Quan, H. (2018). Revisiting the marshmallow test: A conceptual replication investigating links between early delay of gratification and later outcomes. *Psychological Science, 29*, 1159–1177.

Way, B. M., Creswell, J. D., Eisenberger, N. I., & Lieberman, M. D. (2010). Dispositional mindfulness and depressive symptomatology: Correlations with limbic and self-referential neural activity during rest. *Emotion, 10*, 12–24.

Weinberg, R., & Comar, W. (1994). The effectiveness of psychological interventions on competitive sports. *Sports Medicine, 18*, 406–418.

Weinberg, R. S. (1992). Goal setting and motor performance. A review and critique. In G. C. Roberts (Ed.), *Motivation in sport and exercise* (pp. 177–197). Human Kinetics.

Williams, K. J., Donovan, J. J., & Dodge, T. L. (2000). Self-regulation of performance: Goal establishment and goal revision processes in athletes. *Human Performance, 13*, 15.

Wolf, S. A., Harenberg, S., Tamminen, K., & Schmitz, H. (2018). "Cause you can't play this by yourself": Athletes' perceptions of team influence on their precompetitive psychological states. *Journal of Applied Sport Psychology, 30*, 185–203. https://doi.org/10.1080/10413200.2017.1347965

Yerkes, R. M., & Dodson, J. D. (1908). The Relation of Strength of Stimulus to Rapidity of Habit Formation. *Journal of Comparative Neurology & Psychology, 18*, 459–482.

Cognitive Training in Sports

Jan Mayer, Hans-Dieter Hermann and Adam Beavan

Contents

J. Schüler et al. (eds.), *Sport and Exercise Psychology*, https://doi.org/10.1007/978-3-031-03921-8_21

Learning Objectives

Basic:
- Knowing what cognitive training means and what its goals are
- To know various methods of cognitive training
- To be able to explain differences between fast and slow thinking and their interaction in sports

Advanced:
- To be able to explain the relevance of the executive functions and their central processes
- Being able to demonstrate how competence conviction can be constructed

Experts:
- Ability to describe the process of mental training
- Understanding the development of positive and goal-oriented thoughts through the regulation of self-talk
- Understand the interplay between fast and slow thinking and in which situations they are most appropriately used
- Understand how specific gaming interventions may improve the underlying processes of decision-making and which specific processes are benefitted

21.1 Sport Psychology in the Practice of Competitive Sports

Sport Practice

The sprinter Asafa Powell set the world record in the 100-m race several times between 2005 and 2007. However, the fastest man in the world at that time had not been able to win a major individual title (World Championship or Olympic Games). He is considered the uncrowned sprinter hero. A television documentary 'In the Body of the Top Athletes' (arte, programm.ARD.de) investigated, among other things, the reasons why it was not possible for Asafa to recall his record performance at a major event. Scientists have attempted to answer this question by means of functional diagnostics (i.e. electromyography examinations) of the leg muscles. Based on the observation that Asafa's record runs involved a very finely tuned, automated and intuitive coordination of the leg muscles (i.e. perfect intermuscular coordination), the scientists' analysis revealed that Asafa tried to consciously intervene in the movement with pure willpower (in attempt to run faster) at the World Championships. This conscious process disrupted his normal coordinated and automated movement sequences. This was evident as each of his steps was 20 cm shorter than in the record runs. Notably, Asafa commented on his disastrous run: 'I just wanted to be as fast as possible—and that was the fatal mistake!'

In addition to general mental health and fitness, supporting an athlete's individual performance in a competitive situation is the central objective of a sport psychologist. The goal is to complete an optimal performance at a predefined date (Eberspaecher et al., 2002; Immenroth et al., 2008; Sly et al., 2020). In order to achieve this, sport psychologists have a wide range of scientifically based intervention techniques at their disposal, depending on the given material (i.e. budget), temporal (i.e. selective or continuous work), personnel (i.e. individual or group work) and activity-specific (i.e. training, competition) conditions. Through cognitive training, athletes should be enabled to regulate themselves, especially in competition situations, in such a way that optimal performance can be achieved (Mayer & Hermann, 2011; Gonzalez & McVeigh, 2013). The ability to actively shape both thought and imagination processes in demanding situations that require decisive actions can be acquired and is the subject of cognitive training.

Cognitive Training

The content of **cognitive training** is the active design of both thought and imagination processes so that performance-enhancing cognitions can be retrieved according to the situation.

Particularly in the decisive phases of the competition, the behaviour of the athlete must not be negatively influenced by disturbing thoughts such as constant negative thinking, doubts or 'wanting' too much. The basis for understanding cognitive training is primarily a scientific examination of human thinking. In the following section, the 'dual systems theory' by Kahneman (2011) will be briefly discussed.

21.2 Dual Systems Theory by Kahneman

Within the framework of the dual systems theory, cognitive psychologist and Nobel Prize winner Daniel Kahneman (2011) distinguishes between **fast** and **slow thinking**. This refers to the interaction between subconscious thinking that intrinsically and reliably controls our learned and automated behaviour and conscious thinking being activated when the situation is important or difficult. The subconscious system runs fast and is accordingly called 'fast thinking'. However, the conscious system needs relatively more time to process information and to consider what to do and is therefore called 'slow thinking'.

Fast thinking works automatically, intuitively, largely effortlessly, without voluntary control and is a subconscious process. It enables efficient, automatic, intuitive action, which happens largely without thinking.

Fast Thinking

Fast thinking refers to automatic, intuitive thought processes that occur effortlessly and without conscious control.

In conscious experience, our actions are characterized by control, freedom of decision and concentration (slow thinking). One could also say that slow thinking is our mind, which we can actively use and strive for when it seems important to us. According to Kahneman (2011), a central ability of slow thinking is (higher) executive control or executive function. Slow thinking 'can program the memory to obey an instruction that overrides the usual reactions' (Kahneman, 2011, p. 52).

The executive functions include problem-solving competence, action competence, strategic competence as well as insight, impulse control and frustration tolerance (Kubesch, 2008; Barenberg et al., 2011; Meltzer, 2007), based on the three core executive functions of working memory, inhibition and cognitive flexibility.

Working memory enables the active maintenance of task-relevant information required for further operations, making it easier to remember one's action plans or instructions from other individuals and thus to take action alternatives into account to a greater extent (Kubesch, 2008; Diamond et al., 2007). In addition, an increased capacity of the working memory reduces mental wandering, supports concentration (Kane et al., 2007) and promotes problem-solving competence (Klingberg, 2009).

Inhibition is the ability to suppress behaviour. Attention and behaviour can be better controlled by a well-functioning inhibitory control and are therefore less susceptible to external conditions, one's own emotions or entrenched behaviour (Diamond et al., 2007). Inhibition thus supports self-disciplined behaviour.

Cognitive flexibility, which is related to working memory, makes it possible to adapt quickly to new demands, view situations and conditions from different, new perspectives and the ability to switch between these perspectives (Diamond et al., 2007).

Typical for slow thinking/executive functions is that its operations involve effort, and it is characterized by lethargy, the tendency to make only the effort that is absolutely necessary for the respective task.

Study Box

The explanation of how athletes are able to navigate and act within their environment using their perceptual-cognitive abilities matches closely with how previous researchers have described executive functions being engaged within a sporting environment (Beavan et al., 2020; Jacobson & Matthaeus, 2014). For example, a football player is good at being adaptive to the ever-changing and unpredictable environment, such as switching between offensive and defensive roles (i.e. matching closely to executive function cognitive flexibility), processing the information relative to an extensive procedural and declarative knowledge base (i.e. working memory), and suppressing an intended action such as a pass if a player becomes marked by a defender but also stopping an inappropriate verbal response in situations such as a discussion with the referee or fan (i.e. inhibition). Often, executive functions are described as 'game intelligence' in a sports (Stratton et al., 2004).

Slow Thinking

Slow thinking refers to more rational thought processes, the executive functions of thinking. It requires effort, energy and is time-consuming.

The separation of effort between fast and slow thinking is highly efficient because fast thinking normally is utilised and is extremely reliable. Fast thinking is not rational, hardly constrained by logic and is therefore not susceptible to doubt. It suppresses contradictions and ambiguity and spontaneously constructs 'solutions' that are as coherent as possible given the time constraints to decide (Kahneman, 2011). Contrastingly, slow thinking is constantly presented with interpretations of the perceived facts from the subconscious system, (fast thinking) and usually, the mind accepts these offers as true.

The importance of fast thinking in everyday life is immense. More than 90% of our behaviour is controlled by this 'autopilot'—although we usually experience ourselves permanently under constant conscious control. In some situations, we become aware of the dominance of fast thinking, for instance, while driving a car. Although we consciously deal with very different things (i.e. using a telephone while driving), the motor requirements (i.e. accelerating, clutch, steering) are generally handled by the fast thinking system [▶ Side Story: The Bat and Ball Problem (According to Kahneman, 2011)].

Side Story

The Bat and Ball Problem (According to Kahneman, 2011)

To become aware of how often we fall back and rely on our fast thinking, try to solve the following task: A racket and a ball together cost $1.10. The racket costs $1 more than the ball. How much does the ball cost?

Most people answer spontaneously '10 cents'. However, this would mean that the racket alone costs $1.10 and the ball costs an additional 10 cents. In total, both items would cost $1.20. Nevertheless, the answer '10 cents' seems to be intuitively correct. Many people prefer to trust this intuition, i.e. their fast thinking system, rather than resorting to their slow thinking system to solve this more logically. The problem can be solved very quickly by writing it down as an equation:

$$1.10 = (1 + 0.05) + 0.05$$

According to this, the ball costs 5 cents. If you add $1, you get the price of the racket of $1.05.

21.2.1 Fast and Slow Thinking in Elite Sports

In many situations, especially in the context of elite sports, the speed at which decisions are made is often crucial. In many sports such as boxing, fencing, or tennis, one has to react at such speed that the decision to execute a specific action can only be sourced from the intuition processes (fast thinking).

Reflection

Why You Should Not Think Consciously When Returning a Serve (After a Serve from the Opponent) in Tennis—Processes in the Brain During Returning a Serve (Carter, 2014)

- 0 ms: Attention is directed towards the opponent. Possibly the perception is compared with previous experiences.
- 70 ms: The ball is on its way (flown about 3 m). The player does not yet see the ball consciously, but unconsciously his brain is already planning the actions necessary for the return. At this stage, the player mainly uses information about the movements of the opponent to plan their own movements.
- 250 ms: The ball has almost crossed the net. The player's brain combines the information gathered so far to design a reaction to the rapidly approaching ball. This plan incorporates information about the body language of the server, the subconscious knowledge about the speed and trajectory of the ball and activated memories.
- 285 ms: Conscious thinking sets in. Subconsciously, the real-time position of the ball is already calculated. The player thinks he sees the ball where it actually is.
- 355 ms: The ball lands in the own half of the field. The motor areas fire. Arm and bat are brought into position so that the player can hit the ball.
- 500 ms: The ball is directly in front of the player. If the conscious perception of the trajectory of the ball deviates significantly from the previous subconscious prediction, the player can discard the older planning and form an alternative. However, to do this, the player needs another 200–300 ms; meaning the player will then no longer be able to hit the ball.

In elite sports, a systematic interchange between slow and fast thinking is often important in order to avoid disturbing the highly automated movement sequences but while still being able to accurately grasp the demands of the current situation. This interplay between fast and slow thinking can be illustrated using the example of a golf player.

After teeing off, the golfer approaches his ball on the fairway. Now it is a matter of analyzing the distance to the hole, the further course of the fairway, the wind conditions and possible obstacles (bunkers, water) as well as the possible flight of the ball with concentration and focus. This is strenuous and requires concentration, i.e. slow thinking. External advice—from the caddy (the carrier of the club bag and advisor regarding club selection and stroke strategy)—is obtained and integrated. However, as soon as the shot is struck, the golfer must be able to 'let go' and allow the automated processes to take control. Fast, highly complex and perfect movements must be left to fast thinking (which requires a correspondingly long phase of practice and training to shift what was once an effortful process into a relatively effortless action). The mind would be too slow for such a task; it would even interfere with the automated sequences and prevent the optimal execution of the movement.

After the golf swing, slow thinking must be reactivated. It has to be reflected upon whether the golf swing was successful and what must be done next. The prac-

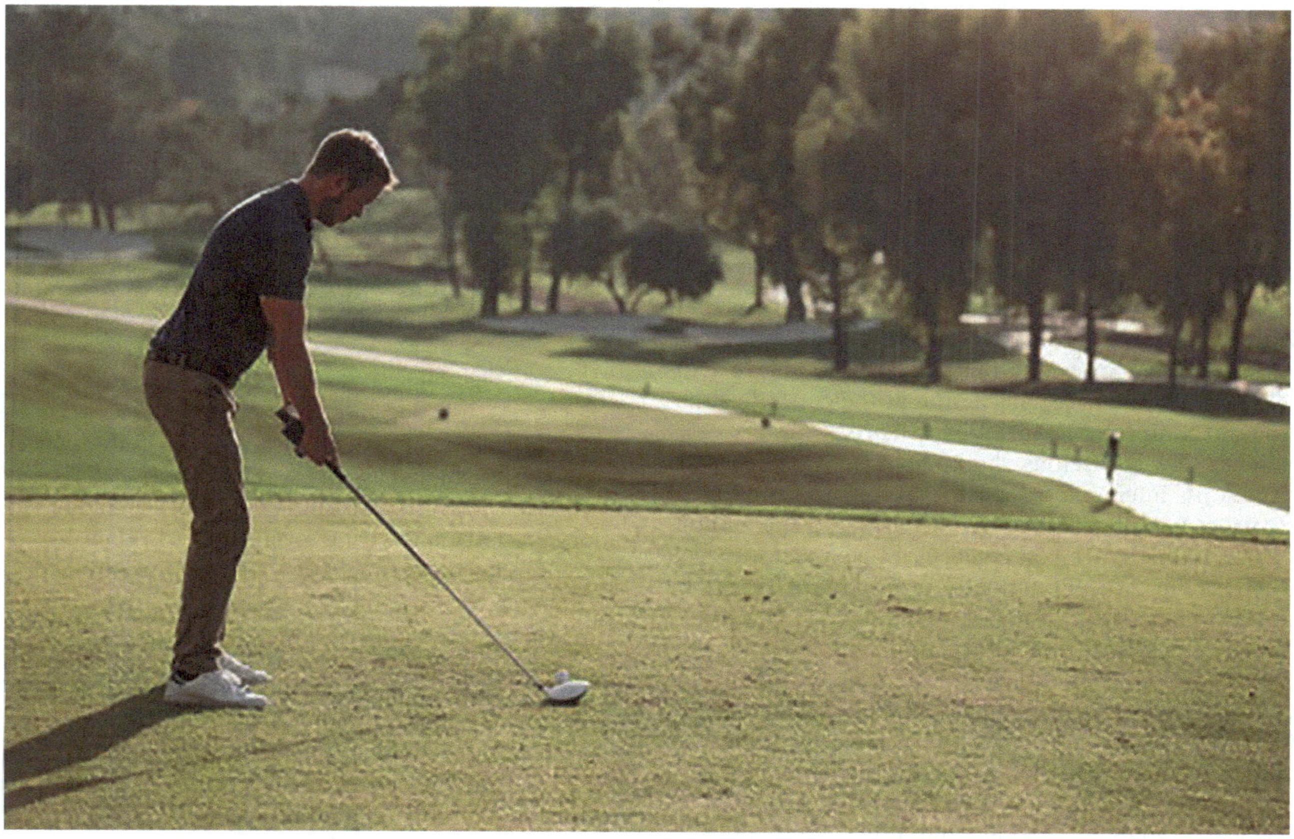

Fig. 21.1 The interchange between fast and slow thinking as the key to sporting success (© Monkey Business/▶ stock.adobe.com)

tised rituals (i.e. for relaxation and stroke preparation) have to be carried out (Fig. 21.1).

21.2.1.1 Interplay of Fast and Slow Thinking

Fast thinking is responsible for the execution of automated, long-time trained movement patterns that are necessary for maximum performance. In many sporting situations, however, it is not enough to leave control solely to fast thinking. The deliberate use of slow thinking (i.e. executive functions) alternating smoothly with fast thinking is the key to success.

Evidence in favour of using this dual system is reported during the development of working memory into adolescence, resulting in a better ability to perform more complex tasks, control distraction and be more adaptable (Furley & Wood, 2016). In turn, abstract thought (i.e. creativity) and decision-making benefit from a more efficient and flexible working memory system (Luna, 2009) and would be expected to lead to better in-game decision-making performance (Voss et al., 2010).This is supported by a study in ice hockey athletes that reported players with a better working memory capacity were better able to adjust their decision-making behaviour to the situational demands of the game (Furley & Memmert, 2012).

Not wanting to intervene in the movement process (i.e. trusting in fast thinking and letting the movement process happen without over-thinking) can be a successful strategy. An important basis for this is competence conviction.

21.2.2 Competence Conviction

In the concept of competence conviction (according to Bandura, 1977), a distinction is made between **competence conviction** (the term is used synonymously with the term self-efficacy conviction in the literature) and **consequence expectation**. Consequence expectation is the assessment of a person that a certain behaviour leads to a certain result (i.e. in football, the assessment of a player that he/she generally can safely convert a penalty kick). Competence conviction, on the other hand, includes the certainty that the actions necessary for a certain result can be implemented in the concrete situation (i.e. a penalty kick in the final of the World Cup).

Consequence Expectation and Competence Conviction

The **consequence expectation** is the personal assessment that a certain behaviour leads to a certain event. This expectation must be distinguished from **competence conviction**, which additionally includes the certainty of having the necessary competences in the specific situation.

A person may be convinced that a certain behaviour leads to a certain result and generally believes that he/she can do so. However, if this person is not able to actually perform the necessary action in the concrete situation, no competence conviction will arise.

The slow, conscious thinking, is activated in such situations, intervening with the automated movement sequence and disturbs it. This means that a lack of conviction in one's own competence can be a major reason for the failure of elite athletes in important situations during competition.

There is a wealth of information that indicates that competence conviction is a very central and important component in the development of elite performance. Corresponding empirical studies also confirm this. The connection between one's belief in competence and sporting performance has been the subject of numerous scientific studies (Feltz et al., 2008). A meta-analysis by Moritz et al. (2000) showed a moderate mean correlation ($r = 0.38$). Other studies have indicated that competence conviction is the strongest predictor of athletic performance (Feltz et al., 2008).

? In the systematic development of a competence conviction, a person can use four starting points or sources of information (Bandura, 1977) (Fig. 21.2):
- Mastery experiences: individual personal experience in successfully coping with the requirement; successful practice of carrying out the skill in the real world
- Vicarious learning: representative experience: successful practice in the mind
- Verbal persuasion
- Emotional and physiological states, appropriate activation

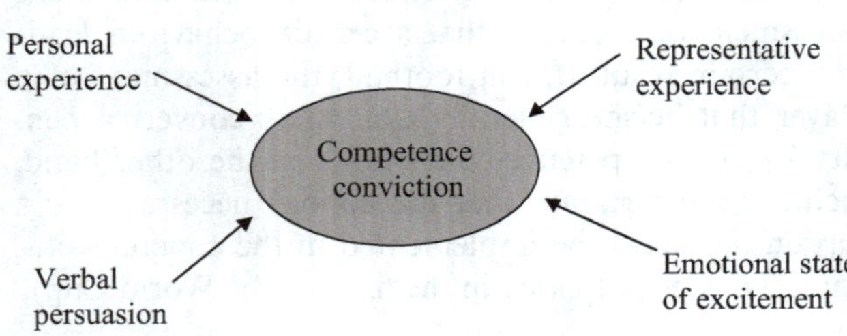

Fig. 21.2 Information sources of competence conviction

- **Mastery Experiences; Individual Personal Experience in Successfully Meeting the Challenge: Successful Practice in the Real World**

Many years of training in addition to successful past performances of the respective activity within competitions are required to build up adequate confidence in one's own abilities. Successfully and repeatedly mastering challenging situations will forge a strong connection between one's own ability and the success achieved. Positive expectations with regard to one's own competence will slowly build up.

- **Vicarious Learning; Representative Experience: Successful Practice in the Mind**

The observation of people who successfully master demanding situations can lead to the observer also expecting to be able to act successfully in the given demanding situation. From the underlying social comparison processes, conclusions are drawn about one's own competence.

- **Verbal Persuasion**

The third source for building up a competence conviction is verbal persuasion. Within verbal persuasion, it can further be distinguished between the source of the belief. The source of the conviction can be an external source, such as from the coach, who provides verbal persuasion for the athlete, and also as an internal source (i.e., self-talk) (▶ Sect. 21.3.2).

- **Emotional and Physiological States, Appropriate Activation**

Situations that are demanding usually evoke activation states that can have an informative value in terms of personal competence (Immenroth et al., 2008; Shatil, 2013). If the activation state that is experienced is unsuitable for the current requirement of the task, it weakens the belief in one's competence. For example, in situations where the activation level is too high—one might feel too shaky and excessively nervous. In situations where the individual has too low of an emotional activation—they tend to feel lethargic and tired.

Development of a Competence Conviction

The development of a competence conviction can be achieved through four different sources. The most important and most stable way is the repeated experience of one's own successful actions. Alternatively, competence convictions can be generated both by observing and imagining successful actions and by verbal persuasion from external and internal sources. In addition, an emotional activation level appropriate to the situation supports the own competence conviction.

In summary, it can be stated that the following effects must be achieved through appropriate cognitive training methods so that—as initially defined as the objective of cognitive training—the athlete is able to regulate himself/herself in such a way that optimum performance can be called upon, especially in competition situations:

- In demanding situations in which learned and automated movement sequences are retrieved, it is important that the athlete can allow fast thinking and that slow thinking does not intervene. This seems to succeed above all with an existing strong competence conviction
- Slow thinking should be designed to accompany and optimize actions before, during, and after the requirements situation
- Slow thinking should work as fast as possible in certain demanding situations in sport

21.3 Methods of Cognitive Training

Among the cognitive training methods described in the following, **mental training** occupies a special position since this psychological training modality has been the subject of scientific research for many years and has been used in the early stages of sport psychological practice (Immenroth et al., 2008; Shatil, 2013). Relatively new, however, is the approach to enhance an individual's executive functions by using gaming procedures.

21.3.1 Mental Training

According to Eberspaecher (2001), mental training is defined as the planned repeated and conscious imagining of a movement without its simultaneous practical execution.

Mental training should include as many sensory modalities as possible. The imagination of the feeling of movement is of fundamental importance. For adequate movement imagination, it is therefore always a matter of incorporating the most intensive kinaesthetic movement information possible.

These ideas can also be understood as test and command variables of human action (Eberspaecher, 2001; Gonzalez & McVeigh, 2013). The development of an appropriate movement concept is, therefore, an essential prerequisite for mental training. The practice of incorrect or inappropriate ideas also has a training effect—but here the incorrect or unwanted movements or action patterns are trained.

> **Mental Training**
>
> Mental training describes the planned repeated and conscious imagining of movement sequences without their actual execution.

It was Paivio (1985) who already distinguished different dimensions of mental training (cognitive/motivational and specific/general). In general, with the goal of optimizing competition performance, a distinction can be made between a more rational-action controlling and a motivational-emotional function of mental training.

The two basic objectives of mental training can be derived by the:

1. Optimization of competence conviction (motivational-emotional function)
2. Optimization of the learning and automation process of actions (rational-action control function)

21.3.1.1 Mental Training to Optimize the Competence Conviction

The most effective source for building up a competence conviction is the self-experienced effectiveness (mastery experience = success) in the requirement situation. The second most effective source is the vicarious learning. The observation of people who successfully master requirement situations can lead the observer to the expectation that they themselves can also act successfully in the given requirement situation. Various studies have shown that the equality between model and observer and, accordingly, the fit of the model's execution of action is the decisive component for positive changes in competence conviction.

Previous work on mirror neurons reveals interesting and relevant findings. For example, neurons were found in the premotor cortex of monkeys, which are already activated when an activity is merely observed as if they were performing this action themselves (Rizzolatti et al., 1996). While the monkey sees how another monkey takes a peanut and eats it, it imitates this situation inside its brain. The monkey reflects the motor behaviour of his conspecific. The fact that humans also activate motor brain regions solely by observing movements could be shown by measuring the brain activity of subjects who observed finger movements (Iacoboni et al., 1996). Actions that are perceived by viewing other people also activate a motor schema of their own in the brain of the observer; exactly the same schema that would be responsible if the observer was to perform the observed action himself/herself. In order to have a positive effect on the observer's competence conviction, it is therefore recommended to watch videos of one's own successful performance. Many athletes prepare themselves for important competitions by watching video material of their own successful actions intensively again and again.

Representative experiences can also take place in the pure imagination of individuals. In fact, the person observed does not have to be someone else, but an individual can mentally visualize how they themselves successfully master an upcoming challenge.

Previous research provides supporting evidence for the motivational-emotional effect of mental training. For example, Page et al. (1999) found in a study of 40 elite swimmers that mental training reduces the perceived fear of competition and leads to an increase in self-confidence. The influence of mental training on competition-related competence conviction has been the subject of scientific research on several occasions. Positive effects are described consistently (Morris et al., 2005; Weinberg, 2008; Feltz et al., 2008). These effects on performance-relevant psychological variables can certainly also be explained by the fact that the successful presentation of one's own actions leads to the elimination of negative consequence thinking, which is often seen as a trigger for fear of competition or insufficient competence conviction.

Competence Conviction Through Mental Training
An appropriate idea of what to do in order to successfully accomplish a specific situation (i.e. an important competition) has a positive effect on competence conviction in the context of representative experience.

Compared to the motivational-emotional functions, the rational action-controlling functions of mental training have a much higher relevance for basic sport psychology (see Immenroth et al., 2008; Shatil, 2013). Accordingly, the available empirical results on the rational action-controlling function of mental training are much more elaborated.

21.3.1.2 Mental Training to Optimize the Learning and Automation Process of Actions

Regarding the rational-action-controlling function, the question arises of how effective mental training compares to **practical training**. Can one train just as effectively in the mind or does practical training have decisive advantages?

To investigate the effectiveness of mental training, the four-group repeated measurement paradigm (Fig. 21.3) has become the established methodological approach. Within the framework of this research paradigm, the effect of mental training has been demonstrated for several movement tasks.

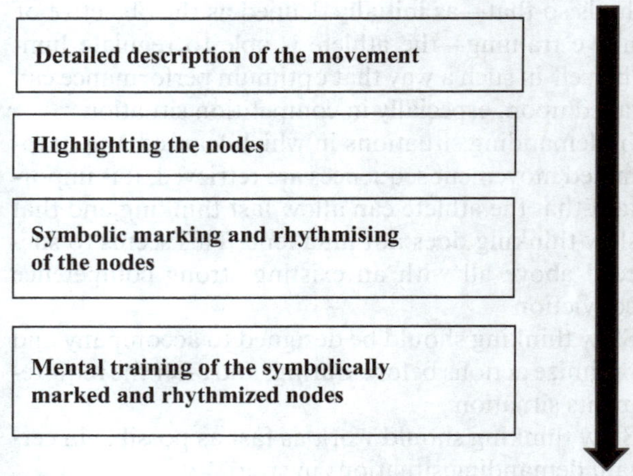

Fig. 21.3 Four-group measurement repetition paradigm

With the aim of increasing the effect of learning and performance, the following results can be determined by this paradigm across tasks (Murphy, 1994; Munzert, 2001):

- Mental training is more effective than no training. This means there is a fundamental effect of mental training. This is especially relevant for all areas of application where no practical training is possible (i.e. during non-training periods in sports, regeneration periods, injury or rehabilitation phases).
- The effect of mental training is less than the effect of practical training. This is central to the practical use of mental training; mental training cannot and should not replace practical training but rather supplement it.
- The combination of mental training and practical training provides the greatest increase in performance. In this respect, it is also clear that mental training should be an additional training in practice. Only in a few exceptions should mental training also replace practical training (i.e. in order to reduce physical load).

According to Munzert (2001), from an application-oriented perspective, it is interesting to be able to demonstrate and determine the 'pure' effect of mental training. For this purpose, several meta-analyses were carried out in which a large number of experimental studies were collectively analyzed to determine cross-task related effects. The most frequently cited meta-analyses by Feltz and Landers (1983), [later extended by Feltz et al. (1988)], attests to mental training's fundamental effectiveness, with the restriction, however, that mental training is more effective for movement tasks that contain more cognitive components than for tasks with a larger motor component. This has also been confirmed by the most comprehensive meta-analysis to date presented by Driskell et al. (1994). A more cognitive movement task is one in which, for example, certain temporal and spatial parameters must be passed through, such as passing through a labyrinth or a slalom. A more motor-related task would be, for example, sitting in a racing kayak without tipping over.

In a meta-analysis, Feltz and Landers (1983) report an average effect size of 0.48. In the methodologically optimized revision of the meta-analysis by Feltz et al. (1988) an effect size of 0.43 was calculated. Driskell et al. (1994) found larger effect sizes in cognitive movement tasks (0.69) than in motor-related tasks (0.34).

Comparison Between Mental Training and Practical Training

Mental training is more effective than no training but less effective than practical training. The combination of mental and practical training achieves the greatest performance improvements. Therefore, cognitive movement tasks benefit more from mental training than motor tasks.

Studies that have focused on the exploration of the brain in connection with movement imagination and mental training provide fundamental findings for understanding the mechanisms of mental training and creating an essential foundation.

Two studies with functional magnetic resonance imaging (fMRI) from 1996 (Roth et al., 1996; Porro et al., 1996) specifically address the role of premotor area (PMA) and supplementary motor area (SMA) and especially the role of the primary motor cortex during presented and executed finger-thumb movements. Both studies could show that the contralateral primary motor cortex is actively involved in the presentation of movements in addition to PMA and SMA. The studies conclude that mental training and practical movement performance are based on the same neural networks. The primary motor cortex plays an important role during the imagination of movements while participating in as much as all stages of motor control represented as a primarily executive cortex area.

In summary, neuroscientific studies on mental training have shown that large neuronal areas are activated during imagined and practical movement. In a review, Munzert et al. (2009) listed 43 studies that could provide evidence for activation of the primary motor cortex during mental training. In this respect, the assumption of a **functional equivalence** of imagined and practical movements can be mostly confirmed (Sharma & Baron, 2013). The corresponding effects of mental training on learning and the automation process of actions are considered proven, meaning that mental training can be attributed to the development of functional fast thinking in many specific requirement situations.

Functional Equivalence

During mental training, the same areas of the brain (PMA, SMA and primary motor cortex) are activated as during the practical execution of the movement. This allows the assumption that mental training facilitates learning processes and accelerates the optimization of motor task processes.

21.3.1.3 Practice

As previously discussed, the prerequisite for mental training is the development of a correspondingly intensive and differentiated idea of action. The mere invitation to imagine actions or movements cannot yet ensure the quality and differentiation of the idea, which leads to an increase in learning or performance or to the development of competence conviction. Therefore, a systematic approach to the development of a concept of action is recommended.

There are various approaches to this. In practice, the following approaches are generally used (differentiated here in the terminology according to Heuer, 1985):

- Linguistic-symbolic approaches
- Spatially visualized approaches
- Kinaesthetic approaches

Linguistic-Symbolic Approaches

In the case of linguistic-symbolic approaches, the content of the presentation is verbalized and, if necessary, put down in writing. A well-known procedure frequently used for the rational action controlling function of mental training is the Eberspaecher (2001) step model [▶ Methods: Step Model of Mental Training (According to Eberspaecher, 2001)].

Methods: Stage Model of Mental Training (According to Eberspaecher, 2001)

First of all, it is important that the athlete becomes aware of the movement sequence to be trained by addressing as many sensory modalities as possible, **describing** it **comprehensibly** and putting it into words (◘ Fig. 21.4). The next step includes the elaboration of the **central points** of the movement sequence, the so-called nodal points of the movement. Nodal points of a movement are the decisive points of a movement sequence, which must be passed through without fail. In the next step, the **nodes** of the movement to be trained are **marked symbolically**. For example, they are renamed into individual short formulas. The aim is to compress the information (known as chunking). In this way, the imagination is to be approximated to the dynamics and the temporal sequence of the real movement. Finally, the developed idea of movement is **mentally trained**.

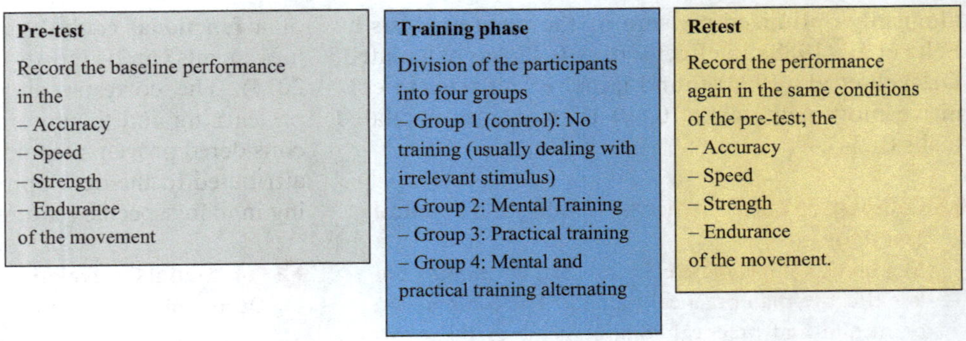

Fig. 21.4 Process of developing an idea

One advantage of the linguistic-symbolic approach in the step-by-step model is that by writing down the movement concept, the coach and the athlete can improve their communication in the training process. However, it should be highlighted that some athletes have difficulties in verbalizing non-visual concepts, especially kinaesthetic experiences. In practice, it is often noticeable that in such cases, only spatial-temporal movement information is included in the movement description. In this case, it is more appropriate to approach the structure of the movement concept via spatial-imagery or kinaesthetic approaches.

Spatial-Visual Approaches

Spatial-visual approaches attempt to develop ideas for action with the help of video recordings. This is based on the findings on mirror neurons, which go back to the work of Rizzolatti et al. (1996). According to Bauer (2006) the observation of actions is particularly suitable for the development of an idea of movement.

Kinaesthetic Approaches

In kinaesthetic approaches, an attempt is made to generate an idea of movement by remembering certain intense experiences of the movement. They are particularly suitable for on-site use, such as at the training location itself. Immediately after an optimal real execution of movement, the athlete is asked to repeat the movement experience through imagery. According to Wriessnegger et al. (2014), mental training is particularly effective after previous practical achievements, also because the athletes report that this method of generating mental imagery of the movement is very easy for them.

Often a combination of the three approaches is used in practical application. In sports, for example, descriptions of movements are written down, and further attempts are made to differentiate them through intensive video analysis. Frequent requests by the coaches for successful action sequences and the athlete's sensations during the course of the movement should help to ensure that the **idea of movement** is constantly adapted to the current performance development.

Building Up a Movement Concept

In sport psychology practice, three different approaches, usually in combination, are used to build up a movement concept. In the linguistic-symbolic approach, the sequence of movements is verbalized, reduced to nodes and rehearsed. The spatial-imagery approach usually uses video recordings to generate ideas of movement. In the kinaesthetic approach, movement sensations are used to build up a mental movement-image, ideally as soon as possible after the optimal execution of a movement.

How can it be determined whether all important aspects are included in the athlete's idea of movement?

The 'PETTLEP Imagery Model' (Holmes & Collins, 2001) is a successful approach to test whether all relevant aspects of an athlete's movement perception are included. Accordingly, the following factors should be included in mental training:

- Physical: refers to the physical and kinaesthetic properties of movement
- Environment: refers to the typical circumstances of the environment
- Task: refers to the task type and the objective
- Timing: refers to the temporal aspect
- Learning: refers to the differentiation of the imagination content and its regular evaluation
- Emotions: refers to the accompanying emotion
- Perspective: refers to the perspective of the imagination (internal perspective or observation perspective)

In mental training, one can distinguish between two perspectives/variants:

- External: Mental training from the **observer's perspective**
- Internal: Mental training from an **internal perspective**

Regarding mental training from the observer's perspective, the trainee observes themselves through their mind's eye while performing the movement. This form of mental training is comparable to watching a video recording of their own action from the perspective of an observer. In mental training from the inner perspective, one calls the inner perspective of a movement into consciousness. This means that you experience the execution of the movement and reproduce it by using as many sensory modalities as possible.

In sport psychology practice, it is noticeable that athletes usually prefer one of the perspectives (observer perspective or internal perspective). Some can also switch arbitrarily between the two (Munzertz & Möllman, 1997; Bertollo et al., 2009). The kinaesthetic sensations associated with this are to be fundamentally separated from the visual perspective of the imagination (Munzert et al., 2000; Munzert & Zentgraf, 2009).

This remark seems to be extremely relevant since in practice; many athletes prefer the observer's perspective and are still able to integrate kinaesthetic information into the movement perception. This corresponds to the study by Munzert et al. (2000), reporting that no stronger kinaesthetic perceptions can be demonstrated for the internal view or not necessarily less intense ones for the observer's perspective. In summary, it can be discussed in the context of Munzert et al. (2000)'s work that it does not seem sensible to prefer a priori one of the imaginary perspectives (observer perspective/internal perspective). For the intensity of mental training, the development of kinaesthetic imagination content is, therefore, central (i.e. Stinear et al., 2006; Guillot et al., 2009).

Observer Perspective and Internal Perspective

In mental training, a distinction can be made between the observer's and the internal perspective (external and internal). Most people prefer one of the two perspectives. However, for an intensive movement, the actual perception itself is not the decisive factor but the intensity of the kinaesthetic information.

21.3.2 Self-Talk Regulation

Self-talk in the sense of self-talk regulation refers to the thoughts that precede, accompany or follow the action. It is not necessary for these thoughts to be spoken aloud. The athlete formulates action plans, gives his or herself instructions, structures their thoughts or comments on their own actions. Self-talk is one of the cognitive strategies most frequently used by elite athletes (Gould et al., 1992; Park, 2000; Shannon et al., 2012; Thelwell et al., 2008).

What Is Self-Talk?

- Any thought that a person has about a certain subject (Zinsser et al., 2006)
- A statement addressed to the person themselves (Hardy et al., 1996)
- It can be either external (observable from outside) or internal (not observable) (Theodorakis et al., 2000)
- A syntactic, perceptible statement of an internal position expressed either loudly or softly, with sender and receiver being the same (van Raalte et al., 2016)

Self-talk is a central element in many sport psychology training programs (i.e. Hanton & Jones, 1999; Thelwell & Greenlees, 2001). It is used in many different forms, which Hardy et al. (2001) investigated in a descriptive study with 150 athletes from different sports. The authors posed four open questions (Hardy et al., 2001, p. 308):

- Where do you use self-talk?
- When do you use self-talk?
- What do you say to yourself?
- Why do you use self-talk?

Although athletes reported that they used self-talk regulation much more often in sport-related environments, at home was the second most frequently cited place (Hardy et al., 2001, p. 310). Of 497 responses to the question of when athletes used self-talk regulation, 279 were 'in competition', with this number referring to self-talk before (136), during (131) and after (12) the competition. When asked what the content of the self-talk was, most of the answers fell into the category *structure*, which in turn was divided into keywords (55), phrases (281) and sentences (30). The second-largest category was the group *task instructions*. This refers to content-related within self-talk in the form of instructions, which were divided into special, technical and general instructions. When asked about the 'why' of self-talk, most of the answers fell into the category 'motivational function' and only about one third into the rational, action-directing function.

Use of Self-Talk

Most self-talk is done by athletes in sport-related environments and at home. Self-talk is mainly of an action-structuring or action-instructing nature and is used more often in its motivational function than in its rational-controlling function.

According to the 'Dual Systems Theory' (Kahneman, 2011), self-talk can be distinguished according to whether it arises from slow thinking or fast thinking (Van Raalte et al., 2016). As previously mentioned, slow thinking requires effort, acts as a monitor of thoughts and actions and is rationally and emotionally neutral. From this point of view, self-talk from slow thinking also requires mental effort and is influenced by different perspectives and newly arriving information. Such self-talk can help to control focus and attention and thereby increases performance. When talking to yourself through the use of slow thinking, a distinction can also be made between proactive and reactive self-talk. The latter occurs as a direct response to an emotional and cognitively distorted fast thinking self-talk (i.e. 'I'm the worst, I should stop'). Once these cognitions have arrived in consciousness, they can also be processed by slow thinking. Proactive self-talk, on the other hand, is used with a specific intention/output. It can either be consistent with the assessment of fast thinking (i.e. 'I can do this' when I actually feel I can do the task) or inconsistent (i.e. 'I can do this' when I do not feel I can complete the task). The former is called consonant, and the latter dissonant self-talk. Due to its inconsistency, it can cause strong cognitive dissonance and requires a change in one's own cognitions as well as a strong use of cognitive resources to reduce dissonance (van Raalte et al., 2016).

In stressful, demanding situations, self-talk is provided by fast thinking. As a result, self-talk is influenced by emotional/intuitive interpretations and arises spontaneously. These conversations are very difficult to control because they react slowly, if at all, to logic and new information. Especially negative self-talk is created in this way, but also positive self-talk, for example, after a goal/victory (see van Raalte et al., 2016).

The model by van Raalte et al. (2016) offers an explanatory approach to the training effects with regard to both systems. Through training, the handling of self-talk becomes more familiar and routine and requires less and less cognitive resources, meaning less slow thinking and more fast thinking instead. This ultimately leads to better performance since more remaining resources can be used for execution. Self-talk is influenced by behaviour, context and personality (van Raalte et al., 2016).

Behaviour Emotions and impressions evoked by behaviour directly affect fast thinking (i.e. a missed ball or pass that arouses anger and rage in the athlete). They are used either directly for self-talk (i.e. 'That was terrible', 'I'm bad') or for modelling and processing slow thinking (i.e. 'I have to be careful', 'The next one will be better').

Contextual Factors External circumstances or contextual factors are conditions that determine the 'when' and 'where'. They require constant rational analysis (slow thinking) and can evoke spontaneous, emotional responses (fast thinking). Context factors include, for example, the time of training or competition, weather, temperature, difficulty, etc. Self-talk can also change the situation or its interpretation and can, for example, contribute to seeing the opponent as a challenge or as not taking them seriously (i.e. 'I am the greatest', 'I cannot take him seriously').

Personal Factors Personal factors directly influence the working methods of slow and fast thinking and, through these, affect behaviour and self-talk. People with high self-esteem, for example, benefit much more from positive self-talk and statements than people with low self-esteem as they find such a positive self-image uncomfortable.

21.3.2.1 Empirical Evidence

Many athletes confirm the relevance of self-talk for athletic performance. Nevertheless, the empirical evidence for its actual learning and performance-enhancing influence in sport-specific situations has not been sufficiently solid and is characterized by many limitations (Immenroth et al., 2008; Shatil, 2013).

In some cases, the investigations of self-talk were carried out in the context of case studies. In De Franscesco and Burke (1997), Gould et al. (1992) and Park (2000), the frequency of use of the athletes' self-talk was analyzed descriptively. Correlation studies were conducted to examine the relationship between an athlete's sporting success and the frequency of self-talk (Van Raalte et al., 1994). An experimental study (Hatzigeorgiadis et al., 2014) found a different use of self-talk during training and in competition situations. Accordingly, athletes (i.e. swimmers) use both task-specific and motivational self-instruction during training. During competition, the focus is on motivational self-instruction.

In some studies, self-instruction has been investigated in relation to the movement task (Weinberg et al., 1984). According to the results of Theodorakis et al. (2000), Boroujeni and Shahbazi (2011) and Chang et al. (2014), task-specific self-instructions improve performance, especially in more fine-motor tasks (i.e. badminton serve, basketball and softball passing accuracy). Performance in strength or endurance tasks can also be improved by means of a positively motivating self-instruction (Boroujeni & Shahbazi, 2011; Chang et al., 2014). A meta-analysis by Hatzigeorgiadis et al. (2011) was also able to show that in studies in which the participants received extensive/intensive training, the improvements achieved were significantly higher than with only brief explanations and instructions. Without training, however, self-talk seems to achieve positive effects so that it can be used for immediate events and results even in the short term.

21.3.2.2 Practice

The cognitive strategy of self-talk regulation uses the self-talk of slow thinking. It is necessary to control and actively manage them. There are various techniques for constructively regulating self-talk. However, not every athlete is aware of his or her self-talk (slow thinking self-talk). Therefore, the first step is to alert the athlete to his or her self-talk. In most cases, the observation of action-accompanying self-talk is recommended as a first step.

Which Techniques for the Regulation of Self-Talk can be Applied and Distinguished?

- Thought stop technique
- Transformation from negative to positive self-talk
- Reframing
- Combating irrational thought processes
- Affirmations

The **thought stopping technique** is a method to interrupt or eliminate unwanted rumination (self-talk of fast thinking). The technique of thought stopping can be helpful for the athlete, assuming the athlete realizes that he or she is burdened with negative thoughts (Kellmann & Beckmann, 2004; Kellmann et al., 2017). For example, clenching the hand into a fist can amplify the stop signal and interrupt stressful thoughts. A positive alternative thought can also be agreed on and the fist can be loosened again. If the athlete can perform the method on themselves, the final goal is achieved. The method was originally developed for therapeutic purposes and has been successfully used for obsessive thoughts, hallucinations and addictions (Hartig, 1974; Kanfer & Karoly, 1972).

Eberspaecher (2001) recommends the following procedure for successful **transformation from negative to positive self-talk**: First of all, all negative thoughts that affect the sporting performance or lead to undesirable behaviour should be listed. The aim of this step is to identify situations and causes of negative thoughts. Then the negative statement should be replaced by a positive one and the statements should be compared in a table.

If you keep a diary or a training book about your self-talk, you can easily recognize negative self-talk and become sensitized for the active design of self-talk. Zinsser et al. (2006) recommend transforming the unwanted thought into a positive and more appropriate thought immediately after it is perceived. Immenroth et al. (2008) recommend the following procedure:

- Step 1: Observation of the movement-accompanying self-talk
- Step 2: Identification of the movement disturbing self-talk
- Step 3: Rephrasing to movement-supporting self-talk
- Step 4: Training of the generated self-talk

Watzlawick et al. (1974) describe a similar procedure with the so-called technique of reorientation or **reframing**. With this technique, one takes a different perspective or viewpoint and confronts one's supposed weakness or difficulty. Almost every negative thought can be put into a different light or interpreted differently so that it helps the athlete instead of hindering them. By realigning, nothing should be downplayed. Rather, the negative thought should be used to the athlete's own advantage. If the athlete struggles with learning a new demanding technique or is in a supposedly difficult situation, he/she can use this situation to his advantage by changing his attitude. For example, he/she could consider the opportunities and possibilities of an improved or new technique (Zinsser et al., 2006).

To identify and **combat irrational thoughts**, 'rational emotive therapy' (RET), according to Ellis (1977), is used. Within the framework of RET, emerging fears are to be countered with a cognitive coping strategy. Zinsser et al. (2006) describe possible irrational thoughts in the context of competitive sports:

- 'I must perform exceptionally well every time'
- 'Others who seem important to me must like me'
- 'Everyone must treat me fairly and kindly'

In the discourse, the sportsman should come to a new formulation. It is about exposing irrational/dysfunctional beliefs and realizing that they lack logical consistency.

Affirmation means approval or assurance. According to Syer and Connolly (1988), the most effective affirmations are credible and vivid. They often arise spontaneously and reflect a feeling experienced in a particularly satisfying and successful situation. 'I am as strong as a bull!' or 'I'm flying towards the finish line!' are examples of such affirmations. Note that these statements contain current, personal, positive messages. Team slogans can also serve as affirmations (Syer & Connolly, 1988).

Strategies of Self-Talk Regulation

The thought stop technique is intended to inhibit and stop negative and inappropriate thoughts. By taking a different perspective, irrational thoughts can be revealed, and negative ones can be reinterpreted into helpful ones. Such thoughts can be transformed into positive and purposeful thoughts through verbalization.

21.3.3 Gaming

Playing sports such as football require quick and permanent adaptation to changing game situations. Sport-specific cognitive abilities, therefore, appear to be important determinants of athletic performance (Mann et al., 2007). A recent meta-analysis on nine studies that have investigated the executive functions of high-level athletes reported that there is a statistically significant effect for high-performance level populations to perform better on assessments that measure executive functions compared to lower-level and non-sporting populations (Scharfen & Memmert, 2019). More specifically, Vestberg et al. (2012) and Verburgh et al. (2014) showed that the executive functions of talented and higher-level footballers are better developed than lower-level counterparts and norm population values. Seemingly, there are many demanding sporting situations in which slow thinking at a high speed seems to make a decisive difference. How can slow thinking be made faster?

'Gaming' refers to the playful training of the executive functions on device such as a computer, tablet or virtual reality with the help of software that is designed to train specific functional areas of the executive functions in a non-sport-specific way. This form of cognitive training is still relatively new. For instance, gaming attempts to train the underlying cognitive processes that set the foundation to which decision-making processes rest upon, such as executive functions. Training one's core cognitive processes through gaming may positively translate into making more accurate and faster decisions in one's respective sport (Mayer et al., 2019). In turn, the use of gaming may enhance the athlete's in-game performance and their confidence in their own abilities to keep up with the cognitive demands of the game.

Nevertheless, there are now some studies that show remarkable effects. A certain trend seems to be emerging; therefore, we will also briefly discuss this here.

21.3.3.1 Effects of Gaming on Executive Functions

Most research is available on the effects of **action video games**. To be considered an action video game, the game must meet several criteria. The criteria are not unimportant because the effects of the games depend on their content, structure and requirements.

? What makes an action video game stand out?

- High perceptual load (many details, objects)
- High speed (of the action and moving objects)
- Cognitive load (What is my current task? How do I fulfil it and what do I have to do afterwards? What happens when I do this or that?)
- Motor challenge (various possible motor actions)
- Spatial and temporal unpredictability (suddenly appearing opponents)
- High degree of peripheral processes (focus is not only at one position)

Some studies show that video game players (VGP) are better at recording and processing spatial information than non-video game players (NVGP). For visual search tasks, VGP are more accurate and faster, regardless of age. However, NVGP can improve their performance after training in video games (Feng et al., 2007; Green & Bavelier, 2003, 2006a; Spence et al., 2009). Since neither the stimuli used nor their localization within the video games and the visual search tasks were identical in the studies, this speaks on the one hand for a causal link between video games and better cognitive performance and on the other hand for a generalization of the effects. In addition, VGP showed a sharper spatial resolution, which was evident in the recognition of smaller letters (Green & Bavelier, 2007), and better contrast sensitivity (Li et al., 2009). In sports, especially in team sports such as football, handball or hockey, it is advantageous to be able to keep the entire playing field in focus.

Further studies indicate that not only the spatial and temporal aspects of attention but also its capacity and distribution, (i.e. working memory), are altered by video games. For example, in a *multiple object tracking* (MOT) task, VGP were able to identify on average two more objects than NVGP (Dye & Bavelier, 2010; Trick et al., 2005). A training study of NVGP, in which their performance improved, also suggests a causal relationship in this respect (Green & Bavelier, 2006b). In addition, VGP showed better performance in a listing task of short flashing stimuli, with VGP scoring more correct results even for a high number of stimuli (Green & Bavelier, 2006b).

Studies on cognitive flexibility showed that VGP and trained NVGP can switch between different tasks much faster (Colzato et al., 2010; Strobach et al., 2012). In addition, multitasking tasks seem to hardly affect VGP performance (Green & Bavelier, 2006a).

Training of Executive Functions
Studies have shown that action video games can train and modify both the spatial and temporal aspects of attention as well as its capacity and distribution. Furthermore, they can also improve working memory and cognitive flexibility (executive functions).

21.3.3.2 Transfer

In this context, the question arises whether non-specific training of executive functions can have a positive influence on sport-specific skills. Is this transfer possible and useful? The basis of the discussion is from when a transfer can be considered a transfer. Which contextual changes must be present for a transfer to be considered as such? It is generally accepted that a very specific ability is more difficult to transfer than a general ability. The more similar the training and the transfer task is, the easier and quicker a transfer is. The more unspecific a task is learned, the more successful a transfer is (Brown, 1989). However, the more the tasks differ from the context, the more difficult the transfer becomes.

Providing an athlete with a training tool that replicates the cognitive demands of their sport without the additional physical load has value. Specifically, these off-pitch training tools can be used for athletes that are wanting to gain an edge on their mental performance or for players who are injured that miss out on the cognitive stimulation regular training (Beavan et al. (2019). Supporting evidence suggests that training the underlying mechanisms that support decision-making (i.e. processing speed or anticipation, etc.) may transfer into athletes having a better cognitive toolkit that can be used to make more informed decisions (Voss et al., 2010).

Back to gaming: Is it possible to train executive functions through gaming, and is a transfer to the sport-related requirement profile proven here? The far transfer hypothesis states that prolonged experience in activities such as sports and video gaming can improve the individual's cognitive abilities that underlie their expertise (Voss et al., 2010). A far transfer is between two seemingly related, but quite distinct contexts or variations. For example, attempting to transfer the effects of an object tracking task on a computer into helping players tracks players on the field during game play. There are already isolated studies that attempt to measure the effect of gaming on sport-specific requirements. Romeas et al. (2016), for example, were able to show that three-dimensional object tracking (*3D-MOT*) had a positive effect on the passing decision-making accuracy in football players (see ▶ Study Box: Improvement of the Pass Decision by 3D Object Tracking Training).

Improving the Pass Decision Through 3D Object Tracking Training

Most research on video games and executive functions is available on the effects of action video games. However, less research has been done on the direct effects of action video games on athletic performance. In one study (Romeas et al., 2016), footballers were examined in their pass decision quality. The passing quality was assessed in standardized *small-sided games* (SSG) with 5 × 5 players on a 30 × 40-metre pitch by an independent, qualified football coach. The footballers played eight games of 5 min each before and after the training phase. The players were randomly assigned to either the training group (3D-MOT), the active control group (3D football videos: 3D-SV) or the passive control group (without training). Training took place twice across 5 weeks. The 3D-MOT training group was able to improve passing decision quality by 15%, while no improvements in passing decision quality were observed in the two control groups. This was the first study to show a transfer from non-contextual, perceptual-cognitive training to sports situations.

Gaming can be used to place the athlete in a stimulating environment that exercises and trains their cognitive abilities all while keeping the athletes engaged and willing to continue to challenge themselves in the game (Beavan et al., 2019). The enhanced level of stimulus presentation keeps the athletes engaged at a cognitively demanding level for long durations of time, which also may have important benefits especially for helping athletes concentrate throughout the entire game, where the first play of the game is as important as the last. Although promising, further studies on the effects of sport-specific transfers are necessary to substantiate the quite plausible use of gaming to optimize executive functions in sports.

Overall, there is a tendency for gaming to improve executive functions. The improvements are probably due to an increased integration rate of sensory information. Other parallels of video games for learning in the context of competitive sports are a certain level of activation and a form of reward for having mastered or won the game. In addition, video games can represent many different situations, making a greater transfer more likely.

21.4 Conclusion

The goal of a sport psychologist is to ensure that athletes under their supervision execute an optimal performance at a pre-defined date. Sport psychologists can work towards this goal with their athletes in the lead up to a certain event by using the range of techniques for mental and cognitive training provided in this chapter. Successful training outcomes may help athletes learn to more appropriately alternate between the deliberate use of slow and fast thinking, improve regulation of self-talk, and strengthen the confidence of one's performance.

Learning Control Questions

Basic:

1. How are executive functions and performance related in competition?
2. What is the difference between training and competition and what does that lead to in sports?
3. What is the goal of cognitive training and by which methods can this be achieved?
4. Briefly explain Kahneman's 'Dual Systems Theory'.
5. How do fast and slow thinking interact in competition?

Advanced:

6. How can competence conviction and consequence expectation be differentiated?
7. How does competence conviction affect the mastering of problems?
8. Which methods can be used to build up competence conviction? Which of them is most effective?
9. What are the key executive functions? Choose one team sport (i.e. volleyball) and one individual sport (i.e. fencing) and explain how each core executive function may help these athletes perform in their respective sport.
10. What is mental training and how does it work?
11. What is a self-talk, and what environments do athletes most often report using this technique?
12. What methods of self-talk regulation do you know?
13. Create an argument as to why athletes with a strong skill set of executive functions have a stronger chance to become elite level athletes.

Experts:

14. What does functional equivalence mean in the context of mental training and how does it affect movement learning?
15. By which methods can movement concepts be built up? Explain them briefly.
16. What cognitive areas can video games train?
17. What basic characteristics that are important for everyday life are trained in video games and what advantage do they provide?
18. What critical roles do nature and nurture play in the development of executive functions in athletes?
19. What are the advantages and disadvantages of using a video game that is decontextualized from any sporting context within reference towards the 'broad transfer hypothesis' for near and far transfer?
20. Place yourself in the shoes of a practitioner working with an Olympic diver. In the final 4 weeks before the Olympics, which mental and cognitive trainings would you focus your efforts on, and why? Justify which intervention techniques you would choose for your athlete, while keeping in mind the opportunity cost associated with each technique.
21. Which intervention techniques are more suitable for closed-skilled sports versus open-skill sports? With reference to question 20, would your intervention techniques for the Olympic diver also work for a volleyball player? Justify the changes in intervention techniques, if any, with respect to the unique constraints of the different sports.

References

Bandura, A. (1977). Self-efficacy: Toward a unifying theory of behavioural change. *Psychological Review, 84*, 191–215.

Barenberg, J., Berse, T., & Dutke, S. (2011). Executive functions in learning processes: Do they benefit from physical activity? *Educational Research Review, 6*(3), 208–222.

Bauer, J. (2006). *Warum ich fühle, was Du fühlst, Intuitive Kommunikation und das Geheimnis der Spiegelneuronen [Why I feel what you feel, Intuitive communication and the secret of mirror neurons]* (10th ed., pp. 7–56). Heyne.

Beavan, A., Spielmann, J., & Mayer, J. (2019). Taking the first steps toward integrating testing and training cognitive abilities within high-performance athletes; insights from a professional German football club. *Frontiers in Psychology, 10*, 2773.

Beavan, A., Spielmann, J., Mayer, J., Skorski, S., Meyer, T., & Fransen, J. (2020). The rise and fall of executive functions in high-level football players. *Psychology of Sport and Exercise, 49*, 101677.

Bertollo, M., Saltarelli, B., & Robazza, C. (2009). Mental preparation strategies of elite modern pentathletes. *Psychology of Sport and Exercise, 10*(2), 244–254.

Boroujeni, S. T., & Shahbazi, M. (2011). The effect of instructional and motivational self-talk on performance of basketball's motor skill. *Procedia Social and Behavioral Sciences, 15*, 3113–3117.

Brown, A. L. (1989). Analogical learning and transfer: What develops? In S. Vosniadou & A. Ortony (Eds.), *Similarity and analogical reasoning* (pp. 369–412). Cambridge University Press.

Carter, R. (2014). *Das Gehirn: Anatomie, Sinneswahrnehmung, Gedächtnis, Bewusstsein, Störungen, [The Brain: Anatomy, Sensory Perception, Memory, Consciousness, Disorders]*. Dorling Kindersley.

Chang, Y.-K., Ho, L.-A., Lu, F. J.-H., Ou, C.-C., Song, T.-F., & Gill, D. L. (2014). Self-talk and softball performance: The role of self-talk nature, motor task characteristics, and self-efficacy in novice softball players. *Psychology of Sport and Exercise, 15*, 139–145.

Colzato, L. S., van Leeuwen, P. J., van den Wildenberg, W. P., & Hommel, B. (2010). DOOM'd to switch: Superior cognitive flexibility in players of firstperson shooter games. *Frontiers in Psychology, 1*, 8.

De Franscesco, C., & Burke, K. L. (1997). Performance enhancement strategies used in a professional tennis tournament. *International Journal of Sport Psychology, 28*, 185–195.

Diamond, A., Barnett, W. S., Thomas, J., & Munro, S. (2007). Preschool program improves cognitive control. *Science, 318*, 1387–1388.

Driskell, J. E., Copper, C., & Moran, A. (1994). Does mental practiceenhance performance? *Journal of Applied Psychology, 79*(4), 481–492.

Dye, M. W., & Bavelier, D. (2010). Differential development of visual attention skills in school-aged children. *Vision Research, 50*, 452–459.

Eberspaecher, H. (2001). *Mentales Training. Ein Handbuch für Trainer und Sportler [Mental training. A handbook for coaches and athletes] (5th, rev. ed)*. Copress Sport.

Eberspaecher, J., Immenroth, M., & Mayer, J. (2002). Sportpsychologie—Ein zentraler Baustein im modernen Leistungssport [Sports psychology—A central building block in modern competitive sports]. *Leistungssport, 32*, 5–10.

Ellis, A. (1977). *Die Rational-Emotive Therapie: Das innere Selbstgespräch bei seelischen Problemen und seine Veränderungen [Rational-emotive therapy: Inner self-talk in mental problems and its changes]*. J Pfeiffer.

Feltz, D. L., Short, S. E., & Sullivan, P. J. (2008). *Self efficacy in sport*. Human Kintics.

Feltz, D. L., & Landers, D. M. (1983). The effects of mental practice on motor skill learning and performance: A meta-analysis. *Journal of Sport Psychology, 5*, 25–57.

Feltz, D. L., Landers, D. M., & Becker, B. J. (1988). A revised meta-analysis of the mental practice literature on motor skill learning. In D. Druckmann & J. A. Swets (Eds.), *Enhancing human performance: Issues, theories, and techniques*. National Academy Press.

Feng, J., Spence, I., & Pratt, J. (2007). Playing action video game reduces gender differences in spatial cognition. *Psychological Science, 18*, 850–855.

Furley, P., & Memmert, D. (2012). Working memory capacity as controlled attention in tactical decision making. *Journal of Sport & Exercise Psychology, 34*(3), 322–344.

Furley, P., & Wood, G. (2016). Working memory, attentional control, and expertise in sports: A review of current literature and directions for future research. *Journal of Applied Research in Memory and Cognition, 5*(4), 415–425.

Gonzalez, D. C., & McVeigh, A. (2013). The art of mental training: A guide to performance excellence. .

Gould, D., Eklund, R. C., & Jackson, S. (1992). Coping strategies used by more versus less successful Olympic wrestlers. *Research Quarterly for Exercise and Sport, 64*, 83–93.

Green, C. S., & Bavelier, D. (2003). Action video game modifies visual selective attention. *Nature, 423*, 534–537.

Green, C. S., & Bavelier, D. (2006a). Effect of action video games on the spatial distribution of visuospatial attention. *Journal of Experimental Psychology: Human Perception and Performance, 32*, 1465–1478.

Green, C. S., & Bavelier, D. (2006b). Enumeration versus multiple object tracking: The case of action video game players. *Cognition, 101*, 217–245.

Green, C. S., & Bavelier, D. (2007). Action-video-game experience alters the spatial resolution of vision. *Psychological Science, 18*, 88–94.

Guillot, A., Nadrowska, E., & Collet, C. (2009). Using motor imagery to learn tactical movements in basketball. *Journal of sport behaviour, 32*(2), 189–206.

Hanton, S., & Jones, G. (1999). The effects of a multimodal intervention program on performers: II. Training the butterflies to fly in formation. *The Sport Psychologist, 13*(1), 22–41.

Hardy, J., Gammage, K., & Hall, C. (2001). A descriptive study of athlete self-talk. *The Sport Psychologist, 15*, 306–318.

Hardy, L., Jones, G., & Gould, D. (1996). *Understanding psychological preparation for sport: Theory and practice of elite performers*. Wiley.

Hartig, M. (1974). Die Anwendung von Techniken der Selbstkontrolle in der Verhaltenstherapie. In C. Kraiker (Ed.), *Handbuch der Verhaltenstherapie*. Reinbek.

Hatzigeorgiadis, A., Galanis, E., Zourbanos, N., & Theodorakis, Y. (2014). Self-talk and competitive sport performance. *Journal of Applied Sport Psychology, 26*, 82–95.

Hatzigeorgiadis, A., Zourbanos, N., Galanis, E., & Theodorakis, Y. (2011). The effects of self-talk on performance in sport: A meta-analysis. *Perspectives on Psychological Science, 6*(4), 348–356.

Heuer, H. (1985). Wie wirkt mentale Übung [How does mental exercise work]? *Psychologische Rundschau, 36*, 191–200.

Holmes, P. S., & Collins, D. J. (2001). The PETTLEP approach to motor imagery: A functional equivalence model for sport psychologists. *Journal of Applied Sport Psychology., 13*(1), 60–83.

Iacoboni, M., Woods, R., Brass, M., Bekkering, H., Mazziotta, J. C., & Rizozolatti, G. (1996). Cortical mechanism of human imitation. *Science, 286*, 2526–2528.

Jacobson, J., & Matthaeus, L. (2014). Athletics and executive functioning: How athletic participation and sport type correlate with cognitive performance. *Psychology of Sport and Exercise, 15*(5), 521–527.

Immenroth, M., Eberspächer, H., & Hermann, H.-D. (2008). *Training kognitiver Fertigkeiten [Cognitive skills training]. Encyclopedia of psychology*. Hogrefe.

Kahneman, D. (2011). *Thinking, fast and slow* (1st ed.). Farrar, Straus and Giroux.

Kane, M. J., Brown, L. H., McVay, J. C., Silvia, P. J., Myin-Germeys, I., & Kwapil, T. R. (2007). For whom the mind wanders, and when: An experience-sampling study of working memory and executive control in daily life. *Psychological Science, 18*(7), 614–621.

Kanfer, F. H., & Karoly, P. (1972). Self-control: A behavioristic excursion into the lion's den. *Behavior Therapy, 3*(3), 398–416.

Kellmann, M., & Beckmann, J. (2004). Sport und Entspannungsverfahren [Sport and relaxation procedures]. D. Vaitl & F.

Kellmann, M., Pelka, M., & Beckmann, J. (2017). Psychological relaxation techniques to enhance recovery in sports. *Sport, recovery, and performance, Routledge*, 247–259.

Klingberg, T. (2009). *The Overflowing Brain. Information overload and the limits of working memory*. Oxford University Press.

Kubesch, S. (2008). *Körperliche Aktivität und exekutive Funktionen [Physical activity and executive functions]. Young sports science series*. Hoffmann.

Li, R., Polat, U., Makous, W., & Bavelier, D. (2009). Enhancing the contrast sensitivity function through action video game training. *Nature Neuroscience, 12*, 549–551.

Luna, B. (2009). Developmental changes in cognitive control through adolescence. *Advances in Child Development and Behavior, 37*, 233–278.

Mann, D., Williams, A. M., Ward, P., & Janelle, C. (2007). Perceptual-cognitive expertise in sport: A meta-analysis. *Journal of Sport & Exercise Psychology, 29*, 457–478.

Mayer, J., & Hermann, H.-D. (2011). *Mentales Training: Grundlagen und Anwendung in Sport, Rehabilitation, Arbeit und Wirtschaft [Mental training: Basics and application in sports rehabilitation, work and business]*. Springer.

Mayer, R. E., Parong, J., & Bainbridge, K. (2019). Young adults learning executive function skills by playing focused video games. *Cognitive Development, 49*, 43–50.

Meltzer, L. (2007). *Executive function in education: From theory to practice*. Guilford Publications.

Moritz, S. E., Feltz, D. L., Fahrbach, K. R., & Mack, D. E. (2000). The relation of self-efficacy measures to sport performance: A meta-analytic review. *Research Quarterly for Ecercise and Sport, 71*, 280–294.

Morris, T., Spittle, M., & Watt, A. (2005). *Imagery in sport*. Human Kinetics.

Munzert, J. (2001). Bewegungsvorstellungen—Bewegungshandlungsvorstellungen [Movement conceptions—Movement action conceptions]. In D. Hackfort (Ed.), *Action psychology research for the theory and practice of sport psychology*. Bps.

Munzert, J., Dültgen, K., & Möllman, H. (2000). Individuelle Merkmale von Bewegungsvorstellungen. Eine explorative Untersuchung im Badminton [Individual characteristics of movement perceptions. An exploratory study in badminton]. *Psychology and Sport, 7*, 15–25.

Munzert, J., Lorey, B., & Zentgraf, K. (2009). Cognitive motor processes: The role of motor imagery in the study of motor representation. *Brain Research Reviews, 60*, 306–326.

Munzertz, J., & Möllman, H. (1997). Zeitliche Dauer mental simulierterBewegungshandlungen im Badminton [Duration of mentally simulated actions in badminton]. *Psychologyand Sport, 4*, 102–113.

Munzert, J., & Zentgraf, K. (2009). Motor imagery and its implications for understanding the motor system. *Progress in Brain Research, 174*, 219–229.

Murphy, S. M. (1994). Imagery interventions in sport. *Medicine and Science in Sports and Exercise, 26*, 486–494.

Page, S. J., Sime, W., & Nordell, K. (1999). The effects of imagery on female college swimmers' perceptions of anxiety. *The Sport Psychologist, 13*(4), 458–469.

Paivio, A. (1985). Cognitive and motivational functions of imagery in human performance. *Canadian Journal of Applied Sport Sciences, 10*, 22–28.

Park, J. K. (2000). Coping strategies used by Korean national athletes. *The Sport Psychologist, 14*, 63–80.

Porro, C. A., Francescato, M. P., Cettolo, V., Diamond, M. E., Baraldi, P., Zuiani, C., Bazzocchi, M., & di Prampero, P. E. (1996). Primary motor and sensory cortex activation during motor performance and motor imagery. *The Journal of Neuroscience, 16*, 7688–7698.

Rizzolatti, G., Fadiga, L., Gallese, V., et al. (1996). "Premotor cortex and the recognition of motor actions". Cognitive Brain Research, 3(2), 131–141.

Romeas, T., Guldner, A., & Faubert, J. (2016). 3D-Multiple Object Tracking training task improves passing decision-making accuracy in soccer players. *Psychology of Sport and Exercise, 22*, 1–9.

Roth, M., Decety, J., Raybaudi, M., et al. (1996). Possible involvement of primary motor cortex in mentally simulated movement: A functional magnetic resonance imaging study. *Neuroreport, 7*(7), 1280–1284.

Scharfen, H. E., & Memmert, D. (2019). Measurement of cognitive functions in experts and elite athletes: A meta-analytic review. Applied Cognitive Psychology, *33*(5), 843–860.

Shannon, V., Gentner, N. B., Patel, A., & Muccio, D. (2012). Striking gold: Mental techniques and preparation strategies used by Olympic gold medallists. *Athletic Insight: The Online Journal of Sport Psychology, 4*, 1–11.

Sharma, N., & Baron, J.-C. (2013). Does motor imagery share neural networks with executed movement: A multivariate fMRI analysis. *Frontiers in Human Neuroscience, 7*, 564.

Shatil, E. (2013). Does combined cognitive training and physical activity training enhance cognitive abilities more than either alone? A four-condition randomized controlled trial among healthy older adults. *Frontiers in Aging Neuroscience, 5*, 8.

Sly, D., Mellalieu, S. D., & Wagstaff, C. R. (2020). "It's psychology Jim, but not as we know it!": The changing face of applied sport psychology. Sport, Exercise, and Performance Psychology, 9(1), 87.

Spence, I., Yu, J. J., Fend, J., & Marshman, J. (2009). Women match men when learning a spatial skill. *Journal of Experimental Psychology. Learning, Memory, and Cognition, 35*, 1097–1103.

Stinear, C. M., Byblow, W. D., Steyvers, M., Levin, O., & Swinnen, S. P. (2006). Kinaesthetic, but not visual, motor imagery modulates corticomotor excitability. *Experimental Brain Research, 168*, 157–164.

Stratton, G., Reilly, T., Williams, A. M., & Richardson, D. (2004). *Youth soccer: From science to performance* (pp. 138–159). Psychology Press.

Strobach, T., Frensch, P. A., & Schubert, T. (2012). Video game practice optimizes executive control skills in dual-task and task switching situations. *Acta Psychologica, 140*(1), 13–24.

Syer, J., & Connolly, C. (1988). *Psychotraining für Sportler [Psychotraining for athletes]*. Rowohlt.

Thelwell, R. C., & Greenlees, I. A. (2001). The effects of a mental skills training package on gymnasium triathlon performance. *The Sport Psychologist, 15*, 127–141.

Thelwell, R. C., Weston, N. J. V., Greenlees, I. A., & Hutchings, N. V. (2008). A qualitative exploration of psychological-skills use in coaches. *The Sport Psychologist, 22*, 38–53.

Theodorakis, Y., Weinberg, R., Natsis, P., Douma, I., & Kazakas, P. (2000). The effects of motivational versus instructional self-talk on improving motor performance. *The Sport Psychologist, 14*, 253–272.

Trick, L. M., Jaspers-Fayer, F., & Sethi, N. (2005). Multiple-object tracking in children. The "Catch the Spies" task. *Cognitive Development, 20*, 373–387.

Van Raalte, J. L., Brewer, B. W., Rivera, P. M., & Petitpas, A. J. (1994). The relationship between observable self-talk and competitive junior tennis players' match performances. *Journal of Sport & Exercise Psychology, 16*, 400–415.

Van Raalte, J. L., Vincent, A., Brewer, B., & W. (2016). Self-Talk: Review and sport-specific model. *Psychology of Sport and Exercise, 22*, 139–148.

Verburgh, L., Scherder, E., van Lange, P., & Osterlaan, J. (2014). Executive functioning in highly talented soccer players. *PLoS One, 9*(3), e91254.

Vestberg, T., Gustafson, R., Maurex, L., Ingvar, M., & Petrovic, P. (2012). Executive functions predict the success of top-soccer players. *PLoS One, 7*(4), e34731.

Watzlawick, P., John, H., Weakland, J. H., & Fisch, R. (1974). *Lösungen. Zur Theorie und Praxis menschlichen Wandels*. Huber.

Voss, M. W., Kramer, A. F., Basak, C., Prakash, R. S., & Roberts, B. (2010). Are expert athletes 'expert'in the cognitive laboratory? A meta-analytic review of cognition and sport expertise. *Applied Cognitive Psychology, 24*(6), 812–826.

Weinberg, R. S., Smith, J., Jackson, A., & Gould, D. (1984). Effect of association, dissociation and positive self-talk strategies on endurance performance. *Canadian Journal of Applied Sport Sciences, 9*(1), 25–32.

Weinberg, R. S. (2008). Does imagery work? Effects on performance and mental skills. *Journal of Imagery Research in Sport and Physical Activity, 3*(1), 1–21.

Wriessnegger, S. C., Steyrl, D., Koschutnig, K., & Müller-Putz, G. R. (2014). Short time sports exercise boosts motor imagery patterns: Implications of mental practice in rehabilitation programs. *Frontiers in Human Neuroscience, 8*, 469.

Zinsser, N., Bunker, L., & Williams, J. M. (2006). Cognitive techniques for building confidence and enhancing performance. In J. M. Williams (Ed.), *Applied sport psychology: Personal growth to peak performance* (5th ed., pp. 349–381). McGraw-Hill.

Applying Group Dynamics to Enhance Sport Teams

Manfred Wegner and M. Blair Evans

Contents

J. Schüler et al. (eds.), *Sport and Exercise Psychology*, https://doi.org/10.1007/978-3-031-03921-8_22

Learning Objectives

Basic:

- Recall key historical works within the study of small groups
- Recognize the key inputs, processes, and outputs that comprise group dynamics

Advanced:

- Recall the predominant approaches to team development
- Recognize seminal models of team development

Experts:

- Develop a skillset to apply team building strategies, based on examples of interventions reported in publications
- Understand how to stimulate team reflections and conduct a debriefing

22.1 Introduction

When we observe a high-performing group in action, it is easy to underestimate the delicate combination of forces necessary for team members to cooperate efficiently. For instance, Hofstätter (1957) described groups using a term that essentially means "person in the plural." Sport teams are nevertheless much more than a plurality of people and instead are dynamic social systems with each team featuring a unique constellation of relationships among members. The field of study involving interactions among teammates is called group dynamics. The study of group dynamics has identified common psychological and social processes that unfold among team members, and the current chapter explores how this knowledge is used to enhance team performance and athlete experiences.

One hallmark of using group dynamics-based approaches is drawing upon theory and deliberately applying the best-available evidence. Theory is therefore important to application, and this chapter builds upon the fundamental principles of group dynamics established in ▶ Chap. 16. For instance, Eys et al. (2020) define small groups using key attributes, such as how (a) team members are aware that they—and their teammates—belong to and represent a "group," (b) team member interactions are guided by social structures like social norms about what behaviors are appropriate, and (c) group members are interdependent, both when pursuing the group's collective outcomes and when pursuing their individual goals. Eys et al. (2020) also established a conceptual framework that distinguishes the elements that contribute to how team members interact with one another.

? Conceptual Framework: Elements That Contribute to How Team Members Interact with One another (Eys et al., 2020)

1. *Inputs*, which are the key characteristics of the group and its members that shape how members interact. This includes member attributes such as personalities or skillsets, as well as features of the group environment such as the number of members in the group, whether members have a collective outcome, and how the training environment is designed.
2. These inputs shape *group structures, group processes, and emergent states*. With time, group members (a) shape group structures that are the shared expectations regarding how their interactions should unfold (e.g., social norms), (b) develop emergent states that include affective and cognitive perceptions regarding the group and fellow teammates over time (e.g., cohesion), and (c) interact in ways that are referred to as group processes—the things that members "do" (e.g., communication).
3. These states and processes come to determine *group and individual outcomes*.

Practitioners use the definition and framework above to identify the goals of an intervention and determine strategies to match those goals. For instance, numerous interventions (e.g., Prapavessis et al., 1996) use the components of this framework to identify aspects of teams that can be modified, including the group structures (e.g., establishing team norms), emergent states (e.g., promoting commitment), or group processes (e.g., teaching leadership skills).

The current chapter introduces key concepts related to group development and characterizes current research approaches to intervene with sport teams. Even though the focus of the current chapter is on sport, we draw from research in other domains and anticipate that approaches described herein may apply to other contexts like workplace teams, students within classrooms, or youth programs. Our chapter concludes by reflecting on how groups develop and emerge with time and how to improve that process.

22.2 Introducing Team Development

Sport researchers and practitioners use group dynamics principles to address many issues. For instance, group dynamics principles can be applied early on when assembling a team (e.g., how can we select personalities who will complement one another?). Despite often being seen as solely a way to get groups off to a "good start," group dynamics principles are also ideally used to maintain a positive environment and promote teamwork throughout a group's lifespan. Team leaders can, for example, use group dynamics principles to address infighting among athletes that may arise throughout a season. To demonstrate the breadth of these issues, the side story provides examples of the "challenges" in teams that we (the chapter authors) have faced in our applied careers working alongside coaches, athlete leaders, sport administrators, and sport organizations. These challenges certainly involve questions focused on how to enhance group functioning but also extend more broadly (see Stumpf & Thomas, 2003). Because groups are ideally a place for athletes to develop positive assets and experience belongingness (Côté et al., 2014; König & Schattenhofer, 2018), group dynamics have also been used to promote athlete well-being, development, and health behaviors.

Side Story

Example reasons for team development

Team development in sport can tackle numerous challenges when trying to enhance the group environment. Below is a non-exhaustive list of common reasons why leaders of sport teams seek out help to develop their teams. Would you add anything else to the list below?

• Helping members feel united	• Developing youths' social skills
• Promoting efficient communication during competition	• Clarify each members' role and their significance for the group
• Promoting commitment to the team	• Selecting members with personalities that complement the group
• Socializing newcomers into the group	• Reducing negative conflict (e.g., infighting)
• Supporting members' mental health	• Fostering positive social norms
• Reducing factions (i.e., cliques)	• Promoting healthy behaviors (e.g., encouraging physical activity)
• Enhancing leadership	• Reducing health-risk behaviors (e.g., discouraging playing while injured)
• Fostering collective understanding of a team's "system" (known formally as a shared mental model; Cannon-Bowers et al., 1993)	• Reducing hazing of newcomers
• Setting group and individual goals	

Sports Practice

As an example of a situation in which group dynamics could inform a solution, consider the following hypothetical scenario involving an adolescent girls' football team competing at the highest level in their region:

> Goal conflicts have created factions among members on the 'Highlands Region Football Club.' Several athletes on this team see their primary goal for being a team member as being recognized by scouts from major clubs and to build their personal skillset to reach the next level. Because this subgroup of athletes uses the group to develop their skills and to be showcased to scouts from more elite teams, they do not invest in fostering relationships with teammates. Other athletes on this team, in contrast, prioritize the group. This second subgroup is dedicated to personal improvement, but they also want to contribute as a unique member of the group and want to achieve team goals. These differing goals are what Stahl views as the driving forces behind members' commitment and satisfaction in the group. Because teammates have formed closer affiliations with others who share their orientation, there are factions of players that are struggling to cooperate and that are producing arguments between teammates away from the field.

Team leaders might intuitively respond to the scenario above in unstructured ways like having social events or hosting general team meetings. Although these strategies may prove effective, an understanding of group dynamics literature may help a coach or sport psychology consultant uncover the source of the conflict in teams. A practitioner with an understanding of the evidence base, for example, may be aware of valid measures to assess members' attitudes about the group, may be aware of strategies for establishing prosocial team norms, or could be trained to deliver specific intervention protocol involving moderated discussions of conflicts. In contrast with the informal strategies and decisions that naturally take place in teams, we will use the term "team development" in this chapter to focus on how group dynamics theories inform strategies, decisions, and interventions that are applied to influence groups (Lacerenza et al., 2018). Team development interventions are the particular focus of the next section of this chapter.

Self-Reflection

Please take a moment to consider a group to which you belong. Perhaps this is your workplace team, an exercise class, or a student club. Consider your personal reasons for belonging to this group—which we describe as your personal goal pool. Using the list below, rank the importance of each goal behind why you are a member of this group from 1 (*most important*) to 10 (*least important*).

Examples:

- Be helpful to others.
- To feel like I "belong" within something.
- Feel accepted.
- Compare my performances or efforts against others.
- Experience being fully engaged in the group tasks.
- Stay committed to my own goals (e.g., training or exercise goals).
- Being recognized by others for the things I am good at.
- Have fun with others in the group.
- Feel good about who I am.
- To feel unique from others in my group.

In what ways do you feel that these reasons influence how to behave in those groups? For instance, how would you respond when you experience others in the group whose priorities differ from your own?

22.2.1 Defining Team Development Interventions

Team development interventions involve combining strategies that are purposefully designed to target specific processes and that use group dynamics theory to do so (see Antons, 2011). Team development interventions are designed and implemented by either (a) a practitioner who is outside of the group's boundaries such as a sport psychology consultant or (b) an existing group leader like a coach. In sport research, team building is the most widespread type of team development intervention (Eys et al., 2020). Birrer and Seiler (2008) describe team building as the set of strategies to facilitate the likelihood that the group will fulfill its collective tasks while satisfying members' needs. Whereas this definition is broad, it does highlight how team building interventions focus on ensuring that members develop positive evaluations regarding the group, their role, and their relationships with teammates.

Archetypal Forms of Team Building

Although team building can practically be delivered through any combination of activities or rituals among members, researchers have identified four "archetypal" forms of team building (Shuffler et al., 2011; Stumpf & Thomas, 2003):

1. *Goal-setting.* Team building measures that bring members together collectively to clarify and agree on group goals, ways for individuals to contribute to group goals, and individual objectives of the group members. Goal-setting also identifies practical ways for members to achieve goals.
2. *Role clarification.* Team building activities to develop an understanding of members' formal and informal roles. These activities may range from clarifying each member's responsibilities to fostering a sense that all members make important contributions to the group.
3. *Interpersonal relationship development.* Team building efforts to improve interpersonal relationships and build trust.
4. *Problem-solving.* Team building strategies that place group members into situations where they face problems and must develop joint solutions, implement them, and review their solution.

There are now dozens of published descriptions or evaluations of team building interventions in sport that include a wide spectrum of approaches including and beyond the four approaches described above (Bruner

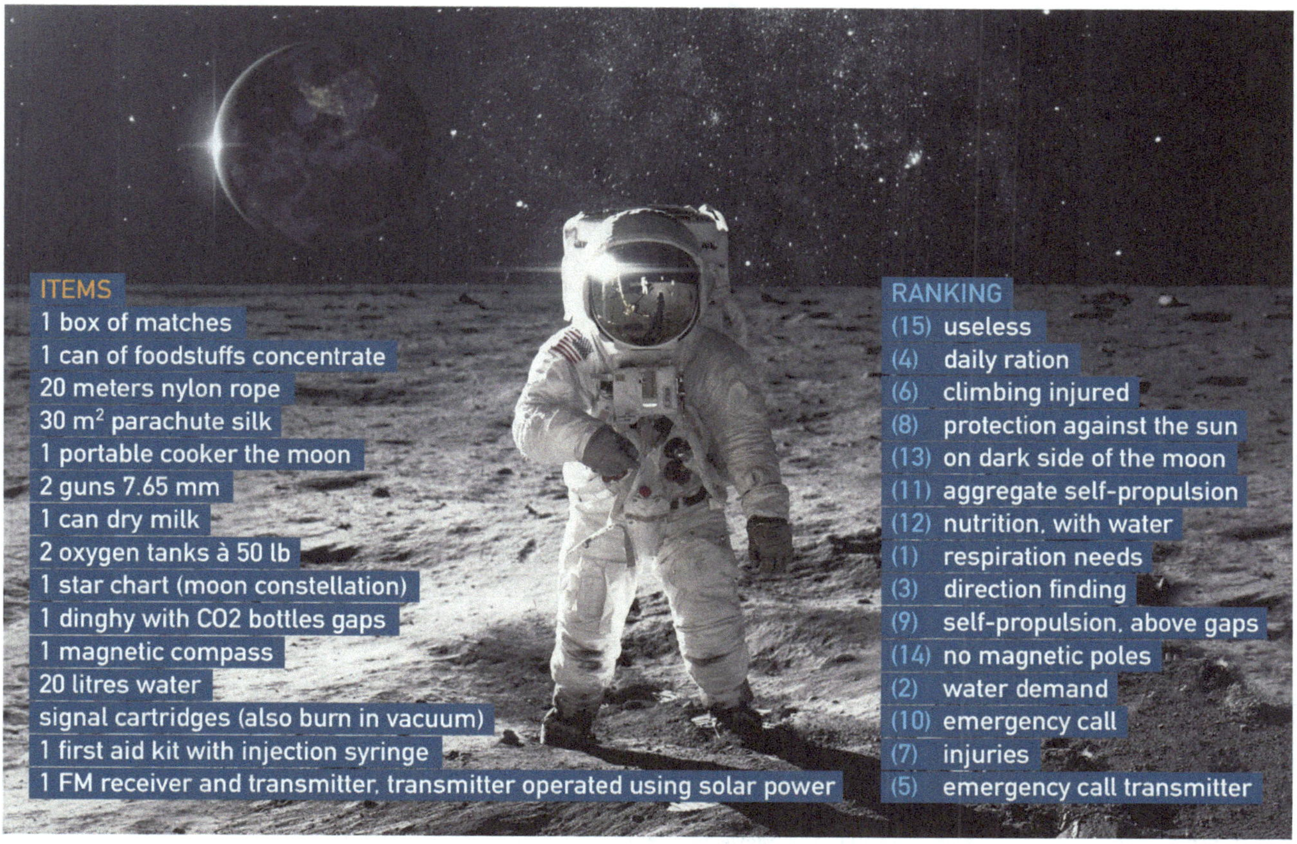

Fig. 22.1 *List of items used within the stranded space team scenario.* On the left is the list of items available to the team to be rated, and on the right is the respective ranking of that item that would be used to score participants' responses (see Pfeiffer & Jones, 1970)

et al., 2013). The box on "Moon survival scenarios…" (accompanied by Fig. 22.1) also provides one example of a problem-solving activity that could be integrated within a team development intervention.

Among the published team building approaches in sport, a review by Bruner et al. (2013) identified one intervention protocol developed by researchers Carron, Spink, and Prapavessis as the most widely applied (e.g., Prapavessis et al., 1996). This protocol focuses on training group leaders (e.g., coaches) to actively deliver strategies that enhance their group environment. A facilitator teaches group leaders about group dynamics and common team building strategies through workshops. Group leaders are educated in group dynamics concepts and then provided with examples that relate to the team environment (e.g., creating some team "swag" for members to wear), structure (e.g., activities to foster norms), and processes (e.g., problem-solving activities; Prapavessis et al., 1996). Subsequently, the facilitator encourages participants to brainstorm and implement strategies for their own groups.

Although early sport literature tended to describe any attempt to intervene on group environments as team building, scholars from organizational psychology (i.e., study of people at work) have more precisely defined team building and distinguished it from additional intervention approaches. Lacerenza et al. (2018) reviewed the evidence base and identified four predominant types of team development interventions, which include team building, teamwork training, leadership training, and team debriefing. These four types each follow different pathways to develop teams, ranging from techniques to help team members coordinate their actions, feel united, and adapt to challenges through group discussion—along with team-based activities to improve the relationships between leaders and followers. Table 22.1 provides clear definitions for each type, describes the focus of that intervention type, and provides an example of each within sport.

Evidence suggests that each of the four intervention approaches can be effective. A meta-analysis aggregating the effects of team building interventions in sport

Table 22.1 Lacerenza et al.' (2018) team development types, applied to sport

Type	Focus	Example
Team building "…a method of helping the group to (a) increase effectiveness, (b) satisfy the needs of its members, or (c) improve work conditions" (Brawley & Paskevich, 1997; p. 13)	**Group as a whole:** All members regularly included in team building **Process- or experience-based:** Members participate in shared activities or rituals	Barker et al. (2014) – **Personal-disclosure mutual-sharing** Adolescent teams participated in group sessions during a major international event. In the first session, rules for disclosure were described, and athletes were prompted to write a speech responding to one or more prompt (e.g., why do you participate in elite sport?). Team members met during two subsequent sessions, and each member presented a speech with their disclosure
Teamwork training Approaches to improve team members' competencies to cooperate as well as their understanding of how to cooperate (Salas et al., 2008)	**Group as a whole:** Members participate in sessions to develop teamwork skills **Learning-based:** Members learn about how to effectively cooperate	McEwan and Beauchamp (2020) – **Teamwork training** Group facilitator hosted two training sessions during the season. During each session, members received feedback regarding their responses to group dynamics surveys and received training. For instance, team members discussed the group goals, completed simulations of critical situations, or completed worksheets about ideal ways to debrief with teammates
Leadership training Approaches to ensure that those appointed to leadership roles use effective behaviors. Includes appointed/formal leaders or informal leaders recognized by others	**Primarily leaders.** Targets leaders' capability to lead. Training can nevertheless include collective activities with all members **Learning-based**. Leaders learn about effective behaviors and about how to self-regulate their actions	Fransen et al. (2020) – **5 Rs of leadership training** Involves workshop sessions with all team members included to identify social and task leaders and subsequently develop leaders' skills to promote a shared team identity. Athlete leaders who are selected by teammates are assigned a role in delivering the workshop, where they lead their team in activities to help their group embody a chosen identity
Team debriefing Members reflect on a performance or shared experience by discussing what happened and reflecting on future actions or goals	**Group as a whole:** All members participate in discussions **Process- or experience-based.** Members engage in discussion	Martin and Eys (2019) Although explicit debriefing interventions are not evident in sport, Martin and Eys described pre- and post-flight briefings among pilots who belonged to an acrobatic flying team. The authors described debriefing among veteran members and recruits. After every group flight, members immediately met for a structured discussion highlighting their successes and mistakes and reflecting on how the group flight unfolded

Note. There can be variability in how much an intervention type focuses on learning or process/experience. For instance, teamwork training and leadership training both target explicit goals for learning but can provide environments for shared experiences that are akin to team building. Likewise, although debriefing is a process-based approach, those leading debriefing may choose to orient discussions around explicit learning goals

reported positive and significant effects on outcomes like perceptions of social cohesion, team performance, and beliefs such as satisfaction with the group (Martin et al., 2009). This meta-analysis did not encompass the additional three types of interventions and was limited to only 17 studies that were of poor methodological quality (i.e., none were experimental and all had small sample sizes). Our understanding of sport team development intervention effectiveness is, therefore, only emerging.

More recent meta-analyses in organizational psychology have clarified our understanding related to team development intervention effectiveness. Notably, researchers who have aggregated effects from across investigations in the workplace continue to report that published studies involving team development interventions report positive effects on numerous team and individual outcomes (DiazGranados et al., 2017). Researchers have, nevertheless, clarified the match between types of team development and key outcomes within organizations. When a practitioner hopes to increase affective outcomes like team members' trust and satisfaction, team building interventions are likely to bring about the greatest improvement. Team building is also most effective for supporting group processes, such as trying to improve communication. In contrast, studies have reported that teamwork training may be the ideal intervention type when practitioners are focused primarily on improving performance, as well as team cognitions (e.g., knowledge of team standards; DiazGranados et al., 2017; McEwan et al., 2017).

22.2.2 Reaching Further Afield to Understand Team Development

To this point, we have primarily drawn upon contemporary work within sport, exercise, and organizational psychology. However, we can learn a great deal by examining the historical roots of team development and by considering team development in other settings. In this section of the chapter, we reflect on (a) the use of T-groups, which emerged alongside early in the history of group dynamics research and (b) how group psychotherapy leaders foster group development. We note that the reader should approach this section with caution because these uses of group dynamics demand training and experience within helping domains (e.g., counselling). Nevertheless, these areas provide insights regarding team development.

T-Groups. The history of group dynamics as a bona fide field of study is commonly drawn back toward the founding of the *Research Center for Group Dynamics* by Kurt Lewin at the Massachusetts Institute for Technology in the 1940s as well as the writing of Austrian psychiatrist Jacob Moreno (see Rechtien, 2007). During these early years, researchers and practitioners began implementing a form of training called "T-groups," which gained popularity as a technique for leadership and management training in organizations (Highhouse, 2002). T-groups encompass a family of strategies (including sensitivity training and encounter groups) that involve discussions in unstructured groups composed of facilitators as well as participants. Participants were often coworkers in organizations or managers attending sessions from several organizations (Rechtien, 2007) who participated in lengthy discussion across extended time periods with the idea that members will engage in experiential learning. T-groups traditionally lacked specific goals or plans for the meeting. Members often entered group discussions with general outcomes in mind like enhancing communication. However, the lack of structure within the groups and ongoing feedback from passive facilitators was designed to prompt personal disclosure. The meetings were designed to foster trust among attendees and encourage personal reflection where members explored internal conflicts as well as conflicts with others, in ways that participants often perceived as profound experiences (Highhouse, 2002).

The T-group intervention approaches of early proponents nevertheless fell out of favor among scholars and practitioners because of several concerns (Highhouse, 2002). As one example, sessions were viewed as unethical to the extent that participants felt coerced to disclose personal information in ways that could damage themselves or their careers. Employees were disclosing personal information in spaces that felt safe but which could damage their standing alongside colleagues.

Modern applications and uses of T-groups are nevertheless evident. Some group dynamics texts do continue to leverage T-group principles (e.g., Antons, 2018; Rechtien, 2007), such as when describing techniques to address conflict among members. Techniques recommended in these texts do include some psychotherapeutic strategies for the use of T-groups that are risky and inadvisable without safeguards in place. For instance, Antons (2018) advocate marathon training sessions lasting over 24 h that stress and deplete members (e.g., lack of sleep, physical exhaustion) with the purported aim of providing more open exchanges among group members. Notwithstanding these concerns, the authors make a strong case for several techniques that sport leaders could apply to team development. Wegner and Dawo (2013), for instance, emphasize the value of *skill training* that involves developing social skills and awareness of others—commonly through perspective taking. Within sport, this might involve placing defense experts from football into attacking roles or vice versa. Another option is role-playing where a facilitator assigns players with roles and places them into scenarios with teammates. These situations can be fictitious, such as where athletes role-play responding to the injury of a star player. This situation could also be more immediate, such as having a discussion where members are assigned to play different roles when discussing team goals for the upcoming season or about decisions facing the group.

The history of T-groups is also the foundation for many principles in common team building strategies used by sport psychology consultants. As an example, personal disclosure team building interventions published in sport literature encourage disclosure as a tool to strengthen interpersonal bonds among members (see Barker et al., 2014). T-groups have also informed the planning for team development meetings, especially when disclosure is a goal. One particularly powerful focus is on breaking social habits (König & Schattenhofer, 2018), where the facilitator hosts a team development meeting in a new setting that disrupts habits in the group. Novel settings "shake up" the typical expectations in groups and may disrupt the status hierarchy to provide low-status members with opportunities to contribute.

Group Psychotherapy Group dynamics principles are also a critical component within group psychotherapy, even though sport and organizational psychologists rarely draw upon theories and findings from clinical or counselling psychology (Parks, 2021). In group psychotherapy, members who are united by a common problem or life experience (e.g., individuals experiencing depression) interact within groups facilitated by counsellors, clinical psychologists, or psychiatrists. The prevailing technique is cognitive behavioral therapy, where participants form consistent groups to openly discuss their goal pursuit in a group that shares feedback and support throughout the process of personal change (Burlingame & Jensen, 2017). As interpersonal relationships form over numerous sessions, group cohesion is one of the most powerful predictors of clinical outcomes in group psychotherapy (Crowe & Grenyer, 2008).

Many insights from group psychotherapy are limited to the use of trained therapists in controlled settings. For instance, the box (▶ For Sports Practice) describes one exemplar methodology used in group psychotherapy. Nevertheless, there are also many practical insights that can be useful when leading sport groups, involving structuring group discussions, setting group goals, managing conflict, selecting members for groups, and fostering a positive group environment. As one example, member-to-member feedback is particularly critical in group psychotherapy, as group members describe their feelings or reactions in response to the actions of another member (Burlingame & Jensen, 2017). Morran et al. (1998) have identified several best practices when structuring feedback during sessions—particularly focused on providing positive feedback (e.g., support and encouragement) and corrective feedback (e.g., reflecting on the feedback receiver's need to change).

Group Psychotherapy Protocol Involving Group Dynamics Concepts

The main text discusses general insights that can be translated from psychotherapy to team development. However, group psychotherapy practitioners have also established protocol and standardized tools that implement group dynamics concepts. One example is systems-centered training—an approach toward psychotherapy that carries numerous assumptions that guide how groups are developed and managed. As one assumption, this approach focuses on subgroups that naturally emerge in groups and uses techniques that leverage *functional subgrouping* (Agazarian, 2004).

Functional subgrouping involves identifying the subgroups that underpin conflict experienced by the group. As opposed to setting out to merge or combine the subgroups, conflict is addressed first within each functional subgroup—where the two factions falling on either side of an issue first discuss the issue within their own subgroup. For instance, a counsellor might first separate the larger group so that members are placed alongside other members of their subgroups and are prompted to discuss their attitudes toward a conflict. This discussion integrates strategies like prompting members of a subgroup to take the perspective of the other subgroup. After lengthy discussion, the group is finally united. The approach to first use the functional subgroups for discussion is because (a) this is a comfortable environment to discuss the issues, (b) members begin to recognize that attitudes in their group are heterogeneous, and (c) members can take perspective of other groups. Imagine as one example a track and field team where the "field" event members (e.g., throwers) are conflicting with track event athletes (e.g., runners) about how to use team resources. Functional subgrouping might first involve separating the group where members only meet with teammates in their same event to discuss the issue while using certain strategies to prepare for a more fruitful large group discussion with all events in attendance.

O'Neill et al. (2013) used this approach as a team development approach in a large organization, where discussions were hosted across many subgroups using functional subgrouping principles. One could also imagine how this could be integrated in sport teams where subgroups are conflicting.

Best Practices for Structuring Feedback During Team Sessions

- Initial attempts to provide feedback should be exclusively positive in nature.
- When corrective feedback is encouraged during discussion, it should be sandwiched or shared alongside positive feedback.
- All feedback should focus on the actions and observable behaviors of the feedback target.
- Those providing feedback need to focus on how receptive others are to feedback.
- Discussion facilitators must guide the process by providing examples of effective feedback and reinforcing group members who correctly use it.

Alongside the best practices like those above, group psychotherapy counsellors are also trained to actively regulate feedback such as by being aware of the ideal timing to "cut off" feedback that is not going well (e.g., Antons,

2018; Morran et al., 1998). Just as psychotherapy might involve providing feedback, sport groups likely integrate feedback in goal-setting, role communication, and when resolving conflict. Insights about prompting effective peer feedback in groups are therefore one example of an application from psychotherapy toward working within sport teams.

22.2.3 Five Key Considerations When Developing Teams

Practitioners who are developing teams must confront several issues that ultimately shape how their intervention is implemented. Below, we present a series of considerations that have emerged in the decades of research and practice in this area (Eys et al., 2020). These considerations include decisions when implementing interventions that involve timing, the facilitator, the contexts where activities take place, the educational process of interventions, and how to measure outcomes. We list these considerations, below, as a series of five questions posed toward a practitioner developing a team development intervention.

Five Key Considerations for Implementing a Team Intervention

1. When will team development be implemented?
2. Who will be implementing strategies in the team?
3. Where will team members participate in interventions?
4. Will your intervention educate team members?
5. How will you measure the group environment and the effectiveness of team development?

22.2.3.1 *When* Will Team Development Be Implemented?

Anecdotally, sport team leaders like coaches often use team development strategies as a short-term or band-aid solution. For instance, some leaders traditionally host activities to enhance interpersonal relationships early in their competitive season (e.g., team meals where everyone contributes). Sport psychology consultants also might choose to deliver team building activities as "one-off" activities upon invitation from a team. Even within organizations, Dyer Jr et al. (2013) observed that most workplaces or organizations implement team development at only singular or acute points of time. Short-term or one-off activities likely *do* benefit teams. However, they may not have a sustained influence when compared to team development that is implemented regularly over the course of a season. Interventions applied throughout a season might integrate aspects like monitoring member's perceptions of the team on a regular basis, responding when members violate team norms, and using team meetings when needed to address ongoing challenges.

Team development should also be deliberate, designed to achieve specific aims related to the group. Lau (2005) outlined a pathway for team development throughout a sport season where the group leader or consultant chooses activities that match aims that may vary in salience throughout a season. Lau (2005) articulated the following aims, which may be relevant at varying points in the season:

- **Team design**. Takes place at the outset of the season to integrate members. Activities and group meetings focus on the transition into a new season, including integrating new members, clarifying leadership, and developing symbols or rituals for the team.
- **Team-starting measures.** Takes place early in the season to speed the development of the group's structure and includes activities like defining team goals and establishing team norms.
- **Team diagnosis and team review.** Takes place throughout the season to monitor the group environment. Strategies involve monitoring satisfaction, institutionalizing feedback between players and coaches, and monitoring goal progress.
- **Team time-out.** This involves activities akin to "pulling an emergency break" to address specific topics that are relevant when responding to situations in the team (e.g., interpersonal conflict, weakening commitment to the team). The activities that might constitute a "time-out" may vary depending upon the team situation to which a group leader is responding.
- **Promoting a positive team climate.** Ongoing activities, often throughout the season, to foster social ties among members and commitment to the group.

The underlying message of this framework is that facilitators or group leaders should thoughtfully select strategies to match the needs of the group at differing points in time.

- *Who* **Will Be Implementing Strategies in the Team?**

Another consideration involves indicating who is most appropriate to implement team development. One approach—termed a direct approach—involves activities developed and implemented directly with the team by a consultant, facilitator, or other outside leaders. For example, imagine a team development workshop delivered to an entire team by a sport psychology consultant. The three sport interventions described in Table 22.1 are direct approaches (i.e., Barker et al., 2014; Fransen et al., 2020; McEwan et al., 2020). In contrast, the consultant or facilitator can take a different approach by working "through" the coach or another existing group leader and may never personally meet with the team as a group. This is called an indirect approach and is where group leaders are trained in team development by a facilitator, and then these group leaders implement and deliver the activities. An indirect approach was used in the Carron and colleagues' framework described above (Prapavessis et al., 1996).

There is no "ideal" regarding who should deliver team development. Direct approaches can be valuable because consultants have extensive education and experience, making it more likely that interventions will be delivered as intended. For instance, trained consultants have skillsets to help ensure that group meetings are productive. Indirect approaches are valuable, in contrast, because they are sustainable and accepted by members. Regarding sustainability, teaching group leaders to manage the group can have a lasting impact even after a consultant is no longer with the group. Regarding acceptability, some activities that involve group discussions might gain more acceptance when delivered by existing team members or a consultant who has become embedded in the group.

▪ *Where* Will Team Members Participate in Interventions?

Practitioners also must determine whether team development should take place within the sport context of the training field, competition, or during group meetings focused on sport tasks. Examples of team development that commonly happens in the sport context include setting norms during group meetings, challenging members with difficult team training sessions, and describing members' roles during practice. There is value, however, in conducting team development interventions outside of the sport environment by taking members "off site." Baumann (2002) argues that out-of-sport contexts provide an environment where members become better acquainted socially and team development is prioritized as an immediate goal.

Decisions around context are optimally framed around transfer, in that team development should ultimately be transferred to guide teammate interactions when members perform or train. Because of this transfer, Wegner and Dawo (2013) advocate that team development activities traditionally conducted in outside settings can be adapted and integrated within sport training. For example, problem-solving is a common team building task delivered in outside settings like having members travel to complete challenging obstacle courses. Similar problem-solving team building activities can be designed and implemented during training sessions, followed by debriefing to discuss experiences and any conflicts in the training environment (see Wegner & Dawo, 2013).

▪ Will Your Intervention *Educate* Team Members?

Team development interventions often depend upon educating members about team dynamics principles. For instance, teamwork training and leadership training interventions explicitly educate participants (see ◘ Table 22.1). In these cases, team development is an educational process, as characterized by literature working in contexts of handball teams (Kleinmann, 2005) and more generally toward sport (e.g., Wegner & Dawo, 2013).

Wegner and Dawo (2013) advocate for these types of team development interventions to progress through a series of educational phases. Activities should begin with an *information and education phase*, where team members learn about why specific aspects of groups are important and assess and discuss their own group environment. Activities in this phase might range from discussing the importance of the team to outlining why a consultant will be leading the group through specific activities. This phase should also emphasize to all members that everyone in the team is important. Next is the *appropriation phase*, where members participate in specific forms of team development. Specific activities vary depending upon the goals of the intervention but should ensure that members have opportunities to interpersonally connect with one another. Finally, the *consolidation phase* is when education from earlier phases is put into practice during training or competition.

? Educational Phases of Team Development (Wegner & Dawo, 2013)

1. *Information and education*: Members learn about group dynamics and discuss their own group environment.
2. *Appropriation*: Team members participate in specific forms of team development.
3. *Consolidation*: Education from earlier phases is put into practice.

As an example, consider how a consultant delivering a role clarification intervention might educate team members. Initial activities might involve a workshop defining the range of roles that members possess, discussing the meaning of a member's roles for group dynamics, and describing how role understanding influences group performance (education). Subsequently, the facilitator may provide some homework for members to write about their role and then participate in a second session where all members describe one another's roles and share feelings about why each member is important (appropriation). Finally, the facilitator might ensure that role communication continues by developing a weekly online survey to monitor members' perceptions of their own role and to provide a way for coaches to provide feedback (consolidation). These phases align with tactics to foster psychological skills, where athletes often progress through initial education phases and then into acquisition and finally implementation (e.g., see ▶ Chap. 20 regarding basic and psychological skill training).

We acknowledge that some types of team building do not entail this explicit learning approach because they impact the group through shared experiences. For instance, social events and problem-solving activities are two examples of team building interventions where the goal is to engage members in a shared experience or process. It can nevertheless be valuable to ensure that members learn from their experience. As such, debriefing can be a critical tool that prompts participants to reflect and share their experiences (Kriz & Nöbauer, 2008). The box (▶ For Sports Practice) provides insights regarding how to lead group members through debriefing.

Key Phases in Debriefing

Debriefing can be an important activity to help ensure that discrete team building activities have their intended influence on the group. Often, debriefing is most successful if key topics are planned by the discussion leader beforehand. The planning for a debriefing session can be structured around one (or more) of the following six phases (see Kriz & Nöbauer, 2008):

Phase 1: How did you feel? Participants are prompted to express their current emotions and feelings about the event that just took place. Members can respond to the feelings of others.

Phase 2: What happened? Members describe the event that took place and highlight critical moments. Debriefing leader can target topics like how effective leaders were.

Phase 3: What have you learned? Members identify the most important lessons learned.

Phase 4: How are task and reality related? Team discusses how the recent event could shape how they behave in the future.

Phase 5: What would have been if…? Members can reflect on hypothetical scenarios that involve what would happen if event unfolded differently.

Phase 6: What happens now? Team establishes clear goals that stem from this event. This includes concrete actions that members can take.

These six phases can shape debriefing that members complete after sport performances but are also useful to help team members learn from a team building activity.

How Will You *Measure* the Group Environment and the Effectiveness of Team Development?

Measurement is valuable for evaluating impact and producing change throughout team development. First, practitioners can monitor the properties of a given group to help guide efforts to intervene upon a given group. Second, practitioners can evaluate the effectiveness of team development activities by regularly monitoring outcomes that they are hoping to change. Third, the mere act of measurement has the potential to produce change. Some of the earliest psychological studies conducted on group dynamics (e.g., 1920s' organizational research involving the Hawthorne plant) revealed that merely observing workplace teams can improve members' interactions and increase performance (Sundstrom et al., 2000).

One comprehensive assessment tool was created by Bruner et al. (2020). The tool includes items that members can complete to describe their perceptions of the group environment (e.g., distinctiveness, togetherness), group structure (e.g., group norms, role clarity), and group processes (e.g., communication, cooperation). The tool includes 11 items that ask about topics such as the extent to which athletes feel that team members accept their roles on the team, the extent that team members conform to norms established by leaders, and the extent that athletes are openly communicating with one another. Items like these could either be completed on a regular basis throughout the season to track the group environment or to evaluate team development interventions.

Other scales and tools used by group researchers also hold value in application. Sociometry is an example of an approach to monitor groups using social networks that convey relationships between members in the group (see Antons, 2018). Although social networks can be derived from any approach that identifies how individuals are connected (e.g., observing video recordings to track how often a pair of teammates interact), the most common approach in sport involves peer nomination items where individuals rate each teammate using a roster.

Sports Practice

As an example using Eberspächer's (1993) distinction between the social- and task-related aspects of teammate relationships, social nominations could involve items such as the following:

- From the following roster, list the top 3 individuals with whom you would most want to sit beside on the team bus.
- One a scale from 1 (not at all) to 5 (every day), indicate how often you send text messages to chat with each team member.

Meanwhile, task nomination items might look like:
- List the three members of your team who you see as most likely to step forward as leaders during competition this year.
- For each member of the team, rate the likelihood that you would ask them for advice about how you could improve using a scale from 1 (not at all likely) to 5 (very likely).

Researchers or practitioners could also use sociometric peer nominations to evaluate how central a member is within their network (i.e., which players from the team receive the most nominations?). The density of the network also represents the social/task integration across the entire team and can be estimated by dividing the number of nominations between teammates by the highest possible number among all members. Finally, nominations can be used to construct a sociogram to depict the group structure and can help identify specific patterns like cliques of close-knit members. ◘ Figure 22.2 illustrates sociograms published in recent sport research. The sociograms depict real-life sport teams and members' interactions away from training—with one team (a) being relatively sparse regarding members' interactions relative to another team (b).

There are of course many tools available for monitoring the group environment, but we hope that readers consider the use of self-report items that comprehensively assess the group environment or those that track the structure of relationships among members of the group.

22.3 Applying Models Describing How Groups Develop

Among the conceptual frameworks used to understand group life, it seems fitting that *team development* interventions are often guided by *group development* theories. Group development (as a process) refers to the changes in how members interact and perceive their group, as they unfold over time. As defined by Saari and Galinsky (1974), group development can be observed through changes in how members structure their interactions (e.g., emergence of norms), how members interact with one another (e.g., more efficient communication),

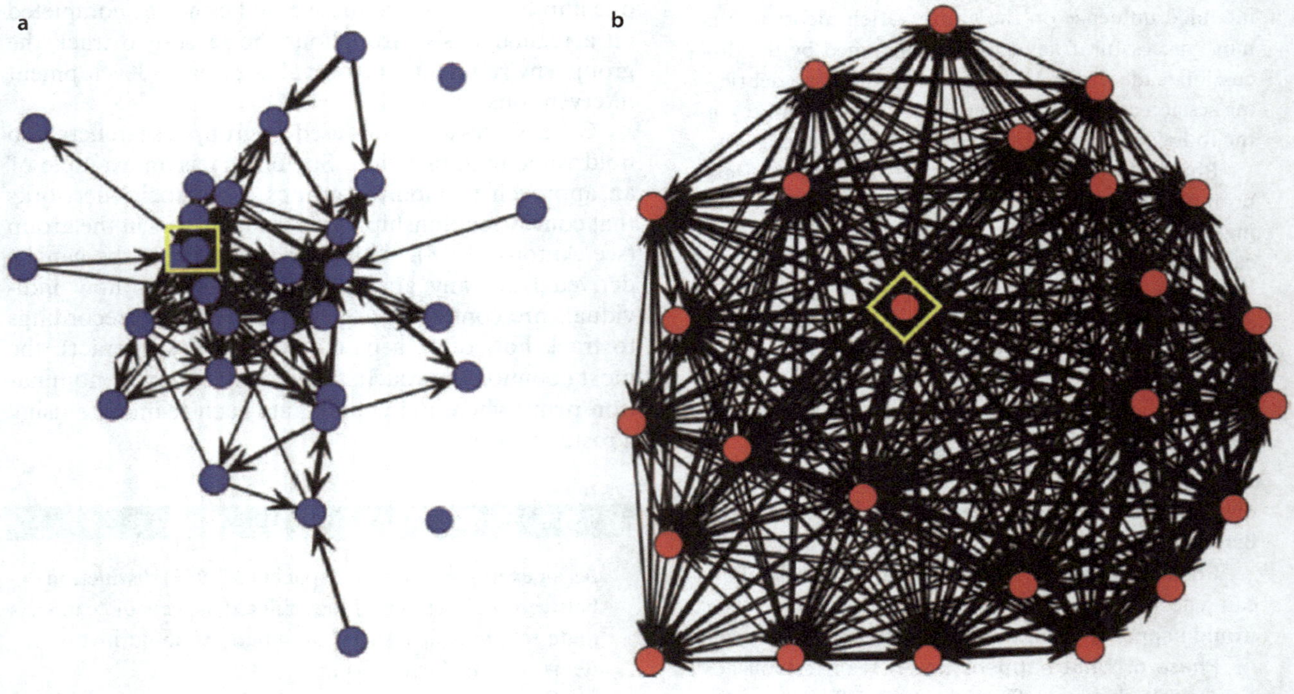

◘ **Fig. 22.2** *Illustration of two team social networks produced from sport team research.* These social network figures are from a study where members of college club sport teams indicated how frequently they interacted with each teammate outside of competition. Lines indicate that one teammate nominated another (arrow dictates direction), with thicker lines indicating ratings of higher levels of interaction. Figures (**a**, **b**) demonstrate differing levels of density in how frequently members in the team interacted as a whole (i.e., group A has low density, and group b has high density) and also indicate which members are the most central within their team's interaction network (i.e., yellow boxes). Note. From "Network centrality, group density, and strength of social identification in college club sport teams." by S. Graupensperger, M. Panza, & M. B. Evans, 2020, Group Dynamics: Theory, Research, and Practice, 24, p. 64. CC BY-NC and how members perceive the group (e.g., perceiving a team's culture). Through the process of sport team development, shared experiences across a season create a transformation where the team that we see at the end of a competitive season fundamentally differs from what the team was at the outset. Amidst the chaos of this transformation, theories of group development seek to identify patterns that hold true across many (or most) groups.

Self-Reflection

Think about a sport team or other groups to which you belonged, where the team's structure seemed to fall apart. In other words, think of a time when it became difficult or impossible to perform the group's function and where members no longer committed. What event(s) triggered this dissolution? Was there anything that the group members could have done to respond to changes in the group before the "wheels fell off"

Phase models of group development characterize how groups progress through common stages. Tuckman's (1965) phase model of team development is the most recognizable in sport (see Weinberg & Gould, 2015) and describes five stages that groups develop through progressively. As members gather they experience the *forming* stage, characterized by members becoming acquainted and often feeling optimistic about the group. Nevertheless, forming is also characterized by ambiguity about the role that each member plays and how the group should operate. Subsequently, groups are expected to enter a *storming* stage as members experience frequent conflicts, negotiating over team norms and roles. *Norming* is then characterized by a period of stability and calm as members accept the group structure and commit to the group—and ultimately the *performing* stage is when groups are seen to be most highly integrated and cooperative. Finally, sport teams approaching the end of their season dissolve in a sense during the transition phase, *adjourning*. One key message when applying this model is that the time shortly after combining members (i.e., forming, storming, norming) is a critical period to establish norms, roles, and shared goals (see also ▸ Chap. 16).

Certain aspects that Tuckman (1965) highlighted are also a starting point for developing interventions (see Birrer & Seiler, 2008). Volk et al. (2014) reported on one long-term intervention using phase-based models of team development to create a group-based physical education module that was hypothesized to be more effective than traditional approaches by promoting cooperation. In a randomized trial with a sample of nearly 100 fifth-grade students ranging from 10 to 14 years of age, the researchers delivered 17 sessions of movement activities to two separate groups. One group was the experimental group receiving sessions designed to promote team development, while other students received a traditional physical education program. Each lesson for the experimental class was designed to promote group processes in line with the sequential stages of Tuckman's model. Whereas the experimental and control groups did not differ early in the intervention, differences emerged within the final five module sessions. Participants in the experimental group reported more engagement in learning tasks, more commitment toward the team, and fewer conflicts with classmates. The experimental group also performed better on cooperative tasks like cooperatively working as a team to take steps on large wooden planks. It is clearly possible, then, that leaders can help their groups progress through phases of development effectively.

Whereas Tuckman's (1965) model is intuitively sensible and can be useful, this model is merely hypothetical and paints a picture that differs from the more turbulent path along which many groups develop. Beyond phase-based models, Arrow et al. (2004) identified four other types of models that address the more chaotic trajectories of group development: (a) adaptive response models, (b) repeating cycles/pendulum models, (c) robust equilibrium models, and (d) punctuated equilibrium models.

Types of Models of Group Development (Arrow et al., 2004)

(a) Adaptive response models, which emphasize that development of every group is unique and shifts as obstacles are faced and overcome.
(b) Repeating cycles or pendulum models that emphasize constant shifts in relationships among members. From this perspective, groups may progress toward unity and a stable group structure—but this state is temporary as groups vacillate between cohesion, stability, and unity versus differences, discord, and change.
(c) Robust equilibrium models, which highlight that after an initial flurry of development, groups develop relatively stable structures that members actively regulate and maintain.
(d) Punctuated equilibrium models (e.g., Gersick, 1988) that resemble the aforementioned equilibrium model but are termed "punctuated" because of a focus on how certain events disrupt the group. These are events that prompt the group into a period of change (e.g., losing streak, change of coach).

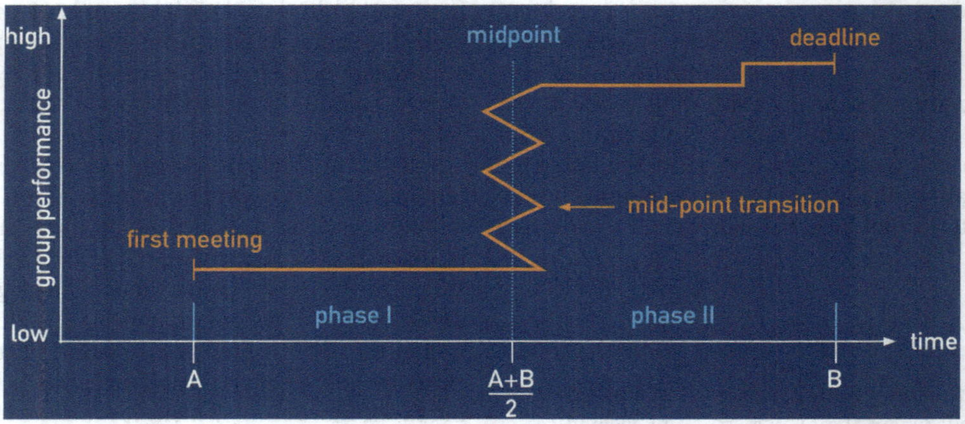

Fig. 22.3 *Hypothetical depiction of group decision-making according to the punctuated equilibrium model* (Gersick, 1988). This figure demonstrates a prototypical pattern in the teamwork behaviors observed among research participants completing cooperative tasks in a research environment and with a time limit. In these settings, teams often fail to coordinate effectively early on; leadership doesn't emerge, members are not communicating effectively, and the team is performing poorly. There is nevertheless a flurry of communication and performance increases around the temporal midpoint of the task as members come to terms with the time-limited nature of their task. Despite not being a clear parallel to many sport tasks, this model does highlight how team development is a dynamic process and not a set of phases

These models differ in part because they have been developed in different settings. For instance, punctuated equilibrium models were tested by studying members who were working in teams on decision-making tasks, where the investigators examined the influence of varying conditions on teamwork and cooperation (see Gersick, 1988). As illustrated in Fig. 22.3, one demonstration of the punctuated equilibrium model is evident in how members cooperate differently as they approach the time limit on a group task. This is demonstrated in findings that members brought together to complete a cooperative task in a research lab or course project often progress slowly toward their goals when they first begin the task but cooperate in the earnest after they pass the temporal midpoint (Gersick, 1988).

Despite their differences, readers of this chapter are likely most interested in shared insights from all four of the more dynamic development models. Most significantly, these models emphasize that development is often a transient state, as opposed to being a progressive path toward actualization. An implication is therefore that group leaders should regularly monitor the group and adapt their team development approaches throughout a season. Group leaders should be particularly vigilant amidst certain events that change the group environment (e.g., injury that removes key player from competition; Surya et al., 2015), which might help them quickly use strategies to intervene before group effectiveness is impacted.

Socialization Among the events that can prompt change in a team's development, the entrance of new members to teams is a particularly important process to address. Sport is of note in relation to the socialization of new members because team composition can shift both (a) at predictable intervals (e.g., beginning of a new season) and (b) amidst competitive seasons (e.g., acquiring or adding a new player). It is not only the newcomers who need to be socialized into a group when these shifts in membership take place. During substantial changes in membership like the beginning of a new season, returning members experience uncertainty about their role in the team in ways that can impact the group (Benson et al., 2016). In this light, even returning veteran members need to be socialized into their role within the "new" team when starting another competitive season.

Socialization into groups refers to the process whereby new (or returning) members learn about their group. Chiefly, this involves learning about norms and values alongside the responsibilities in their own personal roles (Van Maanen & Schein, 1979). Moreland and Levine (1982) characterized how members proceed through socialization in a series of phases. When individuals become new group members, groups are often focused on assimilation, and newcomers are focused on accommodation. A primary focus for the group is asserting their influence and integrating the newcomer (assimilation), whereas the newcomer tries to convince the group that they belong (accommodation). Newcomers who successfully navigate this socialization process become full members, and their focus shifts toward maintaining their role. However, events also might occur that rekindle socialization where the focuses on assimilation and accommodation again become more salient.

Sport research involving socialization has focused on exploring the ways that teams integrate new members. How do existing team members and coaches effectively help newcomers build their knowledge of the responsibilities of all members while also helping newcomers feel socially included? Benson and Eys (2017) surveyed competitive athletes and identified three prevailing types of approaches. First, they identified tactics that involved *coach-initiated role communication*. This would be evident, for example, when a coach describes a newcomer's role and identifies the performances that a newcomer would need to demonstrate if they want a more prominent role (i.e., what is needed to become a "starter"). Second, they identified *serial socialization*, which is when more experienced members are involved in teaching newcomers about the group and helping them to learn their role. Serial socialization can be formally identified where veterans are linked to newcomers and prompted to adopt mentor roles or could be more subtly promoted by group leaders (e.g., when creating pairings for physical training or travel, veterans are assigned alongside newcomers). Finally, athletes described *social inclusionary tasks* where all members were integrated. This would include, for example, a party that every member can attend.

Types of Integration of New Team Members (Benson & Eys, 2017)

1. *Coach-initiated role communication*: Coach describes a newcomer's role and the coach's expectations.
2. *Serial socialization*: More experienced members teach newcomers.
3. *Social inclusionary tasks*: For all members.

Research has demonstrated the value of these socialization tactics, as athletes report higher group cohesion and intentions to return to their team when their teams used relatively higher levels of all three forms of socialization early in the season (Leo et al., 2020). Early season socialization is therefore a critical time to intervene with groups. Teams should integrate multidimensional strategies including direct communication from the coach about one's roles, relationships between veteran and rookie team members, and social activities that include all members.

22.4 Conclusion

The emerging foundation of group dynamics theories and empirical findings (described in ▶ Chap. 16) has produced numerous insights that can be directly applied to enhance sport teams. This evidence base can improve group leaders' decisions in action, such as how they integrate new members into the team or how they ensure that members remain committed. This evidence base has also generated specific intervention protocols that are designed to improve certain parts of groups. These interventions have traditionally included team building activities like having teams face and overcome problems. There is, however, a broader menu of tools to intervene with groups that includes team training, debriefing, and leadership training. This menu of approaches can include theories and strategies from domains outside of sport, such as organizational psychology or psychotherapy.

Learning Control Questions

Basic:

1. List and briefly describe the four common types of team development interventions.
2. What are T-groups?
3. What are three things that teams can implement to ensure that newcomers are effectively socialized into the group?

Advanced:

4. Briefly describe the four common team building approaches (i.e., goal-setting, role clarification, interpersonal relationship development, and problem-solving). For each approach, create hypothetical examples of an activity that a group leader could implement that would demonstrate each approach. For your hypothetical example, try describing an activity that is not already presented in this chapter (e.g., recall team building from your own sport history or that you find through an online search).
5. Describe the three educational phases of team development activities.
6. What is one insight about group development the chapter authors outline as stemming from all four of the non-linear group development models (e.g., adaptive, pendulum, equilibrium, punctuated equilibrium)?

Expert:

7. If you were to describe five key actionable insights from this chapter that you would want every sport coach to know, what would they be?

References

Agazarian, Y. M. (2004). *Systems-centered therapy for groups*. Karnac.

Antons, K. (2011). Die SOL-Saga. *Gruppendynamik und Organisationsberatung*, 42(3), 307–325.

Antons, K. (2018). *Practice of group dynamics: Exercises and techniques*. Hogrefe.

Arrow, H., Poole, M. S., Henry, K. B., Wheelan, S., & Moreland, R. (2004). Time, change, and development: The temporal perspective on groups. *Small Group Research, 35*, 73–105.

Barker, J. B., Evans, A. L., Coffee, P., Slater, M. J., & McCarthy, P. J. (2014). Consulting on tour: A dual-phase personal-disclosure mutual-sharing intervention and group functioning in elite youth cricket. *The Sport Psychologist, 28*, 186–197.

Baumann, S. (2002). *Team psychology: Methods, and techniques*. Meyer & Meyer.

Benson, A. J., & Eys, M. (2017). Understanding the consequences of newcomer integration processes: The Sport Team Socialization Tactics Questionnaire. *Journal of Sport and Exercise Psychology, 39*, 13–28.

Benson, A. J., Eys, M. A., & Irving, P. G. (2016). Great expectations: How role expectations and role experiences relate to perceptions of group cohesion. *Journal of Sport and Exercise Psychology, 38*, 160–172.

Birrer, D., & Seiler, R. (2008). Group dynamics and teambuilding. In J. Beckmann & M. Kellmann (Eds.), *Encyclopedia of psychology: Sport psychology* (pp. 311–392). Hogrefe.

Brawley, L. R., & Paskevich, D. M. (1997). Conducting team building research in the context of sport and exercise. *Journal of Applied Sport Psychology, 9*, 11–40.

Bruner, M. W., Eys, M., Carreau, J. M., McLaren, C., & Van Woezik, R. (2020). Using the Team Environment AssessMent (TEAM) to enhance team building in sport. *The Sport Psychologist, 34*, 62–70.

Bruner, M. W., Eys, M. A., Beauchamp, M. R., & Côté, J. (2013). Examining the origins of team building in sport: A citation network and genealogical approach. *Group Dynamics: Theory, Research, and Practice, 17*, 30–41.

Burlingame, G. M., & Jensen, J. L. (2017). Small group process and outcome research highlights: A 25-year perspective. *International Journal of Group Psychotherapy, 67*, S194–S218.

Cannon-Bowers, J. A., Salas, E., & Converse, S. (1993). Shared mental models in expert team decision making. In N. J. Castellan (Ed.), *Individual and group decision making: Current issues* (pp. 221–246). Erlbaum.

Côté, J., Turnnidge, J., & Evans, M. B. (2014). The dynamic process of development through sport. *Kinesiologia Slovenica, 20*, 14–26.

Crowe, T. P., & Grenyer, B. F. (2008). Is therapist alliance or whole group cohesion more influential in group psychotherapy outcomes? *Clinical Psychology & Psychotherapy, 15*, 239–246.

DiazGranados, D., Shuffler, M. L., Wingate, J. A., & Salas, E. (2017). Team development interventions. In E. Salas, R. Rico, & J. Passmore (Eds.), *The Wiley Blackwell handbook of the psychology of team working and collaborative processes* (pp. 555–586). Wiley.

Dyer, W. G., Jr., Dyer, J. H., & Dyer, W. G. (2013). *Team building: Proven strategies for improving team performance*. Wiley.

Eberspächer, H. (1993). *Sports psychology*. Rowohlt.

Eys, M., Evans, M. B., & Benson, A. (2020). *Group dynamics in sport*. Fit Publishing.

Fransen, K., Haslam, S. A., Steffens, N. K., Peters, K., Mallett, C. J., Mertens, N., & Boen, F. (2020). All for us and us for all: Introducing the 5R shared leadership program. *Psychology of Sport and Exercise, 51*, 101762.

Gersick, C. J. (1988). Time and transition in work teams: Toward a new model of group development. *Academy of Management Journal, 31*, 9–41.

Highhouse, S. (2002). A history of the T-group and its early applications in management development. *Group Dynamics: Theory, Research, and Practice, 6*, 277–286.

Hofstätter, P. R. (1957). *Group dynamics: The critique of mass psychology*. Rowohlt.

Kleinmann, A. (2005). *Ability to work in a team*. Hofmann.

König, O., & Schattenhofer, K. (2018). *Introduction to group dynamics* (9th ed.). Carl-Auer.

Kriz, W. C., & Nöbauer, B. (2008). *Team competence: Concepts, training methods, practice*. Vandenhoeck & Ruprecht.

Lacerenza, C. N., Marlow, S. L., Tannenbaum, S. I., & Salas, E. (2018). Team development interventions: Evidence-based approaches for improving teamwork. *American Psychologist, 73*, 517–532.

Lau, A. (2005). *Collective performance in sports games: An interdisciplinary analysis* [Unpublished thesis]. Martin-Luther University, Halle.

Leo, F. M., López-Gajardo, M. A., González-Ponce, I., García-Calvo, T., Benson, A. J., & Eys, M. (2020). How socialization tactics relate to role clarity, cohesion, and intentions to return in soccer teams. *Psychology of Sport and Exercise, 50*, 101735.

Martin, L. J., Carron, A. V., & Burke, S. M. (2009). Team building interventions in sport: A meta-analysis. *Sport and Exercise Psychology Review, 5*, 3–18.

Martin, L. J., & Eys, M. A. (2019). Setting the conditions for success: A case study involving the selection process for the Canadian Forces Snowbird demonstration team. *Journal of Applied Sport Psychology, 31*, 116–133.

McEwan, D. (2020). The effects of perceived teamwork on emergent states and satisfaction with performance among team sport athletes. *Sport, Exercise, and Performance Psychology*, 9(1), 1.

McEwan, D., & Beauchamp, M. R. (2020). Teamwork training in sport: A pilot intervention study. *Journal of Applied Sport Psychology, 32*, 220–236.

McEwan, D., Ruissen, G. R., Eys, M. A., Zumbo, B. D., & Beauchamp, M. R. (2017). The effectiveness of teamwork training on teamwork behaviors and team performance: A systematic review and meta-analysis of controlled interventions. *PLoS One, 12*(1), e0169604.

Moreland, R. L., & Levine, J. M. (1982). Socialization in small groups: Temporal changes in individual-group relations. *Advances in Experimental Social Psychology, 15*, 137–192.

Morran, D. K., Stockton, R., Cline, R. J., & Teed, C. (1998). Facilitating feedback exchange in groups: Leader interventions. *Journal for Specialists in Group Work, 23*, 257–268.

O'Neill, R., Murphy, V., Mogle, J., MacKenzie, M. J., MacGregor, K. L., Pearson, M., & Parekh, M. (2013). Are systems-centered teams more collaborative, productive and creative? *Journal of Team Performance Management, 19*, 201–221.

Parks, C. D. (2021). A review of research synergies (and lack thereof) between group psychology and group psychotherapy. In C. D. Parks & G. A. Tasca (Eds.), *The psychology of groups: The intersection of social psychology and psychotherapy research* (pp. 11–28). American Psychological Association.

Pfeiffer, J. W., & Jones, J. E. (1970). *A handbook of structured experiences for human relations training*. University Associates Press.

Prapavessis, H., Carron, A. A., & Spink, K. S. (1996). Team building in sport. *International Journal of Sport Psychology, 27*, 269–285.

Rechtien, W. (2007). *Applied group dynamics. A textbook for students and practitioners*. Beltz.

Saari, R. C., & Galinsky, M. J. (1974). A conceptual framework for group development. In P. Glasser, R. Saari, & R. Viner (Eds.), *Individual change through small groups* (pp. 71–88). Free Press.

Salas, E., DiazGranados, D., Klein, C., Burke, C. S., Stagl, K. C., Goodwin, G. F., & Halpin, S. M. (2008). Does team training improve team performance? A meta-analysis. *Human Factors, 50*, 903–933.

Shuffler, M. L., DiazGranados, D., & Salas, E. (2011). There's a science for that: Team development interventions in organizations. *Current Directions in Psychological Science, 20*, 365–372.

Stumpf, S., & Thomas, A. (2003). Introduction. In S. Stumpf & A. Thomas (Eds.), *Teamwork and team development* (pp. IX–XXXV). Hogrefe.

Sundstrom, E., McIntyre, M., Halfhill, T., & Richards, H. (2000). Work groups: From the Hawthorne studies to work teams of the 1990s and beyond. *Group Dynamics: Theory, Research, and Practice, 4*, 44–52.

Surya, M., Benson, A. J., Balish, S. M., & Eys, M. A. (2015). The influence of injury on group interaction processes. *Journal of Applied Sport Psychology, 27*, 52–66.

Tuckman, B. W. (1965). Development sequence in small groups. *Psychological Bulletin, 63*, 384–399.

Van Maanen, J., & Schein, E. H. (1979). Toward a theory of organizational socialization. *Research in Organizational Behavior, 1*, 209–264.

Volk, A., Wegner, M., & Scheid, V. (2014). *Team development in physical education*. Logos.

Wegner, M., & Dawo, O. (2013). Handball. In D. Beckmann-Waldenmayer & J. Beckmann (Eds.), *Handbook of sport psychological practice* (pp. 237–250). Spitta.

Weinberg, R. S., & Gould, D. (2015). *Foundations of sport and exercise psychology*. Human Kinetics.

Talent Identification and Development in Sport

Oliver Höner, Paul Larkin, Thorsten Leber, and Philip Feichtinger

Contents

J. Schüler et al. (eds.), *Sport and Exercise Psychology*, https://doi.org/10.1007/978-3-031-03921-8_23

Learning Objectives

Basic:

- Understand and classify the processes of talent identification and development.
- Distinguish between conceptual approaches of sport psychology talent research.

Advanced:

- Be familiar with theoretical frameworks of giftedness and expertise research, and determine their relevance to talent identification and development.
- Understand relevant psychological characteristics of sport psychology talent diagnostics.
- Be able to reflect on the possibilities and limits of talent identification through sport psychology diagnostics.

Experts:

- Be familiar with approaches to develop cognitive performance and personality-related factors.

23.1 Introduction

High-performance sports require athletes to prepare for the best possible performance during competition. To achieve this, short- and medium-term training plans are developed to reach peak performance at specifically defined time points (e.g., championships, tournaments). This is a key responsibility of a coach who is also supported by an interdisciplinary team consisting of, among others, athletic trainers, physiotherapists, sports medicine specialists, and, increasingly, sport psychologists.

Given the high density in top-class sport, it is important for sporting federations and clubs that wish to remain sustainably competitive to expand the planning perspective to periods of weeks or years. Only in this way, the performance potential of promising youth athletes can be developed in the long term. The identification of talented youth athletes is generally attributed to an "ability" in a specific area that enables them to develop into an "expert" at a high level of performance.

23.1.1 Ability and Expertise

Ability

Ability is defined as the possession of highly developed, partially genetic, natural proficiencies and skills in at least one area of competence (e.g., intelligence or motor activity; Heller & Perleth, 2008).

Expertise

Expertise indicates the capability to yield outstanding performance in one area of performance (e.g., sport, music, or art) through sustainable and replicated skill (in other words, not a coincidence or one-off) (Janelle & Hillman, 2003; Posner, 1988).

The tasks of talent detection, identification, selection, and development are differentiated during the process of youth promotion toward senior high-performance sport (Koopmann et al., 2020; Vaeyens et al., 2013; Williams et al., 2020; Williams & Reilly, 2000). In the initial step of *detection*, youth athletes who have not yet participated or are competing at a low level in the specified sport are detected. Then, athletes should be *identified* who hold the potential to produce peak performance in senior/adult sports. Building on this, it is important to *select* youth athletes for specific groups or teams (e.g., development squads, academy groups) and provide them with a suitable learning environment to *develop* their potential.

Personal, financial, and material resources for the promotion of talent are limited in sports associations and clubs. Therefore, it is imperative to use these resources for athletes who demonstrate the greatest potential to be successful over the long term in high-level sports. In practice, the selection process is typically based on the subjective opinions of coaches and scouts (Ford et al., 2020). Talent identification research, however, strives to scientifically ground such decisions in sports medicine, training sciences, sport sociology, and sport psychology. From a sport psychology perspective, the following questions remain:

- How is talent identification and development researched?
- What is the current understanding of the relevant psychological characteristics?
- Which assessments support/identify the relevant psychological characteristics?

This chapter presents sport psychology perspectives on these central questions of talent research. First, "paradigmatic" approaches will be outlined, with which talent phenomenon is researched (▶ Sect. 23.2). Next, frameworks that consider talent phenomenon from a sport psychology perspective will be introduced. This includes the assessments from ability and expertise research that clarify different phenomena to explain the development of ability and the acquisition of expertise (▶ Sect. 23.3). The main section of the chapter outlines the relevant characteristics of talent identification and development and considers the meaning of *cognitive performance factors* and *personality-related factors*. Selected sport psychological findings of talent research are presented, which deal with the empirical prognostic relevance of potential talent characteristics (► Sect. 23.4). Subsequently, assessments that develop or support cognitive performance factors and personality-related factors are summarized (► Sect. 23.5). Finally, considerations for the identification and development of sporting talent are discussed (► Sect. 23.6).

23.2 Conceptual Approaches to Talent Research in Sport

Talents in sports

Talents in sports are individuals who:

- Still find themselves developing toward their highest performance level.
- Considering their practical experience, are athletically above average in comparison to athletes at a similar biological stage of development and with similar living habits.
- Can be justifiably trusted to achieve athletic peak performance in a later stage of development, taking into account internal performance conditions and available contextual conditions of support (cf. Cobley et al., 2012; Güllich, 2013; Hohmann, 2009; Huijgen et al., 2014).

Building on this underlying definition of the term "talent," we will examine the question of talent based on diverse concepts. As various understandings and perspectives will arise, it is important to reflect on the different approaches of talent research in sport psychology.

Varied Approaches to Sport Psychology Talent Research

- Prospective versus retrospective
- Narrow versus broad
- Static versus dynamic
- Universal versus area-specific
- Person-oriented versus variable-oriented

Prospective Versus Retrospective

Talent research in sport implements *prospective* (future-oriented) and *retrospective* (past-oriented) views of the phenomenon "talent." Talent studies normally follow either one approach or the other, despite recommendations of a combination of prospective and retrospective approaches (Hohmann, 2009).

Prospective talent research in sport psychology is based on pedagogical-psychological giftedness research, guided by the question "Where are the gifted individuals headed?" *Retrospective* talent research is based on cognitive psychological expertise research and is based on the question "Where do the experts come from?" and examines the development of successful athletes (Heller, 2002).

Athletes who will most likely end up having success in their respective sports are identified as "talents" from a prospective viewpoint. In this case, the focus is on the prediction of expected peak performance in the specific sport. This research approach benefits from longitudinal prognosis studies, whereby the *prognostic relevance* of one or more predictors (e.g., achievement motivation, ► Sect. 23.4.2) is evaluated to determine the statistical correlation of a variable (predictor) at youth ages with the athletes' future performance level (criterion, e.g., national team).

From a retrospective perspective, investigations evaluate athletes who have already achieved peak performance and the pathway they undertook to reach this level of performance. This approach aims to identify the characteristics which differentiate skilled athletes (i.e., experts) from less-skilled athletes (i.e., intermediates or novices). Expertise research in sport psychology particularly considers cognitive performance characteristics (e.g., anticipation skills, ► Sect. 23.4.1) and environmental factors (e.g., training style and scale, ► Sect. 23.3.2).

Narrow Versus Broad

An additional conceptual difference in the definition of talent concerns the breadth of the spectrum. Traditionally, a *narrow* concept of talent identifies athletes who achieve outstanding results in competitive performance in a specific sport at a certain time point. However, performance during childhood and youth ages seems to be weak predictors of future success during adulthood, because (among other reasons) the conditions under which the performances are produced are not completely known. However, a broad spectrum of personal factors (e.g., physical maturity, relative age) and/or environmental influences (e.g., expenses already provided for training, access to resources) are not often considered when evaluating current performance levels (Hohmann, 2009).

Due to the multitude of factors that can influence whether or not a youth athlete will eventually become successful, current talent research is based on a *broad* understanding of talent. In addition to competitive performance, anthropometric (e.g., body size), physiological (e.g., aerobic capacity), sociological (e.g., parental support), and psychological (e.g., decision-making ability, motivation) factors are also considered (Vaeyens et al., 2013).

Static Versus Dynamic

> Given changes in performance and their underlying conditions, it is necessary to view the question of talent not only from a *static* (with one-time inquiries) but also from a *dynamic* development perspective. Therefore, diagnostics of talent development should be introduced and measured at multiple time points (longitudinally).

Support for youth athletes takes place primarily during adolescence, the phase of development where a lot of physical, social, and psychological changes occur. For example, the outstanding motor skills of a 12-year-old gymnast may be assessed as merely average later after puberty. *Differential stability*—the stability of differences between individuals over time—seems to be comparable between personality-related dispositions, psychological skills, and motor characteristics in early adolescence (Feichtinger & Höner, 2015). Average correlations between characteristic values of youth athletes between the ages of 11 and 15 highlight sufficient stability in significant and relevant behavioral predictors. However, these correlations also point to the fact that changes in the relative ranking of youth athletes can occur in both characteristic areas. Furthermore, the rate of competition performance change and its conditions count as potentially independent talent predictors (e.g., relative speed of development; Hohmann, 2009); however, the consideration of the process of change poses a complex challenge. This complexity arises from the multitude of relevant factors (personal and environmentally related) that influence the progression of development. In addition, the predictors of talent vary in interrelatedness, between each other as well as in chosen performance criteria (► Side Story: Influences on the Prognostic Relevance).

Side Story

Influences on the Prognostic Relevance (Cf. Hohmann, 2009; Höner & Votteler, 2016; Murr et al., 2018b)

The prognostic relevance of talent predictors (e.g., achievement motivation) for future success cannot be universally quantified for all development phases, sports, and performance levels. A range of phenomena contribute to contextual conditions that can alter the respective prognostic relevance:

- *Emphasis fluctuation*: Predictors' relevance to prognosis can be weighted differently depending on the stage of development (e.g., stress resistance during childhood may be less significant than during adolescence in which demands on youth athletes are noticeably higher).
- *Compensability*: A varied combination of predictors can lead to an identical level of performance, and individual predictors can be compensated differently over time (e.g., some athletes can compensate for a lack of speed through technical or cognitive skills).
- *Group specificity*: The significance and meaning of the predictors can be dependent on sport, age, or athlete performance level (e.g., achievement motivation within a selected group of athletes with high motor skills can be an important predictor of future success, while the predictive strength of achievement motivation is less impactful in athletes with noticeably different motor skills).

Universal Versus Area-Specific

> Talented people are not normally "universal talents" who are gifted at everything. Most are talented in a specific area with specific characteristics.

An important foundation of the modern term "talent" consists of its area specificity (Beckmann et al., 2008). This results from the finding that only very few people are simultaneously highly talented in multiple skill areas such as sport, music, science, etc. (Williams et al., 2020; Williams & Reilly, 2000). This area-specific understanding of talent should also be taken into consideration in the diagnostics of relevant characteristics (► Study Box: Sport-Specific Diagnostics). Furthermore, the specifics of each sport should also be considered within sport psychology talent research (Singer, 2000; Vaeyens et al., 2008). For example, sports like handball, gymnastics, and swimming are differentiated by their structure and requirements, so that different performance factors can be relevant to future success in each sport (Hohmann, 2009).

Study Box

Sport-Specific Diagnostics

Elbe et al. (2003) show that performance prognoses are possibly more reliable with sport-specific diagnostics than with a general psychological questionnaire. They compared the correlation between general and sport-specific achievement motives (hope of success, fear of failure) of students attending an elite sport school with the students' athletic performance (various sports such as swimming, gymnastics, rowing, canoeing, handball, soccer). No meaningful associations were found between general achievement motives and performance in sport. Interestingly, significant correlations emerged between sport-specific achievement motivation in early adolescence and the performance level recorded 3 years later. These findings point toward the superiority of area-specific inquiry to general diagnostics.

Person-Oriented Versus Variable-Oriented

The conceptual difference between person-oriented and variable-oriented approaches has been introduced into the sport psychology discussion (Conzelmann et al., 2016; Zuber et al., 2015).

The *variable-oriented approach* to talent identification and development makes characteristics such as performance endurance and willpower relevance and evaluates in what way these variables make predictions of youth athletes' future success. The strength of this approach is that it offers information about the prognostic relevance of certain characteristics or diagnostics.

A basic feature of the *person-oriented approach* that arose from dynamic interactionism (Magnusson, 1990; Magnusson & Stattin, 1998) is the holistic approach. According to this approach, the individual and their environment constitute inseparable components of an integrated and dynamic system with multiple subsystems. According to this perspective, a single characteristic holds only limited significance for an athlete's future level of performance, independent of other personal and environmental aspects.

In the person-oriented approach, talent identification focuses on the type of people (i.e., patterns of characteristic combinations) that show an unusually high possibility of later success during adulthood.

Thus, the person-oriented approach offers a conceptually convincing supplement to the established variable-oriented approach. However, constraints are also set in the empirical implementation of this approach, because of the limited selection of characteristics in empirical studies, conflicting with the holistic approach.

23.3 Frameworks of Talent Research

Building on the broadly dynamic concept of "talent," frameworks help us consider the process of talent development from the beginning of childhood to peak performance as adults. Frameworks function as an orientation to professional behavior in practice and offer an array of starting points for scientific research (▶ Side Story: Types of Models in Talent Research).

Side Story

Types of Models in Talent Research

Subotnik et al. (2012) identify three types of models which can be used in talent research:

- Models which describe *how potential converts into performance* and bring constructs such as ability or talent, personal or environmental factors, or performance into a sequential context to this end, without further differentiating the development process (e.g., Gagné, 2000; Heller & Perleth, 2008; cf. ◘ Figs. 23.1 and 23.2).
- Models which divide the *course of performance sport careers* into various phases and outline the relevance of individual factors dependent on various stages of development (e.g., Bloom, 1985; Côté, 1999; cf. ◘ Fig. 23.3).
- Models that *list and categorize characteristics* relevant for the conversion of talent into performance (e.g., Tannenbaum, 2003; Williams & Franks, 1998). These models are particularly profitable when evaluating the ability of a single talent characteristic to predict future success (e.g., cf. ◘ Fig. 23.4).

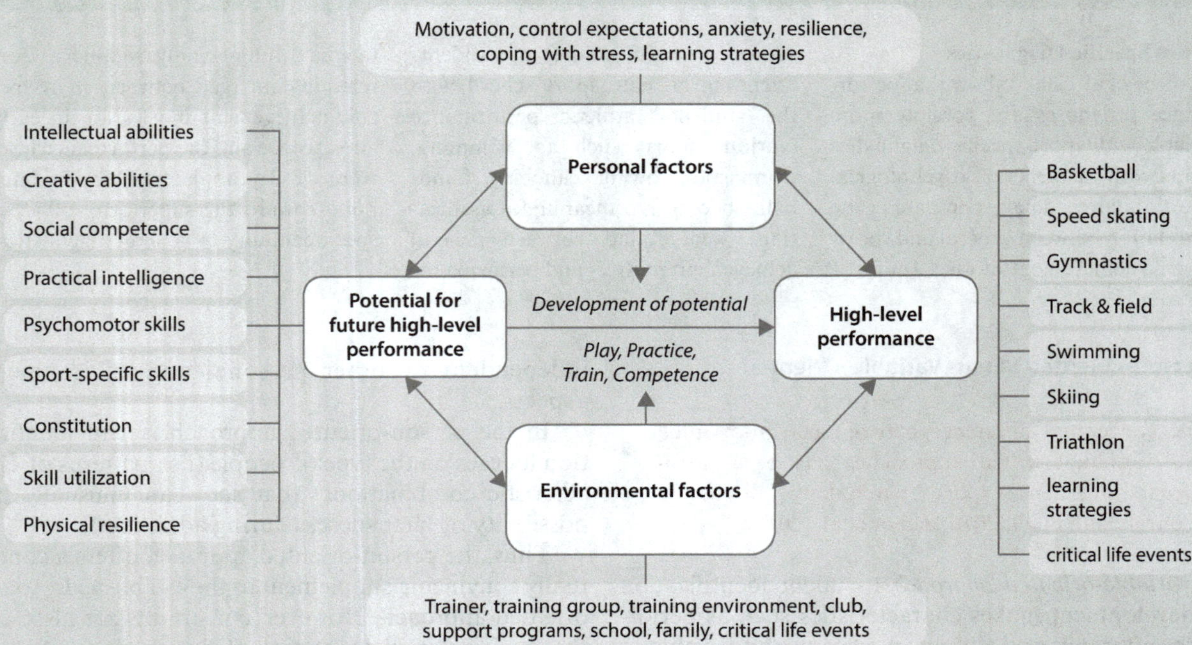

Fig. 23.1 Talent development in sport according to the MMG by Heller and Perleth (modified by Güllich, 2013, p. 630; Hohmann, 2009, p. 311). (With kind permission from Andreas Hohmann)

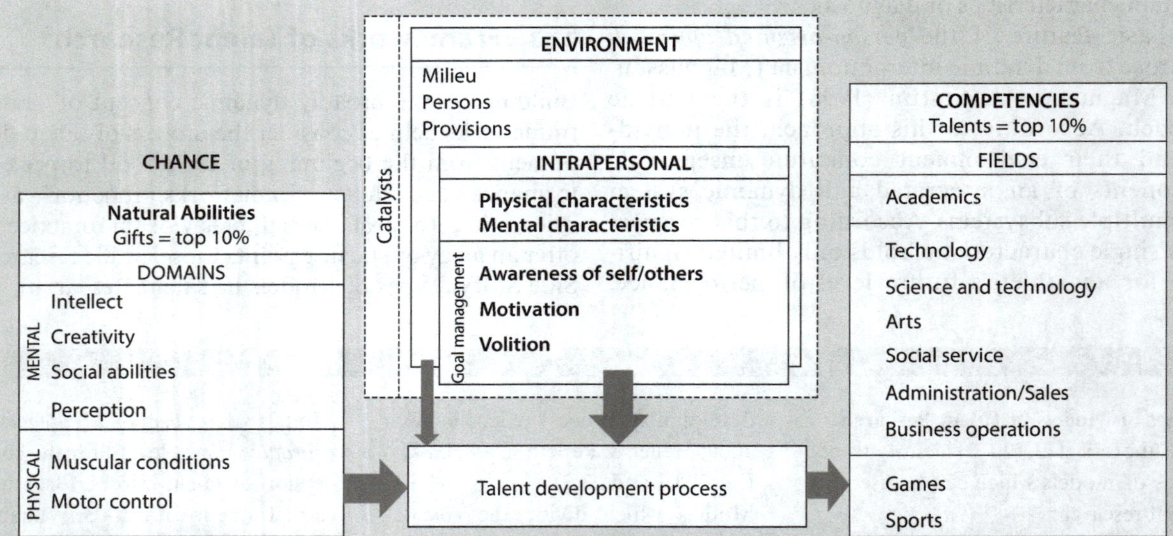

Fig. 23.2 The DMGT (simplified from Gagné, 2010, p. 83). (Reprinted with permission from the publisher Taylor & Francis Ltd)

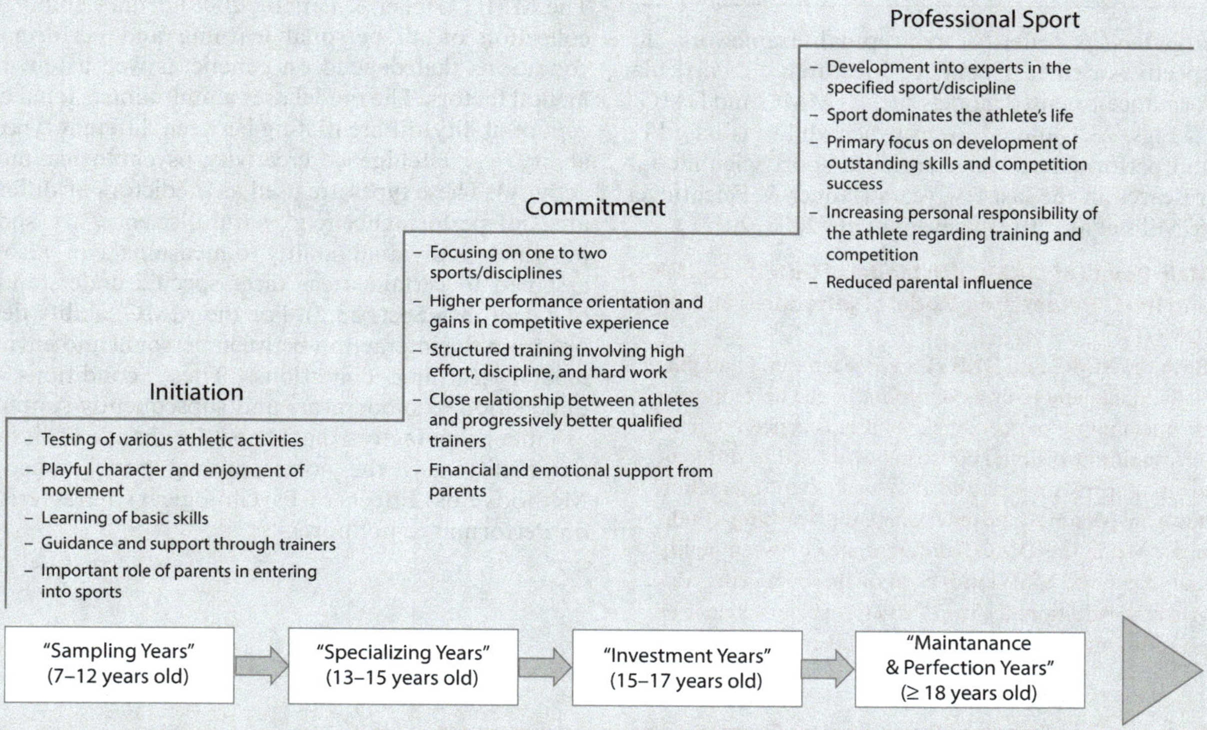

Fig. 23.3 Levels of career development in high-level athletes and age-dependent phases of expertise development (according to Bloom, 1985; Côté, 1999; in the style of Hohmann, 2009, p. 78). (With kind permission from Andreas Hohmann)

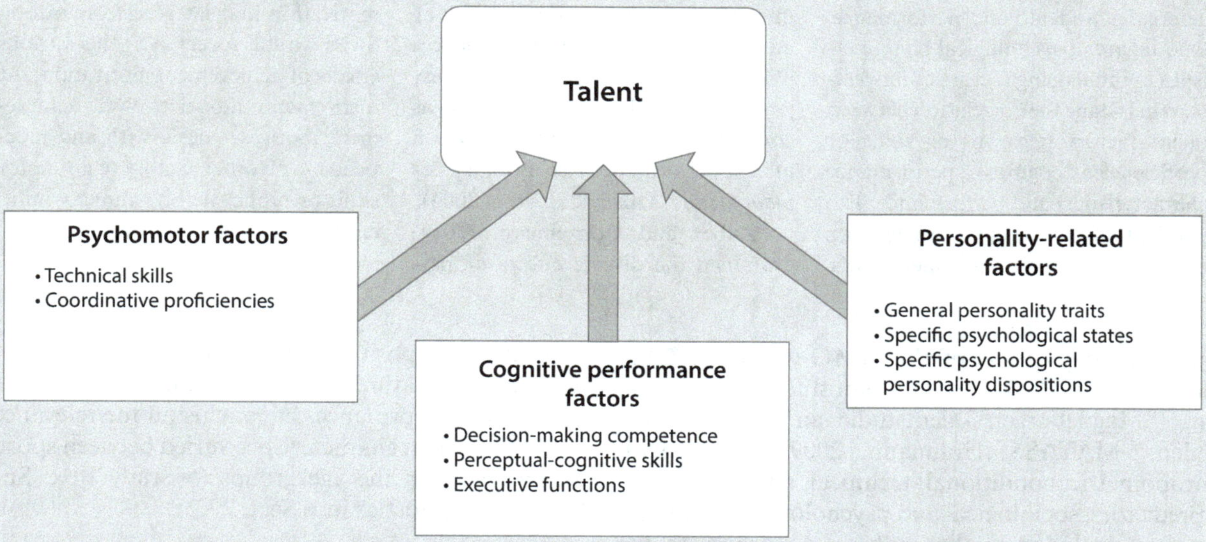

Fig. 23.4 Predictors of talent from a sport psychology perspective

Four of the most well-known frameworks or concepts in sport psychology talent research will be discussed below. The "Munich Model of Giftedness" (MMG) and the "Differentiated Model of Giftedness and Talent" (DMGT) portray two models of prospective giftedness research, while the concepts of the models of *Deliberate Practice* and *Deliberate Play* are associated with retrospective expertise research.

23.3.1 Giftedness Research

Ability models offer a conceptual framework for prospective-oriented talent research. Particular performance-oriented models such as MMG and DMGT (cf. ◘ Figs. 23.1 and 23.2), in which ability is based on certain performances, have enriched sport scientific talent research in the last few years (Höner & Feichtinger, 2016; Mills et al., 2012; Vaeyens et al., 2008, 2013;).

Main Points of the Munich Model of Giftedness (MMG) and the Differentiated Model of Giftedness and Talent (DMGT)

Both the MMG and DMGT assume a natural and partially innate ability as a condition for the development of outstanding performance. Ability is conceptualized as a multidimensional construct expressed in different areas of performance and develops as an interaction between personal and environmental learning conditions. While the DMGT differentiates between ability and talent, the MMG uses both of these concepts congruently. Additionally, the DMGT considers chance as an additional factor that influences talent development.

23.3.1.1 Munich Model of Giftedness (MMG)

The MMG (Heller & Perleth, 2008) defines ability as a collection of all personal learning and performance conditions that depend on genetic as well as environmental factors. The model uses a multidimensional concept of ability, differentiating between different types of ability (e.g., intelligence, creativity, psychological motor activity). These types are used as predictors of different areas of performance (e.g., natural science, art, sport), in which individual ability dimensions can also be assigned to certain areas (area-specific understanding of talent in ► Sect. 23.2). For the MMG, ability develops from the interaction between personal and environmental learning conditions. These conditions are understood as moderators and subsequently simplified as influencing factors that shape the change of individual ability into the corresponding performance (► Methods Box: Effects of Psychological Characteristics on Performance in Sport).

Methods Box: Effects of Psychological Characteristics on Performance in Sport

Various perspectives exist in talent research about the nature of the correlation between psychological characteristics and athletic performance. One regards psychological characteristics as influencing factors or *moderators* that shape the correlation between talent factors (e.g., motor skills or proficiencies, cognitive performance characteristics) and performance. The effect of psychological characteristics can also be indirect, in other words, conveyed through *mediator* variables (Abbott & Collins, 2004). In this way, a high level of motivation can determine the frequency and regularity of athletic training and thus influences athletic performance. Furthermore, psychological characteristics such as concentration and anxiety control can affect performance as primary or *main factors* (Baker & Horton, 2004).

Zuber and Conzelmann (2014) examined the diverse effects of psychological characteristics on athletic performance. The authors analyzed the correlation between achievement motivation and later performance in Swiss youth soccer. Of the various effects of achievement motivation, the main factor model showed achievement motives—along with and independent of other factors (e.g., motor skills or proficiencies)—directly influence athletic performance.

A sport-specific version of the MMG (cf. ◘ Fig. 23.1) underlies one of the largest German studies of sporting talent ("Magdeburger Talentstudie an Sportbetonten Schulen," MATASS; Hohmann, 2009). Along with anthropometric, conditional, technical, and tactical talent predictors, sociological and psychological characteristics were included in the analysis. According to the MMG, the latter characteristics influence the long-term development of complex competition performance from childhood through adulthood. The talent characteristics were explored with youth athletes in swimming, track and field, and handball, to verify the empirical pertinence of performance prediction with adult age groups. Concerning psychological characteristics, the varying relevance of motivational (i.e., achievement motive), volitional (i.e., action control), and endurance-dependent dispositions (i.e., stress resistance) was noticeable in all three sports regarding the future development of performance. In conclusion the relevance of individual talent characteristics varied between sports as well as between the age groups (► Study Box: Sport-Specific Diagnostics in ► Sect. 23.2).

23.3.1.2 Differentiated Model of Giftedness and Talent (DMGT)

The DMGT (Gagné, 2000, 2010) combines essential concepts of sport psychology talent research including the six components of ability, talent, talent development, chance, intrapersonal, and environmental catalysts. Central to the model is the difference between *ability* (i.e., a high level of untrained and spontaneously demonstrated natural proficiencies that are to a certain extent genetically determined) and *talent* (i.e., outstanding, systematically developed competencies, such as knowledge and skills). Similar to the MMG, the DMGT conceptualizes ability as a multidimensional construct that can be expressed in intellectual, creative, social, or motor skills areas and can be manifested in various areas of competence (e.g., academics, art, sport).

Ability is an essential component of talent in the DMGT, so the existence of talent always implies high ability. However, a person with high ability will not necessarily develop into a talent (*underachiever*). The conversion of ability into talent can be influenced by intrapersonal and environmental catalysts. The DMGT explicitly regards chance as the third catalyst of talent development (cf. Fig. 23.2).

Talent development describes the dynamic process of the conversion from natural ability to talent. This process takes place when a gifted individual is put through a systematic learning or training program. However, development should be referred to not only as the formal learning processes (e.g., institutionally in schools or support programs) but also to informal learning (e.g., in everyday life) and growth in general.

Physical and psychological characteristics fit into the category of *intrapersonal catalysts*. The *environmental influences* stem from a broader milieu (e.g., cultural, social, and familiar) or a series of significant persons (e.g., parents, teachers, and friends) as well as specific provisions (e.g., learning plans, support programs, or systems). *Chance factors* include environmental variables such as place of birth, socioeconomic status, and uncontrollable incidents such as accidents or injuries.

The DMGT was developed in education research and is used in sport science both as a heuristic framework model (e.g., Vaeyens et al., 2008) and as a foundation for empirical studies. Mills et al. (2012) explored potential influencing factors relevant to the talent development of youth soccer players transitioning into professional careers. The authors used semi-structured interviews to understand professional youth coaches' (working at clubs in the top 2 English leagues) perceptions of intrapersonal and environmental catalysts (e.g., "Which personality characteristics do youth players need to become professionals?" and "Which parental figures play an important role in the development process of youth players?"). The results showed that awareness, resilience, goal-oriented attributes, intelligence, sport-specific attributes, and environmental factors are considered as important factors by the coaches. This study thereby supports the multidimensional definition of talent and provides indications to the interconnectedness of influencing factors (cf. Mills et al., 2012).

Influencing Factors on Talent Development (Mills et al., 2012)

- Awareness (e.g., self-awareness, awareness of others)
- Resilience (e.g., coping with setbacks, optimistic attitude)
- Goal-oriented attributes (e.g., passion, professional attitude)
- Intelligence (e.g., sport intelligence, emotional competence)
- Sport-specific attributes (e.g., coachability, competitiveness)
- Environmental factors (e.g., significant others, culture of the game)

23.3.2 Expertise Research

Models of giftedness research consider partially innate proficiencies as important conditions for the achievement of high-level performance. Contrastingly, approaches of expertise research explain differences in performance at the highest level especially in relation to the environmental factor of training or practice.

Since the 1990s, researchers have increasingly sought to explore the acquisition of expertise in various areas such as music or sport (Ericsson et al., 2009; Ford et al., 2015). Expertise research is based on diverse investigation approaches (Ericsson, 1996), including (among others) the "laboratory approach," in which cognitive processes that form the basis of high-level performances are analyzed in laboratory studies (▶ Sect. 23.4.1 for cognitive characteristics that according to such analyses mark experts and correspondingly count as relevant characteristics of talent identification). A further/broader approach is the "developmental approach," which is devoted to the analysis of expertise development.

Researchers have proposed various theoretical frameworks to understand the development of high-level performance. These models aim to describe the process of expertise development into different levels and age-related phases (cf. ▶ Sect. 23.1; for similar subdivisions, cf. Salmela, 1995). In this respect, Bloom (1985) proposed a three-step model of general, non-subject-specific expertise development as the initiation, development, and mastery phases. To adapt this model for a sporting population, Côté's sport-specific model (Côté, 1999; see Fig. 23.3) differentiates between *sampling*, *specializing*, *investment*, *maintenance*, and *perfection years*. Specific characteristics are attributed to the various levels or phases, for example, the relationship of youth athletes to coaches or parents or the intention and the extent of sport participation.

In addition to individual development phases, theoretical concepts such as *Deliberate Practice* and *Deliberate Play* were identified to outline beneficial training and learning conditions for individual levels of expertise development. While *Deliberate Play* has a role especially in early development phases of youth athletes (*sampling years*), the main aspect of later phases of development lies primarily with *Deliberate Practice*.

Primary Assertions of Deliberate Practice and Deliberate Play

Highly structured learning processes, regarded as *Deliberate Practice*, facilitate the systematic improvement of area-specific skills, where activities are highly structured and strenuous, with the explicit goal to improve performance, but not inherently enjoyable (Ericsson et al., 1993). This approach assumes under the principle "practice makes perfect" that at least 10 years of such intensive training is required to develop athletic expertise.

In contrast, *Deliberate Play* follows the assumption that early, informal, and playful participation in athletic activities, which are primarily intrinsically motivated (through fun and joy), contributes to the development of expertise in sport.

23.3.2.1 Deliberate Practice

Intentional, purposeful practice constitutes a central factor of expertise development and is known as *Deliberate Practice* (Ericsson et al., 1993). Underlying this concept is highly structured, goal-directed, intensive practice, with the specific aim to improve one's area-specific skills and performances to overcome current performance weaknesses. This approach assumes that high-level performance (i.e., expertise) during adulthood directly relates to the degree of purposeful practice in domain-specific activities (Ward et al., 2004). In consequence the achievable level of performance is not limited by natural ability factors, but rather expertise is acquired through training and purposeful effort. This assumption can be expressed as the "10,000-hour rule" or the "10-year rule" (Ericsson, 1996). According to these rules, individuals must train intensively for at least 10 years in their domain to acquire area-specific expertise (e.g., Coyle, 2009). According to Ericsson and Crutcher (1990), most experts at an international level of performance have begun intensive practice in their domain by the age of 6.

Learning in the *Deliberate Practice* framework is especially effective when mistakes can be recognized and corrected through constructive feedback during exercises. Therefore, exercises should be clearly defined, implemented at a challenging level of difficulty, and repeated frequently (Ericsson et al., 1993).

Deliberate Practice is primarily aligned with the improvement of central performance factors. Rewards or incentives (personal, social, financial) do not result in motivational incentives for the learner when executing the exercises given by the coach. Along these lines, Ericsson et al. (1993) define three conditions for expertise acquisition.

Conditions for Expertise Acquisition (Ericsson et al., 1993)

1. As *Deliberate Practice* is not perceived as fun, the learner must be *motivated* to improve his or her performance; otherwise, his or her commitment during training could quickly diminish.
2. In order to concentrate throughout the entire learning process, *Deliberate Practice* requires a high degree of *effort*, fast recovery after individual exercise sessions, and adequate regulation of the increasing requirements during the training and learning process.
3. The learners require supporting *resources* for the best possible development. These can be adequate equipment/facilities or training possibilities but also support services from family, coaches, or teachers.

Deliberate Practice in sport describes the methodical and consistent analysis of strenuous, sport-specific activities that lead to the systematic improvement of specific aspects of competition performance (Ford et al., 2015). These training activities can strengthen power, fitness, or mental skills but can also include specific activities to improve technique or tactical knowledge.

Many sport scientists have used the *Deliberate Practice* approach as an opportunity to compare training or activity profiles of successful athletes. As in the original studies with musicians (Ericsson et al., 1993), various analyses in sport showed a linear relationship between *Deliberate Practice* and performance level (Helsen et al., 1998; Ward et al., 2007). To further understand this relationship, Macnamara et al. (2016) conducted a meta-analysis whereby the influence of *Deliberate Practice* was seen as marginal when comparing differences in high-level competition performance (from a national level). In addition to general methodological problems in the underlying studies (e.g., operationalization of what *Deliberate Practice* should be), the fact that high-level athletes can generally draw upon *Deliberate Practice* to a large extent is responsible for the small degree of influence. This characteristic, therefore, does not demonstrate a significant force in separating differences in performance at a high level.

23.3.2.2 Deliberate Play

The *Deliberate Play* approach was introduced to expertise research as an alternative model to *Deliberate Practice* (◘ Table 23.1). *Deliberate Play* contains modified versions of competition-oriented sports with flexible and age-appropriate rules, such as small-sided games that can be played and organized by the participants themselves (Berry et al., 2008; Ford et al., 2015). This approach is based on the belief that early and informal participation in athletic activities contributes to the development of expertise in sport (Côté, 1999; Côté et al., 2003). These early, play-oriented types of activity are intrinsically motivating, offer direct rewards, and maximize fun and joy (e.g., street soccer; Berry et al., 2008; Côté & Fraser-Thomas, 2008).

Although play-oriented activities are not characterized as directly advantageous to athletic development (Ericsson et al., 1993), researchers such as Côté (1999) emphasize the importance of play-oriented activities, especially during an athlete's early development. *Deliberate Play* promotes various cognitive and motor experiences beneficial to athletic performance and later *Deliberate Practice* (Ford et al., 2009; Roca et al., 2012). Through the joy of *Deliberate Play*, athletes develop relevant, area-specific proficiencies and skills that stimulate athletic motivation and can later guide *Deliberate Practice* (Côté, 1999; Côté & Fraser-Thomas, 2008).

◘ Table 23.1 Differences between Deliberate Play and Deliberate Practice (simplified from Côté et al., 2007, p. 186)

Deliberate Practice	Deliberate Play
Motivational incentive: Future objectives	Motivational incentive: Current performance
Does not afford much joy	Affords joy
Focus on results of conduct	Focus on conduct
Explicit rules	Flexibility
Adult involvement often required	Adult involvement not required
Takes place in (sports) facilities	Takes place in multiple environments

Furthermore, *Deliberate Play* enables youth athletes to test their creativity (regarding decision-making and movement) without competition or pressure from coaches. This creativity would not necessarily be accepted or encouraged in an organized setting (Côté et al., 2008).

> Play-oriented activities can also lead to better sport-specific performance because athletes develop skills applicable to an array of athletic contexts (Baker & Young, 2014; Côté et al., 2007). Besides, these activities offer an implicit approach to the development of skills. This brings a greater degree of stability to competition, so athletes have a higher likelihood of retrieving learned information (Côté & Fraser-Thomas, 2008).

Various sport scientists have quantified *Deliberate Play* with talented athletes and in doing so highlighted *Deliberate Play*'s positive contributions to expertise development. Retrospective surveys established that professional athletes had spent more time per week playing specific sports during their childhoods than non-professional athletes (Ford & Williams, 2012; Haugaasen et al., 2014). Additionally, it was shown that soccer players who signed professional contracts later in adolescence took part in soccer-specific *Deliberate Play* more often than players without a contract offer (Ford et al., 2009).

23.4 Talent Identification

The identification of talent is an important task in sport, to allocate clubs' and organizations' limited resources (e.g., training time, coaches) as efficiently as possible to youth athletes worthy of promotion. But, to what extent do certain characteristics of youth athletes offer evidence as to whether these athletes will have future success? Defining the concept of talent as broad and dynamic, these diagnostics should consider environmental as well as personal characteristics longitudinally over multiple measurement points (Till & Baker, 2020). Mostly for pragmatic reasons, research from the last few years has presented prospective studies in which singularly, particularly personal characteristics are assessed, and it is examined whether these characteristics can be applied for talent identification purposes.

Sport scientific frameworks can be consulted for the systematizing of existing research findings, in order to categorize the potential predictors of athletic talent (e.g., Vaeyens et al., 2013). In line with the MMG and DMGT (► Sect. 23.3.1), such frameworks distinguish environmental and personal factors at the highest level. According to the DMGT, environmental factors (e.g., parental support, the coach's behavior, conditions of support) are grouped into milieu, persons, and provisions of support (cf. ◘ Fig. 23.2; an overview of the importance of environmental characteristics offered by Li et al., 2014). Regarding personal characteristics, anthropometric (e.g., body size), physiological (e.g., conditional proficiencies), and psychological characteristics are differentiated from one another.

The following considerations of talent identification and development (► Sects. 23.4 and 23.5) focus on psychological predictors. These cover *cognitive performance factors* (e.g., decision-making competence) and *personality-related factors* (e.g., achievement motivation). In this case, cognitive factors apply as direct performance factors, especially in situational sports (e.g., game sports), while personality-related factors influence both performance and general talent development. Furthermore, *psychomotor factors* (e.g., technical skills) are also sport psychological talent predictors (cf. ◘ Fig. 23.4) that are covered in ► Methods Box: The Problem of Insufficient Sensitivity in Talent Diagnostics.

Methods Box: The Problem of Insufficient Sensitivity in Talent Diagnostics

Technical skills (e.g., dribbling, ball control) are normally analyzed through motor performance tests and are considered psychomotor talent predictors (cf. ◘ Fig. 23.4; for a recent review on the prognostic validity of technical skills in talented youth athletes, see Koopmann et al., 2020). However, the prognostic relevance of motor tests to future success is controversial, due to the complexity of performance factors in sports and varying motor development of youth athletes (Lidor et al., 2009). An important distinction in this discussion is whether the prognostic relevance of certain diagnostics is viewed based on the *group average* or the *individual value*.

Based on this distinction, Höner and Votteler (2016) explored the prognostic relevance of motor diagnostics in which technical skills (dribbling, ball control, shooting) as well as speed-related abilities (sprinting, agility) were assessed (cf. Lottermann et al., 2003). The study investigated the motor test performances of over 20,000 U-12 players selected for competence centers within the German Soccer Association talent development program (Deutscher Fußball-Bund, DFB). The analysis examined which players were selected for youth national teams (U-16 to U-19) and what performance factors at the U-12 tests identified these players as talented.

Classic comparisons of group averages showed U-12 players who were selected for youth national teams (U-16 to U-19) demonstrated notably better test scores (by almost one standard deviation) than U-12 players who never made it to that level of performance. This highlights the *general prognostic validity* of motor diagnostics; however, these measures should not be the sole instrument of talent identification. Further analyses revealed that talent prediction based on single examples is inconsistent. On the one hand, even competence center players with outstanding test scores (the test's top 1%) only had a 6% chance to be selected for youth national teams (U-16 to U-19). On the other hand, analyses of *sensitivity* (proportion of correctly identified talents) showed that only 90% of future youth national team players would have remained in the development program if the bottom 30% of U-12 players (according to motor diagnostics performance) had been cut (Höner & Votteler, 2016). Such a process would, therefore, have "weeded out" every tenth potential youth national team player!

This example shows that diagnostics—with an entirely acceptable effect size—can be prognostically valid but problematic regarding their sensitivity. Appropriate diagnostics, therefore, do not justify stand-alone decisions in the selection of talent. Thus, they should be used merely as an additional piece of information (e.g., in addition to the holistic, subjective judgment of the coach) and not as the sole "decision instrument." Furthermore, the added value of a prognostically relevant diagnostic exists in its ability to identify relevant characteristics of talent development whose promotion appears to be especially meaningful (► Sect. 23.5).

23.4.1 Cognitive Performance Factors

Athletes in all sports perform in constantly changing situations under the pressure of time, precision, and complexity. It is therefore important to recognize various options for action and their underlying conditions. For example, a tennis player should recognize early on when his or her opponent goes up to the net, in order to select an appropriate response action.

Selecting and executing an appropriate action requires a decision by the athlete. The athlete generates options and implements a situational problem-solving process in which they identify the best possible options with respect to the current situation (e.g., in handball, the pass to the circle instead of the throw to the goal). The relevant cognitive performance factor for this process is described as decision-making competence and is viewed as a potential talent predictor (cf. ◘ Fig. 23.4).

Decision-Making Competence

Decision-making competence describes an athlete's ability to select the best action for the optimal use of his or her abilities in a specific situation under the pressure of time, precision, and complexity. The decision is a direct interplay between the potential of one's motor ability (implementation of the intended action) and the people involved in the situation (teammates and opponents).

Multiple (cross-sectional) studies provide evidence that experts and youth athletes at high-performance levels make better decisions in video-simulated decision-making tests than intermediate and novice athletes (e.g., Helsen & Starkes, 1999; Höner, 2005; Woods et al., 2016). However, there are a limited number of longitudinal studies that examine the significance of cognitive factors for talent development. Several studies have demonstrated that dimensions of decision-making competence (such as *positioning and deciding* or *acting in changing situations*) may be significant influencing factors on the future success of youth players in Dutch and Finnish soccer (Forsman et al., 2016; Huijgen et al., 2014; Kannekens et al., 2011). However, the findings should be considered with caution as this assessment used a self-evaluation questionnaire rather than objective testing procedures (cf. Nortje et al., 2014).

The basis of an athlete's decision-making competence is formed by various cognitive factors that support the perception of information and subsequent processing during the decision-making process. In sport psychology two main research approaches analyze these processes:

While the "Expert Performance Approach" considers an athlete's context-specific (i.e., sport-specific), perceptual-cognitive skills, the "Cognitive Component Skill Approach" analyzes context-nonspecific (general) executive functions (Romeas et al., 2016).

23.4.1.1 Expert Performance Approach

The *perceptual-cognitive skills* considered in the "Expert Performance Approach" help athletes identify and acquire environmental information and integrate existing knowledge in order to make an appropriate decision (O'Connor et al., 2016; Ward & Williams, 2003). These skills thereby support processes of perceiving information and processing during action in sport. The most well-known perceptual-cognitive skills include anticipation, pattern recognition, and knowledge of situational probabilities.

Anticipation

Anticipation enables athletes to predict events before they happen. It is based on processes of perception, attention, and memory and serves athlete decision-making.

Pattern Recognition

Pattern recognition enables athletes to recognize relevant stimuli in sport-specific situations not only as isolated pieces of information but also within a holistic structure (e.g., a 3-2-1 defensive formation in handball).

Knowledge of Situational Probabilities

Knowledge of situational probabilities enables athletes to assess probabilities of imminent events or alternatives in a sport-specific situation. This is based on the athlete's previous knowledge and the processing of (imminent) information before entering the situation (Farrow & Abernethy, 2007; Williams & Ford, 2013).

The importance of perceptual-cognitive skills has been evaluated as part of the "Laboratory Approach of Expertise Research" (► Sect. 23.3.2), whereby laboratory settings facilitate an analysis of cognitive factors, despite the complexity of athletic actions (Abernethy et al., 2005). In highly standardized settings, video presentations are given to athletes in order to present the most representative tasks as possible (e.g., recognition of the direction of a badminton shot shown in the video). The cognitive processes that form the basis of experts' performances are thereby analyzed in detail with classic methods of cognitive psychology (including reaction time measurements, eye-tracking, temporal and spatial occlusion technique; cf. Hadlow et al., 2018).

The laboratory-based sport psychology expertise research has highlighted cognitive performance factors that differentiate between athletes at various performance levels in *context-specific* or *sport-specific tasks* (Larkin et al., 2016; Roca et al., 2013).

According to Williams et al. (2011), when considering perceptual-cognitive skills, experts are especially skilled at:

- Identifying task-relevant cues about the movements of other athletes (e.g., cues in the wrist for a slice in table tennis) and deploying efficient actions under time pressure (i.e., anticipation)
- Quickly and precisely recognizing structures relevant to the game (e.g., patterns such as tactical formations in sports)
- Assessing the progress of game situations based on the probability of individual options moving forward (e.g., diagonal ball or spike in volleyball) that assist to quickly adapt to changes within the situational conditions of the game environment (▶ Study Box: Perceptual-Cognitive Proficiencies and Executive Functions).

23.4.1.2 Cognitive Component Skill Approach

The prefrontal control and regulation mechanisms, described in neuropsychology as *executive functions*, are some of the most well-known situational, *nonspecific cognitive functions* in the "Cognitive Component Skill Approach."

Executive Functions

Executive functions describe the (volitional) skill to coordinate cognitive, emotional, and motor processes in the sense of higher-level action goals, thereby suppressing unwanted reactions or motivational tendencies in certain circumstances. These functions can be divided into the components of working memory, inhibition control, and cognitive flexibility (Diamond, 2013).

Working Memory

Updating in working memory serves to retain and integrate relevant information (e.g., verbal and visuospatial information).

Cognitive Flexibility

Cognitive flexibility means the ability to switch between different tasks, operations, or rules.

Inhibition

Processing inhibition is used to avoid automatic behavioral responses or distractions (attentional and self-control processes).

Suitable cognitive control of a goal-oriented behavior requires *working memory*, in which current information can be perceived and processed, *cognitive flexibility* to adjust to new situations, and *inhibition control* to suppress action tendencies that conflict with current action goals. These executive functions are assessed through general (not sport-specific), psychological testing procedures (cf. Diamond, 2013 for an overview).

The findings of the "Cognitive Component Skill Approach" are less clear when considering the question of whether athletes of different performance levels differ in terms of coping with nonspecific cognitive tasks. A meta-analysis by Voss et al. (2009) suggests experts coping with non-sport-specific cognitive requirements do not have performance advantages in comparison to less-skilled athletes. However, studies have found differences between athletes of different performance levels in unspecified cognitive tests (▶ Study Box: Perceptual-Cognitive Proficiencies and Executive Functions). According to these studies, talented youth athletes focus and maintain their attention as well as suppress unwanted motor reactions. This offers initial clues that knowledge of youth athletes' executive functions could support the process of talent identification and development, especially when considering executive functions as differential or relatively stable over the lifespan (McCrory et al., 2004). To understand how non-sport-specific cognitive training programs can be used for talent development further research is required (for a general overview of executive function support, see Diamond & Ling, 2016; for initial empirical findings, see Romeas et al., 2016).

Study Box

Perceptual-Cognitive Proficiencies and Executive Functions

The *temporal occlusion technique* is the primary method used to analyze *anticipation*. Athletes receive presentations of game sequences with varying amounts of information, due to the video being cut off at different time points (e.g., shortly before and shortly after contact of an anticipated stroke in badminton). Experts have shown better anticipation skills in various sports (e.g., badminton, soccer, squash, tennis) compared to less-skilled athletes. In particular, experts are able to identify cues earlier in action situations (*advanced cue utilization*) and use these cues to anticipate future events (e.g., stroke direction in badminton) (Cañal-Bruland & Williams, 2010; Huys et al., 2008; Schultz, 2014; Williams & Ericsson, 2005). Anticipation performance can therefore also be fostered through an appropriate, visual searching action (*visual search strategy*) that is characterized by the expert fixing his or her gaze on the opponent as opposed to the ball (Roca et al., 2013; Vaeyens et al., 2007).

The skill of *pattern recognition* is evaluated primarily with the *Recall-Paradigm*. A classic study in the area stems from chess (Chase & Simon, 1973), where chess masters and novices were shown various chess formations for a few seconds, after which they were asked to recreate the formations on a chessboard, implying a retrieval of memory content. Experts had a recall advantage when typical (i.e., structured) chess formations were shown. However, when the chess pieces were set up in an atypical (random) way, the experts had no advantage. Sport psychology research adopted this analysis approach and was able to show for various sports (hockey, basketball, Australian football) that experts can identify structured game patterns and recall them better compared to less-skilled athletes. This advantage is substantiated by the fact that experts perceive individual formations (e.g., individual players) in the form of holistic information chains (*chunks*) when typical game structures are presented to them (Farrow et al., 2010; Garland & Barry, 1991). This advantage does not exist in atypical game situations (i.e., walking off the court at a timeout or leaving the pitch at half time), in which experts can also only recall a limited amount of individual pieces of information from their short-term memory and therefore do not hold a performance advantage over novices. Furthermore, it is possible to find performance differences in pattern recognition skills even between top-level elite players whose coaches rated them as good or less-than-good decision-makers (Berry et al., 2008). Further, findings have indicated pattern recognition skills can transfer between sports with similar structures (e.g., hockey, soccer), but not unrelated structures (e.g., hockey, volleyball) (Smeeton et al., 2004).

To analyze the *knowledge of situation-dependent probabilities*, game excerpts are shown, and the videos are paused at a critical moment (e.g., just before an attacking player passes the ball to a teammate) (Crognier & Féry, 2005; Larkin et al., 2016; Ward et al., 2013). In invasion sports, athletes identify action options and rank the options from most to least dangerous for the defense. With this *situational probability paradigm*, Ward and Williams (2003) showed that 17- to 19-year-old elite youth soccer players demonstrated better situational understanding than players at lower levels. The elite players were more precise in identifying task-relevant information from game situations and could connect this information with prior experience, in order to recognize the best possible options. Further studies suggest differences in skill are also found between variably talented players within the same performance level (O'Connor et al., 2016; Williams et al., 2012).

The importance of *executive functions* was evaluated by Huijgen et al. (2015) with 13- to 17-year-old elite (top 0.5%) or sub-elite (top 12%) Dutch youth soccer players. It was shown in various cognitive psychology tests that elite players did not demonstrate performance advantages at *lower-level* cognitions (e.g., nonspecific reaction skills and visual perception). However, *higher-level* cognitions such as *inhibition control* ("Stop-Signal Task"; Sanchez-Cubillo et al., 2009) and *cognitive flexibility* ("Trail Making Test"; Crowe, 1998) demonstrated a performance advantage for elite youth players (for comparable findings, see Vestberg et al., 2012, Verburgh et al., 2014; for a recent review, see Scharfen & Memmert, 2019).

23.4.2 Personality-Related Factors

To analyze personality-related factors, sport psychology talent research often considers the relationship between personality and performance in sport (for an overview of sport science personality research, cf. Morris, 2000). This specific issue relates to what extent personality-related characteristics in childhood and at youth ages provide evidence of later success in adulthood.

In the last few decades—as a consequence of sport science personality research—there has been a trend to move from exploring *general personality traits* to more *specific psychological states*. Currently, researchers focus on the relevance of *specific psychological personality dispositions* to talent identification.

While comprehensive constructs such as mental strength (e.g., Gerber, 2011) or resilience (e.g., Hohmann, 2009) have been discussed in the framework of talent. These constructs can be understood as the product of various psychological aspects and are therefore not explained further here.

23.4.2.1 General Personality Traits

General Personality Traits

General personality traits are relatively broad, consistently occurring (in various situations), and temporally stable tendencies toward certain behaviors (e.g., Roberts, 2009).

Studies of general personality traits (e.g., extroversion or neuroticism) claim to portray the overall personality and are based on inventories such as the "16 Personality Factor Questionnaire" (Cattell, 1966) or the "Eysenck Personality Inventory" (Eysenck & Eysenck, 1975). This research, however, has not found any clear evidence of a connection between personality and performance. In addition to the methodological weaknesses of the respective studies (e.g., low sample size, varying definitions of "success"), the focus on general personality traits was determined to be the main cause of the ambiguous findings.

This led to the conclusion that "the" one single personality type of a top athlete does not exist (Vealey, 2002). Nevertheless, researchers are still examining this area (e.g., Allen et al., 2013) and use the *Big Five* Model (McCrae & Costa, 2008; McCrae & John, 1992) to initiate further research in this area.

23.4.2.2 Specific Psychological States

State Variables

State variables arise from the interaction between personal and situational factors in specific situations. In comparison to general personality traits, such situation-specific characteristics should offer better predictors of performance (Conzelmann, 2009).

Research in this area explores *state measurements* of anxiety and self-awareness (e.g., "Competitive State Anxiety Inventory"; Martens et al., 1990) and was shown to be more successful in differentiating between athletes of various performance levels compared to the general trait approach (Durand-Bush & Salmela, 2001; Gould et al., 2002). However, a criticism of these findings is that state measures do not reflect the relationship between personality and future performance, because such state variables can by definition change from day to day or from situation to situation (Morris, 2000).

Despite the criticism of state variables' situational dependence, (state-based) psychological skills in talent research have an important practical implication (Abbott & Collins, 2004). Building on this, a series of studies exploring mental techniques such as goal setting, coping strategies, or imagination were implemented (e.g., Macnamara & Collins, 2013). These techniques exemplify the goal of state regulation and the importance of providing youth athletes with appropriate psychological abilities (►Sect. 23.5.2). However, researchers are yet to determine the prognostic relevance of such mental competencies for long-term success.

23.4.2.3 Specific Psychological Personality Dispositions

Specific Psychological Personality Disposition

Specific psychological personality dispositions last through time and situation and refer to the pattern of a person to evaluate individual situations (Gabler, 2000). In contrast to general trait approaches, specific dispositions only represent parts of the personality relevant to sport performance. Further, these characteristics are stable across situations and over time and therefore more suitable for long-term prognoses than state variables.

This research approach is based on sport-specific measurements of psychological personality dispositions (e.g., trait anxiety and achievement motivation; Jones & Swain, 1995; Wenhold et al., 2009). As a foundation for the selection of potentially relevant characteristics, sport psychology talent research is oriented on general giftedness models such as the DMGT or MMG (cf. ▶ Sect. 23.3) and regards specific personality aspects such as motivation (e.g., achievement motivation), volition (e.g., willpower), self-esteem (e.g., self-concept) or emotion (e.g., anxiety).

Important Personality Dispositions

Sport psychology talent research and giftedness models consider specific aspects of personality such as:

- Achievement motivation
- Action orientation and self-control (Volition)
- Self-concept/self-efficacy
- Anxiety

Talent researchers have evaluated the relationship between potentially relevant psychological dispositions with current sporting performance in numerous cross-sectional studies (e.g., Coelho e Silva et al., 2010; Jonker et al., 2010; Reilly et al., 2000). Overall, the results suggest a broad spectrum of characteristics significantly relate to current performance and therefore specific psychological dispositions (e.g., goal orientation, self-confidence) are relevant to performance capability.

The number of prospective studies is significantly lower and considers mostly motivational characteristics (Murr et al., 2018a). These studies point to the prognostic relevance for future success (▶ Study Box: Prognostic Relevance of Motivational Characteristics). In other characteristic areas, only a few prognostic studies exist and highlight the importance of *willpower*, *self-esteem*, and *emotions*. For example, analyses of athletes from individual and team sports highlight that volitional competencies can be important for the achievement of sporting success. These findings deal with characteristics that focus on action-relevant aspects of a certain situation in goal tracking and action implementation (e.g., self-regulation, self-optimization, action orientation; Hohmann, 2009; Höner & Feichtinger, 2016). In this sense, willpower (see also ▶ Chaps. 10 and 20) is considered especially important for individuals who are required to partake in large and difficult training plans throughout a career (Elbe et al., 2005).

> Based on the current research, specific personality dispositions—and similarly, cognitive performance factors (▶ Sect. 23.4.1)—should not be used as the sole assessment criteria for talent identification. Currently, there is no clear evidence for the correlation between psychological characteristics and future athletic success. In addition, the testing methods used can only explain a relatively small portion of the differences in performance between skilled and less-skilled athletes. Nevertheless, psychological testing methods can provide a valuable supplement for coaches and sport psychologists. Furthermore, study results offer a scientific basis for the application of psychological diagnostics as part of talent development.

Study Box

Prognostic Relevance of Motivational Characteristics

Prognostic studies in soccer with variable-oriented (e.g., Höner & Feichtinger, 2016) as well as person-oriented (e.g., Zuber et al., 2015) approaches have shown that both achievement motive components *hope for success* and *fear of failure* significantly predict future success. These findings confirm previous approaches on the importance of achievement motivation in sport (Gabler, 2004), whereby success-oriented athletes show more functional behavior patterns than athletes with a fear of failure (e.g., more effort, self-worth promoting attribution, realistic goal setting, etc.). Furthermore, it has been shown that hope for success demonstrates greater prognostic relevance than fear of failure. Similar correlations have also been shown in other sports (e.g., track and field, swimming) (e.g., Elbe et al., 2003; Hohmann, 2009). Schorer et al. (2010) however found no significant correlations between achievement motive and future success in their prospective studies in handball.

Regarding the prognostic relevance of motivational orientations, sport psychology talent research delivers a more heterogeneous position on the findings. Studies have found motivational orientations to individual (e.g., goal orientation) or social (e.g., competition orientation) reference standards could differentiate between athletes of different performance levels (Höner & Feichtinger, 2016; Zuber et al., 2015). Conversely, other studies have been unable to find significant differences between skilled and less-skilled athletes concerning motivational orientations (e.g., ego-orientation and task-orientation) (Figueiredo et al., 2009; Huijgen et al., 2014). Furthermore, some of these studies report somewhat contradictory results: For example, Elferink-Gemser et al. (2015) found a positive correlation between ego-orientation and performance enhancement for speed skaters throughout a competitive season. However, Cervelló et al. (2007) found track and field athletes and tennis players, who withdrew from a talent promotion program the following season (drop-outs), showed a higher emphasis on ego-orientation (i.e., social reference standard) than those who remained in the program.

23.5 Talent Development

Starting from a broad and dynamic understanding of talent (► Sect. 23.2), psychological variables and their development are increasingly important in talent development. This applies especially to *cognitive performance factors* and *personality-related factors* described in ► Sect. 23.4.

> The training of cognitive performance factors and the systemic-holistic development of personality-related factors in youth athletes are important points of emphasis for sport psychology talent development.

It should be noted that especially in promoting personality-related variables a strictly "evidence-based" approach in sport psychology practice appears limited. Sport psychology measures in talent development are, therefore, not identified with a high level of evidence deduced from, for example, long-term randomized control studies. This assessment should not be attributed to the measures themselves, but rather results from studies with often (overly) ambitious methodological conditions.

Regardless, sport psychology is an essential building block of fundamental talent development in sport federations and clubs. For example, in Germany, the increasing importance of sport psychology support is demonstrated by the fact that, among other factors, sport psychologists have become firmly integrated into institutions such as Olympic training centers or youth academies of professional soccer.

23.5.1 Cognitive Performance Factors

Cognitive performance factors such as *decision-making competence* are especially important for sporting talent (► Sect. 23.4.1). Despite the high relevance of the underlying processes of information collection and processing, it seems there is less focus on developing these skills than other performance factors such as physical conditioning or technical skills. Regarding endurance training, for which physiological stress parameters can be recommended based on scientific studies, coaches have relatively concrete conceptions of the physiological requirements needed in training (e.g., frequency, intensity, and duration of a run). In order to teach technical-tactical skills, exercises with many repetitions (e.g., "technique drills" or "automation" of standard game plays) are often introduced in sports, consistently in line with the *Deliberate Practice* approach (► Sect. 23.3.2.1). These are often taught through simplifying the situation, so the skills are trained in isolation from the game's context (Pill, 2012). Such exercises help develop and stabilize basic techniques and are thereby able to form the foundation for more complex conditions. However, these exercises support replication more than understanding of game actions, because they do not have a direct link to actual game performance, in which decisions/answers are sought to ever-changing situations (Kidman & Lombardo, 2010).

Despite suitable approaches, there are few concrete concepts in practice to support the development of cognitive performance factors (cf. Zentgraf & Munzert, 2014). Fundamentally, cognitive requirements should be a focus of youth training programs to ensure athletes to experience the various decision-making game situations (Davids et al., 2012; Höner, 2012). Outlined below are examples of approaches that have been introduced for the development of cognitive performance factors in youth players.

> In the training of cognitive performance factors, youth athletes:
>
> - Are placed in typical game situations. These can be realistic situations (e.g., *small-sided games*) or simulated situations, where cognitive processes can be trained without physical strain (*video-based training*).
> - Should develop a reflective understanding of the context of relevant game situations through explicit questions recapping the contextual meaning of the situation (*discovery learning*), rather than explicit instructions by the coach.
> - Should learn tangible strategies for the exploration of game situations (*pre-orientation through an adequate field of view alignment*).

23.5.1.1 Small-Sided Games

> Small-sided games are modified games, most often with alternative rules, that are played with fewer players than in standard competition (Halouani et al., 2014; Vilar et al., 2014). Most small-sided games promote actions in tight situations, where players must make situational decisions and convert their intentions (psychological and motor) into action.

Through small-sided games, learning conditions are created in which technical, tactical, and decision-making skills can be developed simultaneously (Davids et al., 2013; Travassos et al., 2012). The variability of these situations, as well as the required situational skills, supports decision-making in various game situations. Small-sided games thereby make recurring learning opportunities possible, in order to develop an implicit—almost incidental and subconscious—understanding of which alternatives are functional in the game. With an adequately open training design by the coach (avoidance of restrictive conditions, "positive culture of mistakes"), small-sided games offer youth players the opportunity to experiment—to an extent at their own pace—with their decision-making and technical skills. For example, in these types of games, athletes interpret cues for themselves to explore new options for action and make their own decisions. There are similarities of this approach with *Deliberate Play* (▶ Sect. 23.3.2.2) or with the development of intrinsic motivation (see ▶ Chap. 8). The motto "play makes perfect" (Roth, 1996) takes precedence over the motto of the *Deliberate Practice* approach, "practice makes perfect."

23.5.1.2 Video-Based Training

> In video-based training, athletes watch video clips that present sport-specific information, with the aim to identify relevant pieces of information to inform decisions on possible successful game actions, with coaches providing appropriate feedback (Berry et al., 2008; Johnson, 2006; Larkin et al., 2014).

Sport-specific video-based training, developed from sport psychology expertise research, uses similar methodological approaches (e.g., temporal occlusion) to the diagnostics of relevant cognitive performance factors (▶ Sect. 23.4.1). Decision-making and perceptual-cognitive skills are thereby trained off-field and implemented without physical stress. As youth athletes often reach physiological limits due to a high volume of conventional training, this form of training constitutes a promising possibility of additional training.

In their systematic review, Larkin et al. (2015) showed video-based training can be implemented as an effective strategy in the development of decision-making capabilities. Video-based programs were found to improve *anticipation performance* (handball: Abernethy et al., 2012; squash: Abernethy et al., 1999; badminton: Hagemann et al., 2006) and *decision-making quality* (soccer: Cañal-Bruland et al., 2007; tennis: Farrow & Abernethy, 2002; basketball: Gorman & Farrow, 2009; cricket: Hopwood et al., 2011; hockey: Williams et al., 2003).

23.5.1.3 Discovery Learning

> In discovery learning, athletes are presented with relevant action situations without providing them with a solution in advance. This promotes independent, reflective understanding of action options in competitive situations (Gréhaigne et al., 2001).

The principle of discovery learning is originally based on the "Socratic method" and is discussed today in the context of the contrast between "structured" and "discovery allowance" teaching in didactics (Klauer & Leutner, 2007). In sport, various teaching approaches (e.g., "teaching games for understanding"; Bunker & Thorpe, 1982) employ this teaching and learning principle and use it to teach game sports during childhood and youth ages.

According to Vickers (2007), discovery learning can be promoted within a training situation through the targeted coach questioning related to meaningful action solutions. This promotes athletes to develop their own solutions independently and critically, without instructions from the coach. Furthermore, targeted questioning regarding possible solutions to problems should lead to sustainable learning processes because:

- Personal responsibility to decisions made by athletes is strengthened (Butler, 2005; Kidman, 2010).
- The athletes are less reliant on feedback from the coach and learn more at their own pace.
- The athletes become better at problem-solving and analyzing their own performances (Potrac & Cassidy, 2006; Williams & Hodges, 2004).

Sport psychology and sport pedagogy studies show that a less "structured" and more "discovery allowing" training approach with a high amount of questioning can improve decision-making because players are encouraged toward higher-order (e.g., strategies for information processing) problem-solving processes (Chambers & Vickers, 2006; Harvey et al., 2010; McNeill et al., 2008; Partington & Cushion, 2013). Therefore, a significant challenge for youth coaches is to use appropriate questions and feedback to guide players toward a solution as independently as possible (Kidman, 2010; Potrac & Cassidy, 2006).

For Sports Practice

Example: Discovery Allowance in Table Tennis
For example, a table tennis coach who instructs a player directly toward potential improvement or points out a mistake after the exercise is practicing structured learning ("More distance!" or "Play the backhand with more backspin!"). In contrast, a coach implementing a discovery allowance training method would guide the athlete to the potential improvement by asking questions such as "What can you do better the next time?" or "What did you notice about your backhand?"

23.5.1.4 Pre-orientation Through Adequate Field of View Alignment (Visual Exploratory Activity)

Adequate athlete decision-making requires appropriate perception (O'Connor & Larkin, 2015). For example, decisions in sports are based on the perception of relevant environmental information such as the location of teammates and opponents, the body position of the most immediate opponent, or the condition of the playing surface (i.e., ski slope, soccer pitch).

> In order to be aware of the important characteristics in a given game situation, an appropriate orientation of one's field of view is required. This field of view can, for example, be altered by a look over the shoulder and is described as "pre-orientation." This process can be trained through certain exercises.

Jordet (2005) evaluated the importance of the field of view orientation in soccer. He defined a player's *visual exploratory activity* as movements of the body or head to perceive information in moments before trapping the ball and also when not in possession of the ball. These movements serve as prerequisites for being able to act appropriately and without delay when trapping the ball. The observational study found that professional players implement these glances more than amateur players and "superstar players" (e.g., Frank Lampard) exhibited these behaviors even more than other professional players. Furthermore, positive correlations were found between visual exploratory activity and subsequent pass quality, providing initial indications that an effective field of view orientation can influence game performance (Fagereng, 2010; Jordet & Bloomfield, 2009; Nyland, 2010).

To support the development of this important skill (► For Sports Practice: Xavi's Greatest Strength: Pre-orientation), coaches should design exercises that promote searching for visual information in the game environment. Coaches can achieve this by designing exercises that focus on the perception of the environment or that make use of certain hints or prompts to remind players to "visually explore" the game environment before trapping the ball. For example, the player must recognize signs in the periphery in addition to their main tasks and report or be explicitly asked to orient their body position as openly as possible to the game situation that arises.

For Sports Practice

Xavi's Greatest Strength: Pre-orientation

Xavi Hernández (Spanish World Cup 2010 champion, among other honors) describes his greatest strength:

When I receive a pass, I have already looked around and know if I have space, can turn, or if I have an opponent behind me. When I am under pressure, I try to play with one or two touches and to receive and take the ball so that the defender cannot steal it. In essence, I try to gain a few meters of space so that I cannot lose the ball and put myself in a position to develop our play. It sounds simple but having command of these skills is very difficult. That is how I survive the game, although I am not physically strong or large. You have to consider the game situation…!

(This quotation is taken from the following link, in which pre-orientation exercises are presented in German: ► https://www.dfb.de/trainer/a-juniorin/artikel/vororientierung-macht-den-igel-zum-hasen-2316/.)

23.5.2 Personality-Related Factors

Currently, there is a considerable debate between different psychological schools of thought (e.g., behavioral psychology methods, systemic counseling) in relation to how objectives (performance optimization, holistic development) and the athletes' spheres of life (school, sport, family) influence personality-related factors and their use in talent development. In talent development, different levels of personality characteristics and their differences in demonstrable performance orientation (► Sect. 23.4.2), as well as their stability, must be taken into account when developing new measures: the more general the personality characteristics, the more difficult the direct interference. This section will discuss the development of general personality traits (► Sect. 23.5.2.1) and specific psychological dispositions and competencies (► Sect. 23.5.2.2).

23.5.2.1 General Personality Traits

> The design of conditional frameworks is more significant than direct interference in the development of general personality traits. General personality trait development should be considered in multi-year periods and often entail extensive changes. The task in this context is therefore not primarily to "develop" but rather much more "allow to develop."

Relevant institutions of sports, such as the German Olympic Sports Confederation, highlight the role of personality development in youth programs with a claim that clearly exceeds the direct contribution to performance. Therefore, performance sports should be mindful to operate under conditions that protect the individual and meet high ethical and moral standards, despite the focus on performance.

Through such claims, responsible organizations bear not only their own expectations of future top-level performers but also their responsibility toward the multitude of athletes who do *not* eventually make it into professional programs and competition that provide a living wage. Personality development is therefore also an important source of support for de-selected athletes (Park et al., 2013).

> In personality-related talent development, there are two relevant higher objectives: the goal of *successful* but also *healthy development* of athletes inside and outside of competitive sports should be taken into account, in addition to performance optimization.

According to Havighurst (1956), an important basis for positive *personality development* involves the successful confrontation of so-called developmental tasks. Hidden behind this concept are certain tasks that are significant for the completion of everyday tasks. Therefore, interventions and conditional frameworks should provide a relevant contribution to coping with important *developmental tasks at youth ages* (▶Side Story: Developmental Tasks at Youth Ages). Based on empirical findings in standard populations (McCormick et al., 2011; Oerter, 2006), it can be assumed that successful coping with developmental tasks leads to an important basis for stable athletic performance in the long term.

A high level of coping efforts is expected during the adolescence phase of talent development (phase of extensive physiological, emotional, and cognitive changes). In addition, it can be assumed that various developmental tasks are more difficult for athletes to overcome or must already be dealt with earlier in life in comparison with young people who do not engage in performance sports. These tasks include independence (e.g., the change from the parents' home to a sport boarding school) or an earlier, intentional analysis of one's professional career. The chances of successful coping with such topics depend not only on each individual but also on the context or environment in which the individual lives.

> Interventions for personality development regard not only the athletes themselves but also their *athletic* (e.g., trainers) and *extracurricular environment* (e.g., family, friends, school) (Henriksen & Stambulova, 2017; Wolfenden & Holt, 2005) in order to create development promoting conditional frameworks.

Side Story

Developmental Tasks at Youth Ages

According to Havighurst (1956), developmental tasks denote learning processes that result from real conditions and whose solution leads to the acquisition of important competencies. Successful mastery of these tasks leads to constructive and satisfactory mastery of life as part of a community. Developmental tasks during adolescence are shaped by changes on widely varied levels (Dreher & Oerter, 1986; Oerter, 2006). ◘ Table 23.2 lists examples of general and sport-related developmental tasks of adolescence. Despite formal differences within study frameworks, the content of these categories is not clearly separated. An interaction between general and area-specific developmental tasks can be assumed, especially during childhood. Ohlert and Kleinert (2015) evaluated the importance of self-defined, sport-related developmental tasks in elite youth handball players in comparison to general developmental tasks. The interviewed athletes set the relevance of athletic and general developmental tasks as roughly equal, which, from the view of the athletes, speaks for the most holistic support as possible.

▪ **Athletic Environment**

Some developmental tasks during childhood can primarily be coped with through independent exploration of possibilities and boundaries (Oerter, 2006). Therefore, a good balance should be maintained in the athletes' environment between preset structures and free space for individual experiences. Furthermore, holistic personality development can only be trained conditionally, which is why its support is primarily related to the formation of conditional frameworks. This is also confirmed by youth performance athletes who recognize their environment as an important factor in their talent development (Ivarsson et al., 2015).

The *coach* plays a key role in talent development since he or she is normally the most important parental figure in the performance sport environment (Rynne et al., 2017).

Besides the coach, other supporting staff such as physiotherapists and career advisors should be considered. This group of people can take on important tasks during development by promoting the analysis of competition and everyday experience. This includes, following pedagogical approaches (e.g., Reimann & Mandl, 2006), designing learning processes as described in ◘ Table 23.3. The quality of interaction in the context of such processes is also directly related to the characteristics of the people in the environment. For example, team sport athletes' self-efficacy is linked to their coach's self-confidence (Feltz et al., 2008). Further, athletes' motivation is also developed through their relationship with important social parental figures in the athletic environment (e.g., the coach) (Vallerand & Losier, 1999). Numerous studies have shown autonomy-promoting interactions with these people (i.e., with as little pressure and control as possible) lead to a higher degree of self-determined motivation within athletes. This correlation is mediated by the basic needs of autonomy, experiences of competence, and relatedness (e.g., Amorose & Anderson-Butcher, 2007; Hollembeak & Amorose, 2005), the three components of self-determination theory, according to Deci and Ryan (1985) (see also ▸Chap. 8).

▪ **Non-athletic Environment**

Regarding the non-athletic environment, findings have shown the relevance of the institution or school, as well as the influence of people in an athlete's private life, can influence development. In the latter case, a distinction can be made between *adults* (especially parents) and *contemporaries* (peers and partners in later adolescence).

Parents are normally the most important non-athletic reference for youth athletes in the adolescent stage of life. However, parental influence tends to decrease as athletes grow older.

23

According to a study with youth tennis players, the influence of adults on talent development can be divided into the areas of emotional support, material support, hardships, pressure, and social relationships (Wolfenden & Holt, 2005). Among adults, parents—above all, in a supportive function—appear to be especially relevant. According to Sheridan et al. (2014), parents have an important influence on youth athlete's motivation, participation in sport, and further individual development. They have also been shown to influence the early withdrawal from a career in performance sports.

During an athlete's development, parents take on multiple hardships and show a variety of competencies. Harwood and Knight (2015) acknowledge that parental competencies must cover a broad range of requirements in talent development (◘ Table 23.3). Parent information sessions may be a platform to help parents understand the talent development and the role they play in this process. Steps should be taken to ensure continual parent engagement with their child's development. This could be achieved through continued communication via virtual platforms and regular information sessions with key representatives from the athletic environment.

As youth athletes mature, the importance of contemporaries (peers) and partners in "couple relationships" grows.

The influence of contemporaries appears to mirror the influence of parents (e.g., motivation, withdrawal from a career in performance sport). It is important when dealing with the shift in relationships that these people also maintain access to relevant knowledge regarding personality development. Therefore, an offer of support equivalent to the aforementioned parent sessions can also be helpful.

The environmental factor of *school* is managed by high-level sports organizations through the promotion of appropriate forms of schooling (e.g., elite sport schools of the German Olympic Sport Federation; Borggrefe & Cachay, 2012), which ensure a continual dialogue between coaches and teachers. The danger of overstress or overload and the resulting risks can be minimized through coordination between the education system and training regimes.

When reflecting on their time at school, many athletes perceive deficits in terms of their academic careers, strategic career planning, and material support (Holt & Mitchell, 2006). An important factor in this perception is the increasing effort and investment required for a career in high-performance sport, which almost invariably results in conflicts between athletic and academic goals (Brettschneider, 1999; Christensen & Sørensen, 2009). For example, exam preparation is often shortened due to the significant investment in training or attendance at training camps and thus absence from regular school classes. This conflict is contrary to the desire to strengthen identities outside of performance sport. This is important because it would ensure that de-selected talents are able to be successful in other areas of life (Cartigny et al., 2019). However, a suitable vocational or academic career path can also be important for athletes who succeed in high-performance sports. In both cases, schooling lays the foundation for success.

Table 23.2 Examples of general and sport-related developmental tasks during adolescence

General developmental tasks (Havighurst, 1956)	Sport-related developmental tasks (Ohlert & Kleinert, 2015)
• More mature relationships with peers	• Expedite athletic development
• Adoption of gender roles	• Develop self-organization
• Acceptance and use of own body	• Develop emotional control
• Emotional independence from parents and other adults	• Find ones' role in a group
• Preparation for a professional career	• Find a balance between stress and rest
• Own values and social responsibility	• Manage the conditional frameworks of performance sport
With kind permission from Hogrefe, Jeannine Ohlert and Jens Kleinert	

Table 23.3 Examples for tasks and requirements of people in a talent's athletic and non-athletic environment

Tasks of people in the athletic environment (Reimann & Mandl, 2006)	Requirements of parents as representatives of the non-athletic environment (Harwood & Knight, 2015)
• Positive reinforcement/encouragement	• Select appropriate training possibilities
• Demonstrate/be a role model	• Provide emergency support
• Explain/convey understanding	• Understand and use appropriate parenting styles
• Support self-experience	• Deal with emotional challenges in competitive situations
• Give impulses/coach	• Adapt to one's own involvement in the personal and athletic development of one's children

23.5.2.2 Specific Personality Dispositions and Competencies

Specific psychological dispositions relate to defined and relatively stable constructs. Changes and developments to these dispositions are possible but are usually intermediate or long term in their nature. Contrastingly, current states (e.g., competitive anxiety) emerge in the short term and can be directly influenced with the help of appropriate strategies (e.g., concerning behavior or perception). Both for the influence on states and the development of dispositions, athletes should acquire competencies that enable them to deal with their tasks and goals—actively and in a regulating manner.

Competencies

Competencies span cognitive, motivational, volitional, and social skills (Weinert, 2001). They are learnable and serve as the solutions to tasks in training, games, or situations in everyday life. This concept of competence also includes willpower or readiness to actively apply competencies in relevant situations.

Present findings of the prognostic importance of personality-related dispositions confirm the importance of individual characteristics (e.g., achievement motivation, motivational orientations, willpower, self-concept, self-efficacy, competitive anxiety) toward future athletic success (▶ Sect. 23.4.2). Despite these findings, the relative stability of these characteristics allows for the systematic development of the characteristics.

Personality dispositions are relatively stable while at the same time are also able to be influenced (Bandura, 1997). Competencies in handling such personality characteristics offer a possibility to constructively deal with their impacts at relatively short notice. They can also be used to develop intermediate- and long-term dispositions in the desired direction.

Someone's interaction with his or her environment leads to experiences that continuously influence on the nature of personality characteristics but also on the development of competencies for handling current states (e.g., coping, self-regulation). Therefore, interventions that foster competencies in the person-environment interaction seem to be another important facet of talent development (Ivarsson et al., 2015; Mayer & Hermann, 2014).

Regarding *achievement motivation*, in performance situations, it can be ascertained that the dimension *hope for success* constitutes a facilitative personality characteristic, while a high disposition toward *fear of failure* is often seen as dysfunctional (Gabler, 2004). These respective characteristics can be influenced by the help of various interventions in the appropriate direction (see also ▶ Chap. 6). These interventions (cf. Rheinberg & Engesser, 2010) draw on some of the following measures to build appropriate competencies:

- Strengthening of experiences of success or promotion of satisfaction following good performances
- Systematic confrontation between ideas of self-worth and simultaneously realistic information about one's own skills
- Training shifts in perceptual and cognitive focus to controllable performance factors (e.g., skills and freedom to act)
- Structural frameworks and external feedback to promote realistic goal setting
- Attribution training, (i.e., learning to attribute a proportion of successes and failures to factors in one's control)

An intervention to promote confidence in one's own skills and proficiencies in performance situations will be explained in more detail in the ▶ For Sports Practice: Fostering Self-Efficacy.

For Sports Practice

Fostering Self-Efficacy

Self-efficacy describes the confidence in one's own skills and proficiencies in a performance situation. Self-efficacy can be understood as general or specific (e.g., sport-specific). According to Bandura (1997), the nature of this characteristic stems from four sources:

- One's own experiences: mastery of challenges and experiences of success.
- Vicarious experiences: successes of appropriate role models.
- Verbal encouragement: effective attribution, positive feedback from relevant people in the environment.
- Emotional arousal: an individual can conclude their current self-efficacy through the level and interpretation of emotional arousal.

One's own experiences are the strongest source of self-efficacy, which can be developed through *prognostic training* (Feltz et al., 2008; Immenroth et al., 2008). This form of training facilitates athlete development through the implementation of training conditions similar to the competition and by analyzing their own goals as well as related expectations and consequences, even before the actual performance situation. For example, a typical sequence for a tennis player practicing her serve could look like the following:

1. *Task definition (by the coach):* 30 min to warm up; then the first 10 serves are served toward a reduced and appropriately marked zone.
2. *Objective (by the player or coach):* 8 out of 10 serves must land in the marked zone.
3. *Agreement on consequences:* Failure to achieve the objective results in an agreed-upon unpopular task (e.g., collecting all balls at the end of the session).
4. *Autonomous warm-up equivalent to real game warm-up.*
5. Punctual *start to the agreed-upon task.*
6. *Determination of the results* (number of accurate serves).
7. *Analysis* of factors leading to success and failure.
8. *Execution of agreed-upon consequences*, if required.

If the athlete is successful, direct effects of this type of training on self-efficacy are assumed. If the athlete is unsuccessful, an improvement in terms of future requirements can be achieved through appropriate action recommendations as well as inspecting one's own attitude. For the athlete, it is important to emphasize the agreement of consequences is not primarily about punishment, but rather about learning to handle the pressure.

Athletes should be able to independently regulate current psychological states or task-related dispositions (e.g., competitive anxiety, self-efficacy) in the short term. Relevant competencies are often correlated with various mental skills and one's own experience. Therefore, these competencies are positively influenced to an extent through the process introduced in ▶ Sect. 23.5.1. Furthermore, self-regulation competencies are particularly suitable (Mayer & Hermann, 2014) for:

- Production of task-related concentration (e.g., regulated self-talk)
- Building of self-efficacy (e.g., training to handle pressure situations)
- Regulation of activation (e.g., relaxation techniques) and emotions such as anxiety (e.g., development of emotional coping routines)

Recommendations for teaching such strategies in youth sport (e.g., Mayer & Hermann, 2014) distinguish three levels that build on each other and show clear parallels to the phases of development according to Bloom (1985) and Côté (1999) (cf. ◘ Fig. 23.1). In the *foundation* (entry) phase, the goal is primarily to elicit curiosity and understanding of individual sport psychology training techniques. The *building and performance stages* (development and performance phase) contain increasingly complex training activities that lead the athletes through performance and pressure situations and enable them to acquire appropriate strategies and proficiencies. As a result, the practice needs to be designed for the individual's requirements.

23.6 Conclusion and Further Discussion

Sport psychology talent research has been able to significantly enrich opinions about talent identification and development in sport over the last few years (Mann et al., 2017). This has been helped by conceptual principles associated with the broad and dynamic concept of talent (▶ Sect. 23.2), in addition to expertise and giftedness in sport (▶ Sect. 23.3). While empirical research findings underline the importance of psychological characteristics in talent identification (▶ Sect. 23.4), there is still a limited understanding of the influence of general psychology measures for talent development (▶ Sect. 23.5).

> The findings from sport psychology talent research highlight the need for strong integration between psychological testing procedures and intervention approaches in talent promotion (Beckmann et al., 2008).

It is therefore not surprising that those responsible for talent identification, such as individual federations (e.g., Swiss Olympic), have a growing interest in sport psychology talent research (Fuchslocher et al., 2016; Jonker et al., 2019) and incorporate psychological diagnostics in their talent identification and selection guidelines to determine factors such as achievement motivation or motivational goal orientation (▶ Study Box: Prognostic Relevance of Motivational Characteristics in ▶ Sect. 23.4.2). This increased importance of sport psychology talent factors is gratifying. However, it should also be accompanied by a sense of responsibility to clarify the practice and what science can and cannot accomplish.

23.6.1 Talent Identification

Cognitive factors, derived from expertise research (▶ Sect. 23.4.1), are of great importance in the selection of talents, especially within situational sports. However, the validity of testing procedures and the extent to which these diagnostics reliably predict the future success of young athletes are still relatively low (Bergkamp et al., 2019). Current objective testing methods are primarily investigated using cross-sectional laboratory studies, where the validity for prognoses and transfer into actual practice can only be inferred indirectly (cf. Murr et al., 2018a).

One significant merit of the approaches to giftedness research (▶ Sect. 23.3.1) is to show the importance of (non-cognitive, non-motor) psychological factors for talent development. Although through more cross-sectional rather than longitudinal studies, sport psychology talent researchers have presented important evidence of the prognostic relevance of dispositions and competencies (e.g., motivational and volitional) (▶ Sect. 23.4.2), and overall characteristics such as courage, resistance, or resilience (Mann et al., 2017). The findings have demonstrated the correlation between individual psychological talent characteristics in youth athletes with their future athletic performance.

> The importance of content and—to a certain extent—proven prognostic relevance of cognitive performance factors and specific psychological dispositions should not tempt us to overestimate the practical relevance of these characteristics for talent identification.

Even diagnostics that show acceptable effect sizes regarding prognostic relevance do not normally justify decisions in individual cases in the identification of talents (▶ Methods Box: The Problem of Insufficient Sensitivity in Talent Diagnostics in ▶ Sect. 23.4). Therefore, from a statistical perspective, sport psychology diagnostics for talent identification only makes sense as an (important) supplement to a coach's holistic, subjective judgment. This is true because athletes can compensate for weaknesses in one characteristic through exceptional strengths in another (compensation; Vaeyens et al., 2008). Furthermore, it is important to consider that most personality-related diagnostics are based on subjective self-assessment questionnaires and not objective performance tests. Therefore, socially desirable response tendencies can be expected, especially in the context of talent advancement where youth athletes wish to present themselves in a particularly positive light (e.g., regarding their achievement motivation) (Feichtinger & Höner, 2014). Applying diagnostics of personality dispositions in the identification of talent could strengthen such tendencies, and diagnostics that use self-assessment questionnaires could thereby lose their value.

23.6.2 Talent Development

Concerning the development of talent, the empirical foundation of sport psychology measures, which promote characteristics such as cognitive performance factors or specific psychological dispositions (▶ Sect.

23.5.2.2), is simpler than measures directed toward general expertise (▶ Sect. 23.3.2) or personality development (▶ Sect. 23.5.2.1). Nevertheless, there is a consensus in practice and science that both approaches should be supported by sport psychology measures.

> The development of cognitive factors as well as specific psychological dispositions of youth athletes should be founded on the application of sport psychology diagnostics.

Prognostic valid diagnostics are needed to ensure a tailored program for talent support. This includes standardized reference values in order to identify strengths and weaknesses, as well as to perform interventions that fit a player's profile of relevant characteristics (Beckmann et al., 2008). The prognostic relevance of such diagnostics could be proven at least somewhat (▶ Sect. 23.4), and sport-specific questionnaire diagnostics with standard values now exist (▶ Study Box: Sport-Specific Diagnostics in ▶ Sect. 23.2). However, it should be noted that most of these measures are only available in one specific language.

Researchers have started to develop some promising measures of cognitive factors of decision-making (▶ Sect. 23.5.1) and psychological dispositions or competencies (▶ Sect. 23.5.2) to promote the development of psychological talent factors. Such measures should be regularly implemented and accompanied by process diagnostics to ensure their sustainability. Furthermore, research is required to assess the effects of psychological factors (▶ Methods Box: Effects of Psychological Characteristics on Performance in Sport in ▶ Sect. 23.3.1.1) to establish and apply sport psychology measures of talent development.

Concerning the general development of expertise in sport, *Deliberate Practice* and its resulting conditions (e.g., motivation, willpower, and available resources) are an imperative requirement for improvement in performance (Ford et al., 2015). Regardless of this, features of *Deliberate Play* such as intrinsic motivation (◘ Table 23.1) are also important elements for the entire phase of talent development and serve as the foundation for a sustainable performance-oriented athletic career. Overall, whether *Deliberate Practice* or *Deliberate Play* is more important for the development of athletes remains unclear (Côté & Fraser-Thomas, 2008). Further, the question, in which development phase youth talents should concentrate on their primary sport, is also difficult to determine from the current retrospective studies, as various development phases and positive circumstances may differ greatly from sport to sport. For a deeper understanding of sport psychology—along with more precise analyses of the training content which exceeds the simplicity of the breadth of training ("10,000-hour rule")—experimental and longitudinal studies that explore the effects of changes to development and environmental factors are required (Baker & Young, 2014). The implementation of these studies into practice poses a very large or even insurmountable, challenge, and, therefore, current recommendations for optimal development should emphasize a balance between *Deliberate Play* and *Deliberate Practice*, especially in the early development phase (Ford et al., 2009). Accordingly, concerning the acquisition of expertise in sport, "many roads lead to Rome: (Güllich, 2014, p. 770).

> Despite the lack of scientific evidence of sport psychology measures, no doubt should exist over the importance of talents' *holistic personality development* in sport—if only because of the responsibility to youth athletes.

This is based on the fact that most youth athletes in talent development programs will not make it to the highest levels of sport. Thus, personality development—which is also important in the world outside sport—is one of the core tasks of a youth development program (Abbott & Collins, 2004). Furthermore, it is evident that generally successful adolescent development influences a person's long-term stability and endurance and is thus also relevant for mental health as well as in high-performance sport.

As the development of a personality results from the interaction between a person and his or her environment, people in the immediate vicinity of talented athletes should be aware of their possible influence and be involved accordingly. It is important to create a framework that reinforces helpful personality traits and active engagement with the environment, for example, by encouraging talents to reflect on their own behavior in as many everyday situations as possible and by paying particular attention to the challenges that arise from dual careers in sport and school (Henriksen & Stambulova, 2017; Mayer & Hermann, 2014). This can be realized within the framework of long-term sport psychology support that considers a talent's stage of psychosocial development and concentrates on relevant developmental tasks.

Learning Control Questions

Basic:

1. What are the most important differences between the prospective and retrospective approaches to talent research?

2. The modern concept of "talent" is broad, dynamic, and area-specific. What do these terms mean in the context of talent identification and development?

Advanced:

3. Different types of models can be used in sport psychology talent research. Discuss their main differences. Include examples.
4. Decision-making is based on several perceptual-cognitive skills. List these skills with a definition and example.
5. How are personality-related characteristics relevant to the development of athletic talents?

Experts:

6. Outline the *Deliberate Practice* and *Deliberate Play* theories, and discuss how both are important for talent development?
7. How can youth coaches develop perceptual-cognitive skills without the physical demands of on-field training? Include examples.
8. What opportunities and approaches should those responsible for the personality development of talents promote?

References

Abbott, A., & Collins, D. (2004). Eliminating the dichotomy between theory and practice in talent identification and development: Considering the role of psychology. *Journal of Sports Sciences, 22*(5), 395–408. https://doi.org/10.1080/02640410410001675324

Abernethy, B., Baker, J., & Côté, J. (2005). Transfer of pattern recall skills may contribute to the development of sport expertise. *Applied Cognitive Psychology, 19*, 705–718. https://doi.org/10.1002/acp.1102

Abernethy, B., Schorer, J., Jackson, R. C., & Hagemann, N. (2012). Perceptual training methods compared: The relative efficacy of different approaches to enhancing sport-specific anticipation. *Journal of Experimental Psychology: Applied, 18*(2), 143–153. https://doi.org/10.1037/a0028452

Abernethy, B., Wood, J. M., & Parks, S. (1999). Can the anticipatory skills of experts be learned by novices? *Research Quarterly for Exercise and Sport, 70*(3), 313–318. https://doi.org/10.1080/02701367.1999.10608050

Allen, M. S., Greenlees, I., & Jones, M. (2013). Personality in sport: A comprehensive review. *International Review of Sport and Exercise Psychology, 6*(1), 184–208. https://doi.org/10.1080/1750984X.2013.769614

Amorose, A. J., & Anderson-Butcher, D. (2007). Autonomy-supportive coaching and self-determined motivation in high school and college athletes: A test of self-determination theory. *Psychology of Sport and Exercise, 8*(5), 654–670. https://doi.org/10.1016/j.psychsport.2006.11.003

Baker, J., & Horton, S. (2004). A review of primary and secondary influences on sport expertise. *High Ability Studies, 15*(2), 211–228. https://doi.org/10.1080/1359813042000314781

Baker, J., & Young, B. (2014). 20 years later: Deliberate practice and the development of expertise in sport. *International Review of Sport and Exercise Psychology, 7*(1), 135–157. https://doi.org/10.1080/1750984X.2014.896024

Bandura, A. (1997). *Self-efficacy: The exercise of control*. W H Freeman/Times Books/Henry Holt.

Beckmann, J., Elbe, A.-M., & Seidel, I. (2008). Talent und Talententwicklung [talent and talent development]. In J. Beckmann & M. Kellmann (Eds.), *Enzyklopädie der Psychologie, Sportpsychologie (Bd. 2): Anwendungen der Sportpsychologie [Encyclopedia of psychology, sport psychology (Vol. 2): Applications of sport psychology]* (pp. 257–309). Hogrefe.

Bergkamp, T. L., Niessen, A. S. M., Den Hartigh, R. J., Frencken, W. G., & Meijer, R. R. (2019). Methodological issues in soccer talent identification research. *Sports Medicine, 49*(9), 1317–1335. https://doi.org/10.1007/s40279-019-01113-w

Berry, J., Abernethy, B., & Côté, J. (2008). The contribution of structured activity and deliberate play to the development of expert perceptual and decision-making skill. *Journal of Sport and Exercise Psychology, 30*(6), 685–708. https://doi.org/10.1123/jsep.30.6.685

Bloom, B. S. (Ed.). (1985). *Developing talent in young people*. Ballantine Books.

Borggrefe, C., & Cachay, K. (2012). "Dual careers": The structural coupling of elite sport and school exemplified by the German Verbundsysteme. *European Journal of Sport and Society, 9*(1–2), 57–80. https://doi.org/10.1080/16138171.2012.11687889

Brettschneider, W.-D. (1999). Risks and opportunities: Adolescents in top-level sport—Growing up with the pressures of school and training. *European Physical Education Review, 5*(2), 121–133.

Bunker, D., & Thorpe, R. (1982). A model for the teaching of games in secondary schools. *Bulletin of Physical Education, 18*(1), 5–8.

Butler, J. I. (2005). TGfU pet-agogy: Old dogs, new tricks and puppy school. *Physical Education and Sport Pedagogy, 10*(3), 225–240. https://doi.org/10.1080/17408980500340752

Cañal-Bruland, R., Hagemann, N., & Strauß, B. (2007). Videobasierte Wahrnehmungstrainings-praktischer Nutzen für Sportler und Schiedsrichter [video-based perception training—Practical benefits for athletes and referees]. *Spectrum der Sportwissenschaften [Spectrum of Sports Science], 19*(1), 51–64.

Cañal-Bruland, R., & Williams, A. M. (2010). Recognizing and predicting movement effects: Identifying critical movement features. *Experimental Psychology, 57*(4), 320–326. https://doi.org/10.1027/1618-3169/a000038

Cartigny, E., Fletcher, D., Coupland, C., & Taylor, G. (2019). Mind the gap: A grounded theory of dual career pathways in sport. *Journal of Applied Sport Psychology, 33*, 280–301. https://doi.org/10.1080/10413200.2019.1654559

Cattell, R. B. (1966). *The scientific analysis of personality* (2nd ed.). Aldine Press.

Cervelló, E., Santos Rosa, F. J., Calvo, T. G., Jiménez, R., & Iglesias, D. (2007). Young tennis players' competitive task involvement and performance: The role of goal orientations, contextual motivational climate, and coach-initiated motivational climate. *Journal of Applied Sport Psychology, 19*(3), 304–321. https://doi.org/10.1080/10413200701329134

Chambers, K. L., & Vickers, J. N. (2006). Effects of bandwidth feedback and questioning on the performance of competitive swimmers. *The Sport Psychologist, 20*(2), 184–197. https://doi.org/10.1123/tsp.20.2.184

Chase, W. G., & Simon, H. A. (1973). The mind's eye in chess. In W. G. Chase (Ed.), *Visual information processing* (pp. 215–281). Academic Press.

Christensen, M. K., & Sørensen, J. K. (2009). Sport or school? Dreams and dilemmas for talented young Danish football players. *European Physical Education Review, 15*(1), 115–133. https://doi.org/10.1177/1356336X09105214

Cobley, S., Schorer, J., & Baker, J. (2012). Identification and development of sport talent: A brief introduction to a growing field of research and practice. In J. Baker, S. Cobley, & J. Schorer (Eds.),

Talent identification and development in sport-international perspectives (pp. 1–10). Routledge/Chapman & Hall.

Coelho e Silva, M., Figueiredo, A., Simões, F., Seabra, A., Natal, A., Vaeyens, R., et al. (2010). Discrimination of U-14 soccer players by level and position. *International Journal of Sports Medicine, 31*(11), 790–796. https://doi.org/10.1055/s-0030-1263139

Conzelmann, A. (2009). Differentielle Sportpsychologie—Sport und Persönlichkeit [differential sport psychology—Sport and personality]. In W. Schlicht & B. Strauß (Eds.), *Grundlagen der Sportpsychologie [Basics of sport psychology]* (pp. 375–439). Hogrefe.

Conzelmann, A., Zibung, M., & Zuber, C. (2016). Das Ganze ist mehr als die Summe seiner Teile—ein Plädoyer für eine personorientierte Talentdiskussion [The whole is more than the sum of it's parts—A plea for a person-oriented talent discussion]. In *3. DFB-Wissenschafts-Kongress 2016 [3rd DFB science congress 2016]* (pp. 48–50). Deutscher Fussball-Bund.

Côté, J. (1999). The influence of the family in the development of talent in sport. *The Sport Psychologist, 13*(4), 395–417. https://doi.org/10.1123/tsp.13.4.395

Côté, J., Baker, J., & Abernethy, B. (2003). From play to practice: A developmental framework for the acquisition of expertise in team sport. In J. Starkes & K. A. Ericsson (Eds.), *The development of elite athletes: Recent advances in research on sport expertise* (pp. 89–113). Human Kinetics.

Côté, J., Baker, J., & Abernethy, B. (2007). Play and practice in the development of sport expertise. In G. Tenenbaum & R. C. Eklund (Eds.), *Handbook of sport psychology* (3rd ed., pp. 184–202). Wiley.

Côté, J., & Fraser-Thomas, J. (2008). Play, practice, and athlete development. In D. Farrow, J. Baker, & C. MacMahon (Eds.), *Developing elite sport performance: Lessons from theory and practice* (pp. 17–28). Routledge.

Côté, J., Strachan, L., & Fraser-Thomas, J. (2008). Participation, personal development and performance through youth sport. In N. Holt (Ed.), *Positive youth development through sport* (pp. 34–45). Routledge.

Coyle, D. (2009). *The talent code: Greatness isn't born. It's grown. Here's how*. New York.

Crognier, L., & Féry, Y. A. (2005). Effect of tactical initiative on predicting passing shots in tennis. *Applied Cognitive Psychology, 19*(5), 637–649. https://doi.org/10.1002/acp.1100

Crowe, S. F. (1998). The differential contribution of mental tracking, cognitive flexibility, visual search, and motor speed to performance on parts A and B of the trail making test. *Journal of Clinical Psychology, 54*(5), 585–591. https://doi.org/10.1002/(SICI)1097-4679(199808)54:5<585::AID-JCLP4>3.0.CO;2-K

Davids, K., Araújo, D., Correia, V., & Vilar, L. (2013). How small-sided and conditioned games enhance acquisition of movement and decision-making skills. *Exercise and Sport Sciences Reviews, 41*(3), 154–161. https://doi.org/10.1097/JES.0b013e318292f3ec

Davids, K., Araújo, D., Hristovski, R., Passos, P., & Chow, J. Y. (2012). Ecological dynamics and motor learning design in sport. In A. M. Williams & N. Hodges (Eds.), *Skill acquisition in sport: Research, theory & practice* (pp. 112–130). Routledge.

Deci, E. L., & Ryan, R. M. (1985). *Intrinsic motivation and self-determination in human behaviour*. Plenum.

Diamond, A. (2013). Executive functions. *Annual Review of Psychology, 64*, 135–168. https://doi.org/10.1146/annurev-psych-113011-143750

Diamond, A., & Ling, D. S. (2016). Conclusions about interventions, programs, and approaches for improving executive functions that appear justified and those that, despite much hype, do not. *Developmental Cognitive Neuroscience, 18*, 34–48. https://doi.org/10.1016/j.dcn.2015.11.005

Dreher, E., & Oerter, R. (1986). Children's and adolescents' conceptions of adulthood: The changing view of a crucial developmental task. In R. K. Silbereisen, K. Eyferth, & G. Rudinger (Eds.), *Development as action in context* (pp. 109–120). Springer.

Durand-Bush, N., & Salmela, J. H. (2001). The development of talent in sport. In R. N. Singer, H. A. Hausenblas, & C. Janelle (Eds.), *Handbook of sport psychology* (2nd ed., pp. 269–289). Wiley.

Elbe, A.-M., Beckmann, J., & Szymanski, B. (2003). Entwicklung der allgemeinen und sportspezifischen Leistungsmotivation von Sportschüler/–innen [development of the general and sport-specific achievement motivation in young elite athletes]. *Psychologie und Sport, 10*(4), 134–143.

Elbe, A.-M., Szymanski, B., & Beckmann, J. (2005). The development of volition in young elite athletes. *Psychology of Sport and Exercise, 6*(5), 559–569. https://doi.org/10.1016/j.psychsport.2004.07.004

Elferink-Gemser, M. T., De Roos, I., Torenbeek, M., Fokkema, T., Jonker, L., & Visscher, C. (2015). The importance of psychological constructs for training volume and performance improvement. A structural equation model for youth speed skaters. *International Journal of Sport Psychology, 46*(6), 726–744.

Ericsson, K. A. (1996). The acquisition of expert performance: An introduction to some of the issues. In K. A. Ericsson (Ed.), *The road to excellence: The acquisition of expert performance in the arts and sciences, sports, and games* (pp. 1–50). Lawrence Erlbaum.

Ericsson, K. A., & Crutcher, R. J. (1990). The nature of exceptional performance. In P. B. Baltes, D. L. Featherman, & R. M. Lerner (Eds.), *Life-span development and behavior* (Vol. 10, pp. 187–217). Lawrence Erlbaum.

Ericsson, K. A., Krampe, R. T., & Tesch-Römer, C. (1993). The role of deliberate practice in the acquisition of expert performance. *Psychological Review, 100*(3), 363–406. https://doi.org/10.1037/0033-295X.100.3.363

Ericsson, K. A., Nandagopal, K., & Roring, R. W. (2009). Toward a science of exceptional achievement. *Annals of the New York Academy of Sciences, 1172*(1), 199–217. https://doi.org/10.1196/annals.1393.001

Eysenck, H. J., & Eysenck, S. B. G. (1975). *Manual of the Eysenck personality questionnaire*. Hodder & Stoughton.

Fagereng, K. (2010). *A real game examination of visual perception in soccer: Testing the relationship between exploration frequency and performance in young and talented players* [Unpublished Master's thesis]. Norwegian School of Sport Sciences, Oslo.

Farrow, D., & Abernethy, B. (2002). Can anticipatory skills be learned through implicit video based perceptual training? *Journal of Sports Sciences, 20*(6), 471–485. https://doi.org/10.1080/02640410252925143

Farrow, D., & Abernethy, B. (2007). Wahrnehmung von Expertinnen und Experten im Sport: Einige Kernfragen und -probleme [Perception of experts in sport: Some key questions and problems]. In N. Hagemann, M. Tietjens, & B. Strauß (Eds.), *Psychologie der sportlichen Höchstleistung [Psychology of sporting peak performance]* (pp. 71–92). Hogrefe.

Farrow, D., McCrae, J., Gross, J., & Abernethy, B. (2010). Revisiting the relationship between pattern recall and anticipatory skill. *International Journal of Sport Psychology, 41*, 91–106.

Feichtinger, P., & Höner, O. (2014). Psychological diagnostics in the talent development program of the German football association: Psychometric properties of an internet-based test battery. *Sportwissenschaft [Sports Science], 44*, 203–213. https://doi.org/10.1007/s12662-014-0341-0

Feichtinger, P., & Höner, O. (2015). Talented football players' development of achievement motives, volitional components, and self-referential cognitions: A longitudinal study. *European*

Journal of Sport Science, 15(8), 748–756. https://doi.org/10.1080/17461391.2015.1051134
Feltz, D. L., Short, S. E., & Sullivan, P. J. (2008). *Self-efficacy in sport*. Human Kinetics.
Figueiredo, A. J., Gonçalves, C. E., Coelho e Silva, M. J., & Malina, R. M. (2009). Characteristics of youth soccer players who drop out, persist or move up. *Journal of Sports Sciences, 27*(9), 883–891. https://doi.org/10.1080/02640410902946469
Ford, P. R., Bordonau, J. L. D., Bonanno, D., Tavares, J., Groenendijk, C., Fink, C., et al. (2020). A survey of talent identification and development processes in the youth academies of professional soccer clubs from around the world. *Journal of Sports Sciences, 38*, 1269–1278. https://doi.org/10.1080/02640414.2020.1752440
Ford, P. R., Coughlan, E., Hodges, N., & Williams, A. M. (2015). Deliberate practice in sport. In J. Baker & D. Farrow (Eds.), *The Routledge handbook of sport expertise* (pp. 347–362). Routledge.
Ford, P. R., Ward, P., Hodges, N. J., & Williams, A. M. (2009). The role of deliberate practice and play in career progression in sport: The early engagement hypothesis. *High Ability Studies, 20*(1), 65–75. https://doi.org/10.1080/13598130902860721
Ford, P. R., & Williams, A. M. (2012). The developmental activities engaged in by elite youth soccer players who progressed to professional status compared to those who did not. *Psychology of Sport and Exercise, 13*(3), 349–352. https://doi.org/10.1016/j.psychsport.2011.09.004
Forsman, H., Gråstén, A., Blomqvist, M., Davids, K., Liukkonen, J., & Konttinen, N. (2016). Development and validation of the perceived game-specific soccer competence scale. *Journal of Sports Sciences, 34*(14), 1319–1327. https://doi.org/10.1080/02640414.2015.1125518
Fuchslocher, J., Romann, M., Birrer, D., Baer, C., Müller, L., Pürro, D., et al. (2016). *Manual Talentidentifikation und -selektion [Manual of talent identification and selection]*. Swiss Olympic.
Gabler, H. (2000). Motivationale Aspekte sportlicher Handlungen [Motivational aspects of sporting activities]. In H. Gabler, R. Nitsch, & R. Singer (Eds.), *Einführung in die Sportpsychologie, Teil I: Grundthemen [introduction to sport psychology, part I: Basic topics]* (Vol. 3, pp. 197–246). Hofmann.
Gabler, H. (2004). Motivationale Aspekte sportlicher Handlungen [motivational aspects of sporting activities]. In H. Gabler, J. R. Nitsch, R. Singer, & J. Munzert (Eds.), *Einführung in die Sportpsychologie, Teil I: Grundthemen [introduction to sport psychology, part I: Basic topics]* (pp. 197–245). Hofmann.
Gagné, F. (2000). Understanding the complex choreography of talent development through DMGT-based analysis. In K. A. Heller, F. J. Mönks, R. J. Sternberg, & R. F. Subotnik (Eds.), *International handbook of giftedness and talent* (2nd ed., pp. 67–79). Pergamon Press.
Gagné, F. (2010). Motivation within the DMGT 2.0 framework. *High Ability Studies, 21*(2), 81–99. https://doi.org/10.1080/13598139.2010.525341
Garland, D. J., & Barry, J. R. (1991). Cognitive advantage in sport: The nature of perceptual structures. *The American Journal of Psychology, 104*(2), 211–228. https://doi.org/10.2307/1423155
Gerber, M. (2011). Mentale toughness im sport [Mental toughness in sport]. *Sportwissenschaft [Sports Science], 41*(4), 283–299. https://doi.org/10.1007/s12662-011-0202-z
Gorman, A. D., & Farrow, D. (2009). Perceptual training using explicit and implicit instructional techniques: Does it benefit skilled performers? *International Journal of Sports Science and Coaching, 4*(2), 193–208. https://doi.org/10.1260/174795409788549526
Gould, D., Dieffenbach, K., & Moffett, A. (2002). Psychological characteristics and their development in Olympic champions. *Journal of Applied Sport Psychology, 14*(3), 172–204. https://doi.org/10.1080/10413200290103482
Gréhaigne, J.-F., Godbout, P., & Bouthier, D. (2001). The teaching and learning of decision making in team sports. *Quest, 53*(1), 59–76. https://doi.org/10.1080/00336297.2001.10491730
Güllich, A. (2013). Talente im Sport [Talents in sport]. In A. Güllich & M. Krüger (Eds.), *Sport: Das Lehrbuch für das Sportstudium [Sport: The textbook for the study of sport]* (Vol. 1, pp. 623–653). Springer Spektrum.
Güllich, A. (2014). Many roads lead to Rome—Developmental paths to Olympic gold in men's field hockey. *European Journal of Sport Science, 14*(8), 763–771. https://doi.org/10.1080/17461391.2014.905983
Hadlow, S. M., Panchuk, D., Mann, D. L., Portus, M. R., & Abernethy, B. (2018). Modified perceptual training in sport: A new classification framework. *Journal of Science and Medicine in Sport, 21*(9), 950–958. https://doi.org/10.1016/j.jsams.2018.01.011
Hagemann, N., Strauss, B., & Cañal-Bruland, R. (2006). Training perceptual skill by orienting visual attention. *Journal of Sport and Exercise Psychology, 28*(2), 143–158. https://doi.org/10.1123/jsep.28.2.143
Halouani, J., Chtourou, H., Gabbett, T., Chaouachi, A., & Chamari, K. (2014). Small-sided games in team sports training: A brief review. *The Journal of Strength & Conditioning Research, 28*(12), 3594–3618. https://doi.org/10.1519/JSC.0000000000000564
Harvey, S., Cushion, C. J., & Massa-Gonzalez, A. N. (2010). Learning a new method: Teaching games for understanding in the coaches' eyes. *Physical Education and Sport Pedagogy, 15*(4), 361–382. https://doi.org/10.1080/17408980903535818
Harwood, C. G., & Knight, C. J. (2015). Parenting in youth sport: A position paper on parenting expertise. *Psychology of Sport and Exercise, 16*(1), 24–35. https://doi.org/10.1016/j.psychsport.2014.03.001
Haugaasen, M., Toering, T., & Jordet, G. (2014). From childhood to senior professional football: A multi-level approach to elite youth football players' engagement in football-specific activities. *Psychology of Sport and Exercise, 15*(4), 336–344. https://doi.org/10.1016/j.psychsport.2014.02.007
Havighurst, R. J. (1956). Research on the developmental-task concept. *The School Review, 64*(5), 215–223. https://doi.org/10.1086/442319
Heller, K. A. (2002). Theoretische Ansätze und empirische Befunde zur Hochbegabungs- und Expertiseforschung unter besonderer Berücksichtigung sportlicher Talente [Theoretical approaches and empirical finding on the research of giftedness and expertise with special regard to sporting talent]. In A. Hohmann, D. Wick, & K. Carl (Eds.), *Talent im Sport [Talent in sports]* (pp. 52–66). Hofmann.
Heller, K. A., & Perleth, C. (2008). The Munich high ability test battery (MHBT): A multidimensional, multimethod approach. *Psychology Science Quarterly, 50*(2), 173–188.
Helsen, W. F., & Starkes, J. L. (1999). A multidimensional approach to skilled perception and performance in sport. *Applied Cognitive Psychology, 13*(1), 1–27. https://doi.org/10.1002/(SICI)1099--0720(199902)13:1<1::AID-ACP540>3.0.CO;2-T
Helsen, W. F., Starkes, J. L., & Hodges, N. J. (1998). Team sports and the theory of deliberate practice. *Journal of Sport and Exercise Psychology, 20*(1), 12–34. https://doi.org/10.1123/jsep.20.1.12
Henriksen, K., & Stambulova, N. (2017). Creating optimal environments for talent development: A holistic ecological approach. In J. Baker, S. Cobley, J. Schorer, & N. Wattie (Eds.), *Routledge handbook of talent identification and development in sport*. Routledge.
Hohmann, A. (2009). *Entwicklung sportlicher Talente an sportbetonten Schulen: Schwimmen, Leichtathletik, handball [Development of sports talents at elite sport schools: Swimming, track and field, handball]*. Imhof.

Hollembeak, J., & Amorose, A. J. (2005). Perceived coaching behaviors and college athletes' intrinsic motivation: A test of self-determination theory. *Journal of Applied Sport Psychology, 17*(1), 20–36. https://doi.org/10.1080/10413200590907540

Holt, N. L., & Mitchell, T. (2006). Talent development in English professional soccer. *International Journal of Sport Psychology, 37*(2), 77–98.

Höner, O. (2005). *Entscheidungshandeln im Sportspiel Fußball: Eine analyse im Lichte der Rubikontheorie [Decision-making in the sports game of football: An analysis in the light of the Rubicon theory]*. Hofmann.

Höner, O. (2012). Entscheidungshandeln im Fußball: Eine sportpsychologische Betrachtung [Decision-making in football: A sport psychological view]. In B. D. Fußball-Lehrer (Ed.), *Neue Trends bei der Euro 2012: Entscheidungskompetenz in Abwehr und Angriff (Internationaler trainer-Kongress 2012) [New Trends at the EURO 2012: Decision-making competence in defense and attack (International Trainer Congress 2012)]* (pp. 16–23). Dinges & Frick.

Höner, O., & Feichtinger, P. (2016). Psychological talent predictors in early adolescence and their empirical relationship with current and future performance in soccer. *Psychology of Sport and Exercise, 25*, 17–26. https://doi.org/10.1016/j.psychsport.2016.03.004

Höner, O., & Votteler, A. (2016). Prognostic relevance of motor talent predictors in early adolescence: A group-and individual-based evaluation considering different levels of achievement in youth football. *Journal of Sports Sciences, 34*(24), 2269–2278. https://doi.org/10.1080/02640414.2016.1177658

Hopwood, M. J., Mann, D. L., Farrow, D., & Nielsen, T. (2011). Does visual-perceptual training augment the fielding performance of skilled cricketers? *International Journal of Sports Science and Coaching, 6*(4), 523–535. https://doi.org/10.1260/1747-9541.6.4.523

Huijgen, B. C. H., Elferink-Gemser, M. T., Lemmink, K. A. P. M., & Visscher, C. (2014). Multidimensional performance characteristics in selected and deselected talented soccer players. *European Journal of Sport Science, 14*(1), 2–10. https://doi.org/10.1080/17461391.2012.725102

Huijgen, B. C. H., Leemhuis, S., Kok, N. M., Verburgh, L., Oosterlaan, J., Elferink-Gemser, M. T., & Visscher, C. (2015). Cognitive functions in elite and sub-elite youth soccer players aged 13 to 17 years. *PLoS One, 10*(12), e0144580. https://doi.org/10.1371/journal.pone.0144580

Huys, R., Smeeton, N. J., Hodges, N. J., Beek, P. J., & Williams, A. M. (2008). On the dynamical information underlying visual anticipation skill. *Perception & Psychophysics, 70*, 1217–1234. https://doi.org/10.3758/PP.70.7.1217

Immenroth, M., Eberspächer, H., & Hermann, H.-D. (2008). Training kognitiver Fertigkeiten [Cognitive skills training]. In J. Beckmann & M. Kellmann (Eds.), *Enzyklopädie der Psychologie, Sportpsychologie (Bd. 2): Anwendungungen der Sportpsychologie [encyclopedia of psychology, sport psychology (Vol. 2): Applications of sport psychology]* (pp. 119–176). Hogrefe.

Ivarsson, A., Stenling, A., Fallby, J., Johnson, U., Borg, E., & Johansson, G. (2015). The predictive ability of the talent development environment on youth elite football players' well-being: A person-centered approach. *Psychology of Sport and Exercise, 16*(1), 15–23. https://doi.org/10.1016/j.psychsport.2014.09.006

Janelle, C. M., & Hillman, C. H. (2003). Expert performance in sport: Current perspectives and critical issues. In J. L. Starkes & K. A. Ericsson (Eds.), *Expert performance in sports: Advances in research on sport expertise* (pp. 19–49). Human Kinetics.

Johnson, J. G. (2006). Cognitive modeling of decision making in sports. *Psychology of Sport and Exercise, 7*(6), 631–652. https://doi.org/10.1016/j.psychsport.2006.03.009

Jones, G., & Swain, A. (1995). Predispositions to experience debilitative and facilitative anxiety in elite and nonelite performers. *The Sport Psychologist, 9*(2), 201–211. https://doi.org/10.1123/tsp.9.2.201

Jonker, L., Elferink-Gemser, M. T., & Visscher, C. (2010). Differences in self-regulatory skills among talented athletes: The significance of competitive level and type of sport. *Journal of Sports Sciences, 28*(8), 901–908. https://doi.org/10.1080/02640411003797157

Jonker, L., Huijgen, B. C. H., Heuvingh, B., Elferink-Gemser, M. T., & Visscher, C. (2019). How youth football players learn to succeed. In E. Konter, J. Beckmann, & T. M. Loughead (Eds.), *Football psychology: From theory to practice* (pp. 297–311). Routledge.

Jordet, G. (2005). Perceptual training in soccer: An imagery intervention study with elite players. *Journal of Applied Sport Psychology, 17*(2), 140–156. https://doi.org/10.1080/10413200590932452

Jordet, G., & Bloomfield, J. (2009). *Visual exploration in premier league footballers*. Norwegian School of Sport Sciences/University of Groningen.

Kannekens, R., Elferink-Gemser, M., & Visscher, C. (2011). Positioning and deciding: Key factors for talent development in soccer. *Scandinavian Journal of Medicine & Science in Sports, 21*(6), 846–852. https://doi.org/10.1111/j.1600-0838.2010.01104.x

Kidman, L. (2010). *Athlete-centred coaching: Developing decision makers* (2nd ed.). IPC.

Kidman, L., & Lombardo, B. (2010). *Athlete-centred coaching: Developing decision makers*. IPC.

Klauer, K. J., & Leutner, D. (2007). *Lehren und Lernen [Teaching and learning]*. Beltz.

Koopmann, T., Faber, I., Baker, J., & Schorer, J. (2020). Assessing technical skills in talented youth athletes: A systematic review. *Sports Medicine, 50*(9), 1593–1611. https://doi.org/10.1007/s40279-020-01299-4

Larkin, P., Mesagno, C., Berry, J., & Spittle, M. (2014). Development of a valid and reliable video-based decision-making test for Australian football umpires. *Journal of Science and Medicine in Sport, 17*(5), 552–555. https://doi.org/10.1016/j.jsams.2013.08.001

Larkin, P., Mesagno, C., Spittle, M., & Berry, J. (2015). An evaluation of video-based training programs for perceptual-cognitive skill development. A systematic review of current sport-based knowledge. *International Journal of Sport Psychology, 46*(6), 555–586.

Larkin, P., O'Connor, D., & Williams, A. M. (2016). Does grit influence sport-specific engagement and perceptual-cognitive expertise in elite youth soccer? *Journal of Applied Sport Psychology, 28*(2), 129–138. https://doi.org/10.1080/10413200.2015.1085922

Li, C., Wang, C. J., & Pyun, D. Y. (2014). Talent development environmental factors in sport: A review and taxonomic classification. *Quest, 66*(4), 433–447. https://doi.org/10.1080/00336297.2014.944715

Lidor, R., Côté, J., & Hackfort, D. (2009). ISSP position stand: To test or not to test? The use of physical skill tests in talent detection and in early phases of sport development. *International Journal of Sport and Exercise Psychology, 7*(2), 131–146. https://doi.org/10.1080/1612197X.2009.9671896

Lottermann, S., Laudenklos, P., & Friedrich, A. (2003). Techniktraining—Mehr als reine Ballarbeit [Practising technique—More than just ball work]. *Fussballtraining [Soccer Training], 21*(4), 6–15.

Macnamara, A., & Collins, D. (2013). Do mental skills make champions? Examining the discriminant function of the psychological characteristics of developing excellence questionnaire. *Journal of Sports Sciences, 31*(7), 736–744. https://doi.org/10.1080/02640414.2012.747692

Macnamara, B. N., Moreau, D., & Hambrick, D. Z. (2016). The relationship between deliberate practice and performance in sports: A meta-analysis. *Perspectives on Psychological Science, 11*(3), 333–350. https://doi.org/10.1177/1745691616635591

Magnusson, D. (1990). Personality development from an interactional perspective. In L. A. Pervin (Ed.), *Handbook of personality: Theory and research* (pp. 193–222). Guilford.

Magnusson, D., & Stattin, H. (1998). Person-context interaction theories. In R. M. Lerner (Ed.), *Handbook of childpsychology* (Theoretical models of human development) (Vol. 1, 5th ed., pp. 685–759). Wiley.

Mann, D. L., Dehghansai, N., & Baker, J. (2017). Searching for the elusive gift: Advances in talent identification in sport. *Current Opinion in Psychology, 16*, 128–133. https://doi.org/10.1016/j.copsyc.2017.04.016

Martens, R., Burton, D., Vealey, R. S., Bump, L. A., & Smith, D. E. (1990). Development and validation of the competitive state anxiety inventory. In R. Martens, R. S. Vealey, & D. Burton (Eds.), *Competitive anxiety in sport* (pp. 117–190). Human Kinetics.

Mayer, J., & Hermann, H.-D. (2014). *Sportpsychologie im Nachwuchsfußball. Mentale Fertigkeiten entwickeln und trainieren [Sport psychology in elite youth football. Developing and training mental skills]*. Philippka.

McCormick, C. M., Kuo, S. I.-C., & Masten, A. S. (2011). Developmental tasks across the life span. In K. L. Fingerman, C. A. Berg, J. Smith, & T. C. Antonucci (Eds.), *Handbook of life-span development* (pp. 117–139). Springer Publishing Company.

McCrae, R. R., & Costa, P. T. (2008). The five-factor theory of personality. In O. P. John, R. W. Robins, & L. A. Pervin (Eds.), *Handbook of personality: Theory and research* (3rd ed., pp. 159–181). Guilford.

McCrae, R. R., & John, O. P. (1992). An introduction to the five-factor model and its applications. *Journal of Personality, 60*(2), 175–215. https://doi.org/10.1111/j.1467-6494.1992.tb00970.x

McCrory, P., Collie, A., Anderson, V., & Davis, G. (2004). Can we manage sport related concussion in children the same as in adults? *British Journal of Sports Medicine, 38*(5), 516–519. https://doi.org/10.1136/bjsm.2004.014811

McNeill, M. C., Fry, J. M., Wright, S. C., Tan, C. W., & Rossi, T. (2008). Structuring time and questioning to achieve tactical awareness in games lessons. *Physical Education and Sport Pedagogy, 13*(3), 231–249. https://doi.org/10.1080/17408980701345766

Mills, A., Butt, J., Maynard, I., & Harwood, C. (2012). Identifying factors perceived to influence the development of elite youth football academy players. *Journal of Sports Sciences, 30*(15), 1593–1604. https://doi.org/10.1080/02640414.2012.710753

Morris, T. (2000). Psychological characteristics and talent identification in soccer. *Journal of Sports Sciences, 18*(9), 715–726. https://doi.org/10.1080/02640410050120096

Murr, D., Feichtinger, P., Larkin, P., O'Connor, D., & Höner, O. (2018a). Psychological talent predictors in youth soccer: A systematic review of the prognostic relevance of psychomotor, perceptual- cognitive and personality-related factors. *PLoS One, 13*(10), e0205337. https://doi.org/10.1371/journal.pone.0205337

Murr, D., Raabe, J., & Höner, O. (2018b). The prognostic value of physiological and physical characteristics in youth soccer: A systematic review. *European Journal of Sport Science, 18*(1), 62–74. https://doi.org/10.1080/17461391.2017.1386719

Nortje, L., Dicks, M., Coopoo, Y., & Savelsbergh, G. J. P. (2014). Put your money where your mouth is: Verbal self-reported tactical skills versus on-line tactical performance in soccer. *International Journal of Sports Science and Coaching, 9*(2), 321–334. https://doi.org/10.1260/1747-9541.9.2.321

Nyland, N. (2010). *Visual perception in soccer: A study of elite and sub-elite defenders* [Unpubslihed Master's thesis]. Norwegian School of Sport Sciences, Oslo.

O'Connor, D., & Larkin, P. (2015). Decision making and tactical knowledge, an Australian perspective to their development in youth players. In T. Favero, B. Drust, & B. Dawson (Eds.), *International research in science and soccer II* (pp. 204–214). Routledge.

O'Connor, D., Larkin, P., & Williams, A. M. (2016). Talent identification and selection in elite youth football: An Australian context. *European Journal of Sport Science, 16*(7), 837–844. https://doi.org/10.1080/17461391.2016.1151945

Oerter, R. (2006). Entwicklungspsychologische Grundlagen [basics of developmental psychology]. In H. U. Wittchen & J. Hoyer (Eds.), *Klinische Psychologie [Clinical psychology]* (pp. 281–294). Springer.

Ohlert, J., & Kleinert, J. (2015). Entwicklungsaufgaben jugendlicher elite-Handballerinnen und -Handballer [Development tasks of elite youth handball players]. *Zeitschrift für Sportpsychologie, 21*, 161–172.

Park, S., Lavallee, D., & Tod, D. (2013). Athletes' career transition out of sport: A systematic review. *International Review of Sport and Exercise Psychology, 6*(1), 22–53. https://doi.org/10.1080/1750984X.2012.687053

Partington, M., & Cushion, C. (2013). An investigation of the practice activities and coaching behaviors of professional top-level youth soccer coaches. *Scandinavian Journal of Medicine & Science in Sports, 23*(3), 374–382. https://doi.org/10.1111/j.1600-0838.2011.01383.x

Pill, S. (2012). Teaching game sense in soccer. *Journal of Physical Education, Recreation and Dance, 83*(3), 42–52. https://doi.org/10.1080/07303084.2012.10598746

Posner, M. I. (1988). Introduction: What is it to be an expert? In M. T. H. Chi, R. Glaser, & M. J. Farr (Eds.), *The nature of expertise* (pp. 29–36). Erlbaum.

Potrac, P., & Cassidy, T. (2006). The coach as 'a more capable other'. The sports coach as educator. In R. L. Jones (Ed.), *Reconceptualising sports coaching* (pp. 39–50). Routledge.

Reilly, T., Williams, A. M., Nevill, A., & Franks, A. (2000). A multidisciplinary approach to talent identification in soccer. *Journal of Sports Sciences, 18*(9), 695–702. https://doi.org/10.1080/02640410050120078

Reimann, G., & Mandl, H. (2006). Unterrichten und Lernumgebungen gestalten [Teaching and designing learning environments]. In A. Krapp & B. Weidenmann (Eds.), *Pädagogische Psychologie. Ein Lehrbuch [Educational psychology. A textbook]* (pp. 613–658). Beltz.

Rheinberg, F., & Engesser, S. (2010). Motive training and motivational competence. In O. C. Schultheiss & J. C. Brunstein (Eds.), *Implicit motives* (pp. 510–548). Oxford University Press.

Roberts, B. W. (2009). Back to the future: Personality and assessment and personality development. *Journal of Research in Personality, 43*(2), 137–145. https://doi.org/10.1016/j.jrp.2008.12.015

Roca, A., Ford, P. R., McRobert, A. P., & Williams, A. M. (2013). Perceptual-cognitive skills and their interaction as a function of task constraints in soccer. *Journal of Sport and Exercise Psychology, 35*(2), 144–155. https://doi.org/10.1123/jsep.35.2.144

Roca, A., Williams, A. M., & Ford, P. R. (2012). Developmental activities and the acquisition of superior anticipation and decision making in soccer players. *Journal of Sports Sciences, 30*(15), 1643–1652. https://doi.org/10.1080/02640414.2012.701761

Romeas, T., Guldner, A., & Faubert, J. (2016). 3D-multiple object tracking training task improves passing decision-making accuracy in soccer players. *Psychology of Sport and Exercise, 22*, 1–9. https://doi.org/10.1016/j.psychsport.2015.06.002

Roth, K. (Ed.). (1996). *Techniktraining im Spitzensport. Alltagstheorien erfolgreicher trainer [Practising technique in top-class sport. Everyday theories of successful coaches]*. Strauß.

Rynne, S. B., Crudgington, B., Dickinson, R. K., & Mallett, C. J. (2017). On the (potential) value of coaching. In J. Baker, S. Cobley, J. Schorer, & N. Wattie (Eds.), *Routledge handbook of talent identification and development in sport* (pp. 285–300). Routledge.

Salmela, J. H. (1995). Learning from the development of expert coaches. *Coaching and Sport Science Journal, 2*(2), 3–13.

Sanchez-Cubillo, I., Perianez, J., Adrover-Roig, D., Rodriguez-Sanchez, J., Rios-Lago, M., Tirapu, J., & Barcelo, F. (2009). Construct validity of the trail making test: Role of task-switching, working memory, inhibition/interference control, and visuomotor abilities. *Journal of the International Neuropsychological Society, 15*(3), 438–450. https://doi.org/10.1017/S1355617709090626

Scharfen, H.-E., & Memmert, D. (2019). Measurement of cognitive functions in experts and elite athletes: A meta-analytic review. *Applied Cognitive Psychology, 33*(5), 843–860. https://doi.org/10.1002/acp.3526

Schorer, J., Baker, J., Lotz, S., & Büsch, D. (2010). Influence of early environmental constraints on achievement motivation in talented young handball players. *International Journal of Sport Psychology, 41*(1), 42–57.

Schultz, F. (2014). Antizipation von Fußballtorhütern—Untersuchung zur Konzeption einer kognitiven Leistungsdiagnostik im Kontext der sportwissenschaftlichen Talentforschung [Anticipation of football goalkeepers—Investigation on the conception of cognitive performance diagnostics in the context of sports science talent research]. : Dr. Kovač.

Sheridan, D., Coffee, P., & Lavallee, D. (2014). A systematic review of social support in youth sport. *International Review of Sport and Exercise Psychology, 7*(1), 198–228. https://doi.org/10.1080/1750984X.2014.931999

Singer, R. (2000). Sport und Persönlichkeit [Sport and personality]. In H. Gabler, J. R. Nitsch, & R. Singer (Eds.), *Einführung in die Sportpsychologie, Teil I: Grundthemen [Introduction to sport psychology, part I: Basic topics]* (pp. 289–336). Hofmann.

Smeeton, N. J., Ward, P., & Williams, A. M. (2004). Do pattern recognition skills transfer across sports? A preliminary analysis. *Journal of Sports Sciences, 22*(2), 205–213. https://doi.org/10.1080/02640410310001641494

Subotnik, R. F., Olszewski-Kubilius, P., & Worrell, F. C. (2012). A proposed direction forward for gifted education based on psychological science. *The Gifted Child Quarterly, 56*(4), 176–188. https://doi.org/10.1177/0016986212456079

Tannenbaum, A. J. (2003). Nature and nurture of giftedness. In N. Colangelo & G. A. Davis (Eds.), *Handbook of gifted education* (3rd ed., pp. 45–49). Allyn & Bacon.

Till, K., & Baker, J. (2020). Challenges and [possible] solutions to optimizing talent identification and development in sport. *Frontiers in Psychology, 11*, 664. https://doi.org/10.3389/fpsyg.2020.00664

Travassos, B., Araújo, D., Davids, K., Vilar, L., Esteves, P., & Vanda, C. (2012). Informational constraints shape emergent functional behaviours during performance of interceptive actions in team sports. *Psychology of Sport and Exercise, 13*(2), 216–223. https://doi.org/10.1016/j.psychsport.2011.11.009

Vaeyens, R., Coelho e Silva, M. J., Visscher, C., Philippaerts, R. M., & Williams, A. M. (2013). Identifying young players. In A. M. Williams (Ed.), *Science and soccer: Developing elite performers* (3rd ed., pp. 289–306). Routledge.

Vaeyens, R., Lenoir, M., Williams, A. M., & Philippaerts, R. M. (2007). Mechanisms underpinning successful decision making in skilled youth soccer players: An analysis of visual search behaviors. *Journal of Motor Behavior, 39*(5), 395–408. https://doi.org/10.3200/JMBR.39.5.395-408

Vaeyens, R., Lenoir, M., Williams, A. M., & Philippaerts, R. M. (2008). Talent identification and development programmes in sport: Current models and future directions. *Sports Medicine, 38*(9), 703–714. https://doi.org/10.2165/00007256-200838090-00001

Vallerand, R. J., & Losier, G. F. (1999). An integrative analysis of intrinsic and extrinsic motivation in sport. *Journal of Applied Sport Psychology, 11*(1), 142–169. https://doi.org/10.1080/10413209908402956

Vealey, R. S. (2002). Personality and sport behavior. In T. S. Horn & T. S. Horn (Eds.), *Advances in sport psychology* (2nd ed., pp. 43–74). Human Kinetics.

Verburgh, L., Scherder, E. J., van Lange, P. A., & Oosterlaan, J. (2014). Executive functioning in highly talented soccer players. *PLoS One, 9*(3), e91254. https://doi.org/10.1371/journal.pone.0091254

Vestberg, T., Gustafson, R., Maurex, L., Ingvar, M., & Petrovic, P. (2012). Executive functions predict the success of top-soccer players. *PLoS One, 7*(4), e34731. https://doi.org/10.1371/journal.pone.0034731

Vickers, J. N. (2007). *Perception, cognition, and decision training: The quiet eye in action*. Human Kinetics.

Vilar, L., Esteves, P. T., Travassos, B., Passos, P., Lago-Peñas, C., & Davids, K. (2014). Varying numbers of players in small-sided soccer games modifies action opportunities during training. *International Journal of Sports Science and Coaching, 9*(5), 1007–1018. https://doi.org/10.1260/1747-9541.9.5.1007

Voss, M. W., Kramer, A. F., Basak, C., Prakash, R. S., & Roberts, B. (2009). Are expert athletes 'expert' in the cognitive laboratory? A meta-analytic review of cognition and sport expertise. *Applied Cognitive Psychology, 24*(6), 812–826. https://doi.org/10.1002/acp.1588

Ward, P., Ericsson, K. A., & Williams, A. M. (2013). Complex perceptual-cognitive expertise in a simulated task environment. *Journal of Cognitive Engineering and Decision Making, 7*(3), 231–254. https://doi.org/10.1177/1555343412461254

Ward, P., Hodges, N. J., Starkes, J. L., & Williams, M. A. (2007). The road to excellence: Deliberate practice and the development of expertise. *High Ability Studies, 18*(2), 119–153. https://doi.org/10.1080/13598130701709715

Ward, P., Hodges, N. J., Williams, A. M., & Starkes, J. L. (2004). Deliberate practice and expert performance: Defining the path to excellence. In A. M. Williams & N. J. Hodges (Eds.), *Skill acquisition in sport: Research, theory and practice* (pp. 231–258). Routledge.

Ward, P., & Williams, A. M. (2003). Perceptual and cognitive skill development in soccer: The multidimensional nature of expert performance. *Journal of Sport and Exercise Psychology, 25*(1), 93–111. https://doi.org/10.1123/jsep.25.1.93

Weinert, F. E. (2001). Vergleichende Leistungsmessung in Schulen—Eine umstrittene Selbstverständlichkeit [Comparative performance measurement in schools—A controversial matter of course]. In F. E. Weinert (Ed.), *Leistungsmessung in Schulen [Performance measurement in schools]*. Weinheim.

Wenhold, F., Elbe, A.-M., & Beckmann, J. (2009). *Fragebogen zum Leistungsmotiv im sport (AMS-sport) [Questionnaire assessing achievement motives in sport (AMS-sport)]*. Sportverlag Strauss.

Williams, A. M., & Ericsson, K. A. (2005). Perceptual-cognitive expertise in sport: Some considerations when applying the expert performance approach. *Human Movement Science, 24*(3), 283–307. https://doi.org/10.1016/j.humov.2005.06.002

Williams, A. M., & Ford, P. R. (2013). 'Game intelligence': Anticipation and decision making. In A. M. Williams (Ed.), *Science and soccer: Developing elite performers* (pp. 105–121). Routledge.

Williams, A. M., Ford, P. R., & Drust, B. (2020). Talent identification and development in soccer since the millennium. *Journal of Sports Sciences, 38*, 1199–1210. https://doi.org/10.1080/02640414.2020.1766647

Williams, A. M., Ford, P. R., Eccles, D. W., & Ward, P. (2011). Perceptual-cognitive expertise in sport and its acquisition: Implications for applied cognitive psychology. *Applied Cognitive Psychology, 25*(3), 432–442. https://doi.org/10.1002/acp.1710

Williams, A. M., & Franks, A. (1998). Talent identification in soccer. *Sports, Exercise and Injury, 4*(4), 159–165.

Williams, A. M., & Hodges, N. J. (2004). *Skill acquisition in sport: Research, theory and practice*. Routledge.

Williams, A. M., & Reilly, T. (2000). Talent identification and development in soccer. *Journal of Sports Sciences, 18*(9), 657–667. https://doi.org/10.1080/02640410050120041

Williams, A. M., Ward, P., Bell-Walker, J., & Ford, P. R. (2012). Perceptual-cognitive expertise, practice history profiles and recall performance in soccer. *British Journal of Psychology, 103*(3), 393–411. https://doi.org/10.1111/j.2044-8295.2011.02081.x

Williams, A. M., Ward, P., & Chapman, C. (2003). Training perceptual skill in field hockey: Is there transfer from the laboratory to the field? *Research Quarterly for Exercise and Sport, 74*(1), 98–103. https://doi.org/10.1080/02701367.2003.10609068

Wolfenden, L. E., & Holt, N. L. (2005). Talent development in elite junior tennis: Perceptions of players, parents, and coaches. *Journal of Applied Sport Psychology, 17*(2), 108–126. https://doi.org/10.1080/10413200590932416

Woods, C. T., Raynor, A. J., Bruce, L., & McDonald, Z. (2016). Discriminating talent-identified junior Australian football players using a video decision-making task. *Journal of Sports Sciences, 34*(4), 342–347. https://doi.org/10.1080/02640414.2015.1053512

Zentgraf, C., & Munzert, J. (2014). *Kognitives training im sport [Cognitive training in sports]*. Hogrefe.

Zuber, C., & Conzelmann, A. (2014). The impact of the achievement motive on athletic performance in adolescent football players. *European Journal of Sport Science, 14*(5), 475–483. https://doi.org/10.1080/17461391.2013.837513

Zuber, C., Zibung, M., & Conzelmann, A. (2015). Motivational patterns as an instrument for predicting success in promising young football players. *Journal of Sports Sciences, 33*(2), 160–168. https://doi.org/10.1080/02640414.2014.928827

Sleep, Recovery and Rest

Daniel Erlacher, David W. Eccles and Sarah Jakowski

Contents

J. Schüler et al. (eds.), *Sport and Exercise Psychology*, https://doi.org/10.1007/978-3-031-03921-8_24

Learning Objectives

Basic:
- To understand different measures of sleep
- To describe sleep behavior in different sports and sport situations
- To understand different strategies to promote sleep

Advanced:
- To define different facets of recovery
- To describe recovery modalities

Experts:
- To understand the necessity of monitoring sleep and recovery-stress states in athletes
- To explain the importance of rest for athletes
- To learn the benefits of mental rest
- To recognize different resting experiences of athletes

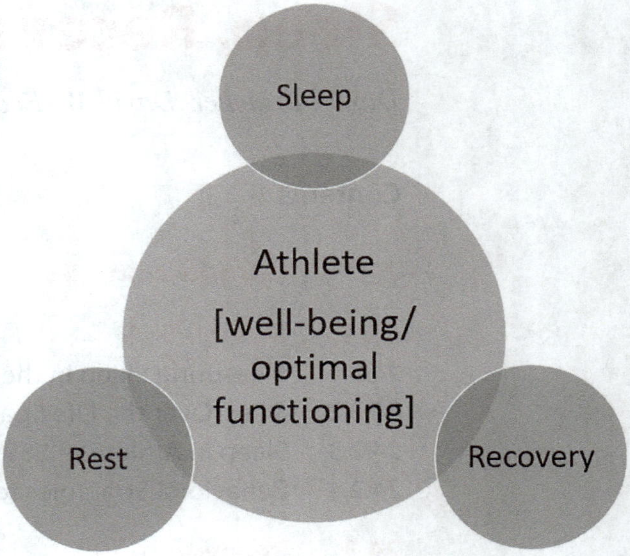

Fig. 24.1 Overall framework of sleep, recovery and rest

24.1 Introduction

The focus of the psychology of sport is often on the activity itself. However, several important processes relevant to that activity rely on the interval between those activities. For example, after learning a new motor skill like a basketball free throw, the acquired skill needs time to consolidate. Similar, after an intensive strength training session, the body needs time to recover and to initiate anabolic processes. The question is if the time interval per se is sufficient for consolidation and recovery or if the process is also state dependent (e.g. sleep) or if specific behaviors (e.g. massage) might shorten the required time for homeostatic balance.

While sleep may be considered the most natural and essential recovery strategy in every human being, it is worthwhile to regard waking activities that serve the restoration of physical and psychological resources as equally important for athletes. Sleep is generally regarded as a valuable resource for psychological and physiological well-being (Kölling et al., 2019). In recent years, sleep as a resource of recovery has increasingly been recognized as part of the preparation of peak performance—not only by athletes but also by coaches.

However, as sleep is highly vulnerable in high-performance sports populations, effective daytime recovery processes and strategies can promote sleep behavior and maintain the biopsychosocial well-being in the long term. Moreover, recovery should be incorporated into comprehensive training agendas, since athletes actually spend a much greater proportion of their time recovering than they do in training (Bishop et al., 2008). From the sport psychological view, recovery is far more than the absence of stress or training, and the recovery process is more complex than randomly executing relaxation techniques and enjoying holidays. Different perspectives need to be considered, while the general aim is to maintain the optimal balance of recovery and stress.

In this context, rest is often overlooked, even though it plays an essential role at the level of practice. Not only within conceptualizations of recovery but also for motor skill learning and expert performance, rest is considered a key component. Most importantly, effective rest exceeds the basic idea of physical inactivity (Fig. 24.1).

24.2 Sleep

[1]Sport and sleep are like peak performance and paralysis. At the first glance, a contrast could hardly be greater. With the second, it becomes apparent that sleep and sport are linked in a reciprocal process (Chennaoui et al., 2015). One affects the other on multiple physiological and psychological levels. It is therefore surprising that the interaction between daytime performance and nighttime rest has been given so little attention—neither in practical fields such as competitive sports nor in the corresponding scientific research. Therefore, the goal of this section is to give a general introduction to the method of sleep research and some basic findings. Afterwards, the focus will be on the athletes' sleep in different sports. Finally, several behavioral strategies to promote sleep will be discussed.

1 Parts of this chapter were adapted from Erlacher (2019). Sport und Schlaf. Berlin: Springer.

Reflection

Looking at top-level sport, the waking state can be considered in a simplified—and not entirely serious—way as a temporary hyperactive catabolic phase, which serves training and competition. But why do we sleep? Why has evolution shaped a state in which an organism is completely inactive and defenceless? The function of sleep must be tremendously important, because it has become evolutionarily accepted despite serious disadvantages—for example, that we cannot save ourselves from sabre-toothed tigers. Thereby, humans sleep for a third of their lives, and they need sleep as much as they need food and water—but still, sleep remains a scientific enigma (Krueger et al., 2016). Nature has given us even more riddles with the nocturnal dream experience. Why does our sleeping brain produce a fantasy world in which we sometimes have bizarre adventures, not even knowing that we are dreaming and rarely remembering the contents after awakening? At the age of 40, we have spent a good 3 years on the "holodeck" in our head. And yet, the function of dreaming is even more obscure than the function of sleep (cf. Erlacher, 2019).

So what does all this have to do with sport? During a gymnastics lesson, a young athlete practises a front tuck dismount from the highbar for the first time, and at the end of the lesson, the new element is yet to be adopted. Later that afternoon, they want to meet for a second training session. Is it worth taking a midday nap to consolidate the newly learnt element? A girl dreams at night of throwing balls and spears as far as possible. The next day she goes to the school championships. Does she achieve a new personal best with the additional "training" at night? The Olympic hopeful in swimming is facing an important qualification race. However, the night before the competition, the athlete doesn't get a wink of sleep. Will the missed sleep affect her performance?

Try to identify other examples where sleep may play an important role in your sport.

24.2.1 Measuring Sleep in the Laboratory and in the Field

Sleep is a unique state: Output and input are virtually switched off. The skeletal muscles relax, so that the body becomes partly paralyzed. One is "unconscious" because the sensory input is limited, so that the experience of the "external world" pauses. The interaction with the environment is reduced to a minimum. Seen from the outside, a sleeping person appears to be "switched off". However, sleep is a complex process, not just a mere "switching off" of the neurons in the central nervous system. Rather, brain activity is constantly changing: from "much" to "little" in recurring cycles. These changes during sleep are measurable. The gold standard of sleep medicine is polysomnography (PSG), which provides a range of sleep parameters. However, there are also alternative methods such as actigraphy and sleep questionnaires, which can also be used in the field of sport (cf. Erlacher, 2019).

Polysomnography In sleep research, sleep is measured by three physiological parameters: brain waves, eye movements and muscle tone. These parameters are recorded by electroencephalography (EEG), electrooculogram (EOG) and electromyography (EMG) (Iber et al., 2007). The polysomnographic measurement of sleep is shown in ▫ Fig. 24.2.

Over one night, this standard recording reveals cyclic changes in the physiological parameters. Based on these variations, sleep can be divided into different stages. The determination of sleep stages is based on the criteria of the American Academy of Sleep Medicine (AASM) of 2007 (Iber et al., 2007).

According to the AASM criteria, five sleep stages are defined including the waking state:
- Stage *W* (waking state)—The EEG contains alpha activity. In non-alpha producers, eye movements, blinks and high tonic submentalis EMG activity are present.
- Sleep stage *N1*—Characterized by a relatively low-amplitude, mixed-frequency EEG often accompanied by slow, rolling eye movements (SEM = slow eye movements). Decreasing muscle tone.
- Sleep stage *N2*—Characterized by sleep spindles and K-complexes on the background of relatively low-amplitude mixed-frequency EEG activity. Sleep spindles are spindle-shaped wave accumulations of 12–14 Hz with a maximum above the central EEG lead and a duration of more than 500 ms. K-complexes are sharp rashes with a negative and positive component, a maximum above the frontal EEG lead and a duration of more than 500 ms.
- Sleep stage *N3*—Characterized by slow-wave activity (SWS = slow-wave sleep or delta waves) of 0.5–2 Hz and an amplitude greater than 75 μV in the frontal EEG lead. An epoch must have 20% or more slow waves.
- Sleep stage *R*—Characterized by a relatively low-amplitude mixed-frequency EEG in combination with episodically occurring rapid eye movements (REM = rapid eye movement) and a low-amplitude EMG.

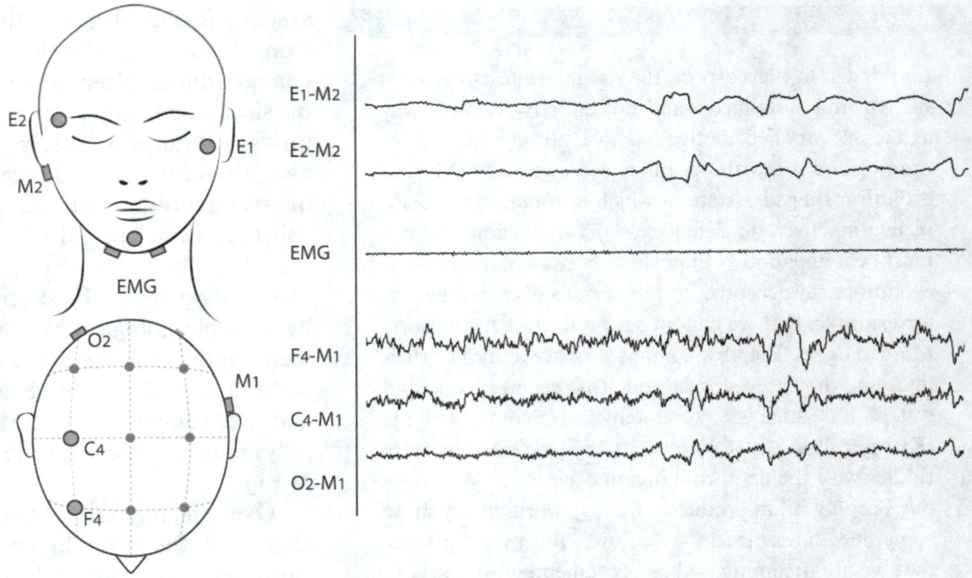

Fig. 24.2 Polysomnographic measurement of sleep. Figure adapted from Erlacher (2019)

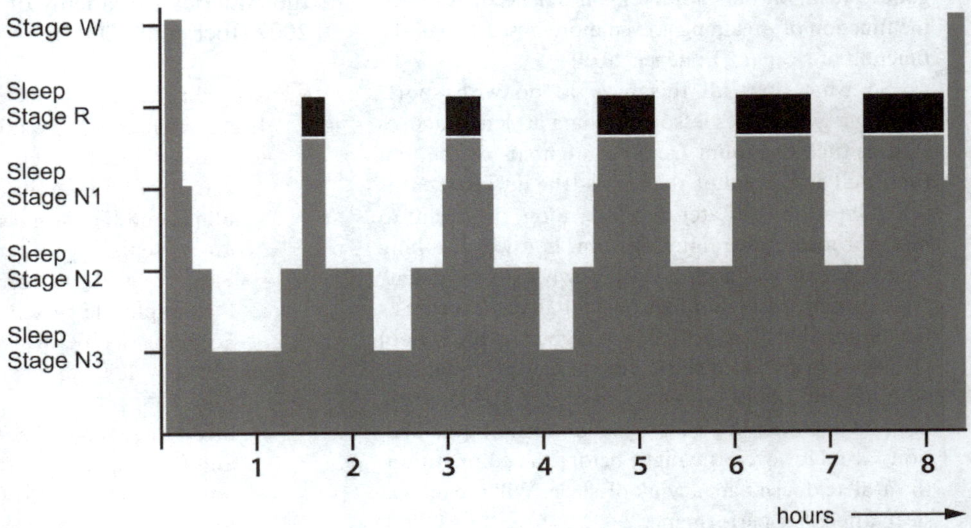

Fig. 24.3 A standardized sleep profile for night sleep. Figure adapted from Erlacher (2019)

The sleep recording is divided into 30-s epochs and assigned to one of the five stages. The stages N1, N2 and N3 taken together are also called NREM stages (non-REM) and are in contrast to stage R or REM sleep. The polysomnographic measurement of one night shows that NREM and REM sleep follow each other cyclically within about 90 min. Stage N3 (deep sleep) is dominant in the first half of the night and stage R (REM sleep) in the second half. Per night, an average of five to six of these cycles results from a sleep time of 8 h. The representation of the sleep stages over one night is done in a sleep profile or hypnogram (Fig. 24.3).

> With polysomnography (PSG), sleep can be characterized by brain waves, eye movements and muscle activity and is divided into five different sleep stages.

The sleep stages can also be differentiated on a functional level. Stage N1 is also called drowsiness which is seen as a transition between wakefulness and sleep. Stage N2 accounts for the largest percentage of the night and is therefore called stable sleep (see Stuck et al., 2018). In stage N3, sleep is very deep, the muscles are deeply relaxed and heart and breathing rates are slow and regular. This stage is often referred to as deep sleep. Characteristic for stage R is completely paralzsed muscles, whereas cortical activation is increased. If one wakes people from this stage, they are very likely to report a vivid dream. Therefore, REM sleep is often referred to as dream sleep, although dreams are also remembered in other stages (Schredl, 2018).

> Sleep is an active (cyclically recurring) process that is divided into REM-NREM stages, with REM stage being the longest in the early morning hours.

Sleep Characteristics

On the basis of sleep measurement and evaluation, night sleep can be described using various parameters relevant to sleep medicine. The parameters are also recommended by the American Academy of Sleep Medicine (AASM) and include time and percentage data (AASM, 2008).

Bedtime (time in bed, TIB). Includes the period from "light off" to "light on". In the sleep laboratory, this time is given, and a typical night would be 8 h.

Sleep onset latency (SOL). Describes the time in minutes required to fall asleep. Normally, falling asleep refers to the first occurrence of sleep stage N2. In sleep medicine, the parameter stands for the ability of a person to fall asleep.

Awake after the start of sleep (wake after sleep onset, WASO). Describes the total duration in minutes of waking phases that occur after falling asleep until "light on". A special case is the morning awakening and describes the duration from the final awakening until "light on".

Sleep period time (SPT). Describes the period from falling asleep to the final awakening.

Total sleep time (TST). Describes the period of time actually slept during the sleep period. For this purpose, the nocturnal waking phases and the morning awakening are subtracted from the sleep period duration.

Sleep efficiency (SE). Indicates the ratio of total sleep time to total bedtime. It is expressed as a percentage. Sleep efficiency is a measure of the ability to sleep at night. Values above 85% are considered to be normal, although no clear limits are defined in sleep medicine.

In sleep reports, absolute and relative information on the individual sleep stages are usually given. The minute data depend on the individual sleep duration and are, therefore, sometimes unsuitable for comparison between people. Relative figures, on the other hand, are good for comparison. For example, the proportion of stage R sleep remains fairly stable at 15–20% over the life span.

> Polysomnography is used to calculate various sleep parameters that can then be used to characterize sleep.

Actigraphy Actigraphy is an alternative tool for determining objective sleep data. The activity monitor is a small accelerometer that is sensitive to movement direction and intensity. The basic idea of actigraphy is that movement is correlated with alertness, and long periods of inactivity are correlated with sleep (Sargent et al., 2016). Activity monitors, which are often worn on the non-dominant wrist, have the advantage that they are suitable for field studies because they are easy to use for participants. However, they are limited because they cannot really distinguish between sleep (or even different sleep stages) and alertness (e.g. Marino et al., 2013). The question about the validity of actigraphy measures has been investigated in different studies with different populations, and generally sleep measures with wrist actigraphy compared to PSG are quite accurate for normal sleepers. However, they suffer from insufficient *specificity*, e.g. the amount of sleep scored by PSG as wake epochs that are correctly classified as wake epochs by actigraphy, in people with sleep problems (Erlacher & Ehrlenspiel, 2018).

Sleep Questionnaires The easiest way to learn about sleep is to ask a person about it: How long did it take you to fall asleep? Were you awake at night? In addition, questioning is the only way to learn about the subjective sensations of sleep: How restful was your sleep? Did you sleep deeply? Because the experience of whether the night's sleep was restful or was felt to be deep is only accessible to the sleeping person him- or herself. For example, deep sleep is only partially related to the feeling of being refreshed after sleep. In order to query certain sleep characteristics in a standardized way, one can either use sleep questionnaires or sleep diaries. As the title of the book published by Azmeh Shahid and colleagues in 2012 suggests, there are a number of different sleep scales: *STOP, THAT and One Hundred Other Sleep Scales* (Shahid et al., 2012).

The questionnaires vary in scope and whether specific or different sleep disorders are to be surveyed. For example, the *STOP-Bang* questionnaire comprises eight items and is a screening method for recording obstructive sleep apnoea. The individual letters of the questionnaire name stand for the items (e.g. snoring, tiredness). The *Landecker Inventory for Sleep Disorders* (LISST) is a screening questionnaire that includes 75 items and asks about different sleep disorders (e.g. insomnia, narcolepsy) (Weeß et al., 2002). In the box, two frequently used questionnaires and the sleep diary will be briefly introduced.

Methods Box

- A good example of a subjective measure of sleep is the Pittsburgh Sleep Quality Index (PSQI) by Buysse et al. (1989), which is a self-assessment questionnaire that assesses sleep quality and sleep disorders over the past month. Nineteen items add up to seven component scores (e.g. subjective sleep quality). The sum of the scores for these seven subscales generates a global score of overall sleep quality and ranges from 0 to 21, with higher scores indicating a higher level of sleep-related symptoms. According to Buysse et al. (1989), a global score of more than 5 (cut-off) divides the participants into "bad" and "good" sleepers. The PSQI is a widely used tool and has also the advantage that there are several validated translations for different languages. However, the PSQI evaluates sleep in a feature-based perspective over a period of 1 month and is not able to measure the subjective sleep parameter for a single night.
- This issue is resolved, for example, by a German questionnaire: *Sleep Questionnaire A and B* (Görtelmeyer, 2011). The two versions of the validated self-assessment scale capture the characteristic components of subjective sleep quality of the last 2 weeks (SF-B) and the state component of sleep and sleep quality of the last night (SF-A). The SF-A comprises 25 items that measure composite scores of five factors: sleep quality, feeling refreshed in the morning, emotional balance in the evening, mental exhaustion in the evening, and sleep-related somatic symptoms during sleep.
- In the meantime, several sleep questionnaires for athletes have been developed (e.g. Driller et al., 2018 or Samuels et al., 2016).
- Another way to measure subjective sleep variables is to keep a *daily sleep diary* (Liendl et al., 2004). The sleep diary provides an additional source of sleep information with daily variability as well as progress and outcome monitoring. Sleep diaries can contain either a single item or a varying number of questions.

Sleep characteristics can be calculated from polysomnography, actigraphy or the sleep questionnaire and must be interpreted against this background.

24.2.2 Sleep Over the Life Span

A frequently asked question is as follows: How much sleep does a person need? A quick glance at Fig. 24.4 reveals that the answer to this question is not that simple. The figure shows data from two publications. The solid line with the squares represents cross-sectional sleep laboratory data on life span (Roffwarg et al., 1966). The two dotted lines with the circles are longitudinal questionnaire data collected over 36 years of life (Strauch, 2010).

If we first look at the *cross-sectional sleep lab data*, we notice that a newborn baby sleeps two-thirds of the day. The sleep rhythm is polyphasic, so that several sleep episodes occur every 24 h: The baby wakes up after 2–6 h of sleep, drinks milk and soon after falls asleep again and so on. After 3 months, waking periods during the night are rare, so that a nightly main sleep phase and a midday nap become established. At the end of infancy, there are 12–13 h of sleep, whereas in infancy, sleep decreases mainly during the day. In early childhood, sleep duration is 10–11 h, and when children start school, they are usually awake all day, so that a monophasic sleep-wake pattern has developed during the first 6 years. From late childhood through puberty to adolescence, the sleep duration decreases again significantly, so that it is about 7–8 h in young adulthood. The total sleep time continues to decrease moderately over adulthood. Older people also often sleep during the day and wake up more often during the night. Thus, sleep in old age is similar to polyphasic sleep.

The figure also shows that the distribution of sleep stages changes rapidly, especially in infancy. While in the newborn infant, half of the total sleep consists of sleep stage R, the REM sleep duration decreases to 30% in the first year of life, while the NREM stages remain the same. In toddlers, the proportion of stage R is already between 18 and 20% and thus as high as in young adults.

The dotted lines in the figure are questionnaire data collected by Inge Strauch every 2 years starting in 1975 to 1991 from 61 boys/men and 67 girls/women (Strauch, 2010). In 2008, she carried out a further follow-up survey with the same persons. The *longitudinal questionnaire data* reflect almost exactly the cross-sectional sleep laboratory data. The decrease in adolescence is clearly visible, which can be explained by a later bedtime. During this period, the parents' bedtime control decreases significantly, so that sleep is determined more autonomously. The second dotted line shows sleeping duration during the holidays, showing that if you have more available total sleep time, as is during the holidays, you sleep longer. This is an indication of the intra-individual fluctuations in sleep duration. However, it

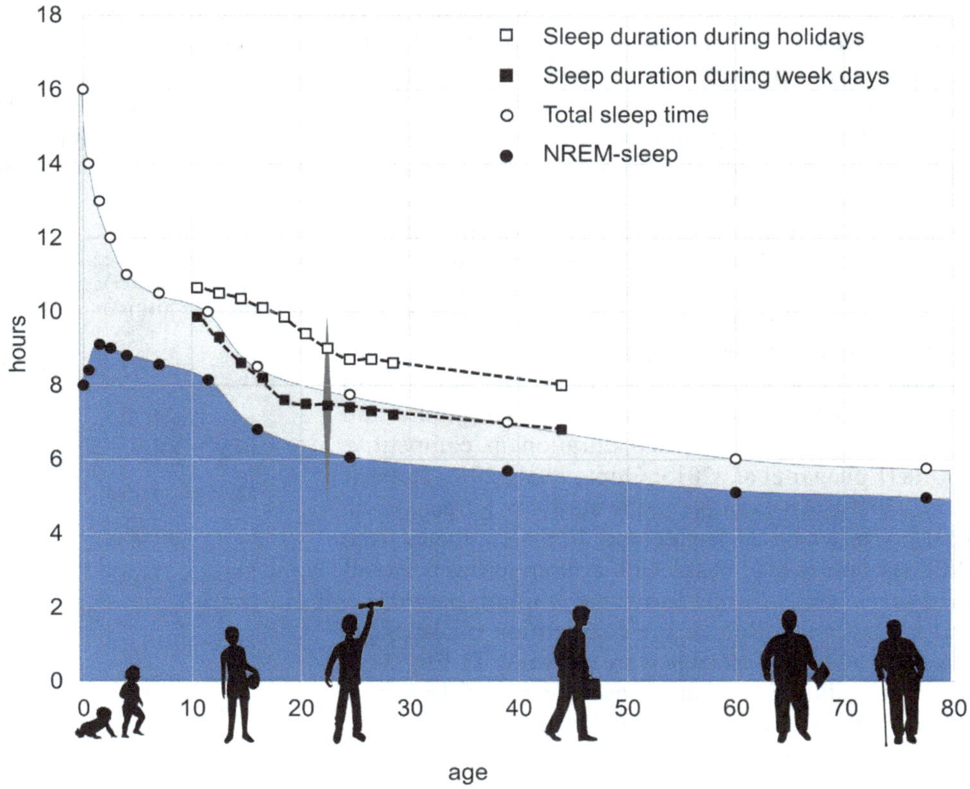

Fig. 24.4 Sleep duration over the life span. Data from Roffwarg et al. (1966) and Strauch (2010). Figure adapted from Erlacher (2019)

also raises the question of whether, for example, 14-year-old children who sleep 10.3 h during the holidays and only 8.6 h during the school days are suffering from an excessive sleep deficit. Evidence of the inter-individual variations in sleep duration can be found in the grey error bars at the age of 22 to 23 years. On average, total sleep time in that age group is 7.5 h but ranges from 5.5 to 10 h. Almost 18% were identified as short sleepers (6.5 or less hours) and 13% as long sleepers (8.5 or more hours) (Strauch, 2010). Longitudinal data reveal that there are no constant short or long sleepers and, at least for the second and third decades of life, no overarching characteristics can be found for such a distinction.

In view of this intra- and inter-individual variation in the indicated total sleep time, sleep research has been investigating the question of how many hours of sleep a person actually needs in order to function well.

Sleep Regulation

The sleep-wake continuum is regulated by the interaction of *homeostatic mechanisms*, which monitor the duration of wakefulness and sleep periods, and *circadian processes*, which determine the optimal time for sleep (Erlacher, 2019). Furthermore, these processes underlie endogenous functions, such as thermoregulation, as well as exogenous mechanisms, such as the light-dark cycle. One of the most prominent models of this linkage is the two-process model of sleep regulation by Borbély et al. (2016).

24.2.3 Sleep in Athletes

The positive effect of physical activity on sleep is generally well documented (Wang & Boros, 2019). It is therefore assumed that athletes tend to sleep longer and better than people who are physically inactive. For example, competitive swimmers in training phases with increased intensity and volume showed longer slow-wave sleep, while the total sleep duration remained the same (Taylor et al., 1997). However, other studies showed opposite results with regard to sleep duration in competitive sports. In a questionnaire study by Swinbourne et al. (2016), 175 team athletes (rugby, cricket) were asked about their sleep behavior during different training periods. In total, 22% said they received less than 7 h of sleep, with less sleep during training and competition than during non-training. In another questionnaire study involving 383 female and 507 male athletes from various team sports (hockey, netball, soccer, rugby) in

South Africa, three-quarters of the respondents stated that they slept on average between 6 and 8 h per night. Furthermore, on weekends as many as 11% of the respondents said they slept less than 6 h (Venter et al., 2010). Although sleep duration is only one of many parameters for a healthy sleep pattern, the general recommendations of the National Sleep Foundation in the USA, for example, assume 7–9 h of sleep per night for adults (Hirshkowitz et al., 2015; Fullagar et al., 2015).

In the meantime, the scientific production on sleep research in athletes has seen a significant growth with over 300 publications (Lastella et al., 2020). A huge number of those studies have been carried out to record the sleep behavior of athletes using actigraphy and partly support the low sleep duration in competitive sports (Fullagar et al., 2015; Gupta et al., 2017; Roberts et al., 2019). An example is the study by Sargent et al. (2014a), in which 24 female and 46 male athletes from different sports (e.g. basketball, swimming) were examined for 2 weeks during a normal training period, i.e. outside a competition or pre-competition phase. Sleep duration and sleep efficiency are shown in ◘ Fig. 24.5. The figure illustrates that on average only 6 to 7 h of sleep were achieved. In 37% of the cases, the sleep efficiency is below 85%.

In another study by Lastella et al. (2015a), the sleep-wake behavior was examined over an average period of 11 days. The bedtime and sleep duration broken down by the individual sports are shown in ◘ Table 24.1. The average sleep duration over all persons was 6 h and 48 min with an average sleep efficiency of 86%. The athletes from the individual sports slept half an hour less than the persons in team sports with 6 h and 30 min. The lowest total sleep times were measured in the sport triathlon with almost 6 h. It is noticeable, for example, that the average bedtime of triathletes was just under 8 h, so that the persons would have been awake in bed for 2 h.

In the study by Nédélec et al. (2019), the average sleep duration for top footballers on the training day was also 6 h and 23 min. Here too, the bedtime was just

◘ **Table 24.1** Bedtime, sleep duration and sleep efficiency in different sports. Data from Sargent et al. (2014b). Table from Erlacher (2019)

	Bedtime (h)	**Total sleep time (h)**	**Sleep efficiency (percentage)**
Individual sports			
Cycling ($n = 29$)	8.0 (1.0)	6.7 (0.9)	86.5 (5.5)
Mountain bike ($n = 5$)	8.8 (0.8)	7.0 (0.7)	83.7 (5.4)
Racewalking ($n = 6$)	8.2 (1.1)	7.1 (1.0)	91.1 (5.7)
Swimming ($n = 18$)	8.5 (1.4)	6.4 (1.5)	84.4 (6.7)
Triathlon ($n = 8$)	7.9 (0.8)	6.1 (0.9)	83.8 (4.1)
Team sports			
Australian rules Football ($n = 19$)	8.4 (1.2)	6.7 (1.2)	85.0 (4.9)
Basketball ($n = 11$)	8.9 (1.1)	7.5 (1.0)	88.1 (3.8)
Rugby union ($n = 22$)	8.3 (1.6)	6.9 (1.5)	87.3 (5.2)
Football ($n = 6$)	8.3 (1.6)	6.9 (1.5)	86.7 (4.2)

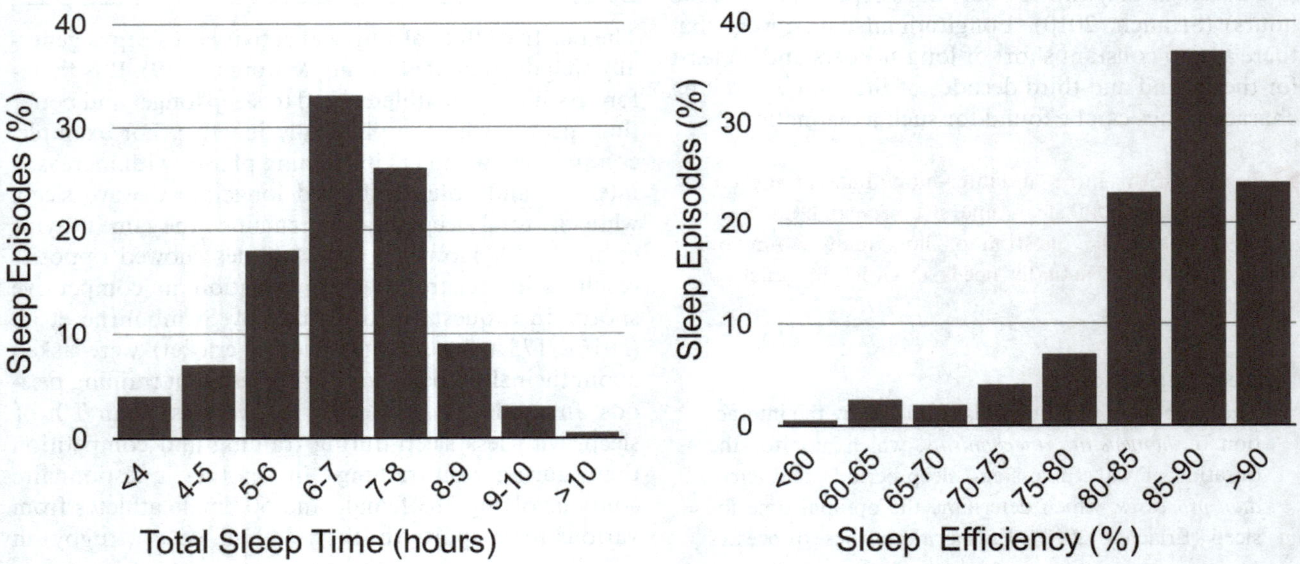

◘ **Fig. 24.5** Distribution of sleep duration and sleep efficiency for athletes. Data from Sargent et al. (2014b)

over 8 h. These long nightly waking hours are hardly imaginable for competitive sports, neither in triathlon nor in football, so that in these cases the waking hours may be overestimated by the actigraphy.

In several reviews from the past years, up to 54 studies have been included that examined sleep during training and competition periods (Fullagar et al., 2015; O'Donnell et al., 2018; Roberts et al., 2019). The summarized data actually indicate that athletes do not get enough sleep and that they might also have sleep problems (Gupta et al., 2017). However, it should not be forgotten that people who do not do sport can also have sleep problems (e.g. insomnia), for example, a study in which 107 professional ice hockey players were screened for sleep problems and 23 were medically suspicious. The sleep medical examination of these 23 athletes showed the following sleep disorders (cf. ICSD-3, 2014): obstructive sleep apnoea (n = 14), insomnia (n = 13), restless legs syndrome and periodic leg movements (n = 4), parasomnia (n = 1) and delayed sleep phase (n = 1). One athlete was diagnosed with three different sleep disorders, 9 athletes were diagnosed with two disorders each and 13 athletes received only one diagnosis (Tuomilehto et al., 2017).

The requirements of individual sports seem to interfere with sleep behavior, so that reduced sleep duration and sleep efficiency can often be observed in these athletes.

24.2.3.1 Sleep During Training Periods

The general conditions in competitive sports place high demands on professional athletes. Depending on the type of sport, up to four training units with up to 6 h of training must be completed during intensive training phases (e.g. Kölling et al., 2016a). It would be ideal if the athletes sleep well after training so that the physiological adaptation processes and the corresponding regeneration can proceed well. However, some of the training factors interfere with sleep behavior.

Training Times Sleep or swim? This was the question posed by Sargent et al. (2014a), who examined one female and six male athletes during a 2-week training phase with high exercise intensities. The study lasted 2 weeks, during which one training session was scheduled for 6:00 a.m. on 12 days, plus further training phases spread over the day. There were no training sessions on Sundays. Early-morning training severely restricts sleep, so that on average only just under 5 h and 30 min were slept—well below the recommended sleep duration. In some cases, the lack of sleep was even compensated for by a midday nap. Sleep was also made up for on the non-training days by extending the bedtime to 9 h and 20 min. Similar results were obtained in a group of 55 junior national rowers who were investigated via sleep logs and actigraphy during a 4-week training camp. The impact of sleep on subjective recovery measures was clearly interfered with the setting of a training camp (Kölling et al., 2016a).

Morning and Evening Types The training times in the different sports lead to the assumption that the chronotype will also be distributed differently, i.e. the "larks" and the "owls" will choose a sport that suits their biorhythm. In a study by Lastella et al. (2016), 114 athletes from five sports (cricket, cycling, hockey, football and triathlon) completed a questionnaire to determine their chronotype. Morning types are more common in sports that require morning training (e.g. triathlon), and evening types are more common in sports that require evening training (e.g. cricket).

Training Forms In a study by Kölling et al. (2016b), 42 athletes had to undergo either intensive strength training or intensive intermittent training (high-intensity interval training = HIIT) for 1 week. The sleep parameters in the strength group did not change during the entire period. In contrast, the HIIT group showed a decrease in sleep efficiency during the training phase compared to the baseline nights. The authors concluded that intensive intermittent exercise results in a higher recovery requirement than strength training—and therefore increased sleep time—compared to baseline. Since strength training and HIIT require different adaptation processes, the question of whether more sleep is required after certain training units or in certain sports (weightlifting vs. long-distance running) is very exciting. Further investigations would therefore be urgently required. Another aspect concerns training under specific conditions such as hypoxia training at altitude. These training conditions could also influence sleep (Hoshikawa et al., 2014).

Overtraining Too much training over a long period of time with insufficient recovery can lead to a loss of performance and chronic maladjustment (overtraining syndrome, ▶ Sect. 24.3.2). Interestingly, sleep disorders are often described as one of the many symptoms of overtraining, such as persistent muscle soreness or clinical disorders (Lastella et al., 2018). For example, sleep efficiency is significantly reduced in the transition from symptoms of overuse to overtraining. These results are often interpreted to mean that sleep disorders occur in parallel with overtraining. Whether there is a direct effect of overtraining on sleep needs to be investigated in further studies.

After-Lunch Nap As the studies on sleep behavior during intensive training periods show (cf. O'Donnell et al., 2018), naps seem to be a suitable method for athletes to reduce sleep debt. Waterhouse et al. (2007) investigated the effects of naps on sprinting performance after partial sleep deprivation to 4 h of night sleep. After a 30-min nap, 20-m sprint performance was increased, alertness increased and sleepiness decreased compared to the control condition without nap. Thus, naps can be beneficial in learning skills, strategies or tactics. Taking a nap can also be beneficial for athletes who need to wake up early for training or competition. When taking a nap, however, care must be taken not to sleep too long, so that the sleep pressure is then too low in the evening, which can affect the night's sleep.

Nutrition Nutritional behavior, which is very important for sports, can also have an influence on sleep. For example, carbohydrates that can be quickly absorbed by the body (high glycemic index) seem to be more supportive of sleep if they are taken about an hour before going to bed. On the other hand, high amounts of fat seem to reduce the total sleeping time (Halson, 2014). Glucose metabolism and neuroendocrine function as a result of chronic partial sleep deprivation can lead to changes in carbohydrate metabolism, appetite, food intake and protein synthesis. While there is some research that studies sleep and nutrition in sports, due to the complex interaction, there is still research needed to highlight the importance of nutritional behavior and diets to improve sleep (Halson, 2014).

> During training periods, sleep can be affected by various factors (training type, overtraining, nutrition, etc.).

24.2.3.2 Sleep During Competitions

In any athletic career, competitions are special highlights, and therefore sleep in combination with a competition could be of special interest. In particular, the night before an important competition or game can have an impact on the athlete's performance. In addition to anecdotal reports and retrospective studies, evidence suggesting that athletes may have poor sleep quality before a competition is quite rare. Recent research underlines the importance of sleep for competition performance indicating relationships between poor sleep quality and loss and between sleep duration and performance, respectively (e.g. Silva & Paiva, 2016).

Sleep Before a Competition In large-scale cross-sectional studies, more than 60% of the samples of German (Erlacher et al., 2011b), Australian (Juliff et al., 2015) and Japanese (Erlacher, 2019) elite and college athletes answered "yes" when asked if they had slept worse than normal at least once in the previous 12 months before a competition. Of the German athletes who had slept poorly before a competition, most (60%) reported that their impaired sleep had no effect, with only about 30% reporting that they felt sleepy all day long, i.e. they may have experienced less restful sleep effects (Erlacher et al., 2011b). Similar figures were found in a study that examined sleep before a specific event (Lastella et al., 2014). In the morning of a marathon run, 68% of athletes reported that they slept worse the night before compared to a normal night. While retrospective self-reports indicate impaired sleep quality, studies with repeated measurements of self-reported sleep quality found no support for previous retrospective studies. For example, no differences were found when comparing sleep quality scores for normal nights measured with a single item with those for nights before competitions in a small sample of female netball players (Romyn et al., 2016) and a sample of racing cyclists (Lastella et al., 2015b).

In a study by Erlacher et al. (2009), in addition to the subjective sleep quality, the participants also recorded their competitive anxiety in the morning of a sport test. While the somatic proportion of the competitive anxiety did not correlate with subjective sleep quality, there was a clear correlation between the feeling of recovery after sleep and the anxiety components and confidence. In a second longitudinal study, subjective sleep quality and competitive anxiety were now measured in professional athletes in the morning of a competition and 4 days before (Ehrlenspiel et al., 2018). In this study, too, there was no correlation between competitive anxiety and subjective sleep quality, but rather with the feeling of relaxation after sleep. Contrary to the anecdotal examples, subjective sleep quality seems to be weakly, if at all, related to somatic and cognitive aspects of competitive anxiety. On the other hand, the perceived effects of sleep ("having slept in") may show substantial correlations.

Beside the internal factors in professional sport, more and more external factors related to competitions interfere with optimal sleep. For example, games and competitions often take place in the early or late evening (Nédélec et al., 2019). The increase in sport events in the evening (e.g. Champions League soccer matches) poses various problems. For organizational reasons alone, the time for sleeping is strongly shifted to the rear. In addition, activating substances (e.g. caffeine) or the physical and mental activation of the competition itself can negatively influence sleep. In the previously mentioned study by Nédélec and colleagues (2019), the sleeping time for the top soccer players after an evening game was on average just 4 h and 51 min. Therefore, it seems that not only the night before a competition but also after a competition should be further investigated.

Jet-Lag Most professional sports engage in competition which makes regular short-haul (domestic) and long-haul (international) travel a necessity. As discussed before, the competition itself is a factor in disturbed sleep, and the concomitant domestic or international travel associated with competition demands can further interfere with sleep behavior (Duffield & Fowler, 2018). Either because of the length or the extent of flight, a combination of jet-lag and/or travel exhaustion can interrupt sleep habits (Waterhouse et al., 2004). More specifically, travel by plane in seated and crowded environments and in a loud and hypoxic atmosphere can make it difficult to sleep. On the other hand, the crossing of time zones results in the desynchronization of the internal clock with external daytime "zeitgeber"—resulting in disturbed sleep/waking behavior in the new time zone (Reilly et al., 2007). Either way, when athletes are required to travel to or from competition, there is a risk of disrupted sleeping patterns, although most short-haul flights result in minimal disruption to sleep quantity or quality (Duffield & Fowler, 2018). Rather, long-haul or overnight travel is more likely to result in disrupted sleep behaviors and poorer sleep quantity and quality (Fowler et al., 2015). A limited number of studies investigated the effects of jet-lag in athletes indicating rather indirect effects on performance (Kölling et al., 2016a). To support the recovery processes and to enhance the adaptation to the destination, behavioral strategies, such as arranging sleep-wake and meal times according to the target time, should be preferred over medications (Reilly et al., 2007).

Competitions or Tournaments Lasting Several Days Sport events that last more than 1 day are very common in competitive sports. Usually the competition time in such competitions is limited to a part of the day—be it for a game (e.g. European Championship in soccer), one or two preliminary heats (e.g. World Championship in swimming) or multiple stages (e.g. in a cycling tour). Between the individual competitions, there is at least one or more nights during which normal sleep is possible (Lastella et al., 2015b). For example, a road cycling season lasts from February to October covering between 50 and 70 competitions, a competition lasts between several days or up to 3 weeks with multiple stages from up to 290 kilometres. During this period, the riders are not given a day off, except for the 3-week national tours such as the Tour de France. In addition, there is a constant change of surroundings or places to stay overnight and a variation of starting times, which have a negative effect on the quality and duration of sleep (Lastella et al., 2015c).

Another form of competitions lasting several days is extreme endurance sports without stages. Leger et al. (2008), for example, recorded sleep data with mobile measuring units for sailors during a boat race lasting several days. The sailors who had the better sleep management strategies, i.e. who were able to ensure sufficient sleep, also had a better result in the race. Because such sport events are becoming more and more popular, it would be interesting to further investigate the impact of sleep deprivation in such situations on performance.

Distressing Dreams Dreaming defined as mental experiences (perceptions, thoughts and emotion) occurring during sleep provides another interesting access to the athletes' internal status on recovery and performance. The dream usually reflects waking activities. For example, sport students who are frequently involved in sport activities during the day show higher active participation in sport or sport themes in dreams compared to psychology students (Erlacher & Schredl, 2004). Especially stressful situations, such as competitions, might alter the dream content of athletes and consequently evoke disturbed dreaming. In a questionnaire study, about 15% of the athletes ($n = 840$) stated that they experienced at least one distressing dream before an important competition or game during the preceding 12 months (Erlacher et al., 2011a). Dream content might also mirror the need for recovery or recovery-related processes; however, so far no study looked at dream content in athletes after high intensive workouts (Erlacher, 2019).

24.2.4 Behavioral Strategies to Promote Sleep

In view of the fact that sleep plays an important role in recovery and thus in the success of training, the question arises as to how optimum conditions for sleep can be achieved in athletes. In fact, some factors, such as reduced sleep duration during intensive training camps, can be quickly recognized and thus also changed. Although the early-morning start for coaches and top athletes in sports (e.g. swimming, rowing, triathlon) is common, there are no scientific findings on whether early-morning training is beneficial (e.g. Sargent et al., 2014a). Sargent et al. speculate that the early-morning start is a legacy from a time in which non-professional athletes had to train before work or school. So, an obvious strategy is to start the first training 2 or 3 h later. Another example would be that in sport academies, it would be beneficial, in order to promote sports performance, to organize the school start later.

Early-morning exercise sessions can shorten usual sleep durations and therefore cause sleep problems in the long view—especially in athletes with a chronotype of the evening type. Therefore, training sessions should not only be postponed, but may also be adapted to circadian rhythms (e.g. Vitale et al., 2019), whereby these temporal adjustments raise organizational problems. However, such a change would also accommodate potential athletes who choose sports that correspond to their chronotype but not necessarily to their sporting inclination. The coaching staff could also take the chronotype more into account for talent selection (cf. Lastella et al., 2016).

As the previous studies show, measuring sleep-wake cycles by means of actigraphy is a possibility that can be realized in competitive sports. Individual sleep-wake data could indicate possible improvements in sleep-wake times during training phases by measurements in training-free periods (longitudinal data). Both coaches and athletes must be careful when evaluating the data obtained, in order not to prematurely suspect an insomniac disorder in an athlete, especially if the sleep is only considered at one point in time (cross-sectional data). Rather, it is important to find the optimal sleep-wake rhythm for each athlete. If abnormalities are present, it should be analyzed how, when and why the sleep problems occur. Regardless of this, attention should be paid to good sleep hygiene (e.g. darkened, cool and quiet sleeping environment) (cf. Fullagar et al., 2015).

For this reason, additional bedtime could be tried—sleep extension through longer night sleep or midday nap—to improve sleep. A few studies show positive effects on, for example, the motor learning performance or the recovery (e.g. Bonnar et al., 2018). But also caution is required, because the nap can reduce the sleep pressure for the night's sleep and, therefore, the subsequent sleep might possibly be impaired. Likewise, the longer bedtimes should be shortened again, if it is not possible to sleep during this time, as this decreases the sleep efficiency and thus sleep problems can arise. These few examples show that sleep coaching is advisable. If sleep problems persist, a sleep expert should be consulted.

A restful sleep is important, for example, to be able to sleep confidently before an important game or competition. Therefore, general and specific recommendations to optimize sleep are needed. A sports-tailored sleep reduction must be adapted to the special conditions of the respective sports and orient itself around the sleeping possibilities given there. In order to prevent sleep disorders, and not to be helpless in the face of it, the so-called sleep training and sleep reduction were developed. Training for a healthy restful sleep follows the rule of thumb "less is more", i.e. instead of lying awake, preferring a shorter bedtime to increase sleep efficiency and taking into account individual sleep needs. Sleep hygiene (regular bedtimes, sleep rituals, no late trainings or cognitive preparations) causes changes in sleep habits and an optimization of the sleeping environment.

To implement these measures in sports, special attention may be required. Simple strategies, such as implementation of consistent sleep-wake patterns and non-stimulating pre-bedtime routines, can be applied to improve individual sleep (Caia et al., 2018).

Implementing a sleep education with athletes therefore seems to be a useful strategy, whereas several methods are available for such an intervention (■ Fig. 24.6).

? Motor Learning in Lucid Dreams

Sleep might be not only a passive state which serves recovery, for example, when a sleeping person is aware of dreaming, a state of lucid dreaming is achieved in which the person is capable of actively influencing the contents of the dream (Dresler et al., 2016; Erlacher & Ehrlenspiel, 2018). Experimental research could show that lucid dream practice has a positive effect on waking performance. Recently, Stumbrys et al. (2016) instructed participants to practise a finger-tapping task in their dreams and compared the pre- to post-test performance change with a practical, mental training and a control group, respectively (Stumbrys et al., 2016). The lucid dream practice group showed higher effects in finger tapping compared to mental imagery. However, this technique does not seem very common among athletes (Erlacher et al., 2012). More experimental research is required in terms of techniques to induce lucid dreaming and the effect of this on performance and physiology (Erlacher & Schredl, 2008a, 2008b; Erlacher & Stumbrys, 2020). On the other hand, as sleep supports the regeneration processes and aims to purposely detach athletes from their sport, lucid dreaming may interfere with this process. Even though athletes applying lucid dream practice did not mention such problems (Schädlich & Erlacher, 2018), athletes and staff could carefully schedule "dream practice" apart from designated recovery nights or even encourage lucid dream activities which possibly improve recovery (e.g. relaxation).

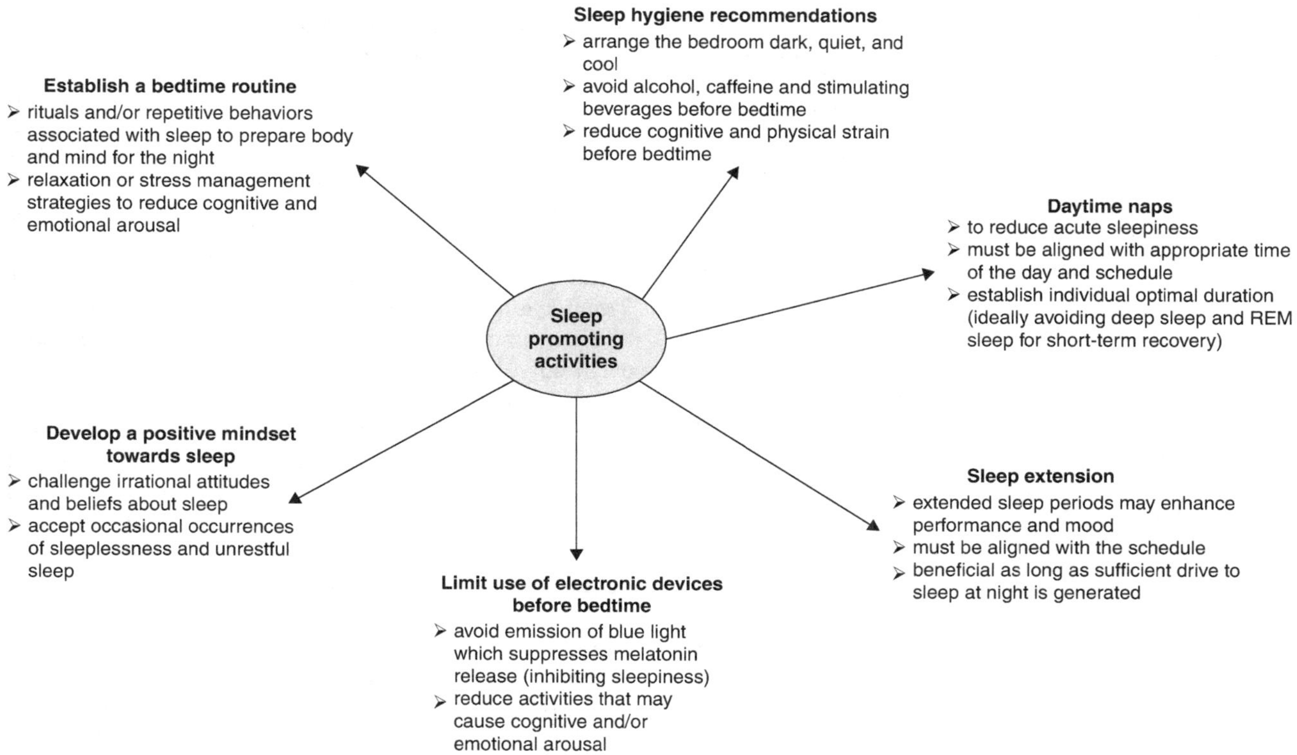

Fig. 24.6 Sleep-promoting activity considerations and objectives for athletes to maximize sleep. Based on the recommendations of Fullagar et al. (2015), Nédélec et al. (2015) and Irish et al. (2015)

24.3 Recovery

Apart from sleep, recovery in general plays an important role in the training continuum and, in particular, in maintaining athletes' health and well-being.

24.3.1 Conceptualization of Recovery

The re-establishment of depleted resources and regaining homoeostasis is the aim of recovery, and therefore, it can be described from a physiological, psychological, behavioral, social and environmental perspective (Heidari & Kellmann, 2019). In that sense, *recovery* is an umbrella term which comprises multifaceted activities. Relevant components are, for instance, *regeneration*, *relaxation* and *rest*, while these terms are frequently used interchangeably in different areas of sport science (Kellmann et al., 2018). On the micro level, recovery is achieved through physiological processes that take place to restore the hormonal, cellular and fluid balance, among others, to undo the fatigue or damage which is induced by training and competition. This is more aptly described as *regeneration* (Kölling & Kellmann, 2019). In addition, the dimensions of time play an important role for regeneration and for recovery as a whole. Bishop et al. (2008) differentiate between *immediate recovery*, which takes place between rapid, time-proximal finite efforts (e.g. recovery phases of one leg within alternating walking strides); recovery between training sets (i.e. *short-term recovery*), with different work-to-rest ratios that are suggested; and the *training/competition recovery*, which refers to the time between separate sessions or bouts. Numerous strategies and activities can be applied for those different purposes. For instance, Hausswirth and Mujika (2013) describe stretching, hydration, nutrition, sleep, massage and physiotherapy, compression garments, local thermal applications, variations in thermal ambience and water immersion therapy to enhance performance in sport. From a more holistic perspective, recovery modalities can be characterized by *passive*, *active* and *pro-active activities* (Kellmann, 2002), where different levels of self-determination and self-regulation can be observed (Beckmann & Kellmann, 2004). For instance, while the application of compression garments is genuinely a passive strategy, the perceived effectiveness may be influenced by the degree of the self-determined decision behind this approach. Even if the use of compression garments is directed by the coach, one athlete may be convinced of the beneficial effect, whereas another athlete may feel highly uncomfortable wearing them. Therefore, it is important to note that the recovery experience is individual to a great extent. This concerns physical as well as emotional, mental and cognitive aspects of recovery (Loch et al., 2019). According to an occupational conceptualization, psychological detachment, relaxation, mastery and control are relevant domains of recovery experience to unwind from work-related demands (Sonnentag & Fritz, 2007). Not only professional athletes but also athletes for whom their sport is the main purpose in life need to establish recovery routines outside the sport context.

Recovery

"Recovery describes a restorative, psychophysiological process that aims at the reestablishment of depleted resources. It can be described from a physiological, psychological, behavioral, social, and environmental perspective, whereas the importance of each aspect for comprehensive recovery varies across individuals and situations" (Heidari & Kellmann, 2019, p. 242).

Regeneration

"Within the field of sport and exercise science, regeneration refers to the physiological processes of restoration following training or competition induced fatigue" (Kölling & Kellmann, 2019, p. 245).

What Are Your Top Three Recovery Strategies?

Several situations require different recovery strategies so that you need a diverse and flexible "tool box". Reconsider activities and resources which were useful in the past. Do you know how to (re-)activate them and adapt them to current situations if necessary?

- Physical recovery strategies (e.g. cool-down activities, stretching)
- Psychological strategies (e.g. relaxation techniques, systematic breathing)
- Social recovery (e.g. visiting family/friends, phone, messaging)
- Pro-active recovery (e.g. mindfulness practices, purposeful breaks, changing task/environment)

24.3.2 The Interrelation of Recovery and Stress in Sport

The balance effective training load and recovery demands is an essential component of optimal athlete preparation. While most exercise-induced adaptations take place during the recovery phase, this process is barely complete between workouts due to high training volume or intensity in elite sports (Bishop et al., 2008). *Training* is a process of overload that is deliberately used to disturb homoeostasis, which causes acute *fatigue* and eventually leads to an improvement in performance after recovery (Meeusen et al., 2013). Thus, short-term decrements in performance are intentionally anticipated in terms of *functional overreaching* to achieve the effect of supercompensation. An imbalance between training load and recovery will lead to *non-functional overreaching*, where the first signs of psychological and hormonal disturbances will occur. Additionally, confounding factors regarding inadequate nutrition, immunology, psychosocial stressors and disordered sleep may be observed (Meeusen & De Pauw, 2018; Meeusen et al., 2013). When the procedure of overtraining is maintained over a longer period, these symptoms will manifest and aggravate so that the *overtraining syndrome* will be developed. This state is characterized by prolonged maladaptation of several biological, neurochemical, hormonal and psychological regulation mechanisms. However, intensified training alone is not a sufficient explanation, as non-sport-related factors play also a significant role in the aetiology of the overtraining syndrome (Kellmann et al., 2018). *Underrecovery* is considered as a precondition which is characterized by an imbalance between life demands and recovery (Altfeld & Kellmann, 2014).

According to Kellmann (2002) increasing stress requires increasing recovery, while both are limited by an individual's stress capacity and recovery resources. The boundaries of the recovery-stress balance become apparent, when stress accumulates and the recovery demands cannot be met appropriately. For instance, one night of reduced sleep might be tolerated easily and compensated by lighter training intensity or a daytime nap. When training overload is maintained over a longer period, the habitual sleep duration may not be sufficient. At the same time, unlimited sleep extension is barely a feasible option. Additional recovery activities are necessary to meet the increased demands. The *scissors model* explains that the-more-the-better is not recommended at both sides of the recovery-stress continuum (Kallus & Kellmann, 2000; Kellmann, 2002). Analogous to the concept of the *individual zones of optimal functioning* (Hanin, 2000), the performance optimum can be achieved as long as an individual is capable of managing the current stress level and the associated recovery demands within his or her individual capacity.

Overtraining Syndrome

Overtraining as a verb indicates a process of intensified training with possible outcomes of short-term (functional) overreaching, non-functional overreaching or overtraining syndrome. "By using the expression 'syndrome', we emphasize the multifactorial aetiology and acknowledge that exercise (training) is not necessarily the sole causative factor of the syndrome" (Meeusen et al., 2013, p. 187).

Underrecovery Syndrome

Periods of excessive psychosocial and physical demands eventually overstrain an individual's resources and increase the need of recovery. Underrecovery is a precondition of the overtraining syndrome which describes short-term as well as long-term consequences of the imbalance between life demands and recovery of an individual (Altfeld & Kellmann, 2014).

Recovery is an umbrella term to describe the restoration of biopsychosocial homoeostasis. In accordance with (Kellmann (2002) and Kallus and Kellmann (2000), the following key characteristics can be conceptualized:

- Different recovery demands result from different characteristics of previous activities/stressors (e.g. duration, intensity, timing).
- The recovery process is gradual and cumulative.
- Recovery experience is determined by the individual's perception and appraisal of the personal recovery capacity in relation to the situational demands.
- Recovery can be achieved through the cessation, reduction or change of stress.
- Recovery takes place on various levels, such as physiological, emotional, cognitive, behavioral, social or environmental.
- Passive recovery includes automated processes of biological and psychological restoration, and active recovery requires a purposeful action, whereas pro-active recovery constitutes self-initiated and self-determined activities.

Rowing Over the Edge: Non-functional Overreaching and Overtraining Syndrome as Maladjustment: Diagnosis and Treatment from a Psychological Perspective

Birrer (2019) presents a case study of a 21-year-old rower who revealed signs of non-functional overreaching/overtraining syndrome. The multifactorial aetiology of the maladaptation is reflected in his challenging personal and situational characteristics.

Training-related factors:

- Significant increase in weekly training volume
- Change from the open category to lightweight rowing (individual weight limit 72.5 kg, team mean limit 70 kg)
- Change of discipline (scull to one oar)
- Change of training environment (from the club level to the A-National team)
- Disagreement with national coach concerning the required weight limits

Personal features:

- Suicide of a close friend
- Breakup with girlfriend
- End-of-term school examinations
- Perfectionistic personality with very high personal standards

The rower developed signs of non-functional overreaching within several weeks, beginning from calendar week 13. In weeks 25 and 26, symptomology included cough, low sleep quality, fatigue, feeling powerless, performance inability, headache, diarrhoea, indisposition and asthma.

Intervention

The goals of the sport psychological treatment were to:

- Enhance the awareness of his basic biopsychosocial processes.
- Facilitate his acceptance of unpleasant physical and emotional sensations.
- Tackle his overreaching athlete identity.
- Attend to his predominant performance-related sources of self-esteem.

The intervention also involved weekly mood and *recovery-stress monitoring*. As he disclosed many negative emotions, his task was to engage consciously in a mood-repair mode in which he would deliberately choose activities, music and readings with a mood-enhancing impact; in addition, he was encouraged to explore *activities outside the sport* that he perceives as fun and fulfilling. Moreover, Birrer (2019) used a mixture of elements of several approaches, such as cognitive behavior therapy, psychological skills training, mindfulness-based and acceptance-based interventions. The latter two, for instance, comprised methods to consciously be in the present moment and viewing thoughts and emotions as acceptable as they are, with no need to alter or reduce them (Birrer et al., 2012; Gardner & Moore, 2017; Hayes, 2004). These processes, which were accompanied by psychoeducation on the function of mood, enabled the athlete to *increase his awareness* of training intensity and recovery aspects. He was also taught *autogenic training* to support the re-establishment of his emotional balance and enhance his recovery capacity. Among other approaches and aims of the intervention, an important element was to enhance training quality and his self-awareness regarding signs of stress and recovery. The weekly mood monitoring was helpful in estimating the physical as well as psychological development, which also supported the decision to integrate leisure physical activity into the intervention.

The rower's personal advice to other athletes is that "sometimes it takes more courage to skip a workout than to just stubbornly go through the training plan" (Birrer, 2019, p. 58).

24.3.3 Assessing and Monitoring Recovery and Stress States

In research and practice, the assessment of the current as well as chronic recovery-stress state of an athlete is necessary to determine the effect of training and non-training-related stimuli, which guides future decision-making. *Monitoring* the training process has evolved as a growing area of research in the last decades (Bourdon et al., 2017). Considerations of monitoring issues comprise the dosage (e.g. training and competition load, life load), athlete characteristics (e.g. physical, psychological, technical, tactical) and the response (e.g. performance) (McGuigan, 2017). Apparently, performance is the criterion marker of recovery, as it is the most important variable in sports (Bishop et al., 2008). At the same time, its assessment is often too complex, costly and time-consuming in many types of sport to be suitable for the daily monitoring routine. This also holds true for other physiological and biochemical measures. *Self-report measures* serve as surrogate as well as direct indicator of an athlete's recovery-stress state and performance readiness. Subjective measures reflect acute and chronic training loads even with superior sensitivity and consistency than objective measures (Saw et al., 2016). Since psychological disturbances, especially mood, are critical characteristics of the overtraining syndrome, coaches, sport psychologists and support staff need to be aware of those changes and detect non-functional developments as early as possible (Meeusen et al., 2013). For this purpose, standardized and validated psychometric tools may be useful (Saw et al., 2017). Either for individual or team assessments, questionnaires can be applied in a non-invasive and economic way.

Successful implementation and application of psychometric monitoring tools require careful considerations. Saw et al. (2017) recommend the following steps to select an instrument:
- What dimensions align with the intended purpose (e.g. sleep, mood, stress, recovery, emotions) and what is the theoretical basis for the chosen dimension(s)?
- What is the psychometrically strongest measure aligned with the chosen theoretical basis?
- If more than one is available, select the most feasible empirical measure.
- If the data is intended to be used for applied research, ensure the measure has acceptable psychometric properties, and establish these for the cohort/context if not pre-existing.

Monitoring the Athlete Training Response: Subjective Measures Trump Commonly Used Objective Measures

In a systematic review, Saw et al. (2016) compared subjective self-report measures and objective measures in the context of monitoring athletes' training response and well-being. They included objective measures which were taken at rest (e.g. blood markers, heart rate) or during exercise (e.g. oxygen consumption, heart rate response). In particular, markers of the endocrine, immune and inflammation systems, erythrocytes and muscle damage were analysed. Submaximal and maximal physiological parameters as well as short and sustained performance measures were also included. Subjective self-report measures with published validity and reliability were chosen which assess athletes' well-being, mood or perceived stress. The authors examined associations between subjective and objective measures and their responsiveness to training on the basis of 54 articles.

Consistently, the subjective measures identified impaired well-being with acute increases as well as in response to chronic training load and improved well-being with an acute reduction in training load. Twenty-two out of the 54 studies revealed higher sensitivity, consistency and responsiveness for subjective measures. There was moderate evidence of a typical response to acute changes in training load in the objective measures of creatine kinase, short and sustained performance. Moderate to strong evidence of responsiveness to ongoing training was found for five objective measures. Based on the results, the facets of well-being depicting vigour/motivation, physical symptoms/injury, non-training stress, fatigue, physical recovery, general health/well-being and being in shape may be useful to monitor acute changes. Furthermore, conflicts/pressure, self-regulation and lack of energy seem to be useful dimensions for ongoing training monitoring. Overall, the lack of association between subjective and objective measures provides support for the combined use.

Questionnaires

Self-report measures can be considered as a valuable source of information for sport science research as well as sport practice, since athlete monitoring has become an integral component of training and preparation. Several questionnaires are available which assess different dimensions.

One-Dimensional Measures of Stress and/or Recovery

One-item scales are economic tools to assess one dimension. Within training and exercise monitoring, the most common are *Borg's Rating of Perceived Exertion* (RPE) (Borg, 1998) and its derivate, the *Session-*RPE (Foster, 1998) to evaluate the effect of training load. The global recovery state can be assessed on a similar scale using the *Total Quality Recovery Scale* (TQR Scale) (Kenttä & Hassmén, 1998). However, this scale of perceived recovery is expanded through the TQR-*Action Scale* within the framework of Kenttä and Hassmén (1998, 2002). Athletes can collect recovery points by performing pre-defined recovery activities over a 24-h period. Actions include (a) nutrition and hydration, (b) sleep and rest, (c) relaxation and emotional support and (d) stretching and warm down. This method helps raising athletes' awareness and the promotion of adequate recovery.

Mood

Since the manifestation of the overtraining syndrome is closely connected to detecting mood disturbances, the *Profile of Mood States* (POMS) by McNair et al. (1992) is one of the most applied questionnaires in this field. Several derivatives and adaptations to the sport context exist. Originally, six mood dimensions are assessed: *tension*, *depression*, *anger*, *vigour*, *fatigue* and *confusion*.

Emotion

The *Emotional Recovery Questionnaire* (EmRecQ) was developed by Lundqvist and Kenttä (2010) to assess positively toned emotional states experienced by athletes in relation to their response to training load and recovery. In total, 22 items are rated on a 5-point rating scale describing their current state. These are summarized to the five subscales *happiness*, *security*, *harmony*, *love* and *vitality*.

Sources and Symptoms of Stress

Rushall (1990) developed a tool for measuring stress tolerance in elite athletes. The *Daily Analyses of Life Demands for Athletes* (DALDA) consists of two parts, with nine sources of life stress (Part A) and 25 symptoms of stress (Part B), which are evaluated as either (a) worse than normal, (b) normal or (c) better than normal. The need to take corrective actions is indicated by marked increases of "worse-than-normal" responses in either part of the inventory.

Multidimensional Measures of the Recovery-Stress State

The *Recovery-Stress Questionnaire for Athletes* (RESTQ-Sport) (Kellmann & Kallus, 2016) retrospectively assesses recovery activities and stressful events experienced in the past 3 days and nights. With 76 items, a comprehensive recovery-stress balance can be captured which comprises a total of 19 scales. These divide into general stress (*general stress*, *emotional stress*, *social stress*, *conflicts/pressure*, *fatigue*, *lack of energy*, *physical complaints*), general recovery (*success*, *social recovery*, *physical recovery*, *general well-being*, *sleep quality*) as well as sport-specific stress (*disturbed breaks*, *emotional exhaustion*, *injury*) and sport-specific recovery scales (*being in shape*, *personal accomplishment*, *self-efficacy*, *self-regulation*).

Another multidimensional and more economic tool is the *Acute Recovery and Stress Scale* (ARSS) (Kellmann & Kölling, 2019; Kellmann et al., 2016; Kellmann & Kölling, 2020) which consists of a 32-item adjective list. These cover the scales *physical performance capability*, *mental performance capability*, *emotional balance*, *overall recovery*, *muscular stress*, *lack of activation*, *negative emotional state* and *overall stress*. A derivative of the ARSS is the *Short Recovery and Stress Scale* (SRSS) where these eight scales are directly rated as items and the corresponding adjectives are used as descriptors. In both questionnaires, the current state is assessed on a 7-point rating scale.

24.3.4 Recovery Management in Sport

In general, recovery can be realized through either terminating or reducing stress or through change of activities (Kallus & Kellmann, 2000). Recovery needs to be tailored to the specific characteristics of the situation and adapted to current demands. But, most importantly, recovery strategies should always be implemented purposefully and in accordance with the individual's preferences. As insufficient knowledge on recovery and/or individually inadequate recovery activities as well as insufficient self-regulation are major contributors to underrecovery, these issues need to be addressed equally by athletes and coaches (Frank et al., 2018). The individual needs to be aware of the need for recovery and the main source of stress as well as to be able to identify available recovery strategies (Balk & Englert, 2020). *Self-monitoring* is, therefore, an important self-regulatory skill. Keeping a diary and using standardized questionnaires are tools to support the athlete's understanding and awareness of the interrelation between stress demands and need for recovery. In addition, cognitions and emotions need to be regulated, particularly those related to past activities. Thus, selecting and implementing an adequate recovery strategy is the initial challenge, while its initiation and effective execution may become the subsequent barrier (Beckmann & Kellmann, 2004). In many situations, *self-control* is needed to initiate appropriate recovery strategies, which even may be effortful and require additional resources (Balk & Englert, 2020). This may lead to an ironic situation. When there is an increased necessity to recover in the face of high stressors, but the likelihood to actually recover under these circumstances is reduced, Sonnentag (2018) termed this the *recovery paradox*. For instance, people may delay going to bed despite their intentions while there are no external circumstances to be made accountable for Kroes et al. (2016). To achieve high athletic goals, not only training but also recovery needs to be prioritized by the athletes as well as coaches.

At the physiological level, the concept of training periodization may be likewise applied to recovery. According to Mujika et al. (2018), withholding recovery at certain times (most commonly in preparation phase) serves to maximize adaptation to training in the long term (*chronic recovery*). In terms of *acute recovery*, increased recovery should be used to decrease acute fatigue during the competition phase or to prepare for certain training sessions.

Recovery Self-Regulation

"Recovery self-regulation can be defined as the act of identifying one's current state, one's desired future state and undertaking actions to minimize the discrepancy between both states during the recovery phase (e.g. between training sessions or competitions)" (Balk & Englert, 2020, p. 274).

❯ There is no "one-size-fits-all" approach; consideration of the sport and its demands, as well as the individual needs of the athlete, should be at the forefront when periodizing recovery (Mujika et al., 2018, p. 546).

? Depending on the main aim of the recovery activity, strategies can be differentiated on several dimensions; clear distinctions are difficult, as one strategy may fulfil several purposes on different levels at the same time:

- Regeneration and physical recovery: adequate sleep, re-hydration, nutrition, cold-water immersion, cool-down, stretching, foam rolling
- Cognitive/mental recovery: breathing techniques, power napping, imagery, relaxation techniques
- Emotional recovery: mindfulness-based practice, debriefing, expressive writing
- Social recovery: enjoyable activities with family and friends

Acute Effects of Psychological Relaxation Techniques Between Two Physical Tasks

In many sports, quick recovery is a necessity due to several competitions or training sessions within one day. Pelka et al. (2017) examined the acute effects of psychological relaxation techniques between two repeated sprint test protocols. These consisted of six sprints of 4-s duration with 20 s breaks in between, which were performed on a non-motorized treadmill. In a counterbalanced cross-over study, 27 athletic participants completed the physical tasks once per week and executed one of the five relaxation techniques in the 25-min recovery interval. The interventions included progressive muscle relaxation which consisted of a standardized protocol of tensing and relaxing specific muscle groups, a standardized yoga practice, breathing exercises where the exhalation phase was twice as long as the inhalation period (3:6 or 4:8 s rhythms) and a power nap condition. The fifth intervention was a sedentary control condition providing the possibility to read or go through a collection of comics. Each session was scheduled at the same day of the week at the same time to ensure comparable baseline conditions and to avoid distortion through chronobiological influences. Before each sprint test, a standardized warm-up procedure was applied. Following the first 6 x 4 s sprint test, participants performed additional 4 x 4 s sprints to induce fatigue.

The need for recovery was depicted in the subjective ratings (◘ Fig. 24.7). Perceived *overall recovery* declined after each sprint. On the subjective level, each recovery condition seemed to be effective, as ratings increased post-relaxation. Regarding the repeated-sprint ability, an interaction between treatment and measurement points was observed. Compared to the control condition, only breathing exercises and power napping had a positive effect on the average maximum speed in the post-relaxation repeated-sprint test. Apparently, these strategies can be applied without prior practice, and they seem to be better suited for this specific setting.

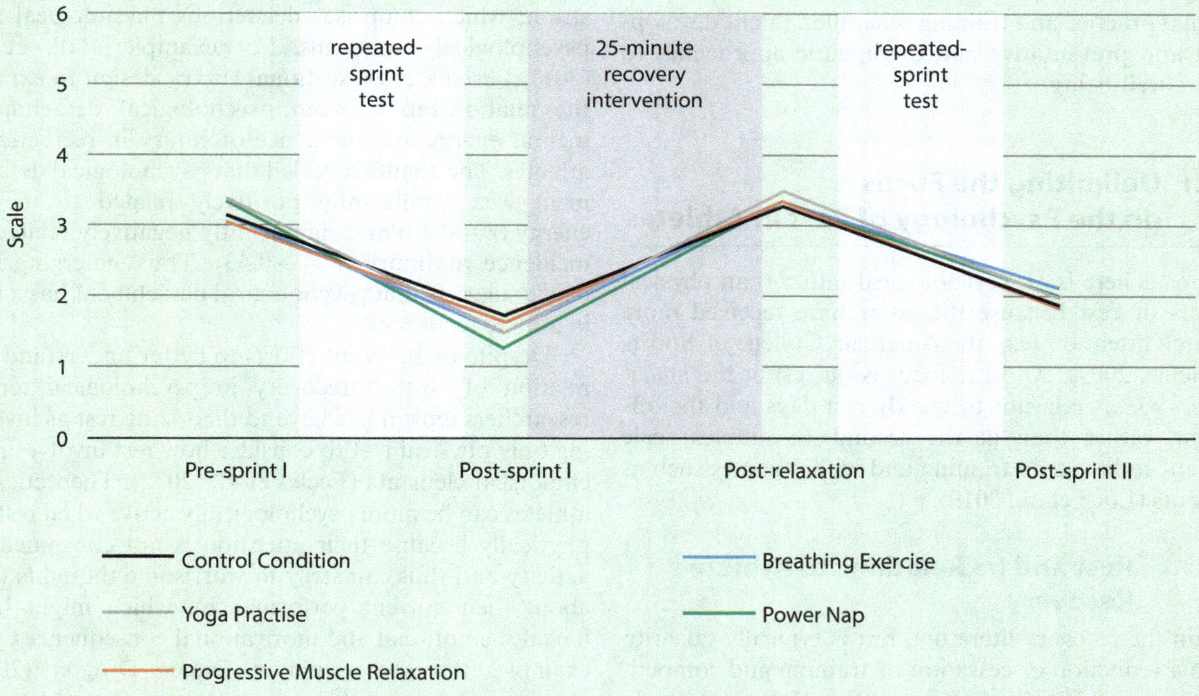

◘ **Fig. 24.7** Recovery ratings during the experimental set-up (modified and adapted from Pelka et al., 2017)

24.4 Rest

Rest appears critical to sustained high performance in sports and other human performance contexts. For example, Quarterback Brett Favre reported that he obtained needed breaks during his career by escaping from the cities in which he played to "hide" at his home in Mississippi (NFL Network, n.d.). Despite the importance placed on rest by athletes, little attention has been paid to the concept of rest and specifically to psychological aspects of rest. Rest is considered as a key component within conceptualizations of *recovery* (Kellmann et al., 2018), *motor skill learning* (Shea et al., 2000) and *expert performance* (Ericsson et al., 1993). However, rest is rarely the main focus of research on these topics. Consequently, conceptualizations of rest seldom extend beyond physical inactivity (Eccles & Riley, 2014). At the level of practice, rest is considered the most effective means to prevent and treat the overtraining and burnout syndromes (Goodger & Kentta, 2010). However, little useful information is available about the best practice concerning rest. Thus, advances in the understanding of rest will provide a stronger foundation for optimal practice and training schedules, talent development and preventative and therapeutic approaches to athlete well-being.

24.4.1 Delimiting the Focus on the Psychology of Rest in Athletes

The focus here is on psychological rather than physical aspects of rest because the latter have received more research attention (e.g. the American College of Sports Medicine, 2009). Another focus is on rest at the *hours-to-weeks scale* relevant to weekly rest days and the off-season, rather than at the seconds-to-minutes scale relevant to breaks in training and within games such as timeouts (Loch et al., 2019).

24.4.1.1 Rest and Its Relations to Athlete Recovery

Within the recovery literature, rest is typically taken to mean a reduction or cessation of training and competition activities (Eccles & Riley, 2014; Kellmann et al., 2018). In their consensus statement on recovery, Kellmann et al. (2018) propose, in a section on definitions of central terms, that rest is a "method" for achieving recovery, is a "passive" rather than "active" recovery method (e.g. cool-down jogging) and is "characterized by inactivity", where "inactivity" is implicitly considered as physical inactivity. Thus, the proposed primary function of rest within the recovery literature is to facilitate recovery from physical and psychological fatigue caused by training and competition.

However, much remains unknown about relationships between rest and recovery. Notwithstanding Kellmann's et al. (2018) definition, rest is rarely defined in the recovery literature and often conflated with recovery itself. Also, defining rest as physical inactivity is problematic because stopping physical activity does not ensure that psychological activity stops. Various sport-related stressors lead athletes to experience anxiety outside of training and competition, including during rest days (Woodman & Hardy, 2001). Traditionally, little concern has been given within sport psychology to theorizing rest as "psychological inactivity" and to pinpointing the relationship between this form of rest and athlete recovery. However, exceptions include recent research on *psychological detachment* in athletes by Balk et al. (2017a, 2017b). Psychological detachment is considered a recovery experience that involves stopping thinking about stressful elements of sport when away from sport, thoughts that would otherwise lead to strain, which comprises deleterious physiological and psychological symptoms. For example, Balk et al. (2017a) used a cross-sectional survey design to explore the relationship between psychological detachment, mental energy and incidence of injury in recreational athletes. The results revealed that psychological detachment was significantly positively related to mental energy ($r = 0.44$) and significantly negatively related to incidence of injury ($r = -0.43$). Thus, emerging evidence suggests that psychological detachment has a role in athlete recovery.

Despite these recent efforts to better understand the relation of rest to recovery in psychological terms, researchers must move beyond theorizing rest as involving only physical rest to consider how rest involves psychological elements (Eccles et al., 2022). Theoretically, athletes can be more psychologically active when resting physically because their attention is not consumed by activity and thus can stray to worrisome thoughts (e.g. about their current performance), which might have harmful emotional and motivational consequences. For example, the soccer player Didier Drogba (2015) describes in his autobiography how he thought that a vacation before an upcoming season was going to be enjoyable but in fact he spent much of the free time provided worrying about the upcoming season.

The understanding of athlete recovery also will be increased by further research on rest in the form of psychological detachment. Researchers must identify factors affecting the ease with which athletes can achieve psychological detachment.

Insights are also needed into how athletes achieve rest in the form of psychological detachment. In the absence of research in this area, researchers have presented recommendations for detachment based on lay theories; for example, Balk et al. (2017b) recommended that coaches support athletes' efforts to detach by organizing breaks in training schedules. It is possible that there are a variety of psychologically based methods of aiding psychological detachment. For example, workers who are better able to achieve a state of *mindfulness* during work are better able to psychologically detach after work (e.g. Hulsheger et al., 2014). Similarly, Kudlackova et al. (2013) showed that athletes reporting a greater use of *mental relaxation strategies* such as meditation are more likely to report being able to cope with athlete lifestyle stressors such as whether they will be picked to start, an ability consistent with the concept of psychological detachment. Future research should involve intervention studies to pinpoint psycho-regulative strategies, such as mindfulness, that promote psychological detachment in athletes following training and competition (see also ► Chap. 20).

Finally, future research should identify if rest involves any other qualities that function to enhance recovery beyond psychological detachment. Can rest be described fully as "not thinking about one's sport" (i.e. detachment), or does rest involve additional psychological states or experiences?

24.4.1.2 Rest and Its Relations to Acquiring Movement Skills

A general finding within the field of motor learning is that *distributed practice*, which involves practice sessions separated by rest periods of seconds to days, results in better learning than massed practice, which involves little or no rest between practice sessions (Shea et al., 2000). Shea et al. (2000) studied the effects of distributing practice across days, compared to within days. In one experiment, participants practised a continuous balance task during two sessions. For one group, the sessions were separated by 20 min of rest, and, for another group, the rest period between sessions was 24 h. Participants in both groups completed a retention test 24 h after the completion of the second session. The findings showed that the 24-h rest period resulted in better learning than the 20-min rest period.

A key explanation for benefits of distributed practice is better *memory consolidation* (Shea et al., 2000), which involves the neurobiological metamorphosis of memories from relatively unstable states into a more permanent form, a process lasting hours to days. New repetitions of the criterion task during this process disrupt the consolidation of the memory of the original repetition of that task, resulting in a weaker memory. However, separating two practice sessions with a rest period, during which the criterion task is not attempted, allows for memories created in the first session to be consolidated, at least in part, before the second session. Nonetheless, important questions remain about how the qualities of these rest periods affect the learning process. First, many studies of distributed practice involve rest periods containing not only wakeful rest but also sleep, which is known to promote memory consolidation for motor activity (Schmid et al., 2020). Sleep is inevitable when practice is distributed across multiple days, but there has been no research on the relative contributions of wakeful rest and sleep to the consolidation process. Such studies would have implications for understanding post-practice factors contributing to motor learning.

Second, there have been few considerations of how qualities of wakeful rest within distributed practice schedules affect motor learning. Research on effects of post-practice rest on the learning of cognitive tasks (Craig et al., 2018) has revealed that learning is greater when practice is followed immediately by a rest period that is quiet and relaxing than when it is followed by engagement in mentally effortful tasks. The proposed explanation for this *quiescent effect* is that effortful tasks disrupt memory consolidation, resulting in a poorer memory; thus, the more quiescent the rest period, the better the learning. Humiston and Wamsley (2018) recently conducted the first study of this effect in the motor domain, using a simple motor sequence task involving button-presses. The results indicated that task performance was significantly better for a quiescent condition than for a mentally effortful condition on an immediate post-test, but there was no significant difference in performance between conditions on a retention test. This result contrasts with the studies involving cognitive tasks described above, where quiescent rest benefited performance on both immediate and retention tests. However, the study by Humiston and Wamsley is the first to explore quiescent effects in the motor domain, and further research is needed to identify the extent to which the quiescent effect holds in the motor domain.

24.4.1.3 Rest and Its Relations to the Development of Expert Sports Performance

Research on the development of expert sports performance has been heavily influenced by Ericsson et al.'s (1993) *deliberate practice* framework, within which rest plays a central role. Ericsson et al. (1993) posited that "deliberate" practice is necessary to achieve expert levels in a given domain and can be differentiated from alternate practice types by its emphasis on highly focused attempt to enhance current performance. These authors also proposed a monotonic benefit assumption, which is that the amount of time an individual engages in deliberate practice is monotonically related to their acquired performance level. Thus, experts have on average accumulated more time engaged in deliberate practice than their less-skilled counterparts and typically have accumulated over a decade of such practice from childhood before reaching the expert level. Ericsson et al.'s framework also features an *effort* constraint on engaging in deliberate practice. Deliberate practice requires much effort because it places great demands on the attentional and physical systems. Therefore, daily deliberate practice must be limited to about 4 h per day, and these hours of deliberate practice must be divided into individual practice sessions of lasting no more than about 80 min. The remainder of the individual's time must be spent resting to enable complete recovery prior to the following day's engagement in deliberate practice. While researchers have applied the deliberate practice framework to the sport domain (e.g. Baker & Young, 2014; Eccles et al., 2009), their interest has concerned engagement in practice activities. In contrast, little research attention has been paid to the rest periods that necessarily accompany such practice according to the theorized effort constraint, and future research should target enhancing our understanding in this area (Eccles, 2020).

? According to the extant literature, there are three functions of rest in relation to athlete performance and well-being:

- Rest is fundamental in the process of recovery following training and competition.
- Rest facilitates learning by enhancing memory consolidation following practice of novel technical and tactical skills.
- The development of expertise depends on years of daily engagement in only a few hours of maximum-quality deliberate practice followed by many hours of resting.

24.4.2 The Eccles-Kazmier Model of the Psychology of Rest in Athletes

Eccles and Kazmier (2019) undertook a study aimed directly at understanding the psychology of rest in athletes. Given the dearth of previous research on this topic, Eccles and Kazmier worked inductively from interview data to produce a descriptive model of the psychology of rest in athletes. Specifically, these researchers interviewed all 22 members of a high-level women's field hockey squad at a UK university. The researchers used a semi-structured interview guide with open-ended questions, beginning with "What does rest mean to you?" An inductive content analysis was conducted, where the aim was to identify concepts within textual data. Concept identification was aided by informal note-taking, memo writing and construction of concept hierarchies, which were useful in understanding relationships between concepts and the overall structure and coherence of the model. As the model created constitutes an unprecedented effort at understanding the psychology of rest in athletes, we describe it here in some detail.

24.4.2.1 An Athlete's Current Level of Rest and the Process of Resting

The model distinguishes between two key concepts: (a) the extent to which an athlete currently feels rested (also referred to here as *rest level*) and (b) a *process of resting*. Athletes conceive of feeling rested as involving a physical aspect and a mental aspect, which they consider as largely independent. The primary focus in the model is on the mental aspect, which has several characteristics. Mentally rested athletes feel fresh; poorly rested athletes feel tired. Compared to poorly rested athletes, mentally rested athletes value their sport and feel more motivated to participate in their sport and accordingly apply more effort to it. Athletes enjoy their sport more when well rested than poorly rested.

An athlete's level of mental rest is increased via engagement in a process of resting, which encompasses (a) sleep and (b) resting while awake (hereon, wakeful resting). The emphasis in the model is on wakeful resting. Research indicates that wakeful resting comprises six psychological experiences, called resting experiences.

? Description of the Six Resting Experiences That Constitute the Process of Resting:

- Resting experience 1: Getting a break from always thinking about one's sport
- Resting experience 2: Getting a break from any kind of effortful thinking
- Resting experience 3: Getting a break from feeling life is controlled by one's sport
- Resting experience 4: Getting a break from the monotony of the daily routine
- Resting experience 5: Being able to catch up on important work tasks
- Resting experience 6: Being able to have a personal life outside of one's sport

Resting Experience 1: Getting a Break from Always Thinking About One's Sport

The resting experience and why it is needed. Athletes often feel like they are always thinking about their sport, especially in-season, because they feel constantly engaged in their sport. When they are not doing things directly related to their program, like training, then they are doing things to support their program activities like preparing meals and studying game plans. Constantly thinking in this way is mentally effortful, which, over time, leads athletes to feel mentally tired and in turn less motivated to engage in their sport. Thus, a psychological experience comprising the process of resting is the experience of not thinking about one's sport. Plainly, if an athlete can "switch off" from thinking about their sport for a while on a rest day, they will feel more rested for it.

Strategies that help athletes obtain this resting experience. Switching-off is aided by achieving a focus on a subject unrelated to one's sport, which makes it difficult to think concurrently about one's sport. Achieving this focus is facilitated by engaging in activities different from one's sport such as watching TV. Switching-off is also facilitated by *avoiding cues* serving as reminders of one's sport, including artefacts (e.g. sport equipment) and physical (e.g. training facilities) and social (e.g. teammates) environments. A key means of avoiding these cues is to achieve a perception of distance or escape from them, which is aided by geographically distancing oneself from the cues or "leaving town".

Resting Experience 2: Getting a Break from Any Kind of Effortful Thinking

The resting experience and why it is needed. Because always thinking about one's sport is mentally fatiguing, athletes not only need to switch off from thinking about their sport, but they also need a break from effortful thinking generally. Thus, a psychological experience comprising the process of resting is the experience of not engaging in effortful thinking. Plainly, if an athlete can spend some time on a rest day "not thinking hard", they will feel more rested for it.

Strategies that help athletes obtain this resting experience. Athletes can obtain this resting experience by engaging in activities and environments that impose few mental demands. Research indicates that *low-demand activities* undertaken by athletes on rest days to obtain mental rest include watching a favourite TV show, reading fiction, taking a bath and jogging outdoors. *Low-demand physical environments* include being at home, especially in one's own bedroom with the door closed, in nature and in relatively quiet venues such as cafes or restaurants (vs. noisy venues such as nightclubs). *Low-demand social environments* include spending time alone or with a few close friends or family, which contrasts with being with a large group of friends.

Resting Experience 3: Getting a Break from Feeling Life Is Controlled by One's Sport

The resting experience and why it is needed. Athletes often feel that their lives are controlled by their sport. They must adhere to fixed schedules of training sessions and meetings and coach-imposed guidelines on eating, sleeping and socializing. These experiences of being controlled are detrimental to feeling well rested because athletes want to feel they have control over their lives. Perceptions of being controlled therefore reduce their motivation to engage in their program. Thus, a key psychological experience that comprises the process of resting is the experience of assuming increased *control* over one's life. Plainly, if an athlete can spend some time on a rest day doing what they want, and without regard for any external commitments, they will feel more rested for it.

Strategies that help athletes obtain this resting experience. Busy sport and study or work commitments provide few opportunities for athletes to feel free from external commitments, especially during the season. However, in our research, athletes have reported *planning ahead* so that rest days include a period of "me time" during which the athlete can do what they want and when they want. Athletes often spend at least some of this time alone, in part because this removes obligations to consider others' needs, which further heightens feelings of control.

Resting Experience 4: Getting a Break from the Monotony of the Daily Routine

The resting experience and why it is needed. Athletes spend much time in-season following the same routines. They walk or drive the same routes to training, operate in the same venues (e.g. gym) and train, socialize and even reside with the same people: teammates and coaches. These invariant routines become monotonous, which is detrimental to feeling rested. Thus, a psychological experience comprising the process of resting is the experience of *variety* in one's routines and physical and social environments. Plainly, if an athlete can spend some time on their rest day doing something different from normal, in a location different from normal and with people different from normal, they will feel more rested for it.

Strategies that help athletes obtain this resting experience. In our research, athletes have described deliberate attempts to "break the monotony" by switching up their normal routines. Examples of switching-up activities include reading a fiction book for leisure and going shopping. Examples of switching-up locations include jogging on a different route and taking a day trip to a new location. Examples of switching-up people include meeting with friends they see less often than their teammates.

Resting Experience 5: Being Able to Catch Up on Important Work Tasks

The resting experience and why it is needed. Due to sport commitments, athletes often feel unable to pay enough attention to work tasks outside their sport, such as paid work, studying and chores. Athletes feel stress when unable to attend to work tasks, particularly when these tasks have deadlines and their completion is repeatedly postponed due to sport commitments. These experiences of stress are detrimental to feeling rested. Thus, a psychological experience comprising the process of resting is the experience of removing this form of stress, and the athlete can only remove this form of stress by completing their outstanding work tasks. Plainly, if an athlete gets an opportunity on a rest day to complete a postponed work task that has become "a weight on their mind", they will feel more rested for it.

Strategies that help athletes obtain this resting experience. In our research, athletes have reported deliberately scheduling time and then carefully protecting this *scheduled time*, early on a rest day to complete a pressing work task that has been postponed due to sport commitment. This strategy enables athletes to remove this "weight from their mind" and thus feel more rested. Doing work tasks early on a rest day removes these "weights" early in the day, allowing athletes to obtain other resting experiences more easily later in the day. For example, attempts to obtain a break from an effortful thinking by jogging outdoors will be less effective if an outstanding work task is weighing on your mind during the jog.

Resting Experience 6: Being Able to Have a Personal Life Outside of One's Sport

The resting experience and why it is needed. Athletes often feel they do not have enough of a personal life outside of sport. Due to their sport commitments, they cannot spend the time they want with friends and family, and engaged in hobbies, which leads to frustration. These experiences of frustration are detrimental to feeling rested. Thus, a key psychological experience comprising the process of resting is the experience of removing these frustrations, and the athlete can only remove these frustrations by *indulging their personal life*. Plainly, if an athlete gets the opportunity on a rest day to do a personal activity that they have become frustrated about not being able to do due to their sport, they will feel more rested for it.

Strategies that help athletes obtain this resting experience. In our research, athletes have reported deliberately scheduling time and then carefully protecting this scheduled time, on a rest day to engage in personal activities. This strategy enables athletes to reduce frustrations associated with feeling that they cannot have a personal life outside of sport, which makes them feel more rested.

Putting Wakeful Resting Experiences Together to Illustrate Ineffective and Effective Mental Resting: Examples with Student-Athletes

Consider these prototypical cases of two student-athletes, Jacque and Dorothy, who spend an in-season rest day in different ways.

Jacque's rest day. Over breakfast, Jacque reads news about his sport and interacts with teammates via social media. He leaves home for a team meeting at his gym. The meeting was called at short notice by his coach, which meant Jacque needed to postpone facetiming an old friend. Jacque drives to the gym via his usual route. In the meeting, his coach asks the team to solve a problem they have on offense. The team cannot fix the problem during the meeting, so the coach asks the team to consider the problem overnight and revisit it at morning training. Jacque thinks about the problem while driving home and getting ready for a team night out. He meets his teammates for dinner, and they go on to a nightclub.

Why Jacque's rest day is ineffective. Let us interpret this day using the wakeful resting experiences outlined above. First, Jacque had few opportunities to stop thinking about his sport during his rest day; for much of the day, he was focused on his sport and surrounded by cues to think about his sport (e.g. sport news, social media, teammates, coaches, gym). Second, the offense problem involved effortful thinking and left little time for low-demand activities, and his night out with a large group of friends, while fun, was not a low-demand activity. Third, the meeting and subsequent directive to think about the offense problem meant that part of the day was controlled by his program; Jacque had relatively few opportunities to do exactly what he wanted. Fourth, he followed a regular routine by driving to and from and spending time at his gym, and his only companions during the day were his coaches and teammates; opportunities for variety were few. Finally, Jacque was eager to facetime his old friend, but this personal activity was postponed due to a sporting commitment, which enhanced (vs. reduced) frustrations around not having enough of a personal life.

Dorothy's rest day. Dorothy drives early to a cafe she does not normally visit to work on a school project with an imminent deadline. Dorothy has been itching to work on the project but has not been able to due to her busy competitive schedule. Dorothy had planned after completing this work to "take some time off" before meeting a friend later in the day. So, on her drive home from the cafe, she decides on impulse to stop at a park she has been meaning to check out and take a walk on the park trails. Getting home, she puts her smartphone away and spends the afternoon in her bedroom catching up on a favourite TV show unrelated to her sport. Later, she meets a good friend who does not play her sport at a restaurant she has been wanting to try. The two friends then go bowling, which is not Dorothy's sport.

Why Dorothy's rest day provides her with considerable mental rest. In contrast to Jacque, Dorothy's day involved activities unrelated to her sport, which reduced opportunities to think about this sport. She also did not visit her training facility or spend time with coaches or teammates and even put away her phone for a while, thereby avoiding cues to think about her sport. Following her early work on the application, she got a break from effortful thinking by spending time doing activities (walk, TV, dinner with a good friend, bowling) and in environments (nature, bedroom, restaurant) imposing few cognitive demands. Dorothy took advantage of some scheduled time to do just what she wanted (walk, TV), thereby achieving a break from feeling controlled. She broke up her usual routines and experienced some variety by going to different venues (cafe, park, restaurant) and with different people (her non-sport friend). Finally, Dorothy got a pressing work item out of the way, reducing her stress over this, and spent time on a favourite TV show and catching up with a friend, which reduced frustrations around not having enough of a personal life.

24.4.2.2 Implications of the Eccles-Kazmier Model for Theory

The Eccles and Kazmier (2019) model of the psychology of rest has implications for key theories in sport psychology and thus for future research in this area. For example, theories of recovery should consider that recovery depends not only on a process of resting physically, which is the traditional focus within the recovery literature, but also on a process of resting mentally. Second, this mental resting process not only involves sleep, another traditional focus of the recovery literature, but also wakeful resting involving specific resting experiences. Third, the functions of rest extend beyond promoting recovery from training- and competition-induced physical and psychological fatigue, which has been the function of traditional focus within the recovery literature. One additional function of rest is to afford athletes' perceptions of internal control, which helps alleviate athletes of frustrations arising from perceptions of enduring external control by their sport program. Thus, theories of recovery might need to be revised to include multiple psychological processes: Recovery might involve both resource restoration following mental fatigue (Loch et al., 2019) and psychological need satisfaction following frustration of the need for autonomy (Ryan & Deci, 2000). Research is now needed to establish the generalizability of the model proposed by Eccles and Kazmier given that athletes in their study were female, collegiate and from one country.

24.4.3 Why Has Rest Been Overlooked?

First, rest might be overlooked due to a natural tendency to focus on the physical actions of athletes because physical action is a fundamental component of sport and typically what makes sport exciting. In contrast, rest, which is traditionally considered to involve physical inactivity, is of little inherent interest. Second, competition outcomes (e.g. goals), which are important to all sport stakeholders, are readily apparent as the direct consequences of physical actions taken during competitions. By comparison, engagement in rest occurs some hours before and after a competition, and some distance away from the competition venue. Thus, it might be relatively unapparent that competition outcomes depend in part on rest. Third, relative to rest, the physical actions inherent to sport might be considered observable and concrete and thus lend themselves to definition and measurement, whereas rest is a less tangible concept, and behaviors associated with rest as more covert, happening often literally behind closed doors (Eccles et al., 2021). These qualities make rest appear challenging to understand and research. Fourth, it is equally plausible that rest is considered as simple and self-explanatory, which deemphasizes the need for an analysis of this concept.

Fifth, rest is undervalued at cultural and societal levels. Cultural norms and values operate subconsciously to influence attitudes, emotions and behaviors of members of these cultures (Tibbert et al., 2015). The pressures for sport organizations to deliver results have spawned a sport subculture characterized by a "performance narrative" (Douglas & Carless, 2015), which places much value on relentless effort and resilience, which in turn fosters a quantity-over-quality approach training (Coulter et al., 2016). Athletes operating within these subcultures may feel that their willingness to adopt these values is being monitored by their sport organization and failures to adopt them will be punished (Manley et al., 2016). These pressures can lead athletes to eschew rest and engage in extra training, with deleterious consequences for performance and well-being (Brustad & Ritter-Taylor, 1997).

Sport subcultures are located within larger societies, and thus the values held within sport subcultures may be extensions of values inherent within these societies (Coulter et al., 2016). Researchers in various disciplines have proposed that rest is undervalued within contemporary societies, which instead place much value on being busy and hard-working (Bellezza et al., 2017). This value system has been attributed to broader historical cultural influences including religions within which hard work is considered virtuous (Weber, 1930). These influences also include social reactions to traditional hierarchical class systems, which have spawned anti-elitist attitudes that promote the need for individuals to demonstrate membership of an "everyman" class by being a "man of action" (Rigney, 1991). In addition, meritocratic socio-political ideologies that stress individual agency and responsibility have fostered notions that "exceptionally lofty goals are… well within reach" for all, striving towards lofty goals is highly valued, goals are obtained via hard work and failure is temporary and overcome by working harder still (Luthar & Kumar, 2018).

Five reasons why rest has been overlooked:

- There is a natural tendency to focus on action over inaction.
- Competition outcomes (e.g. goals) apparent as direct consequences of physical actions.
- Rest occurs covertly, making it challenging to research.
- Rest is considered as simple and self-explanatory.
- Rest is undervalued at cultural and societal levels.

24.4.4 Implications for Practice

The extant research on the psychology of rest in athletes provides an initial foundation for deriving strategies for the best practice. These strategies should be viewed cautiously because research is needed to test their efficacy in applied settings. Nonetheless, in the meantime, practitioners will benefit from considering how these strategies can inform their work.

In relation to recovery, we propose four principles for consideration. First, recovery does not just involve recovering physically; it involves recovering mentally. Second, providing physical rest days (i.e. a break from physical training) does not guarantee athletes the mental rest they need (e.g. stopping thinking about sport). Third, athletes can achieve the mental rest they need if they have the time, and can obtain the social and physical environmental conditions, required for high-quality (a) sleep and (b) wakeful resting. Fourth, high-quality wakeful resting involves specific resting experiences, as discussed above.

In relation to motor learning, memory consolidation following the practice of novel tasks appears to be facilitated by immediate post-task activities imposing low (vs. high) cognitive demands. Therefore, practitioners should avoid creating a schedule whereby practice sessions focused on learning new technical and tactical game skills are immediately followed by other forms of demanding mental activity (e.g. game film analysis, studying). By contrast, learning may benefit from explicitly scheduling low-demand activities (e.g. taking a quiet bath) for at least 15 min following such practice.

Practitioners should avoid using narratives that devalue rest and should challenge others' use of them. Examples include "rest is not for the dead; rest is for the smart". Practitioners should also avoid simplistic descriptions of the value of (a) extensive practice (e.g. Ericsson et al., 1993), (b) attributing gains to outstanding effort rather than talent (e.g. Dweck, 2006) and (c) being highly mentally resilient and tough (e.g. Bryan et al., 2019). Research on these concepts indicates that "more is not better". For example, expert performance in sport is theorized to be developed by engaging daily in a limited period of high-quality practice that is followed by extensive rest (Ericsson et al., 1993).

Conclusions

The Complex Field of Sleep, Recovery and Rest in Sports

While sleep can be considered as universal human requirement, its implementation and conditions are highly individual making it a challenging issue for elite athletes. Considering that the need for sleep and the response to training stimuli as well as to sleep loss are inter-individually different, practitioners should generally prefer an individual approach to sleep promotion interventions (Fullagar & Bartlett, 2016). Regular monitoring of sleep behavior (objective as well as subjective assessment) and routine assessment of training parameters and recovery-stress responses are, therefore, important in elite sports (Heidari et al. 2018). On the one hand, this allows for detecting irregularities (e.g. due to travel or illness) and deriving interventions at an early stage. On the other hand, implementation of recovery modalities and sleep management strategies can be evaluated. Moreover, feedback of the data can be used to coach the athletes in terms of the importance of regular sleep habits and increasing awareness of the mutual relationship between training stress and sufficient recovery.

Recovery constitutes an umbrella term to describe different modalities of waking activities which serve the restoration of resources on physiological as well as psychological levels. As training and life stress can accumulate from acute fatigue over functional and non-functional overreaching to underrecovery and the development of the overtraining syndrome, appropriate and timely recovery has to take place. Monitoring the recovery-stress state is a useful method to observe and manage the balance between current demands and the psycho-physiological well-being of athletes. Recovery activities need to match with the characteristics of the specific situation and the individual preferences. Knowledge on recovery and self-regulatory skills, such as self-monitoring and self-control, are important requirements for the selection and implementation of recovery activities.

The extant literature indicates that there are at least three possible functions of rest in relation to athlete performance and well-being. First, rest is fundamental in the process of recovery following training and competition. Second, rest facilitates learning by enhancing memory consolidation following practice of novel technical and tactical skills. Third, the development of expertise depends on years of daily engagement in only a few hours of maximum-quality deliberate practice followed by many hours of resting. In addition, recent research aimed at understanding the nature of rest suggests that recovery does not just involve recovering physically; it involves recovering mentally. In addition, providing physical rest days (i.e. a break from physical training) does not guarantee athletes the mental rest they need (e.g. stopping thinking about sport). This research also indicates that athletes can achieve the mental rest they need if they have the time and can obtain the social and physical environmental conditions, required for high-quality (a) sleep and (b) wakeful resting, where high-quality wakeful resting involves specific resting experiences.

Learning Control Questions

Basic:

1. Name different methods for sleep.
2. Name the different stages of sleep.
3. How and why do sleep durations change over the life span?

Advanced:

4. Name and explain different sleep-promoting activities for athletes.
5. Why is recovery important for an athlete's health and well-being?
6. Name and explain different recovery dimensions and techniques.
7. What is the difference between recovery and rest?

Experts:

8. Explain mental rest and give examples for mental rest strategies.
9. What are the benefits of rest? How does rest affect an athlete's performance?

References

AASM (Ed.). (2008). *Das AASM-Manual zum Scoring von Schlaf und assoziierten Ereignissen: Regeln, Technologie und technische Spezifikationen [The AASM manual for scoring sleep and associated events: Rules, technology, and technical specifications]*. Steinkopff.

Altfeld, S., & Kellmann, M. (2014). Underrecovery syndrome. In R. C. Eklund & G. Tenenbaum (Eds.), *Encyclopedia of sport and exercise psychology* (pp. 773–775). Sage.

American College of Sports Medicine. (2009). American College of Sports Medicine position stand. Progression models in resistance training for healthy adults. *Medicine and Science in Sports and Exercise, 41*, 687–708. https://doi.org/10.1249/MSS.0b013e3181915670

Baker, J., & Young, B. W. (2014). 20 years later: Deliberate practice and the development of expertise in sport. *International Review of Sport & Exercise Psychology, 7*, 135–157. https://doi.org/10.1080/1750984X.2014.896024

Balk, Y. A., & Englert, C. (2020). Recovery self-regulation in sport: Theory, research, and practice. *International Journal of Sports Science and Coaching*. https://doi.org/10.1177/1747954119897528

Balk, Y. A., de Jonge, J., Oerlemans, W. G. M., & Geurts, S. A. E. (2017a). Physical recovery, mental detachment and sleep as predictors of injury and mental energy. *Journal of Health Psychology*, 24, 1828–1838. https://doi.org/10.1177/1359105317705980

Balk, Y. A., de Jonge, J., Oerlemans, W. G. M., & Geurts, S. A. E. (2017b). Testing the triple-match principle among Dutch elite athletes: A day-level study on sport demands, detachment, and recovery. *Psychology of Sport and Exercise, 33*, 7–17. https://doi.org/10.1016/j.psychsport.2017.7.006

Beckmann, J., & Kellmann, M. (2004). Self-regulation and recovery: Approaching an understanding of the process of recovery from stress. *Psychological Reports, 95*, 1135–1153.

Bellezza, S., Paharia, N., & Keinan, A. (2017). Conspicuous consumption of time: When busyness and lack of leisure time become a status symbol. *Journal of Consumer Research, 44*, 118–138. https://doi.org/10.1093/jcr/ucw076

Birrer, D. (2019). Rowing over the edge: Nonfunctional overreaching and overtraining syndrome as maladjustment—Diagnosis and treatment from a psychological perspective. *Case Studies in Sport and Enxercise Psychology, 3*, 50–60. https://doi.org/10.1123/cssep.2019-0006

Birrer, D., Röthlin, P., & Morgan, G. (2012). Mindfulness to enhance athletic perforance: Theoretical considerations and possible impact mechanisms. *Mindfulness, 3*, 235–246. https://doi.org/10.1007/s12671-012-0109-2

Bishop, P. A., Jones, E., & Woods, A. K. (2008). Recovery from training: A brief review. *Journal of Strength Conditioning Research, 22*, 1015–1024. https://doi.org/10.1519/JSC.0b013e31816eb518

Bonnar, D., Bartel, K., Kakoschke, N., & Lang, C. (2018). Sleep interventions designed to improve athletic performance and recovery: A systematic review of current approaches. *Sports Medicine, 48*, 683–703.

Borbély, A. A., Daan, S., Wirz-Justice, A., & Deboer, T. (2016). The two-process model of sleep regulation: A reappraisal. *Journal of Sleep Research, 25*(2), 131–143. https://doi.org/10.1111/jsr.12371

Borg, G. (1998). *Borg's Perceived Exertion and Pain Scale*. Human Kinetics.

Bourdon, P. C., Cardinale, M., Murray, A., Gastin, P. B., Kellmann, M., Varley, M. C., Gabbett, T. J., Coutts, A. J., Burgess, D. J., Gregson, W., & Cable, N. T. (2017). Monitoring athlete training loads: Consensus statement. *International Journal of Sports Physiology and Performance, 12*(S2), 161–170. https://doi.org/10.1123/IJSPP.2017-0208

Brustad, R. J., & Ritter-Taylor, M. (1997). Applying social psychological perspectives to the sport psychology consultancy process. *The Sport Psychologist, 11*, 107–119. https://doi.org/10.1123/tsp.11.1.107

Bryan, C., O'Shea, D., & MacIntyre, T. (2019). Stressing the relevance of resilience: A systematic review of resilience across the domains of sport and work. *International Review of Sport and Exercise Psychology, 12*, 70–111. https://doi.org/10.1080/1750984X.2017.1381140

Buysse, D. J., Reynolds, C. F., Monk, T. H., Berman, S. R., & Kupfer, D. J. (1989). The Pittsburgh Sleep Quality Index: A new instrument for psychiatric practice and research. *Psychiatric Research, 28*, 193–213.

Caia, J., Kelly, V. G., & Halson, S. L. (2018). The role of sleep in maximising performance in elite athletes. In M. Kellmann & J. Beckmann (Eds.), *Sport, recovery and performance: Interdisciplinary insights* (pp. 151–167). Routledge.

Chennaoui, M., Arnal, P. J., Sauvet, F., & Leger, D. (2015). Sleep and exercise: A reciprocal issue? *Sleep Medicine Reviews, 20*, 59–72. https://doi.org/10.1016/j.smrv.2014.06.008

Coulter, T. J., Mallett, C. J., & Singer, J. A. (2016). A subculture of mental toughness in an Australian Football League club. *Psychology of Sport and Exercise, 22*, 98–113. https://doi.org/10.1016/j.psychsport.2015.06.007

Craig, M., Ottoway, G., & Dewar, M. (2018). Rest on it: Awake quiescence facilitates insight. *Cortex, 109*, 205–214. https://doi.org/10.1016/j.cortex.2018.09.009

Douglas, K., & Carless, D. (2015). *Life story research in sport. Understanding the experiences of elite and professional athletes through narrative*. Routledge.

Dresler, M., Erlacher, D., Czisch, M., & Spoormaker, V. I. (2016). Lucid dreaming. In M. Kryger, T. Roth, & W. C. Dement (Eds.), *Principles and practice of sleep medicine* (6th ed., pp. 539–545). Elsevier.

Driller, M., Mah, C., & Halson, S. (2018). Development of the athlete sleep behavior questionnaire: A tool for identifying maladaptive sleep practices in elite athletes. *Sleep Science, 11*, 37–44.

Drogba, D. (2015). *Commitment: My autobiography*. Hodder and Stoughton.

Duffield, R., & Fowler, P. (2018). Domestic and international travel: Implications for performance and recovery in team-sport athletes. In M. Kellmann & J. Beckmann (Eds.), *Sport, recovery, and performance: Interdisciplinary insights* (pp. 183–197). Routledge.

Dweck, C. S. (2006). *Mindset: The new psychology of success*. Random House.

Eccles, D. W., & Riley, K. (2014). Rest. In R. C. Eklund & G. Tenenbaum (Eds.), *Encyclopedia of sport and exercise psychology* (pp. 598–600). Sage.

Eccles, D. W. (2020). Expertise: The state of the art. In G. Tenenbaum & R. C. Eklund (Eds.), *Handbook of sport psychology* (Vol. 1, 4th ed., pp. 467–486). Wiley.

Eccles, D. W., & Kazmier, A. (2019). The psychology of rest in athletes: An empirical study and initial model. *Psychology of Sport and Exercise, 44*, 90–98. https://doi.org/10.1016/j.psychsport.2019.05.007

Eccles, D. W., Balk, Y., Gretton, T., & Harris, N. (2022). "The forgotten session": Advancing research and practice concerning the psychology of rest in athletes. Journal of Applied Sport Psychology, 34(1), 3–24. https://doi.org/10.1080/10413200.2020.1756526.

Eccles, D. W., Kazmier, A., & Erhardt, A. (2021). Solitude as means of obtaining mental rest in skilled athlete populations. In R. J. Coplan, J. C. Bowker, & L. J. Nelson (Eds.), *The handbook of solitude: Psychological perspectives on social isolation, social withdrawal, and being alone* (2nd ed.) (pp. 280−293). Wiley.

Eccles, D. W., Ward, P., & Woodman, T. (2009). The role of competition-specific preparation in expert sport performance. *Psychology of Sport and Exercise, 10*, 96–107.

Ehrlenspiel, F., Erlacher, D., & Ziegler, M. (2018). Changes in subjective sleep quality before a competition and their relation to competitive anxiety. *Behavioral Sleep Medicine, 16*(6), 553–568. https://doi.org/10.1080/15402002.2016.1253012

Ericsson, K. A., Krampe, R. T., & Tesch-Romer, C. (1993). The role of deliberate practice in the acquisition of expert performance. *Psychological Review, 100*, 363–406. https://doi.org/10.1037/0033-295X.100.3.363

Erlacher, D. (2019). *Sport und Schlaf. Angewandte Schlafforschung für die Sportwissenschaft [Sport and sleep. Applied sleep research for sports science]*. Springer.

Erlacher, D., & Ehrlenspiel, F. (2018). Sleep, dreams, and athletic performance. In M. Kellmann & J. Beckmann (Eds.), *Sport, recovery, and performance: Interdisciplinary insights* (pp. 168–182). Routledge.

Erlacher, D., & Schredl, M. (2004). Dreams reflecting waking sport activities: A comparison of sport and psychology students. *International Journal of Sport Psychology, 35*(4), 301–308.

Erlacher, D., & Schredl, M. (2008a). Cardiovascular responses to dreamed physical exercise during REM lucid dreaming. *Dreaming, 18*, 112–121.

Erlacher, D., & Schredl, M. (2008b). Do REM (lucid) dreamed and executed actions share the same neural substrate? *International Journal of Dream Research, 1*(1), 7–13.

Erlacher, D., & Stumbrys, T. (2020). Wake up, work on dreams, back to bed and lucid dream: A sleep laboratory study. *Frontiers in Psychology, 11*(1383). https://doi.org/10.3389/fpsyg.2020.01383

Erlacher, D., Ehrlenspiel, F., & Schredl, M. (2011a). Frequency of nightmares and gender significantly predict distressing dreams of German athletes before competitions or games. *The Journal of Psychology, 145*(4), 331–342. https://doi.org/10.1080/00223980.2011.574166

Erlacher, D., Ehrlenspiel, F., Adegbesan, O., & Galal El-Din, H. (2011b). Sleep habits in German athletes before important competitions or games. *Journal of Sports Sciences, 29*(8), 859–866. https://doi.org/10.1080/02640414.2011.565782

Erlacher, D., Schredl, M., Ehrlenspiel, F., & Bosing, M. (2009). Subjective sleep quality and state anxiety of high-school students prior to a final sport exam. In A. M. Columbus (Ed.), *Advances in psychology research* (pp. 179–186). Nova Science Publishers.

Erlacher, D., Stumbrys, T., & Schredl, M. (2012). Frequency of lucid dreams and lucid dream practice in German athletes. *Imagination, Cognition and Personality, 31*(3), 237–246. https://doi.org/10.2190/IC.31.3.f

Foster, C. (1998). Monitoring training in athletes with reference to overtraining syndrome. *Medicine and Science in Sports and Exercise, 30*, 1164–1168.

Fowler, P. M., Duffield, R., & Vaile, J. (2015). Effects of simulated domestic and international air travel on sleep, performance, and recovery for team sports. *Scandinavian Journal of Medicine and Science in Sports, 25*(3), 441–451. https://doi.org/10.1111/sms.12227

Frank, R., Nixdorf, I., & Beckmann, J. (2018). Stress, underrecovery, and health problems in athletes. In M. Kellmann & J. Beckmann (Eds.), *Sport, recovery, and performance: Interdisciplinary insights* (pp. 119–131). Routledge.

Fullagar, H. H. K., & Bartlett, J. D. (2016). Time to wake up: Individualising the approach to sleep promotion interventions. *British Journal of Sports Medicine, 50*, 143–144.

Fullagar, H. K., Skorski, S., Duffield, R., Hammes, D., Coutts, A., & Meyer, T. (2015). Sleep and athletic performance: The effects of sleep loss on exercise performance, and physiological and cognitive responses to exercise. *Sports Medicine, 45*, 161–186.

Gardner, F. L., & Moore, Z. E. (2017). Mindfulness-based and acceptance-based interventions in sport and performance contexts. *Current Opinion in Psychology, 16*, 180–184. https://doi.org/10.1016/j.copsyc.2017.06.001

Goodger, K., & Kentta, G. (2010). Professional practice issues in athlete burnout. In S. Hanton & S. Mellalieu (Eds.), *Professional practice in sport psychology: A review* (pp. 133–165). Routledge.

Görtelmeyer, R. (2011). *SF-A/R und SF-B/R. Schlaffragebogen A und B. Revidierte Fassung [SF-A/R and SF-B/R. Sleep questionnaires A and B. Revised version]*. Göttingen: Hogrefe.

Gupta, L., Morgan, K., & Gilchrist, S. (2017). Does elite sport degrade sleep quality? A systematic review. *Sports Medicine, 47*, 1317–1333.

Halson, S. L. (2014). Sleep in elite athletes and nutritional interventions to enhance sleep. *Sports Medicine, 44*(Suppl. 1), S13–S23.

Hanin, Y. L. (2000). Individual Zones of Optimal Functioning model: Emotion-performance relationships in sport. In Y. L. Hanin (Ed.), *Emotions in sport* (pp. 65–89). Human Kinetics.

Hausswirth, C., & Mujika, I. (2013). *Recovery for performance in sport*. Human Kinetics.

Hayes, S. C. (2004). Acceptance and Commitment Therapy, Relational Frame Theory, and the Third Wave of Behavioral and Cognitive Therapies. *Behavior Therapy, 35*, 639–665. https://doi.org/10.1016/j.beth.2016.11.006

Heidari, J., Kölling, S., Pelka, M., & Kellmann, M. (2018). Monitoring the recovery-stress state in athletes. In M. Kellmann & J. Beckmann (Eds.), Sport, recovery, performance. *Interdisciplinary insights* (pp. 3–18). Routledge.

Heidari, J., & Kellmann, M. (2019). Recovery. In D. Hackfort, R. J. Schinke, & B. Strauss (Eds.), *Dictionary of sport psychology* (pp. 242–243). Elsevier Inc.

Hirshkowitz, M., Whiton, K., Albert, S. M., Alessi, C., Bruni, O., DonCarlos, L., et al. (2015). National Sleep Foundation's updated sleep duration recommendations: Final report. *Sleep Health, 1*, 233–243. https://doi.org/10.1016/j.sleh.2015.10.004

Hoshikawa, M., Uchida, S., Ganeko, M., Sumitomo, J., Totoki, M., Kojima, T., et al. (2014). Sleep quality under mild hypoxia in men with low hypoxic ventilatory response. *European Journal of Sport Science, 14*(Suppl 1), S205–S212. https://doi.org/10.1080/17461391.2012.681805

Hulsheger, U. R., Lang, J. W. B., Depenbrock, F., Fehrmann, C., Zijlstra, F. R. H., & Alberts, H. J. E. M. (2014). The power of presence: The role of mindfulness at work for daily levels and change trajectories of psychological detachment and sleep quality. *Journal of Applied Psychology, 99*, 1113–1128. https://doi.org/10.1037/a0037702

Humiston, G. B., & Wamsley, E. J. (2018). A brief period of eyes-closed rest enhances motor skill consolidation. *Neurobiology of Learning and Memory, 155*, 1–6. https://doi.org/10.1016/j.nlm.2018.06.002

Iber, C., Ancoli-Israel, S., Chesson, A., & Quan, S. F. (Eds.). (2007). *The AASM manual for the scoring of sleep and associated events: Rules, terminology and technical specifications* (1st ed.). American Academy of Sleep Medicine.

Irish, L. A., Kline, C. E., Gunn, H. E., Buysse, D. J., & Hall, M. H. (2015). The role of sleep hygiene in promoting public health: A review of empirical evidence. *Sleep Medicine Reviews, 22*, 23–36.

ICSD-3. (2014). *International Classification of sleep disorders* (3rd ed.). American Academy of Sleep Medicine.

Juliff, L. E., Halson, S. L., & Peiffer, J. J. (2015). Understanding sleep disturbance in athletes prior to important competitions. *Journal of Science and Medicine in Sport, 18*(1), 13–18. https://doi.org/10.1016/j.jsams.2014.02.007

Kallus, K. W., & Kellmann, M. (2000). Burnout in athletes and coaches. In Y. L. Hanin (Ed.), *Emotions in sport* (pp. 209–230). Human Kinetics.

Kellmann, M., & Kallus, K. W. (2016). The recovery-stress questionnaire for athletes. In K. W. Kallus & M. Kellmann (Eds.), *The recovery-stress questionnaires: User manual* (pp. 89–134). Pearson.

Kellmann, M., & Kölling, S. (2019). *Recovery and stress in sport: A manual for testing and assessment*. Routledge.

Kellmann, M., & Kölling, S. (2020). *Das Akutmaß und die Kurzskala zur Erfassung von Erholung und Beanspruchung für Erwachsene und Kinder/Jugendliche [The Acute Measure and the Short Scale of Recovery and Stress for Adults and Children/Adolescents]*. Sportverlag Strauß.

Kellmann, M. (2002). Underrecovery and overtraining: Different concepts—Similar impact? In M. Kellmann (Ed.), *Enhancing recovery: Preventing underperformance in athletes* (pp. 3–24). Human Kinetics.

Kellmann, M., Bertollo, M., Bosquet, L., Brink, M., Coutts, A. J., Duffield, R., et al. (2018). Recovery and performance in sport: Consensus statement. *International Journal of Sports Physiology and Performance, 13*, 240–245. https://doi.org/10.1123/ijspp.2017-0759

Kellmann, M., Kölling, S., & Hitzschke, B. (2016). *Das Akutmaß und die Kurzskala zur Erfassung von Erholung und Beanspruchung im Sport—Manual [The Acute and the Short Recovery and Stress Scale for Sports—Manual]*. Sportverlag Strauß.

Kenttä, G., & Hassmén, P. (1998). Overtraining and recovery. A conceptual model. *Sports Medicine, 26*, 1–16.

Torkild, G., & Hassmén, P. (2002). Underrecovery and overtraining: A conceptual model. In M. Kellmann (Ed.), *Enhancing recovery: Preventing underperformance in athletes* (pp. 57–79). Human Kinetics.

Kölling, S., & Kellmann, M. (2019). Regeneration. In D. Hackfort, R. J. Schinke, & B. Strauss (Eds.), *Dictionary of sport psychology* (pp. 245–246). Elsevier Inc.

Kölling, S., Duffield, R., Erlacher, D., Venter, R., & Halson, S. L. (2019). Sleep-related issues for recovery and performance in athletes. *International Journal of Sports Physiology & Performance, 14*(2), 144–148. https://doi.org/10.1123/ijspp.2017-0746

Kölling, S., Steinacker, J. M., Endler, S., Ferrauti, A., Meyer, T., & Kellmann, M. (2016a). The longer the better: Sleep–wake patterns during preparation of the World Rowing Junior Championships. *Chronobiology International, 33*, 73–84.

Kölling, S., Wiewelhove, T., Raeder, C., Endler, S., Ferrauti, A., Meyer, T., & Kellmann, M. (2016b). Sleep monitoring of a six-day microcycle in strength and high-intensity training. *European Journal of Sport Science, 16*, 507–515.

Kroes, F. M., Evers, C., Adriaanse, M. A., & de Ridder, D. T. D. (2016). Bedtime procrastination: A self-regulation perspective on sleep insufficiency in the general population. *Journal of Health Psychology, 21*, 853–862. https://doi.org/10.1177/1359105314540014

Krueger, J. M., Frank, M. G., Wisor, J. P., & Roy, S. (2016). Sleep function: Toward elucidating an enigma. *Sleep Medicine Reviews, 28*, 46–54.

Kudlackova, K., Eccles, D. W., & Dieffenbach, K. (2013). Use of relaxation skills by differentially skilled athletes. *Psychology of Sport and Exercise, 14*, 468–475. https://doi.org/10.1016/j.psychsport.2

Lastella, M., Lovell, G. P., & Sargent, C. (2014). Athletes' precompetitive sleep behaviour and its relationship with subsequent precompetitive mood and performance. *European Journal of Sport Science, 14*(sup1), S123–S130. https://doi.org/10.1080/17461391.2012.660505

Lastella, M., Memon, R. A., & Vincent, E. G. (2020). Global Research Output on Sleep Research in Athletes from 1966 to 2019: A Bibliometric Analysis. *Clocks & Sleep, 2*(2). https://doi.org/10.3390/clockssleep2020010

Lastella, M., Roach, G. D., Halson, S. L., & Sargent, C. (2015a). Sleep/wake behaviours of elite athletes from individual and team sports. *European Journal of Sport Science, 15*, 94–100.

Lastella, M., Roach, G. D., Halson, S. L., & Sargent, C. (2016). The chronotype of elite athletes. *Journal of Human Kinetics, 54*, 219–225.

Lastella, M., Roach, G. D., Halson, S. L., Martin, D. T., West, N. P., & Sargent, C. (2015b). Sleep/wake behaviour of endurance cyclists before and during competition. *Journal of Sports Sciences, 33*(3), 293–299. https://doi.org/10.1080/02640414.2014.942690

Lastella, M., Roach, G. D., Halson, S. L., Martin, D. T., West, N. P., & Sargent, C. (2015c). The impact of a simulated grand tour on sleep, mood, and well-being of competitive cyclists. *Journal of Sports Medicine and Physical Finess, 55*(12), 1555–1564.

Lastella, M., Vincent, G. E., Duffield, R., Roach, G. D., Halson, S. L., Heales, L. J., & Sargent, C. (2018). Can sleep be used as an indicator of overreaching and overtraining in athletes? *Frontiers in Physiology, 9*, 436.

Leger, D., Elbaz, M., Raffray, T., Metlaine, A., Bayon, V., & Duforez, F. (2008). Sleep management and the performance of eight sailors in the Tour de France a la voile yacht race. *Journal of Sports Sciences, 26*, 21–28.

Liendl, S., Lauer, C. J., & Hoffmann, R. M. (2004). Pre-screening via sleep logs in sleep-disordered patients—Adaptational effects, yes or no? *Somnologie, 8*, 67–70.

Loch, F., Ferrauti, A., Meyer, T., Pfeiffer, M., & Kellmann, M. (2019). Rest the mind: A novel topic with scare insights. Considering potential mental recovery strategies for short rest periods in sports. *Performance Enhancement & Health, 6*, 148–155. https://doi.org/10.1016/j.peh.2019.04.002

Lundqvist, C., & Kenttä, G. (2010). Positive emotions are not simply the absence of the negative ones: Development and validation of the Emotional Recovery Questionnaire (EmRecQ). *The Sport Psychologist, 24*, 468–488. https://doi.org/10.1123/tsp.24.4.468

Luthar, S., & Kumar, N. (2018). How can you help children thrive in a world focused on success? In T. McCullough & K. Whitaker (Eds.), *Wealth of wisdom: The top 50 questions wealthy families ask* (pp. 149–155). Wiley. https://doi.org/10.1002/9781119331568.ch22

Manley, A., Roderick, M., & Parker, A. (2016). Disciplinary mechanisms and the discourse of identity: The creation of "silence" in an elite sports academy. *Journal of Culture and Organization, 22*, 221–244. https://doi.org/10.1080/14759551.2016.1160092

Marino, M., Li, Y., Rueschman, M. N., Winkelman, J. W., Ellenbogen, J. M., Solet, J. M., et al. (2013). Measuring sleep: Accuracy, sensitivity, and specificity of wrist actigraphy compared to polysomnography. *Sleep, 36*, 1747–1755.

McGuigan, M. (2017). *Monitoring training and performance in athletes*. Human Kinetics.

McNair, D. M., Lorr, M., & Droppleman, L. F. (1992). *Revised manual for the Profile of Mood States*. Educational and Industrial Testing Service.

Meeusen, R., & De Pauw, K. (2018). Overtraining—What do we know? In M. Kellmann & J. Beckmann (Eds.), *Sport, recovery, and performance: Interdisciplinary insights* (pp. 51–62). Routledge.

Meeusen, R., Duclos, M., Foster, C., Fry, A., Glesson, M., Nieman, D., Raglin, J., Rietjens, G., Steinacker, J. M., & Urhausen, A. (2013). Prevention, diagnosis and treatment of the overtraining syndrome: Joint consensus statement of the European College of Sport Science (ECSS) and the American College of Sports Medicine (ACSM). *Medicine and Science in Sports and Exercise, 45*, 186–205. https://doi.org/10.1249/MSS.0b013e318279a10a

Mujika, I., Halson, S. L., Burke, L. M., Balagué, G., & Farrow, D. (2018). An integrated, multifactorial approach to periodization for optimal performance in individual and team sports. *International Journal of Sports Physiology and Performance, 13*, 538–561. https://doi.org/10.1123/ijspp.2018-0093

Nédélec, M., Halson, S. L., Abaidia, A.-E., Ahmaidi, S., & Dupont, G. (2015). Stress, sleep and recovery in elite soccer: A critical review of the literature. *Sports Medicine, 45*, 1387−1400.

Nédélec, M., Dawson, B., & Dupont, G. (2019). Influence of night soccer matches on sleep in elite players. *The Journal of Strength & Conditioning Research, 33*, 174–179.

NFL Network. (n.d.). A football life: Favre leaves Green Bay. Retrieved from http://www.nfl.com/videos/a-football-life/0ap3000000724859/A-Football-Life-Favre-leaves-Green-Bay

O'Donnell, S., Beaven, C. M., & Driller, M. W. (2018). From pillow to podium: A review on understanding sleep for elite athletes. *Nature and Science of Sleep, 10*, 243–253.

Pelka, M., Kölling, S., Ferrauti, A., Meyer, T., Pfeiffer, M., & Kellmann, M. (2017). Acute effects of psychological relaxation techniques between two physical tasks. *Journal of Sports Sciences, 35*, 216–223. https://doi.org/10.1080/02640414.2016.1161208

Reilly, T., Atkinson, G., Edwards, B., Waterhouse, J., Åkerstedt, T., Davenne, D., et al. (2007). Coping with jet-lag: A Position Statement for the European College of Sport Science. *European Journal of Sport Science, 7*(1), 1–7. https://doi.org/10.1080/17461390701216823

Rigney, D. (1991). Three kinds of anti-intellectualism: Rethinking Hofstadter. *Sociological Inquiry, 61*, 434–451. https://doi.org/10.1111/j.1475-682x.1991.tb00172.x

Roberts, S. S. H., Teo, W.-P., & Warmington, S. A. (2019). Effects of training and competition on the sleep of elite athletes: A systematic review and meta-analysis. *British Journal of Sports Medicine, 53*, 513–522.

Roffwarg, H. P., Muzio, J. N., & Dement, W. C. (1966). Ontogenetic development of the human sleep-dream cycle. *Science, 152*, 604.

Romyn, G., Robey, E., Dimmock, J. A., Halson, S. L., & Peeling, P. (2016). Sleep, anxiety and electronic device use by athletes in the training and competition environments. *European Journal of Sport Science, 16*(3), 301–308. https://doi.org/10.1080/17461391.2015.1023221

Rushall, B. S. (1990). A tool for measuring stress tolerance in elite athletes. *Journal of Applied Sport Psychology, 2*(1), 51–66. https://doi.org/10.1080/10413209008406420

Ryan, R. M., & Deci, E. L. (2000). Self-determination theory and the facilitation of intrinsic motivation, social development, and well-being. *American Psychologist, 55*, 68–78. https://doi.org/10.1037/0003-066X.55.1.68

Samuels, C., James, L., Lawson, D., & Meeuwisse, W. (2016). The Athlete Sleep Screening Questionnaire: A new tool for assessing and managing sleep in elite athletes. *British Journal of Sports Medicine, 50*, 418–422.

Sargent, C., Halson, S. L., & Roach, G. D. (2014a). Sleep or swim? Early-morning training severely restricts the amount of sleep obtained by elite swimmers. *European Journal of Sport Science, 14*(Suppl. 1), S310–S315.

Sargent, C., Lastella, M., Halson, S. L., & Roach, G. D. (2014b). The impact of training schedules on the sleep and fatigue of elite athletes. *Chronobiology International, 31*, 1160–1168.

Sargent, C., Lastella, M., Halson, S. L., & Roach, G. D. (2016). The validity of activity monitors for measuring sleep in elite athletes. *Journal of Science and Medicine in Sport, 19*, 848–853.

Saw, A. E., Kellmann, M., Main, L. C., & Gastin, P. B. (2017). Athlete self-report measures in research and practice: Considerations for the discerning reader and fastidious practitioner. *International Journal of Sports Physiology and Performance, 12*(S2), 127–135.

Saw, A. E., Main, L. C., & Gastin, P. B. (2016). Monitoring the athlete training response: Subjective self-report measures trump commonly used objective measures: A systematic review. *British Journal of Sports Medicine, 50*, 281–291. https://doi.org/10.1136/bjsports-2015-094758

Schädlich, M., & Erlacher, D. (2018). Practicing sports in lucid dreams—Characteristics, effects, and practical implications. Current Issues in Sport. *Science, 3*(7). https://doi.org/10.15203/CISS_2018.007

Schmid, D., Erlacher, D., Klostermann, A., Kredel, R., & Hossner, E.-J. (2020). Sleep-dependent motor memory consolidation in healthy adults: A meta-analysis. *Neuroscience and Biobehavioral Reviews, 118*, 270–281. https://doi.org/10.1016/j.neubiorev.2020.07.028

Schredl, M. (2018). *Reserching Dreams. The Fundamentals*. Palgrave Macmillan.

Shahid, A., Wilkinson, K., Marcu, S., & Shapiro, C. (2012). *STOP, THAT and one hundred other sleep scales*. Springer.

Shea, C. H., Lai, Q., Black, C., & Park, J. H. (2000). Spacing practice sessions across days benefits learning of motor skills. *Human Movement Science, 19*, 737–760. https://doi.org/10.1016/S0167-9457(00)00021-X

Silva, M. R. G., & Paiva, T. (2016). Poor precompetitive sleep habits, nutrients' deficiencies, inappropriate body composition and athletic performance in elite gymnasts. *European Journal of Sport Science, 16*(6), 726–735. https://doi.org/10.1080/17461391.2015.1103316

Sonnentag, S., & Fritz, C. (2007). The Recovery Experience Questionnaire: Development and validation of a measure for assessing recuperation and unwinding from work. *Journal of Occupational Health Psychology, 12*, 204–221. https://doi.org/10.1037/1076-8998.12.3.204

Sonnentag, S. (2018). The recovery paradox: Portraying the complex interplay between job stressors, lack of recovery, and poor well-being. *Research in Organizational Behavior, 38*, 169–185. https://doi.org/10.1016/j.riob.2018.11.002

Strauch, I. (2010). *Schlafgewohnheiten und Schlafqualität. Von der Kindheit bis ins Erwachsenenalter*. Schattauer.

Stuck, B. A., Maurer, J. T., Schlarb, A. A., Schredl, M. & Weeß, H.-G. (2018). *Praxis der Schlafmedizin. Diagnostik, Differentialdiagnostik und Therapie bei Erwachsenen und Kindern (3. Aufl.) [Practice of sleep medicine. Diagnosis, differential diagnosis and therapy in adults and children, 3rd ed.]*.: Springer Medizin.

Stumbrys, T., Erlacher, D., & Schredl, M. (2016). Effectiveness of motor practice in lucid dreams: A comparison with physical and mental practice. *Journal of Sports Sciences, 34*(1), 27–34. https://doi.org/10.1080/02640414.2015.1030342

Swinbourne, R., Gill, N., Vaile, J., & Smart, D. (2016). Prevalence of poor sleep quality, sleepiness and obstructive sleep apnoea risk factors in athletes. *European Journal of Sport Science, 16*, 850–858.

Taylor, S. R., Rogers, G. G., & Driver, H. S. (1997). Effects of training volume on sleep, psychological, and selected physiological profiles of elite female swimmers. *Medicine and Science in Sports and Exercise, 29*, 688–693.

Tibbert, S. J., Andersen, M. B., & Morris, T. (2015). What a difference a "mentally toughening" year makes: The acculturation of a rookie. *Psychology of Sport and Exercise, 17*, 68–78. https://doi.org/10.1016/j.psychsport.2014.10.007

Tuomilehto, H., Vuorinen, V.-P., Penttilä, E., Kivimäki, M., Vuorenmaa, M., Venojärvi, M., et al. (2017). Sleep of professional athletes: Underexploited potential to improve health and performance. *Journal of Sports Sciences, 35*, 704–710.

Venter, R. E., Potgieter, J. R., & Barnard, J. G. (2010). The use of recovery modalities by elite South African team athletes. *South African Journal for Research in Sport, Physical Education and Recreation, 32*, 133–145.

Vitale, J. A., Banfi, G., Sias, M., & La Torre, A. (2019). Athletes' rest-activity circadian rhythm differs in accordance with the sport discipline. *Chronobiology International, 36*, 578–586.

Wang, F., & Boros, S. (2019). The effect of physical activity on sleep quality: A systematic review. *European Journal of Physiotherapy*, 1–8. https://doi.org/10.1080/21679169.2019.1623314

Waterhouse, J., Atkinson, G., Edwards, B., & Reilly, T. (2007). The role of a short post-lunch nap in improving cognitive, motor, and sprint performance in participants with partial sleep deprivation. *Journal of Sports Sciences, 25*, 1557–1566.

Waterhouse, J., Reilly, T., & Edwards, B. (2004). The Stress of Travel. *Journal of Sport Sciences, 22*, 946–966.

Weber, M. (1930/2005). The Protestant ethic and the spirit of capitalism. Routledge.

Weeß, H.-G., Schürmann, T., & Steinberg, R. (2002). Das Landecker Inventar für Schlafstörungen [The Landeck inventory for sleep disorders] (III-2.3.2). In H. Schulz (Ed.), *Kompendium Schlafmedizin [Sleep Medicine Compendium]* (pp. 1–3). Ecomed.

Woodman, T., & Hardy, L. (2001). A case study of organizational stress in elite sport. *Journal of Applied Sport Psychology, 13*, 207–238. https://doi.org/10.1080/10413200175314989

Exercise and Health

Contents

Models to Explain and Change Health Behavior and Physical Activity

Ines Pfeffer, Kyra Hamilton, Thomas Hannan and Mirko Wegner

Contents

J. Schüler et al. (eds.), *Sport and Exercise Psychology*, https://doi.org/10.1007/978-3-031-03921-8_25

Learning Objectives

Basic:

- Describe the major theories and models used to explain and change health behavior.
- Describe and explain the motivational and volitional phases of stage-based models.
- Define the terms "self-efficacy expectation" and "implementation intentions," and discuss their influence on changing health behavior.
- Explain and name the stages and strategies of behavior change within the transtheoretical model.

Advanced:

- Describe and explain the categorization of the major theories and models into the four model types: models of motivation, models of action execution, stage and process models, and dual-process theories.
- Explain the key assumptions of dual-process theories of physical activity behavior.
- Distinguish and describe the postulated type 1 and type 2 processes of the affective-reflective theory of physical inactivity and exercise.

Experts:

- How does the physical activity adoption and maintenance model extend the assumptions of the affective-reflective theory?
- Describe and explain the use of integrated models of health behavior.

People's health and illness are strongly influenced by their "lifestyle" behaviors. Chronic conditions and diseases such as high blood pressure, cardiovascular disease, obesity, diabetes mellitus, back pain, osteoporosis, and arthrosis are often the result of prolonged engagement in unhealthy behavior. For example, it is empirically well established that having an inactive lifestyle is a key risk factor for the development of cardiovascular diseases. Consequently, to prevent the development of chronic disease or slow down disease progression, decreasing engagement in unhealthy behaviors and promoting engagement in more healthy lifestyle behaviors are needed. Health, regarded as a positive bio-psycho-social state (WHO, 2000), and health behaviors, defined as behaviors that contribute to a person's health and well-being, are often influenced by individuals' self-regulation efforts (Schwarzer, 1997). Health self-regulation refers to the motivational, volitional, and behavioral processes of abandoning health-risk behaviors in favor of adopting and maintaining health-enhancing behaviors. Physical activity, for example, promotes physical fitness, physical self-concept, and subjective well-being. Regular physical activity can therefore be seen as a resource that can promote both our physical and mental health.

When discussing the impact that health behaviors have on a person's health and well-being, it is useful to distinguish between health-enhancing behaviors and health-risk behaviors. Health-enhancing behaviors, such as physical activity and healthy eating, can help prevent chronic disease as well as prevent physical damage (e.g., age-related muscle loss), promote cardiovascular fitness, and increase life expectancy. In contrast, health-risk behaviors, such as physical inactivity and prolonged sitting, can increase the risk of chronic disease and ill health and reduce life expectancy. Although health-enhancing behaviors and health-risk behaviors impact individuals' health differently, both fall under the generic term of "health behavior" (Schwarzer, 2004).

In the case of physical activity, in order to receive the associated health benefits, it is important that individuals perform some form of moderate to vigorous intensity physical activity on a regular basis, engage in muscle-strengthening activities, and limit prolonged sedentary behavior (see WHO for current physical activity guidelines; Bull et al., 2020). Yet, despite global interest in increasing physical activity engagement, epidemiological studies show that a substantial percentage of the adult population are not meeting the current recommendations for physical activity and exercise (► Chap. 15). For example, 43% of people in North America, 35% in Europe, and 17% in Southeast Asia are not sufficiently active to gain health benefits (Hallal et al., 2012; Sallis et al., 2016). As a result, a focus of health psychology and behavioral medicine research is to provide a better understanding of the factors influencing people's decisions to engage in regular physical activity and exercise.

In recent decades, researchers have been continuously working on developing models of health behavior and behavior change to help understand why, for example, some people engage in cancer screening behaviors, eat a healthy diet, or are physically active on a regular basis, and others do not. In addition, these models attempt to provide insight into how unfavorable health behaviors can be successfully changed, and more healthful behaviors can be adopted and maintained. Because of the impact that health behaviors have on individuals' health and well-being, a multitude of theoretical models have been proposed that try to explain such differences in health behavior (for an overview, see Conner & Norman, 2015; Hagger et al., 2020b). The aim of this chapter is to provide a descriptive overview, rather than a comprehensive account of the current state of research, of the main models of health behavior and how they specifically apply to physical activity. The models presented below can be divided into four broad categories: (1) motivational models, (2) theories of action execution, (3) stage/process models, (4) dual-process theories, and integrated models of health behavior.

In regard to *motivation models*, this chapter will describe and explain prominent motivational determinants that influence individuals' decision-making to engage or not engage in a certain health behavior. The primary aim of these models is to identify the constructs that influence a person's intention to perform a health behavior. In the context of the present overview, the theory of planned behavior (▸ Chap. 15; Ajzen, 1991), health belief model (Rosenstock, 1974), and social-cognitive theory (Bandura, 1986) will be discussed, although it should be noted that other theories and models of motivation, such as self-determination theory (Deci & Ryan, 1985; see ▸ Chap. 8), have been shown to provide explanatory power for physical activity behavior. The motivation models presented in this chapter focus on the question that follows: Which factors (or constructs) contribute to the development of a health behavior intention? As such, the common focus of each of these models is primarily on explaining and predicting the formation of an intention which, in turn, is poised to predict actual behavior.

For theories of action execution, it is suggested that these theories have a primary focus on examining constructs that bridge the gap between the intention (as outlined in motivational models) and the implementation of this intention into subsequent action. They therefore have a focus on volitional and self-control processes that help an individual regulate their thoughts, emotions, and behavior to help realize their intention. The theory of action control (Kuhl & Goschke, 1994) is one such model that falls in this category and is discussed in detail in ▸ Chap. 10. Other factors shown to explain the intention-behavior gap, such as implementation intentions (Gollwitzer, 1999; Gollwitzer & Brandstätter, 1997) and action planning and coping planning (Sniehotta et al., 2005), are explained in more detail in this chapter.

Stage and process models to explain health behavior represent a more complex approach to understanding health behavior and behavior change. As outlined by these models, individuals are assumed to progress through several qualitatively distinct stages during the behavior change process. Specifically, in this chapter, the transtheoretical model (Prochaska & DiClemente, 1983), health action process approach (Health Action Process Approach; Schwarzer, 2008; Schwarzer & Hamilton, 2020), and the motivation-volition process model (Fuchs, 2007; Fuchs et al., 2011) are discussed as stage or process models. The Rubicon model of action phases (Achtziger & Gollwitzer, 2018; Heckhausen & Heckhausen, 2010) as a stage model is described in ▸ Chaps. 7 and 10.

Dual-process theories such as the affective-reflective theory of physical inactivity and exercise (Brand & Ekkekakis, 2018) and the physical activity adoption and maintenance model (Strobach et al., 2020) are introduced and discussed. These models assume that human behavior is regulated by two different types of information processing that can be distinguished based on the levels of automaticity or reflectiveness of actions. Dual-process approaches provide an innovative theoretical framework for explaining and examining health behaviors (such as physical activity). Finally, we end with a discussion of *integrated models of behavior* and their role in addressing the limitations in explanatory power of the existing theory to arrive at models that afford testing of more comprehensive predictions of behavior.

This chapter deals with models that explain health behavior and, more specifically, physical activity and provides an initial introduction to the health chapters of this textbook. The following chapter, ▸ Chap. 26, examines the question of the conditions under which sport and physical activity have positive effects on mental health. Chapter 27 then deals with the foundations and development of stress, its harmful consequences, and the health-promoting potential of sport and physical activity. Finally, the concluding chapter on health, ▸ Chap. 28, outlines the benefits of sport and physical activity for mental and physical illnesses and discusses the negative side effects associated with sport, such as sports addiction or injuries.

25.1 Motivation Models

25.1.1 Theory of Planned Behavior

The *theory of planned behavior* (Ajzen, 1985, 1991) is one of the most commonly used social cognition models and identifies various constructs that are believed to explain the (health) behavior of people. In this model, the *intention* construct (i.e., the extent to which an individual is motivated to perform a given target behavior in the future) is considered to be the most important determinant of behavioral action. Intention is proposed to be predicted by three belief-based constructs: *attitude*, *subjective norm*, and *perceived behavioral control* (◘ Fig. 25.1).

Attitude reflects the positive or negative evaluations of the behavior in question and is an aggregate of behavioral beliefs—beliefs about the likely consequences (instrumental behavioral beliefs) and experiences (experiential behavioral beliefs) resulting from performance of the behavior—for example, the belief that exercising (the behavior) improves physical fitness (the outcome) or is fun (the experience). A person will develop a stronger intention to perform the target behavior if they evaluate the behavior, which may be a discreet and single

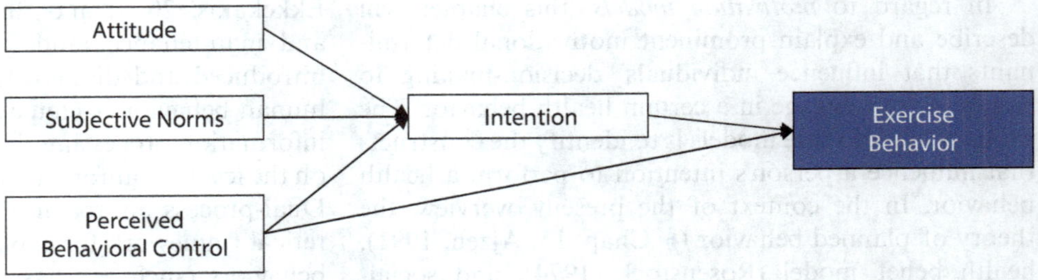

Fig. 25.1 The theory of planned behavior (Ajzen, 1991)

occurrence or a continuous change in their health behavior, as positive (e.g., as useful, good, joyful, interesting, or pleasant).

Subjective norm reflects an aggregate of normative beliefs—beliefs about the expectations (injunctive normative beliefs) and behaviors (descriptive normative beliefs) of significant social referents. An injunctive normative belief is the expectation or subjective probability that a given referent individual or group (e.g., friends, family, partner, doctor) approves or disapproves of performing the target behavior. Descriptive normative beliefs are beliefs as to whether important others themselves perform the behavior. The stronger the perceived subjective norm, the stronger the intention is to perform the target behavior.

Lastly, *perceived behavioral control* reflects an individual's belief in their ability and confidence to perform the target behavior. Perceived behavioral control is considered an aggregate of control beliefs—beliefs about factors that may facilitate or impede performance of the behavior. Control factors include considerations that make the behavior easy or difficulty to perform, of required skills and abilities, and of access and availability to required resources. This construct is conceptually similar to *self-efficacy* (Bandura, 1986) and is presumed to influence behavior both directly (reflecting actual behavioral control) and indirectly via behavioral intention. Original theory of planned behavior theorizing posited perceived behavioral control to moderate the intention-behavior relationship, as the greater the individuals actual control over the behavior, the more likely it is that the intention will be carried out (Ajzen, 1985). However, only recently has research continued to test this moderation effect (Hagger et al., n.d., under review; Phipps et al., 2021; Yang-Wallentin et al., 2004).

> *Intention* is a conscious decision to achieve a certain result or to perform a certain behavior. Whether a person ultimately behaves accordingly depends on the strength of this intention. In the theory of planned behavior, the strength of intention is, in turn, determined by three factors: attitude, subjective norm, and perceived behavioral control (Ajzen, 1991).

A meta-analysis by Hagger et al. (2002), which includes more than 72 publications in the field of sports and physical activity, confirmed previous meta-analytical findings by Hausenblas et al. (1997). Specifically, Hagger et al. revealed that attitude, subjective norm, and perceived behavioral control all contributed to intention, which, in turn, significantly predicted behavior. Although support for the theory of planned behavior in health behavior more broadly has been demonstrated (Hamilton et al., 2020a; 2020b; McEachan et al., 2011), the use of randomized controlled studies where the individual constructs of the theory of planned behavior are specifically manipulated and in which the effect on physical activity is examined remains scarce. Experimental testing of the theory of planned behavior as an intervention approach is an important next step that needs to be pursued more vigorously to identify concrete and effective ways to increase physical activity engagement.

25.1.2 Health Belief Model

According to Rosenstock's *health belief model* (Rosenstock, 1974), the performance of a health behavior is influenced by several underlying beliefs. *Perceived health threat* reflects beliefs about the perceived *severity* (seriousness) of a particular illness, as well as beliefs about one's own subjective *vulnerability* (susceptibility) to that illness. *Perceived effectiveness of health behavior* reflects beliefs about the perceived *benefits* versus *costs* of performing the respective behavior. Lastly, *general health motivation* reflects an individual's general willingness to address a particular health issue, while *cues to action* reflect environmental or situational factors that may prompt the performance of a behavior (Fig. 25.2).

For example, a person who experiences their first heart attack may be assessed by their doctor and is told that without performing regular physical activity, they are at risk of having a second and more severe heart attack (*high susceptibility* and *high severity*). In this instance, the individual would be more likely to start exercising than a person who is not faced with such concrete threats. At the same time, the likelihood of the health behavior (performing regular physical activ-

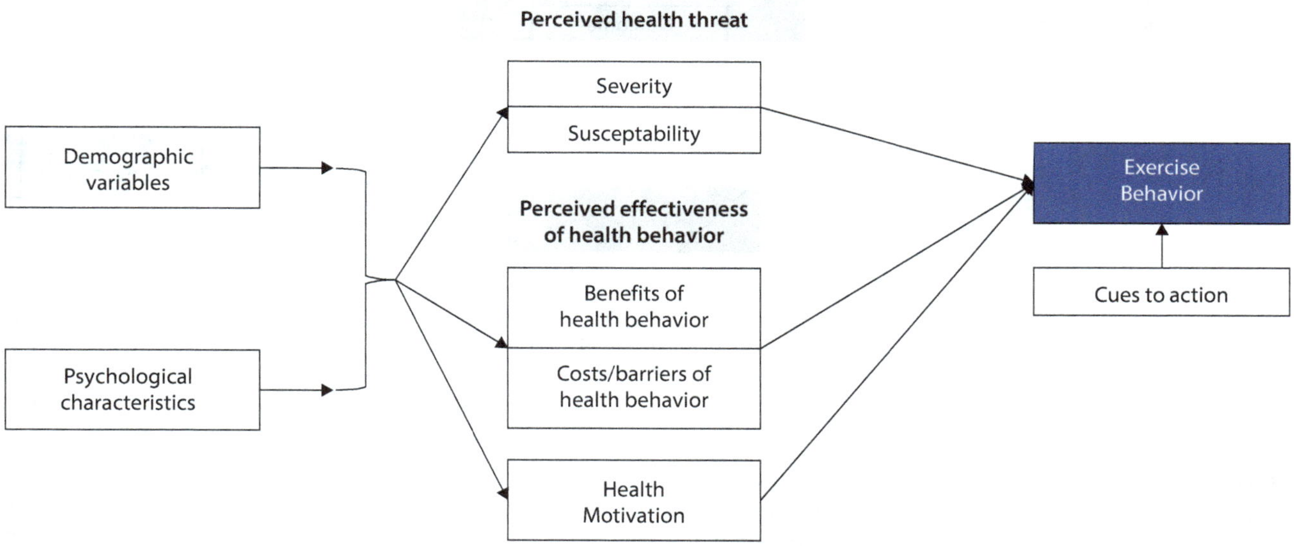

Fig. 25.2 The health belief model (Rosenstock, 1974)

ity) can be increased if a person is convinced of its effectiveness. For instance, if the individual is informed about statistics on how physical activity reduces the likelihood of a second heart attack, they may recognize more clearly the *benefits* of exercising. Behavior can also be facilitated by removing *barriers* to initiating the health behavior—for example, when opportunities to be sedentary are less readily available because a person has removed the television from their apartment. In addition, ensuring that health is a high priority in this person's life can increase their *health motivation* to behave in a healthy way and facilitate the initiation and maintenance of health behavior. Lastly, the presence of certain *cues to action* can influence the probability of the occurrence of health behavior and may include cues such as physical symptoms (e.g., stabbing in the chest), advertising for health or support groups, campaigns encouraging health behaviors (e.g., gym ads), or even conversations about health behavior change that remind the person of their health-related goals. Overall, it is assumed that all six determinants in the model of health beliefs independently influence health behavior (Abraham & Sheeran, 2015). The constructs mentioned are also influenced by sociodemographic variables (such as age and sex) as well as personality variables (psychological characteristics).

The health belief model assumes that cost-benefit analysis (subjectively perceived advantages compared to disadvantages), perceived threat (beliefs about susceptibility to and severity of disease), general health motivation (wanting to maintain positive health), and situational or environmental cues to action (behavioral prompts) determine whether a person adopts a health behavior (e.g., regular physical activity) or not.

The health belief model has stimulated extensive research on different health behaviors. Importantly, the concepts of vulnerability and the cost-benefit ratio of health behavior are also taken into account in more recent theories (e.g., in the transtheoretical model or health action process approach, see ► Sects. 25.3.1 and 25.3.2). However, various theoretical and empirical weaknesses of the health belief model have been pointed out and intensively discussed. In particular, the model's poor predictive power with regard to behavioral change has been criticized (Harrison et al., 1992), which has resulted in the diminished use of the model today in the context of physical activity behavior.

25.1.3 Social-Cognitive Theory

According to the *social-cognitive theory* (Bandura, 1986), health behavior is mainly influenced by *self-efficacy expectations* and *outcome expectations* of a person in relation to a certain health behavior. Self-efficacy expectations refer to a person's beliefs about their own ability to successfully and independently master the desired actions (e.g., maintaining a sporting activity or taking part in a yoga class), on the basis of their own skills, even potential barriers may exist (e.g., time constraints). As mentioned above (► Sect. 25.1.1), there are conceptual similarities between the perceived behavioral control construct in the theory of planned behavior and Bandura's self-efficacy construct (Bandura, 1986).

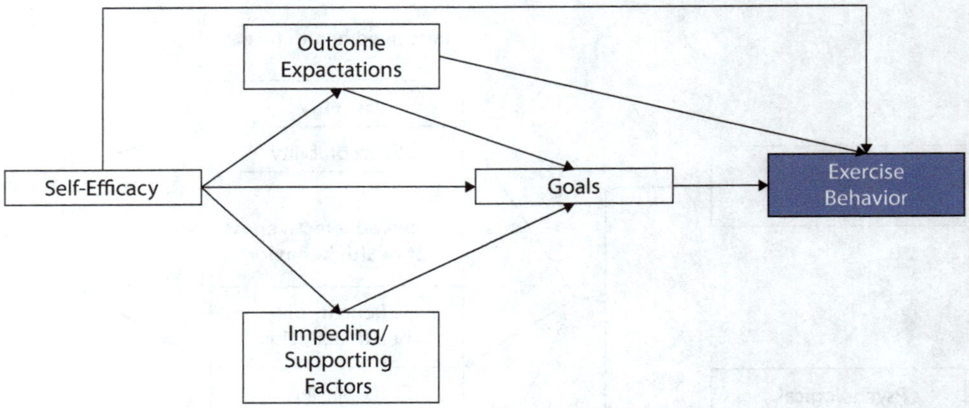

Fig. 25.3 The social-cognitive theory (Bandura, 1986)

Outcome expectations reflect an individual's beliefs about the effectiveness of the planned action with regard to the health goal to be achieved, as well as possible disadvantages that may arise from the execution of the behavior. For example, if an elderly patient expects that a fall prevention program will help them avoid future accidents, they will be more likely to participate in such a program. Importantly, environmental and social factors also play a role and may support or impede a person's motivation to perform the behavior (Fig. 25.3). For example, the fact that a friend has also decided to take part in such a fall prevention program could encourage the patient to set the goal of participating in the program. An obstacle could be, for example, that this program takes place in another city and the patient therefore would need to rely on private transportation because public transportation is unavailable or the program may require a significant financial outlay.

Persons with high self-efficacy expectations set themselves higher goals, initiate their actions more quickly, and show greater persistence in pursuing their goals despite potential barriers and difficulties that may arise. They do not give up so quickly in the event of defeat and are better able to deal with failure.

Together, social-cognitive theory suggests that self-efficacy, expectations, outcome expectations, and supportive/impeding factors can facilitate or inhibit the formation of goals and that goals are an important prerequisite for the execution of behavior. Self-efficacy beliefs are one of the most important resources for behavioral change. Notably, the special importance of a person's self-efficacy beliefs for health behavior changes has been demonstrated in various studies, including research on dealing with stress (Lazarus & Folkman, 1987) and dealing with illness (Bandura et al., 1988). For this reason, self-efficacy beliefs are also an important component in other health behavior models (e.g., health action process approach; ► Sect. 23.3.2; Schwarzer, 2008; Excursus: Four Sources of Self-Efficacy Expectations).

Side Story

Four Sources of Self-Efficacy Expectations

Bandura names four concrete sources from which a person's beliefs regarding their self-efficacy can be enhanced: (1) the successful own execution of an action, (2) substitute experiences (learning vicariously through observation of a model), (3) symbolic experiences (verbal information), and (4) emotional arousal. Each of these four factors can increase a person's self-efficacy and will be discussed in the following section in the context of a participant attending a yoga course:

Successful own execution of an action: Self-efficacy can be enhanced through successfully performing a desired action. For example, if an individual successfully attends a yoga class and experiences no difficulty in performing the required movements, their belief in their ability to meet the requirements of the course (e.g., physical abilities) will increase, which will strengthen their expectations of being able to participate successfully in this course in the future.

Substitute experience (vicarious learning): Self-efficacy can also be enhanced through observational (vicarious) learning. For instance, after watching a friend participate in the yoga class and experience no difficulty, it is possible that the participant may come to believe that they themselves might also be able to participate successfully in such a course.

Verbal information: If this person is encouraged by the trainer and other participants in their movement competence (e.g., through positive feedback during the exercise) and encouraged to continue participating in the course, they may also be convinced that they have the required skills to continue participating.

Emotional arousal: Since people draw conclusions about their competence from their own level of emotional arousal (Bandura, 1986), it is possible that the participant is very much looking forward to the upcoming yoga class and concludes that they will be able to meet the demands of the course. On the other hand, this person might also be nervous (e.g., experiencing palpitations, sweaty palms) and conclude that their physical ability or skill level might not be sufficient to successfully participate in the yoga class.

25.2 Theories of Action Execution

Theories of action execution are primarily focused on understanding why individuals fail to translate their health behavior intentions into subsequent action. In this way, models of action execution largely address the well-documented *intention-behavior gap*. These models can be considered *volition models* as they focus on the realization of intentions after the completion of intention formation and, thus, address action control. The central question that these models attempt to address is which processes are required in order for a person to successfully realize their goals or objectives. In the chapter on volition in sport (▶ Chap. 10), the theory of action control (Kuhl & Goschke, 1994) is discussed in detail. In this section, the focus is on the concepts of implementation intentions (Gollwitzer, 1990, 1999) and planning (Schwarzer, 2008; Sniehotta et al., 2005) which assist in intention realization after the motivational phase has been completed. The focus is thus on the self-regulatory abilities of a person after the goal has been set and the processes needed to facilitate the translation of intentions into action.

Volition describes the conscious, voluntary translation of intentions (goals and motives) into results and involves the effortful self-regulation of one's own cognitions, emotions, motives, and actions in a targeted manner.

The intention-behavior gap (◘ Fig. 25.4) describes the phenomenon that not every intention is translated into observable behavior. Health behavior can often only be predicted partially on the basis of a person's intention. For example, many individuals often form New Year's Eve resolutions or intentions but rarely translate these goals into observable behavior. Understanding what processes facilitate intention translation is therefore a primary focus of models of action execution.

Implementation Intentions, Action Planning, and Coping Planning

Implementation intentions are effective self-regulation strategies that facilitate goal attainment and the translation of intentions into action (Gollwitzer, 1999; Gollwitzer et al., 2004). An implementation intention is a formulated "if-then" plan that pairs a desired action with a specified scenario (e.g., *if* situation Y arises, *then* I will do X). As Gollwitzer notes, it is important that *implementation intentions* are distinguished from general *goal intentions*. Specifically, as outlined above (▶ Sect. 23.1) and in common motivation theories (e.g., theory of planned behavior; Ajzen, 1991), goal intentions reflect a person's willingness to act in order to execute a behavior or to achieve a general goal ("I intend to achieve X"). In this context, "X" can be a behavior or a result. However, Gollwitzer points out that the formation of strong intentions is often not sufficient for the successful implementation and maintenance of a health behavior, as the distance between intention and goal achievement can be very long and often requires great persistence and pronounced goal striving. Intentions may also vary in stability from the time they are formed to the time they are acted upon. Implementation intentions are thus subordinate in time to goal intentions. They effectively help individuals make the transition from the motivational to the volitional phase (e.g., to anticipate possible actions) and increase the likelihood of an intention being translated into concrete action ("When situation Y occurs, I do X").

Initial research into implementation intentions first focused on less complex behaviors that were performed

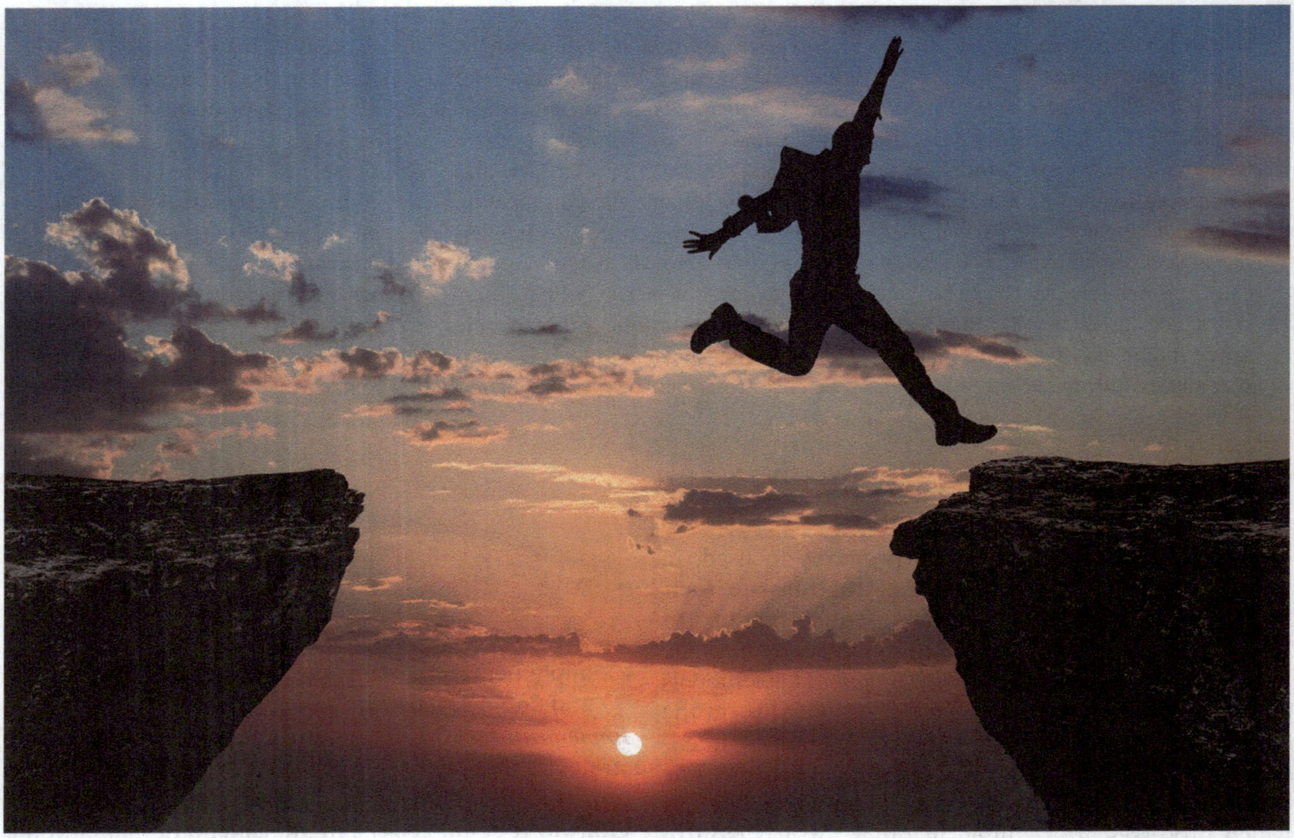

Fig. 25.4 Illustration of the intention-behavior-gap (© es0lex/stock.adobe.com)

in laboratory studies (e.g., computer tasks). However, Schwarzer and colleagues extended the concept to more complex behaviors in the field of health behavior, which lead to an increased focus on the role of *planning* in health behavior interventions. Sniehotta et al. (2005) emphasize that in the case of complex health behaviors, it is useful to distinguish between *action planning,* a task-facilitating strategy that considers how an individual prepares to perform a behavior, and *coping planning,* a distraction-inhibiting strategy that considers how an individual prepares to avoid foreseen barriers and obstacles that may arise when performing a specific behavior and potentially competing behaviors that may derail the behavior. (Pfeffer et al., 2020; Schwarzer & Hamilton, 2020).

In action planning, targeted actions are linked to situational information or stimuli by specifying when, where, and how a specific action is to be performed. In this way, an important distinction between planning and implementation intentions is that planning strategies provide more detailed linkages between situational cues and behavioral responses. Action plans are effective because through pairing an action with specific situational cues, the performance of that action becomes more likely upon encountering that cue, even when a person is distracted (Gollwitzer, 1999). Action planning works by identifying a targeted behavior (e.g., going for a brisk walk) and then linking this behavior to a predefined situation regarding when (e.g., getting home from work), where (e.g., around the neighborhood), and how (e.g., walking for at least 30 min). It is assumed that this enables an automated execution (stimulus-response linking) of the planned behavior in the situation. The execution of the action is then fast and effective, with limited additional conscious intention/resources required. Thus, a plan only works if a clear representation of the situation is linked to an equally clear representation of the response reaction (Gollwitzer & Oettingen, 1998) and formulated in terms of a detailed "if-then" linkage (Hagger & Luszczynska, 2014; Excursus: Action plans and coping plans).

Action Plans and Coping Plans

Examples of Action Plans
- When the lectures are over on Tuesdays and Fridays (when?), then I will go straight to the gym on my way home (where?) and do 45 min (how long?) of strength training (what?).
- If I go to university early on Mondays and Thursdays (when?), then I will take the bike (what?) with my girlfriend (with whom?) and ride 20 min (how long?) along the river (where?) to the university and back in the evening.
- When it is 10 o'clock on Sundays (when?), then I will go jogging (what?) with my partner (with whom?) in the city park (where?) for 30 min (how long?).

Examples of Coping Plans
- If it rains early on Mondays or Thursdays and I can't ride my bike, then I will take my swimsuit and go to the indoor swimming pool right after university and swim for 30 min.
- If I have too much to do on Tuesdays and Fridays, then I will tell myself that engaging in 30 min of sport will help me concentrate better afterward.
- If I don't feel like going jogging on Sundays, then I will tell myself that I will feel much better afterward.

Reflection

In the following, check the effectiveness of implementation intentions (planning) on yourself. Make a simple table with two columns. In the left column, name goals (goal intentions) that you have not yet translated into behavior (e.g., "I want to go swimming 3 days a week," "I want to eat meat on only 2 days of the week," "I want to use reusable bags when I go shopping to avoid plastic waste"). Then translate these goal intentions into action plans (e.g., "When I come home from university on Mondays, Wednesdays, and Fridays, then I will go straight to the swimming pool for swimming 1000 m," "When I am in the supermarket doing my weekly shopping, then I will buy only two meals of meat," "When I go to the regional greengrocer's shop on Saturday, then I will take a basket to put my groceries in").

Goal Intentions I want to ...	**Action Plans (= Implementation Intentions)** If ... then ...	**Degree of goal attainment after one week**

Check after 1 week: Have I been able to implement my goals better? If not, what obstacles interfered with your action plans? In addition to your action plans, form coping plans (see below). Use action planning and coping planning as effective self-regulation strategies in the future.

Coping planning refers to the anticipation of potential obstacles and possible coping actions (Sniehotta et al., 2006). This involves identifying challenging situations that could derail the implementation of the intention and mental representation of ways to overcome them. The structure of coping plans ("If it rains on Monday, then I will go to the swimming pool instead of jogging") corresponds to the structure of the underlying implementation plans ("If I come home from work on Monday, then I will go jogging"). The coping plan takes into account a person's own experiences with such situations and can be especially helpful for maintaining a planned activity. Empirical evidence suggests that younger people benefit more from independent coping planning and older people more from guided coping planning (Sniehotta et al., 2006). Implementation intentions and action planning, on the other hand, are considered more important for the acquisition of a regular sports or physical activity (Study Box: Effects of a Planning Intervention on Physical Activity Behavior).

Study Box

Effects of a Planning Intervention on Physical Activity Behavior

In a randomized controlled trial with experimental and control group, Pfeffer and Strobach (2019) investigated the effects of a planning intervention (action and coping planning) on physical activity behavior (see study model in ◘ Fig. 25.5). They examined for whom a planning intervention is most effective and how such interventions work. Specifically, it was questioned whether the specificity of the action plan and coping plan that was formed and the coping-related self-efficacy (the confidence to be able to constructively deal with relapses into physical inactivity) mediated the effect of the planning intervention on physical activity behavior. In addition, intention strength (to be physically active on a regular basis) was examined as a moderator of the intervention effect as well as a moderator of the mediation effects (moderated mediation; for moderators and mediators in general, see ► Chap. 15).

The results showed that the planning group significantly increased its physical activity behavior compared to the control group and that the effect of the planning intervention on physical activity behavior was moderated by intention strength. Specifically, persons with weak physical activity intentions benefited most from the planning intervention. Furthermore, the mediator effect of the action planning, the coping planning, and the coping-related self-efficacy was found to be moderated by the strength of intention. For subjects with strong intentions, the formation of action plans and their coping self-efficacy contributed to higher levels of physical activity, whereas for subjects with low intentions, the formation of coping plans was most relevant. Accordingly, persons with strong intentions benefit from action plans and high coping-related self-efficacy, while persons with weak intentions benefit from coping plans. Overall, the results indicate that a planning intervention may effectively increase physical activity engagement but that the effects of the intervention may vary between individuals.

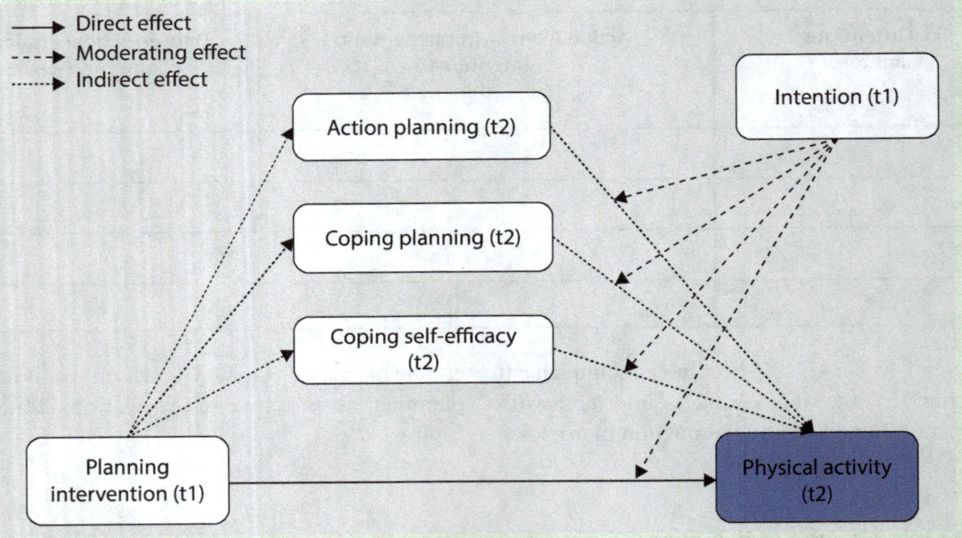

◘ **Fig. 25.5** Research model of the planning study (Pfeffer & Strobach, 2019)

Reflection

Here is an opportunity to measure the degree of your own physical activity planning.

How can it be assessed whether someone has generated specific action and coping plans?

Within the framework of the health action process approach (► Sect. 25.3.2), a standardized questionnaire (Schwarzer et al., 2007) was developed by Schwarzer and colleagues, which depicts the two theoretically distinguishable planning components of action planning and coping planning. Subjects are asked to assess the extent to which they agree with the following statements on a four-level scale (from 1 = "not correct" to 4 = "exactly right").

"Now please think of the coming weeks. How exactly have you already planned your daily physical activity (lasting for at least 30 min)?" "I already have concrete plans regarding...

1. ...what physical activities to engage in."
2. ...how to be physically active."
3. ...when to be physically active."
4. ...where to be physically active."
5. ...how often to be physically active."
6. ...with whom to be physically active."
7. ...how I will continue to be physically active, even though I feel physically challenged."
8. ...how I will continue to be physically active, even if I have to stop several times."
9. ...how I will continue to be physically active, despite my other obligations and interests."
10. ...how I will continue to be physically active, even if something comes up in the meantime."

(Items 1–6 represent action planning, and items 7–10 coping planning.)

Empirical literature provides evidence for the conceptual distinction between the two planning constructs (Carraro & Gaudreau, 2013; Kwasnicka et al., 2013; Scholz et al., 2008); however, more convergent than discriminant validity of these two concepts is often observed. That noted, keeping action planning and coping planning as two distinct constructs is useful for the design of interventions (Schwarzer & Hamilton, 2020).

Hagger and Luszczynska (2014) derive recommendations for future research efforts in the field of health behavior planning. In particular, the implementation of randomized controlled intervention studies, which additionally investigate mediators (mechanisms of action) and moderators of the effects of plans on physical activity behavior and use objective measuring instruments to record physical activity, is in demand. In addition, the effectiveness of planning interventions should be investigated for different *stages of behavioral change* (▸ Sect. 25.2) and for persons with different levels of intention within these stages (Schwarzer & Hamilton, 2020).

For Sports Practice

Hagger and Luszczynska (2014) summarize the current state of research on the effectiveness of planning in the context of health behavior and provide concrete recommendations for the design of planning interventions to promote health behavior change:

1. Plans should always be formulated as "if-then" links, not in general terms.
2. Plans should refer to individually relevant situational cues that need to be identified first.
3. The formulation of action plans should always be supplemented by coping plans.
4. The formulation of plans should be guided by a trained consultant.
5. Ideally, plans should be created dyadically or collaboratively.
6. Subjects should receive a reminder of their plans ("booster" reminders).
7. For the formulation of plans, especially for persons with low intentions and high resistance to change, additional measures are taken to promote motivation and (volitional) self-efficacy expectations.

25.3 Stage and Process Models

Stage and process models assume that human behavior can be characterized by two phases: a motivational phase, in which the decision or intention to behave or change behavior is made (intention formation), and a volitional phase, in which the intention is translated into appropriate behavior (Hagger & Chatzisarantis, 2005; Schwarzer & Hamilton, 2020). In this way, these models assume that the behavior change process involves an individual passing through qualitatively different stages. However, the observable change in behavior is not the first stage. Changes in a person's thinking and experience start long before changes in behavior can be observed (Prochaska & DiClemente, 1983). The dynamic process of behavioral change extends over an extended period of time and occurs in stages that differ in qualitative characteristics. The following section will present stage and process models that have been applied to the context of physical activity and exercise, namely, (1) the transtheoretical model (Prochaska & DiClemente, 1983), (2) the health action process approach (Schwarzer, 2008), and (3) the motivation-volition process model (Fuchs et al., 2011).

25.3.1 Transtheoretical Model of Behavior Change

The *transtheoretical model* of behavior change (DiClemente & Graydon, 2020; Prochaska & DiClemente, 1983) is focused on the process of *intentional behavior change* that leads to successful sustained change and was originally developed and empirically tested in the field of smoking cessation. It has subsequently been successfully applied to other health behaviors including alcohol and drug abuse, help-seeking behaviors (e.g., preventive medical checkups), sun-safe behaviors, risky sexual behavior, and—crucial for this textbook—physical activity (DiClemente & Graydon, 2020; Prochaska & Marcus, 1994).

The model is called "transtheoretical" because it uses different explanatory approaches and integrates the mechanisms of action of different (psycho-)therapeutic schools. According to Prochaska and DiClemente (1982), behavior change occurs through different *stages of change* (descriptive level) and through the use of different *strategies of change* (procedural level). In addition to these stages and strategies of behavioral change, the model emphasizes the importance of other cognitive variables (*markers of change*), such as the *self-efficacy expectations* and the expected positive (pros) and negative (cons) consequences of maintaining a problem behavior and behavior change (decisional balance; advantages and disadvantages). The further people progress in the stages, the higher the self-efficacy expectation and the perceived advantages (pros) with regard to the target behavior—i.e., at the level of unintentional behavior the lowest, at the level of maintenance the highest. In contrast, the perceived disadvantages (cons) decrease over the stages. Furthermore, the *context of change* is also considered in the transtheoretical model as health behavior change always occurs within the life context of a person, which can enhance or interfere with change. Relevant life contexts are life situations and symptoms, belief systems, dyadic interpersonal relationships, systems issues (family, work, and social network), and more sustained characterological or identity issues (DiClemente & Graydon, 2020).

The five discrete stages proposed by the *transtheoretical model* represent the time dimension (◘ Fig. 25.6). In order for a health-risk behavior (e.g., excessive sedentary behavior) to be successfully stopped or a health-enhancing behavior (e.g., regular physical activity) to be successfully maintained, an individual must progress through all stages in the model. Each of the stages of the model will be discussed in the following section and will be applied to the uptake of regular physical activity.

In the first stage of the model, *precontemplation*, an individual displays no motivation or intention to change their current behavior (e.g., physical inactivity) in the near future (i.e., in the next 6 months). The person may lack information and problem awareness regarding their current level of physical inactivity. At this point, it is often not possible to move on to the next level without active intervention targeted at problem awareness and intention formation. At the next stage, *contemplation*, the individual may be at least aware of the advantages and disadvantages of the planned behavior change, but they may still be in a state of ambivalence such that the person cannot decide on a concrete plan of action. However, a person at this stage has at least formed an intention to change their behavior within the next 6 months. In stage 3, *preparation* (◘ Fig. 25.7), the person is highly motivated to do physical activity on a regular basis. Characteristic for this phase is that an intention to act has already been formed and the decision in favor of the behavior (e.g., to do regular physical activity) has been made. In addition, initial steps have already been taken to realize the intention (e.g., information has been obtained, sports shoes have been purchased, or offers of advice have been accepted). Individuals at this stage may feel enticed by concrete offers such as sports, exercise, or nutrition courses. Often the preparation stage is characterized as a "transition stage" to the next, lasting for approximately 1 month and in which the behavior is not yet fully demonstrated (e.g., not exercising regularly, but doing so a couple of times a week for at least 30 min). From stages 2 and 3, a regression to previous stages can take place at any time (◘ Table 25.1). Next comes stage 4, *action*

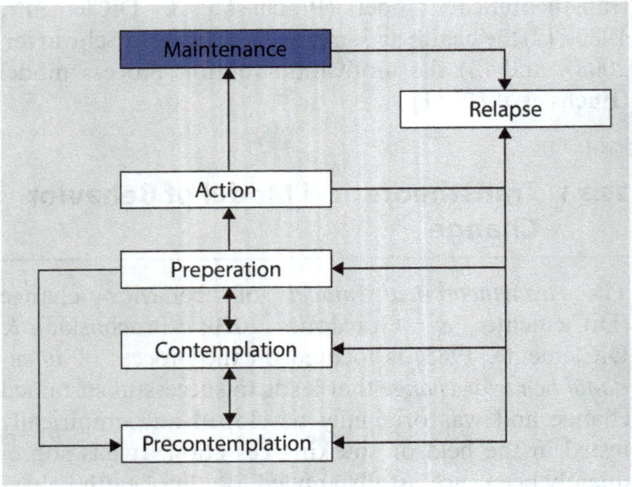

◘ **Fig. 25.6** Stages of change in the transtheoretical model (Prochaska & DiClemente, 1983)

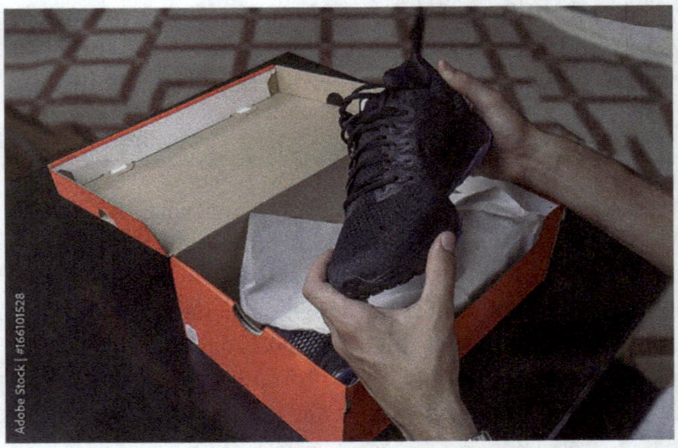

◘ **Fig. 25.7** Preparation to become physically active (© Nicola/stock.adobe.com)

Table 25.1 Cognitive-affective and behavioral processes of change in the transtheoretical model (Prochaska & DiClemente, 1982)

Cognitive-affective processes	
Consciousness raising	Conscious perception of the resulting consequences and awareness of possible change paths from problem behavior
Dramatic relief	Creating an emotional connection and personal involvement with the problem behavior and its consequences
Environmental reevaluation	Conscious perception of emotional/ cognitive consequences of problem or target behavior for the personal environment
Self-reevaluation	Conscious perception of emotional and cognitive consequences of the problem or target behavior for oneself
Social liberation	Active perception and awareness of environmental conditions that facilitate the change in problem behavior
Behavioral processes	
Self-liberation, commitment	The conviction that change is possible and the commitment to implement this change
Stimulus control	Remove triggers for problem behavior and/ or provide incentives for favorable alternative behavior
Countercondi-tioning	Replace unfavorable behaviors by favorable behavior in the sense of a problem solution
Helping relationships	Actively asking for and demanding concrete social support, but also the ability to accept help
Reinforcement management	Conscious use of rewards (material or immaterial) for steps that lead in the desired direction

stage, in which the target behavior is carried out and the problematic behavior is reduced or the health-promoting behavior is built up. At this stage, an individual has performed the target behavior regularly (compared to the preparation stage) but has maintained the behavior for less than 6 months. As the self-regulation of the person is very important in this phase, this phase is prone to relapse into physical inactivity. If the target behavior (e.g., exercising daily for at least 30 min) has been shown for more than 6 months, the person is in stage 5, *maintenance*. In this stage, efforts must continue to be directed toward preventing a relapse into earlier stages where problematic behavioral patterns are present.

For an individual to successfully change a problematic behavior, they should successfully progress through stages 1–5. However, Prochaska and DiClemente (1983) emphasize that probable regression to previous stages or relapse into physical inactivity is the rule rather than the exception and that the stage transition is rarely linear. They also stress that such a change in behavior usually requires more than one attempt and takes time. Moreover, it is not yet clear whether the periods of time proposed in the transtheoretical model for the respective stages in the context of physical activity behavior are as long as those for smoking cessation. It is also important to consider individual differences in personal resources (e.g., access to gym facilities) that may impede a person's progression through each of the stages.

In addition to the levels of behavior change, Prochaska and DiClemente (1983) distinguish a total of ten *strategies of behavioral change* (Table 25.1), which can be divided into two dimensions that each describe five self-regulation strategies: cognitive-affective strategies (experiential processes) and behavioral strategies (behavioral processes). The *cognitive-affective strategies* mainly refer to subjective evaluations of the self or the target behavior (e.g., thinking about their sense of self as someone who is physically active or how their current state of physical inactivity impacts on others). They are primarily used in the early phases of behavioral change when an individual may lack the motivation to change or is in the process of forming new physical activity intentions. The *behavioral strategies*, on the other hand, are more action-oriented and relate to the translation of the motivation formed in the first stages into observable behavior (e.g., substituting unhealthy thoughts and behaviors with healthy thoughts and behaviors, modifying the environment to support behavior change). They are therefore more relevant in the later stages of behavior change, from preparation to maintenance.

> The *cognitive-affective* and *behavioral* change strategies together with the stages of behavioral change form the core of the "transtheoretical model." They allow the planning of stage-specific interventions that are adapted to the needs of the persons in a particular stage. In this way, the motivation to change can be promoted in relation to the willingness to change, and consulting resources can be used efficiently.

Existing evidence on the use of behavior change strategies in the context of physical activity and movement is mixed. In their meta-analysis based on physical activity-related transtheoretical model studies, Marshall and Biddle (2001) conclude that all ten proposed strategies of behavior change are relevant to changes in physical activity behavior. In particular, they found that cognitive-affective strategies seem to be most often used in the action stage, while behavioral strategies are mainly used in the maintenance stage. By contrast, a meta-analysis

Table 25.2 The use of change strategies alongside the stages of behavior change

Precontemplation	Contemplation	Preparation	Action	Maintenance
• Consciousness raising				
• Environmental reevaluation				
	• Dramatic relief			
	• Self-reevaluation			
	• Social liberation			
		• Self-liberation, commitment		
		• Employing helpful relationships		
			• Self-reinforcement management	
			• Counter-conditioning	
			• Stimulus control	

by Rosen (2000) specifically examined the order of change strategies used across the stages and found that for physical activity, the cognitive-affective strategies seemed to be used most frequently in both the action and maintenance stages (Table 25.2; Pfeffer & Alfermann, 2008; Prochaska & DiClemente, 1983).

Overall, the role of cognitive and behavioral strategies in the process of physical activity change does not seem to be entirely clear. Nevertheless, there is increasing evidence that sequential and stage-specific use is not given in the same way in physical activity behavior as, for example, in smoking cessation (Marshall & Biddle, 2001; Pfeffer & Alfermann, 2008; Rosen, 2000).

Based on their systematic review of the effectiveness of transtheoretical model-based interventions to change physical activity behavior, Hutchison et al. (2009) concluded that it is not possible to make statements on the effectiveness of such interventions, as only a few studies are available that have used the model to derive interventions in its entirety by including both the stages and strategies of behavior change, self-efficacy expectations, as well as accounting for the advantages and disadvantages of the model. It is clear that further research is needed that utilizes all components of the model when developing interventions and that the effectiveness of these interventions is examined using randomized controlled trials.

However, the transtheoretical model has generally proven its worth as a theoretical basis for describing and explaining changes in behavior, and previous research results have supported the core assumptions of the model largely independently of the behavior under study. On the one hand, it provides a theoretical framework for explaining change processes in health behavior and, on the other hand, can be used to derive stage-specific interventions to promote change processes. This makes the model interesting for both research and practice.

25.3.2 Health Action Process Approach

The *health action process approach* (Schwarzer, 2008) is a hybrid model that combines features of stage and continuum social cognition models. The health action process approach specifies six constructs as the core antecedents of behavior: intention, risk perception, outcome expectancies, self-efficacy, planning, and action control (Fig. 25.8). A key feature of the health action process approach is the distinction it makes between a motivational phase (where individuals are in a deliberative mindset while forming a goal intention) and a volitional phase (where individuals are in an implementation mindset while pursuing their goal) (Schwarzer & Hamilton, 2020). Goal setting and goal pursuit therefore represent two distinct processes that require self-regulatory effort, with intention operating as a bridge between the initial goal setting phase (motivational phase) and subsequent goal pursuit phase (volitional phase).

In the motivational phase of the health action process approach, outcome expectancies, risk perceptions, and action self-efficacy are constructs that make

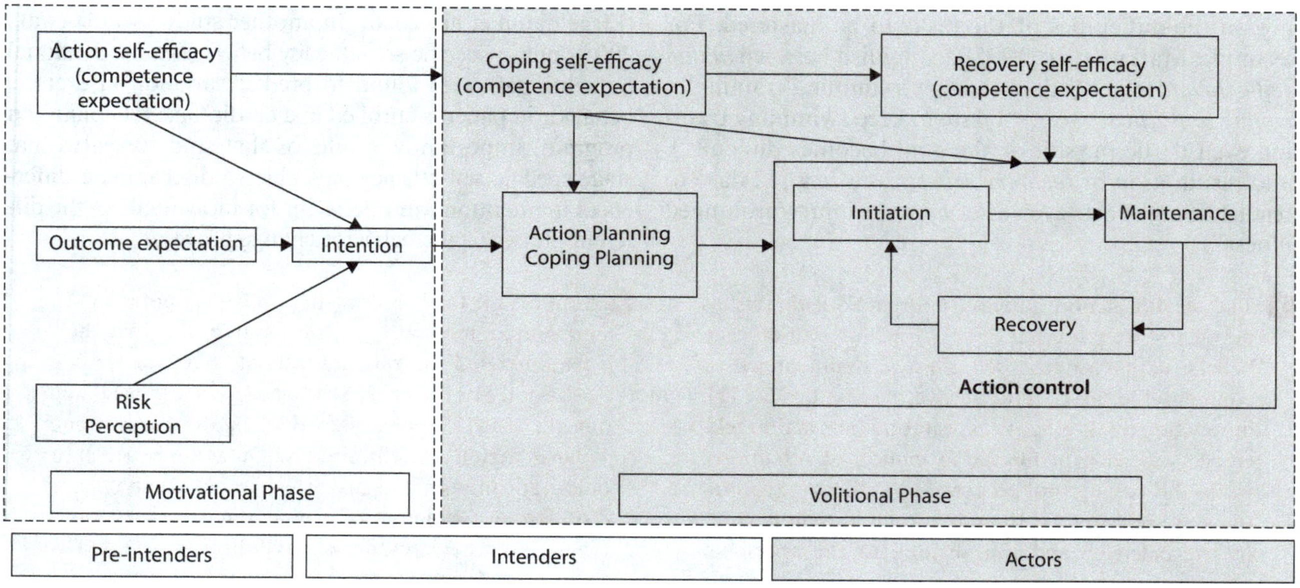

Fig. 25.8 The health action process approach (Schwarzer, 2008)

formation of intentions more likely (Schwarzer & Hamilton, 2020). *Outcome expectancies* refer to a person's beliefs that performing the target behavior will lead to outcomes that have utility for the individual and is the result of rational decision-making of balancing the pros and cons of certain behavioral outcomes—similar to attitudes in the theory of planned behavior (e.g., "If I exercise five times per week, I will reduce my cardiovascular risk"). *Risk perceptions* refer to a person's belief in the severity of a health condition that may arise from not performing the target behavior and their vulnerability toward it. It is suggested that risk perceptions may be sufficient for developing a motivation to change, but later on, other variables may be more influential in the self-regulation process. Lastly, *action self-efficacy* (sometimes referred to as task self-efficacy) represents optimistic beliefs about personal agency during the pre-actional, motivational phase.

In the *volitional phase* of the health action process approach, action planning, and coping planning are important determinants of behavior, with behavioral maintenance determined by action control (Schwarzer & Hamilton, 2020). As discussed earlier in this chapter, *action planning* and *coping planning* are important self-regulation strategies. Action plans are detailed plans about *when*, *where*, and *how* the behavior is to be executed in the future, while coping plans are detailed plans about what to do should one encounter a potential threat or challenge that may impede goal attainment. *Action control* comprises three facets: self-monitoring (e.g., "I consistently monitor when, where, and how long I exercise"), awareness of standards (e.g., "I have always been aware of my exercise training program"), and self-regulatory effort (e.g., "I took care to exercise as much as I intended to"). Keeping records of behaviors (e.g., diary entries, activity monitors) is a useful action control strategy that can help people be more aware of their behavioral gains and deficits and, therefore, encourages continued action or alternative action if needed (Schwarzer, 2008). Action control is a useful behavior change technique that has been applied to a variety of health behaviors (Reyes Fernández et al., 2016; Zhou et al., 2015a, 2015b), including physical activity (e.g., Parschau et al., 2013).

> The health action process approach differentiates between a motivational phase and a volitional phase in the process of changing health behavior. In addition, this model distinguishes between persons who have not (yet) formed an intention to take up or change health behavior and are correspondingly inactive (*non-intenders*); persons who have already formed an intention and are motivated to act, but have not yet done so (*intenders*); and persons who are motivated to act and have already taken up or changed the specified health behavior (*actors*).

An important feature of the health action process approach is the varying types of self-efficacy beliefs. Specifically, self-efficacy beliefs are suggested to vary according to the situational demands that a person faces at a particular point in the change process and depending on the difficulties of the tasks to be mastered. For example, Marlatt et al. (1995) distinguish between *action self-efficacy* (e.g., "I dare to start swimming training"), *coping self-efficacy* (e.g., "I dare to keep swimming training even if the pursuit of the goal becomes difficult"), and resumption or *recovery self-efficacy* (e.g., "I dare to restart doing sports even after a sports injury/prolonged illness").

> The health action process approach distinguishes between three stage-specific forms of self-efficacy beliefs: action or task self-efficacy, maintenance or coping self-efficacy, and recovery self-efficacy. The motivational self-efficacy expectation (i.e., action self-efficacy) is relevant for the formation of intentions, while the coping and recovery self-efficacy expectations are relevant for the initiation and maintenance of the behavior and thus belong to the volitional phase.

As briefly mentioned above, self-efficacy is proposed to be important in both the motivational and volitional phases of the health behavior change process and, therefore, considered to be phase-specific. This is because during the course of health behavior change different tasks have to be mastered and different self-efficacy beliefs are required to master these tasks successfully (Schwarzer & Hamilton, 2020). Action self-efficacy beliefs play a role in the motivational phase of the change process and describe the confidence of a person to be able to initiate and complete a desired behavior. In contrast, coping and recovery self-efficacy belong in the volitional phase, where coping self-efficacy is posited to be an important determinant of behavior and recovery self-efficacy important in behavioral maintenance. Coping self-efficacy, sometimes referred to as maintenance self-efficacy, refers to an individual's optimistic beliefs in their ability to be able to overcome obstacles and barriers that may stand in the way of maintaining the desired goal. For example, an exercise program might turn out to be much more difficult to adhere to than expected, but a self-efficacious person responds confidently with better strategies, more effort, and prolonged persistence to overcome the challenges. Recovery self-efficacy addresses the experience of failure and recovery from setbacks and refers to an individual's confidence in their ability to get back on track after setbacks and missteps and effectively resume control of the behavior (Scholz et al., 2005; Schwarzer, 2008).

In the field of rehabilitation sports, findings demonstrate that implementing a brief 5- to 10-min planning intervention can have positive effects on the maintenance of physical activity following inpatient rehabilitation (Ziegelmann et al., 2006). In another study (Scholz et al., 2005), phase-specific self-efficacy beliefs (i.e., motivational or volitional) were found to predict variation in exercise behavior in patients enrolled in a cardiologic rehabilitation program. Importantly, results of that study revealed that stage-specific self-efficacy was able to discriminate differences in intentions and behavior for individuals in the different phases of the behavior change process.

> Support for the health action process approach as an integrated motivational-volitional model has been demonstrated in the context of physical activity behavior. For instance, a recent meta-analysis (Zhang et al., 2019) demonstrated that for the motivational phase, action self-efficacy and outcome expectatancies (advantages and disadvantages of the behavior) are strong predictors of physical activity intentions, while risk perception (vulnerability) was found to have a weaker effect. For the volitional phase, the formation of strong intentions, action and coping plans, as well as volitional self-efficacy (coping and recovery self-efficacy) were all important predictors of behavior (Zhang et al., 2019).

25.3.3 Motivation-Volition Process Model

The *motivation-volition process model* (Fuchs et al., 2007, 2011) is a framework concept that integrates motivational and volitional phases and variables that can be applied to continuous sports and exercise behaviors and was developed specifically for the area of physical activity.

In the motivational phase of the motivation-volition process model, similar to the health action process approach, the formation of an *intention* is influenced by two factors (Fig. 25.9). First, *perceived behavior control* (self-efficacy beliefs) and the *outcome expectations* (expected advantages and disadvantages) of regular physical activity influence whether an *intention* is formed and how strong this intention is. In this instance, to form strong intentions to exercise, an individual must believe that the expected benefits of initiating regular physical activity will exceed the expected costs and the person must be convinced they have the required ability and resources to carry out the target behavior. A unique feature of the motivation-volition process model, however, is that it presumes that motivation is not only determined by outcome expectations and perceived behavioral control but also by the amount of *self-concordance* that is present. Self-concordance is introduced as an important prerequisite for intrinsic motivation in ► Chap. 8. In essence, self-concordance reflects the extent to which

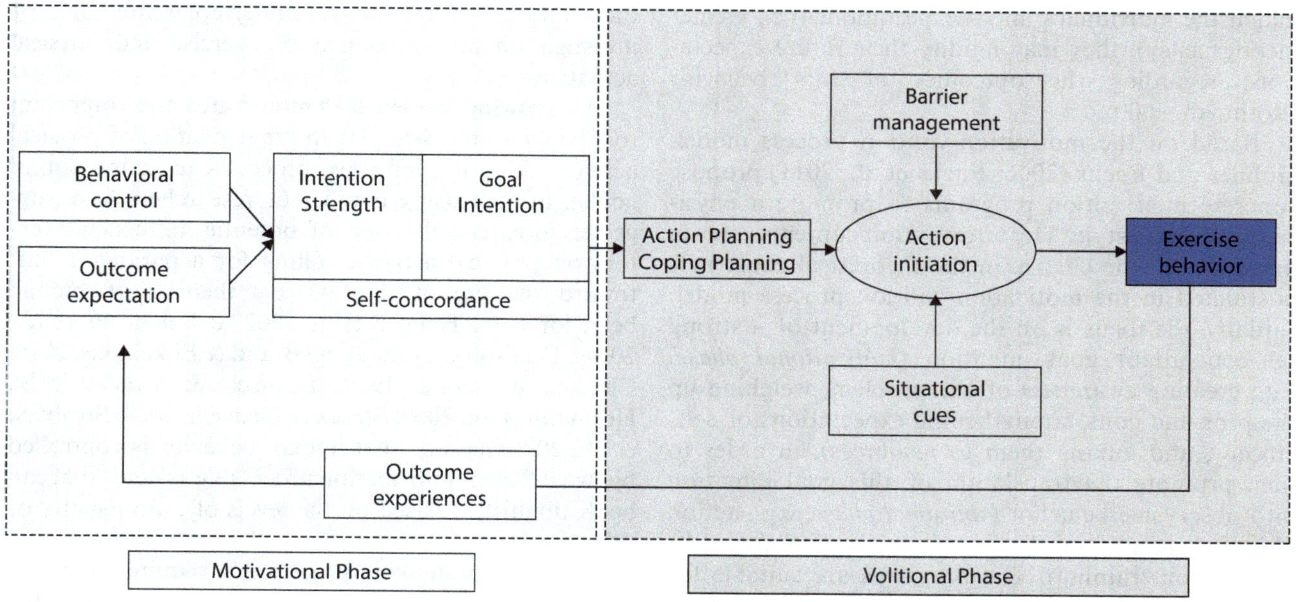

Fig. 25.9 The motivation-volition process model (Fuchs, 2007)

an individual's intention or goal (e.g., "I intend to be physically active on a regular basis") corresponds to their own personal interests and personally held values (Fuchs et al., 2017; Seelig & Fuchs, 2006).

> *Self-concordance* describes the degree of ego proximity with a target intention. The more the target intention is in harmony with the personal interests and values of a person, the higher self-concordance there is. By contrast, the more an individual's intention is pursued due to external constraints or possible anticipated sanctions, the lower self-concordance there is (Fuchs et al., 2017; Seelig & Fuchs, 2006).

If behavioral intentions are strong and there is a high degree of self-concordance with the goal intention, volitional strategies and steering mechanisms can then be used to translate those intentions into subsequent action. *Implementation intentions* and *action planning* (Gollwitzer, 1999; Gollwitzer et al., 2004; Hagger & Luszczynska, 2014) can be helpful here. Implementation intentions and action plans involve deciding the *when*, *how*, *where*, and *with whom* of future physical activity. For instance, one may form the following action plan: "I intend to go for a one-hour run in the city forest on Fridays after work at 5 pm." If there are potential obstacles or barriers that may arise which will interfere with performing that action, formulating plans to overcome those barriers (*coping planning*) is an important volitional strategy that can increase the likelihood of taking up and maintaining physical activity (► Sect. 25.2).

In addition to the formation of action plans, other volitional control strategies can be utilized to help shield the planned behavior from internal and external barriers. Similar to the health action process approach, these self-regulatory abilities fall under the *action initiation* stage of the motivation-volition process model and can be utilized to help protect one's health-related intentions from factors that may impede goal attainment (e.g., competing intentions or an invitation from a family member to perform a counter-intentional behavior). The *action control theory* (Kuhl & Goschke, 1994), for example, mentions attention control, emotion control, coping with failure, environmental control, motivation control, and economical information processing as such action control strategies.

In addition, Fuchs et al. (2011) emphasize that *outcome experiences* are also important as they can provide feedback to the individual and contribute to sustainable behavioral change. When deciding to perform a behavior, an individual may believe that performing that behavior will result in a particular outcome or consequence. For instance, a person may have the expectation that by doing sport they will lose 5 kg. Once the behavior has been performed, the experienced consequences of that behavior will be compared to the expectations that were initially placed on that behavior (e.g., "Have my expectations of losing 5 kg been fulfilled by doing sport?"). If their body weight has actually been reduced by 5 kg, this experience is positive. When there is greater congruency between the consequences of the experience and the individual's expectations, and they are satisfied with the consequences compared to their expectations, the more likely it is that this experience will have a positive effect on their motivation to continue playing sport. In contrast, if the experienced consequences do not match the individual's initial expectations (i.e., greater incongruency), they may modify their future expectations regarding the outcomes of that behavior (Rothman, 2000).

Based on the motivation-volition process model, Göhner and Fuchs (2006; Fuchs et al., 2011) propose concrete intervention programs to promote a physically active lifestyle. The intervention contents refer in particular to the change in the theoretical constructs postulated in the motivation-volition process model. Initially, the focus is on the development of a strong self-concordant goal intention (*motivational phase*, e.g., creating awareness of the problem, weighing up the pros and cons, strengthening expectations of self-efficacy, and linking them to resources), in order to then promote the translation of this goal intention into observable behavior (*volitional phase*, e.g., action planning, identifying barriers, coping planning, self-observation training). The programs are suitable for prevention and rehabilitation settings and the effectiveness of these programs has been empirically proven (Fuchs et al., 2011).

25.4 Dual-Process Theories of Physical Activity Behavior and Integrated Models of Health Behavior

As evidenced by the sections above, understanding the motivation to initiate physical activity behavior has dominated research interest over the last several decades. The theory of planned behavior (Ajzen, 1991) and social-cognitive theory (Bandura, 1986), for example, focus on the cognitive antecedents of behavioral intentions and specify which factors lead to strong intentions (e.g., intentions to be physically active). These traditional models conceptualize a person as a thinking and rationally acting organism (Norman & Conner, 2005). For instance, these models posit that individuals' decision-making is primarily driven by the rational evaluation of information, such as weighing up the positive and negative consequences of a behavior. These models, therefore, focus heavily on the role of constructs that govern reflective, explicit cognitive processes. However, one criticism of these models is that they are too restrictive in their view of the processes that govern our actions, as a solid evidence base is growing that shows automatic or implicit processes also play a role in guiding health behavior (Hofmann et al., 2008), including physical activity behavior (e.g., Chevance et al., 2017; Hannan et al., 2019; Phipps et al., 2021). Despite this increasing evidence, research examining the constructs that represent implicit, automatic processes, such as implicit attitudes and habits, remains an underrepresented area of investigation in the context of exercise and physical activity.

As growing evidence demonstrates the important role implicit processes play in the regulation of physical activity alongside reflective processes (e.g., intentions, goals), an increasing number of researchers have suggested to extend the view of potential influencing factors on physical activity, calling for a paradigm shift toward the use of dual-process theories of human behavior (e.g., Hagger et al., 2020a; Sniehotta et al., 2014). Dual-process theories (Brand & Ekkekakis, 2018; Chaiken & Trope, 1999; Deutsch & Strack, 2020; Hofmann et al., 2009; Strack & Deutsch, 2004; Strobach et al., 2020) assume that human behavior is controlled by two different information processing systems that can be distinguished based on the levels of automaticity or reflectiveness of actions. The *reflective system* uses an explicit decision-making process that requires cognitive resources and is therefore effortful and slow, while the *impulsive system* uses more automatic processes that are fast and effortless and occur automatically without overly drawing on cognitive resources. Dual-process approaches provide an innovative theoretical framework for explaining and examining health behaviors, such as physical activity, and how the interplay of constructs that underpin reflective, deliberative, and implicit, automatic processes can affect behavior. In the following section, we will briefly describe two exercise-specific dual-process theories: (1) the affective-reflective theory of physical inactivity and exercise (Brand & Ekkekakis, 2018) and (2) the physical activity adoption and maintenance model (Strobach et al., 2020).

25.4.1 Affective-Reflective Theory of Physical Inactivity and Exercise

The *affective-reflective theory* (Brand & Ekkekakis, 2018; ◻ Fig. 25.10) of physical inactivity and exercise is a dual-process model which focuses largely on automatic affective valuations and automatic processes to explain physical activity behavior. Broadly, the affective-reflective theory distinguishes between default *type 1 processes* (i.e., those that are fast, automatic, effortless and requiring minimal cognitive resources) and *type 2 processes* (i.e., those that are reflective, slow, effortful, controlled, and dependent on the availability of self-control resources) in the regulation of physical activity and sedentary behavior (Brand & Ekkekakis, 2018). However, a distinct feature of the affective-reflective theory model is that it considers the individual's momentary state of physical (in)activity at which an exercise-

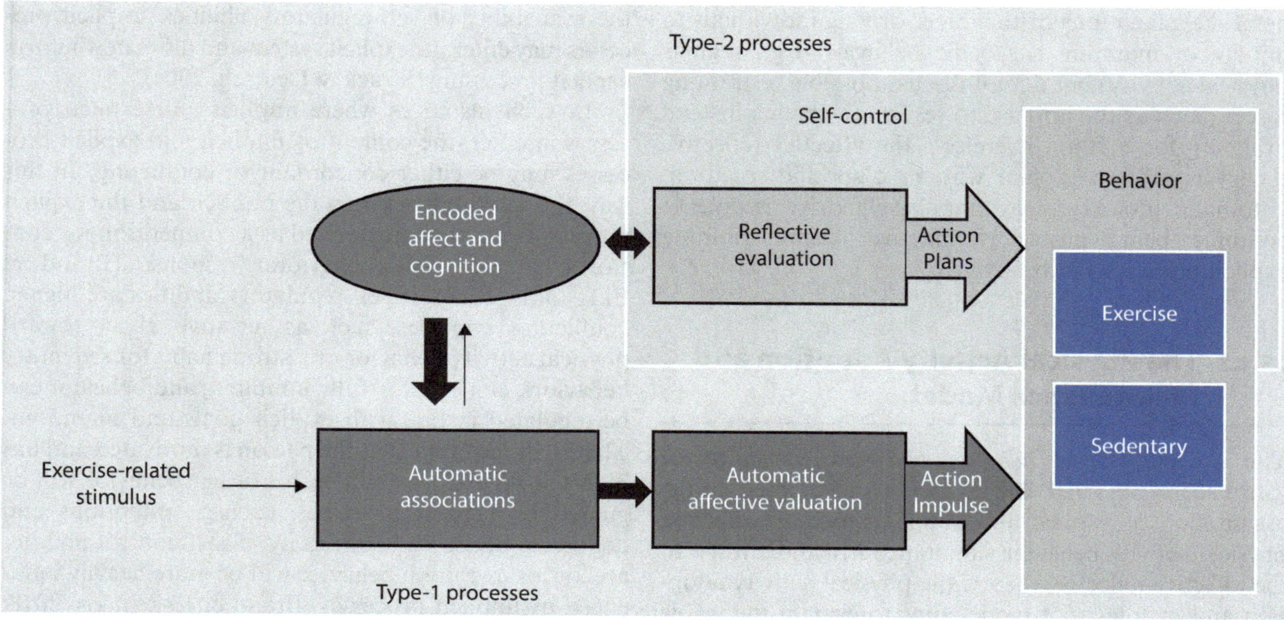

Fig. 25.10 The affective-reflective theory of physical inactivity and exercise (Brand & Ekkekakis, 2018)

related stimulus is perceived. For example, an individual watching television might perceive an exercise-related stimulus from an external source (e.g., seeing people riding a bicycle on the screen) and/or an internal source (e.g., remembering their partner's advice to be more physically active), which activates automatic associations in long-term memory. These mental associations are pre-existing links between the target stimuli, for example, the perceived physical activity cue or the individual's current sedentary behavior and positive/pleasant or negative/unpleasant valuations. Once activated, these automatic affective valuations can result in a discrete approach (e.g., forces driving the individual to change the present state and to become active) or avoidance impulse (e.g., forces restraining an individual from changing the present state).

The *automatic affective valuation* provides the basis and can "color" the subsequent controlled processes (e.g., encoded affect and cognition). For example, the immediate impulse to relax on the couch (type 1 process) might weaken or interfere with a person's plans to go for an afternoon walk (type 2 process). According to the affective-reflective theory, the availability of self-control resources determines whether type 1 or type 2 processing will prevail and guide behavior. In situations where self-control resources or abilities are readily available (Hofmann et al., 2008), a slower and more effortful type 2 process (Strack & Deutsch, 2004) will follow the automatic affective valuation and will have a greater influence on behavior. Higher-level cognitive operations as proposed in traditional models of social behavior (e.g., weighting the positive and negative consequences of adopting a behavior, deliberative reasoning about one's needs and values) can result in action planning (e.g., formation of behavioral goals, intentions, and generating action and coping plans) (Schwarzer & Hamilton, 2020). Action plans, as well as action impulses, can represent a driving or restraining force with respect to a potential alternative to the individual's ongoing behavior.

It is important to note that the content and result of type 2 processing (e.g., forming the intention to perform a behavior or generating detailed action plans) and the result of type 1 processing may be concordant (e.g., the spontaneous impulse for a brisk walk in the sun and the intention to follow one's partner's advice to be more physically active) or discrepant (e.g., the action impulse is to rest on the couch despite having the intention to be more physically active). It is proposed that the action impulse will generally prevail in situations where self-regulatory resources or abilities are low or impaired (Baumeister & Heatherton, 1996; Englert, 2016; Hofmann et al., 2008). For instance, where an individual may be distracted or they are under high cognitive load, their actions will be influenced more strongly by type 1 than by type 2 processes (Friese et al., 2008).

The assumption of a possible approach-avoidance conflict (i.e., automatic affective valuation and the result of the controlled processes can be contradicting) is a significant improvement of the affective-reflective theory compared to traditional theories of physical activity behavior (i.e., motivational theories and stage theories; Ajzen, 1991; Schwarzer, 2008). These theories provide helpful explanations of the forces driving individuals to initiate or maintain a specific behavior (e.g., regular physical activity) but do not discuss possible restraining forces (such as the impulse to rest on the couch instead of going for a run). Therefore, the affective-reflective theory is able to explain why, in a specific situation, automatic processes may impulsively drive people to continue being physically inactive despite holding explicit intentions to be active.

25.4.2 The Physical Activity Adoption and Maintenance Model

The *physical activity adoption and maintenance model* (Strobach et al., 2020; ◘ Fig. 25.11) is also based on the assumption of explicit and implicit processes affecting physical activity behavior simultaneously. In contrast to the affective-reflective theory, the physical activity adoption and maintenance model aims to explain the whole process of adoption and maintenance of physical activity behavior and is therefore not only focused on the single situation at which an exercise-related stimulus is perceived, but nevertheless comprises this point of view. In line with the reflective-impulsive model (Strack & Deutsch, 2004) and the affective-reflective theory (Brand & Ekkekakis, 2018), implicit processes are considered the default response upon which explicit processes are based on. Depending on the intensity of implicit processes and the availability of self-regulatory abilities, implicit processes may enter the explicit system and ultimately inform explicit processing (Strack & Deutsch, 2004).

In such instances where implicit and explicit processes interact, the content of implicit and explicit processes may be either concordant or conflicting. In this way, the interplay between the implicit and the explicit processes can be characterized as a competition for control over the overt behavioral response (Brand & Ekkekakis, 2018). If self-regulatory abilities are higher, conflicting impulses, such as negative affect toward physical activity behavior or a strong habit for sedentary behaviors, can be effortfully inhibited, and behavior can be regulated in line with explicit goals and intentions. That is, in the event that the person is motivated and has high self-regulatory abilities, his or her behavior will be guided by explicit processes, such as intentions and deliberate decisions. Conversely, if self-control abilities are low or impaired, behavior will be more heavily influenced by implicit processes (Brand & Ekkekakis, 2018; Pfeffer & Strobach, 2020; Strack & Deutsch, 2004). As outlined in the physical activity adoption and maintenance model, the most prominent explicit processes include physical activity intention, trait self-regulation, and executive functions, while the implicit processes are represented by automatic affective reactions and habit (Strobach et al., 2020). These variables and how they are intertwined in the regulation of physical activity behavior are described in detail below (◘ Fig. 25.11).

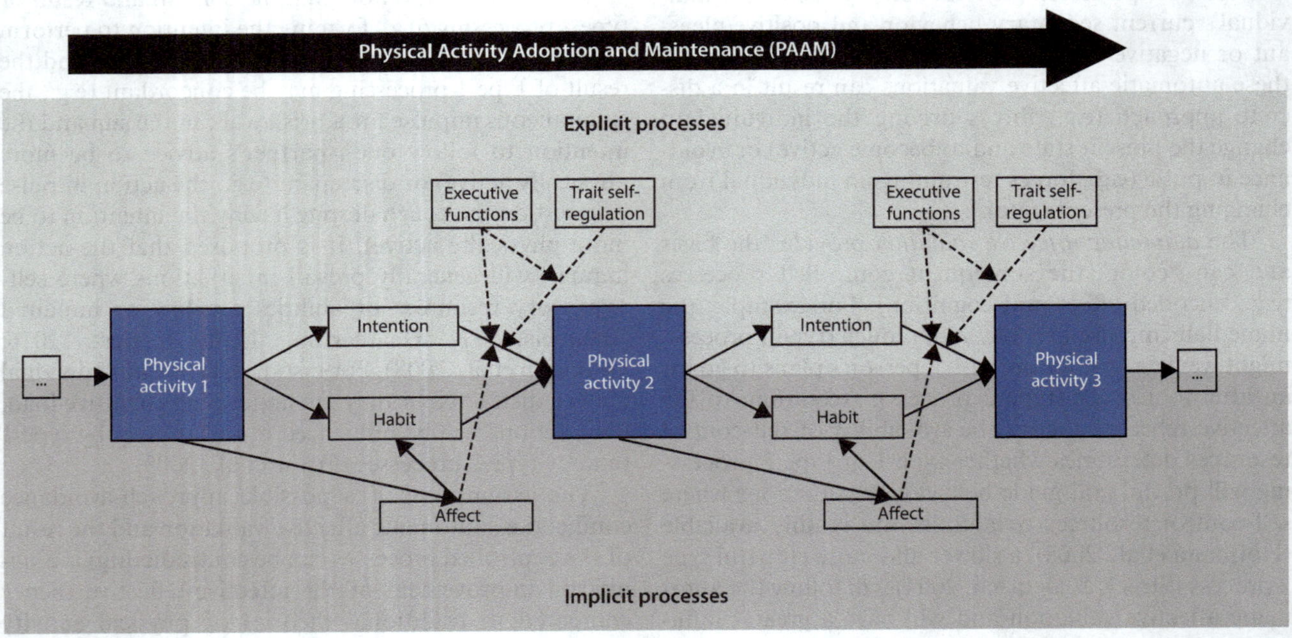

◘ **Fig. 25.11** The physical activity adoption and maintenance model (Strobach et al., 2020)

Explicit Processes

In line with previous research, *explicit processes* are defined as deliberative, effortful, and intentional processes (e.g., Chaiken & Trope, 1999). The basic feature of explicit processes is the guidance of intentional and goal-directed behavior. Explicit processes rely on the availability of cognitive resources to control behavior, and, as such, they are slow and inefficient (Baumeister & Vohs, 2007). In the physical activity adoption and maintenance model, explicit processes include social cognition variables (i.e., intentions and trait self-regulation; Baumeister et al., 1998; Rhodes et al., 2019) as well as self-regulatory processes such as executive functions (e.g., inhibition, updating, shifting; Hofmann et al., 2012).

In regard to the link between social cognition variables and physical activity, individuals are more likely to form physical activity *intentions* when they believe that physical activity is beneficial and that they are actually capable of being physically active (Rhodes et al., 2019). As discussed earlier in this chapter, empirical studies support the central role of intentions for physical activity enactment (Hagger et al., 2002), even though a substantial amount of variance in physical activity behavior remains unexplained by the intention construct alone (Rhodes & de Bruijn, 2013; Sheeran & Webb, 2016).

Regulating the self allows individuals to resist impulses and immediate gratifications in order to initiate behaviors directed at long-term goals and intentions (e.g., Duckworth & Kern, 2011). Empirical research has reliably shown that *trait self-regulation* is crucial in health-related domains (Englert, 2016; Hagger et al., 2019a, 2019b) and there are inter-individual differences in the ability to self-regulate (Tangney et al., 2004). Apart from *inhibiting* certain behavioral tendencies (i.e., *inhibitory self-regulation*), the *initiation* of goal-directed behavior to achieve a desirable long-term goal is an additional central aspect of trait self-regulation (i.e., *initiatory self-regulation*). Saunders et al. (2018) and de Ridder et al. (2011) argue that performing a desired behavior and refraining from an undesired behavior are separate dimensions, which are both functions of trait self-regulation (de Ridder et al., 2012). With regard to physical activity behavior, the physical activity adoption and maintenance model proposes that *initiatory self-regulation* is the more relevant aspect, as physical activity is a positive health behavior that has to be initiated continuously to reach and maintain the desired (health) benefits (de Ridder et al., 2011). Thus, the authors assume that individuals with lower levels of initiatory trait self-regulation are less likely to bridge the intention-behavior gap than individuals with higher levels of initiatory trait self-regulation (Pfeffer & Strobach, 2017).

Executive functions are the mental processes, mainly supported by the prefrontal cortex, which regulate lower-level processes (e.g., individual's perceptions and beliefs), and thereby enable self-regulation through the explicit organization of complex information and the regulation of thoughts, feelings, and behaviors in favor of long-term goals (Buckley et al., 2014; Dohle et al., 2017; Hall & Fong, 2007; Hofmann et al., 2012). A widely accepted concept of executive functions considers three distinct but overlapping executive domains: (1) *inhibition*, (2) *updating*, and (3) *shifting* (Miyake & Friedman, 2012; Miyake et al., 2000). The physical activity adoption and maintenance model identifies updating and shifting as particularly important for *initiating* health behavior. Specifically, the *updating function* can support goal achievement through various mechanisms, as successful self-regulation requires keeping the representation of goals and goal-relevant information active in one's mind for further processing while also downregulating unwanted affect that is incompatible with goal attainment (Hofmann et al., 2011; Hofmann et al., 2012; Kruglanski et al., 2002). While it can be helpful to keep a self-regulatory goal in working memory (supported by the updating function), it can be counterproductive to continuously apply the same rigid plans or means for goal attainment. For example, barriers and difficulties may arise that might impede pre-existing action plans, or new opportunities may arise that might be more effective for achieving the intended goal (Hofmann et al., 2011). Self-regulation can therefore benefit from the *shifting function* by flexibly adapting plans and means to changing circumstances (Vallacher & Wegner, 1987). Individuals with higher cognitive flexibility (i.e., shifting) may be better at adapting their means for goal attainment to rapidly changing environments, which may lead to more adapted behavior in relation to the self-regulatory goal (Buckley et al., 2014).

In line with Wilkowski and Robinson (2016), the physical activity adoption and maintenance model assumes that motivation *and* cognitive ability may be important to consider when predicting self-regulatory outcomes. Self-report measures of self-regulation (such as *trait* self-regulation) may reflect the *motivation* or *willingness* to exert self-regulation across a wide range of situations and behaviors (Karremans et al., 2015; Wilkowski & Robinson, 2016), while executive functions represent the *cognitive ability* to exert self-regulation in more process-oriented terms (Hofmann et al., 2012; Wilkowski & Robinson, 2016). In line with this assumption, a meta-analysis by Duckworth and Kern (2011) revealed only a small correlation between measures of executive functions and trait self-regulation (r = .10).

This suggests that both measures share little common variance even though they convincingly argue to assess self-regulation.

▪ Implicit Processes

Implicit processes can be conceptualized as automatic processes that represent well-learned, spontaneous, and non-conscious influences which are triggered by environmental or internal cues (e.g., Chaiken & Trope, 1999). Compared to explicit processes, implicit processes are fast and effortless, but their response is rather rigid and inflexible (Kahneman, 2017). Implicit processes are based on the principles of associative activation, which is related to classical and operant conditioning (Dickinson, 2016) and typically influence impulsive and intuitive behaviors that involve little deliberation (Rhodes et al., 2019). The two implicit processes included in the physical activity adoption and maintenance model are affective reactions and habits.

Affects refer to subjective experiences that represent simple, non-explicit, and rapid feelings (Frijda, 1986). Russell (2003, p. 147) defined core affect as "a neurophysiological state that is consciously accessible as a simple, non-explicit feeling that is an integral blend of hedonic (pleasure–displeasure) and arousal (sleepy–activated) values." Affects are differentiated on the basis of their valence, that is, how positive or negative the experiences are, and support the activation of approach or avoidance behavior. Unlike core emotions, like anger and happiness, affect refers to simple automatic valuations that something is good or bad (Baumeister et al., 2007). When people experience positive feelings while performing a certain behavior, they are more likely to repeat this behavior than when the behavior is associated with negative feelings (Backhouse et al., 2007). The physical activity adoption and maintenance model therefore assumes that positive affective states towards physical activity increase the probability of successfully translating intentions into behavior, whereas negative affective states might increase the intention-behavior gap.

Habits are automatic impulses to perform an action in response to environmental cues and develop when a specific behavior is consistently performed in stable environmental contexts. Because the automatic nature of habits means that the behavior does not rely on the use of explicit processes (Ouellette & Wood, 1998), and behaviors that have become habitual are more resistant to change. The physical activity adoption and maintenance model assumes that habit formation is characterized by a gradual shift in the regulation of behavior from the use of effortful and explicit (i.e., intentional) cognitive processes, to the implicit regulation of behavior via effortless and automatic (i.e., automatically triggered by environmental cues) processes (Gardner et al., 2011; Gardner & Lally, 2018; Nilsen et al., 2012). While some evidence indicates that habits and intentions have a complementary influence on behavior (Hamilton et al., 2017a, 2017b, 2020a, 2020b; Phipps et al., 2020), research is still on-going into which processes and conditions better facilitate habit formation (Brown et al., 2020; Hagger, 2016). In the context of physical activity, the physical activity adoption and maintenance model assumes that positive affective reactions during physical activity are important for promoting habit formation, whereas pairing physical activity with negative affective states may interfere with the habit formation process (Colwill & Rescorla, 1985).

In sum, the authors assume that explicit and implicit processes operate simultaneously and that the implicit processes will prevail when self-regulatory abilities (i.e., trait self-regulation, executive functions) are lower. In line with habit formation theory, we assume that the probability that a situation will elicit a behavior automatically is associated with the frequency of behavior enactment in a stable environment. By repeating a behavior frequently in the same context, the control of behavior *gradually* shifts from being explicitly controlled (e.g., intention) to being predominantly implicitly controlled (i.e., automatically triggered by situational or contextual cues) due to habit formation. According to our physical activity adoption and maintenance model, this shift will be supported by positive affective reactions during physical activity and/or high trait self-regulation and executive function abilities.

25.4.3 Integrated Models of Health Behavior

As presented above, innumerable psychological theories have been applied to predict physical activity behavior, often with the purpose to identify viable targets for behavior change interventions. A key problem of these theories, and the constructs of which they comprise, is that they often fail to account for a substantive proportion of the variance in behavior, including physical activity. A solution to this may be to integrate constructs from multiple theories to arrive at a new theory that provides more effective behavioral prediction with optimal parsimony. Theory integration can therefore help address the gaps of the theory in its capacity to explain behavior (Trafimow, 2012) and also assist in managing redundancy of constructs across theories by identifying core constructs shown to be effective in predicting behavior (Hagger, 2009).

Although there are numerous approaches to theory integration, Hagger and Hamilton (2020) outline four common approaches: (a) additional constructs approach, (b) core constructs approach, (c) consensus-based approaches, and (d) utility-based approaches.

An *additional constructs approach* is perhaps the most basic and is where constructs are added to an existing theory to address shortcomings in prediction of the existing theory. A classic example is the theory of reasoned action (Fishbein & Ajzen, 1975) which was augmented to include self-efficacy from social-cognitive theory (Bandura, 1986) to produce the theory of planned behavior (Ajzen, 1991). A myriad of papers over the past few decades have been published that claim to have extended a theory by adding constructs, including in the physical activity domain (Allom et al., 2016; Arnautovska et al., 2019; Cowie et al., 2018; Hamilton et al., 2013, 2017a, 2017b). However, it is important to note that when adding constructs to an existing theory clear theoretical specification of how the additional constructs relate to existing constructs is needed; otherwise it constitutes a "weak" theory (Davis et al., 2015).

The *core constructs approach* aims to summarize and then condense key constructs from theories with similar conceptualization but different labels (e.g., attitudes from the theory of planned behavior and outcome expectancies from the health action process approach) into core categories. This approach is best viewed as being informative in the process of integration rather than in the development of a specific integrated theory.

Expert consensus approach is another approach that can be used to identify commonalities and redundancy across theories. For example, Michie et al. (2011) applied expert consensus to specify links between constructs from identified theories and specific behavior change techniques, which yielded a searchable database of links between constructs and techniques (Connell et al., 2018). The database can help inform further theory integration and intervention development by identifying potential means to change target constructs from the various theories.

A final approach to integration is a *utility-based approach*, which is premised on reducing redundancy and increasing complementarity (Hagger, 2009). Reducing redundancy is similar to the core constructs approach and addresses the so-called *déjà-variable* phenomenon: the feeling of having seen a construct with similar definition and content but different label (Hagger, 2014). Increasing complementarity is about identifying how constructs and processes from different theories provide complimentary explanations of behavior. This may help determine the extent to which particular theoretical constructs or processes are relevant to predicting and explaining the particular behavior and those that may be redundant. For example, risk perception is common to many social cognition theories (e.g., health action process approach); however, research has shown the construct to be irrelevant in determining behavior in those who do not perceive themselves to be at risk, e.g., perceived risk of cardiovascular disease as a determinant of physical activity participation in younger populations (e.g., perceived risk of cardiovascular disease as a determinant of physical activity participation in younger populations; Zhang et al., 2019). In this case, examining risk perception is perhaps not useful in a theory applied to that particular population.

A myriad of *integrated theories* have been developed and tested based on the approaches outlined above (e.g., Bagozzi & Warshaw, 1990; Borland, 2017; de Vries et al., 2005; Gerrard et al., 2005; Hagger & Chatzisarantis, 2014; Hall & Fong, 2007; Hamilton et al., 2012; Maher & Conroy, 2016; Montaño & Kasprzyk, 2015; Perugini & Conner, 2000). Two examples specifically developed in the physical activity domain include the *trans-contextual model* of Hagger et al. (2003) and the *integrated behavior change model* for physical activity (Hagger & Chatzisarantis, 2014).

Trans-contextual Model

The trans-contextual model was originally developed to explain the constructs and processes that link school students' motivation for participation in physical activity in school physical education to their motives and beliefs toward and participation in leisure time physical activity. The model draws on self-determination theory (Deci & Ryan, 1985), the hierarchical model of intrinsic and extrinsic motivation (Vallerand et al., 1997), and the theory of planned behavior (Ajzen, 1991) to outline the processes involved (see Hagger et al., 2003, for a full description of the model). In brief, based on self-determination theory, the model predicts that the classroom environment fostered by physical education teachers (e.g., engaging in autonomy-supportive behaviors) determines the type or *form* of motivation (e.g., autonomous motivation, controlled motivation) students experience when performing physical activities in their physical education classes and, importantly, their persistence on tasks. Research demonstrates that autonomously motivated individuals are more likely to persist on tasks and experience greater interest and engagement. Thus, fostering school students' autonomous motivation toward physical activity in physical education contexts through teachers engaging in autonomy-supportive behaviors is therefore considered adaptive and desirable. This autonomous motivation toward physical activities in the physical education context is suggested to transfer across contexts (i.e., to the leisure time context), based on Vallerand's (1997) hierarchical model. Finally, the model posits that autonomous motivation toward physical activities in a leisure time context will be related to students' beliefs and intentions toward, and future participation in, physical activity. This process is modeled by the sets of beliefs from the theory of planned behavior. The trans-contextual model has received meta-analytic support for model predictions across multiple studies (Hagger & Chatzisarantis, 2016), as well as replications of the model predictions across national groups (Hagger et al., 2005) and in other educational contexts (Chan et al., 2015; Hagger & Hamilton, 2018; Hagger et al., 2016).

▪ Integrated Behavior Change Model

The integrated behavior change model (Hagger & Chatzisarantis, 2014) was originally designed to explain the complexity of physical activity behavior and integrates constructs and pathways that represent multiple processes (motivational, volitional, implicit) to provide a more comprehensive explanation of physical activity behavior, as well as the mechanisms involved. The model derives its predictions from social cognition (e.g., theory of planned behavior; Ajzen, 1991), dual-process (e.g., reflexive-impulsive model; Deutsch & Strack, 2020), and dual-phase (e.g., health action process approach; Schwarzer & Hamilton, 2020) theories. The integrated behavior change model specifies three key behavioral processes: (a) a conscious, deliberative route to behavior represented by effects of social cognition constructs (attitude, subjective norm, perceived behavioral control) from the theory of planned behavior on behavior mediated by intentions; (b) a non-conscious, automatic route to behavior represented by direct effects of implicit attitudes and motives, as well as habit; and (c) two action phases, a motivational phase in which intention formation is determined by constructs identified in (a) and a volitional phase in which intentions are implemented via planning (Hagger & Chatzisarantis, 2014; Hagger & Hamilton, 2020). In addition, the model specifies autonomous forms of motivation from self-determination theory as determinants of the social cognition constructs, as outlined in the theorizing of the trans-contextual model (see Hagger & Chatzisarantis, 2009). Although relatively new, numerous studies across a variety of behaviors have provided support for many of the component pathways of the model (Caudwell et al., 2019; Hagger et al., 2017; Hamilton et al., 2017a, 2017b; Phipps et al., 2020).

25.5 General Conclusion

Numerous models explaining physical activity behavior have been developed in the last decades. These models have strengthened our understanding about the relevant predictors and processes that influence people's exercise and physical (in)activity behavior. However, they have advantages and disadvantages that have to be considered when choosing a model for research or health promotion practice.

Motivation models can be used to understand and predict a person's intention to be physically active. However, although intention is often a good predictor of behavior, results of meta-analyses reveal that a large amount of variance in physical activity behavior remain unaccounted for when measuring intention alone (Rhodes & de Bruijn, 2013; Sheeran & Webb, 2016). Despite holding strong intentions to exercise, many individuals often fail to translate their intentions into subsequent action. This phenomenon is also referred to in the literature as the "intention-behavior gap" (► Chaps. 10 and 15). The unsatisfactory explanatory power of motivation models could be based on the insufficient consideration of volitional mechanisms that promote the translation of an intention into concrete action.

This insight has led to the development of more theoretical approaches to action execution. In contrast to motivation models, theories of action execution place less emphasis on identifying the processes that influence the formation of behavioral intentions (Gollwitzer & Oettingen, 1998). Instead, models of action execution focus on the volitional processes and mechanisms through which behavioral intentions can be successfully translated into action. However, neither the motivation models presented in the first section of this chapter nor the theories of action execution presented in the second section of this chapter seem to explain the behavioral change process sufficiently. An integration of motivational and volitional explanation models may serve to better explain the processes and mechanisms that lead to behavior change.

For the investigation of physical activity, stage models have become increasingly accepted in recent years as they are able to describe and differentiate the behavioral change processes that occur at various stages. The two central assumptions of stage models are that (1) individuals behave differently at different stages and differ in various characteristics and that (2) information and interventions must be planned and implemented in a stage-specific manner in order to achieve a successful stage transition and thus a successful change in behavior (Armitage & Conner, 2000; Conner & Norman, 2015). In various studies it has been shown that interventions that take into account aspects of models of action performance can make better predictions of health behavior (e.g., physically active lifestyle; Milne et al., 2002; Prestwich et al., 2003; Sheeran & Silverman, 2003). However, there is still a lack of meaningful longitudinal studies that examine the sustainability of such interventions over several months and years. Such longitudinal research may provide greater insight into how specifically cognitions and behavior change over the various stages and also help identify how potential lapses in behavior can be identified and avoided.

An additional problem with stage models is that it is not yet sufficiently well specified which constructs influence the behavior change process and how (causality). In particular, the process of volition (apart from the concepts of planning and volitional self-efficacy expectation) is not yet sufficiently differentiated and empirically specified in stage models. This is an important task for future research which can help identify at which stage volitional processes may be most effective. This will help create more effective stage-specific interventions, which will be beneficial for creating lasting behavior change (Sutton, 2000).

Side Story

Future Directions

In their recent paper, Rothman and Sheeran (2020) summarized challenges of the current health behavior change research and provided suggestions for future directions. They criticize that although research on health behavior change is still growing, the progress that was made in the past decades has been smaller than expected. Therefore, they describe the obstacles investigators currently must navigate around when planning and evaluating behavior change programs. The authors raised six higher-order questions that should be addressed to increase the impact of health behavior change research not least for practitioners and policymakers:

1. How do we identify targets for interventions (e.g., What principles determine which targets are important for a health behavior?)?
2. Why isn't there a periodic table of health behavior change constructs (e.g., What drives investigators' choice of theories and constructs?)?
3. How do we know if a target is valid (e.g., Should experiments be deemed the "gold standard" for testing target validity?)?
4. How do intervention strategies engage targets (e.g., What strategies can be used if targets are difficult or impossible to change?)?
5. What are the best ways to change targets (e.g., Why are there so few competitive tests of different strategies to change the same target?)?
6. How do we embrace the conditional nature of intervention effects on behavior change (e.g., What are the implications of embracing the assertion that "context matters" for interventions to promote health behavior change)? (Rothman & Sheeran, 2020, p. 949)

The authors aim to prompt a commitment to strategies that address these challenges in order to accelerate knowledge about healthy lifestyles and advances in health behavior change.

The models and theories briefly presented here illustrate a variety of possible explanations for health behavior and behavioral changes in physical activity. The assessment of explanatory power and predictive value is only one criterion. Another criterion should be how well the respective theories can actually be used to implement effective interventions to promote physical activity. Dual-process theories provide a promising and future-oriented approach to examine the adoption and maintenance of physical activity behavior by differentiating between implicit and explicit processes. However, to date there is only preliminary empirical evidence for the complex interplay of these processes in the context of physical activity behavior, and empirical studies testing these models more comprehensively are required, even though empirical evidence for the individual paths already exists. Future research will bring further insights into the complex regulation of physical activity behavior based on implicit and explicit processes. The consideration of affective variables as proposed in the affective-reflective theory and the physical activity adoption and maintenance model may further improve previous theories. Thus, the picture of relevant variables guiding physical activity adoption and maintenance might become more complete, which subsequently allows to derive more effective interventions to promote physical activity initiation and adherence.

While empirical literature is expanding on the use of integrated theories to behavior change, evidence is limited, and further testing of such models is needed across different behaviors, contexts, and populations. Notwithstanding, theory integration offers an elegant way forward to explaining physical activity behavior to arrive at new theories that provide improved predictive capability with minimum expense to parsimony. While existing tests of integrated theories show promise, more research is needed. Future research adopting cross-lagged panel, experimental, or intervention designs is required in order to make better inferences of change and causation in integrated theory components.

25

Learning Control Questions

Basic:

1. What is the most important determinant of health behavior change according to the theory of planned behavior? Which three components influence this determinant?
2. Which determinants influence health behavior in Bandura's social-cognitive model?
3. Which four sources help build self-efficacy expectations? Which is the most important source for developing self-efficacy expectation?
4. What stage-specific forms of self-efficacy expectation does the health action process approach model specify?
5. Describe and provide an example of self-concordance.
6. Which are the two information processing types distinguished in dual-process theories?

Advanced:

7. Which determinants influence behavioral change in the health belief model? Describe each of these components in more detail.
8. What distinguishes implementation intentions from goal intentions? Formulate a goal and an implementation intention using an example of your own choice.
9. Name and describe the stages of behavioral change in the transtheoretical model.
10. What are the main variables identified in the motivation-volition process model? How does this model differ from the affective-reflective theory of physical inactivity and exercise?
11. Outline and describe four common approaches of theory integration.

Experts:

12. What types of models for health behavior change do you know? What are the defining features that differentiate these model types from each other?
13. What is meant by the intention-behavior gap? What strategies or factors help bridge the gap?
14. Name a questionnaire to measure a relevant construct to explain health behavior. What exactly does this questionnaire measure? Describe.
15. Identify and describe the various cognitive-affective and behavioral processes that are important for starting and maintaining physical activity.
16. Describe relevant explicit and implicit processes that are involved in physical activity regulation, and specify how they might act in parallel and interact in predicting physical activity behavior.
17. Explain the integrated behavior change model, and describe which approach of theory integration was used.

References

Abraham, C., & Sheeran, P. (2015). The health belief model. In M. Conner & P. Norman (Eds.), *Predicting and changing health behaviour: Research and practive with social cognition models* (3rd ed., pp. 30-69). : Open University Press.

Achtziger, A., & Gollwitzer, P. M. (2018). Motivation and volition in the course of action. In J. Heckhausen & H. Heckhausen (Eds.), *Motivation and action* (pp. 485–527). : Springer.

Ajzen, I. (1985). From intentions to actions: A theory of planned behavior. In J. Kuhl, & J. Beckmann (Eds.), *Action-control: From cognition to behavior* (pp. 11-39). : Springer.

Ajzen, I. (1991). The theory of planned behavior. *Organizational Behavior & Human Decision Processes, 50*(2), 179–211. https://doi.org/10.1016/0749-5978(91)90020-T

Allom, V., Mullan, B., Cowie, E., & Hamilton, K. (2016). Physical activity and transitioning to college: The importance of intentions and habits. *American Journal of Health Behavior, 40*(2), 280–290.

Armitage, C. J., & Conner, M. (2000). Social cognition models and health behaviour: A structured review. *Psychology and Health, 15*(2), 173–189.

Arnautovska, U., Fleig, L., O'callaghan, F., & Hamilton, K. (2019). Older adults' physical activity: The integration of autonomous motivation and theory of planned behaviour constructs. *Australian Psychologist, 54*(1), 46–54.

Backhouse, S. H., Ekkekakis, P., Biddle, S. J., Foskett, A., & Williams, C. (2007). Exercise makes people feel better but people are inactive: paradox or artifact? *Journal of Sport and Exercise Psychology, 29*(4), 498–517.

Bagozzi, R. P., & Warshaw, P. R. (1990). Trying to consume. *Journal of Consumer Research, 17*(2), 127–140. https://doi.org/10.1086/208543

Bandura, A. (1986). *Social foundations of thought and action: A social cognitive theory*. Prentice-Hall, Inc..

Bandura, A., Cioffi, D., Taylor, C. B., & Brouillard, M. E. (1988). Perceived self-efficacy in coping with cognitive stressors and opioid activation. *Journal of Personality and Social Psychology, 55*(3), 479.

Baumeister, R. F., Bratslavsky, E., Muraven, M., & Tice, D. M. (1998). Ego depletion: Is the active self a limited resource? *Journal of Personality and Social Psychology, 74*(5), 1252–1265.

Baumeister, R. F., & Heatherton, T. F. (1996). Self-regulation failure: An overview. *Psychological Inquiry, 7*(1), 1–15.

Baumeister, R. F., & Vohs, K. D. (2007). Self-regulation, ego depletion, and motivation. *Social and Personality Psychology Compass, 1*(1), 115–128.

Baumeister, R. F., Vohs, K. D., Nathan DeWall, C., & Zhang, L. (2007). How emotion shapes behavior: Feedback, anticipation, and reflection, rather than direct causation. *Personality and Social Psychology Review, 11*(2), 167–203.

Borland, R. (2017). CEOS theory: A comprehensive approach to understanding how to maintain behaviour change. *Applied Psychology: Health and Well-Being, 9*(1), 3–35. https://doi.org/10.1111/aphw.12083

Brand, R., & Ekkekakis, P. (2018). Affective–reflective theory of physical inactivity and exercise. *German Journal of Exercise & Sport Research, 48*(1), 48–58.

Brown, D. J., Hagger, M. S., & Hamilton, K. (2020). The mediating role of constructs representing reasoned-action and automatic processes on the past behavior-future behavior relationship. *Social Science & Medicine, 258*, 113085.

Buckley, J., Cohen, J. D., Kramer, A. F., McAuley, E., & Mullen, S. P. (2014). Cognitive control in the self-regulation of physical activity and sedentary behavior. *Frontiers In Human Neuroscience, 8*, 747–747. https://doi.org/10.3389/fnhum.2014.00747

Bull, F. C., Al-Ansari, S. S., Biddle, S., Borodulin, K., Buman, M. P., Cardon, G., Carty, C., Chaput, J. P., Chastin, S., & Chou, R. (2020). World Health Organization 2020 guidelines on physical activity and sedentary behaviour. *British Journal Of Sports Medicine, 54*(24), 1451–1462.

Carraro, N., & Gaudreau, P. (2013). Spontaneous and experimentally induced action planning and coping planning for physical activity: A meta-analysis. *Psychology of Sport & Exercise, 14*, 228–248.

Caudwell, K. M., Keech, J. J., Hamilton, K., Mullan, B. A., & Hagger, M. S. (2019). Reducing alcohol consumption during pre-drinking sessions: Testing an integrated behaviour-change model. *Psychology & Health, 34*(1), 106–127. https://doi.org/10.1080/08870446.2018.1518527

Chaiken, S., & Trope, Y. (1999). *Dual-process theories in social psychology*. Guilford Press.

Chan, D. K. C., Yang, S. X., Hamamura, T., Sultan, S., Xing, S., Chatzisarantis, N. L. D., & Hagger, M. S. (2015). In-lecture learning motivation predicts students' motivation, intention, and behaviour for after-lecture learning: Examining the trans-contextual model across universities from UK, China, and Pakistan. *Motivation and Emotion, 39*(6), 908–925. https://doi.org/10.1007/s11031-015-9506-x

Chevance, G., Héraud, N., Varray, A., & Boiché, J. (2017). Change in explicit and implicit motivation toward physical activity and sedentary behavior in pulmonary rehabilitation and associations with postrehabilitation behaviors. *Rehabilitation Psychology, 62*(2), 119.

Colwill, R. M., & Rescorla, R. A. (1985). Instrumental responding remains sensitive to reinforcer devaluation after extensive training. *Journal of Experimental Psychology: Animal Behavior Processes, 11*(4), 520.

Connell, L. E., Carey, R. N., de Bruin, M., Rothman, A. J., Johnston, M., Kelly, M. P., & Michie, S. (2018). Links between behavior change techniques and mechanisms of action: An expert consensus study. *Annals of Behavioral Medicine*. https://doi.org/10.1093/abm/kay082

Conner, M., & Norman, P. (2015). *Predicting and changing health behaviour: Research and practice with social cognition models*. Open University Press.

Cowie, E., White, K., & Hamilton, K. (2018). Physical activity and parents of very young children: The role of beliefs and social-cognitive factors. *British Journal of Health Psychology, 23*(4), 782–803.

Davis, R., Campbell, R., Hildon, Z., Hobbs, L., & Michie, S. (2015). Theories of behaviour and behaviour change across the social and behavioural sciences: A scoping review. *Health Psychology Review, 9*(3), 323–344. https://doi.org/10.1080/17437199.2014.941722

de Ridder, D. T. D., de Boer, B. J., Lugtig, P., Bakker, A. B., & van Hooft, E. A. (2011). Not doing bad things is not equivalent to doing the right thing: Distinguishing between inhibitory and initiatory self-control. *Personality and Individual Differences, 50*(7), 1006–1011.

de Ridder, D. T. D., Lensvelt-Mulders, G., Finkenauer, C., Stok, F. M., & Baumeister, R. F. (2012). Taking stock of self-control: A meta-analysis of how trait self-control relates to a wide range of behaviors. *Personality and Social Psychology Review, 16*(1), 76–99. https://doi.org/10.1177/1088868311418749

de Vries, H., Mesters, I., van de Steeg, H., & Honing, C. (2005). The general public's information needs and perceptions regarding hereditary cancer: An application of the Integrated Change Model. *Patient Education and Counseling, 56*(2), 154–165. https://doi.org/10.1016/j.pec.2004.01.002

Deci, E. L., & Ryan, R. M. (1985). *Intrinsic motivation & self-determination in human behavior*.

Deutsch, R., & Strack, F. (2020). Changing behavior using the reflective-impulsive model. In M. S. Hagger, L. D. Cameron, K. Hamilton, N. Hankonen, & T. Lintunen (Eds.), The handbook of behavior change (pp. 164-177). : Cambridge University Press.

Dickinson, A. (2016). *Instrumental conditioning revisited: updating dual-process theory*. Paper presented at the Associative learning and cognition: homage to professor NJ Mackintosh. In Memoriam (1935–2015).

DiClemente, C., & Graydon, M. (2020). Changing Behavior Using the Transtheoretical Model. In M. S. Hagger, L. Cameron, K. Hamilton, N. Hankonen, & T. Lintunen (Eds.), *The handbook of behavior change* (pp. 136-149). : Cambridge University Press.

Dohle, S., Diel, K. & Hofmann, W. (2017). Executive functions and the self-regulation of eating behavior.A ppetite, 30, 1e6.

Duckworth, A. L., & Kern, M. L. (2011). A meta-analysis of the convergent validity of self-control measures. *Journal of Research in Personality*, 45(3), 259–268. https://doi.org/10.1016/j.jrp.2011.02.004

Englert, C. (2016). The strength model of self-control in sport and exercise psychology. *Frontiers in Psychology, 7*, 314.

Fishbein, M., & Ajzen, I. (1975). *Belief, attitude, intention and behavior*. Addison-Wesley.

Friese, M., Hofmann, W., & Wänke, M. (2008). When impulses take over: Moderated predictive validity of explicit and implicit attitude measures in predicting food choice and consumption behaviour. *British Journal of Social Psychology, 47*(3), 397–419.

Frijda, N. H. (1986). *The emotions*. Cambridge University Press.

Fuchs, R. (2007). Das MoVo-Modell als theoretische Grundlage für Programme der gesundheitsverhaltensänderung [The MoVo-Process Model as theoretical basis of health behavior change programs]. In R. Fuchs, W. Göhner, & H. Seelig (Eds.), *Aufbau eines körperlich-aktiven Lebensstils [Development of a physically active lifestyle]* (pp. 317-325). : Hogrefe.

Fuchs, R., Goehner, W., & Seelig, H. (2011). Long-term effects of a psychological group intervention on physical exercise and health: The MoVo concept. *Journal of Physical Activity & Health, 8*(6), 794–803.

Fuchs, R., Göhner, W., & Seelig, H. (2007). *Aufbau eines körperlich-aktiven Lebensstils: Theorie, Empirie und Praxis*. Hogrefe Verlag.

Fuchs, R., Seelig, H., Göhner, W., Schlatterer, M., & Ntoumanis, N. (2017). The two sides of goal intentions: Intention self-concordance and intention strength as predictors of physical activity. *Psychology & Health, 32*(1), 110–126.

Gardner, B., de Bruijn, G.-J., & Lally, P. (2011). A systematic review and meta-analysis of applications of the Self-Report Habit Index to nutrition and physical activity behaviours. *Annals of Behavioral Medicine, 42*(2), 174–187.

Gardner, B., & Lally, P. (2018). Modelling habit formation and its determinants. In B. Verplanken (Ed.), *The psychology of habit. Theory, mechanisms, change, and contexts* (pp. 207–229). Springer.

Gerrard, M., Gibbons, F. X., Stock, M. L., Lune, L. S. V., & Cleveland, M. J. (2005). Images of smokers and willingness to smoke among African American pre-adolescents: An application of the prototype/willingness model of adolescent health risk behavior to smoking initiation. *Journal of Pediatric Psychology, 30*(4), 305–318. https://doi.org/10.1093/jpepsy/jsi026

Göhner, W., & Fuchs, R. (2006). Änderung des Gesundheitsverhaltens: MoVo-Gruppenprogramme für körperliche Aktivität und gesunde Ernährung [Health behavior change]. *Hogrefe Verlag*.

Gollwitzer, P. M. (1990). Action phases and mind-sets. In E. Higgins & R. M. Sorrentino (Eds.), *Handbook of motivation and cognition. Foundations of social behavior*. 2nd ed. pp. 53-92). : The Guilford Press.

Gollwitzer, P. M. (1999). Implementation intentions: Strong effects of simple plans. *American Psychologist, 54*(7), 493–503. https://doi.org/10.1037/0003-066X.54.7.493

Gollwitzer, P. M., & Brandstätter, V. (1997). Implementation intentions and effective goal pursuit. *Journal of Personality & Social Psychology, 73*(1), 186–199.

Gollwitzer, P. M., Fujita, K., & Oettingen, G. (2004). Planning and the implementation of goals. In R. F. Baumeister & K. D. Vohs (Eds.), *Handbook of self-regulation: Research, theory, and applications* (pp. 211–228). : Guilford Press.

Gollwitzer, P. M., & Oettingen, G. (1998). The emergence and implementation of health goals. *Psychology and Health, 13*(4), 687–715.

Hagger, M. S. (2009). Theoretical integration in health psychology: Unifying ideas and complimentary explanations. *British Journal of Health Psychology, 14*(2), 189–194. https://doi.org/10.1348/135910708X397034

Hagger, M. S. (2014). Avoiding the "déjà-variable" phenomenon: Social psychology needs more guides to constructs. *Frontiers in Psychology, 5*, 52.

Hagger, M. S. (2016). Non-conscious processes and dual-process theories in health psychology. *Health Psychology Review, 10*(4), 375–380.

Hagger, M. S., Cameron, L. D., Hamilton, K., Hankonen, N., & Lintunen, T. (2020a). Changing behavior: A theory-and evidence-based approach. In M. S. Hagger, L. D. Cameron, K. Hamilton, N. Hankonen, & T. Lintunen (Eds.), *The handbook of behavior change* (pp. 1-14). Cambridge University Press.

Hagger, M. S., Cameron, L. D., Hamilton, K., Hankonen, N., & Lintunen, T. (2020b). *The handbook of behavior change*. Cambridge University Press.

Hagger, M. S., & Chatzisarantis, N. (2005). *The social psychology of exercise and sport*. McGraw-Hill Education.

Hagger, M. S., & Chatzisarantis, N. (2014). An integrated behavior change model for physical activity. *Exercise and Sport Sciences Reviews, 42*(2), 62–69.

Hagger, M. S., & Chatzisarantis, N. L. D. (2009). Integrating the theory of planned behaviour and self-determination theory in health behaviour: A meta-analysis. *British Journal of Health Psychology, 14*(2), 275–302. https://doi.org/10.1348/135910708X373959

Hagger, M. S., & Chatzisarantis, N. L. D. (2016). The trans-contextual model of autonomous motivation in education: Conceptual and empirical issues and meta-analysis. *Review of Educational Research, 86*(2), 360–407. https://doi.org/10.3102/0034654315585005

Hagger, M. S., Chatzisarantis, N. L. D., Barkoukis, V., Wang, C. K. J., & Baranowski, J. (2005). Perceived autonomy support in physical education and leisure-time physical activity: A cross-cultural evaluation of the trans-contextual model. *Journal of Educational Psychology, 97*(3), 376–390. https://doi.org/10.1037/0022-0663.97.3.376

Hagger, M. S., Chatzisarantis, N. L. D., & Biddle, S. J. H. (2002). A meta-analytic review of the theories of reasoned action and planned behavior in physical activity: Predictive validity and the contribution of additional variables. *Journal of Sport & Exercise Psychology, 24*(1), 3–32. https://doi.org/10.1123/jsep.24.1.3

Hagger, M. S., Chatzisarantis, N. L. D., Culverhouse, T., & Biddle, S. J. (2003). The processes by which perceived autonomy support in physical education promotes leisure-time physical activity intentions and behavior: A trans-contextual model. *Journal of Educational Psychology, 95*(4), 784.

Hagger, M. S., Cheung, M., Ajzen, I., & Hamilton, K. (n.d., under review). Moderation effects in the theory of planned behavior: A meta-analysis in the health behavior domain.

Hagger, M. S., Gucciardi, D. F., Turrell, A. S., & Hamilton, K. (2019a). Self-control and health-related behaviour: The role of implicit self-control, trait self-control, and lay beliefs in self-control. *British Journal of Health Psychology, 24*(4), 764–786.

Hagger, M. S., & Hamilton, K. (2018). Motivational predictors of students' participation in out-of-school learning activities and academic attainment in science: An application of the trans-contextual model using Bayesian path analysis. *Learning and Individual Differences, 67*, 232–244. https://doi.org/10.1016/j.lindif.2018.09.002

Hagger, M. S., & Hamilton, K. (2020). Changing Behavior Using Integrated Theories. In M. S. Hagger, L. D. Cameron, K. Hamilton, N. Hankonen, & T. Lintunen (Eds.), *The handbook of behavior change* (pp. 208–224). : Cambridge University Press.

Hagger, M. S., Hankonen, N., Kangro, E. M., Lintunen, T., Pagaduan, J., Polet, J., Ries, F., & Hamilton, K. (2019b). Trait self-control, social cognition constructs, and intentions: Correlational evidence for mediation and moderation effects in diverse health behaviours. *Applied Psychology: Health and Well-Being, 11*(3), 407–437.

Hagger, M. S., & Luszczynska, A. (2014). Implementation intention and action planning interventions in health contexts: State of the research and proposals for the way forward. *Applied Psychology: Health & Well-Being, 6*(1), 1–47. https://doi.org/10.1111/aphw.12017

Hagger, M. S., Sultan, S., Hardcastle, S. J., Reeve, J., Patall, E. A., Fraser, B., Hamilton, K., & Chatzisarantis, N. L. (2016). Applying the integrated trans-contextual model to mathematics activities in the classroom and homework behavior and attainment. *Learning and Individual Differences, 45*, 166–175.

Hagger, M. S., Trost, N., Keech, J., Chan, D. K. C., & Hamilton, K. (2017). Predicting sugar consumption: Application of an integrated dual-process, dual-phase model. *Appetite, 116*, 147–156. https://doi.org/10.1016/j.appet.2017.04.032

Hall, P. A., & Fong, G. T. (2007). Temporal self-regulation theory: A model for individual health behavior. *Health Psychology Review, 1*(1), 6–52. https://doi.org/10.1080/17437190701492437

Hallal, P. C., Andersen, L. B., Bull, F. C., Guthold, R., Haskell, W., Ekelund, U., & Lancet Physical Activity Series Working Group. (2012). Global physical activity levels: Surveillance progress, pitfalls, and prospects. *Lancet, 380*(9838), 247–257.

Hamilton, K., Cox, S., & White, K. M. (2012). Testing a model of physical activity among mothers and fathers of young children: Integrating self-determined motivation, planning, and theory of planned behavior. *Journal of Sport and Exercise Psychology, 34*(1), 124–145.

Hamilton, K., Fleig, L., Henderson, J., & Hagger, M. S. (2017a). Being active in pregnancy: Theory-based predictors of physical activity among pregnant women. *Women & Health, 9*(2), 213–228.

Hamilton, K., Gibbs, I., Keech, J. J., & Hagger, M. S. (2020a). Reasoned and implicit processes in heavy episodic drinking: An integrated dual-process model. *British Journal of Health Psychology, 25*(1), 189–209.

Hamilton, K., Kirkpatrick, A., Rebar, A., & Hagger, M. S. (2017b). Child sun safety: Application of an Integrated Behavior Change model. *Health Psychology, 36*(9), 916.

Hamilton, K., Thomson, C. E., & White, K. M. (2013). Promoting active lifestyles in young children: Investigating mothers' decisions about their child's physical activity and screen time behaviours. *Maternal and Child Health Journal, 17*(5), 968–976.

Hamilton, K., van Dongen, A., & Hagger, M. S. (2020b). An extended theory of planned behavior for parent-for-child health behaviors: A meta-analysis. *Health Psychology, 39*(10), 863.

Hannan, T. E., Moffitt, R. L., Neumann, D. L., & Kemps, E. (2019). Implicit approach–avoidance associations predict leisure-time exercise independently of explicit exercise motivation. *Sport, Exercise, and Performance Psychology, 8*(2), 210.

Harrison, J. A., Mullen, P. D., & Green, L. W. (1992). A meta-analysis of studies of the health belief model with adults. *Health Education Research, 7*(1), 107–116.

Hausenblas, H. A., Carron, A. V., & Mack, D. E. (1997). Application of the theories of reasoned action and planned behavior to exercise behavior: A meta-analysis. *Journal of Sport and Exercise Psychology, 19*(1), 36–51.

Heckhausen, J., & Heckhausen, H. (2010). Motivation und Entwicklung. In J. Heckhausen & H. Heckhausen (Eds.), *Motivation und Handeln* (pp. 427-488). : Springer.

Hofmann, W., Friese, M., Schmeichel, B. J., & Baddeley, A. D. (2011). Working memory and self-regulation. In M. Boekaerts, P. R. Pintrich, & M. Zeidner (Eds.), *Handbook of self-regulation: Research, theory, and applications* (Vol. 2, pp. 204–225).

Hofmann, W., Friese, M., & Strack, F. (2009). Impulse and self-control from a dual-systems perspective. *Perspectives on Psychological Science, 4*(2), 162–176. https://doi.org/10.1111/j.1745-6924.2009.01116.x

Hofmann, W., Friese, M., & Wiers, R. W. (2008). Impulsive versus reflective influences on health behavior: A theoretical framework and empirical review. *Health Psychology Review, 2*(2), 111–137.

Hofmann, W., Schmeichel, B. J., & Baddeley, A. D. (2012). Executive functions and self-regulation. *Trends in Cognitive Sciences, 16*(3), 174–180. https://doi.org/10.1016/j.tics.2012.01.006

Hutchison, A. J., Breckon, J. D., & Johnston, L. H. (2009). Physical activity behavior change interventions based on the transtheoretical model: A systematic review. *Health Education & Behavior, 36*(5), 829–845.

Kahneman, D. (2017). *Thinking, fast and slow*. Penguin.

Karremans, J. C., Pronk, T. M., & van der Wal, R. C. (2015). Executive control and relationship maintenance processes: An empirical overview and theoretical integration. *Social and Personality Psychology Compass, 9*(7), 333–347.

Kruglanski, A. W., Shah, J. Y., Fishbach, A., Friedman, R., Chun, W. Y., & Sleeth-Keppler, D. (2002). A theory of goal systems. *Advances in Experimental Social Psychology, 34*, 331–378.

Kuhl, J., & Goschke, T. (1994). A theory of action control: Mental subsystems, modes of control, and volitional conflict-resolution strategies. In J. Kuhl & J. Beckman (Eds.), *Volition and Personality: Action versus state orientation* (pp. 93–124). : Hogrefe & Huber.

Kwasnicka, D., Presseau, J., White, M., & Sniehotta, F. F. (2013). Does planning how to cope with anticipated barriers facilitate health-related behaviour change? A systematic review. *Health Psychology Review, 7*, 129–145.

Lazarus, R. S., & Folkman, S. (1987). Transactional theory and research on emotions and coping. *European Journal of Personality, 1*(3), 141–169.

Maher, J. P., & Conroy, D. E. (2016). A dual-process model of older adults' sedentary behavior. *Health Psychology, 35*(3), 262–272. https://doi.org/10.1037/hea0000300

Marlatt, G. A., Baer, J. S., & Quigley, L. A. (1995). Self-efficacy and addictive behavior. In A. Bandura (Ed.), *Self-efficacy in changing societies* (pp. 289-315). : Cambridge University Press.

Marshall, S. J., & Biddle, S. J. H. (2001). The transtheoretical model of behavior change: A meta-analysis of applications to physical activity and exercise. *Annals of Behavioral Medicine, 23*(4), 229–246.

McEachan, R. R. C., Conner, M., Taylor, N. J., & Lawton, R. J. (2011). Prospective prediction of health-related behaviours with the theory of planned behaviour: A meta-analysis. *Health Psychology Review, 5*(2), 97–144.

Michie, S., Ashford, S., Sniehotta, F. F., Dombrowski, S. U., Bishop, A., & French, D. P. (2011). A refined taxonomy of behaviour change techniques to help people change their physical activity and healthy eating behaviours: The CALO-RE taxonomy. *Psychology & Health, 26*(11), 1479–1498.

Milne, S., Orbell, S., & Sheeran, P. (2002). Combining motivational and volitional interventions to promote exercise participation: Protection motivation theory and implementation intentions. *British Journal of Health Psychology, 7*(2), 163–184.

Miyake, A., & Friedman, N. P. (2012). The nature and organization of individual differences in executive functions four general conclusions. *Current Directions in Psychological Science, 21*(1), 8–14. https://doi.org/10.1177/0963721411429458

Miyake, A., Friedman, N. P., Emerson, M. J., Witzki, A. H., Howerter, A., & Wager, T. D. (2000). The unity and diversity of executive functions and their contributions to complex "frontal lobe" tasks: A latent variable analysis. *Cognitive Psychology, 41*(1), 49–100. https://doi.org/10.1006/cogp.1999.0734

Montaño, D. E., & Kasprzyk, D. (2015). Theory of reasoned action, theory of planned behavior, and the integrated behavioral model. In K. Glanz, B. K. Rimer, & K. Viswanath (Eds.), *Health behavior and health education: Theory, research, and practice* (5th ed., pp. 95-124). : Jossey-Bass.

Nilsen, P., Roback, K., Broström, A., & Ellström, P.-E. (2012). Creatures of habit: accounting for the role of habit in implementation research on clinical behaviour change. *Implementation Science, 7*(1), 53.

Norman, P., & Conner, M. (2005). The theory of planned behavior and exercise: Evidence for the mediating and moderating roles of planning on intention-behavior relationships. *Journal of Sport & Exercise Psychology, 27*(4), 488–504. https://doi.org/10.1123/jsep.27.4.488

Ouellette, J. A., & Wood, W. (1998). Habit and intention in everyday life: The multiple processes by which past behavior predicts future behavior. *Psychological Bulletin, 124*(1), 54.

Padin, A. C., Emery, C. F., Vasey, M., & Kiecolt-Glaser, J. K. (2017). Self-regulation and implicit attitudes toward physical activity influence exercise behavior. *Journal of Sport and Exercise Psychology, 39*(4), 237–248.

Parschau, L., Fleig, L., Koring, M., Lange, D., Knoll, N., Schwarzer, R., & Lippke, S. (2013). Positive experience, self-efficacy, and action control predict physical activity changes: A moderated mediation analysis. *British Journal of Health Psychology, 18*(2), 395–406.

Perugini, M., & Conner, M. (2000). Predicting and understanding behavioral volitions: The interplay between goals and behaviors. *European Journal of Social Psychology, 30*(5), 705–731. https://doi.org/10.1002/1099-0992%28200009/10%2930%3A5<705%3A%3AAID-EJSP18>3.0.CO%3B2-%23

Pfeffer, I., & Alfermann, D. (2008). Initiation of physical exercise: an intervention study based on the transtheoretical model. *International Journal of Sport Psychology, 39*(1), 41–58.

Pfeffer, I., Englert, C., & Müller-Alcazar, A. (2020). Perceived stress and trait self-control interact with the intention–behavior gap in physical activity behavior. *Sport, Exercise &*

Performance Psychology, 9(2), 244–260. https://doi.org/10.1037/spy0000189

Pfeffer, I., & Strobach, T. (2017). Executive functions, trait self-control, and the intention-behavior gap in physical activity behavior. *Journal of Sport & Exercise Psychology, 39*(4), 277–292. https://doi.org/10.1123/jsep.2017-0112

Pfeffer, I., & Strobach, T. (2019). Effects of a planning intervention on physical activity behavior in an RCT: Intention strength as moderator and action planning, coping planning and coping self-efficacy as mediators. *Sport, Exercise & Performance Psychology, 8*(2), 192–209.

Pfeffer, I., & Strobach, T. (2020). Physical activity automaticity, intention, and trait self- control as predictors of physical activity behavior—a dual-process perspective. *Psychology, Health & Medicine.*

Phipps, D. J., Hagger, M. S., & Hamilton, K. (2020). Predicting limiting 'free sugar'consumption using an integrated model of health behavior. *Appetite, 150*, 104668.

Phipps, D. J., Hannan, T. E., Rhodes, R. E., & Hamilton, K. (2021). A dual-process model of affective and instrumental attitudes in predicting physical activity. *Psychology of Sport and Exercise, 54*, 101899.

Prestwich, A., Lawton, R., & Conner, M. (2003). The use of implementation intentions and the decision balance sheet in promoting exercise behaviour. *Psychology and Health, 18*(6), 707–721.

Prochaska, J. O., & DiClemente, C. C. (1982). Transtheoretical therapy: toward a more integrative model of change. *Psychotherapy: Theory, Research & Practice, 19*(3), 276–288.

Prochaska, J. O., & DiClemente, C. C. (1983). Stages and processes of self-change of smoking: Toward an integrative model of change. *Journal of Consulting and Clinical Psychology, 51*(3), 390–395. https://doi.org/10.1037/0022-006X.51.3.390

Prochaska, J. O., & Marcus, B. H. (1994). The transtheoretical model: Applications to exercise. In R. K. Dishman (Ed.), *Advances in exercise adherence* (pp. 161–180). : Human Kinetics.

Reyes Fernández, B., Knoll, N., Hamilton, K., & Schwarzer, R. (2016). Social-cognitive antecedents of hand washing: Action control bridges the planning–behaviour gap. *Psychology & Health, 31*(8), 993–1004.

Rhodes, R. E., & de Bruijn, G.-J. (2013). How big is the physical activity intention-behaviour gap? A meta-analysis using the action control framework. *British Journal of Health Psychology, 18*(2), 296–309. https://doi.org/10.1111/bjhp.12032

Rhodes, R. E., McEwan, D., & Rebar, A. L. (2019). Theories of physical activity behaviour change: A history and synthesis of approaches. *Psychology of Sport and Exercise, 42*, 100–109.

Rosen, C. S. (2000). Is the sequencing of change processes by stage consistent across health problems? A meta-analysis. *Health Psychology, 19*(6), 593.

Rosenstock, I. M. (1974). The health belief model and preventive health behavior. *Health Education Monographs, 2*(4), 354–386.

Rothman, A. (2000). Toward a theory-based analysis of behavioral maintenance. *Health Psychology, 19*(1), 64–69.

Rothman, A. J., & Sheeran, P. (2020). What is slowing us down? Six challenges to accelerating advances in health behavior change. *Annals of Behavioral Medicine*, 54(12), 948–959.

Russell, J. A. (2003). Core affect and the psychological construction of emotion. *Psychological Review, 110*(1), 145–172.

Sallis, J. F., Bull, F., Guthold, R., Heath, G. W., Inoue, S., Kelly, P., et al. (2016). Progress in physical activity over the Olympic quadrennium. *The Lancet, 388*(10051), 1325–1336.

Saunders, B., Milyavskaya, M., Etz, A., Randles, D., & Inzlicht, M. (2018). Reported self-control is not meaningfully associated with inhibition-related executive function: A Bayesian analysis. *Collabra: Psychology, 4*(1), 39.

Scholz, U., Schüz, B., Ziegelmann, J. P., Lippke, S., & Schwarzer, R. (2008). Beyond behavioural intentions: Planning mediates between intentions and physical activity. *British Journal of Health Psychology, 13*(3), 479–494. https://doi.org/10.1348/135910707X216062

Scholz, U., Sniehotta, F. F., & Schwarzer, R. (2005). Predicting physical exercise in cardiac rehabilitation: The role of phase-specific self-efficacy beliefs. *Journal of Sport & Exercise Psychology, 27*(2), 135–151. https://doi.org/10.1123/jsep.27.2.135

Schwarzer, R. (1997). *Gesundheitspsychologie: Ein Lehrbuch [Health psychology: A textbook]*. Hogrefe Verlag.

Schwarzer, R. (2004). *Psychologie des Gesundheitsverhaltens: Einführung in die Gesundheitspsychologie [Psychology of health behavior: An introduction to health psychology]*. Hogrefe Verlag.

Schwarzer, R. (2008). Modeling health behavior change: How to predict and modify the adoption and maintenance of health behaviors. *Applied Psychology, 57*(1), 1–29.

Schwarzer, R., & Hamilton, K. (2020). Changing behavior using the health action process approach. In M. Hagger, L. D. Cameron, K. Hamilton, N. Hankonen, & T. Lintunen (Eds.), *The handbook of behavior change* (pp. 89-103). : Cambridge University Press.

Schwarzer, R., Schüz, B., Ziegelmann, J. P., Lippke, S., Luszczynska, A., & Scholz, U. (2007). Adoption and maintenance of four health behaviors: Theory-guided longitudinal studies on dental flossing, seat belt use, dietary behavior, and physical activity. *Annals of Behavioral Medicine, 33*(2), 156–166. https://doi.org/10.1007/BF02879897

Seelig, H., & Fuchs, R. (2006). Messung der sport-und bewegungsbezogenen Selbstkonkordanz. *Zeitschrift für Sportpsychologie, 13*(4), 121–139.

Sheeran, P., & Silverman, M. (2003). Evaluation of three interventions to promote workplace health and safety: evidence for the utility of implementation intentions. *Social Science & Medicine, 56*(10), 2153–2163.

Sheeran, P., & Webb, T. L. (2016). The intention–behavior gap. *Social & Personality Psychology Compass, 10*(9), 503–518. https://doi.org/10.1111/spc3.12265

Sniehotta, F. F., Presseau, J., & Araújo-Soares, V. (2014). Time to retire the theory of planned behaviour. *Health Psychology Review, 8*(1), 1–7.

Sniehotta, F. F., Scholz, U., & Schwarzer, R. (2006). Action plans and coping plans for physical exercise: A longitudinal intervention study in cardiac rehabilitation. *British Journal of Health Psychology, 11*(1), 23–37. https://doi.org/10.1348/135910705X43804

Sniehotta, F. F., Schwarzer, R., Scholz, U., & Schüz, B. (2005). Action planning and coping planning for long-term lifestyle change: Theory and assessment. *European Journal of Social Psychology, 35*(4), 565–576. https://doi.org/10.1002/ejsp.258

Strack, F., & Deutsch, R. (2004). Reflective and impulsive determinants of social behavior. *Personality & Social Psychology Review, 8*(3), 220–247.

Strobach, T., Englert, C., Jekauc, D., & Pfeffer, I. (2020). Predicting adoption and maintenance of physical activity in the context of dualprocess theories. *Performance Enhancement and Health, 8*(1), 100162.

Sutton, S. (2000). Interpreting cross-sectional data on stages of change. *Psychology and Health, 15*(2), 163–171.

Tangney, J. P., Baumeister, R. F., & Boone, A. L. (2004). High self-control predicts good adjustment, less pathology, better grades, and interpersonal success. *Journal of Personality, 72*(2), 271–322. https://doi.org/10.1111/j.0022-3506.2004.00263.x

Trafimow, D. (2012). The role of auxiliary assumptions for the validity of manipulations and measures. *Theory & Psychology, 22*(4), 486–498. https://doi.org/10.1177/0959354311429996

Vallacher, R. R., & Wegner, D. M. (1987). What do people think they're doing? Action identification and human behavior. *Psychological Review, 94*(1), 3.

Vallerand, R. J. (1997). Towards a hierarchical model of intrinsic and extrinsic motivation. *Advances in Experimental Social Psychology, 29*, 271–360. https://doi.org/10.1016/S0065-2601(08)60019-2

Vallerand, R. J., Fortier, M. S., & Guay, F. (1997). Self-determination and persistence in a real-life setting: Toward a motivational model of high school dropout. *Journal of Personality and Social Psychology, 72*, 1161–1176.

WHO. (2000). *The world health report 2000: Health systems: Improving performance*. World Health Organization.

Wilkowski, B., & Robinson, M. (2016). Cognitive control processes underlying individual differences in self-control. In E. R. Hirt, J. J. Clarkson, & L. Jia (Eds.), Self-regulation and ego control (pp. 301-324). Elsevier.

Yang-Wallentin, F., Schmidt, P., Davidov, E., & Bamberg, S. (2004). Is there any interaction effect between intention and perceived behavioral control. *Methods of Psychological Research Online, 8*(2), 127–157.

Zhang, C. Q., Zhang, R., Schwarzer, R., & Hagger, M. S. (2019). A meta-analysis of the health action process approach. Health Psychology, Advance online publication.

Zhou, G., Gan, Y., Miao, M., Hamilton, K., Knoll, N., & Schwarzer, R. (2015a). The role of action control and action planning on fruit and vegetable consumption. *Appetite, 91*, 64–68.

Zhou, G., Sun, C., Knoll, N., Hamilton, K., & Schwarzer, R. (2015b). Self-efficacy, planning and action control in an oral self-care intervention. *Health Education Research, 30*(4), 671–681.

Ziegelmann, J. P., Lippke, S., & Schwarzer, R. (2006). Adoption and maintenance of physical activity: Planning interventions in young, middle-aged, and older adults. *Psychology & Health, 21*(2), 145–163. https://doi.org/10.1080/14768320500018891

Physical Activity, Subjective Well-Being and Mental Health

Gorden Sudeck, Ansgar Thiel and Kelley Strohacker

Contents

J. Schüler et al. (eds.), *Sport and Exercise Psychology*, https://doi.org/10.1007/978-3-031-03921-8_26

Learning Objectives

Basic:

- Be able to describe psychological components of health and well-being
- Be familiar with methods for assessing well-being used in exercise psychology

Advanced:

- Being able to summarize research findings regarding how physical activity (primarily exercise) affects well-being and mental health

Experts:

- Be able to explain why and under what conditions positive effects of physical activity occur
- Be able to describe starting points for the targeted promotion of well-being and mental health through physical activity and exercise

26.1 Introduction

Physical activity enhances well-being and improves quality of life! This statement sounds so familiar that we may believe it to already be evident. Physically active individuals report that their experiences support this statement, health and fitness companies advertise with similar slogans, and comparable statements regularly appear in print and digital media. In this chapter, we will discuss, from a scientific perspective, if this connection is indeed clear and under which circumstances it might exist.

First, we must clarify key terminology to prevent conflation of related, but distinct constructs. "Physical activity" is an umbrella term that refers to any bodily movement that is produced by skeletal muscle and that increases metabolic rate above that of rest (Caspersen et al., 1985). Physical activity can be accumulated through activities occurring in all domains—transportation, occupational, domestic, and leisure-time. In this chapter, we will often refer to "exercise," which is a form of leisure-time physical activity that is planned, structured, and repeatedly performed with the intent to maintain or improve one or more components of health- or skill-related physical fitness.

Despite the widely advertised positive associations between physical activity and numerous health outcomes, a considerable proportion of people are insufficiently active, with some reporting no physical activity at all. This discrepancy is quite surprising, as one might assume that people would have a primary interest in improving their well-being and quality of life, as well as optimizing their own mental health through appropriate activities, such as structured exercise or sport. Yet the many anecdotal reports regarding the positive effects of physical activity on mental health are seemingly countered by a variety of excuses as to why people are not active on a regular basis. Motivation is lacking. Access to good-quality resources and suitable training partners are missing. Most commonly, people indicate that they simply do not have the time to dedicate to additional activities beyond their everyday obligations. While this phenomenon of physical inactivity is dealt with in other parts of this textbook (► Chaps. 10, 15, and 25, Intention-Behavior-Gap; ► Chap. 25, Models of Health Behavior), we take a closer look here at the opening statement in particular: we examine if the assumption that physical activity positively impacts well-being and mental health is scientifically well-founded.

To best preface this chapter, it is important to note that physical activity does not have the same effect on everyone's well-being and mental health. Further, context matters, effects are dependent on the type of activity undertaken, the settings in which they are performed, and ultimately on the subjective experience of the individual. In addition, well-being and mental health are multilayered constructs; physical activity may have differing effects on their various subcomponents. Taken together, the advertised messaging fails to capture the complexity of the relationships between physical activity, subjective well-being, and mental health.

In the following sections, we will first discuss what is meant by mental health and well-being and how these constructs are embedded in a holistic, biopsychosocial health model (► Sect. 26.2). Building on this, we present what is known regarding relationships specifically between exercise (including sporting activities) and mental health (► Sect. 26.3), followed by explanations of these relationships from different scientific perspectives. These explanations, in turn, form the basis for identifying starting points for the targeted promotion of well-being and mental health through exercise-related and other physical activity (► Sect. 26.4).

26.2 Psychological Dimensions of Health and Well-Being

26.2.1 Basic Definitions of Health and Health Models

Definitions of health can vary widely. For example, health is defined differently from a biomedical perspective than from a psychological, sociological, or legal perspective. The historical–cultural context also has an influence on the understanding of health. Further, theoretical models in which determinants of health are addressed vary depending on the professional background of the experts (Waller, 2006).

For the purpose of this chapter, we refer to a health definition by the health scientist Klaus Hurrelmann, as this integrates different perspectives and thus makes it possible to identify central components of a multidisciplinary understanding of health.

Health

"Health is the stage of a balance regarding risk factors and protective factors that occurs when a person succeeds in coping with both internal (physical and psychological) and external (social and material) demands. Health is a stage that provides a person with well-being and enjoyment of life." (Hurrelmann, 2000, S. 94; translation by the authors)

Hurrelmann's definition has several advantages for exercise science research on health and well-being:

- Hurrelmann' s definition places the **subjective components of health** at the center of consideration by emphasizing individual categories of well-being and enjoyment of life. In this chapter, these subjective categories represent a central point of reference for understanding the effects of physical activities.
- It is a **positive definition of health**. It is formulated based on the characteristics and determinants of a "healthy state" (e.g., What are the facets of health? What factors must be present for people to feel healthy?). Conversely, traditional medical definitions define health as the absence of disease, a negative perspective that focuses primarily on biological damage, disorders, or injuries (▶ Chap. 28). Thus, the positive understanding of health is dedicated to the question of what constitutes health beyond the absence of disease and how it can be established or maintained.
- Hurrelmann's definition **integrates physical, psychological, and social determinants of health**. This corresponds to the early definition of health by the World Health Organization (WHO) in 1946, whose central aim was to overcome the negatively focused medical definition (i.e., health as the absence of disease).
- Hurrelmann's definition further allows for the integration of different paradigmatic health models that determine the scientific discussion (Faltermaier, 2005). On the one hand, risk factors of impaired health or the onset of disease can be considered, which are typically addressed in **biomedical disease models** (e.g., the effects of high blood pressure, lipid metabolism disorders, or substance use such as nicotine or alcohol) or in **biopsychosocial disease models** (e.g., the effects of stress in studies and/or in work/private life). On the other hand, Hurrelmann's definition is also compatible with a salutogenetic understanding of health, which was developed by the medical sociologist Aaron Antonovsky (1979). For more information on the concept of salutogenesis, see ▶ Side Story: Salutogenesis.

Side Story

Salutogenesis

The "concept of salutogenesis" was developed by the medical sociologist Aaron Antonovsky (1923–1994) as an antithesis to the concept of pathogenesis (How does disease develop?). The concept of salutogenesis has strongly influenced health science by focusing on the question of how health develops and under which conditions people remain healthy. The basic assumption is that people move along a continuum between health and illness across their lifespan as a function of stress situations and coping actions. From this point of view, not only risk factors (e.g., stress at work) are central, allowing the consideration of protective factors or resources that a person can rely on in the physical, psychological, social, or material areas and the extent to which he or she can draw upon them, depending on internal and external demands. For example, stamina and strength (physical), emotional stability and high self-control (psychological), social support (social), and financial resources (material, e.g., for therapies that require payment) can be used as resources to counteract existing health risks or health impairments. Individuals' degree of success in coping with stressful situations depends on the extent to which they can activate such resources. This **sense of coherence**, according to Antonovsky, plays a decisive role in this context. The sense of coherence is understood to be a global feeling of confidence "that, firstly, the demands from the inner or outer world of experience across the lifespan are structured, predictable and explainable, and that, secondly, the resources are available that are necessary to meet the demands. And third, that these demands are challenges that merit investment and commitment" (Antonovsky, 1993, p. 12; translation by the authors).

Thus, stressful situations that are objectively comparable in magnitude or scope can result in very different consequences for health and well-being, depending on the use of protective resources (Bengel et al., 2001). For example, the same sports injury may have catastrophic emotional, physical, and career consequences for some individuals and merely represent a manageable challenge for others.

26

Health

As early as 1948, the World Health Organization (WHO) defined health as a multifaceted phenomenon and proclaimed it as a fundamental human right.

"Health is a state of complete physical, mental and social well-being and not merely the absence of disease or infirmity. The enjoyment of the highest attainable standard of health is one of the fundamental rights of every human being without distinction of race, religion, political belief, economic or social condition" (▶ Side Story: Biopsychosocial Model of Health: Three Dimensions of Health).

26.2.2 Elements of Subjective Well-Being and Mental Health

In line with the health models discussed above, exercise and health science literature identify well-being as an important health component. Fundamental to individual well-being is the psychological processing of one's own livelihood and the perception of psychological and physical sensations. Such processing can concern both general assessments of one's own life and health, as well as specific experiences and evaluations (e.g., regarding one's own body or social relationships).

Side Story

Biopsychosocial Model of Health: Three Dimensions of Health

At some point in their lives, most people have felt that their subjective condition does not correspond, or only partially corresponds, with a doctor's finding ("I don't feel as sick as the doctor diagnosed" and vice versa: "I feel so sick and the doctor says I only have a slight cold"). The theoretical modeling of this phenomenon is referred to as the "orthogonal health concept," in which the (objective) medical finding and the subjective condition are considered as two dimensions of health that are largely independent of each other (Franke, 2010). This relative independence is well illustrated by the example of chronic back pain. The experience of pain leads to discomfort and often to a subjective sense of illness. Frequently, however, there are no medical results to validate these complaints, such as a diagnosed herniated disc or another orthopedic explanation for the pain in the back region. In medical terms, this type of complaint, while it pertains to the physical body, is referred to as a somatoform disorder. Such disorders are primarily characterized by subjectively perceived symptoms, but for which no medical factors, medications, or medically diagnosable disorders can otherwise be used as an explanation. Conversely, people can feel healthy and well even though they have a medical diagnosis of a disease because, for example, they have found a positive coping strategy in dealing with the disease, or they simply ignore it (Thiel et al., 2013; ◘ Fig. 26.1).

In psychiatry, the determination of a medical finding is closely linked to a systematic recording of the subjective condition, such as when affective disorders (e.g., depression) are involved (Scharfetter, 2002; ▶ Chap. 28). In these scenarios, the focus is on subjectively perceived suffering. In other clinical areas pertaining to health research, the importance of well- or ill-being for the subjective perception of (and coping with) illness is accounted for through the increasing use of *patient-reported outcomes* (Brettschneider et al., 2011) or indicators of *subjective well-being and ill-being* to measure well-being, ill-being, and quality of life (Diener, 2005).

The "orthogonal health concept" integrates subjective conditions and medical findings but neglects the social dimension of a "biopsychosocial health concept." The dimension of social health is primarily a

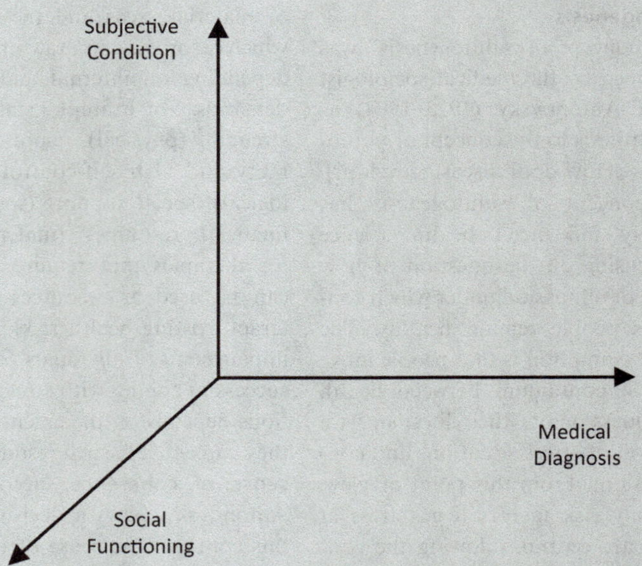

◘ **Fig. 26.1** Three-dimensional model of medical findings, subjective condition, and social functionality (Thiel et al., 2013, p. 114)

question of "functioning" in relevant social contexts, such as school, work, or family. Accordingly, the ability to perform tasks that are linked to a specific social role is accepted as another central component of health. For example, can I meet the expectations set for me as a student? Can I fulfill the responsibilities at work? As a parent, can I care for my children? This component is often considered when assessing health-related quality of life (Radoschewski, 2000).

To integrate this component conceptually, Thiel et al. (2013) complement the "orthogonal health model" with a third, independent dimension that describes functioning in social roles. The independence of this dimension from medical findings and subjective conditions is evident from the fact that people can indeed "function" (at least temporarily) despite diagnosed disease and poor well-being if they still manage to fulfill their tasks and obligations (e.g., as a parent, employee, student) to a sufficient degree, as imposed by the external expectations within each given context. However, an incongruence of subjective condition, medical findings, and functionality can certainly lead to negative consequences in any health-related respect in the medium and long term. More recently, this aspect has been discussed in connection with presenteeism. Presenteeism is defined as people going to work to perform their occupational tasks, regardless of whether they are well or not. It is now known that presenteeism behavior can result in even higher costs (e.g., health costs for the people that experience illness and financial costs for the employer) in the medium term than absenteeism (i.e., when people are absent from work due to illness; Johns, 2010). This finding also extends to professional sports (Mayer & Thiel, 2018). For example, it is very common for elite athletes to enact recovery behaviors too late in the event of injury or illness and to prematurely return to training or competition after (apparent) recovery. This phenomenon of *playing hurt* or *competing hurt* is one of the most important causes of overload problems and frequently results in a long-term absence of the athletes, which in turn can lead to significant performance losses of the team. In their qualitative analysis exploring mental toughness in regular exercisers, Crust et al. (2014) noted that a similar theme emerged, which they labeled "overcommitment." Extending this concern beyond athletes, regularly exercising individuals admitted to not always behaving sensibly (e.g., ignoring signs that a rest day is needed, the tendency to exercise when injured). While this phenomenon remains understudied in health promotion settings, it is reasonable to consider that such behaviors, while not necessarily pathological (i.e., exercise addiction), could impede regular exercise and incur larger healthcare costs in the future.

Considering a biopsychosocial understanding of health, which includes the interactions between the three dimensions of medical findings, subjective condition and social functioning are of particular interest for research into the effects of physical activity. Thus, understanding the effects of physical activity on subjective well-being and mental health can benefit from relating them to objective health parameters and contexts of social functioning.

26.2.2.1 Subjective Well-Being: Definition and Scope

Well-Being

Well-being encompasses evaluations of one's own life and the relationship between pleasant and unpleasant physical and psychological sensations (Lischetzke & Eid, 2005). It is based on cognitive and affective processes that can relate to one's life in general or to specific aspects, such as one's health, body, or social environment.

In numerous publications in health science, researchers have based their studies on the generic concept of subjective well-being (Diener, 2005) to emphasize the subjectivity of perceptions, sensations, and evaluations (Lischetzke & Eid, 2005). In this context, subjectivity means that well-being is always a product of a person's mental system and cannot be isolated from the individual's view of his or her own life, health, etc. (Becker, 1982). Thus, well-being is often characterized using subjective data collected via verbal communication (e.g., interview, questionnaire). Nevertheless, well-being is not completely inaccessible to objective observation. Rather, it can be characterized in various ways, for example, based on nonverbal cues (e.g., posture, facial expression) or based on direct observations of a person's actions (e.g., passivity in the case of sadness), as well as by assessing biological (e.g., neurotransmitters such as serotonin) or cognitive correlates (e.g., faster reaction times in the case of state-congruent words). For this reason, some authors omit the addition of "subjective" (in the case of "subjective" well-being) and just refer to well-being or ill-being (Diener, 2005).

26.2.2.2 Differentiation of Well-Being According to Temporal and Content-Related Aspects

Regarding **temporal aspects**, well-being can be differentiated into state and trait well-being (Becker, 1991). When assessing state well-being, a person would be asked, for example, to rate his or her mood for a singular moment in time (e.g., "right now"). Conversely, when assessing trait well-being, a person would be asked to rate his or her typical mood (e.g., "in general"). State well-being is quite unstable and exhibits fluctuations without necessarily influencing trait well-being because the deviations are relatively short-lived. This means that well-being in the evening can be predicted by certain events during the respective day—which can potentially also include exercise-related activity. However, time-series analyses of well-being have also revealed regular compensatory mechanisms (Fujita & Diener, 2005). Thus, increases in well-being are usually at least partially reversed by opposing changes in well-being on the following day (homeostasis). Accordingly, following short-lived changes, well-being usually settles again at an average level typical for the person concerned (set point). However, the individual set point can change across the lifespan. Thus, in the longer term, a pattern of gradual decline in positive affect at the state level, for example, can lead to a decline in general well-being (Diener et al., 2006).

Different approaches are available for **content-related structuring of well-being**, each with a different emphasis. The previous descriptions are based on the work of Ed Diener, one of the most distinguished well-being researchers of the last decades. He initially based his research on a primarily hedonistic perspective on well-being (Diener et al., 1999). Hedonistic theories assume that people strive for and want to repeat pleasant positive sensations and experiences (e.g., pleasure, joy), whereas they try to avoid negative, unpleasant experiences and sensations (e.g., pain, discomfort) as best they can (Kahnemann, 1999). From this perspective, well-being is thus based on all positive human experiences and sensations, with both cognitive-evaluative components and affective–emotional components determining one's state of well-being. **Cognitive-evaluative components** relate to satisfaction with life in general or with specific aspects such as with one's own health, body, social relationships, or other areas of life (e.g., satisfaction at work). The **affective–emotional component** is closely related to subjective experience of emotions (▶ Chap. 11). Well-being is associated with the presence of positive emotions (e.g., joy, happiness, excitement) and the absence of negative emotions (e.g., sadness, anger, annoyance, fear). In this context, the distinction between subjective feelings on the one hand and emotions as bodily representations of these feelings on the other hand is interesting when considering the effects of physical activity on affective–emotional components of well-being (e.g., Damasio, 1999). From this perspective, body perception can be understood as the background of mental operations in terms of a structurally coupled "mind-body state." Here, feelings are the mental (and verbal) processing of bodily sensations triggered by physiological processes (e.g., generation of muscle force, increased cardiac output, and elevated respiration rate) initiated through physical activity.

> Differentiation of the subjective dimension of health:
> - Refer to the distinction between cognitive-evaluative and affective–emotional components (Diener et al., 1999)
> - Refer to physical, mental, and social areas (e.g., Lehnert et al., 2012)
> - Refer to positive (*well-being*) and negative aspects (*ill-being*)

A categorization of central components of well-being is provided in ◘ Fig. 26.3. In addition to general life satisfaction, body satisfaction (as a facet of physical well-being) and satisfaction with social relationships and with social support (as facets of social well-being) are shown separately.

Affective well-being, as described earlier, is closely related to the subjective experience of emotions. These affective experiences are usually methodologically captured using verbal or written descriptions one's own feeling states using appropriate adjectives. Differentiations of these affective experience categories can be attributed to Wilhelm Wundt (1905), who, at the beginning of the twentieth century, fundamentally distinguished between three basic dimensions labeled as "pleasant–unpleasant," "calm–activated," and "relaxed–tense" (cf. Schlicht & Reicherz, 2012).

In recent work, there is broad consensus that a basal characterization of the affective state requires at least the two basic dimensions of affective valence and activation (Ekkekakis, 2008; Schimmack & Grob, 2000). This characterization, referred to as the "circumplex model of affect," posits that all moods and emotions arise from these two fundamental neurophysiological systems (Russell, 1980). The dimension of affective valence comprises the hedonistic coloring of the affective state from positive, pleasant to negative, unpleasant states. It is assumed that changes in positive affect (e.g., pleased, happy) are not necessarily coupled with reductions of negative affect (e.g., unhappy, sad), in the sense that these feelings exist at opposite ends of a singular continuum. Rather, the occurrences of either positive or negative affect can be relatively independent of each other. This becomes particularly apparent when the affective state is considered over a longer period of time and the fluctuations of the affective well-being are taken into account. For example, various studies report that the reduction of negative affect (e.g., fear, sadness) does not automatically lead to an increase in positive affect (e.g., joy, love) (Diener et al., 1995).

Activation is the second dimension of basic affect. Here, research discusses whether the activation–deactivation aspect by itself can characterize affective well-being (highly activated vs. low activated) or whether statements regarding affective well-being can only be made when activation is combined with the valence dimension (Schimmack & Grob, 2000; Tellegen et al., 1999). The latter combination makes it possible to differentiate between the dimensions "energy vs. tiredness" (e.g., energetic, vital, alert, enthusiastic vs. unenergetic, tired, bored) and "calmness vs. tension" (e.g., restless, anxious vs. calm, relaxed) when describing activation states (▶ Methods: Dimensional and Categorical Approaches to Affective State and Its Measurement).

Methods: Dimensional and Categorical Approaches to Affective State and Its Measurement

For a better understanding of affective well-being, it is helpful to describe and classify the common measurement methods for this field of research. The types of measurement implemented (e.g., the measurement of affective states via questionnaires) can reflect either a dimensional or a categorical approach. Dimensional approaches assume that the subjective experience of the affective state can be mapped with a few basic dimensions. This is usually done with global adjective pairs such as "positive vs. negative," "pleasant vs. unpleasant" (dimension of affective valence), or "highly activated vs. low activated" (dimension of activation).

In exercise psychology research, the Feeling Scale (Hardy & Rejeski, 1989) and the Felt Arousal Scale (Svebak & Murgatroyd, 1985) are widely used instruments for recording the two basic affect dimensions (◘ Fig. 26.2a). They each use only one adjective pair to capture the two dimensions as efficiently and generically as possible (e.g., "good" vs. "bad" anchors for valence, "low" vs. "high" anchors for arousal). These two scales are often used in research that incorporates the "circumplex model" of affective responses to exercise (Ekkekakis, 2008). In the "circumplex model," the activation dimension is positioned perpendicularly to the valence dimension, resulting in four quadrants that demonstrate different manifestations of affective responses.

In other approaches, these combined affect manifestations are represented by three dimensions. Here, activation is differentiated into two subdimensions: feelings of energy vs. tiredness and calmness vs. tension. In the "Multidimensional State of Mood Questionnaire" (Steyer et al., 1997), the polarity of these dimensions becomes clear. Thus, the questionnaire records the affective valence dimension (labeled "good–bad mood" by applying the adjectives "good–bad," "well–unwell," "satisfied–dissatisfied"), energetic arousal dimension (applying the adjectives "wakefulness–tiredness" and "energetic–devoid of energy"), and calmness/tension dimension (applying the adjectives calm–agitated, relaxed–tense) (◘ Fig. 26.2b).

Categorical approaches emphasize concrete emotions such as joy, anger, or depression. The measurement methods place particular emphasis on a reliable recording of the concrete emotional category and usually use several items for one emotion. An example is the "Befindlichkeitsskalen" (BFS ["mood survey scales"]; Abele & Brehm, 1986a), which have been frequently used in exercise psychology in Germany. These scales present adjectives, referred to as "items" in psychometric terms, that are self-assessed to indicate the individual's state well-being asking for the well-being right now or—modifying the prompt—asking for trait well-being. The 40 items refer to eight subscales pertaining to activation, elation, contemplation, calmness, fatigue, depression, anger, and excitement. These emotional categories can also be located in one of the four quadrants of the "circumplex model," although the basic affect dimensions are no longer represented (◘ Fig. 26.2c). Another example, commonly used in English-speaking settings and often applied to sport and exercise research, is the "Profile of Mood States" (POMS; McNair et al., 1981). Here, 65 items are rated and scored to understand the broad categories of tension–anxiety, depression, anger–hostility, vigor, fatigue, and confusion.

Studies in exercise psychology with a specific interest in assessing changes in certain qualities of affective well-being tend to use categorical procedures (e.g., reduction of depressive symptoms or anxiety). However, if the interest instead lies in the broader changes of the affective state, dimensional measurement procedures are suitable. Due to the generally small number of items, the latter are advantageous in terms of low burden of participants. Further, due to their brevity and generalized wording, dimensional approaches are logistically more feasible to implement when measuring "in-task" affective states during exercise (i.e., while an individual is actively under exertion). For further reading on this topic, Ekkekakis (2008) provides an intensive discussion of the advantages and disadvantages of a dimensional and categorical conception and assessment of affective well-being.

26.2.2.3 Physical Well-Being

Physical well-being is characterized by body-related sensations. Antonio Damasio and Gil Carvalho call these sensations "mental experiences of body states" (Damasio & Carvalho, 2013, p. 144). According to Damasio and Carvalho, such "feelings… create an additional level of regulation of behavior" (Damasio & Carvalho, 2013, p. 143). The organism thereby follows the direction (positive or negative) as well as the intensity of the homeostatic deviations mediated by the sensing of body states. In the activation dimension, the affective condition is strongly characterized by psychophysiological aspects, which illustrates the connection to the physical condition.

As early as the 1950s, philosophical anthropology dealt in detail with the experiential entanglement of corporeality and perception. Phenomenologically, physical feeling can be positive as well as negative and conscious as well as unconscious. A positive bodily feeling can manifest itself in such a way that, as Buytendijk puts it, "in full health […] I experience my body as an unconscious mediator of my being in the moment" (Buytendijk, 1958, p. 160; translation by the authors). In this case (e.g., in everyday actions), the body is not consciously perceived, but simply functions with little to no disturbance. Body and mind thereby form an experientially inseparable unity. The German term for "being the body" is *Leib sein*, as opposed to "having a body" (Plessner, 1970). "Having a body" in the sense of a positive body feeling, however, is a conscious process of experiencing (e.g., relaxation after a very strong physical effort). "Having a body" in the sense of a negative

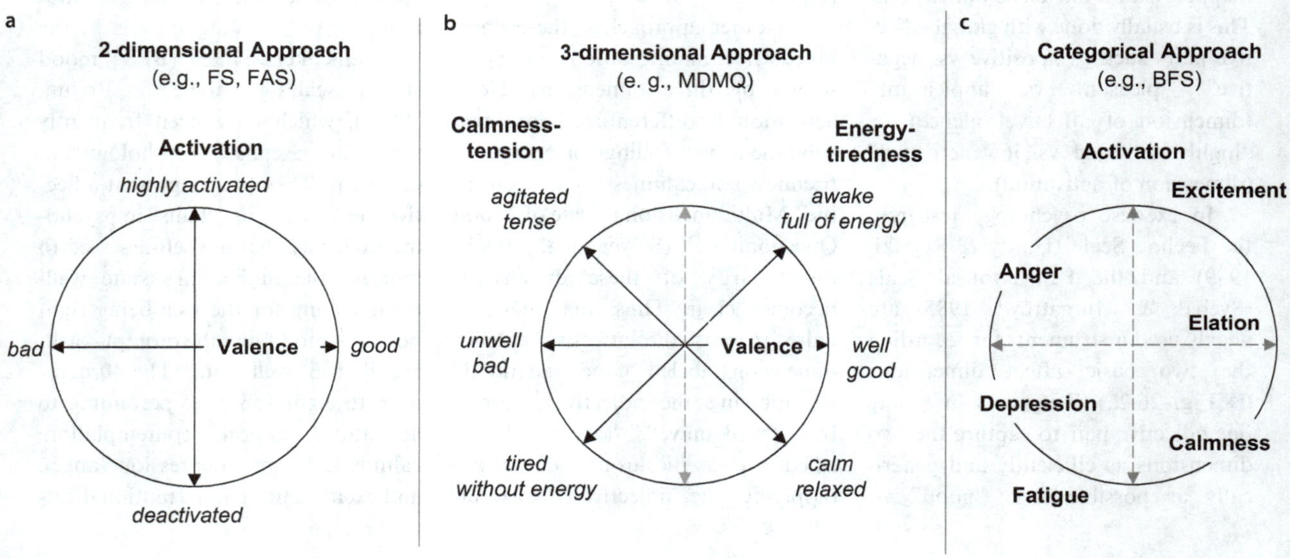

◘ **Fig. 26.2** (a–c) Dimensional and categorical measurement procedures including different adjectives used for assessments (FS, Feeling Scale; FAS, Felt Arousal Scale; MDMQ, Multidimensional Mood Questionnaire; BFS, "Befindlichkeitsskalen" [Mood Survey Scales])

body experience, in turn, is basically characterized as a state of consciously experiencing physical discomfort. Physical discomfort can occur as a subjective experience of objective physical diagnoses as well as represent a physical ill-being without objective diagnoses. In this context, the relative independence of body-related self-evaluations from physical sensation becomes clear.

Satisfaction with one's own body and accepting one's own body (as a cognitive-evaluative process) does not necessarily have to correspond to physical sensations. In this context, self-evaluations in terms of body satisfaction or dissatisfaction go beyond the purely descriptive body image that a person has of him−/herself.

26.2.2.4 Social Well-Being

Social well-being includes sensations corresponding with social reference points. These include, for example, feelings of belonging or being needed and the experience of social support or acceptance by others, but also loneliness or experiences of social neglect. Social well-being thus circumscribes the subjective experience of affection from and towards other persons (Sudeck & Schmid, 2012). In addition to affective components, evaluative aspects are also relevant for social well-being (e.g., satisfaction with affection from other persons, the feeling of being overburdened by tasks imposed by others, or the qualitative assessment of relationships with relevant others). Finally, the subjective self-assessment of one's own social functioning (i.e., the ability to fulfill role expectations) also contributes to social well-being. In this particular context, the intertwining of affective and evaluative aspects becomes apparent, for example, when a person is dissatisfied with the fact that he or she is inadequately able to fulfill parental duties due to work-related obligations (◘ Fig. 26.3).

26.2.2.5 Hedonistic and Eudemonistic Concepts of Subjective Well-Being

For a more differentiated view of the effects of physical activity on well-being and mental health, further research in the context of positive psychology is of interest. A central concern of positive psychology is enhancing mental health beyond average or normal levels, which expands the long-dominant clinical perspective on mental illness, which focuses on restoring mental health to normal levels following a deficit (e.g., Keyes, 2002; Seligman, 2002). Much work in the realm of positive psychology focuses on the hedonistic understanding of well-being noted earlier, that is, the experience of positive affect and the absence of negative affect. In addition, however, some work in this line of research also ask what constitutes a "good life" in the sense of an eudemonistic principle of life. This involves, for example, self-determination and the ability to shape one's

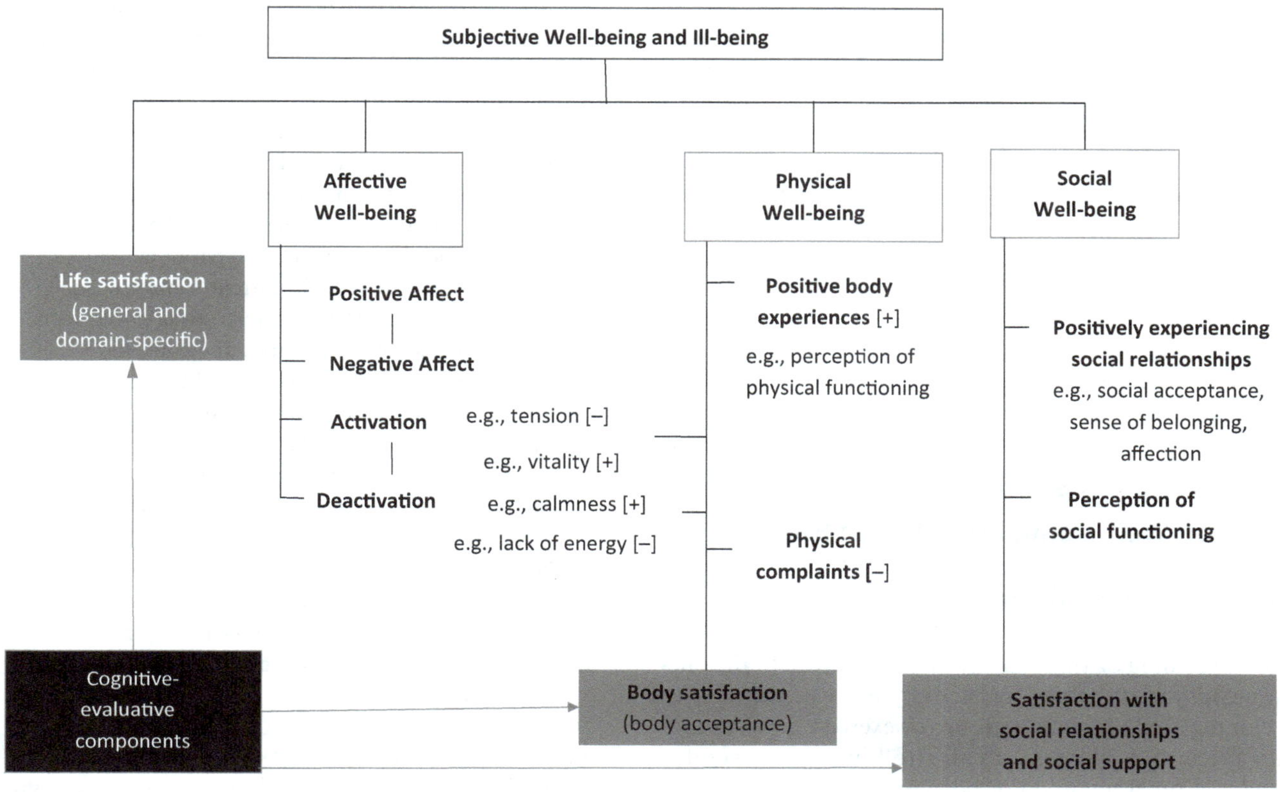

◘ **Fig. 26.3** Overview of components of well-being and ill-being

own life, but also realizing one's own potential, one's own strengths, and accepting one's own weaknesses (Ryff & Singer, 2008).

Even more recent is the construct of flourishing, which has become very influential in the scientific discussion of well-being (cf. Diener et al., 2010; Keyes, 2002; Seligman, 2002). This construct was developed by Corey Keyes (2002) and Barbara Fredrickson (Fredrickson & Losada, 2005). The concept of flourishing refers to a positive view of personal potential and resources as well as a positive life evaluation, which are emotionally associated with a state of inner fulfillment. Sometimes this discussion also emphasizes the functionality aspect (i.e., the subjective experience of positive functioning as well as meaningful, purposeful, and effective engagement in activities; Seligman, 2011). It stands to reason that this approach also includes the sense of coherence described above within the framework of the "salutogenesis approach" (▶ Side Story: Salutogenesis). In summary, the central components of the flourishing concept can be identified as, firstly, the significance and meaningfulness of one's own life; secondly, the committed achievement of life goals and associated experiences of competence, optimism, and resilience; and thirdly, being socially integrated.

Interim Conclusion: The Need for a Precise Concept Specification

Research on well-being and mental health is very multifaceted. Given the multitude of theoretical concepts and terminology, it is often difficult to make generalized statements when analyzing the state of research regarding the effects of physical activity on well-being and mental health. In some cases, very different conceptions and components of well-being and mental health are nevertheless considered together in reviews (Lehnert et al., 2012). If possible, a differentiated analysis of the relationships between physical activity and specific facets of well-being and mental health should be undertaken with adequate conceptual clarity (Schlicht & Schwenkmezger, 1995).

26.3 Effects of Physical Activity on Well-Being and Mental Health

26.3.1 A Heuristic Framework

The beginning of this chapter briefly referred to the phenomenal variety of physical activity, exercise, and sports. I can jog alone or with a group, or exercise on a stationary piece of equipment. I can stroll in a quiet wooded area and quiet my mind or be in an urban area and stay focused to avoid traffic, pedestrians, or other obstacles in my path. I can play fun-oriented volleyball on the beach or compete in a recreational volleyball game with more ambitious teammates. If I need loud motivation, then I might attend an aerobics class led by a boisterous instructor with upbeat music. If I am irritated or distracted by excess noise, then I may seek out a yoga class led by a calm instructor with only ambient noise in the background. Such lists can be continued almost endlessly and illustrate the diversity of exercise and sporting activities, not only regarding the different physical load parameters, but also to the very different psychosocial requirements and incentives. In accordance with this diversity, it can hardly be assumed that all (or even the same) exercise and sporting activities per se produce the same physiological and psychological response (Lehnert et al., 2012).

Following action psychology frameworks (e.g., Nitsch, 2004) and a transdisciplinary model of individual differences in physical activity behavior change (Bryan et al., 2011), we assume that physiological and psychological responses to physical exercise and sporting activities are determined by characteristics of the activity itself, the person, and the environment and temporal characteristics (cf. Lehnert et al., 2012).

Which Parameters Generally Determine the Individual Response to Physical Activity?

- **Activity characteristics:** Which physical load parameters are present (e.g., duration, intensity of the activity, as well as type of activity such as endurance-oriented activity, strength training, ball games) and with which psychosocial demands and incentives can the activity be circumscribed?
- **Personal factors:** What motivation for exercise and sporting activities do people have, and what preferences do they have for certain types of activities or intensities? What is their current biopsychosocial health state and what previous experiences with exercise and sporting activities do people have?
- **Environmental factors:** What are the physical (e.g., nature, fitness center, noise) and social environmental conditions of the activity (e.g., need for cooperation in group activities, opportunities for interaction with training partners and training instructors)?
- **Temporal characteristics:** Is a single exercise session considered with its temporally immediate effects, or is it a matter of physical adaptation and psychological processing of multiple, repeated exercise sessions?

To better understand the effects of exercise and sporting activities on biopsychosocial health, we have begun

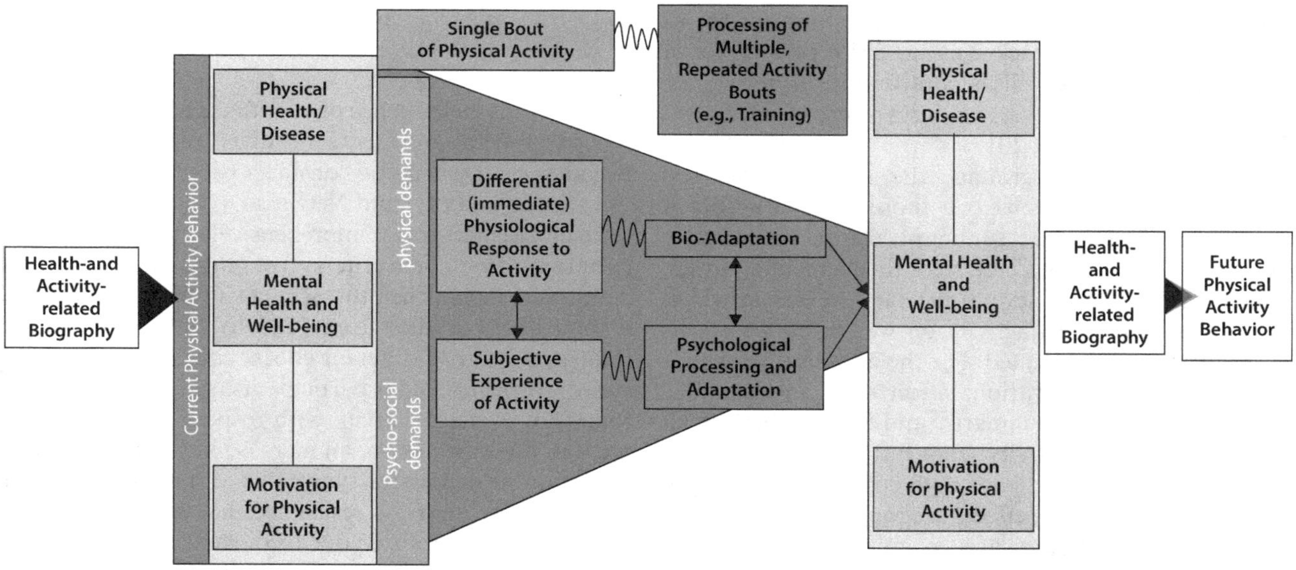

Fig. 26.4 A transdisciplinary framework of the individual response to physical activity

to translate these ideas into a heuristic framework in Fig. 26.4. Underlying this framework are three basic assumptions that are revisited at various points in this paper:

1. Both immediate effects of single sessions and effects of multiple, repeated periods of activity are based on an interplay of physical load parameters, psychosocial demands and incentives of activity, and personal preconditions (e.g., physical preconditions, motivation to exercise, health status).
2. Immediate physiological responses to physical activity (e.g., body temperature, heart rate, stress response) and the subjective experience of the activity (e.g., changes in affect, experience of pain, perceived stress and exertion) are related to each other, but can vary greatly from individual to individual. This potentially also applies to longer-term biological adaptations as well as the psychological processing of repeated activities (e.g., in the context of structured exercise training).
3. This complexity is embedded in the individual activity- and health-related biography, which bundles the subjective health- and activity-related experiences in a meaningful way. Changes in biopsychosocial health status and motivation generated by being active are incorporated into the individual activity and health biographies, thereby helping to determine future activity behavior. The structures of the activity and health biography are thus permanently updated via subjective processing of physiological and psychological responses to the physical activity.

26.3.2 Research Overview on the Effects of Physical Activity on Well-Being and Mental Health

There are now numerous empirical studies that have examined the effects of physical activity on well-being and mental health. Of central importance here are intervention studies in which the aim is to investigate the impact of physical activity on changes in well-being and mental health (e.g., by comparing a physical exercise group and a control group and to attribute these changes to the physical exercise in a causal manner). Interventions can assess efficacy (i.e., outcomes under ideal and controlled circumstances) or effectiveness (i.e., outcomes under "real-world conditions and constraints), depending on study design characteristics (Singal et al., 2014). In addition, longitudinal studies are of interest to observe the extent to which physical activity is related to subsequent well-being and mental health. In cross-sectional studies, on the other hand, in which physical activity as well as mental health parameters is only empirically measured at the same point in time, the question of what is the cause and effect cannot be empirically answered. Thus, well-being and mental health may also be a precondition for physical activity. In this regard, researchers interested in using "readiness to exercise" (i.e., preexercise mental and physical states) to guide person-adaptive programming have provided initial evidence for this relational direction. That is, lack of energy, negative feeling states, and physical discomfort have been cited as underlying perceptions of readiness to exercise (Strohacker et al., 2019; Strohacker & Zakrajsek, 2016), as well as contributors to ratings of exercise-related affective responses (Beaumont et al., 2021; Strohacker et al., 2017).

Against this background, the research overview focuses, wherever possible, on those reviews in which intervention studies are summarized in a quantitative manner. These studies, referred to as meta-analyses, bundle the results of several primary studies in which the effects of physical activity on well-being and mental health were investigated. For the quantitative assessment of the results, various effect sizes are available, which can be used to summarize and evaluate the overall effects of physical activity from different studies (e.g., despite different methods of data collection or exercise programs). In this way, effects are roughly distinguished with small, medium, and large magnitudes (▶ Methods: Effect Sizes).

Methods: Effect Sizes

The term "effect size" indicates the magnitude of a statistical effect. Various effect size measures are used to assess this. One example is "Cohen's d" (Cohen, 1988). It is the effect size for mean differences between two groups (e.g., intervention group vs. control group) with the same group sizes as well as the same group variances.

- Small effect: $d = 0.2$
- Medium effect: $d = 0.5$
- Large effect: $d = 0.8$

Furthermore, meta-analyses typically identify moderators of the attainable effects that involve important characteristics of the individual (e.g., gender, health status), the activity itself (e.g., endurance activities vs. strength training, duration of sessions), or environmental conditions (e.g., group activity vs. individual training).

Differentiated Findings for Effects on Well-Being and Mental Health

- A general review of studies clearly shows that the effects of physical activity on well-being and mental health must be viewed in a very differentiated manner (e.g., Lehnert et al., 2012; Wagner & Brehm, 2008).
- Generally, the effects depend on which component of well-being or mental health is considered.
- Moreover, consistent findings usually emerge only when certain forms of physical activities (e.g., endurance activity) are considered with specific load parameters (e.g., specific duration or intensity) or among specific target groups (e.g., women, people of older age).

The fact that the evidence on the effects of physical activity on well-being and mental health is quite differentiated becomes clear when one considers two early meta-analyses. Schlicht (1995) and Netz et al. (2005) compiled the state of research very comprehensively by using a broad spectrum of outcome criteria from the domains of well-being and mental health. Schlicht (1995) summarized a total of 39 studies from 1980 to 1990, from which information on 44 different effects could be determined based on nearly 9,000 participants. A small effect was found for exercise activity with respect to an improvement in life satisfaction, an increase in positive affect, a reduction in depressive symptoms and anxiety, and an improvement in stress resistance. However, this effect could not be generalized due to the heterogeneity of the results in the included studies. Only when the analysis was differentiated according to age, gender, and type of activity consistent, positive effects emerged. Based on these analyses, women aged between 31 and 50 years benefited the most. In addition, endurance activities were demonstrated to be beneficial for well-being and mental health in persons aged between 31 and 50 years, with a small to medium effect size.

About 10 years later, the meta-analysis by Netz et al. (2005) was published, summarizing the effects of physical activity on mental health in older adults. This meta-analysis included over 400 studies. The mean age of the participants was over 50 years. There was a significant association with mental health with a small effect size for the global effect of the intervention groups that were physically active for several weeks. This was three times as high as in the control groups. However, differentiation by outcome criteria showed significant differences between the intervention and control groups for global indicators of well-being and self-efficacy, such that Cohen's d effect sizes ranged from 0.30 to 0.40 for the intervention group, whereas it was close to 0 for the control group. In contrast, there were no differences between the intervention and control groups for life satisfaction, for example. In addition, age was observed to moderate the effects. The mental health of individuals aged 54–64 benefited most from physical activity, whereas individuals aged 75 and older showed the least positive effects on mental health. Again, endurance-oriented activities were found to be most beneficial for mental health. However, the effects were rather small. Moreover, homogeneous, positive effects were found mainly in those studies in which the physical activities were performed at a moderate intensity. Overall, physiological adaptations, such as an improvement in cardiovascular fitness or muscular strength, were found to be associated with an improvement in well-being.

The above mentioned meta-analyses suggest that the effects of physical activity on mental health must be analyzed separately for specific subdomains, as otherwise hardly any generalizable effects can be expected. The component of well-being and mental health that is studied must be clearly defined (Schlicht & Schwenkmezger, 1995). Furthermore, the meta-analytic findings suggest that the search for activity-related, personal, and environmental moderators should be further intensified.

In the following research overview, we will take a closer look at the effects of physical activity on different domains of well-being—based on our heuristic framework (► Sect. 26.3.1). The focus is on the effects in apparently healthy individuals (for effects on clinical populations, see ► Chap. 28).

26.3.2.1 Affective Well-Being

When summarizing research results on the effects of physical activity on affective well-being, the temporal aspect of the effect must be taken into account. That is, the immediate effects of single sessions of activity should not be conflated with the effects of multiple, repeated periods of activity.

Immediate Effects of Single Sessions of Structured Physical Exercise

Research in exercise psychology demonstrating an immediate "feel-good effect" of physical exercise has a long tradition. The first studies from the 1970s and 1980s were conducted with a basic hedonistic understanding of well-being. The general conclusion was that "Exercise makes you feel better" (Morgan, 1981), which evolved into a conventionally held belief among researchers and practitioners.

In German-speaking countries, comparable positive effects of single exercise sessions on affective states have been repeatedly found from the 1980s onwards. Based on a categorical approach using the "Befindlichkeitsskalen" (BFS; see above), different fitness and health sport activities (e.g., running, fitness training with equipment, ski gymnastics, swimming, aerobics, step aerobics) were analyzed (Abele & Brehm, 1986b, 1993; Brehm, 1998; Wagner and Brehm, 2008). A prevailing pattern of results emerged across the different exercise activities. Thus, the subjects' affective well-being improved immediately after the exercise sessions compared to that of the measurement immediately before. Positive changes were observed in the affect categories of "good mood," activation, and calmness, with gradual differences in the magnitude of affect improvements comparing activity types (e.g., largest effect with group-based fitness classes and smallest effect with equipment-based fitness training). Similarly, a reduction in negative affect categories was noted relatively consistently. That is, after the exercise sessions, participants reported less anger, agitation, and depression, as well as lower ratings regarding a "lack of energy" (cf. Brehm, 1998). Brehm and colleagues describe this pattern of changes in affect categories, which can be observed in about 75% of exercise participants, as an *equilibration effect*. This is to express that exercise can contribute to a restoration of homeostasis in affective well-being by promoting positive aspects and reducing negative aspects. Brehm and colleagues also found several determinants of changes in well-being. For example, stronger effects were observed following moderate exercise intensities and in individuals who presented with a worse state of well-being before the exercise sessions began. Finally, positive changes in well-being were associated with more favorable perceptions of competence with regards to the experience.

Meanwhile, more contemporary research from national and international groups has considerably expanded the state of knowledge. An exemplary insight is provided by a comprehensive meta-analysis by Reed and Ones (2006). Here, the authors included studies that had examined the effects of endurance activity on the positive activated affect using measurement procedures for positive affect, vitality, joy, and energetic activation. In the "circumplex model," these measures correspond to the quadrant between high activation and positive affective valence (◘ Fig. 26.2). The meta-analysis identified 158 studies with a total of 13,000 participants from the period between 1979 and 2005. The global comparison of affect values before and after exercise demonstrated a medium, relatively robust effect ($d = 0.45$).

◘ Table 26.1 summarizes the main findings on the effect of physical exercise on positive activated affect, considering different physical load parameters. On average, the greatest effects were found for endurance activities with light intensities, a duration of up to 35 min, and a low or moderate activity dose (where activity dose is defined as specific combinations of duration and intensity). In contrast, the few studies examining very high activity doses and longer activity duration over 75 min showed negative affective responses.

A personal factor that could be consistently identified as a moderator, in line with the findings of Brehm's research group, is the state of well-being before the activity (see upper part of ◘ Table 26.1). Thus, the increase in positively activated affect was consistently strongest when participants reported low baseline levels. However, it is important to consider that low baseline levels, by default, have greater potential for improvement and that ceiling effects due to scale constraints likely play a role as well.

With regard to the heuristic framework explained above (◘ Fig. 26.4), the findings make it plausible that physical load parameters influence immediate physiological responses and, thus in turn, predetermine the extent

Table 26.1 Simplified presentation of meta-analytic findings on effects on positive activated affect after single sessions of endurance activity (Reed & Ones, 2006) and after multi-week endurance-oriented exercise programs (Reed & Buck, 2009)

Immediate effects of single aerobic exercise sessions (*single bout*)				Effects of multi-week aerobic exercise programs (*multiple bouts*)			
Moderator	*k*	*N*	d_{corr}	Moderator	*k*	*N*	d_{corr}
Baseline positive activated affect (preexercise)							
<–0.5 z	75	2861	0.63	<–0.5 z	35	1171	0.81
–0.5 z to 0.5 z	66	2159	0.34	–0.5 z to 0.5 z	38	1125	0.45
>0.5 z	49	1686	0.39	>0.5 z	24	592	0.26
Intensity							
Light	23	748	0.57	Light	16	483	0.72
Moderate	91	2732	0.35	Moderate	56	1455	0.50
High	60	1679	0.31	High	20	645	0.68
Session duration							
7–15 min	33	1317	0.56	15–25 min	30	504	0.55
20–28 min	69	2063	0.46				
30–35 min	62	1940	0.57	30–35 min	36	1051	0.68
40–60 min	35	1323	0.37	40–60 min	34	1327	0.49
>75 min	12	331	–0.72				
Activity dose (defined as a combination of intensity and duration)							
Low	73	2447	0.45	Low	31	688	0.60
Moderate	82	2146	0.46	Moderate	28	808	0.56
High	15	279	0.09	High	29	997	0.65
Very high	6	216	–0.98				
				Frequency			
				<3 days/week	20	713	0.57
				3 days/week	61	1776	0.52
				>3 days/week	18	415	0.79
				Program duration			
				4–9 weeks	30	995	0.51
				10–12 weeks	45	1208	0.63
				13–32 weeks	27	879	0.36

Notes: *k* number of independent effect sizes, *N* number of participants, d_{corr} standardized mean change from pre-to-post measurements corrected for sample size. Conventional classification of effect sizes: $d_{corr:}$ 0.2 = small effect, 0.5 = medium effect, 0.8 large effect. *z* = values transformed to the standard normal distribution: the mean value of this distribution is zero (so this corresponds to a mean baseline level here). Values <0.5 *z* correspond to baseline values that deviate negatively from the mean by more than half a standard deviation (lower PAA at baseline) and values >0.5 *z* deviate positively from the mean (higher PAA at baseline)

to which well-being is positively influenced. However, Reed and Ones' meta-analysis provides only descriptive evidence in this regard, which is why the authors point to the importance of theory-driven research to better understand and explain the specific constellations of personal and activity-related characteristics and their significance for affective well-being. The lack of empirical clarity is also reflected in Panteleimon Ekkekakis' statements regarding immediate affective responses to exercise activities. Ekkekakis, who has initiated several reviews and edited books on the topic, expresses substantial doubts about an overly optimistic evaluation that exercise positively impacts affective well-being, largely due to the methodological weaknesses of existing research designs (e.g., Van Landuyt et al., 2000). ▶ Section 26.4 will deal in more detail with the explanation of the effects of physical activity on affective well-being.

What Methodological Problems May Lead to an Overestimation of Immediate Positive Effects of Exercise on Well-Being?

- **Limitations of before-and-after comparisons:** The mere consideration of pre- to postexercise comparisons overlooks potentially negative effects during the session, when an individual is actively under exertion. For example, the relatively homogeneous increase in well-being after the end of the exercise activity may be generated by a *rebound effect*, which primarily reflects a reaction to the termination of the activity (i.e., finally ending an exercise session that felt aversive) rather than reflecting the response to the activity itself.
- **Selection bias:** Numerous study results were obtained from people who were already physically active and participated in exercise and sports programs. On average, positive findings have limited generalizability to sample populations of inactive or physically unfit individuals.
- **Measurement of affect:** The majority of existing studies used categorical measurement procedures that strongly emphasize negative affect categories. For example, the Profile of Mood State (POMS; McNair et al., 1981), which has been widely used internationally to assess immediate effects of exercise, was developed in the clinical psychiatric setting. As a result, the basic dimensions of affect may be inadequately covered (Backhouse et al., 2007).

Ekkekakis (2015) therefore cautions against the undifferentiated assumption "Exercise makes you feel better" (i.e., that *most* people feel better through exercise alone). On the basis of current research findings, he rather concludes:

- *Certain* exercise doses can lead to improvements in well-being for *some* people (e.g., Ekkekakis et al., 2011).
- Most inactive people feel worse with exercise (e.g., Ekkekakis et al., 2010).
- The highest interindividual variability in the direction and magnitude of affective response (including negative responses) exists *during* exercise (e.g., Ekkekakis et al., 2005; Sudeck & Conzelmann, 2014). This is even more significant, because affective responses *during* exercise have predictive significance for future behavior (Rhodes & Kates, 2015).

Ekkekakis strongly urges researchers to consider using dimensional measurement procedures to record the spectrum of affect changes repeatedly and economically during an exercise activity, in addition to capturing pre- and postexercise ratings. In particular, such procedures are likely to allow more robust analyses of the interplay between subjective experience of the activity and changes in motivation for future exercise behavior.

Effects of Multi-Week Exercise Programs

The effects of single sessions contribute to our understanding of exercise-related affective responses from a theoretical point of view, but for practical purposes, repeated exercise sessions are of particular interest. It is reasonable to consider that individuals who are habitually active achieve this degree of behavioral maintenance by repeating certain types of activity (via sports clubs or fitness center attendance) rather than frequently engaging in many different "one-off" sessions. The latter behavioral pattern may more commonly occur in the novice exerciser as he or she explores possible modes to determine likes and dislikes. However, it is important to remember that it is physiologically advantageous for exercise training to achieve a degree of specificity, as well as regularity, to experience desired adaptations in health and fitness parameters in a timely manner. To summarize the effects of multiple bouts of exercise on affective well-being, Reed and Buck (2009) analyzed 105 original studies on the effects of multiple weeks of endurance activity on positive activated affect from the period between 1980 and 2009, pooling a total of 370 effect sizes in 9,840 subjects without specific health conditions or diseases. A global examination of the pre–post comparisons of the exercise groups showed a moderate positive effect of the multi-week exercise programs. In contrast, as expected, no significant changes in positive activated affect were observed in participants of control groups. A direct comparison of the exercise and control groups after the intervention period showed a moderate effect in favor of the exercise groups.

Regarding the activity-related moderators, ◘ Table 26.1 shows that the differences depending on the physical load parameters are smaller for the multi-week interventions compared to that of the immediate affective responses (Reed & Ones, 2006). This is particularly noticeable for activity dose, which is not a significant moderator of longer-term effects on positive activated affect. No clear trend emerges for intensity levels. Thus, moderate intensities yield moderate effect sizes, but smaller effects compared to that of light and vigorous intensities. Furthermore, as with the single exercise sessions, the improvement in affective well-being for multi-week programs is dependent on the baseline level at the beginning of the intervention period (low baseline well-being is associated with greater improvements in well-being). Finally, it should be noted that the

Study Box

Meta-Analysis by Arent et al. (2000)

A meta-analysis on the effects of multi-week exercise programs on affective well-being was conducted by Arent et al. (2000). The authors focused on studies including older adults. The meta-analysis compiled 32 original studies that examined the effects of various preventive exercise programs (cardiovascular endurance training, strength training, or combinations of endurance and strength training) on positive and negative affect. The meta-analysis draws the following conclusions comparing exercise groups and control groups:

- **Overall result:** Overall, it was determined that exercise programs elicited a positive, statistically significant advantage, which was in the small to medium effect range. There were no statistically significant differences between the various types of activity. Thus, both cardiovascular and muscle-strengthening exercise and combinations thereof had positive effects on affective well-being. In addition, the studies indicated substantial heterogeneity in the results, so a moderator analysis was conducted. Moderators, described below, included activity-related characteristics (e.g., frequency per week) and different components of affective well-being (positive vs. negative affect).
- **Frequency per week:** Exercise programs with two or fewer sessions per week were more effective than programs with more than two sessions per week. Thus, in contrast to the analysis by Reed and Buck (2009), the benefit of more frequent weekly exercise sessions could not be confirmed in this age group.
- **Exercise duration:** The strongest effects were found in programs in which the duration of the activity was determined by the participants themselves and was not fixed. In addition, only programs with sessions of more than 45 min were effective, while programs in the range of 30 to 35 min did not produce significant improvements in affective well-being.
- **Program duration:** Analogous to the meta-analysis by Reed and Buck (2009), the largest effects were found for programs lasting up to 12 weeks, whereas longer programs produced only small positive effects.
- **Intensity:** The effect sizes of light-intensity programs were moderate and significantly larger than the effects of medium- and high-intensity programs.
- **Positive vs. negative affect:** Findings were not impacted based on whether the studies examined effects on positive affect or negative affect. For both dimensions, small to medium effect sizes could be summarized.

strongest effects were found in programs with more than three exercise sessions per week and a program duration of 10 to 12 weeks (► Study Box: Meta-Analysis by Arent et al. (2000)).

A third relevant meta-analysis for the effects of multi-week exercise programs on affective well-being is the work of Gillison et al. (2009). They analyzed six intervention studies on the effects of exercise programs on the psychological well-being of healthy adults. In contrast to Reed and Buck (2009), various exercise programs (e.g., muscle strengthening, stretching, and their combinations with endurance training) were included along with endurance activities. This review also showed an overall positive and statistically significant, but small, effect across the different studies (◘ Fig. 26.5).

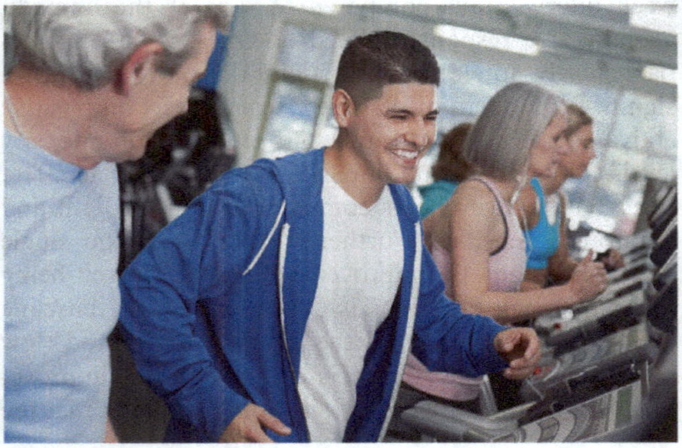

◘ **Fig. 26.5** Exercise can have a positive effect on well-being

Conclusion for the Effects of Multi-Week Exercise Programs on Affective Well-Being

- The meta-analyses consistently conclude that multi-week exercise programs exert a positive effect on affective well-being. The effects vary in magnitude between small and medium effects.
- The moderator analyses show a high differentiation along physical load parameters with inconsistent findings regarding specific parameters. This suggests that personal and other characteristics likely influence the strength of the effect.
- Compared to that of the single exercise sessions, a weaker moderating influence of activity-related characteristics (intensity, duration of activity) was observed for the multi-week programs. This suggests that with repeated physical exercise, the psychological processing of the activity experiences becomes increasingly important and the effects may thus become more independent of physical load parameters.
- The extent to which biological adaptation and fitness improvements are associated with changes in

affective well-being cannot be clearly clarified based on existing research. While the meta-analysis by Netz et al. (2005) indicates an association, the results of the meta-analysis by Arent et al. provide no evidence for a consistent relationship.

- Accordingly, Reed and Buck (2009) call for the advancement of theory-driven research with a stronger focus on the interplay between psychological processing and biological adaptation. In addition, they argue that more research is needed on how the subjective experience of the activity (e.g., in the form of immediate affective responses) relates to longer-term changes in general affective well-being.

26.3.2.2 Additional Components of Well-Being and Ill-Being

For the additional areas of subjective well-being and ill-being (e.g., life satisfaction, physical well-being, social well-being), most research efforts have been directed towards examining the effects of multi-week exercise programs.

Life Satisfaction

Changes in life satisfaction through physical exercise have been studied most frequently in older adults. The aforementioned meta-analysis by Netz et al. (2005) included an extensive study pool for this subdomain of well-being, with 48 effects from intervention groups and 34 effects from control groups. No statistically significant differences were found for older adults who participated in exercise intervention groups compared to those assigned to control groups without exercise.

An earlier review (Rejeski & Mihalko, 2001), on the other hand, provides contradictory results, such that three studies demonstrated positive effects on life satisfaction and three studies demonstrated null effects. In one reviewed study, by Mihalko and McAuley (1996), the observed positive changes in life satisfaction of older adults were attributed to improvements in muscle strength as a result of the strengthening training intervention. Importantly, strength improvements correlated with an increase in the ability to perform activities of daily living. Thus, the improvement in life satisfaction can be described as a complex, multifactorial effect: Increases in muscle strength allow for better performance of and coping with activities of daily living, which ultimately leads to higher life satisfaction. Rejeski and Mihalko (2001) also emphasize the complexity of the relationship between exercise and life satisfaction. For example, the subjective experience of the activity (e.g., enjoyment of the activity, perception of social interaction) is likely to have a mediating role for relationships between exercise and life satisfaction. However, there still exists a lack of research to support an empirical foundation for the interactions between physical adaptation, the psychological processing of activity, and changes in life satisfaction.

The overall striking inconsistency of the findings could stem from the fact that life satisfaction is a relatively stable psychological construct. Particularly among people in older adulthood, studies have described a certain paradox of life satisfaction in old age (e.g., Staudinger, 2000). That is, older persons more often report that they are satisfied and better off than would be expected on the basis of objectively measurable parameters (e.g., physical limitations, decrease in social contacts). This paradox of subjective well-being (Staudinger, 2000) thus expresses only a low correlation of life satisfaction with objective living conditions and circumstances (Diener et al., 1999). The paradox is explained by (not necessarily consciously intended) adaptation processes to objective living conditions. People evaluate their situation differently and in a way that allows them to maintain their life satisfaction.

Physical Well-Being

In the domain of physical well-being, there are some studies on the role of exercise for body image, which address cognitive-evaluative components and partly affective sensations related to the body. Body image encompasses the characteristics a person attributes to his or her body, the importance he or she places on these characteristics, and his or her affective relationship to his or her body, particularly his or her (dis)satisfaction with his or her body (Paulus, 1986; Thiel, 2013). As early as the 1970s and 1980s, various studies found evidence that physical exercise positively influences an individual's body image (for an overview, see Mrazek, 1986). This effect was previously observed with moderate intensities and short program duration, which was explained by an expectancy effect: Due to the belief that "when training will improve one's body in some way, one's attitude will also improve" (Mrazek, 1986, p. 238; translation by the authors).

Campbell and Hausenblas (2009) also reported that exercise-induced changes in body (dis)satisfaction and positive perceptions of the body need not be systematically related to fitness improvements. In their meta-analysis, they summarized 57 intervention studies conducted between 1972 and 2007 that compared groups with multi-week exercise programs versus no-exercise control groups. The studies were conducted almost exclusively with insufficiently active individuals, with studies including sample populations categorized as normal weight and as overweight/obese nearly balanced. Global observations across all studies revealed a small, positive effect of the exercise programs on increasing body satisfaction, reducing body dissatisfaction, and a more favorable perception of one's own body. Detailed examination of the effects revealed moderation by the group under study and specific intervention characteristics. For example, the largest effects were found in adults, and there was a tendency for a positive influence on physical well-being to be more likely in people who were overweight than in those classified as normal weight. Regarding activity characteristics, there were no substantial differences in body image-related effects between endurance activities, muscle strengthening activities, and combined programs. Similarly, physical load parameters (duration, intensity) were not relevant for body image outcomes. However, higher weekly frequency was associated with stronger effects. Finally, Campbell and Hausenblas (2009) observed an advantage for exercise programs that were not combined with other intervention components. With respect to the latter finding, however, a more recent meta-analysis by Alleva et al. (2015) concludes that interventions that focus only on physical exercise in order to increase fitness do not produce improvements in body (dis)satisfaction and body image. These contradictory findings suggest that more research is needed to determine which elements of an exercise program elicit more favorable changes in physical well-being beyond fitness improvement alone and which do not. For example, an exercise program that focuses on improving body-related functionality and experience of competence might be expected to have a different effect on body image than one that focuses primarily on physical appearance (Ginis & Bassett, 2011; Martin & Lichtenberger, 2002).

Research on the effects of physical activity in people with health disorders often focuses on physical well-being and, in particular, on the perception of physical complaints (► Chap. 28; Pahmeier, 2012). The effectiveness of exercise programs (e.g., preventive training for low-back health, fit-and-healthy exercise program, cf. Brehm et al., 2005) for reducing physical complaints has also been studied for preventive exercise programs. Positive effects have been demonstrated in a number of intervention studies (cf. Pahmeier, 2012).

Social Well-Being

For the domain of social well-being, the state of research is still quite limited. There are hardly any intervention studies or longitudinal studies in which the relationship between exercise activities and social-related facets of well-being has been investigated. An additional problem is that, comparatively, there exists fewer established measurement methods for this domain of well-being.

In the meta-analysis by Gillison et al. (2009), for example, social well-being was listed together with social functioning in a common category entitled "social relationships." This review involved a pooled analysis of 15 original papers. The meta-analytic findings showed that exercise activities have no effect on social relationships in healthy adults. Accordingly, it cannot be assumed that exercise has general effects on the evaluation and perception of social relationships. It should be noted, however, that the analysis was based on a rather unspecific aggregation of social characteristics of well-being and social functioning. Assessing particular aspects of social well-being in a more differentiated way, as called for by Sudeck and Schmid (2012), various parameters can be identified that moderate the effects of exercise on well-being. For example, studies suggest that the social context of exercise programs (e.g., group-based training) and positive perceptions of social relationships in the exercise context (e.g., social support in the exercise context, perceived group cohesion) are relevant in determining whether effects on global social well-being are evident (Gillison et al., 2009). There is also evidence that—at least in the field of oncological rehabilitation—group-based exercise programs add value to social well-being due to their socially integrative nature (Emslie et al., 2007; Mutrie et al., 2007). Finally, regarding social facets of well-being, women seem to benefit more from exercise activities than that in men (e.g., Tessier et al., 2007; Wendel-Vos et al., 2004). For example, they feel more socially included and accepted and experience stronger affection and bonding in the group. Moreover, longitudinal studies have demonstrated that there is a relatively consistent relationship between physical activity and an individual's assessment of the potential for functioning in social activities (e.g., Lee & Russell, 2003; Wolin et al., 2007). This is expected to subsequently have a positive effect on the evaluation and perception of social relationships. However, this correlation seems to emerge only over a longer period, possibly several years.

Overall, it must be noted that the phenomena pertaining to social effects of exercise activities are vastly underresearched to date. The initial findings and assumptions mentioned above therefore require further empirical research, with particular attention to be paid to the extent to which exercise programs address the promotion of social facets of well-being (Sudeck & Schmid, 2012).

26.3.2.3 Physical Activity and Well-Being in Everyday Life

The previous sections have primarily focused on structured physical exercise, which is usually carried out during leisure time either in a laboratory, in the "real world" in supervised exercise programs, or as self-directed activities. However, in line with the recommendations for health-promoting physical activity (WHO, 2010), it is also of interest to understand the extent to which low-threshold, everyday physical activities beyond structured exercise are associated with positive effects on well-being. In this context, two lines of research are very important:

1. Studies that distinguish the effects of activities within different domains (e.g., leisure activities, transportation activities, household activities, work-related activities)
2. Studies conducted using the "ambulatory assessment approach" (or "ecological momentary assessment" [EMA]), which provides time-intensive data collected from individuals in their natural, free-living environment

White et al. (2017) addressed the domain-specific effects of physical activity on mental health in their meta-analysis. Outcome criteria ranged from mental health characteristics to psychological well-being, positive affect, and life satisfaction. The available original studies from 1988 to 2015 yielded 53 independent effect sizes that were relatively consistent in indicating a small positive association between leisure-time physical activity and mental health. A similarly small positive association was shown for transportation activities, that is, activities necessary to move from place to place, such as to and from work. However, the variation in the results was larger. This suggests that in this activity domain, the purpose of transportation (e.g., routes to work, active transportation during leisure time) plays an important role in mental health outcomes. In contrast, there were no statistically significant improvements in mental health for physical activities during work as well as at home. These findings suggest that physical activity recommendations aimed at promoting mental health and well-being need to focus more on the context of the activity, rather than total accumulated activity across any and all domains.

In recent years, the relationships between physical activity and well-being in everyday life have increasingly become the focus of research in exercise and health psychology. This shift in focus outside of laboratory settings is due, in part, to the expanded technical possibilities for recording perceptions of well-being and activity in the context of everyday life. On the one hand, everyday physical activities can be increasingly better recorded by accelerometer-based devices (Gabrys et al., 2015). On the other hand, smartphone-based surveys make it possible to assess aspects of well-being repeatedly with high frequency across single or multiple days. As a result, the direct relationship between physical activity and well-being can be studied very close to everyday life and with less bias (Kanning et al., 2013; ◘ Fig. 26.6). As this field continues to evolve, it is important to remember that outcomes from questionnaires and outcomes from processing raw data (via various algorithms) downloaded from accelerometer-based devices are not equivalent or interchangeable. Troiano et al. (2014)

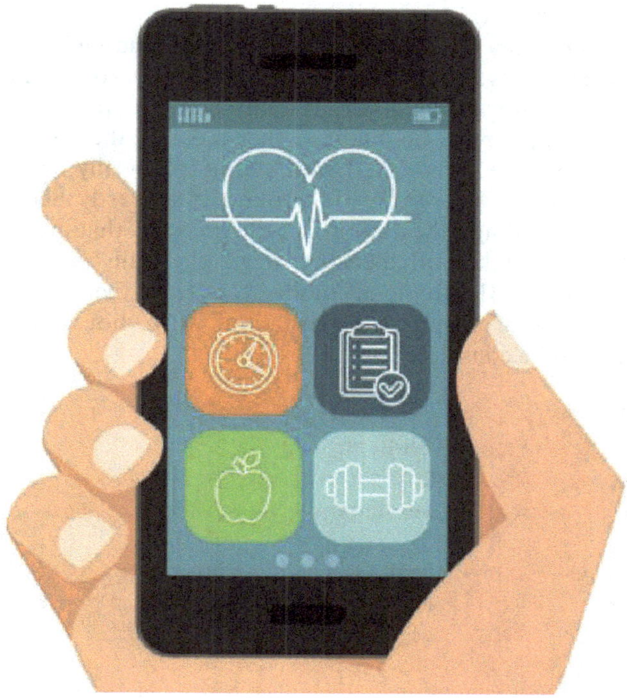

◘ **Fig. 26.6** Physical activity monitoring using smartphones

articulate this distinction in measured constructs, in that accelerometer-based devices quantify bodily movement, whereas self-report instruments capture behaviors and their related constructs. Rather, these outcomes can be *complementary*. For example, a known limitation of self-report instruments is that, because they solely rely on participant recall, they do not sufficiently capture time spent in habitual (i.e., performed automatically and subconsciously), incidental, or intermittent physical activities that are often hard to remember. Conversely, accelerometer-based devices do not sufficiently capture nonambulatory modes of activity and cannot provide insight regarding psychosocial, environmental, or contextual (i.e., exercise vs. occupational activity) factors that may moderate the relationships between physical activity and target outcomes. Thus, researchers should avoid overreaching or incorrect statements when only using one method. Further, researchers should endeavor to integrate both methods in alignment with one another, leveraging their complementary strengths and limitations to more comprehensively measure and describe the performance and experience of physical activity over time.

Meanwhile, the first reviews are available for this research area. Liao et al. (2015) summarize the results from 12 original studies on various dimensions of affective well-being from the period between 1996 and 2015. Overall, quite consistent generalizable effects of everyday physical activity on positive affect (in terms of affective valence) and energy levels (e.g., increase in vitality) emerge. However, inconsistent findings were observed regarding the reduction of negative affect and tension. Regarding generalizability across populations, however, it must be qualified that most of these studies have been conducted with young, physically active individuals. Against the background of the partly inconsistent findings, the authors see the necessity that in further research, both personal (e.g., physically inactive persons) and situational moderators (e.g., the activity domains of leisure, transportation, work, household) should be considered.

Effects of Physical Activities in Everyday Life on Subsequent Well-Being

- **Positive affect**: Physical activity is consistently associated with improvement in subsequent positive affect.
- **Negative affect**: So far, there are rather mixed, inconclusive findings for a reduction of negative affect.
- **Energy/vitality**: An increase in feelings of energy and vitality through physical activity is observed relatively consistently.
- **Calmness vs. tension**: Concerning possible effects on the experience of calmness or the reduction of tension or agitation, mixed results are present so far, which do not allow a clear conclusion.

26.4 Explanatory Approaches

Previous descriptions of the effects of exercise on well-being were provided using primarily empirical findings. However, as theoretical explanations had been referred to at various points, these now will be the focus for the remainder of the chapter.

One explanation is that cognitive factors (e.g., perception, attention, expectations, evaluations) contribute to how physical exercise influences well-being. Research conducted by Rose and Parfitt (2007, 2010) has provided initial insight regarding which cognitive factors impact subjective experience during physical exercise. Their findings are based on verbal and written feedback during and after endurance exercise on an ergometer. The findings reveal a broad range of subjectively experienced factors that were cited as determinants of affective responses to exercise, which in turn can be interpreted as starting points to optimally design exercise activities in ways that promote positive affective experiences.

What Cognitive Factors Encountered During the Activity Positively Influence the Subjective Experience? (Rose & Parfitt, 2010)

- The perception that one is capable of mastering the task at hand (*perceptions of ability*)
- The belief that exercise will result in a significant, desired benefit (*expectancy outcomes*), including the perception that one's own goals will be met (*goal achievement*)
- The ability to redirect attention away from (physical) symptoms provoked by physical exertion (*attentional focus*)
- The experience that one is supported in controlling the means by which the task is accomplished, for example, by being allowed to choose the intensity oneself (*perception of control*)
- The individual's own observation and control of the intensity so that it feels comfortable and is appropriately evaluated from a subjective point of view (*self-monitoring and interpretation of exercise intensity*)
- Perceiving physical symptoms not as discouraging, but as conducive to task accomplishment (*awareness of interoceptive cues*)
- Improving the perception of physical symptoms through specific features of activity design, such as a warm-up, rhythmizing of movement, or experiencing a steady state (*perception of physiological state*)
- The recognition that one is almost finished with a fixed-duration activity (*anticipation of the end*)

The factors identified by Rose and Parfitt mainly focus on the psychological processing of the activity stimulus, with cognitive evaluations of the activity and physical symptoms playing a major role. However, for methodological reasons (supervised ergometer-based exercise), environmental conditions (social, spatial) that might have an influence on the subjective experience of exercise were not addressed. In this respect, the focus is only indirectly placed on the interaction between exercise instructors and exercise participants (e.g., autonomy support, designing an appropriate warm-up).

Exemplary Environmental Conditions That Influence How Physical Exercise Affects Well-Being

- Behavior of instructors, teachers, coaches (e.g., Rose & Parfitt, 2010)
- Outcome in competitive sport (e.g., Alfermann & Stoll, 1996)
- Accompanying music (Karageorghis et al., 2012)

Study Box

Body-Related Stigma Experiences and Their Relevance for Well-Being and Mental Health

Recent research demonstrates that body-related stigmatization and discrimination (e.g., defamation based on obesity or disability) can lead to severe psychological problems for those affected (Puhl & Heuer, 2010). Body-related discrimination against people with obesity begins very early in the lifespan. In an experimental study, children with obesity depicted in photographs were more likely to be labeled as "lazy," "not very attractive," and "not very intelligent" by their peers (Thiel et al., 2008). The degree of stigmatization here correlated strongly with the rejection of children with obesity in their choice of playmates, with stronger effects observed in males. It is reasonable to assume that this latter finding relates to the important role that physical activity plays in the social integration of boys in peer groups. In another experimental study with a comparable design (Giel et al., 2010), we found evidence of very strong discrimination against people with obesity in the workplace. For example, pictures of people with obesity were judged by recruiters to be significantly less successful, willing, and able to perform professionally than people observed to be of normal weight. Only about 6% of respondents favored the people with obesity to be short-listed when applying for a department manager position. Additionally, only a minority (2%) of the personnel managers assigned a prestigious profession to the women with obesity shown in the pictures. It is not surprising that such assessments by others often lead to low self-esteem, body dissatisfaction, and even depression in people with obesity (Puhl & Heuer, 2010).

- Body-related stigma experiences (▶ Study Box: Body-Related Stigma Experiences and Their Significance for Well-Being and Mental Health).
- Natural experiences (*green exercise*; e.g., Gladwell et al., 2013; Thompson Coon et al., 2011)
- Expectancies of *significant others* (e.g., results in competitive sports, body shape; Thiel et al., 2016)

Discrimination against people with obesity is particularly evident in exercise and sports settings. Starting within school settings, students with obesity are regularly laughed at, rejected, discriminated against, and teased in the context of exercise and sports (Puhl et al., 2011). The consequences of such experiences may persist throughout life. For example, in an exploratory experiment with adults, we found that after simply viewing video clips with implicitly body-related stigmatizing content, viewers classified as overweight reported feeling significantly angrier and worn down than that of a comparable normal-weight control group (Carl et al., 2018).

Some of the factors identified by Rose and Parfitt for a positive affective state during exercise can be explained from the perspective of social cognitive theory according to Bandura (1997). In particular, the **"self-efficacy hypothesis"** is an important psychological explanatory approach. Under this model, it is assumed that perceptions of self-efficacy can be enhanced by succeeding in challenging tasks (*mastery experiences*), observing characteristically representative individuals successfully perform similar tasks (*vicarious experiences*), receiving positive feedback from others on one's own abilities (*verbal persuasion*), and experiencing positive psychological activation. Bandura indicated that this latter component is particularly influential when performing tasks that require strength and stamina. Increased confidence to carry out desired tasks, in turn, is associated with a positive state of well-being.

However, as previously explained, to understand the effects of physical exercise on well-being and mental health, it is important to note that physiological and psychological factors are interrelated. Usually, in overviews on explanatory approaches for the psychological effects of exercise, researchers differentiate between physiological, psychological, and mixed model approaches. In German-language textbooks and encyclopedias, the work of Schlicht and Schwenkmezger (1995) has provided initially an important overview, which has been partly modified and supplemented (e.g., Wagner & Brehm, 2008). In ◘ Table 26.2, the different explanations are each briefly outlined to give the reader a preliminary overview. For more in-depth information, please refer to specific sources (see Ekkekakis, 2013, for an overview) or to other chapters in this volume (▶ Chap. 27 on stress). However, explanatory approaches that enable an integration of physiological and psychological explanatory approaches will be singled out as examples.

Table 26.2 Physiological, psychological, and mixed explanations for the effects of physical exercise on well-being (modified and supplemented based on Lehnert et al., 2012)

	Improvement of well-being through/because …	Activity-related specifications	Primary component of well-being	Further reading
(Neuro-)physiological approaches				
Cardiovascular fitness	… improved physical fitness.	Repeated aerobic activity	Unspecific (physical well-being)	Biddle and Ekkekakis (2005)
Thermogenic hypothesis	… raised body temperature.	Primarily aerobic activity	PA-NA	Koltyn (1997)
Cerebral blood flow	… increased cerebral blood flow leading to increased oxygen transport.	Primarily aerobic activity	PA-NA Activation–deactivation	Rogers et al. (1990)
Endorphin hypothesis ("runner's high")	… increased release of endorphins.	Higher intensity/long duration	PA, physical complaints/pain	Hoffmann (1997)
Endocannabinoid hypothesis	… increased endocannabinoid release.		PA	Sparling et al. (2003)
Monoamine hypothesis – Central serotonin – Catecholamines (esp. noradrenalin)	… a change in the specific neurotransmitter systems.		NA, deactivation	Chaouloff (1997) and Dishman (1997)
Transient hypofrontality hypothesis	… reduced neural activity in the prefrontal cortex due to limited resources for brain activity (thereby reducing conscious cognitive processes).		PA-NA Activation–deactivation	Dietrich (2006)
Cross-stressor adaptation hypothesis	… repeated and sufficiently intensive and long-lasting stressors that lead to nonspecific adaptations of the stress reaction; the reduction in stress reactivity can be transferred to other non-exercise-related stressors.	Repeated, intensive aerobic activity	NA, deactivation (stress reactivity)	Sothmann (2006)
(Social-)psychological approaches				
Self-efficacy hypothesis (mastery hypothesis)	… increases in competence expectancies due to mastery experiences.		PA, deactivation, cognitive-evaluative (resources)	Bandura (1997)
Theory of basic psychological needs	… the satisfaction of the basic psychological needs of autonomy, competence, and relatedness.		PA, activation (vitality)	Deci and Ryan (2000)
Distraction hypothesis ("time-out")	… distraction from problems and stress.		NA, deactivation	Bahrke and Morgan (1978)
Meditative consciousness states (flow experience; "flow")	… the fit between skill and challenge level.		PA, activation	Csikzentmihalyi (1982)
Exercise and self-esteem model	… increased self-esteem through changes in physical self-efficacy that exert a positive influence on the two components of self-esteem "physical competence" and "physical acceptance" on a more global level.		Cognitive-evaluative components; physical well-being	Sonstroem and Morgan (1989)

Table 26.2 (continued)

	Improvement of well-being through/because …	Activity-related specifications	Primary component of well-being	Further reading
Social support hypothesis	… experiencing social support and social relatedness.	Social-integrative activities	PA, social well-being	Fox (2000) and Sudeck and Schmid (2012)
Mixed approaches				
Dual-mode theory	… the existence of two affective pathways (cognitive processes and the perception of interoceptive cues).	Depending on intensity	PA-NA	Ekkekakis (2003)
Two-dimensional activation model	… an increase in the energetic arousal level accompanied by a simultaneous decline in tension arousal.	Intensity	PA-NA Activation–deactivation	Thayer (1989)
Green exercise hypothesis	… physiological response to natural environment and the experienced connectedness to nature.	Natural environment	PA-NA Activation–deactivation	Gladwell et al. (2013)

PA positive affect, *NA* negative affect

26.4.1 Dual-Mode Theory

In recent years, the "dual mode theory" has received considerable attention and has been empirically well established (Ekkekakis & Acevedo, 2006). The term "dual mode" implies two principal pathways that determine the immediate affective response to exercise activity. First, the influence of cognitive factors is assumed, which include the previously mentioned factors that influence the subjective experience of exercise (Rose & Parfitt, 2010; e.g., perception of own competence, expectation of positive consequences, and achievement of individual goals). Neurocognitive processes in the prefrontal and sensorimotor cortex are hypothesized to be related to the emotional system. As part of these "high-road" processes (Ekkekakis & Acevedo, 2006), signals are sent primarily to the amygdala, and through it, the perception and interpretation of external stimuli as well as physical symptoms are mediated in an affectively significant way. Second, interoceptive stimuli (e.g., based on muscular fatigue, lactate formation, impaired breathing) are assumed to be directly (i.e., not cognitively mediated) related to the emotional system and to co-determine the affective response. These "low-road" processes are based, for example, on receptors and neuronal areas responsible for the regulation of the cardiovascular, respiratory, and endocrine systems, pain regulation, or the sense of taste (to the point of nausea).

A key assumption of the dual-mode theory is that the degree to which the two principal affective pathways are relevant depends primarily on the exercise intensity (Table 26.3). At intensities occurring below the first ventilatory threshold (VT1), the affective response is assumed to be relatively homogeneous and positive, with cognitive factors having little to moderate influence. When intensities approach VT1, the greatest inter-

Table 26.3 Characteristics of affective response in different ranges of exercise intensity according to the dual-mode theory (Ekkekakis, 2003; Ekkekakis & Acevedo, 2006)

Intensity range	Affective response	Interindividual variability	Influencing factors
Below VT1 ("moderate")	Positive (*pleasure*)	Homogeneity	Low to moderate influence of cognitive factors
At VT1 ("heavy")	Positive to negative (*pleasure, displeasure*)	High variability	Strong influence of cognitive factors
Above VT1 ("severe")	Negative (*displeasure*)	Homogeneity	Strong influence of interoceptive factors

Notes. *VT1* ventilatory threshold 1. It describes the transition from a primarily aerobic energy supply to a mixed aerobic–anaerobic energy supply. In terms of spirometry, it refers to the ratio of an initial disproportionate increase in carbon dioxide output in relation to oxygen uptake (Scharhag-Rosenberger & Schommer, 2013) individual variability of affective responses is observed. In this intensity range, it is mainly cognitive factors that determine whether people experience the activity as pleasant or unpleasant. Finally, for intensities that exceed VT1, interoceptive factors are assumed to exert the most salient influence. This leads to relatively homogeneous, albeit negative, affective responses. The relevance of interoceptive stimuli in this context can be justified by evolutionary theory. Thus, a permanent physical overload signals that the critical and unpleasant bodily state should be terminated as soon as possible, as it would otherwise lead to damage of the body systems (Ekkekakis & Acevedo, 2006). It is particularly important to remember, however, that the level of effort at which VT occurs is a function of both training status and genetics. Thus, the occurrence of this physiological event cannot be accurately predicted for individuals based on the traditional approach of labeling intensity as "light-," "moderate-," or "vigorous-" based percentages of age-predicted maximal heart rate or percentages of maximal oxygen consumption. In other words, performing moderate-intensity exercise, as defined in the traditional manner, would result in some exceeding VT while others do not.

26.4.2 Hypofrontality Hypothesis

The hypofrontality hypothesis (Dietrich, 2006) represents a neurophysiological explanatory approach, but it provides further potential for integrating different explanatory approaches (see also Stoll & Ziemainz, 2012). The hypothesis states that a massive increase in neuronal activity in the motor and sensory cortex results from physical exercise. Therefore, due to limited metabolic capacities in the brain, physical exertion requires a reduction in information processing capacities in the prefrontal cortex. Neuronal activities that are not necessary for the realization of the exercise activity are temporarily downregulated. This includes higher complex cognitive activities as well as emotional information processing, insofar as they are irrelevant for the actual task accomplishment. This process makes it possible, for example, to interrupt ruminating on current problems. In this sense, the hypofrontality hypothesis can be directly linked to psychological approaches that describe a time-out potential of exercise activity that promotes well-being ("distraction hypothesis"; ◘ Table 26.2). As deregulation in the prefrontal cortex can also be accompanied by a loss of the sense of space and time, a feeling of flowing attention, and pain relief, this hypothesis also reveals parallels to the flow hypothesis, which is also used as a psychological approach to explain positive effects of exercise on affective well-being (► Chap. 8 on intrinsic motivation).

Multiple Explanatory Approaches as a Basis for the Optimal Fostering of Well-Being

- The effects of exercise on well-being are a complex phenomenon that cannot be adequately explained by a single approach.
- For a deeper understanding of these effects, an integration of physiological and psychological explanatory approaches is of particular importance.
- An appropriate consideration and methodological integration of the complex set of personal, activity-related, and social factors is a major scientific challenge for explaining the effects of exercise on well-being.
- The systematic and purposeful design of exercise sessions and programs is based, at best, on such complex explanatory approaches for the effects of exercise on well-being.

26.5 Summary and Perspectives

In summary, physical exercise can promote positive effects on well-being. The evidence for this statement is abundant. However, the extent of positive effects and the degree of empirical evidence vary depending on the facet of well-being studied and the type of activity performed.

Summary of Evidence

- On average, moderate positive effects on affective well-being are found both for single exercise sessions and for repeated activities over several weeks.
- Evidence for improvements in physical well-being is quite positive. Positive effects of multi-week exercise programs have been empirically substantiated for body satisfaction and a positive body image as well as for the reduction of physical complaints.
- For life satisfaction, no clear findings can be established based on the various meta-analyses currently available.
- For social well-being, there is emerging evidence that both multi-week exercise programs and regular physical exercise over longer periods of several years have positive effects, with findings indicating a reliance on personal and environmental factors (e.g., on the target group or on socially

integrative activities). However, the level of evidence is still low.

Even though physical exercise can be described as promoting well-being among different individuals, it should be reiterated that future research needs to look more closely at the specific temporal, task-related, and social conditions under which physical exercise takes place. First, the personal preconditions that characterize the individual (biological, cognitive, affective, motivational, social) must be considered. Second, the setting in which activity takes place must be systematically taken into account, starting with the exercise offered and the equipment provided, as well as the group characteristics and the supervisors. The explicit consideration of these factors is likely to allow researchers to then determine interindividual differences in response to exercise. However, to be able to make statements as precisely as possible, researchers should—as we have highlighted in the present chapter—clearly identify the different domains of well-being under study. The scientific perspective should ideally be an integrative, biopsychosocial one. That is, (neuro)physiological approaches should be combined with (social)psychological and sociological approaches. It is expected that such research approaches can provide the knowledge necessary to more pointedly and optimally influence well-being through systematic exercise and sport programs.

Future research should further focus on the educational question of how people can be empowered to make exercise-related decisions that more positively impact their own well-being. In this context, health education elements in exercise programs aimed at building physical activity-related health competence will be of particular importance (Sudeck & Pfeifer, 2016).

The aspect of health education is important, particularly with regard to providing fun and enjoyment in being physically active. How and to what extent affective states and physical activity are related seems to be changeable over the lifespan (Lee et al., 2016). Thus, to find starting points to effectively promote positive affect through physical activity, it is important to examine individual activity biographies. Biographies bundle the various personal experiences in exercise and sport settings. For example, a person enjoyed sports as a child, was active in clubs during childhood and adolescence, but then discontinued activity at times of increased school demands and became more active again as a university student. This person's activity biography is thus characterized by a change in activity behavior and different levels of performance and presumably also by a change in motivation and enjoyment towards activity.

Research into activity biographies makes it possible to make statements about the conditions under which physical activity, exercise, and sports are experienced as meaningful, understandable, and manageable from the individual's point of view, but also about what activity barriers prevail. With this knowledge, exercise and sports programs can be tailored even better to individual needs, which should be of great relevance especially for the promotion of well-being and mental health. Experts now suggest that tuning interventions to the (often dynamic) physical, psychological, contextual, and behavioral requirements of each individual, rather than the broad application of "one-size-fits-all" approaches, is necessary to advance the science of physical activity promotion (Chevance et al., 2021; Conroy et al., 2020).

Overall, the knowledge regarding how individuals can be enabled to effectively regulate their state of well-being and mental health through physical activity is still rather poor. However, starting points for an individual optimization of effects of physical activity have already been described, such as pacing and an appropriate perception of exertion (Thiel et al., 2018), or through flexible programming achieved by routinely monitoring preexercise mental and physical states to dynamically inform person-specific modifications (Strohacker & Beaumont, 2020). In this regard, exercise recommendations from the American College of Sports Medicine (2011) that address the affective state during exercise activity are useful. Here, affective response during exercise activity can be used as a secondary method for controlling the physical load (Ekkekakis et al., 2004), which—according to existing research—is of great importance for the initiation and maintenance of regular exercise behavior (e.g., Brand & Ekkekakis, 2018; Rhodes & Kates, 2015).

Finally, future research will be interested in the question to what extent the affective experience and the psychological processing of exercise depend on (epi) genetic factors. There is increasing evidence that genetic predispositions do not only determine the physiological response to physical activity and that the physiological response is not solely determined by temporally stable genetic preconditions (e.g., Bloch & Zimmer, 2012; Bryan et al., 2011). For example, recent work suggests that the eustress associated with physical activity acts as an epigenetic modulator that promotes positive epigenetic changes and, in turn, reduces the risk of obesity and chronic degenerative diseases (Sanchis-Gomar et al., 2012). However, this line of research is still in its infancy, particularly because too little attention has been paid to the question, central to environmental epigenetics, of how social structure and social regulation are causally linked to genome structure and gene regulation (Landecker & Panofsky, 2013).

Finally, we return to the question posed at the onset of this chapter, namely, to what extent the assumption of a positive effect of physical activity on well-being and mental health is scientifically well-founded. Given the current state of research, we can assume that physical activity, primarily via structured exercise, has a positive effect on affective well-being, both in the short term and immediately after an activity, as well as in the long term in the case of multi-week programs. We also know that the immediate pleasure derived from the activity is an important source of self-determined motivation for the activity behavior. However, due to different psychophysiological preconditions and different social circumstances, these effects vary from individual to individual and potentially within individuals over time. Against this background, many questions remain unanswered, which an interdisciplinary exercise and sport science must address in order to make evidence-based statements about the conditions for a physically active lifestyle to promote outcomes relating to both health and well-being.

Learning Control Questions

Basic:

1. Which health concepts can be distinguished within current health sciences texts that offer terminological definitions of health?
2. What is to be understood by the "biopsychosocial health model," and where does well-being fall into place in such an understanding of health?
3. How can well-being be identified content wise, and what components of well-being can be differentiated from one another?
4. How do categorical and dimensional approaches to affective well-being differ from one another?

Advanced:

5. Which parameters generally determine individual reaction to physical activities?
6. What basic assumptions underlie the "transdisciplinary framework" of the individual response to physical activity?
7. Illustrate the transdisciplinary framework of the individual response to physical activity. Take into account the role that parameters of physical load and subjective experience play.
8. What influence does a biography (in regards to activity and health) have on individual response to physical activities?
9. Sum up in keywords the current findings on the effects of sports activities on affective health. Differentiate the immediate- and long-term effects.
10. Which methodological aspects need to be taken into account when analyzing the effects of physical exercise on affective well-being to avoid superficial conclusions?
11. What has already been found regarding the potential effects of physical exercise on physical and social well-being, and how is the state of the research for these components of well-being to be understood?
12. What are the empirical findings regarding the effects of everyday physical activity on the different dimensions of affective well-being?

Experts:

13. Why is it worthwhile to identify the *everyday* relationship between well-being and the different domains of activity?
14. What explanatory approaches exist for the effects of physical activities on well-being and psychological health, and what is to be understood by a mixed approach in this context?
15. What cognitive factors could influence the well-being during physical activity?
16. What roles do cognitive factors play for well-being during physical exercise dependent on exercise intensity according to the "dual-mode theory?"
17. Based on current explanatory approaches and empirical findings, name the possible components of an optimal structure for physical exercises promoting well-being. Differentiate between immediate and long-term effects.
18. What role can the exercise instructor play in shaping activities to promote well-being, and what role do environmental conditions play?

References

Abele, A. E., & Brehm, W. (1986a). Befindlichkeitsveränderungen im Sport. *Sportwissenschaft, 16*, 288–302.

Abele, A. E., & Brehm, W. (1986b). Zur Konzeptualisierung und Messung von Befindlichkeit—Die Entwicklung der "Befindlichkeitsskalen" (BFS). *Diagnostica, 32*, 209–228.

Abele, A. E., & Brehm, W. (1993). Exercise, mood, well-being, and health. *International Review of Health Psychology, 2*, 53–80.

Alfermann, D., & Stoll, O. (1996). Befindlichkeitsveränderungen nach sportlicher Tätigkeit. *Sportwissenschaft, 26*, 406–423.

Alleva, J. M., Sheeran, P., Webb, T. L., Martijn, C., & Miles, E. A. (2015). Meta-analytic review of stand-alone interventions to improve body image. *PLoS One, 10*(9), e0139177.

American College of Sports Medicine. (2011). Quantity and quality of exercise for developing and maintaining cardiorespiratory, musculoskeletal, and neuromotor fitness in apparently healthy adults. Guidance for prescribing exercise. *Medicine and Science in Sports and Exercise, 43*, 1334–1359.

Antonovsky, A. (1979). *Health, stress and coping*. Jossey-Boss.

Antonovsky, A. (1993). Gesundheitsforschung versus Krankheitsforschung. In A. Franke & M. Broda (Eds.), *Psychosomatische Gesundheit. Versuch einer Abkehr vom Pathogense-Konzept* (pp. 3–14). dgvt-Verlag.

Arent, S. M., Landers, D. M., & Etnier, J. L. (2000). The effects of exercise on mood in older adults: A meta-analytic review. *Journal of Aging and Physical Activity, 8*, 407–430.
Backhouse, S. H., Ekkekakis, P., Biddle, S. J., Foskett, A., & Williams, C. (2007). Exercise makes people feel better but people are inactive: Paradox or artifact? *Journal of Sport and Exercise Psychology, 29*, 498.
Bahrke, M. S., & Morgan, W. P. (1978). Anxiety reduction following exercise and meditation. *Cognitive Therapy and Research, 2*, 323–333.
Bandura, A. (1997). *Self-efficacy: The exercise of control*. Freeman.
Beaumont, C. T., Ferrara, P. M., & Strohacker, K. (2021). Exploring determinants of recalled in-task affective valence during recreational exercise. *Physiology & Behavior, 230*, 113261.
Becker, P. (1982). *Psychologie der seelischen Gesundheit: Theorien, Modelle, Diagnostik*. Hogrefe.
Becker, P. (1991). Wohlbefinden. Theoretische Grundlagen. In A. Abele & P. Becker (Eds.), *Wohlbefinden. Theorie—Empirie—Diagnostik* (pp. 13–51). Weinheim.
Bengel, J., Strittmatter, R., & Willmann, H. (2001). *Was erhält Menschen gesund? Antonovskys Modell der Salutogenese—Diskussionsstand und Stellenwert*. Bundeszentrale für gesundheitliche Aufklärung.
Biddle, S. J. H., & Ekkekakis, P. (2005). Physically active lifestyles and well-being. In F. A. Huppert, B. Keverne, & N. Baylis (Eds.), *The science of well-being* (pp. 140–168). Oxford University Press.
Bloch, W., & Zimmer, P. (2012). Epigenetik und Sport. *Deutsche Zeitschrift fur Sportmedizin, 63*, 163–167.
Brand, R., & Ekkekakis, P. (2018). Affective–reflective theory of physical inactivity and exercise. *German Journal of Exercise and Sport Research, 48*, 48–58.
Brehm, W. (1998). Stimmung und Stimmungsmanagement. In K. Bös & W. Brehm (Eds.), *Gesundheitssport: Ein Handbuch* (pp. 201–211). Hofmann.
Brehm, W., Wagner, P., Sygusch, R., Schönung, A., & Hahn, U. (2005). Health promotion by means of health sport—A framework and a controlled intervention study with sedentary adults. *Scandinavian Journal of Medicine & Science in Sports, 15*, 13–20.
Brettschneider, C., Lühmann, D., & Raspe, H. (2011). *Der Stellenwert von Patient Reported Outcomes (PRO) im Kontext von Health Technology Assessment (HTA)*. Deutsches Institut für Medizinische Dokumentation und Information (DIMDI).
Bryan, A. D., Magnan, R. E., Nilsson, R., Marcus, B. H., Tompkins, S. A., & Hutchison, K. E. (2011). The big picture of individual differences in physical activity behavior change: A transdisciplinary approach. *Psychology of Sport and Exercise, 12*, 20–26.
Buytendijk, F. J. J. (1958). *Das Menschliche*. Koehler.
Campbell, A., & Hausenblas, H. A. (2009). Effects of exercise interventions on body image: A meta-analysis. *Journal of Health Psychology, 14*, 780–793.
Carl, J., Thedinga, H. K., Zipfel, S., & Thiel, A. (2018). Stimulating weight stigma in future experimental designs on physical activity—Development and pilot validation of a video instrument. *Obesity Facts, 11*, 206–220.
Caspersen, C. J., Powell, K. E., & Christenson, G. M. (1985). Physical activity, exercise, and physical fitness: Definitions and distinctions for health-related research. *Public Health Reports, 100*, 126–131.
Chaouloff, F. (1997). The serotonin hypothesis. In W. P. Morgan (Ed.), *Physical activity & mental health* (pp. 179–198). Taylor & Francis.
Chevance, G., Perski, O., & Hekler, E. B. (2021). Innovative methods for observing and changing complex health behaviors: Four propositions. *Translational Behavioral Medicine, 11*, 676–685.
Cohen, J. (1988). *Statistical power analysis for the behavioral sciences*. Erlbaum.
Conroy, D. E., Lagoa, C. M., Hekler, E., & Rivera, D. E. (2020). Engineering person-specific behavioral interventions to promote physical activity. *Exercise and Sport Sciences Reviews, 48*, 170–179.
Crust, L., Swann, C., Allen-Collinson, J., Breckon, J., & Weinberg, R. (2014). A phenomenological exploration of exercise mental toughness: Perceptions of exercise leaders and regular exercisers. *Qualitative Research in Sport, Exercise and Health, 6*, 441–461.
Csikszentmihalyi, M. (1982). Toward a psychology of optimal experience. In L. Wheeler & L. (Eds.), *Review of personality and social psychology* (pp. 13–36). Sage.
Damasio, A. (1999). *The feeling of what happens: Body and emotion in the making of consciousness*. Harcourt.
Damasio, A., & Carvalho, G. B. (2013). The nature of feelings: Evolutionary and neurobiological origins. *Nature Reviews Neuroscience, 14*, 143–152.
Deci, E. L., & Ryan, R. M. (2000). The "what" and "why" of goal pursuits: Human needs and the self-determination of behavior. *Psychological Inquiry, 11*, 227–268.
Diener, E. (2005). *Guidelines for national indicators of subjective well-being and ill-being* [Electronic Version]. https://internal.psychology.illinois.edu/~ediener/Documents/Guidelines_for_National_Indicators.pdf
Diener, E., Lucas, R., & Scollon, C. (2006). Beyond the hedonic treadmill: Revising the adaptation theory of Well-being. *American Psychologist, 61*, 305–314.
Diener, E., Smith, H., & Fujita, F. (1995). The personality structure of affect. *Journal of Personality and Social Psychology, 69*, 130–141.
Diener, E., Suh, E. M., Lucas, R. E., & Smith, H. (1999). Subjective well-being: Three decades of progress. *Psychological Bulletin, 125*, 276–302.
Diener, E., Wirtz, D., Tov, W., Kim-Prieto, C., Choi, D.-W., Oishi, S., & Biswas-Diener, R. (2010). New well-being measures: Short scales to assess flourishing and positive and negative feelings. *Social Indicators Research, 97*, 143–156.
Dietrich, A. (2006). Transient hypofrontality as a mechanism for the psychological effects of exercise. *Psychiatry Research, 145*, 79–83.
Dishman, R. K. (1997). The norepinephrine hypothesis. In W. P. Morgan (Ed.), *Physical activity & mental health* (pp. 199–212). Taylor & Francis.
Ekkekakis, P. (2003). Pleasure and displeasure from the body: Perspectives from exercise. *Cognition & Emotion, 17*, 213–239.
Ekkekakis, P. (2008). Affect circumplex redux: The discussion on its utility as a measurement framework in exercise psychology continues. *International Review of Sport and Exercise Psychology, 31*, 505–553.
Ekkekakis, P. (Ed.) (2013). Routledge Handbook of Physical Activity and Mental Health. *London: Routledge*.
Ekkekakis, P. (2015). *Escape from cognitivism: Exercise as hedonic experience*. Presentation at the FEPSAC congress, 2015 in Berne, Switzerland.
Ekkekakis, P., & Acevedo, E. O. (2006). Affective responses to acute exercise: Toward a psychobiological dose-response model. In E. O. Acevedo & P. Ekkekakis (Eds.), *Psychobiology of physical activity* (pp. 91–109). Human Kinetics.
Ekkekakis, P., Hall, E., & Petruzzello, S. (2004). Practical markers of the transition from aerobic to anaerobic metabolism during exercise: Rationale and a case for affect-based exercise prescription. *Preventive Medicine, 38*, 149–159.
Ekkekakis, P., Hall, E. E., & Petruzzello, S. J. (2005). Variation and homogeneity in affective responses to physical activity of varying intensities: An alternative perspective on dose–response based on evolutionary considerations. *Journal of Sports Sciences, 23*, 477–500.
Ekkekakis, P., Lind, E., & Vazou, S. (2010). Affective responses to increasing levels of exercise intensity in normal-weight, overweight, and obese middle-aged women. *Obesity, 18*, 79–85.
Ekkekakis, P., Parfitt, G., & Petruzzello, S. J. (2011). The pleasure and displeasure people feel when they exercise at different intensities. *Sports Medicine, 41*, 641–671.

Emslie, C., Whyte, F., Campbell, A., Mutrie, N., Lee, L., Ritchie, D., et al. (2007). 'I wouldn't have been interested in just sitting round a table talking about cancer'; exploring the experiences of women with breast cancer in a group exercise trial. *Health Education Research, 22*, 827–838.

Faltermaier, T. (2005). *Gesundheitspsychologie*. Kohlhammer.

Fox, K. R. (2000). The effects of exercise on self-perceptions and self-esteem. In S. J. H. Biddle, K. R. Fox, & S. H. Boutcher (Eds.), *Physical activity and psychological well-being* (pp. 88–117). Routledge.

Franke, A. (2010). *Modelle von Gesundheit und Krankheit* (2nd ed.). Huber.

Fredrickson, B. L., & Losada, M. F. (2005). Positive affect and complex dynamics of human flourishing. *American Psychologist, 60*, 678–686.

Fujita, F., & Diener, E. (2005). Life satisfaction set point: Stability and change. *Journal of Personality and Social Psychology, 88*, 158–164.

Gabrys, L., Thiel, C., Tallner, A., Wilms, B., Müller, C., Kahlert, D., Jekauc, D., Frick, F., Schulz, H., Sprengeler, O., Hey, S., Kobel, S., & Vogt, L. (2015). Akzelerometrie zur Erfassung körperlicher Aktivität. *Sportwissenschaft, 45*, 1–9.

Giel, K. E., Thiel, A., Teufel, M., Mayer, J., & Zipfel, S. (2010). Weight bias in work settings—A qualitative review. *Obesity Facts, 3*, 33–40.

Gillison, F. B., Skevington, S. M., Sato, A., Standage, M., & Evangelidou, S. (2009). The effects of exercise interventions on quality of life in clinical and healthy populations: A meta-analysis. *Social Science & Medicine, 68*, 1700–1710.

Ginis, K. A. M., & Bassett, R. L. (2011). Exercise and changes in body image. In T. F. Cash & L. Smolak (Eds.), *Body image: A handbook of science, practice and prevention* (pp. 378–386). Guilford.

Gladwell, V. F., Brown, D. K., Wood, C., Sanderock, G. S., & Barton, J. L. (2013). The great outdoors: How a green exercise environment can benefit all. *Extreme Physiology & Medicine, 2*, 3.

Hardy, C. J., & Rejeski, W. J. (1989). Not what, but how one feels: The measurement of affect during exercise. *Journal of Sport and Exercise Psychology, 11*(3), 304–317.

Hoffmann, P. (1997). The endorphin hypothesis. In W. P. Morgan (Ed.), *Physical activity & mental health* (pp. 213–232). Taylor & Francis.

Hurrelmann, K. (2000). *Gesundheitssoziologie*. Weinheim.

Johns, G. (2010). Presentism in the workplace: A review and research agenda. *Journal of Organizational Behaviour, 31*, 519–542.

Kahnemann, D. (1999). Objective happiness. In D. Kahnemann, E. Diener, & N. Schwarz (Eds.), *Well-being: Foundations of hedonic psychology* (pp. 3–25). Russell-Sage.

Kanning, M., Ebner-Priemer, U. W., & Schlicht, W. (2013). How to investigate within-subject associations between physical activity and momentary affective states in everyday life: A position statement based on a literature overview. *Frontiers in Psychology, 4*, 187.

Karageorghis, C. I., Terry, P. C., Lane, A. M., Bishop, D. T., & Priest, D. (2012). The BASES Expert Statement on use of music in exercise. *Journal of Sports Sciences, 30*, 953–956.

Keyes, C. L. M. (2002). The mental health continuum: From languishing to flourishing in life. *Journal of Health and Social Behavior, 43*, 207–222.

Koltyn, K. F. (1997). The thermogenic hypothesis. In W. P. Morgan (Ed.), *Physical activity and mental health* (pp. 213–226). Taylor & Francis.

Landecker, H., & Panofsky, A. (2013). From social structure to gene regulation, and back: A critical introduction to environment epigenetics for sociology. *Annual Review of Sociology, 39*, 333–357.

Lee, C., & Russell, A. (2003). Effects of physical activity on emotional well-being among older Australian women: Cross-sectional and longitudinal analyses. *Journal of Psychosomatic Research, 54*, 155–160.

Lee, H., Emerson, J. A., & Williams, D. M. (2016). The exercise-affect-adherence pathway: An evolutionary perspective. *Frontiers in Psychology, 7*, 1285.

Lehnert, K., Sudeck, G., & Conzelmann, A. (2012). Subjective well-being and exercise in the second half of life: A critical review of theoretical approaches. *European Review of Aging and Physical Activity, 9*, 87–102.

Liao, Y., Shonkoff, E. T., & Dunton, G. F. (2015). The acute relationships between affect, physical feeling states, and physical activity in daily life: A review of current evidence. *Frontiers in Psychology, 6*, 1975.

Lischetzke, T., & Eid, M. (2005). Wohlbefinden. In H. Weber & T. Rammsayer (Eds.), *Handbuch der Persönlichkeitspsychologie und Differentiellen Psychologie* (pp. 413–422). Hogrefe.

Martin, K. A., & Lichtenberger, C. M. (2002). Fitness enhancement and changes in body image. In T. F. Cash & L. Smolak (Eds.), *Body image: A handbook of science, practice and prevention* (pp. 414–421). Guilford.

Mayer, J., & Thiel, A. (2018). Presenteeism in the elite sports workplace: The willingness to compete hurt among German elite handball and track and field athletes. *International Review for the Sociology of Sport, 53*, 49–68.

McNair, D. M., Lorr, M., & Droppleman, L. F. (1981). *Profile of mood states*. Educational and Industrial Testing Service.

Mihalko, S. L., & McAuley, E. (1996). Strength training effects on subjective wellbeing and physical function in the elderly. *Journal of Aging and Physical Activity, 4*, 56–68.

Morgan, W. P. (1981). Psychological benefits of physical activity. In F. J. Nagle & H. J. Montoye (Eds.), *Exercise in health and disease* (pp. 299–314). Thomas.

Mrazek, J. (1986). Einstellungen zum eigenen Körper. In J. Bielefeld (Ed.), *Körpererfahrung* (pp. 223–249). Hogrefe.

Mutrie, N., Campbell, A. M., Whyte, F., McConnachie, A., Emslie, C., Lee, L., et al. (2007). Benefits of supervised group exercise programme for women being treated for early stage breast cancer: Pragmatic randomised controlled trial. *BMJ, 334*(7592), 517.

Netz, Y., Wu, M.-J., Becker, B. J., & Tenenbaum, G. (2005). Physical activity and psychological well-being in advanced age: A meta-analysis of intervention studies. *Psychology and Aging, 20*, 272–284.

Nitsch, J. R. (2004). Die handlungstheoretische Perspektive: ein Rahmenkonzept für die sportpsychologische Forschung und Intervention. *Zeitschrift für Sportpsychologie, 11*, 10–24.

Pahmeier, I. (2012). Sportliche Aktivität und psychosomatische Beschwerden. In R. Fuchs & W. Schlicht (Eds.), *Sportliche Aktivität und seelische Gesundheit* (pp. 79–99). Hogrefe.

Paulus, P. (1986). Körpererfahrung und Selbsterfahrung in persönlichkeitspsychologischer Sicht. In J. Bielefeld (Ed.), *Körpererfahrung* (pp. 87–122). Hogrefe.

Plessner, H. (1970). Lachen und Weinen. In H. Plessner (Ed.), *Philosophische Anthropologie* (pp. 11–171). Fischer.

Puhl, R. M., & Heuer, C. A. (2010). Obesity stigma: Important considerations for public health. *American Journal of Public Health, 100*, 1019–1028.

Puhl, R. M., Luedicke, J., & Heuer, C. (2011). Weight-based victimization toward overweight adolescents: Observations and reactions of peers. *Journal of School Health, 81*, 696–703.

Radoschewski, M. (2000). Gesundheitsbezogene Lebensqualität—Konzepte und Maße. *Bundesgesundheitsblatt, Gesundheitsforschung, Gesundheitsschutz, 43*, 165–189.

Reed, J., & Buck, S. (2009). The effect of regular aerobic exercise on positive activated affect: A meta-analysis. *Psychology of Sport and Exercise, 10*, 581–594.

Reed, J., & Ones, D. S. (2006). The effect of acute aerobic exercise on positive activated affect: A meta-analysis. *Psychology of Sport and Exercise, 7*, 477–514.
Rejeski, W. J., & Mihalko, S. L. (2001). Physical activity and quality of life in older adults. *Journal of Gerontology: Series A, 56A*, 23–35.
Rhodes, R. E., & Kates, A. (2015). Can the affective response to exercise predict future motives and physical activity behavior? A systematic review of published evidence. *Annals of Behavioral Medicine, 49*, 715–731.
Rogers, R. L., Meyer, J. S., & Mortel, K. F. (1990). After reaching retirement age physical activity sustains cerebral perfusion and cognition. *Journal of the American Geriatrics Society, 38*, 123–128.
Rose, E. A., & Parfitt, G. (2007). A quantitative analysis and qualitative explanation of the individual differences in affective responses to prescribed and self-selected exercise intensities. *Journal of Sport and Exercise Psychology, 29*, 281.
Rose, E. A., & Parfitt, G. (2010). Pleasant for some and unpleasant for others: A protocol analysis of the cognitive factors that influence affective responses to exercise. *International Journal of Behavioral Nutrition and Physical Activity, 7*, 15.
Russell, J. A. (1980). A circumplex model of affect. *Journal of Personality and Social Psychology, 39*, 1161–1178.
Ryff, C. D., & Singer, B. H. (2008). Know thyself and become what you are: A eudaimonic approach to psychological well-being. *Journal of Happiness Studies, 9*, 13–39.
Sanchis-Gomar, F., Garcia-Gimenez, J. L., Perez-Quilis, C., Gomez-Cabrera, M. C., Pallardo, F. V., & Lippi, G. (2012). Physical exercise as an epigenetic modulator: Eustress, the "positive stress" as an effector of gene expression. *Journal of Strength and Conditioning Research, 26*, 3469–3472.
Scharfetter, C. (2002). *Allgemeine Psychopathologie*. Thieme.
Scharhag-Rosenberger, F., & Schommer, K. (2013). Die Spiroergometrie in der Sportmedizin. *Deutsche Zeitschrift fur Sportmedizin, 64*, 362–366.
Schimmack, U., & Grob, A. (2000). Dimensional models of core affect: A quantitative comparison by means of structural equation modeling. *European Journal of Personality, 14*, 325–345.
Schlicht, W. (1995). *Wohlbefinden und Gesundheit durch Sport*. Hofmann.
Schlicht, W., & Reicherz, A. (2012). Sportliche Aktivität und affektive Reaktionen. In R. Fuchs & W. Schlicht (Eds.), *Sportliche Aktivität und seelische Gesundheit* (pp. 12–33). Hogrefe.
Schlicht, W., & Schwenkmezger, P. (1995). Sport in der Primärprävention: Eine Einführung aus verhaltens- und sozialwissenschaftlicher Sicht. In W. Schlicht & P. Schwenkmezger (Eds.), *Gesundheitsverhalten und Bewegung. Grundlagen, Konzepte und empirische Befunde* (pp. 1–17). Schorndorf.
Seligman, M. (2002). *Authentic happiness: Using the new positive psychology to realize your potential for lasting fulfilment*. Free Press.
Seligman, M. (2011). *Flourish: A visionary new understanding of happiness and well-being*. Simon & Schuster.
Singal, A. G., Higgins, P. D., & Waljee, A. K. (2014). A primer on effectiveness and efficacy trials. *Clinical and Translational Gastroenterology, 5*, e45.
Sonstroem, R. J., & Morgan, W. P. (1989). Exercise and self-esteem: Rationale and model. *Medicine & Science in Sports & Exercise, 28*, 619–625.
Sothmann, M. S. (2006). The cross-stressor adaptation hypothesis and exercise training. In E. O. Acevedo & P. Ekkekakis (Eds.), *Psychobiology of physical activity* (pp. 149–160). Human Kinetics.
Sparling, P. B., Giuffrida, A., Piomelli, D., Rosskopf, L., & Dietrich, A. (2003). Exercise activates the endocannabinoid system. *Neuroreport, 14*, 2209–2211.
Staudinger, U. M. (2000). Viele Gründe sprechen dagegen, und trotzdem geht es vielen Menschen gut: Das Paradox des subjektiven Wohlbefindens. *Psychologische Rundschau, 51*, 185–197.
Steyer, R., Schwenkmezger, P., Notz, P., & Eid, M. (1997). *Der Mehrdimensionale Befindlichkeitsfragebogen (MDBF)*. Hogrefe.
Stoll, O., & Ziemainz, H. (2012). *Laufen psychotherapeutisch nutzen. Grundlagen, Praxis, Grenzen*. Springer.
Strohacker, K., & Beaumont, C. T. (2020). The shared criticisms of periodization models and behavior-change theories for exercise: An opportunity for collaborative advancement? *Kinesiology Review, 9*, 170–178.
Strohacker, K., Boyer, W. R., Smitherman, K. N., Cornelius, E., & Fazzino, D. (2017). Assessing energy level as a marker of aerobic exercise readiness: A pilot investigation. *International Journal of Exercise Science, 10*, 62.
Strohacker, K., & Zakrajsek, R. A. (2016). Determining dimensionality of exercise readiness using exploratory factor analysis. *Journal of Sports Science and Medicine, 15*, 229.
Strohacker, K., Zakrajsek, R. A., Schaltegger, E. T., & Springer, C. M. (2019). Readiness to perform aerobic activity in adults with obesity: A thematic analysis of online surveys. *Research Quarterly for Exercise and Sport, 90*, 619–628.
Sudeck, G., & Conzelmann, A. (2014). Zur interindividuellen Variabilität affektiver Reaktionen im Verlauf von Freizeit-und Gesundheitssportprogrammen. *Zeitschrift für Gesundheitspsychologie, 22*, 89–103.
Sudeck, G., & Pfeifer, K. (2016). Physical activity-related health competence as an integrative objective in exercise therapy and health sports—Conception and validation of a short questionnaire. *German Journal of Exercise and Sport Research, 46*, 74–87.
Sudeck, G., & Schmid, J. (2012). Sportliche Aktivität und soziales Wohlbefinden. In R. Fuchs & W. Schlicht (Eds.), *Sportliche Aktivität und seelische Gesundheit* (pp. 56–77). Hogrefe.
Svebak, S., & Murgatroyd, S. (1985). Metamotivational dominance: A multimethod validation of reversal theory constructs. *Journal of Personality and Social Psychology, 48*, 107.
Tellegen, A., Watson, D., & Clark, L. A. (1999). On the dimensional and hierarchical structure of affect. *Psychological Science, 10*, 297–303.
Tessier, S., Vuillemin, A., Bertrais, S., Boini, S., Le, B. E., Oppert, J. M., et al. (2007). Association between leisure-time physical activity and health-related quality of life changes over time. *Preventive Medicine, 44*, 202–208.
Thayer, R. B. (1989). *The biopsychology of mood and arousal*. Oxford University Press.
Thiel, A. (2013). Altersbilder. In W. Schlicht & N. Schott (Eds.), *Körperlich aktiv altern* (pp. 60–77). Juventa.
Thiel, A., Alizadeh, M., Giel, K., & Zipfel, S. (2008). Stigmatisierung von adipösen Kindern und Jugendlichen durch ihre Altersgenossen. *Psychotherapie, Psychosomatik, Medizinische Psychologie, 58*, 462–270.
Thiel, A., Seiberth, K. & Mayer, M. (2013). Sportsoziologie. Sportsoziologie. In *Ein Lehrbuch in 13 Lektionen*. Meyer & Meyer.
Thiel, A., Thedinga, H. K., Thomas, S. L., Barkhoff, H., Giel, K. E., Schweizer, O., Thiel, S., & Zipfel, S. (2016). Have adults lost their sense of play? An observational study of the social dynamics of physical (in)activity in German and Hawaiian leisure settings. *BMC Public Health, 16*, 689.
Thiel, C., Pfeifer, K., & Sudeck, G. (2018). Pacing and perceived exertion in endurance performance in exercise therapy and health sports. A competence-oriented view. *German Journal of Exercise and Sport Research, 48*, 136–144.
Thompson Coon, J., Boddy, K., Stein, K., Whear, R., Barton, J., & Depledge, M. H. (2011). Does participating in physical activity in outdoor natural environments have a greater effect on physical and mental wellbeing than physical activity indoors? A systematic review. *Environmental Science & Technology, 45*, 1761–1772.

Troiano, R. P., McClain, J. J., Brychta, R. J., & Chen, K. Y. (2014). Evolution of accelerometer methods for physical activity research. *British Journal of Sports Medicine, 48*, 1019–1023.

Van Landuyt, L. M., Ekkekakis, P., Hall, E. E., & Petruzzello, S. J. (2000). Throwing the mountains into the lakes: On the perils of nomothetic conceptions of the exercise-affect relationship. *Journal of Sport and Exercise Psychology, 22*, 208–234.

Wagner, P., & Brehm, W. (2008). Körperlich-sportliche Aktivität und Gesundheit. In J. Beckmann & M. Kellmann (Eds.), *Anwendungen der Sportpsychologie* (pp. 543–608). Hogrefe.

Waller, H. (2006). *Gesundheitswissenschaft*. Kohlhammer.

Wendel-Vos, G. C., Schuit, A. J., Tijhuis, M. A., & Kromhout, D. (2004). Leisure time physical activity and health-related quality of life: Cross-sectional and longitudinal associations. *Quality of Life Research, 13*, 667–677.

White, R. L., Babic, M. J., Parker, P. D., Lubans, D. R., Astell-Burt, T., & London, C. (2017). Domain-specific physical activity and mental health: A meta-analysis. *American Journal of Preventive Medicine, 52*, 653–666.

Wolin, K. Y., Glynn, R. J., Colditz, G. A., Lee, I.-M., & Kawachi, I. (2007). Long-term physical activity patterns and health-related quality of life in U.S. women. *American Journal of Preventive Medicine, 32*, 490–499.

World Health Organization. (1948). Preamble to the constitution of the World Health Organization as adopted by the International Health Conference, New York. *Official Records of the World Health Organization, 2*, 100.

World Health Organization. (2010). *Global recommendations and physical activity on health*. WHO.

Wundt, W. (1905). *Grundzüge der physiologischen Psychologie*. Engelmann.

Sports, Stress, and Health

Markus Gerber and Flora Colledge

Contents

J. Schüler et al. (eds.), *Sport and Exercise Psychology*, https://doi.org/10.1007/978-3-031-03921-8_27

Learning Objectives

Basic:

- After reading the chapter, you can clearly explain the societal relevance of stress.
- You will be able to define stress.
- You can list the most important stress models and can reproduce their main content in your own words.
- You can describe the physiological reactions to stress.
- You can list physical and psychological consequences of stress.
- You can explain how sports can reduce stress and why sports can act as a stressor.
- You will know the main stress sources in performance sports.

Advanced:

- You can reflect about the different perspectives on stress in the domain of sports (stress regulation through sports, stress regulation in performance sports).
- You will know about the bidirectional relationship of physical activity and stress and know how to empirically test them.
- You can answer the question how burnout is related to sports and stress.

Experts:

- You can explain the importance of recovery in performance sports and name strategies to support recovery.
- You will understand the working mechanisms of stress management trainings and know how you would apply it to the sports that you perform yourself.

27.1 Introduction: Stress and Its Societal Relevance

Life can be understood as a constant process of adaptation to the conditions in which one finds oneself. The price of failure to adapt is dissatisfaction and illness (Uchino et al., 2007). Stress increases the risk of failed adaptation; however, not all forms of stress have a negative impact on our health. So long as we are able to physiologically tolerate stress, and the stressors themselves lead us to improve our performance or overcome phases of lethargy, stress is a positive, healthy promoter of adaptation **(eustress)**. On the other hand, when stressors overwhelm our ability to cope and become an excessive drain on our physical resources without adequate recovery time, stress is understood to be something negative **(distress)** (Selye, 1956).

In the past, researchers have variously described stress as a **stimulus** (stressor), a **reaction** (a biological, emotional, cognitive, or behavioral response), or a **cognitive-transactional process** (Semmer & Zapf, 2017). A further well-established distinction is made between **acute** (temporally limited) and **chronic stress**, with chronic stress understood as a result of the presence of long-term stressors (e.g., long-lasting problems in the workplace, care of a family member) and considered to be of particular relevance for health. It is important to note that high levels of perceived stress may also be caused by internal factors, such as a predisposition to endlessly mull over past problems. Cacioppo and Berntson (2011) differentiate between four health-relevant components of stress: exposure, reactivity, recovery, and restoration. **Exposure** refers to the number of stressors a person is confronted with; **reactivity** describes the scale of reaction to a potentially stressful occurrence; **recovery** refers to the length of time required for prestressor, baseline levels to be reached following stress onset; and **restoration** refers to the efficiency of anabolic processes, which are responsible for the replenishment of coping resources or the renewal of damaged physiological structures.

Health-Relevant Components of Stress

1. Exposure (the number of stressors a person is confronted with).
2. Reactivity (the scale of reaction to a potentially stressful occurrence).
3. Recovery (the length of time required for prestressor, baseline levels to be achieved following stress onset).
4. Restoration (the efficiency of anabolic processes, which are responsible for the replenishment of coping resources or the renewal of damaged physiological structures).

When asked about their levels of stress, many people report these to be troublingly high (Staatssekretariat für Wirtschaft, 2011). Findings from the sixth "European Working Conditions Surveys" (EWCS) emphasize that more than a third of employees experience time pressure at work, interruptions, and long working hours (Eurofound, 2016). Furthermore, in the service sector, employees feel that they must keep their emotions in check, and consequently, a high degree of emotion regulation is required of them. According to Elfering et al. (2017), work-related stress has numerous and wide-ranging consequences, and entails both **direct costs** (e.g., societal resources used for treatment, rehabilitation, and care), **indirect costs** (e.g., loss of production or performance due to stress-related employee absence, reduced performance, high employee turnover, early retirement, invalidity, or early death), and **intangible (human) costs** (e.g., suffering of the affected individuals, their family, and/or friends). Studies in various countries conclude that stress-related costs account for between 1% and 2.5% of a nation's gross domestic product (Ramaciotti

& Perriard, 2001). What these facts have to do with physical activity, exercise, and sports will be explained in the subsequent sections, following the definition of a number of key terms.

27

Knowing where and how much stress-related costs arise is of great social importance. On the one hand, it forms the basis for the design of suitable measures and at the same time creates the basis at the political level for the targeted mobilization of financial resources (e.g., prevention, expansion of health services, and research) (Elfering et al., 2017).

27.2 Key Terms

Semmer and Zapf (2017) present a model of stress, stress management, and consequences of stress, which incorporates the majority of fundamental concepts in this field (Fig. 27.1). Such a model is valuable because, while the term "stress" is frequently used in daily life, in the scientific literature it is found in a variety of contexts, sometimes with differing implications. Semmer and Zapf's (2017) model emphasizes that stress is a product of **stressors**, that is, conditions or situations which provoke stress. The term "stressor" refers to a situation that most people would perceive as stressful, much in the way a virus can be said to be dangerous, even though it does not cause sickness in all those infected (Semmer & Zapf, 2017). Whether a stressor does in fact lead to perceived stress depends on **individual appraisal processes** (e.g., How is this situation a challenge for me? What could go wrong? Am I able to manage the situation?). This is coupled with the availability of **protective resources** (e.g., high levels of self-confidence, the presence of trusted and supportive individuals), or, alternatively, aggravating factors (e.g., **vulnerability factors** such as anxiety, irritability, inexperience with the stressor in question). Generally, stressful situations evoke some sort of **coping behavior**. These behaviors allow an individual to avoid stress, reduce or eliminate perceived stress, and minimize the negative consequences of the stressful experience. Although a number of classifications have been made over the years, most models of coping are two-dimensional and encompass problem-focused and emotion-focused coping. **Problem-focused coping** aims to address the stressor itself via external (e.g., discussion) or internal (e.g., adapting one's goals) processes. **Emotion-focused coping** aims to stabilize the emotions that are provoked by a stressor, for example, by distracting oneself, employing relaxation techniques, or through physical activity, exercise, and sports. The efficiency of the coping behavior has an influence on the extent of the **consequences** of the stressful experience. In other words, more or less efficient coping behaviors can influence the degree to which a stressor prompts negative emotions (e.g., irritation, anger, fear, frustration) or physiological reactions (e.g., heightened blood pressure, cortisol production, release of adrenaline or inflammation markers). Whether stress has a long-term impact also depends on whether periods with a high number of stressors (e.g., exams, conflict with a superior at work) are followed by phases of efficient recovery. If

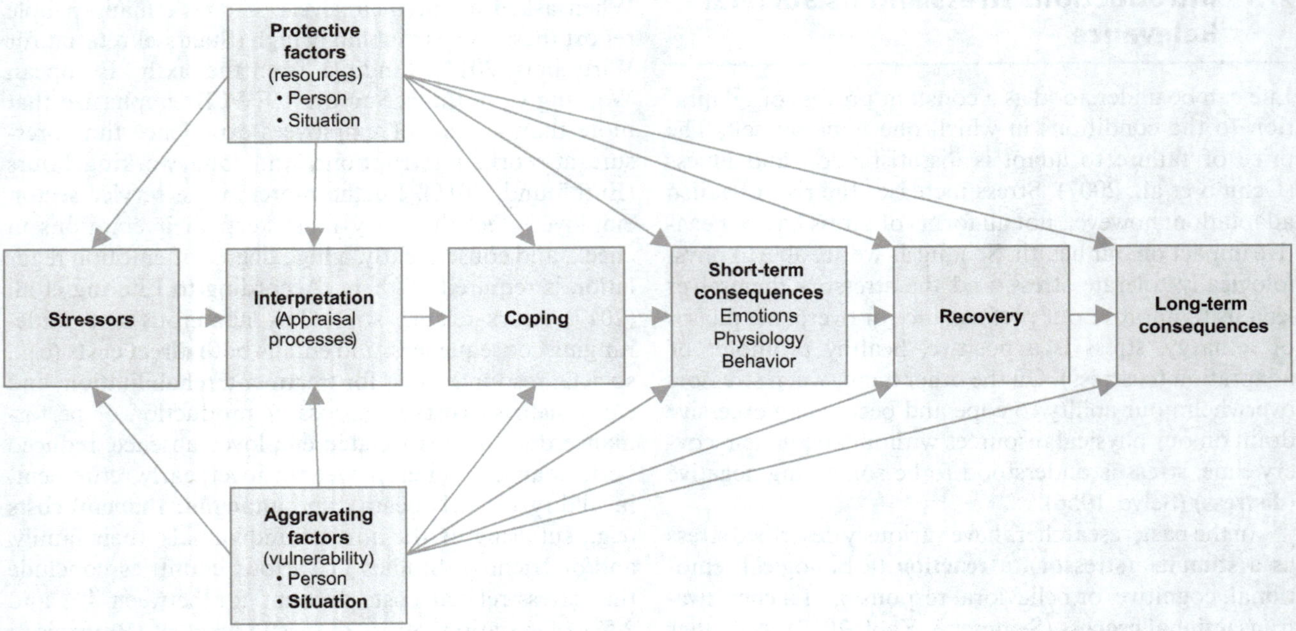

Fig. 27.1 Stress, coping, and the consequences of stress (from Semmer & Zapf, 2017, p. 27)

this is the case, periods of stress can lead to positive adaptations in the longer term, such as increased feelings of self-efficacy, or the development of skills which make future stressors easier to cope with. Maladaptive coping or insufficient recovery, however, can lead to long-term negative consequences, with stress leading to physiological (e.g., disturbed cortisol secretion), morphological (e.g., altered hippocampal volume), and psychological (e.g., distrust, anxiety, exhaustion, feelings of helplessness and hopelessness) changes. Poorer tolerance for stress and a reduced ability to recover are also potential consequences.

Basic Dimensions of Coping

Problem-focused coping aims to address the stressor itself via external (e.g., discussion) or internal (e.g., adapting one's goals) processes.

Emotion-focused coping aims to stabilize the emotions that are provoked by a stressor, for example, by distracting oneself, employing relaxation techniques, or through physical activity, exercise, and sports.

27.3 Stress Models

A number of theoretical approaches to the topic of stress can be found in the scientific literature. A number of these theories include concepts which form part of the model described above. In what follows, the most important stress models are presented.

27.3.1 Reaction-Focused Models

Reaction-focused models take the **reaction of the human body** to unspecified situations as their central point. These models originate in part from the work of French physiologist Claude Bernard, 1974, one of the first researchers to apply a systematic approach to the examination of stress processes (Semmer & Zapf, 2017). He introduced the concept of "dynamic equilibrium," which suggests that any factor which disrupts the equilibrium of the human body should be viewed as negative. His area of research was primarily physiological (e.g., the effects of ambient temperature) and thus still somewhat removed from modern theories integrating psychological stressors. Walter Cannon (1914) further developed Bernard's theory with the concept of "**homeostasis.**" On Cannon's understanding, homeostasis refers to the cohesive totality of reactions which contribute to the maintenance of a stable status quo (steady state) in the human body. Cannon was interested not only in physiological stressors, but also in emotional ones. Accordingly, his suggestion that emotional stress could provoke a fight-or-flight response is still often cited today. Cannon hypothesized that both reactions are determined by the catabolic effects of the sympathetic nervous system, which provides humans with energy in urgent situations.

The Concept of Homeostasis

The concept of homeostasis was originated by Walter Cannon and refers to the cohesive totality of reactions which contribute to the maintenance of a stable status quo (steady state) in the human body.

While Cannon was mainly concerned with the short-term effects of emotional stress, Hans Selye (1956) was interested on the longer-term consequences. His model of a "**general adaptation syndrome**" was based on the observation that animals under chronic stress go through a typical process of behavioral and physiological changes. The first phase (**alarm reaction stage**) primarily involves the sympathetic nervous system. As efforts to manage the stressor increase (**resistance stage**), glucocorticoids (such as cortisol) are released by the hypothalamic-pituitary-adrenal (HPA) axis. Selye believed that extended resistance phases, caused by ineffective coping strategies, would lead to the exhaustion of physiological resources and consequently to impairments in health (**exhaustion stage**).

Cannon's concept of "homeostasis" and Selye's model of a "general adaptation syndrome" form the basis of all modern reaction-focused stress models.

Cannon's and Selye's approaches have been adapted over time, but form the basis of all modern reaction-focused stress models. McEwen and Stellar (1993) have criticized the concept of "homeostasis" for what they see as the unrealistic suggestion that a stable status quo is the natural state of the human body in daily life. They point out that factors such as blood pressure, heart rate, hormone secretion, and neural activity are in fact characterized by their constant variation. McEwen and Wingfield (2003) refer to the human ability to adapt to constantly changing conditions, and if necessary initiate or end specific processes, as "**allostasis.**" This ability is more pronounced in the young and healthy than in the old and unwell. A stress reaction occurs when internal or external influences disrupt the allostasis equilibrium. Long-term effects of chronic stress lead to a higher **allostatic load** or **allostatic overload**. McEwen (2013) further emphasizes that physiological and psychological processes are closely linked and that the regulation of allostatic reactions is controlled by the brain. From a physiological point of view, the sympathetic nervous system, the HPA axis, and the immune system are particularly relevant as **mediators of stress reactivity** and are also responsible for the majority of changes in risk factors for chronic degenerative diseases.

The Concept of Allostasis

The concept of "allostasis" refers to the human ability to adapt to constantly changing conditions and if necessary initiate or end specific processes.

27.3.2 Stimulus-Focused Models

Stimulus-focused models are chiefly concerned with stress-provoking stimuli. In these models, stress is understood as an **external factor** which can lead to an increased allostatic load. External factors which constitute stressors vary widely and include experiences of war, social isolation, imprisonment, or experiencing natural disasters or terrorism. So-called **critical life events**, including problems with family, partners, friends, finances, living conditions, lifestyle, or free-time activities, are also the focus of research in this area. Particularly severe life events include the death of a partner, child, or close family member. Stimulus-oriented models are often employed in conjunction with research on **posttraumatic stress disorder** (Rosenbaum et al., 2017), but are also suited to studies in populations with limited cognitive abilities (e.g., young children), who are not fully able to evaluate the impact of potentially stressful situations. Some researchers focus specifically on regularly occurring everyday problems, so-called **daily hassles**. These include minor arguments, everyday irritations, or pressure situations at school or at work (Gerber et al., 2017a).

27.3.3 Cognitive-Transactional Models

Although reaction- and stimulus-focused models have convincingly shown that stress can lead to increased risk for chronic degenerative diseases and psychiatric disorders, they have not fully explained interindividual differences in the perception of, and reactivity to, stress (Gerber, 2008a, 2008b). For this reason, psychologists have defined stress as a cognitive transaction between internal and external demands, which require a number of **evaluative (appraisal) processes** (Hobfoll, 1998; Lazarus & Folkman, 1984). **Cognitive-transactional stress models** therefore provide an explanation for the fact that the same event (e.g., an exam) is perceived as more or less stressful by different people. These differences are not based solely on the objective relevance of the event (e.g., final exams are generally perceived to be more stressful than midterm exams), but are also determined in large part by internal factors. These include, among others, (a) the subjective relevance of the event, (b) the personal aspirations of the individual (e.g., ambition, tendency to perfectionism), (c) past experiences (e.g., success or failure at exams), (d) stable personality traits (e.g., general anxiety before exams), and (e) the extent of external pressure (e.g., parent's expectations). In stressful situations, it is not only the subjective relevance of the potentially stressful event which is evaluated (**primary appraisal**: What is at stake?). The perception of stressfulness depends more on the evaluation of the resource available for managing the problem (**secondary appraisal**: Do I have the personal and social capacities to deal with this stressor successfully?). Cognitive-transactional theories are based on the premise that every individual has a frame of reference for interpreting stressful situations. This explains why certain people have a higher stress tolerance and are more resilient to stress than others (Luthar et al., 2006; Masten, 2001). Following an individual's attempts to manage stress, the cognitive-transactional approach posits a third appraisal situation (**reappraisal**). During this process, individuals reflect on whether their attempts to reduce the stress they perceive were successful (Lazarus & Folkman, 1984). If the person is unable to find some relief, the problems risk becoming a source of distress, which will have a long-term negative effect on the health and well-being of that person (Gerber & Schilling, 2017).

> Cognitive-transactional stress models explain why the same event can be perceived as more or less stressful by different individuals.

27.3.4 The Reserve-Capacity Model

The reserve-capacity model, presented by Gallo and Matthews (2003), constitutes a framework which explains why illness occurs unequally in populations, disproportionately affecting individuals from lower socioeconomic backgrounds (Marmot, 2003). This model links epidemiological, physiological, and psychological approaches to stress research. According to Semmer and Zapf (2017), this model posits that the ability of an individual to manage a difficult situation depends on their **reserve capacities**. These capacities include material (e.g., financial savings), social (e.g., friendship circles, social support), and personal (e.g., self-efficacy, general knowledge) resources (Kohlmann & Eschenbeck, 2017). Resources contribute to reduced stress perception, and/or improved ability to deal with stressors, in individuals with a high reserve capacity (Siegrist, 2017). The social determinants of stress and stress management are also emphasized by Hobfoll (1989, 1998) in his "**conservation of resources (COR)**" theory. Specifically, he notes that humans generally value the same **resources**, which is why resource-related conflicts can occur between members of a society. The COR theory also suggests that disadvantaged persons are more susceptible to stress, as they typically have fewer resources to manage acute or chronic stress. A lack of resources and/or the fear of losing further resources may also explain why individuals with fewer available resources react defensively or passively in stressful situations. These individuals are chiefly preoccupied with using the resources they have to deal with everyday situations. Without investing resources, however, escaping the threat of a chronic stress-induced downward spiral becomes difficult.

27.3.5 Work-Related Models

The field of occupational psychology has also seen the development of stress models which specifically focus on work-related stress (Semmer & Zapf, 2017; Siegrist, 2017). The most well known of these are the "job demand-control" (JDC) model, the "job demand-reward" (JDR) model, and the "effort-reward imbalance" (ERI) model. In the **JDC model** (Karasek, 1979), a particular job characteristic, in other words, a quantitative challenge (e.g., time pressure), is pitted against the opportunity to make one's own decisions. It is suggested that demanding situations are more likely to have a negative impact when they are combined with low levels of individual control (a combination which is termed "high strain"). The **JDR model** (Bakker & Demerouti, 2007) is an extension of the JDC model. On this new approach, control is seen as only one of many resources (to wit, the sum of all physical, psychological, social, and organizational aspects of work which facilitate the achievement of work-related goals, reduce physical and psychological costs, and promote development and learning). A further distinction is made between motivational and health-related mechanisms. Specifically, it is suggested that employee challenges (e.g., work capacity, time pressure) moderate the relationship between resources and engagement with work. For example, it may be that available resources only positively impact work motivation when the overall burden of stressors is not too high. Resources, conversely, are expected to moderate the relationship between demands and exhaustion. In other words, the likelihood an individual under pressure at work will suffer from exhaustion is increased when their employer provides them with few resources, or when they receive little support from colleagues. While the models presented above focus on demands and resources, the **ERI model** (Siegrist et al., 2004) takes a different approach. This model is concerned not only with job characteristics, but also with contractual relationships in the workplace, in terms of the exchange between effort and reward. In cases where this transaction is perceived to be out of balance, for instance, when high engagement is met with little reward (e.g., salary, promotion opportunities, job security, recognition, and performance valuation), stress is assumed to be the result.

27.4 Physiological Stress Reactions

Stress provokes a number of physiological reactions in the human body. In this section, the most important of these reactions and processes will be described. Particular attention is paid to changes in the central nervous system, the hormonal system, and the immune system. A more detailed description of these mechanisms can be found in the works of von Dawans and Heinrichs (2017), Ehrlenspiel and Strahler (2012), or Gerber (2017).

According to von Dawans and Heinrichs (2017), the central nervous system is the chief control center responsible for managing the response to various stressors. Information from the peripheral nervous system (so-called afferent information) is sent to the central nervous system (CNS) and is processed, so that an appropriate stress reaction is initiated. Of particular relevance in this process are the amygdala, the hippocampus, and the prefrontal cortex, parts of the limbic system which are responsible for emotion processing. The **amygdala** is responsible for the activation of central stress axes, while the **prefrontal cortex** can have an activating or a suppressing role. The **hippocampus** is involved in the negative feedback loop of the HPA axis (see below) and works to suppress excessive or long-lasting stress reactions.

Physiological stress reactions are chiefly regulated by two axes: the **sympathetic-adrenomedullary system (SAM)** and the HPA axis (◘ Fig. 27.2). The SAM is a part of the **autonomic nervous system (ANS)** and is responsible for fast-response stress reactions. It prepares the body for a **fight-or-flight response** within seconds. The ANS comprises the sympathetic, parasympathetic, and intestinal nervous systems and regulates homeostasis in the human body and other essential functions (e.g., respiration, digestion, circulation). The human capacity to consciously influence the ANS is extremely limited, although possible via biofeedback loops (Rief & Bernius, 2011). The sympathetic and parasympathetic systems have an antagonistic relationship, with the **parasympathetic system** chiefly dominant at rest and the **sympathetic system** taking over under conditions of stress. The SAM is responsible for transmitting stress signals directly to the organs via central nervous activation of the sympathetic system and provoking the release of catecholamines (adrenaline, noradrenaline) via the activation of the adrenal medulla. This leads to a state of alarm in the body and is accompanied by rapid adaptations to heart rate and respiration frequency, the

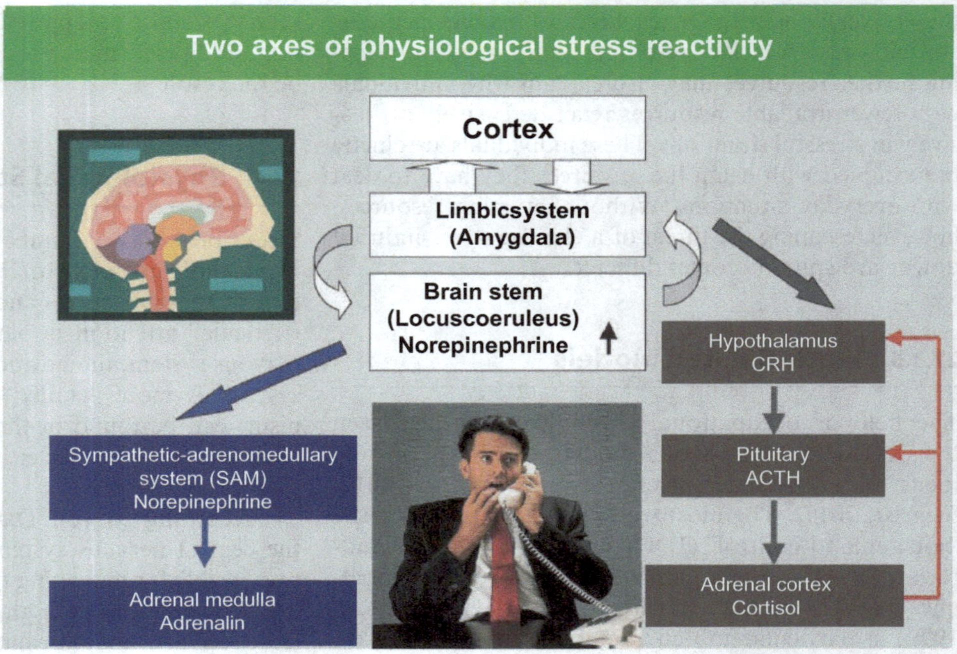

Fig. 27.2 Simplified overview of the two axes of physiological stress reactions (adapted from Kaluza, 2004)

mobilization of energy reserves, and increased blood flow to large muscle groups. Less important processes (e.g., digestion, sexual function) are suppressed. The reduced influence of the parasympathetic system (also known as the "vagal brake") reduces heart rate variability, which can lead to negative consequences in cases of chronic stress.

In comparison with the SAM, the **HPA axis** reacts relatively slowly, as its signals are transmitted via the blood (via the stress hormone cortisol) and not electrochemical signaling. The effects of **cortisol** are mediated by mineral corticoids and glucocorticoid receptors, and its effects first become apparent within minutes. As the term HPA axis suggests, the stress signal begins in the hypothalamus, where **corticotropin-releasing hormone (CRH)** is secreted. The CRH, in turn, is responsible for the secretion of **adrenocorticotropic hormone (ACTH)** in the pituitary, which reaches the adrenal glands via the bloodstream. The adrenal glands release cortisol. Cortisol, due to its fat solubility, can cross the blood-brain barrier. In the brain, it binds to receptors in the hippocampus and via a negative feedback loop can suppress the activity of the HPA axis (which combats an excessive stress response). Cortisol production is regulated not only by stress, but also by ultradian and circadian rhythms, with cortisol levels increasing rapidly upon morning awakening **(the cortisol awakening response [CAR])** and reducing throughout the day after reaching their peak (with a low point around midnight). Chronic dysregulation of the HPA axis (and consequent hyper- or hypocortisolism) can have far-reaching health consequences, as nearly all organs in the human body contain cortisol receptors.

> Chronic dysregulation of the HPA axis (and consequent hyper- or hypocortisolism) can have far-reaching health consequences, as nearly all organs in the human body contain cortisol receptors.

Aside from the two main stress axes described here, the **immune system** is also increasingly being viewed as having an important function in stress reactivity (Cacioppo et al., 1998; Segerstrom & Miller, 2004). von Dawans and Heinrichs (2017) point out that the nervous, hormonal, and immune systems are closely linked and that cortisol and other catecholamines influence immune functioning. In simple terms, acute stress leads to an activation of the immune system, while in the longer term, stress has an immunosuppressive effect. Conversely, proinflammatory cytokines, in other words proteins which cause inflammation, can also influence the stress response via the hypothalamus, the sympathetic nervous system, the pituitary, and the adrenal glands. This prevents an overactive immune response by means of a negative feedback loop.

27.5 Stress-Related Health Consequences

Stress can lead to severe impairments in health. A model of the process of stress-induced illness is depicted in Fig. 27.3.

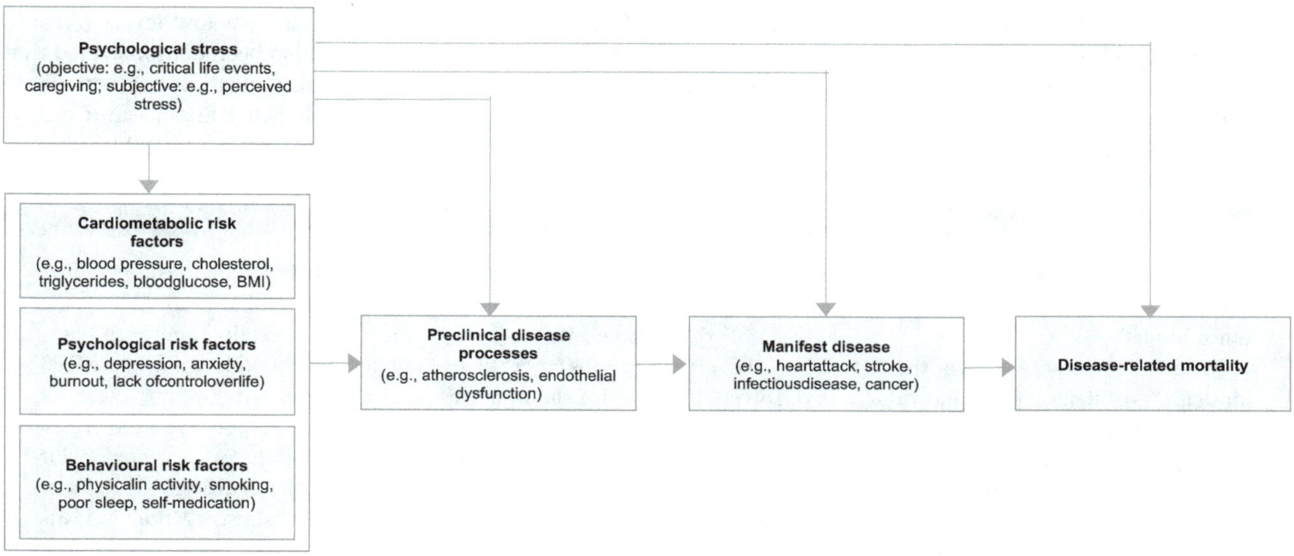

Fig. 27.3 Model of stress-induced illness

27.5.1 Stress and Mortality

In the meantime, several studies are available in which a significant connection between stress levels and an increased risk of premature death could be demonstrated (overview: Gerber & Schilling, 2017). In a meta-analysis of prospective studies in which stress levels were measured using the "12-Item General Health Questionnaire" (GHQ-12), Russ et al. (2012) found that people with high stress levels had almost twice as high a mortality risk as the unexposed reference group (hazard ratio = 1.94; 95% confidence interval: 1.66–2.26). It was also confirmed that the effects of stress on mortality are mediated by lifestyle factors such as smoking, type 2 diabetes, and cardiovascular diseases (Rutters et al., 2014). It is also known that high maternal stress is associated with increased infant mortality and an increased risk of congenital malformations (Class et al., 2013; Hansen et al., 2000).

Chronic stress is associated with a twofold increased risk of premature death.

27.5.2 Stress and Physical Health

To date, several studies have established a relationship between stress exposure and a heightened risk of premature death. The majority of these studies **address cardiovascular disease**. In their review, Gerber and Schilling (2017) show that there is also a wide range of empirical research regarding other forms of disease (e.g., metabolic syndrome, overweight and obesity, cancer, infectious disease, gastrointestinal disease, asthma, and headaches). Due to limitations of space, this article will focus solely on cardiovascular health (Uchino et al., 2007).

Meta-analytical findings from a study on work-related stress indicate that stressed individuals have a 40% higher chance of suffering from cardiovascular disease in the future (Kivimäki et al., 2006). Similar findings have been reported for stress induced by critical life events (Rozanski et al., 2005). Further studies suggest that even stress experiences during childhood can negatively impact heart health (Wegman & Stetler, 2009).

In particular, there are significant associations between stress and **coronary heart disease**, that is, disease of the blood vessels of the heart, usually caused by arteriosclerosis (Hemingway & Marmot, 1999). High levels of stress are associated with a risk of heart attack equal to that of other established risk factors, such as smoking, diabetes, or family history (Yusuf et al., 2004). Studies have also shown that the risk of heart attack is two and a half times higher during times of acute stress, in comparison to stress-free periods (Steptoe & Kivimäki, 2013). Furthermore, stress increases the risk of cardiac arrhythmia, a frequent cause of sudden cardiac death (Lampert et al., 2002).

There is also a wealth of data regarding the stress-related risk of **stroke**, including a meta-analysis indicating that individuals under higher levels of stress have a 33% higher risk (Booth et al., 2015). Here too, stress is understood to be a risk factor as relevant as high blood pressure, smoking, overweight, or excessive drinking (O'Donnell et al., 2010). Overall, research suggests that the increased cardiovascular disease risk of stressed individuals is attributable to, among other factors, higher stress reactivity and/or glucocorticoid resistance (▶ Side

Story: Excerpt: "Reactivity Hypothesis Model" vs. "Glucocorticoid Resistance Model").

Regarding **patients already suffering from cardiovascular disease**, studies have shown that mortality is significantly higher among those with medium or high stress levels, in comparison to those with low levels (Arnold et al., 2012). It has, however, also been demonstrated that stress management and health education can contribute to a 30% reduction in repeat heart attacks and a 35% reduction in mortality (Dusseldorp et al., 1999).

Side Story

Excerpt: "Reactivity Hypothesis Model" Vs. "Glucocorticoid Resistance Model"

The "**Reactivity Hypothesis Model**" postulates that individuals who show a high cardiovascular response to stress (e.g., a sharp increase in blood pressure) are more at risk for cardiovascular diseases (Krantz & Manuck, 1984). This model is generally supported by the current literature (Matthews et al., 2004; Treiber et al., 2003). The model also proposes that, besides stress reactivity, stress exposure plays an important role. Accordingly, it has been shown that individuals exposed to high levels of stress at work, who also have a high stress reactivity, are particularly at risk of developing arteriosclerosis of the arteria carotis over time (Everson et al., 1997). Furthermore, a meta-analysis has shown that not only stress reactivity, but also recovery from stress, must be considered. Schuler and O'Brien (1997) have shown that slow recovery from stress is associated with a higher risk of high blood pressure.

Alternatively, the link between stress and cardiovascular disease can be attributed to altered immune functioning. Although it is believed that numerous stress-induced diseases (e.g., cancer, infectious diseases) can be attributed to immunosuppression, according to Miller et al. (2002), the "immunosuppression approach" cannot adequately explain illnesses which are characterized by an excessive inflammation response (e.g., allergies, rheumatological or cardiovascular disease). Miller et al.'s (2002) "**Glucocorticoid Resistance Model**" posits that chronic stress limits the sensitivity of the immune system to glucocorticoid hormones. In other words, stress leads to a disruption of the negative feedback loop which usually protects against an excessive immune response (von Dawans & Heinrichs, 2017).

27.5.3 Stress and Psychological Health

Deficits in psychological well-being are often closely linked to stress, and it is generally accepted that unpredictable and uncontrollable stress levels have a particularly negative effect on mental health (Kessing et al., 2003). This can be illustrated with the example of stress and **depressive disorders**. According to Paykel (2001), first-time depressive episodes can often be attributed to critical life events. In a systematic review of 12 studies, Siegrist (2008) showed that individuals with high levels of work-related stress had an 80% higher risk of having developed a depressive disorder at follow-up (► Side Story: Excerpt: The Association Between Stress and Depressive Disorders).

Side Story

Excerpt: The Association Between Stress and Depressive Disorders

Researchers have identified a **dysregulation of the HPA axis** as a key mechanism explaining the link between stress and depression: in line with this, individuals with depressive disorders have higher baseline cortisol concentrations, altered circadian cortisol secretion, and higher cortisol levels following phases of acute stress (Ising et al., 2007; Stetler & Miller, 2011). In addition, psychological mechanisms may also play a role. Repeated stressful experiences and depressive episodes can lead to progressive **changes in information processing**, resulting in a reduction in the stress tolerance threshold in affected individuals (Segal et al., 1996). In particular, it is believed that individuals with depression develop **negative expectation patterns** (or networks), which become stronger over time. As these networks are strengthened, even relatively mild stressors can provoke a large reaction (Monroe & Harkness, 2005). It is also possible that **personality changes**, or poorly adapted **emotion regulation**, can lead to reduced stress tolerance (Moriya & Takahashi, 2013). **Sleep disorders** may represent a further link between stress and depressive disorders (Brand, 2017). Studies show that there is a relatively strong association between high stress and poor sleep (Morin et al., 2003). High correlations also exist between depressive disorders and sleep complaints (Taylor, 2008). Insufficient sleep is also associated with reduced immune functioning, which can increase the risk of illness when under stress (Hall et al., 1998).

27.6 Stress Regulation and Sports

The topic of stress regulation and sports can be viewed from two differing perspectives (Gerber & Fuchs, 2017). From the point of view of sports as a health-promoting activity, the focus is on sports as a means to stress regulation ("**stress regulation *through* sports**"). The central question is the degree to which sports and physical activity can help us to cope with daily challenges (such as at work, or with family), so that negative health effects of these stressors can be avoided or reduced. From the point of view of performance sports, on the other hand, the central focus is "**stress regulation *during* sports**." In other words, how can athletes cope with high levels of training and psychological pressure, without suffering a drop in physical performance or psychological complaints? Important factors are those which allow top-level and elite athletes to perform at the highest level under pressure.

These perspectives are linked to differing research traditions (Gerber & Fuchs, 2017). While the disciplines of health psychology, sports medicine, and biopsychological stress research are primarily concerned with the perspective of "stress regulation through sports," "stress regulation during sports" is closely linked to "classic" sports psychology. Key research subjects in this domain are the management of performance pressure and competition anxiety. Both these perspectives will be addressed in more detail below.

> The topic of stress regulation and sports can be viewed from two differing perspectives. From the point of view of sports as a health-promoting activity, the focus is on sports as a means to stress regulation ("**stress regulation *through* sports**"); from the point of view of performance sports, on the other hand, the central focus is "**stress regulation *during* sports**."

27.7 Stress Regulation Through Sports

In the past two decades, several models have been developed to summarize the stress-regulating effects of exercise and sports. Fuchs and Klaperski (2017) make a rough distinction between stress occurrence and coping with stress. During stress occurrence, a further distinction can be made between the **stressor-reducing** and **resource-strengthening effects** of physical activity, exercise, and sports (Fig. 27.4). When stress occurs, a **reactivity-reducing effect** on the coping level is also posited, which can be further subdivided into cognitive, affective, behavioral, and biological effects. In this context, **palliative-regenerative coping** is also discussed. The term "palliative" refers to the potential for physical activity, exercise, and sports to prevent unnecessarily intense or long stress reactions. "Regenerative" refers to the potential of physical activity, exercise, and sports to help stressed individuals quickly return to a stable base-

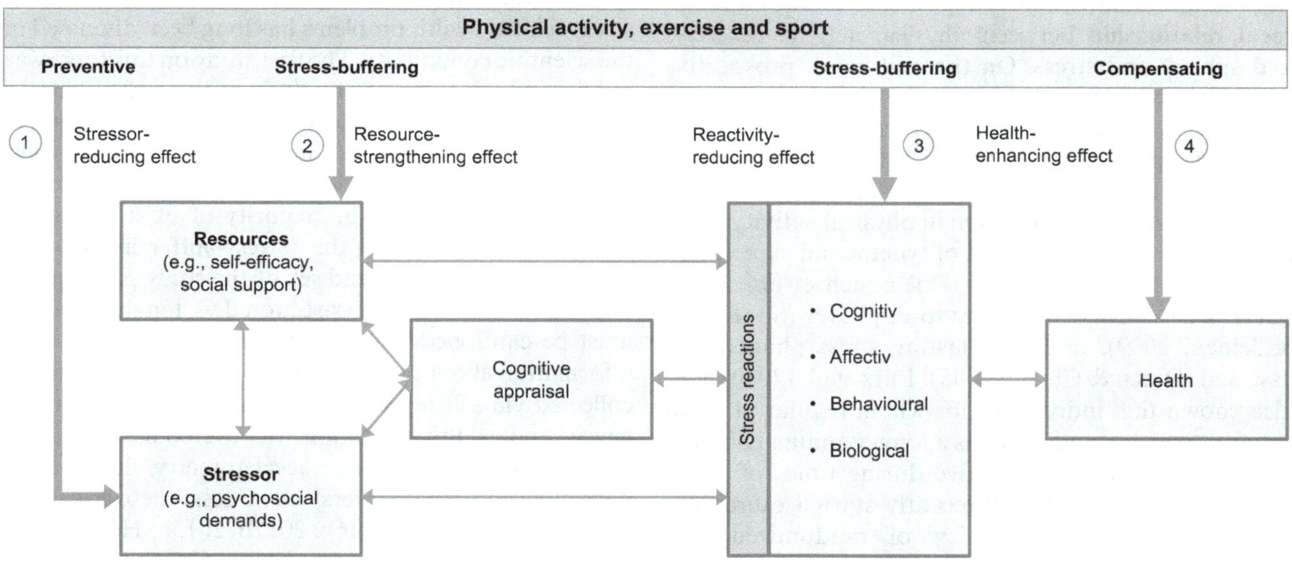

Fig. 27.4 Stress-regulating mechanisms of physical activity

line state following a reaction to stress. All these mechanisms underpin the "**stress-buffering effects**" of physical activity, exercise, and sports. In other words, they offer potential explanations for the fact that individuals with physically active lifestyles suffer fewer negative health consequences during periods of high stress (Gerber & Pühse, 2009; Klaperski, 2017). In addition, a more general health-promoting effect is integrated in the model. This is intended to emphasize that regular participation in physical activity, exercise, and sports is beneficial for health, regardless of the amount of a stress a person is experiencing.

27.7.1 Are Physically Active People Less Stressed, or Does Stress Lead to Reduced Physical Activity?

Several empirical studies address the link between physical activity (exercise and sports) and stress (Klaperski, 2017; Stults-Kolehmainen & Sinha, 2014). While the majority of cross-sectional studies suggest that high levels of physical activity, exercise, or sports are associated with lower perceived stress (e.g., Aldana et al., 1996; Lovell et al., 2015), these findings do not shed light on potential causal mechanisms. In other words, it is not clear whether these associations indicate that participation in physical activity, exercise, and sports reduces stress, or whether individuals under high levels of stress tend not to engage in such activities. Longitudinal studies suggest that there is a **reciprocal relationship** between physical activity (exercise and sports) and stress. On the one hand, prospective studies show that baseline measures of physical activity, exercise, and sports predict levels of perceived stress at follow-up (Jonsdottir et al., 2010; Schnohr et al., 2005). On the other hand, several studies have shown that stress leads to a reduction in physical activity, exercise, and sports, independent of whether an experimental approach was employed (Roemmich et al., 2003), stress was assessed on a day-to-day level (Sonnentag & Jelden, 2009), or longer-lasting stress phases were assessed (Oaten & Cheng, 2005). Lutz et al. (2010) have also shown that individuals for whom regular physical activity, exercise, and sports is a long-standing habit are more easily able to stay active during times of stress than those who have only recently started exercising. Finally, in a literature review of randomized controlled trials, Klaperski (2017) reported that 6 out of 11 trials showed a stress-reducing intervention effect on perceived stress (see ▸ Study Box: The Influence of Stress on People's Physical Activity Behavior: A Meta-Analysis).

Study Box: The Influence of Stress on People's Physical Activity Behavior: A Meta-Analysis

In order to determine the effects of work-related stress on physical activity behavior, Fransson et al. (2012) combined data from 14 European cohort studies. Baseline data for 170,162 people was available. Of these, 56,735 were followed up for a period of between 2 and 9 years. Results from the cross-sectional data indicate that individuals who are stressed at work are 26% more likely to be physically inactive, compared to individuals without high levels of work-related stress. The prospective analyses show similar results, with stressed individuals having a 21% increased risk of becoming physically inactive at follow-up.

27.7.2 Can Physical Activity in Times of Stress Protect Against Negative Health Consequences?

The question of whether physical activity, exercise, and sports have the potential to protect individuals from stress-related health problems has long been discussed in the scientific community. The first study on this topic was published by Kobasa et al. (1982) in the early 1980s. In the following years, many original studies have emerged, which will not be addressed in more detail here. In their review of the literature, Gerber and Pühse (2009) came to the conclusion that the majority of existing studies (at least partly) support the "**stress-buffer hypothesis**," independent of the age and sex of the study participants and the study design (cross-sectional vs. longitudinal). It must be cautioned that in many of the earlier studies, information about physical activity levels and health was collected via self-report from the study participants. In newer studies, this limitation was overcome by the use of objective measures (e.g., accelerometry, fitness tests, physiological risk markers) to assess these variables (Gerber et al., 2016a, 2016b, 2017b, 2013b; Holtermann et al., 2010; Puterman et al., 2010). One of these studies is described in more detail in the following study box (▶ Study Box: Fitness-Related Stress-Buffer Effects). Similarly, one newer study adopted a person-centered approach, in order to determine whether statistical analyses are capable of identifying stress-resilient individuals (that is, individuals who show no physiological symptoms despite being exposed to high levels of stress). The results indicated that, under high levels of stress, resilient individuals report, on average, more sports and physical activity than individuals with numerous symptoms (Gerber et al., 2014b). Recently, a number of interventional studies have been carried out. O'Dougherty et al. (2012) implemented a 16-week aerobic exercise program with 303 American women and reported that, in the endurance exercise group, the influence of critical life events on the development of depressive symptoms could be buffered, which was not the case in the control group. Klaperski et al. (2014) found a similar pattern of results in a study of 149 male participants, although they examined perceived stress in general, rather than critical life events. For further literature on the triangular relationship between (a) stress, (b) physical activity, exercise and sports, and (c) specific health indicators such as overweight/obesity, sleep, cognitive function, and cardiovascular health, see Holmes (2017), Ludyga (2017), Brand (2017), and Deiseroth and Hanssen (2017) (▶ Side Story: Excerpt: Explanation of Stress-Buffering Effects).

Study Box: Fitness-Related Stress Buffer Effects

In order to determine whether a high level of fitness can "buffer" the effects of stress which are detrimental to health, researchers in Switzerland and Sweden carried out a study with approximately 200 health workers (Gerber et al., 2016a). Their fitness levels were objectively assessed with a submaximal fitness test (the Åstrand bicycle test). The participants were divided into three groups categorized as unfit, moderately fit, or highly fit, based on age and sex-specific norm values. Stress levels were assessed with a questionnaire. Based on this, two groups were created (high vs. low stress). In addition, psychological well-being (symptoms of depression, burnout) and risk factors for cardiovascular disease (high blood pressure, BMI, blood lipid values, blood sugar) were measured. The results of the study showed that, among those experiencing low stress levels, there were only minimal differences in health markers between the three fitness groups. However, individuals with high levels of stress and low fitness suffered from more health impairments than their moderately and highly fit counterparts. The findings for depressive symptoms and low-density lipoprotein (LDL) cholesterol are illustrated below as examples of this difference. For LDL cholesterol, a value of ≥3.0 mmol/L is considered to be the clinical cutoff which, according to European guidelines (De Backer et al., 2003), should not be exceeded (◘ Fig. 27.5).

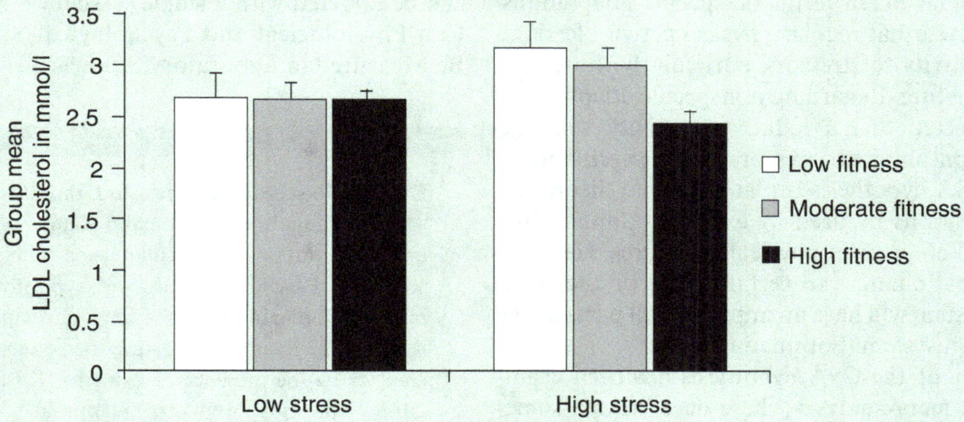

◘ **Fig. 27.5** Differences in LDL cholesterol concentration between individuals with low vs. high stress levels and low, moderate, and high fitness

27

Side Story

Excerpt: Explanation of Stress-Buffering Effects

Stress-buffering effects can be attributed to a stress-reducing, resource-strengthening, or reactivity-reducing mechanism (Fig. 27.4). The first of these is at play when exercise or sports participation contributes to the fact that particular stressors do not even occur (e.g., avoidance of chronic disease or social isolation). The second mechanism is applicable when exercise and sports help us to develop particular resources which impact positively on the stress management process (e.g., the development of mental toughness, the availability of social support systems in times of need; for an overview of the current state of research on this topic, see Fuchs & Klaperski, 2017). The reactivity-reducing mechanism is responsible for physiological, psychological, or behavioral stress reactions being perceived as less severe (receded reactivity), or a quicker return to baseline levels following a stressful episode (improved recovery).

On a physiological level, reduced stress reactivity in active or fit individuals can be explained by the so-called **cross-stressor adaptation hypothesis** (CSA hypothesis). This posits that (a) the physiological reaction to physical, cognitive, and psychosocial stressors leads to an equal activation of the SAM system and HPA axis, and (b) repeated exposure to sufficiently long and intense stressors leads to specific and nonspecific adaptations of the human organism. In terms of specific adaptations, it can be expected that regular physical activity leads to a reduced reactivity to stressors, particularly those of a physiological nature. Regarding nonspecific adaptations, it can be expected that a reduced reactivity will also accompany non-physical stressors (e.g., psychological stress). The CSA hypothesis is plausible on a theoretical level, as adaptations induced by exercise training often lead to general changes in physical structures. Hence, it is suggested that changes to certain parts of the stress modulation system will have an impact on all parts of the stress regulation system (Sothmann, 2006).

The validity of the CSA hypothesis has been examined in several **meta-analyses**; these have yielded somewhat conflicting results (Crews & Landers, 1987; Forcier et al., 2006). While support was found for the CSA hypothesis with regards to cardiovascular markers specifically, evidence for its soundness disappears upon the inclusion of other reactivity indicators (Jackson & Dishman, 2006) (▶ Reflection: How Can Physiological and Psychological Stress Reactions Be Measured in Laboratory Studies?). Jackson and Dishman (2006) conclude that fit individuals do not show reduced reactivity to experimental stressors, when compared to that of an unfit control group. However, they do observe that fitter individuals appear to recover from stress more quickly. It must be noted that this analysis was mainly limited to studies which exposed participants to cognitive stressors. By contrast, more recent studies, which employ psychosocial stressors (▶ Side Story: Excerpt: Psychosocial Stress in Laboratory Studies), indicate that fit individuals display reduced reactivity to stress, particularly with regards to the activity of the HPA axis (Mücke et al., 2018). These studies also emphasize that the stress-relieving effects of regular physical activity, exercise, and sports participation, or high fitness levels, depend on further factors. In a laboratory study by Gerber et al. (2017c), it was found that the protective effects identified in the laboratory, and linked to physical activity, were particularly high for individuals with high levels of stress. Similarly, Puterman et al. (2011) report that physical activity shows a particular association with lower stress reactivity when individuals have a tendency to spend a long time ruminating on problems. To date, the only **intervention study** with healthy individuals to be carried out addressing this topic suggests that reactivity to experimentally induced stress is reduced after several weeks of endurance training (Klaperski et al., 2014). However, no such effect was found among patients suffering from major depressive disorders (Gerber et al., 2020). Strong empirical evidence also shows that stress reactivity to laboratory stressors is reduced when physical exercise is undertaken immediately prior (Hamer et al., 2006). This finding is important, as it shows that the stress-reducing effects of physical activity do not only appear after weeks of training, but can be targeted with a **single session** (▶ Methods: How Can Physiological and Psychological Stress Reactions Be Measured in Laboratory Studies?).

Side Story

Excerpt: Psychosocial Stress in Laboratory Studies

According to Dickerson and Kemeny (2004), socio-evaluative stress in particular leads to higher cortisol secretion. Psychosocial stress is typically induced in laboratory conditions by asking participants to give a speech or interact with study personnel or an audience, or by the presence of cameras (Kasten & Fuchs, 2017). The most well-known approach is the "**Trier Social Stress Test**" (TSST: Kirschbaum et al., 1993), during which a 5-min-long job interview is staged. This is followed by 5 min of mental arithmetic tasks. There is now a TSST designed specifically for children (TSST-C: Buske-Kirschbaum et al., 1997) and one for groups (TSST-G: von Dawans et al., 2011). In light of the fact that carrying out a TSST is a relatively elaborate procedure, more simple approaches, such as the "**Sing-a-Song Test**," have been created (Brouwer & Hogervorst, 2014).

Methods: How Can Physiological and Psychological Stress Reactions Be Measured in Laboratory Studies?

Numerous assessment paradigms can be employed (Kasten & Fuchs, 2017). Cardiovascular indicators (e.g., **heart rate, blood pressure, electrodermal activity**) are often used to measure physiological stress reactivity. SAM activity can be measured via the proxies of heart **rate variability, catecholamines**, or **alpha-amylase**, while activity of the HPA axis is often assessed via **salivary cortisol** measures. Psychological stress can be assessed using cognitive and emotion-based parameters. At the cognitive level, for example, **memory** can be tested (de Quervain et al., 2000), while at the emotional level, questionnaires can be used to assess typical stress emotions such as **anxiety** (Laux et al., 1981) or **anger** (Schwenkmezger et al., 1992). Lists of adjectives can also be employed to assess **current mood** (McNair et al., 1971; Watson et al., 1988).

Practical Implications for Physical Activity, Exercise, and Sports

The stress-reducing effects of a single bout of sports or exercise lasts for approximately 4 h, although it must be noted that the bout itself must last 30 min and be of at least moderate intensity (approximately 50% of VO_2 max). This implies that, ideally, the stress-reducing effects of physical activity, exercise, and sports should be targeted by short, regular activity bouts, rather than a single, long training session and that timing plays an important role. Stressed individuals may want to consider at what point during the day or week they experience most stress and plan their physical activity accordingly, so that they benefit from the "stress-buffer effect" to the greatest degree.

From a methodological point of view, it is worth considering the degree to which **laboratory stressors** can be compared with stressful experiences in real life (Kasten & Fuchs, 2017). Laboratory studies, thanks to their controlled conditions (e.g., the potential to standardize all procedures, experimental manipulation, and randomization), provide a high degree of **internal validity**. However, doubts have been raised about the **ecological validity** of the data, as stress in the laboratory and in daily life are not directly comparable (e.g., due to a lack of subjective relevance or short-term nature of the stressors). Recently, the "**ecological momentary assessment**" (EMA) has emerged as a method of assessing intense and chronic stressors outside of the laboratory, in everyday settings (Beal & Weiss, 2003; Reichert et al., 2020). EMA is usually carried out using smartphones and involves repeatedly answering a number of self-report questions. In addition, continuous assessment of physiological parameters may be carried out using mobile devices (e.g., electrocardiograms, accelerometers). Generally, researchers must specify in advance if data are to be gathered at fixed time points (in other words, the delays between measurements remain constant), or whether this is event-dependent (that is, the measurement begins when a particular event, such as a stressor, occurs). This approach has the advantage that, compared to retrospective stress questionnaires (e.g., Kasten & Fuchs, 2017). However, the analysis of EMA data is fairly complicated, as individual characteristics are measured at several time points, and the "nested" nature of the data means that multilevel modelling must be employed. These approaches have, to date, rarely been used in the context of exercise and sports. In two studies, using ambulatory assessment, researchers examined the effects of a 20-week aerobic training program on **real-life stress reactivity** in inactive university students (von Haaren et al., 2015, 2016). The end-of-semester examination period was chosen as the real-life stressor; the primary outcome was heart rate variability over 2 days. The results indicated that, compared to that of the control group, individuals in the training group improved their cardiorespiratory fitness by 10%. Furthermore, after controlling for relevant covariates, it emerged that fitter students had higher heart rate variability, and lower emotional stress reactivity, during the exam phase (◘ Fig. 27.6). Most recently, in an EMA study with Swiss police officers, Schilling et al. (2020) found lowered physiological stress reactivity to acute work stress in officers with higher levels of cardiovascular fitness.

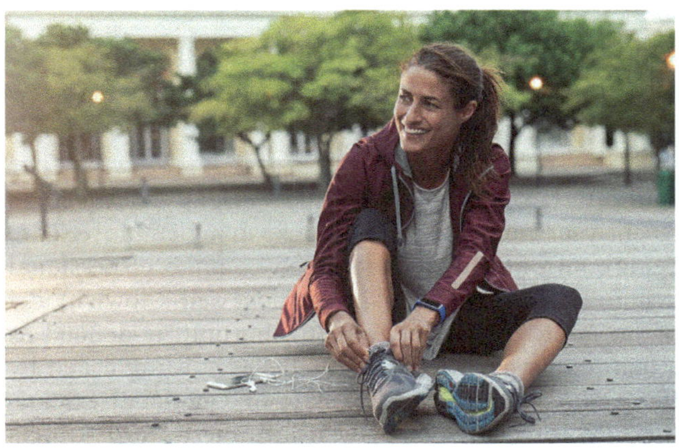

◘ **Fig. 27.6** Physical activity, exercise, and sports serve as a stress-buffers due to various modes of action, e.g., by positively influencing appraisal processes or by reducing physiological stress reactions

Practical Implications for Physical Activity, Exercise, and Sports

An important question for sports and exercise scientists is whether **particular types of physical activity, exercise, and sports** have higher stress-reducing effects than others (Gerber et al., 2014a). There is no general answer to this question. This is due to the fact that the stress-buffering effects of physical and sporting activities are influenced by a number of mechanisms. Fuchs and Klaperski (2017) come to the following conclusion: When a stressor, such as **social isolation**, needs to be reduced, then activities which naturally bring people together, such as team sports or a running group, should be prioritized. If physical activity, exercise, and sports are being used as means to improve **self-efficacy**, then activities which provide a lasting sense of achievement (such as completing a half-marathon) should be considered. If the aim is to have a **mental "time-out"** (a reduction of cognitive activity), then jogging by oneself may not be ideal (it is likely that the individual will be aware of all the thoughts going through their mind and hence not be able to "switch off"); activities which prevent one from dwelling on problems and require full attention (such as games) would be better. As different types of physical activity, exercise, and sports work via different mechanisms, developing standardized physical activity, exercise, or sports programs to improve stress management can be challenging. In other words, such programs are not **personalized**. Consequently, it is the task of exercise and sports therapists and coaches to develop individualized programs which have a high degree of **ecological congruence** (Hobfoll, 1998). This ensures that, by taking into consideration the personal and social circumstances of the individual, the exercise program is as effective as possible.

27.7.3 Can Physical Activity, Exercise, and Sports Prevent and Treat Burnout?

Burnout has gained increasing societal relevance in recent years, in large part because many employees are being confronted with increasingly complex professional demands (Burisch, 2006). In the most well-known model of burnout, by Maslach (1976), burnout is defined as a **multidimensional construct** which is distinguished by three core symptoms: (a) a state of **emotional exhaustion**, (b) a negative or cynical attitude towards others (also known as "**depersonalization**"), and (c) doubt of one's professional capabilities and a subjectively perceived **reduction in performance** at work.

Treatment methods for burnout can be divided into those employed in cases of acute/chronic burnout and those used to prevent burnout. In a review of the literature, Awa et al. (2010) report that in two-thirds of cases, individualized **preventive approaches** are employed, which encompass cognitive behavioral therapy, psychotherapy, adaptive skills training, communication skills training, social support, and relaxation techniques. Workplace-focused approaches (e.g., the restructuring of work processes, performance evaluation, changes in shift work) are employed relatively rarely in comparison. The review reports that in 84% of cases, positive results were achieved, with a combination of individual- and workplace-focused approaches yielding the best results.

The severity of burnout symptoms is important when considering treatment approaches. For mild cases, measures such as changes in lifestyle habits and an improved work-life balance can be prioritized. If symptoms are more severe, psychotherapeutic interventions or drug treatment with antidepressants may be required (Nil et al., 2010).

> For mild cases of burnout, measures such as changes in lifestyle habits and an improved work-life balance can be prioritized. If symptoms are more severe, psychotherapeutic interventions or drug treatment may be required. Physical activity can also have a positive effect.

Studies on the **potential of physical activity, exercise, and sports to prevent and treat burnout** have recently been summarized in a systematic review (Wunsch & Gerber, 2017). A key finding is that a physically active lifestyle is associated with reduced symptoms of burnout in cross-sectional studies. Evidence from longitudinal and intervention studies also now indicates that regular physical activity reduces the risk of burnout in the future (Bretland & Thorsteinsson, 2015; Tsai et al., 2013). Gerber et al. (2013a) demonstrated that 12 weeks of endurance training had a positive effect on symptom severity in a sample of 12 men with high burnout levels. These findings are, however, limited by the fact that no control group was included in the study. Lindegård et al. (2015) reported that treatment effects were longer lasting among formerly inactive burnout patients who became physically active following multimodal therapy. It made no difference whether participants were active only once per week, or more frequently. Even a small increase in activity levels appears to improve the longer-term effects of multimodal treatment.

27.7.4 Can Sports Play a Role in the Treatment of Posttraumatic Stress Disorder?

Posttraumatic stress disorder can emerge as a consequence of exposure to a potentially traumatic experience such as war, torture, physical violence, sexual abuse, or natural disaster. The lifetime prevalence of posttraumatic stress disorder is estimated by researchers to be approximately 7% (Kessler et al., 2005). Posttraumatic stress disorder is associated with a significantly elevated mortality rate (Pietrzak et al., 2011), particularly due to the increased risk for cardiovascular and metabolic disease (Pacella et al., 2013). A further reason for the lower life expectancy is an increase in unhealthy behaviors, including physical inactivity (Zen et al., 2012). To date, little is known about the potential of **physical activity as a treatment method** for posttraumatic stress disorder. According to Rosenbaum et al. (2017), only two randomized controlled trials have tested the effects of a guided sports program as an addition to usual treatment modalities (Powers et al., 2015; Rosenbaum et al., 2015). In both studies, the authors concluded that sports therapy results in improved physical and psychological well-being in this population, particularly when traditional treatment approaches are not attractive to those affected.

27.8 Stress Regulation in Performance Sports

Stress is also a central theme in performance sports. Athletic performance in high-level sports is carried out under **conditions of pressure**; often, there is a lot on the line, not only for the athletes, but also for spectators (Ehrlenspiel et al., 2017). According to Beckmann and Ehrlenspiel (2017), a key question for sports psychologists is how athletes deal with stressful situations and how stress can influence high-performance sports. Sports psychology research has paid particular attention to the issue of **anxiety during competitions**. The triad of physiological reactivity, subjective experience, and behavioral tendencies and impulses has been the subject of specific focus. Researches have approached this topic from three perspectives, namely, (a) the examination of the association between fearful experiences and performance in sports competition situations (the state perspective), (b) research into the psychological mechanisms which explain why anxiety in performance situations leads to poor performance (the general psychological perspective), and (c) the search for personal characteristics which moderate the association between performance situation and emergence of anxiety, or between anxiety and the ability to perform (the trait perspective). A detailed illustration of existing findings on these three perspectives is presented by Ehrlenspiel and colleagues (Ehrlenspiel, 2017; Ehrlenspiel et al., 2017). ▶ Chapter 12 of this book focuses on anxiety in sports in greater detail.

27.8.1 Causes of Stress in Elite Sports

Elite athletes are confronted with a variety of challenges on a daily basis. These include physiological factors (e.g., intense training, frequent travel, illness, injury), social factors (e.g., relationship problems, isolation, financial pressure), and psychological factors (negative thoughts, high expectations), as well as environmental factors (e.g., unfortunate training conditions or bad weather). Beckmann and Ehrlenspiel (2017) provide a comprehensive coverage of the **causes of stress in elite sports**. The authors note that numerous situational and personal factors are involved in the emergence of stress in performance sports, and frequently numerous stressors within and outside of the sports itself can influence athletes simultaneously. For this reason, many athletes employ performance-sports-specific **psychological skills training**, in order to improve competitive performance by reducing anxiety and controlling stress.

Research on stress in competitive sports often centers on the "cognitive-transactional stress model" (Mellalieu et al., 2009). According to Beckmann and Ehrlenspiel (2017), this takes into account the fact that stress processes depend, to a large degree, on personality traits, coping skills, and the stress-recovery balance of the athlete (e.g., Beckmann & Kellmann, 2004). This explains why the same stressor can be perceived differently by different athletes (Fletcher & Sarkar, 2012).

Some studies have identified **stressors** which are reported by performance athletes as being particularly troubling (Fletcher & Fletcher, 2005; Hanton et al., 2005). Distinctions are made between forms of stress which originate in performance sports itself. These include stressors which occur **during or immediately before a competition** (e.g., fear, nervousness, competition density, series of failures), but also organizational stressors (e.g., communication with the coach, dealing with the media). Chronic stress is also an issue for performance athletes, due, for example, to consistently **high-performance pressure, financial uncertainty, or existential worries**. Further sources of stress for performance athletes include problems with partners or family, social isolation due to frequent travel demands, or high training costs (Breuer & Hallmann, 2013). For young athletes, the pressures of sports and school can represent a double burden (Hoffmann & Richartz, 2006; Richartz & Brettschneider, 1996). Furthermore, **transitional phases**, such as the transition from junior to senior competition, have been described as stressful. This is due, on the one hand, to the fact that such changes often coincide with other life transitions (e.g., from school to working life) (Beckmann et al., 2006) and, on the other hand, to the fact that only a few junior athletes are able to translate their achievements into success at the senior level (Vanden Auweele et al., 2004). For adult athletes, the **end of the career** can be a critical life event (Taylor & Ogilvie, 1994). The changes in focus required can lead to considerable levels of stress. This is particularly the case when an athletic career must be ended involuntarily (e.g., due to injury) (Wylleman et al., 2004). In line with this, numerous studies suggest that many former performance athletes experience a depressive episode following the end of their careers (Gouttebarge et al., 2016).

> Elite athletes are confronted with many sources of stress in their sporting lives. One of the biggest challenges is the end of their career.

27.8.2 The Importance of Recovery in Elite Sports

In order to be successful at the highest level in sports, **many years of training at the limits of one's potential** are required. Consequently, high levels of commitment and motivation are necessary (Kellmann et al., 2017; Lemyre et al., 2007). Many elite athletes (particularly younger ones) may go beyond their limits. In such times, there is a **risk of insufficient recovery**. While short phases of insufficient recovery can generally be tolerated fairly well, particularly when targeted recovery strategies and relaxation techniques are employed (Gustafsson et al., 2017; Kellmann et al., 2017), longer phases with higher or excessive training intensity and poor recovery can lead to **overreaching** and **overtraining** (Meeusen et al., 2013). Symptoms of overtraining include performance plateaus or decreases, physiological changes, depressive mood, general apathy, irritability, sleep problems, increased risk of injury and infection, and changes in hormonal profile (Beckmann & Ehrlenspiel, 2017; Kellmann, 2002). Overtraining typically requires a recovery phase of several weeks or even months, and medical and/or psychological treatment is often necessary (Kellmann et al., 2017).

In a "**Joint Consensus Statement**" on the presentation, diagnosis, and treatment of the overtraining syndrome published in 2013 (Meeusen et al., 2013), it is suggested that the balance between stress and recovery can be measured via a number of parameters. These include psychological tests, biochemical markers, and sports-specific performance testing, although none of these methods can give an exact representation of the state of the athlete; rather, such methods should be employed regularly as a means of monitoring athletes, in order to assess the subjective training load and demands currently experienced and, if necessary, prompt an early intervention (Beckmann & Ehrlenspiel, 2017; Kellmann et al., 2017). One of the most well-known tools for measuring the balance between stress and recovery in performance athletes is the "**Recovery-Stress Questionnaire for Athletes**" (Kallus & Kellmann, 2016; see ► Methods: The Recovery-Stress Questionnaire for Athletes). A systematic review of other approaches, including their application, can be found in Kellmann et al. (2017).

Methods: The "Recovery-Stress Questionnaire for Athletes"

The "Recovery-Stress Questionnaire for Athletes" (RESTQ; Kallus & Kellmann, 2016) is used to measure the current recovery-stress status of an athlete. The RESTQ is based on the notion that an accumulation of burdensome events in various areas of life, combined with insufficient recovery, will lead to a critical psychophysiological state. The RESTQ can be used by athletes between the ages of 10 and 88 and presents a full picture of current levels of stress and recovery. The general version of the RESTQ comprises seven load scales and five recovery scales. There is also a specific version for coaches, children, and adolescents, for working environments, and for clinical environments. The questionnaires can be adapted to particular time frames (e.g., 3, 7, or 14 days or nights).

27.8.3 Burnout in Athletes

As shown above, some athletes have difficulties coping with the challenges presented by performance sports. To date little is known about the prevalence of burnout in top-level sports, although it is thought that between 1% and 10% of athletes will experience a **state of extreme and chronic exhaustion**, which can lead to a **premature career end** (Gerber et al., 2018; Gustafsson et al., 2017). If junior athletes enter this state, national programs may lose talented athletes (Gustafsson et al., 2007). Following Maslach's definition (see above), burnout in sports is also understood to be a **multidimensional construct**. The core dimensions are (a) emotional and physical exhaustion, (b) a subjective feeling of failure or inadequacy in sports, and (c) a devaluation of the meaning and importance of performance sports (Raedeke & Smith, 2001).

Burnout in Elite Sports

Burnout in elite sports is understood to be a multidimensional construct. The core dimensions are (a) emotional and physical exhaustion, (b) a subjective feeling of failure or inadequacy in sports, and (c) a devaluation of the meaning and importance of performance sports.

Since the 1980s, numerous models have been developed to try and explain the causes of burnout in high-performance athletes (Coakley, 1992; Raedeke, 1997; Silva, 1990; Smith, 1986). These findings have been synthesized in an **integrated model** by Gustafsson et al. (2011) (see ◘ Fig. 27.7). This model highlights the predisposing conditions, early symptoms, and consequences of burnout. The influence of moderators, which may increase or reduce the risk of burnout, is also addressed. Factors associated with an increased risk include a unidimensional perception of one's identity as an athlete, high levels of investments, social pressure, a feeling of self-worth which is closely linked to athletic success, and a lack of attractive alternatives to continuing with sports. Further, potentially negative factors are a tendency towards perfectionism (particularly an excessive fear of mistakes or failure), a lack of social support, little control over one's athletic career, a limited and inflexible set of coping strategies, and conditions which reduce motivation (e.g., a strong focus on oneself, an excessively performance-oriented training environment). An overview of the current state of research in this field can be found in Gustafsson et al. (2017).

27.8.4 Stress and Injury in Elite Sports

Injuries can be a **stressful life event** for athletes and can sometimes lead to the premature end of an athletic career (Bußmann & Alfermann, 1990). In order to develop effective prevention programs, it is important to identify risk factors which are associated with an increased likelihood of injury in high-performance athletes (Tranaeus et al., 2017). In this context, Williams and Andersen (1998) developed the "**model of stress and athletic injury**" (◘ Fig. 27.8). This model illustrates the influence of psychosocial factors in the emergence of sports injuries. It suggests that an athlete's reaction to a potentially stressful situation depends on a closely linked constellation of personality traits, early experiences of stress, and available coping resources.

Studies examining the influence of stress on injury in performance sports have been carried out since the early 1980s (for an overview, see Tranaeus et al., 2015). Many of these studies support the validity of the model presented in ◘ Fig. 27.8. For example, it has been shown that both critical life events and smaller daily stressors are associated with an increased injury risk (Ivarsson et al., 2014; Rogers & Landers, 2005). This also holds true for higher stress reactivity (Andersen & Williams, 1999). A review of numerous interventions has shown that a variety of **psychological approaches** (e.g., mindfulness-based approaches, psychological skills training) can reduce this injury risk (Tranaeus et al., 2017). In their model, Brewer et al. (2002) point out that the injury recovery process can be influenced by many biopsychosocial factors. Key psychological factors are, among others, motivation to continue one's athletic career, individual pain

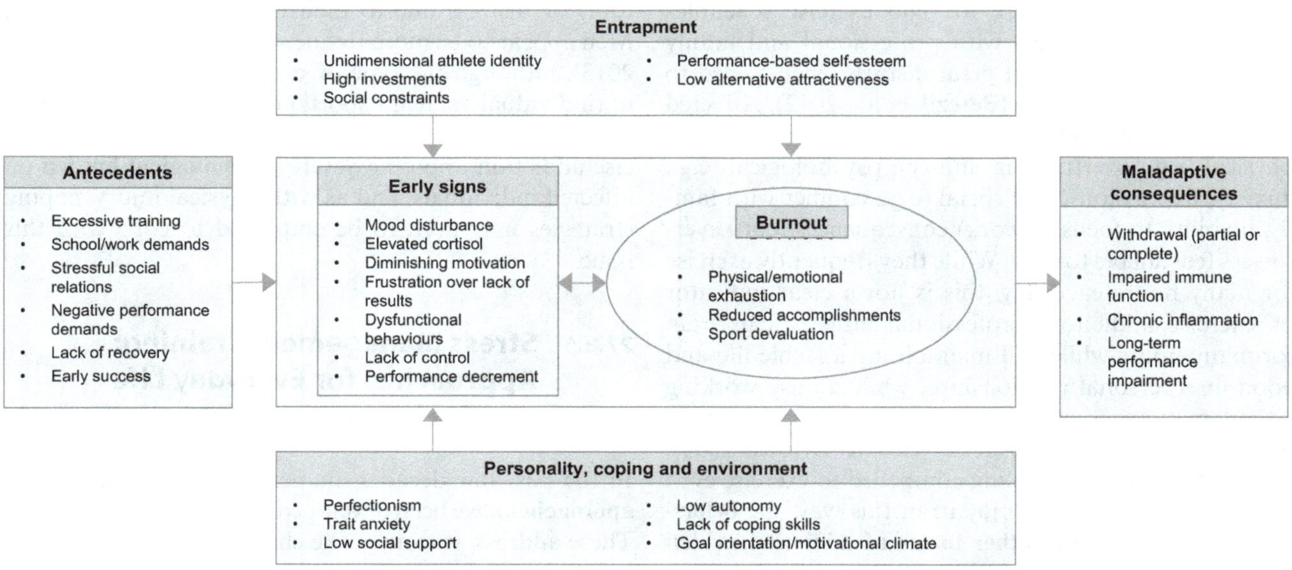

◘ **Fig. 27.7** Integrated model of burnout in athletes (Gustafsson et al., 2011)

27

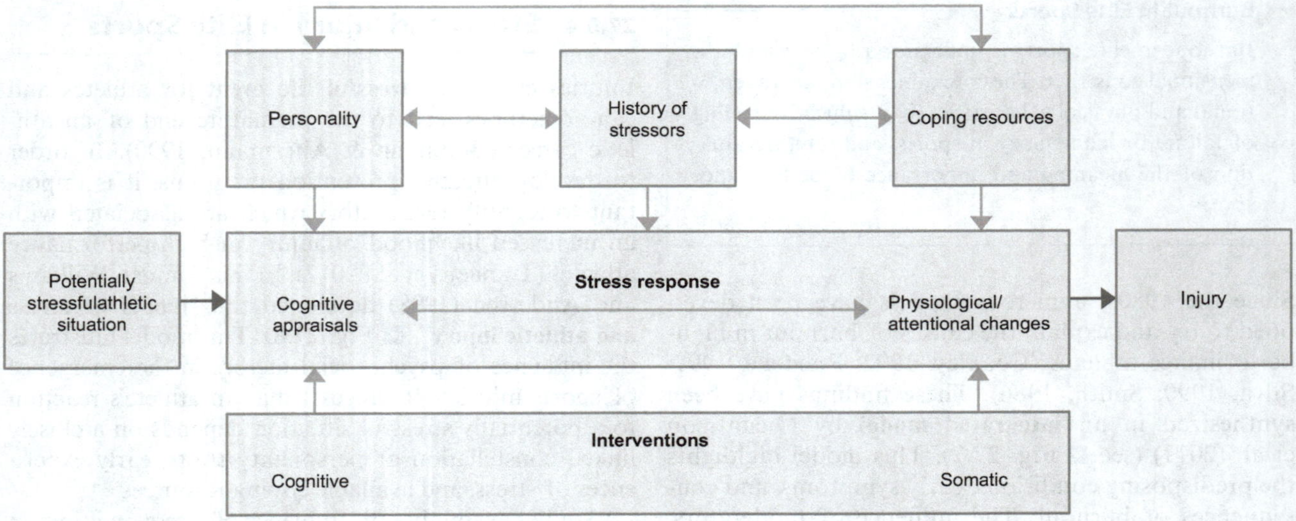

Fig. 27.8 The model of stress and injury in performance sports (Brewer et al., 2002)

tolerance, and the conviction that one can successfully navigate the rehabilitation phase (Brewer, 2010).

27.8.5 Sports and Exercise Addiction

While insufficient recovery can lead to the physiological problems listed above, engaging in **too much sports and exercise** can also have psychological causes and consequences. Since the 1970s, when Baekeland (1970) observed that a group of athletes recruited for a study on sleep refused to stop exercising, there has been evidence that a small number of individuals develop a **compulsive attitude towards sports and exercise** (Cunningham et al., 2016). These individuals exercise through severe injury and illness, adhere to rigid exercise schedules even when this conflicts with professional and family commitments, and report great distress when forced to reduce or stop exercising (Berczik et al., 2012). Affected individuals are aware that this behavior has negative physical (e.g., overtraining, injury), psychological (e.g., anxiety, depression), and social (e.g., conflict with family, inability to focus at work) consequences, but nevertheless feel unable to stop. While they frequently exercise for many hours each day, this is not a clear indicator of exercise addiction; professional athletes can train for many hours while still maintaining a stable life and good interpersonal relationships, while a busy working parent may experience distress when adhering strictly to 90 min per day of exercise (Cox & Orford, 2004). Those affected report feeling compelled to exercise even though they no longer enjoy it; in this way, the **behavior strongly resembles other forms of addiction**, which can result, over time, in a desensitization of the brain's reward pathways (Adinoff, 2004). While in some cases, weight loss may be the goal that causes an individual to exercise compulsively (so-called **secondary exercise addiction**), in other cases exercise is pursued to excess as an end in itself (**primary exercise addiction**) (Cook et al., 2014). As exercise can reduce feelings of stress and depression, exercise addiction is thought to result from an excessive, out-of-control pursuit of this positive experience (Szabo et al., 2015).

However, research in this area is still in its early stages. While prevalence estimates vary, conservative calculations based on literature reviews suggest that between 0.1% (Breuer & Kleinert, 2009) and 8% (Trott et al., 2020) of exercising individuals report marked symptoms of distress due to their excessive exercise habits. Men appear to be more frequently affected (Szabo et al., 2013), although the type of exercise or sports engaged in (individual vs. team sports) does not appear to have an influence (Lichtenstein et al., 2014). Sports and exercise addiction impose a **severe psychological burden** on affected individuals, and as with physical injury, coping strategies may need to be employed to cope with this issue.

27.8.6 Stress Management Training: Approaches for Everyday Life and Performance Sports

In the past few decades, numerous **stress management approaches** have been developed (Hartmann et al., 2014). These address, variously, the challenging situation itself

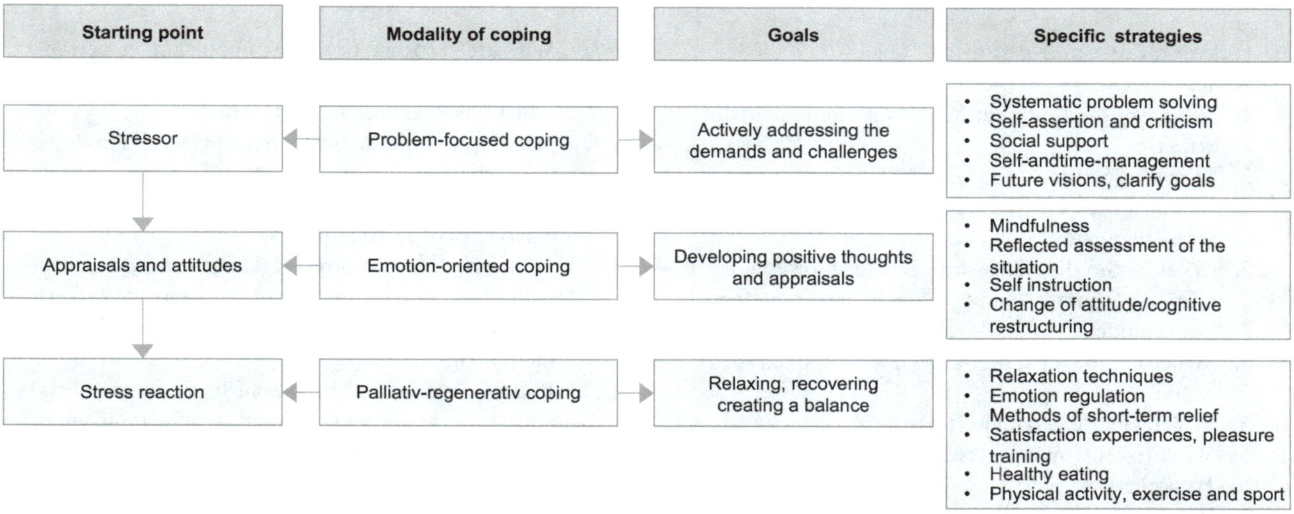

Fig. 27.9 Approaches and strategies for individualized stress management

(problem-focused coping), evaluative processes and attitudes (emotion-oriented coping), or the psychobiological stress reaction (palliative-regenerative coping; Kaluza & Chevalier, 2017). An overview of the implementation of stress management techniques **for adults** in everyday life can be found in Kaluza and Chevalier (2017). More recently, various theory- and evidence-based stress management trainings **for children and adolescents** have been developed, often designed to be applied in a school setting. An overview of programs currently implemented in German-speaking regions can be found in Lohaus (Lohaus, 2017). These programs are highly relevant, as psychosomatic problems often emerge during childhood and adolescence (Gerber & Pühse, 2007), and the ability to manage stress at this age is a key health goal (Jeannin et al., 2005). While the majority of existing programs are carried out during lessons in the classroom, there is also a stress management program specifically designed for physical education lessons (Lang et al., 2017). The creators point out that physical education lessons are often the setting for health-related activities and goals (Pühse et al., 2011). The stress management training program gives physical education teachers guidance on how the topic of health education can be addressed. A further advantage of this approach is that, in physical education class, stress reactions can be experienced on a physical level, and coping strategies can be employed and reflected upon immediately. Evidence for the effectiveness of the training program can be found in Lang et al. (2016, 2017, 2019) (Fig. 27.9).

Several stress management programs have also been developed **specifically for performance athletes**. Sallen (2017) provides a comprehensive review of **stress-resistance training methods**. He emphasizes that the goal of these programs is not to help performance athletes "live a completely stress-free life," but rather to "empower athletes to deal independently with stressors which, due to their intensity or duration, are experienced as unpleasant, limiting, or damaging ("**empowerment approach**"). Stress-resistance interventions for elite athletes are often not completely new inventions. Typically, elements of existing methods are included (e.g., cognitive behavioral therapy, relaxation techniques). Stress-resistance training can also overlap with other interventions commonly used in performance sports (e.g., psychological skills training; Birrer & Morgan, 2010). According to Sallen (2017), existing programs can be differentiated on the basis of whether they aim, primarily, towards a reduction of stress-related influences on mental well-being, or a reduction of stress-related performance decreases in sports. It is concluded that the implementation of such stress-resistance programs in performance sports has positive effects, but these may be limited to certain aspects of performance and are not particularly strong. Such programs are, however, highly recommended, as athletes report benefitting greatly from them.

Learning Control Questions

Basic:

1. What are the four health-relevant components of stress?
2. Describe Semmer and Zapf's (2017) framework model. What are the key terms on the topic of stress regulation?
3. What is the difference between reaction-focused, stimulus-focused, and cognitive-transactional stress models?
4. Which are the most well-known work-related stress models?
5. Which are the two main stress axes?
6. What is the main message of the "Reactivity Hypothesis Model?"
7. What is the "stress-buffering effect?"

Advanced:

8. Is stress associated with a higher risk of cardiovascular disease and depression? Which mechanisms underlie this?
9. Which indicators can be used to calculate the cost of stress?
10. Do stressed people live shorter lives? Why? How is the "reserve-capacity model" linked to Hobfoll's "COR theory?"
11. Which perspectives can be employed to understand stress regulation and sports? Which research traditions are associated with these two perspectives?
12. Which mechanisms in the emergence and management of stress are attributable to physical activity, exercise, and sports?
13. Are physically active people less stressed? Does stress lead to reduced physical activity, exercise, and sports? Or do physical activity and stress interact?
14. What happens during the Trier Social Stress Test? Why do we need research paradigms like the TSST?
15. What are the key premises of the "cross-stressor adaptation hypothesis?" Is this hypothesis supported by empirical evidence?
16. Which factors can lead to burnout in athletes? Describe the model of Gustafsson et al. (2011). Do you agree with all components? Do you miss something? What are the main sources of stress in performance sports? How could they be prevented?

Experts:

17. Why is there no single type of sports which generally reduces stress?
18. Can exercise and sports be used to treat burnout and posttraumatic stress disorder? What are the underlying working mechanisms?
19. Why are recovery processes important in performance sports? How can insufficient recovery in athletes be diagnosed and treated?
20. What signs might indicate that a person is developing exercise addiction?
21. What role do psychological influences play in the emergence of sports injuries?
22. How effective are stress management programs within and outside of the performance sports setting? What could be done to successfully implement them?
23. If being asked for the relationship between sports and stress, could you "answer" with a mind map that structures your answer?

References

Adinoff, B. (2004). Neurobiologic processes in drug reward and addiction. *Harvard Review of Psychiatry, 12*, 305–320.

Aldana, S. G., Sutton, L. D., & Jacobson, B. H. (1996). Relationship between leisure time physical activity and perceived stress. *Perceptual and Motor Skills, 82*, 315–321.

Andersen, M., & Williams, J. (1999). Athletic injury, psychosocial factors and perceptual changes during stress. *Journal of Sports Sciences, 17*, 735–741.

Arnold, S. V., Smolderen, K. G., Buchanan, D. M., Li, Y., & Spertus, J. A. (2012). Perceived stress in myocardial infarction: Long-term mortality and health status outcomes. *Journal of the American College of Cardiology, 60*, 1756–1763.

Awa, W. L., Plaumann, M., & Walter, U. (2010). Burnout prevention: A review of intervention programs. *Patient Education and Counseling, 78*, 184–190.

Baekeland, F. (1970). Exercise deprivation: Sleep and psychological reactions. *Archives of General Psychiatry, 22*, 365–369.

Bakker, A. B., & Demerouti, E. (2007). The job demands-resources model: State of the art. *Journal of Managerial Psychology, 22*, 309–328.

Beal, D. J., & Weiss, H. M. (2003). Methods of ecological momentary assessment in organizational research. *Organizational Research Methods, 6*, 440–464.

Beckmann, J., & Ehrlenspiel, F. (2017). Strategien der Stressregulation im Leistungssport [strategies of stress regulation in elite sport]. In R. Fuchs & M. Gerber (Eds.), *Handbuch Stressregulation und Sport* (pp. 417–433). Springer.

Beckmann, J., Elbe, A.-M., Szymanski, B., & Ehrlenspiel, F. (2006). Chancen und Risiken vom Leben im Verbundsystem von Schule und Leistungssport—Psychologische, soziologische und Leistungsaspekte [Opportunities and risks of life in the network systems of school and competitive sport—Psychological, sociological and performance aspects]. Sport und Buch Strauß.

Beckmann, J., & Kellmann, M. (2004). Self-regulation and recovery: Approaching an understanding of the process of recovery from stress. *Psychological Reports, 95*, 1135–1153.

Berczik, K., Szabó, A., Griffiths, M. D., Kurimay, T., Kun, B., Urbán, R., & Demetrovics, Z. (2012). Exercise addiction: Symptoms, diagnosis, epidemiology, and etiology. *Substance Use and Misuse, 47*, 403–417.

Bernard, C. (1974). *Lectures on the phenomena of life common to animals and plants*. Thomas. (Original work published 1878).

Birrer, D., & Morgan, G. (2010). Psychological skills training as a way to enhance an athlete's performance in high-intensity sports. *Scandinavian Journal of Medicine and Science in Sports, 20*, 78–87.

Booth, J., Connelly, L., Lawrence, M., Chalmers, C., Joice, S., Becker, C., & Dougall, N. (2015). Evidence of perceived psychosocial stress as a risk factor for stroke in adults: A meta-analysis. *BMC Neurology, 15*, 233. https://doi.org/10.1186/s12883-12015-10456-12884

Brand, S. (2017). Sportaktivität, stress und Schlaf [Physical activity, exercise, stress and sleep]. In R. Fuchs & M. Gerber (Eds.), *Handbuch Stressregulation und Sport* (pp. 293–310). Springer.

Bretland, R. J., & Thorsteinsson, E. B. (2015). Reducing workplace burnout: The relative benefits of cardiovascular and resistance exercise. *PeerJ, 3*, e891. https://doi.org/10.7717/peerj.7891

Breuer, C., & Hallmann, K. (2013). *Dysfunktionen des Spitzensports: Doping, Match-Fixing und Gesundheitsgefährdungen aus Sicht von Bevölkerung und Athleten [Dysfunctions of elite sport: Doping, match-fixing and health risk from the perspective of the population and athletes]*. Bundesinstitut für Sportwissenschaften.

Breuer, S., & Kleinert, J. (2009). *Primäre Sportsucht und bewegungsbezogene Abhängigkeit—Beschreibung, Erklärung und Diagnostik*. Springer.

Brewer, B. W. (2010). The role of psychological factors in sport injury rehabilitation outcomes. *International Review of Sport and Exercise Psychology, 3*, 40–61.

Brewer, B. W., Andersen, M. B., & Van Raalte, J. L. (2002). Psychological aspects of sport injury rehabilitation: Towards a biopsychosocial approach. In D. L. Mostofsky & L. D. Zaichkowsky (Eds.), *Medical and psychological aspects of sport and exercise* (pp. 41–54). Fitness Information Technology.

Brouwer, A. M., & Hogervorst, M. A. (2014). A new paradigm to induce mental stress: The sing-a-song stress test (SSST). *Frontiers in Neuroscience, 8*, 141–148.

Burisch, M. (2006). *Das Burnout-Syndrom. Theorie der inneren Erschöpfung [The burnout syndrome: Theory of internal exhaustion]*. Springer.

Buske-Kirschbaum, A., Jobst, S., Wustmans, A., Kirschbaum, C., Rauh, W., & Hellhammer, D. (1997). Attenuated free cortisol response to psychosocial stress in children with atopic dermatitis. *Psychosomatic Medicine, 59*, 419–426.

Bußmann, G., & Alfermann, D. (1990). Aufhören oder Weitermachen? Wenn Athletinnen ihre Laufbahn vorzeitig beenden [To quit or to continue? When athletes end their careers prematurely]. *Sportpsychologie, 4*, 20–26.

Cacioppo, J. T., & Berntson, G. G. (2011). Balancing demands of the internal and external milieu. In H. S. Friedman & R. Cohen Silver (Eds.), *Oxford handbook of health psychology* (pp. 73–91). Oxford University Press.

Cacioppo, J. T., Berntson, G. G., Malarkey, W. B., Kiecolt-Glaser, J. K., Sheridan, J. F., Poehlmann, K. M., Burleson, M. H., Ernst, J. M., Hawkley, L. C., & Glaser, R. (1998). Autonomic, neuroendocrine, and immune responses to psychological stress: The reactivity hypothesis. *Annals of the New York Academy of Sciences, 840*, 664–673.

Cannon, W. (1914). The emergency function of the adrenal medulla in pain and the major emotions. *American Journal of Physiology, 33*, 356–372.

Class, Q. A., Khashan, A. S., Lichtenstein, P., Langström, N., & D'Onofrio, B. M. (2013). Maternal stress and infant mortality: The importance of the preconception period. *Psychological Science, 24*, 1309–1316.

Coakley, J. (1992). Burnout among adolescent athletes: A personal failure or a social problem? *Sociology of Sport Journal, 9*, 271–285.

Cook, B., Hausenblas, H., & Freimuth, M. (2014). Exercise addiction and compulsive exercising: Relationship to eating disorders, substance use disorders, and addictive disorders. In T. D. Brewerton & A. B. Dennis (Eds.), *Eating disorders, addictions and substance use disorders: Research, clinical and treatment perspectives* (pp. 127–144). Springer-Verlag Publishing.

Cox, R., & Orford, J. A. (2004). A qualitative study of the meaning of exercise for people who could be labelled as 'addicted' to exercise—Can 'addiction' be applied to high frequency exercising? *Addiction Research & Theory, 12*, 167–188.

Crews, D. J., & Landers, D. M. (1987). A meta-analytic review of aerobic fitness and reactivity to psychosocial stressors. *Medicine and Science in Sports and Exercise, 19*, 114–130.

Cunningham, H. E., Pearman, S. R., & Brewerton, T. D. (2016). Conceptualizing primary and secondary pathological exercise using available measures of excessive exercise. *International Journal of Eating Disorders, 49*, 778–792.

De Backer, G., Amgrosioni, E., Borch-Johnsen, K., Grotons, C., Cifkova, R., Dallongeville, J., Ebrahim, S., Faergeman, O., Graham, I., Mancia, G., Manger Cats, V., Orth-Gomer, K., Perk, J., Pyörälä, K., Rodicio, J. L., Sans, S., Sansoy, V., Sechtem, U., Silber, S., Thomsen, T., & Wood, D. (2003). European guidelines on cardiovascular disease prevention in clinical practice. *European Journal of Cardiovascular Prevention and Rehabilitation, 2003*, S1–S78.

de Quervain, D. J., Roozendaal, B., Nitsch, R. M., McGaugh, J. L., & Hock, C. (2000). Acute cortisone administration impairs retrieval of long-term declarative memory in humans. *Nature Neuroscience, 3*, 313–314.

Deiseroth, A., & Hanssen, H. (2017). Körperliche Aktivität, Stress und arterielle Gefässsteifigkeit [Physical activity, stress and arterial stiffness]. In R. Fuchs & M. Gerber (Eds.), *Handbiuch Stressregulation und Sport* (pp. 325–342). Springer.

Dickerson, S. S., & Kemeny, M. E. (2004). Acute stressors and cortisol responses: A theoretical integration and synthesis of laboratory research. *Psychological Bulletin, 130*, 355–391.

Dusseldorp, E., van Elderen, T., Maes, S., Meulman, J., & Kraaij, V. (1999). A meta-analysis of psychoeducational programs for coronary heart disease patients. *Health Psychology, 18*, 506–519.

Ehrlenspiel, F. (2017). *Angst im Sport [Anxiety in sport]*. Springer.

Ehrlenspiel, F., Geukes, K., & Beckmann, J. (2017). Stress, Angst und Leistung im Leistungssport [Stress, anxiety and performance in elite sport]. In R. Fuchs & M. Gerber (Eds.), *Handbuch Stressregulation und Sport* (pp. 391–416). Springer.

Ehrlenspiel, F., & Strahler, K. (Eds.). (2012). *Psychoneuroendocrinology of sport and exercise: Foundations, markers, trends*. Routledge.

Elfering, A., Brunner, B., Igic, I., Keller, A., & Weber, L. (2017). Gesellschaftliche Bedeutung und Kosten von Stress [Social relevance and costs of stress]. In R. Fuchs & M. Gerber (Eds.), *Handbuch Stressregulation und Sport* (pp. 123–141). Springer.

Eurofound. (2016). *First findings: Sixth European Working Conditions Survey*. https://www.eurofound.europa.eu/publications/resume/2015/working-conditions/first-findings-sixth-european-working-conditions-survey-resume

Everson, S. A., Lynch, J. W., Chesney, M. A., Kaplan, G. A., Goldberg, D. E., Shade, S. B., Cohen, R. D., Salonen, R., & Salonen, J. T. (1997). Interaction of workplace demands and cardiovascular reactivity in progression of carotid atherosclerosis: Population based study. *BMJ, 314*, 553–558.

Fletcher, D., & Fletcher, J. A. (2005). A meta-model of stress, emotions and performance: Conceptual foundation, theoretical framework, and research directions. *Journal of Sports Sciences, 23*, 157–158.

Fletcher, D., & Sarkar, M. (2012). Psychological resilience: A review and critique of definitions, concepts, and theory. *Psychology of Sport and Exercise, 18*, 12–23.

Forcier, K., Stroud, L. R., Papandonatos, G. D., Hitsman, B., Reiches, M., Krishnamoorthy, J., & Niaura, R. (2006). Links between

27

physical fitness and cardiovascular reactivity and recovery to psychological stressors: A meta-analysis. *Health Psychology, 25*, 723–739.

Fransson, E. I., Heikkilä, K., Nyberg, S. T., Zins, M., Westerlund, H., Westerholm, P., Väänänen, A., Virtanen, M., Vahtera, J., Theorell, T., Suominen, S. B., Singh-Manoux, A., Siegrist, J., Sabia, S., Rugulies, R., Pentti, J., Oksanen, T., Nordin, M., Nielsen, M. L., Marmot, M., Magnusson Hanson, L. L., Madsen, I. E. H., Lunau, T., Leineweber, C., Kumari, M., Kouvonen, A., Koskinen, A., Koskenvuo, M., Knutsson, A., Kittel, F., Jöckel, K.-H., Joensuu, M., Houtman, I. L., Hooftman, W. E., Goldberg, M., Geuskens, G. A., Ferrie, J. E., Erbel, R., Dragano, N., De Bacquer, D., Clays, E., Casini, A., Burr, H., Borritz, M., Bonenfant, S., Bjorner, J., Alfredsson, L., Hamer, M., Batty, G. D., & Kivimäki, M. (2012). Job strain as a risk factor for leisure-time physical inactivity: An individual-participant meta-analysis of up to 170′000 men and women. *American Journal of Epidemiology, 176*, 1078–1089.

Fuchs, R., & Klaperski, S. (2017). Stressregulation durch Sport und Bewegung [Stress regulation through physical activity, exercise and sport]. In R. Fuchs & M. Gerber (Eds.), *Handuch stressregulation und sport* (pp. 205–226). Springer.

Gallo, L. C., & Matthews, K. A. (2003). Understanding the association between socioeconomic status and physical health: Do negative emotions play a role? *Psychological Bulletin, 129*, 10–51.

Gerber, M. (2008a). *Sport, Stress und Gesundheit bei Jugendlichen [Sport, stress and health among adolescents]*. Hofmann.

Gerber, M. (2008b). Sportliche Aktivität und Stressreaktivität: Ein Review [Physical activity, exercis, sport and stress reactivity: A review]. *Deutsche Zeitschrift fur Sportmedizin, 59*, 4–10.

Gerber, M. (2017). Physiologische Wirkmechanismen des Sports unter Stress [Physiological mechanisms of physical activity, exercise and sport under stress]. In R. Fuchs & M. Gerber (Eds.), *Handbuch Stressregulation und Sport* (pp. 251–273). Springer.

Gerber, M., Börjesson, M., Ljung, T., Lindwall, M., & Jonsdottir, I. (2016a). Fitness moderates the relationship between stress and cardiovascular risk factors. *Medicine and Science in Sports and Exercise, 48*, 2075–2081.

Gerber, M., Brand, S., Elliot, C., Holsboer-Trachsler, E., Pühse, U., & Beck, J. (2013a). Aerobic exercise training and burnout: A pilot study with male participants suffering from burnout. *BMC Research Notes, 6*, 78. https://doi.org/10.1186/1756-0500-1186-1178

Gerber, M., Brand, S., Elliott, C., Holsboer-Trachsler, E., & Pühse, U. (2014a). Aerobic exercise, ball sports, dancing, and weight lifting as moderators of the relationship between stress and depressive symptoms: An exploratory cross-sectional study with Swiss university students. *Perceptual and Motor Skills, 119*, 679–697.

Gerber, M., Endes, K., Brand, S., Herrmann, C., Colledge, F., Donath, L., Faude, O., Hanssen, H., Pühse, U., & Zahner, L. (2017a). In 6- to 8-year-old children, cardiorespiratory fitness moderates the relationship between severity of life events and health-related quality of life. *Quality of Life Research, 26*(3), 695–706. https://doi.org/10.1007/s11136-11016-11472-11136

Gerber, M., Endes, K., Herrmann, C., Colledge, F., Brand, S., Donath, L., Faude, O., Pühse, U., Hanssen, H., & Zahner, L. (2016b). Does physical fitness buffer the relationship between psychosocial stress, retinal vessel diameters, and blood pressure among primary schoolchildren. *BMRI Cardiology, 2016*, 6340431. https://doi.org/10.1155/2016/6340431

Gerber, M., Endes, K., Herrmann, C., Colledge, F., Brand, S., Donath, L., Faude, O., Pühse, U., Hanssen, H., & Zahner, L. (2017b). Fitness, stress and body composition in primary schoolchildren. *Medicine and Science in Sports and Exercise, 49*(3), 581–587.

Gerber, M., & Fuchs, R. (2017). Stressregulation und Sport: Ein Überblick zum Stand der Forschung [Stress regulation, physical activity, exercise and sport: An overview of the state of research]. In R. Fuchs & M. Gerber (Eds.), *Handbuch Stressregulation und Sport* (pp. 3–20). Springer.

Gerber, M., Gustafsson, H., Seelig, H., Kellmann, M., Ludyga, S., Colledge, F., Brand, S., Isoard-Gautheur, S., & Bianchi, R. (2018). Usefulness of the Athlete Burnout Questionnaire (ABQ) as a screening tool for the detection of clinically relevant burnout symptoms among young elite athletes. *Psychology of Sport and Exercise, 39*, 104–113.

Gerber, M., Imboden, C., Beck, J., Brand, S., Colledge, F., Eckert, A., Holsboer-Trachsler, E., Pühse, U., & Hatzinger, M. (2020). Effects of aerobic exercise on cortisol stress reactivity in response to the Trier Social Stress Test in inpatients with major depressive disorders: A randomized controlled trial. *Journal of Clinical Medicine, 9*(5), 1419. https://doi.org/10.3390/jcm9051419

Gerber, M., Jonsdottir, I. H., Lindwall, M., & Ahlborg, G. (2014b). Physical activity in employees with differing occupational stress and mental health profiles: A latent profile analysis. *Psychology of Sport and Exercise, 15*, 649–658.

Gerber, M., Lindwall, M., Lindegård, A., Börjesson, M., & Jonsdottir, I. H. (2013b). Cardiovascular fitness protects from stress-related symptoms of burnout and depression. *Patient Education and Counseling, 93*, 146–152.

Gerber, M., Ludyga, S., Mücke, M., Colledge, F., Brand, S., & Pühse, U. (2017c). Low vigorous physical activity is associated with increased adrenocortical reactivity to psychosocial stress in students with high stress perceptions. *Psychoneuroendocrinology, 80*, 104–113.

Gerber, M., & Pühse, U. (2007). Psychosomatische Beschwerden und psychisches Wohlbefinden bei Schülerinnen und Schülern der Sekundarstufe II [Psychosomatic complaints and mental well-being among high school students]. *Psychologie in Erziehung und Unterricht, 54*, 223–235.

Gerber, M., & Pühse, U. (2009). Do exercise and fitness protect against stress-induced health complaints? A review of the literature. *Scandinavian Journal of Public Health, 37*, 801–819.

Gerber, M., & Schilling, R. (2017). Stress als Risikofaktor für körperliche und psychische Gesundheitsbeeinträchtigungen [Stress as a risk factor for physical and mental health impairments]. In R. Fuchs & M. Gerber (Eds.), *Handbuch Stressregulation und Sport* (pp. 93–122). Springer.

Gouttebarge, V., Aoki, H., & Kerkhoffs, G. M. (2016). Prevalence and determinants of symptoms related to mental disorders in retired male professional footballers. *Journal of Sports Medicine and Physical Fitness, 56*, 648–654.

Gustafsson, H., Kentää, G., & Hassmén, P. (2011). Athlete burnout: An integrated model and future research directions. *International Review of Sport and Exercise Psychology, 4*, 3–24.

Gustafsson, H., Kenttä, G., Hassmén, P., & Lundqvist, C. (2007). Prevalence of burnout in competitive adolescent athletes. *The Sport Psychologist, 21*, 21–37.

Gustafsson, H., Madigan, D. J., & Lundkvist, E. (2017). Burnout in athletes. In R. Fuchs & M. Gerber (Eds.), *Handbuch Stressregulation und Sport* (pp. 489–504). Springer.

Hall, M., Baum, A., Buysse, D. J., Prigerson, H. G., Kupfer, D. J., & Reynolds, C. F. (1998). Sleep as a mediator of the stress-immune relationship. *Psychosomatic Medicine, 60*, 48–51.

Hamer, M., Taylor, A., & Steptoe, A. (2006). The effect of acute exercise on stress related blood pressure responses: A systematic review and meta-analysis. *Biological Psychology, 71*, 183–190.

Hansen, D., Lou, H. C., & Olsen, J. (2000). Serious life events and congenital malformations: A national study with coplete follow-up. *Lancet, 356*, 875–880.

Hanton, S., Fletcher, D., & Coughlan, J. (2005). Stress in elite sport performers: A comparative study of competitive and organizational stressors. *Journal of Sports Sciences, 23*, 1129–1141.

Hartmann, T., Gerber, M., & Pühse, U. (2014). Zeig dem Stress die rote Karte. In *Ein bewegungsorientiertes Stressmanagement? [Taking stress out of the game: A movement-oriented stress management training]*. Meyer & Meyer Verlag.

Hemingway, H., & Marmot, M. (1999). Psychosocial factors in the aetiology and prognosis of coronary heart disease: Systematic review of prospective cohort studies. *BMJ, 318*, 1460–1467.

Hobfoll, S. E. (1989). Conservation of resources: A new attempt at conceptualizing stress. *American Psychologist, 44*, 513–524.

Hobfoll, S. E. (1998). *Stress, culture, and community: The psychology and philosophy of stress*. Plenum Press.

Hoffmann, K., & Richartz, A. (2006). Chronische Belastungen im Kinderleistungssport. Eine Analyse protektiver Ressourcen [Chronic stress in child elite sport. An analysis of protective resources]. *Leipziger Sportwissenschaftliche Beiträge, 47*, 1–15.

Holmes, M. (2017). Physical activity, stress and obesity. In R. Fuchs & M. Gerber (Eds.), *Handbuch Stressregulation und Sport* (pp. 311–323). Springer.

Holtermann, A., Mortensen, O. S., Burr, H., Søgaard, K., Gyntelberg, F., & Suadicani, P. (2010). Physical demands at work, physical fitness, and 30-year ischaemic heart disease and all-cause mortality in the Copenhagen male study. *Scandinavian Journal of Work, Environment & Health, 36*, 357–365.

Ising, M., Horstmann, S., Kloiber, S., Lucae, S., Binder, E. B., Kern, N., Künzel, H. E., Pfenning, A., Uhr, M., & Holsboer, F. (2007). Combined dexamethasone/corticotropin releasing hormone test predicts treatment response in major depression—A potential biomarker? *Biological Psychiatry, 62*, 47–54.

Ivarsson, A., Johnson, U., Lindwall, M., Gustafsson, H., & Altemyr, M. (2014). Psychosocial stress as a predictor of injury in elite junior soccer: A latent growth curve analysis. *Journal of Science and Medicine in Sport, 17*, 366–370.

Jackson, E. M., & Dishman, R. K. (2006). Cardiorespiratory fitness and laboratory stress: A meta-regression analysis. *Psychophysiology, 43*, 57–72.

Jeannin, A., Narring, F., Tschumper, A., Inderwildi Bonivento, L., Addor, V., Bütikofer, A., Suris, J.-C., Diserens, C., Alsaker, F., van Melle, G., & Michaud, P.-A. (2005). Self-reported health needs and use of primary health care services by adolescents enrolled in post-mandatory schools or vocational training programmes in Switzerland. *Swiss Medical Weekly, 135*, 11–18.

Jonsdottir, I. H., Rödjer, L., Hadzibajramovic, E., Börjesson, M., & Ahlborg, G. J. (2010). A prospective study of leisure-time physical activity and mental health in Swedish health care workers and social insurance officers. *Preventive Medicine, 51*, 373–377.

Kallus, K. W., & Kellmann, M. (2016). *RESTQ: The recovery-stress questionnaire for athletes: User manual*. Pearson.

Kaluza, G., & Chevalier, A. (2017). Stressbewältigungstrainings für Erwachsene [Coping training programs for adults]. In R. Fuchs & M. Gerber (Eds.), *Handbuch Stressregulation und Sport* (pp. 143–162). Springer.

Kaluza, G. (2004). Stressbewältigung. Trainingsmanual zur psychologischen Gesundheitsförderung. Springer.

Karasek, R. A. (1979). Job demands, job decision latitude, and mental strain: Implications for job-redesign. *Administrative Science Quarterly, 24*, 285–308.

Kasten, N., & Fuchs, R. (2017). Methodische Aspekte der Stressforschung [Methodological aspects of stress research]. In R. Fuchs & M. Gerber (Eds.), *Handbuch Stressregulation und Sport* (pp. 179–201). Springer.

Kellmann, M. (2002). Underrecovery and overtraining: Different concepts—Similar impact? In M. Kellmann (Ed.), *Enhancing recovery: Preventing underperformance in athletes* (pp. 3–24). Human Kinetics.

Kellmann, M., Kölling, S., & Pelka, M. (2017). Erholung und Belastung im Leistungssport [recovery and stress in elite sport]. In R. Fuchs & M. Gerber (Eds.), *Handbuch Stressregulation und Sport* (pp. 435–449). Springer.

Kessing, L. V., Agerbro, E., & Mortensen, P. B. (2003). Does the impact of major stressful life events on the risk of developing depression change throughout life? *Psychological Medicine, 33*, 1177–1184.

Kessler, R. C., Berglund, P., Demler, O., Jin, R., Merikangas, K. R., & Walters, E. E. (2005). Lifetime prevalence and age-of-onset distributions of DSM-IV disorders in the National Comorbidity Survey Replication. *Archives of General Psychiatry, 62*, 593–602.

Kirschbaum, C., Pirke, K. M., & Hellhammer, D. H. (1993). The Trier Social Stress Test: A tool for investigating psychobiological stress responses in a laboratory setting. *Neuropsychobiology, 28*, 76–81.

Kivimäki, M., Head, J., Ferrie, J. E., Shipley, M. J., Brunner, E., Vahtera, J., & Marmot, M. G. (2006). Work stress, weight gain and weight loss: Evidence for bidirectional effects of job strain on body mass index in the Whitehall II study. *International Journal of Obesity, 30*, 982–987.

Klaperski, S. (2017). Exercise, stress and health: The stress-buffering effect of exercise. In R. Fuchs & M. Gerber (Eds.), *Handbuch Stressregulation und Sport* (pp. 227–249). Springer.

Klaperski, S., von Dawans, B., Heinrichs, M., & Fuchs, R. (2014). Effects of a 12-week endurance training program on the physiological response to psychosocial stress in men: A randomized controlled trial. *Journal of Behavioral Medicine, 37*, 1118–1133.

Kobasa, S. C., Maddi, S. R., & Puccetti, M. C. (1982). Personality and exercise as buffers in the stress-illness-relationship. *Journal of Behavioral Medicine, 5*, 391–404.

Kohlmann, C.-W., & Eschenbeck, H. (2017). Stressbewältigung und Persönlichkeit [Coping and personality]. In R. Fuchs & M. Gerber (Eds.), *Handbuch Stressregulation und Sport* (pp. 51–66). Springer.

Krantz, D. S., & Manuck, S. B. (1984). Acute physiologic reactivity and risk of cardiovascular disease: A review and methodologic critique. *Psychological Bulletin, 96*, 435–464.

Lampert, R., Joska, T., Burg, M. M., Batsford, W. P., McPherson, C. A., & Jain, D. (2002). Emotional and physical precipitants of ventricular arrhythmia. *Circulation, 106*, 1800–1805.

Lang, C., Brand, S., Colledge, F., Holsboer-Trachsler, E., Pühse, U., & Gerber, M. (2019). Teaching stress management in physical education: A quasi-experimental study with vocational students. *Scandinavian Journal of Educational Research, 63*, 245–257.

Lang, C., Feldmeth, A. K., Brand, S., Holsboer-Trachsler, E., Pühse, U., & Gerber, M. (2016). Stress management in physical education class: Improved coping skills can mediate stress perceptions in adolescents. *Journal of Teaching in Physical Education, 35*, 149–158.

Lang, C., Feldmeth, A. K., Brand, S., Holsboer-Trachsler, E., Pühse, U., & Gerber, M. (2017). Effects of a physical education based coping training on adolescents' coping skills, stress perceptions and quality of sleep. *Physical Education and Sport Pedagogy, 22*, 213–230.

Laux, L., Glanzmann, P., Schaffner, P., & Spielberger, C. D. (1981). *Das State-Trait-Angst-Inventar: Theoretische Grundlagen und Handweisung [The state-trait-anxiety inventory: Theoretical foundations and manual]*. Beltz.

Lazarus, R. S., & Folkman, S. (1984). *Stress, appraisal, and coping*. Springer.

Lemyre, P.-N., Roberts, G. C., & Stray-Gundersen, J. (2007). Motivation, overtraining, and burnout: Can self-determination predict overtraining and burnout in elite athletes? *European Journal of Sport Science, 7*, 115–126.

Lichtenstein, M. B., Larsen, K. S., Christiansen, E., Støving, R. K., & Bredahl, T. V. G. (2014). Exercise addiction in team sport and

individual sport: Prevalences and validation of the exercise addiction inventory. *Addiction Research & Theory, 22*, 431–437.
Lindegård, A., Jonsdottir, I. H., Börjesson, M., Lindwall, M., & Gerber, M. (2015). Changes in mental health in compliers and non-compliers with physical activity recommendations in patients with stress-related exhaustion. *BMC Psychiatry, 15*, 272. https://doi.org/10.1186/s12888-12015-10642-12883

27

Lohaus, A. (2017). Stressmanagementtrainings für Kinder und Jugendliche [Coping training programs for children and adolescents]. In R. Fuchs & M. Gerber (Eds.), *Handbuch Stressregulation und Sport* (pp. 163–178). Springer.
Lovell, G. P., Huntsman, A., & Hedley-Ward, J. (2015). Psychological distress, depression, anxiety, stress, and exercise in Australian and New Zealand mothers: A cross-sectional survey. *Nursing & Health Sciences, 17*, 42–48.
Ludyga, S. (2017). Sportaktivität, Stress und das Gehirn. In R. Fuchs & M. Gerber (Eds.), *Handbuch Stressregulation und Sport* (pp. 275–291). Springer.
Luthar, S. S., Sawyer, J. A., & Brown, P. J. (2006). Conceptual issues in studies of resilience: Past, present, and future research. *Annals of the New York Academy of Sciences, 1094*, 105–115.
Lutz, R., Stults-Kolehmainen, M., & Bartholomew, J. (2010). Exercise caution when stressed: Stages of change and the stress-exercise participation relationship. *Psychology of Sport and Exercise, 11*, 560–567.
Marmot, M. G. (2003). Understanding social inequalities in health. *Perspectives in Biology and Medicine, 46*, S9–S23.
Maslach, C. (1976). Burned-out. *Human Behavior, 9*, 16–22.
Masten, A. S. (2001). Ordinary magic: Resilience processes in development. *American Psychologist, 56*, 227–238.
Matthews, K. A., Katholi, C. R., McCreath, H., Whooley, M. A., Williams, D. R., Zhu, S., & Markovitz, J. H. (2004). Blood pressure reactivity to psychological stress predicts hypertension in the CARDIA study. *Circulation, 110*, 74–78.
McEwen, B. S. (2013). The brain on stress: Toward an integrative approach to brain, body, and behavior. *Perspectives on Psychological Science, 8*, 673–675.
McEwen, B. S., & Stellar, E. (1993). Stress and the individual. Mechanisms leading to disease. *Archives of Internal Medicine, 153*, 2093–2101.
McEwen, B. S., & Wingfield, J. C. (2003). The concept of allostasis in biology and biomedicine. *Hormones and Behavior, 43*, 2–15.
McNair, D. M., Lorr, M., & Droppleman, L. F. (1971). *Manual of the profile of mood states*. Educational and Industrial Testing Services.
Meeusen, R., Duclos, M., Foster, C., Fry, A., Gleeson, M., Nieman, D., Raglin, J., Rietjens, G., Steinacker, J., & Urhausen, A. (2013). Prevention, diagnosis, and treatment of the overtraining syndrome: Joint consensus statement of the European College of Sport Science and the American College of Sports Medicine. *Medicine and Science in Sports and Exercise, 45*, 186–205.
Mellalieu, S. D., Neil, R., Hanton, S., & Fletcher, D. (2009). Competition stress in sport performers: Stressors experienced in the competition environment. *Journal of Sports Sciences, 27*, 729–744.
Miller, G. E., Cohen, S., & Ritchey, A. K. (2002). Chronic psychological stress and the regulation of pro-inflammatory cytokines: A glucocorticoid-resistance model. *Health Psychology, 21*, 531–541.
Monroe, K. L., & Harkness, S. M. (2005). Life stress, the "kindling" hypothesis, and the recurrence of depression: Considerations from a life stress perspective. *Psychological Review, 112*, 417–445.
Morin, C. M., Rodrigue, S., & Ivers, H. (2003). Role of stress, arousal, and coping skills in primary insomnia. *Psychosomatic Medicine, 65*, 259–267.
Moriya, J., & Takahashi, Y. (2013). Depression and interpersonal stress: The mediating role of emotion regulation. *Motivation and Emotion, 37*, 600–608.
Mücke, M., Ludyga, S., Colledge, F., & Gerber, M. (2018). Influence of regular physical activity and fitness on stress reactivity as measured with the Trier Social Stress Test protocol: A systematic review. *Sports Medicine, 48*, 2607–2622.
Nil, R., Joacobshagen, N., Schächinger, H., Baumann, P., Höck, P., Hättenschwiler, J., Ramseier, F., Seifritz, E., & Holsboer-Trachsler, E. (2010). Burnout—Eine Standortbestimmung [Burnout—A position assessment]. *Schweizer Archiv für Neurologie und Psychiatrie, 161*, 72–77.
O'Donnell, M. J., Xavier, D., Liu, L., Zhang, H., Chin, S., Rao-Melacini, P., Rangarajan, S., Islam, S., Pais, P., McQueen, M. J., Mondon, C., Damasceno, A., Lopez-Jaramillo, P., Hankey, G. J., Dans, A. L., Yusoff, K., Truelsen, T., Diener, H. C., Sacco, R. L., Ryglewicz, D., Czlonkowska, A., Weimar, C., Wang, X., Yusuf, S., & Interstroke investigators. (2010). Risk factors for ischaemic and intracerebral haemorrhagic stroke in 22 countries (the INTERSTROKE study): A case control study. *Lancet, 376*, 112–123.
O'Dougherty, M., Hearst, M. O., Syed, M., Kurzer, M. S., & Schmitz, K. H. (2012). Life events, perceived stress and depressive symptoms in a physical activity intervention with young adult women. *Mental Health and Physical Activity, 5*, 148–154.
Oaten, M., & Cheng, K. (2005). Academic examination stress impairs self-control. *Journal of Social and Clinical Psychology, 24*, 254–279.
Pacella, M. L., Hruska, B., & Delahanty, D. L. (2013). The physical health consequences of PTSD and PTSD symptoms: A meta-analytic review. *Journal of Anxiety Disorders, 27*, 33–46.
Paykel, E. S. (2001). Stress and affective disorders in humans. *Seminars in Clinical Neuropsychiatry, 6*, 4–11.
Pietrzak, R. H., Goldstein, R. B., Southwick, S. M., & Grant, B. F. (2011). Medical comorbidity of full and partial posttraumatic stress disorder in US adults: Results from wave 2 of the National Epidemiologic Survey on Alcohol and Related Conditions. *Psychosomatic Medicine, 73*, 697–707.
Powers, M. B., Medina, J. L., Burns, S., Kauffman, B. Y., Monfils, M., Asmundson, G. J., Diamond, A., McIntyre, C., & Smits, J. A. (2015). Exercise augmentation of exposure therapy for PTSD: Rationale and pilot efficacy data. *Cognitive Behaviour Therapy, 44*, 314–327.
Pühse, U., Barker, D., Brettschneider, W.-D., Feldmeth, A. K., Gerlach, E., McGuaig, L., McKenzie, T. L., & Gerber, M. (2011). International approaches to health-oriented physical education: Local health debates and differing conceptions of health. *International Journal of Physical Education, 3*, 2–15.
Puterman, E., Lin, J., Blackburn, E., O'Donovan, A., Adler, N., & Epel, E. (2010). The power of exercise: Buffering the effect of chronic stress on telomere length. *PLoS One, 5*, e10837.
Puterman, E., O'Donovan, A., Adler, N. E., Tomiyama, A. J., Kemeny, M., Wolkowitz, O. M., & Epel, E. (2011). Physical activity moderates effects of stressor-induced rumination on cortisol reactivity. *Psychosomatic Medicine, 73*, 604–611.
Raedeke, T. D. (1997). Is athlete burnout more than stress? A commitment perspective. *Journal of Sport and Exercise Psychology, 19*, 396–417.
Raedeke, T. D., & Smith, A. L. (2001). Development and preliminary validation of an athlete burnout measure. *Journal of Sport and Exercise Psychology, 23*, 281–306.
Ramaciotti, D., & Perriard, J. (2001). *Les coûts du stress en Suisse [stress-related costs in Switzerland]*. Staatssekretariat für Wirtschaft (SECO).

Reichert, M., Giurgiu, M., Koch, E., Wieland, L., Lautenbach, S., Neubauer, A., von Haaren-Mack, B., Schilling, R., Timm, I., Notthoff, N., Marzi, I., Hill, H., Brüssler, S., Eckert, T., Fiedler, J., Burchartz, A., Anedda, B., Wunsch, K., Gerber, M., Jekauc, D., Woll, A., Dunton, G., Kanning, M., Nigg, C., Ebner-Priemer, U., & Liao, Y. (2020). Ambulatory assessment for physical activity research: State oft he science, best practices and future directions. *Psychology of Sport and Exercise, 50*, 101742.

Richartz, A., & Brettschneider, W. D. (1996). *Weltmeister werden und die Schule schaffen. Zur Doppelbelastung von Schule und Leistungstraining [Becoming world champion and passing the school. The double burden of school and performance training]*. Hofmann.

Rief, W., & Bernius, P. (2011). *Biofeedback: Grundlagen, Indikationen, Kommunikation, Vorgehen [Biofeedback: Basics, indications, communication and procedure]*. Schattauer.

Roemmich, J. N., Gurgol, C. M., & Epstein, L. H. (2003). Influence of an interpersonal laboratory stressor on youths' choice to be physically active. *Obesity Research, 11*, 1080–1087.

Rogers, T., & Landers, D. (2005). Mediating effects of peripheral vision in the life event stress/athletic injury relationship. *Journal of Sport and Exercise Psychology, 27*, 271–288.

Rosenbaum, S., Sherrington, C., & Tiedemann, A. (2015). Exercise augmentation compared with usual care for post-traumatic stress disorder: A randomized controlled trial. *Acta Psychiatrica Scandinavica, 131*, 350–359.

Rosenbaum, S., Stubbs, B., Schuch, F., & Vancampfort, D. (2017). Exercise and posttraumatic stress disorder (PTSD). In R. Fuchs & M. Gerber (Eds.), *Handbuch Stressregulation und Sport* (pp. 375–387). Springer.

Rozanski, A., Blumenthal, J. A., Davidson, K. W., Saab, P. G., & Kubzansky, L. (2005). The epidemiology, pathophysiology, and management of psychosocial risk factors in cardiac practice: The emerging field of behavioral cardiology. *Journal of the American College of Cardiology, 45*, 637–651.

Russ, T. C., Stamatakis, E., Hamer, M., Starr, J. M., Kivimäki, M., & Batty, G. D. (2012). Association between psychological distress and mortality: Individual participant pooled analysis of 10 prospective cohort studies. *BMJ, 345*, e4933. https://doi.org/10.1136/bmj.e4993

Rutters, F., Pilz, S., Koopman, A. D., Rauh, S. P., Te Velde, S. J., Stehouwer, C. D., Elders, P., Nijpels, G., & Dekker, J. M. (2014). The association between psychosocial stress and mortality is mediated by lifestyle and chronic diseases: The Hoorn study. *Social Science and Medicine, 118*, 166–172.

Sallen, J. (2017). Stress-Resistenz-Trainings für Topathleten [Stress resistance trainings for elite athletes]. In R. Fuchs & M. Gerber (Eds.), *Handbuch Stressregulation und Sport* (pp. 505–535). Springer.

Schilling, R., Herrmann, C., Ludyga, S., Colledge, F., Brand, R., Pühse, U., & Gerber, M. (2020). Does cardiorespiratory fitness buffer stress reactivity and stress recovery in police officers? A real-life study. *Frontiers in Psychology, 11*, 594.

Schnohr, P., Kristensen, T. S., Prescott, E., & Scharling, H. (2005). Stress and life dissatisfaction are inversely associated with jogging and other types of physical activity in leisure time—The Copenhagen City Heart Study. *Scandinavian Journal of Medicine and Science in Sports, 15*, 107–112.

Schuler, J. L., & O'Brien, W. H. (1997). Cardiovascular recovery from stress and hypertension risk factors: A meta-analytic review. *Psychophysiology, 34*, 649–659.

Schwenkmezger, P., Hodapp, V., & Spielberger, C. D. (1992). *Das State-Trait-Ärgerausdrucksinventar STAXI: Handbuch [State-Trait-Anger Inventory STAXI: User manual]*. Huber.

Segal, Z. V., Williams, J. M., Teasdale, J. D., & Gemar, M. (1996). A cognitive science perspective on kindling and episode sensitization in recurrent affective disorder. *Psychological Medicine, 26*, 371–380.

Segerstrom, S. C., & Miller, G. E. (2004). Psychological stress and the human immune system: A meta-analytic study of 30 years of inquiry. *Psychological Bulletin, 130*, 601–630.

Selye, H. (1956). *The stress of life*. McGraw-Hill.

Semmer, N. K., & Zapf, D. (2017). Theorien der Stressentstehung und -bewältigung [Theories of stress generation and coping]. In R. Fuchs & M. Gerber (Eds.), *Handbuch Stressregulation und Sport* (pp. 23–50). Springer.

Siegrist, J. (2008). Chronic psychosocial stress at work and risk of depression: Evidence from prospective studies. *European Archives of Psychiatry and Clinical Neuroscience, 258*, 115–119.

Siegrist, J. (2017). Soziale Stressoren und stressbedingte Erkrankungen [Social stressors and stress-related diseases]. In R. Fuchs & M. Gerber (Eds.), *Handbuch Stressregulation und Sport* (pp. 79–92). Springer.

Siegrist, J., Starke, D., Chandola, T., Godin, I., Marmot, M., Niedhammer, I., & Peter, R. (2004). The measurement of effort-reward imbalance at work: European comparisons. *Social Science & Medicine, 58*, 1483–1499.

Silva, J. M. (1990). An analysis of the training stress syndrome in competitive athletics. *The Journal of Applied Sport Psychology, 2*, 5–20.

Smith, R. E. (1986). Toward a cognitive-affective model of athletic burnout. *Journal of Sport Psychology, 8*, 36–50.

Sonnentag, S., & Jelden, S. (2009). Job stressors and the pursuit of sport activities: A day-level perspective. *Journal of Occupational Health Psychology, 14*, 165–181.

Sothmann, M. S. (2006). The cross-stressor adaptation hypothesis and exercise training. In E. O. Acevedo & P. Ekkekakis (Eds.), *Psychobiology of physical activity* (pp. 149–160). Human Kinetics.

Staatssekretariat für Wirtschaft. (2011). Stressstudie 2010. Stress bei Schweizer Erwerbstätigen. Zusammenhänge zwischen Arbeitsbedingungen, Personenmerkmalen, Befinden und Gesundheit [Stress study 2010. Stress among Swiss employees. Associations between working conditions, personality traits, well-being and health]. Staatssekretariat für Wirtschaft (SECO).

Steptoe, A., & Kivimäki, M. (2013). Stress and cardiovascular disease: An update on current knowledge. *Annual Review of Public Health, 34*, 337–354.

Stetler, C., & Miller, G. E. (2011). Depression and hypothalamic-pituitary-adrenal activation: A quantitative summary of four decades of research. *Psychosomatic Medicine, 73*, 114–126.

Stults-Kolehmainen, M. A., & Sinha, R. (2014). The effects of stress on physical activity and exercise. *Sports Medicine, 44*, 81–121.

Szabo, A., Griffiths, M. D., de La Vega Marcos, R., Mervó, B., & Demetrovics, Z. (2015). Methodological and conceptual limitations in exercise addiction research. *The Yale Journal of Biology and Medicine, 88*, 303–308.

Szabo, A. P., De La Vega, R., Ruiz-Barquín, R., & R., O. (2013). Exercise addiction in Spanish athletes: Investigation of the roles of gender, social context and level of involvement. *Journal of Behavioral Addictions, 2*, 249–252.

Taylor, D. J. (2008). Insomnia and depression. *Sleep, 31*, 447–448.

Taylor, J., & Ogilvie, B. C. (1994). A conceptual model of adaptation to retirement among athletes. *Journal of Applied Sport Psychology, 6*, 1–20.

Tranaeus, U., Ivarsson, A., & Johnson, U. (2015). Evaluation of the effects of psy-chological prevention interventions on sport injuries: A meta-analysis. *Science & Sports, 30*, 305–313.

Tranaeus, U., Ivarsson, A., & Johnson, U. (2017). Stress and injuries in elite sport. In R. Fuchs & M. Gerber (Eds.), *Handbuch Stressregulation und Sport* (pp. 451–466). Springer.

27

Treiber, F. A., Kamarck, T., Schneiderman, N., Sheffield, D., Kapuku, G., & Taylor, T. (2003). Cardiovascular reactivity and development of preclinical and clinical disease states. *Psychosomatic Medicine, 65*, 46–62.

Trott, M., Jackson, S. E., Firth, J., Fisher, A., Johnstone, J., Mistry, A., Stubbs, B., & Smith, L. (2020). Exercise addiction prevalence and correlates in the absence of eating disorder symptomology: A systematic review and meta-analysis. *Journal of Additiona Medicine, 14*(6), e321–e329. https://doi.org/10.1097/ADM.0000000000000664

Tsai, H., Yeh, C., Su, C., Chen, C., Peng, S., & Chen, R. (2013). The effects of exercise program on burnout and metabolic syndrome components in banking and insurance workers. *Industrial Health, 51*, 336–346.

Uchino, B. N., Smith, T. W., Holt-Lunstad, J., Campo, R., & Reblin, M. (2007). Stress and illness. In J. T. Cacioppo, G. Tassinary, & G. G. Berntson (Eds.), *Handbook of psychophysiology* (pp. 608–632). Cambridge University Press.

Vanden Auweele, Y., De Martelaer, K., Rzewnicki, R., De Knop, P., & Wylleman, P. (2004). Parents and coaches: A help or harm? Affective outcomes for children in sport. In Y. Vanden Auweele (Ed.), *Ethics in youth sport* (pp. 85–102). Lannoocampu.

von Dawans, B., & Heinrichs, M. (2017). Physiologische Stressreaktionen [Physiological stress reactivity]. In R. Fuchs & M. Gerber (Eds.), *Handbuch Stressregulation und Sport* (pp. 67–78). Springer.

von Dawans, B., Kirschbaum, C., & Heinrichs, M. (2011). The Trier Social Stress Test for Groups (TSST-G): A new research tool for controlled simultaneous social stress exposure in a group format. *Psychoneuroendocrinology, 36*, 514–522.

von Haaren, B., Haertel, S., Stumpp, J., Hey, S., & Ebner-Priemer, U. (2015). Reduced emotional stress reactivity to a real-life academic examination stressor in students participating in a 20-week aerobic exercise training: A randomised controlled trial using Ambulatory Assessment. *Psychology of Sport and Exercise, 20*, 67–75.

von Haaren, B., Ottenbacher, J., Muenz, J., Neumann, R., Boes, K., & Ebner-Priemer, U. (2016). Does a 20-week aerobic exercise training programme increase our capabilities to buffer real-life stressors? A randomized, controlled trial using ambulatory assessment. *European Journal of Applied Physiology, 116*, 383–394.

Watson, D., Clark, L. A., & Tellegen, A. (1988). Development and validation of brief measures of positive and negative affect: The PANAS scales. *Journal of Personality and Social Psychology, 54*, 1063–1070.

Wegman, H. L., & Stetler, C. (2009). A meta-analytic review of the effects of childhood abuse on medical outcomes in adulthood. *Psychosomatic Medicine, 71*, 805–812.

Williams, J. M., & Andersen, M. B. (1998). Psychosocial antecedents of sport injury: Review and critique of the stress and injury model. *Journal of Applied Sport Psychology, 10*, 5–25.

Wunsch, K., & Gerber, M. (2017). Sportaktivität, Stress und Burnout. In R. Fuchs & M. Gerber (Eds.), *Handbuch Stressregulation und Sport* (pp. 343–374). Springer.

Wylleman, P., Alfermann, D., & Lavallee, D. (2004). Career transitions in sport: European perspectives. *Psychology of Sport and Exercise, 5*, 7–20.

Yusuf, S., Hawken, S., Ounpuuz, S., Dans, T., Avezum, A., Lanas, F., McQueen, M., Budaj, A., Pais, P., Varigos, J., Lisheng, L., & INTERHEART Study Investigators. (2004). Effect of potentially modifiable risk factors associated with myocardial infarction in 52 countries (the INTERHEART study): Case-control study. *Lancet, 2004*, 937–952.

Zen, A. L., Whooley, M. A., Zhao, S. J., & Cohen, B. E. (2012). Posttraumatic stress disorder is associated with poor health behaviors: Findings from the Heart and Soul Study. *Health Psychology, 31*, 194–201.

Exercise, Health Disorders, and Injuries

Martin Kopp, Martin Niedermeier and Matthew P. Herring

Contents

J. Schüler et al. (eds.), *Sport and Exercise Psychology*, https://doi.org/10.1007/978-3-031-03921-8_28

28

Learning Objectives

Basic:

- You will know for what mental disorders exercise is a successful intervention and how strong the effects are.
- You will be able to evaluate the effects of exercise on people with physical health disorders.
- You can list mental and physical disorders for which the effects of exercise have been tested empirically.
- You will know about the acute effects of single bouts of exercise and the chronic effects of exercise programs on different aspects of mental and physical health.
- You will be able to list mental and physical risks and side effects connected to exercise.

Advanced:

- You can summarize the effects of exercise at a higher level of abstraction (not just subfindings).
- You can be able to describe the influence of intensity and duration of single bouts of exercise on affective states in persons with health disorders.
- You will know about the importance of exercise in the context of prevention and treatment of mental and physical health disorders.
- You will know why exercise is expected to be effective in the treatment of mental health disorders.

Experts:

- You can be able to explain the importance of considering acute effects of single bouts of exercise.
- You can be able to enumerate and describe adequate assessments of exercise psychology in patient populations.
- You will be able to list hypothesized mechanisms of exercise in persons with disorders.

28.1 Introduction

Exercise is seen as a preventive behavior against various health problems such as cardiovascular diseases or diabetes (Pedersen & Saltin, 2015). Although the preventive effect of exercise is repeated mantra-like, it does not necessarily lead to increased engagement in exercise and thus reduced likelihood of certain health problems occurring. Over the past three decades, there has been a massive increase in knowledge about the potential of exercise in the treatment of a wide range of health disorders. Less research activity in the context of exercise was conducted when disorders had already been diagnosed, where mainly rest and relaxation was prescribed. The aim of the present chapter is to shed more light on the psychological effects of exercise among people with physical or mental health impairments.

Although physical activity (opposed to exercise) has the potential to show preventive and rehabilitative effects, we focus on exercise in the present chapter given the structured nature of the interventions used in the studies (▶ Chapter 25 for further differentiation of physical activity and exercise). An indication of the preventive potential of physical activity in psychosocially challenging periods is illustrated in the Side Story.

Physical Activity and Exercise

Any movement of the human body produced by skeletal muscles that results in energy expenditure is referred to as **physical activity. Exercise** is a subset of physical activity that is planned, structured, and repetitive, for the purpose of enhancing or maintaining one or more components of fitness (Caspersen et al., 1985).

Side Story

The Potential of Physical Activity for Mental Health in the Coronavirus Pandemic

Physical inactivity and mental illness are long-standing pandemics in their own right, which also appear to have worsened during the recent COVID-19 pandemic. For example, cross-sectional data have suggested that reduced physical activity connected to the pandemic restrictions may lead to negative effects on mental health. In a study of more than 3000 adults, among those who met physical activity guidelines prior to the pandemic, no longer meeting physical activity guidelines after the restrictions was associated with depressive symptoms, loneliness, and stress and with lower positive mental health. Although correlational in nature, these data support that maintained or increased physical activity may mitigate negative pandemic-related psychological consequences (Meyer et al., 2020).

Regarding physical health disorders, it is estimated that physical inactivity was responsible for US$ 53.8 billion of direct health care costs worldwide in 2013 (Ding et al., 2016). In addition, the loss of more than 13 million disability-adjusted life years (DALYs; definition: burden of disease) worldwide is attributed to physical inactivity (Ding et al., 2016).

Although the effects of exercise interventions can be discussed in the context of recovery from physical health impairments, including recurrence-free time or survival time, consistent with the aims of this chapter, exercise effects on both symptoms of clinically relevant mental health impairments and affective state and health-related quality of life will be discussed.

Burden of Disease

Various measures are available to quantify the burden of disease or behavior in society. The World Health Organization uses, among others, the measure of *disability-adjusted life years* (DALYs). DALYs are calculated based on the sum of the years of life lost due both to the disease itself and to the disability/disabilities associated with the disease. A lost DALY therefore represents the loss of a "healthy" year of life. The larger the number of DALYs caused by a health disorder, the higher the burden of disease of this disorder.

Perspectives on Exercise and Health

The division into four chapters on health in this book (▶ Chaps. 25, 26, 27, and 28) reflects a simplified principle of order that could be used as a basis for exercise psychology research on the connection between exercise and health. The different priorities can be demonstrated by the contents of various related disciplines that are used for explanation. Practice and research are of course more complex than a simple division into four components and the boundaries between these components are more fluid. This is also partially expressed in overlaps between the chapters in this book.

- "Models explaining health behavior change and physical activity" (▶ Chap. 25): The models outlined here are based on the basic idea that many diseases are caused by behavior and that health can be achieved by changes in behavior. The models include various variables (e.g., predictors of health intention formation) and focus on health intention formation or on the process of intention realization.
- "Sports, well-being, and mental health" (▶ Chap. 26): This area of research in exercise psychology focuses on the interaction between exercise and well-being. Well-being (emotional state, life satisfaction) is mainly considered here in the "normal," i.e., not deviating from the norm, subclinical population. The research findings reported in ▶ Chap. 26 refer to persons considered healthy. The theoretical sources stem from emotion psychology, but also from related disciplines such as public health research. An important focus of research here is on the specifications of how and under which circumstances (duration, frequency) exercise increases positive well-being and reduces negative emotional states. Research in the clinically relevant area (e.g., anxiety disorders, depression) either is connected here (as a quantitative gradation of the reduction of well-being, so to speak) or puts emphasis on the qualitative differences between nonclinical and clinical populations and thus falls into the fourth category "Sports, diseases, and injuries" (▶ Chap. 28).
- "Sports, stress, and health" (▶ Chap. 27): Another area of research in exercise psychology, which is strongly influenced by medical and biological psychology in terms of theory and measurement methods, focuses on the effects of exercise on physical and psychological changes. Stress is understood here as a physiological (e.g., endocrine processes) and psychological phenomenon (e.g., cognitive assessment processes).
- "Sports, diseases, and injuries" (▶ Chap. 28) deals with the effects of exercise in people with clinically relevant health disorders. In contrast to the previous chapters on health, research findings from populations with various physical and mental disorders are reported. Focus is put on the corresponding severity of the disorder (e.g., symptoms of anxiety or depression) or associated psychological symptoms (e.g., health-related quality of life, affective state).

In addition to physical health disorders, the prevalence and incidence rates of **mental health disorders** have increased dramatically in recent decades. The number of lost DALYs caused by mental health problems has increased by almost 40% from 1990 to 2010 (Murray et al., 2012), and frontline treatments have demonstrated limited success. Thus, exercise is more intensively discussed as a relevant treatment option in mental health disorders.

Since it will not be possible to present a comprehensive overview of exercise effects in all mental and physical disorders in the present chapter, disorders were selected according to the available World Health Organization reports on the main causes of death ("Global Burden of Disease") and the availability of controlled studies on exercise effects in the respective disorders (GBD 2015 Mortality and Causes of Death Collaborators, 2016). The highest available level of evidence was referenced to draw the most rigorous and informed possible conclusions. Results of meta-analyses or systematic reviews with randomized controlled trials are included in the highest level of evidence (level 1a evidence; compare Levels of Evidence according to the Oxford Centre for Evidence-Based Medicine, ◘ Table 28.1). Effect sizes (ES) are specified to quantify the magnitude of the effect. The most commonly used effect sizes for metrically scaled variables are Cohen's d (Cohen, 1988) and Hedges' g (Hedges, 1981). The effect sizes are categorized into low (0.2), medium (0.5), and high (0.8). This classification is also used in the present chapter.

28

Table 28.1 Levels of Evidence according to the Oxford Centre for Evidence-Based Medicine (OCEBM Levels of Evidence Working Group, 2009)

1a	Systematic review of randomized controlled studies
1b	Single randomized controlled study
2a	Systematic review of cohort studies
2b	Single cohort study
3a	Systematic review of case-control studies
3b	Single case-control study
4	Series of case studies
5	Expert opinion

Simplified according to the OCEBM Levels of Evidence Working Group (2009)

28.2 Exercise as Intervention and Rehabilitation in Health Disorders

Acute and Chronic Effects of Exercise

Research on exercise as an intervention in health disorders focuses on both acute effects of single bouts of exercise and chronic effects of exercise programs lasting for several weeks. At present, it is not yet possible to answer the question of whether chronic effects are caused by an accumulation of acute effects or whether there is a change in behavior and experience (Taylor & Faulkner, 2008). However, the connection between acute and chronic effects is of clear interest.

The consideration of **acute** effects of single bouts of exercise is important in patients for several reasons:

1. Many health disorders are treated with pharmacological and/or psychological therapy. These treatment options usually take some time to be fully effective. Because the effect of exercise on mood states and mental health outcomes may start immediately, the time until conventional treatment methods are effective may be bridged or augmented by exercise (Cooney et al., 2013; Stark et al., 2012).
2. The subjective assessment and affective state during and immediately following certain types of behavior, such as exercise, may influence the decision to continue this type of behavior in the future (Ekkekakis et al., 2004). This applies both to the decision, e.g., to start a physically active lifestyle and to the decision to maintain this lifestyle in the future (Ekkekakis et al., 2011; Rhodes & Kates, 2015; Williams et al., 2008), which is well supported on a theoretical basis by the "self-determination theory" (▶ Chap. 8) or the "hedonic theory," definition: hedonic theory).
3. The regulation of the affective state plays an important role in the treatment of patients with mental health disorders. It is not only important to know how the affective state develops in the long term, but also how the affective state changes due to single bouts of exercise (Bartholomew et al., 2005; Joormann et al., 2007).
4. Among otherwise healthy adults and adults with physical and mental health impairments, acute exercise has been shown to improve mood states and mental health outcomes, including anxiety (Ensari et al., 2015; Herring et al., 2017a, 2017b, 2019), feelings of depressed mood (Meyer et al., 2016a, 2016b), and feelings of energy (Herring & O'Connor, 2009; Legrand et al., 2018; Loy et al., 2013). Improved mood states and mental health outcomes are directly related to the quality of life and exercise-induced improvements can therefore cumulatively contribute to improve quality of life.

Hedonic Theory

According to the **hedonic theory**, the majority of people act in the sense of maximizing pleasure and avoiding suffering. This means that future behavior is influenced by the affective state during or immediately after behavior. Accordingly, behavior is more likely to start or be maintained if the affective state is assessed positively (Kahneman, 1999).

When considering the acute effects of single bouts of exercise in exercise psychology, effects on the **affective state** are of particular interest. Readers are referred to the detailed description of the connection between exercise and the affective state in ▶ Chap. 26 (where the term "affective well-being" is used).

In addition to the affective state, **craving** for substances and withdrawal symptoms are considered, especially in patients with addiction disorders. The substance demand is usually assessed based on self-report (e.g., MacKillop, 2006). Unidimensional, multidimensional, and language-free procedures are available for the assessment of the self-reported substance demand. An overview of the assessment methods can be found in Sayette et al. (2000). On the one hand, exercise may have the potential to induce acute, short-term reduced craving for substances, and on the other hand, acute effects of exercise on craving are interesting to gain insight into the potential mechanisms for the chronic effects of exercise programs (Roberts et al., 2012).

When considering the **chronic** effects of exercise programs as an intervention in mental health disorders, the effect on the symptoms of the disorder is primarily relevant.

Exercise Programs as an Intervention for Mental Health Disorders

Fox (2000) gives several reasons why exercise can be effective in the treatment of mental health disorders:

1. Exercise is associated with minimal harmful side effects.
2. The positive effects of exercise on markers of physical health are well documented. Therefore, exercise can be recommended solely on this basis, regardless of potential effects on mental health. This aspect is particularly important because mental health problems are often comorbidities in chronically ill patients.
3. Although little is known about dose-response, exercise is largely accessible and can be applied almost endlessly. In contrast, pharmacological or psychological-psychotherapeutic procedures are usually limited in time.
4. Exercise programs are largely associated with low costs compared to that of other treatment options.
5. Exercise programs can also be used by patients who do not have access to other treatment options, e.g., due to waiting lists and/or lack of financial resources.

The presence and severity of mental disorders is usually clinically diagnosed by the attending physician or psychologist using diagnostic interviews, behavioral observation, and if necessary external information. Rating scales as well as standardized, empirically validated psychological inventories (e.g., "Beck Depression Inventory" (Beck et al., 1996), "Hamilton Rating Scale for Depression" (Hamilton, 1967), "State Trait Anxiety Inventory" (Spielberger et al., 1970), "Hospital Anxiety and Depression Scale" (Zigmond & Snaith, 1983), "Centre for Epidemiological Studies Depression Scale" (Radloff, 1977), "Penn State Worry Questionnaire" (Meyer et al., 1990)) are also used as primary outcomes of chronic effects of exercise programs. Usually, the subscale score of these scales is used as a parameter for the severity of symptoms of the disorder, which is compared to other interventions (e.g., control, placebo, pharmacological or psychological interventions) before and after an exercise intervention.

In addition, the construct of **quality of life** is considered as an indicator of the subjective biopsychosocial state of an individual in relation to his or her own culture and value systems.

Quality of Life

Unfortunately, no overall accepted definition of the construct of **quality of life** is available. The World Health Organization defines quality of life as follows: Quality of life is a person's subjective perception of his or her position in life in relation to the culture and value systems in which he or she lives and in relation to his or her goals, expectations, standards, and concerns. It can be described as a multidimensional concept that depends in a complex way on the physical health of the person, psychosocial status, degree of independence, social relationships, personal beliefs, and the relationship to essential characteristics of a person's environment (World Health Organization, 1998a, 1998b).

The perception of the individual plays a major role in the assessment of quality of life; therefore, questionnaires are usually used. The frequently used questionnaires are the World Health Organization (World Health Organization, 1998a, 1998b) and the "Medical Outcome Studies Short Form Health Survey 36" (Ware & Sherbourne, 1992). An overview of potential methods for assessing quality of life, often referred to as patient-reported outcomes (PRO), is presented in Fayers and Machin (2013). The construct of quality of life is considered more consistent and less sensitive to short-term changes compared to affective states.

In patients with chronic disorders, the construct of **fatigue** is also important (Fig. 28.1). Fatigue may be operationalized through the subjective perception of a reduced capacity to complete physical and mental activities and is characterized by a state of tiredness that does not disappear due to sleeping or resting. Fatigue occurs frequently in the context of oncological diseases, but is also discussed as an independent disorder (chronic

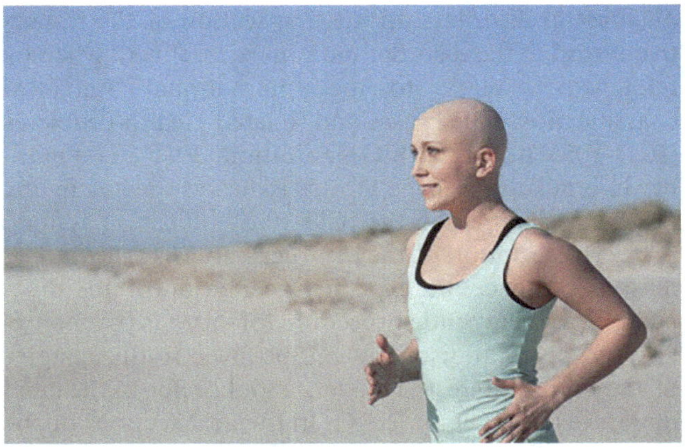

Fig. 28.1 Exercise against fatigue in chronic diseases

fatigue syndrome [CFS]). Similar to the quality of life, fatigue is measured using questionnaires. An overview of frequently used assessment methods for fatigue and their psychometric characteristics can be found in Dittner et al. (2004).

In patients with addiction disorders, the main outcomes in intervention research are the **abstinence or quit rate** or a possible change in the consumption behavior. To be able to consider an intervention successful, it is relevant how many of those affected implement a successful change in behavior and how long the effects last. In addition, effects on psychological constructs such as anxiety or depression are often assessed as secondary parameters.

28.2.1 Exercise as Intervention for Persons with Mental Disorders

First, it should be noted that people with severe mental disorders are likely to die 10 to 20 years earlier compared to that of the general population (Liu et al., 2017). This reduced life expectancy is documented in several meta-analyses and systematic reviews. From a physical health perspective, people with mental disorders have a two to three times higher risk of dying from cardiovascular diseases, respiratory diseases, or infections; in the case of respiratory diseases, this is even true after adjustment for tobacco use and other substance abuse (Liu et al., 2017). In addition to recording the effects of lifestyle modifications such as exercise on mental health, this results in a call for action in psychiatric treatment settings and rehabilitation facilities to improve the general health behavior in people with severe mental disorders. An increase in engagement in exercise is to be considered a central issue in this respect.

The following is a summary of the current literature on the effectiveness of exercise interventions for various mental disorders. In the first section of the respective disorder, the disorder patterns are defined, whereby reference is made to the International Statistical Classification of Diseases and Related Health Problems (ICD-10; World Health Organization, 2015). The number in brackets after the groups indicates the key figure, i.e., the assignment in the ICD-10 classification system. A brief description of the disorder patterns follows. For reasons of space, no explicit presentation of the diagnostic and therapeutic procedure for various psychological and physical disorders can be given in this chapter of the book. Interested readers should refer to the cited literature (Davis et al., 2014). In the next sections of the respective disorder, a distinction is made between acute and chronic effects of exercise. Wherever no level 1a evidence (see above) is available, the results of individual controlled studies are reported.

28.2.1.1 Depressive Disorders

The **depressive episode** and the **recurrent depressive disorder** belong to the group of mood (affective) disorders (F30–F39).

> The term "depression" describes a change in mood, either as a single or as a recurring episode. Affected persons suffer from depressed mood, subjective worthlessness, sleep disturbances, and a reduction in drive and concentration and can also suffer physical health symptoms such as loss of appetite, loss of libido, and weight loss. Depending on the severity of the symptoms, a depressive disorder/episode is classified as mild, moderate, or severe.

The number of documented cases of depressive disorders worldwide in 2010 was 405 million cases. Depressive disorders constitute the largest proportion of mental health disorders and are responsible for more than 40% of lost DALYs due to mental and behavioral disorders worldwide (Whiteford et al., 2013). According to the World Health Organization (2017), depression is the leading cause of disability worldwide, affecting approximately 322 million persons. Because patients frequently do not respond to initial frontline treatments and may need multiple treatments to fully remit (Trivedi et al., 2006), there has been continued interest in alternative and augmentation therapies. Exercise has been recommended as a low-risk augmentation therapy for depression (Trivedi et al., 2011).

Acute Effects of Single Bouts of Exercise

A limited number of studies have supported that exercise of varying intensities improves affective states, including feelings of depressed mood and energy, among people with depression. Bartholomew et al. (2005) reported a larger increase in positive mood states (e.g., vitality) after single bouts of exercise in patients with depressive disorders compared to a control situation without exercise. The exercise bout consisted of 30 min of moderate walking on a treadmill (brisk walking). Both 5 and 30 min after the exercise bout, medium-sized effects were demonstrated (ES > 0.7). However, 1 h after the exercise units, the effect disappeared. In the dimensions of psychological distress, depression, confusion, lack of energy, tension, and anger, no different developments between the resting condition and the exercise unit could be observed. The authors concluded that exercise is suitable for short-term regulation of affective state in patients with depressive disorders.

More recently, Meyer et al. (2016b) reported significant improvements in feelings of depressed mood following counterbalanced 20-min bouts of light-, moderate-, or hard-intensity cycling exercise, compared to seated quiet rest, among 24 women with major depressive disorder. The effect persisted for 30 min following the bout, and findings suggested that exercise intensity was not critically important to the antidepressant response to a single session of exercise. In a separate session, participants manipulated the cycling workload in a "preferred" intensity condition, which was then compared to the light-, moderate-, and high-intensity "prescribed" session that most closely approximated the "preferred" intensity (Meyer et al., 2016a). Reductions in feelings of depressed mood were slightly greater after "prescribed" sessions compared to that of "preferred" sessions, which may have important implications for program development and prescription.

The positive effects may be enlarged if the exercise bout is conducted outdoors. In a study by Frühauf et al. (2016), patients with depressive disorders reported that they felt more energetic during and after the exercise unit compared to that of a resting control situation. The exercise bout consisted of moderate Nordic walking lasting for 60 min. A third exercise bout including moderate activity indoors (cycling) showed less positive affective changes compared to that of the exercise bout outdoors. It was concluded that patients with depressive disorders are likely to benefit directly from additional outdoor exercise bout in the sense of a positive regulation of affective state. However, these findings might be also attributable to the modality of exercise (opposed to the environment). A similar study among participants with mild-to-moderate depression using the identical form of exercise indoor and outdoor (20-min bout of moderate-intensity running) yielded discrepant results (Legrand et al., 2018). Both exercise bouts resulted in large improvements in feelings of energy compared to a sedentary control condition; however, the improvements were not statistically different between outdoor and indoor exercises.

Heggelund et al. (2014) intervened with a single high-intensity interval training bout (4 × 4 min at about 90% of maximal heart rate) and reported larger positive effects on the affective state 3 h after the exercise bout in people with depressive disorders compared to that of a healthy control group. Surprisingly, an exercise bout of only 16 min with high intensity showed positive effects several hours after the exercise bout. High-intensity bouts are usually perceived as unpleasant during exercise (Ekkekakis et al., 2010). High-intensity exercise can effectively increase aerobic performance, which is associated with additional positive health effects. The research team recommended the integration of high-intensity exercise bouts in the treatment of patients with depressive disorders—under appropriate supervision.

Chronic Effects of Exercise Programs Lasting for Several Weeks

More than 40 systematic reviews or meta-analyses have reported on exercise as a therapy for depression, which approximates the number of known trials (Physical Activity Guidelines Advisory Committee, 2018). In the current edition of a Cochrane meta-analysis (a kind of systematic review; Cochrane), Cooney et al. (2013) reported a mean positive effect of exercise interventions on depressive symptoms in patients with depressive disorders compared to that of no treatment control conditions (ES = 0.6) among more than 2300 patients in 39 included trials. When compared directly to psychotherapy and pharmacotherapy, there was no significant difference between the benefits of exercise training and these other empirically supported treatments. Thus, exercise programs can be seen as similarly effective as pharmacological or psychotherapeutic approaches in reducing depressive symptoms. The available data on potential effects on quality of life were not considered in this work.

> **Side Story**
>
> **Cochrane**
>
> Cochrane is an international, nonprofit network of scientists from various disciplines with the aim of generating evidence-based knowledge for the evaluation of medical therapies. Meta-analyses with standardized methodological criteria constitute the basis of the evaluation and Cochrane meta-analyses are seen as a high-quality information for assessing the effectiveness of medical therapies.

Ekkekakis (2015) stated in a critical commentary that the effect sizes successively decreased (~25% between 2009 and 2013 reviews) in the various updates of the Cochrane meta-analysis on exercise and depressive disorders since 2001. This decrease was attributed to methodological deficiencies, including selectivity biases; reanalysis with stricter inclusion criteria showed a recalculated effect size of ES = 0.9, which can be classified as a large effect. Reflections on the methodological approach to chronic effects of exercise programs in patients with depressive disorders can be also found in Schuch et al. (2017), whose updated review adjusted for publication bias and showed an ES = ~1 standard deviation.

Rosenbaum et al. (2014) reported similar findings among studies of patients with mental disorders rather than only depressive disorders. Based on the results of 20 studies and more than 1200 patients, large positive effects of exercise on depressive symptoms (ES = 0.8) and medium positive effects on quality of life (ES = 0.6) were reported. The control condition usually consisted of conventional therapy, but health education and placebo interventions (e.g., sitting on exercise equipment) also were used.

Studies did not permit a rigorous comparison based on exercise modality, frequency, intensity, and duration of exercise. However, studies with exercise programs that met recommended guidelines for aerobic activities and muscle-strengthening exercises according to recent guidelines (see below) showed larger effects compared to programs that did not (Dunn et al., 2005). Therefore, structured and supervised exercise programs that met exercise guidelines are recommended. In the majority of the studies, exercise programs of 10 weeks or more and aerobic exercise training, such as walking or cycling, were used.

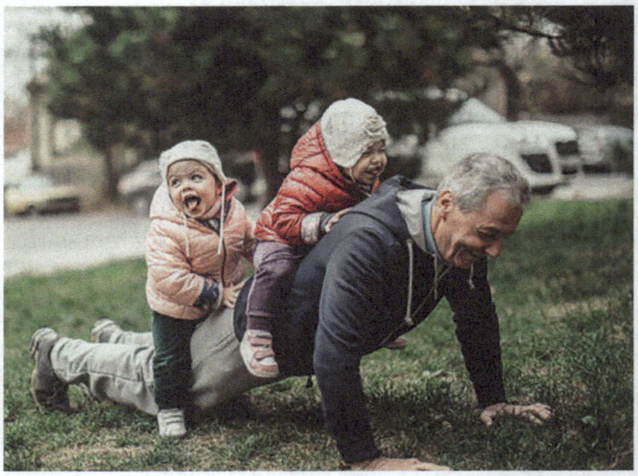

Fig. 28.2 (Playful) muscle-strengthening activities as part of the guidelines of the Physical Activity Guidelines Advisory Committee (2018)

Exercise in Practice

Recommendations According to the Physical Activity Guidelines Advisory Committee (2018)

The Physical Activity Guidelines Advisory Committee published exercise guidelines conducive to health that are based on current state of research. The recommendations for adults are given below (Fig. 28.2):

- Adults should engage in **aerobic activities** of moderate intensity for at least 150 to 300 min per week. Alternatively, adults should engage in 75 to 150 min of vigorous-intensity aerobic physical activity per week, or an equivalent combination of moderate- and vigorous-intensity aerobic activity. These activities should be ideally spread throughout the week.
- Engaging in physical activity of an equivalent longer than 300 min of moderate to vigorous intensity provides additional health benefits.
- In addition to aerobic activities, adults are encouraged to engage in **muscle-strengthening activities** for all major muscle groups on two or more days a week. Preferably, two to three sets of 8–12 repetitions with moderate or greater intensity should be conducted.

People who cannot or do not want to follow these recommendations should try to be physically active, as even lower levels of exercise are better than being physically inactive.

Comparable effects were also observed in adolescent and young adult patients (12 to 25 years; Bailey et al., 2018). Out of 17 studies analyzed, five studies were conducted with a total of 164 patients in a clinical setting. There was a reduction in depressive symptoms due to exercise programs compared to control interventions such as no intervention, waiting list, or treatment as usual (ES = 0.7). The uncertainty of the reported effects due to the lack of high-quality studies is criticized by the authors. Nevertheless, exercise programs in the treatment of depressive disorders in adolescence and young adulthood are considered promising by the authors. Similar to adults, moderate-intensity aerobic activities, which should last 8 weeks or more, are recommended.

The National Institute for Health and Care Excellence recommends structured and supervised programs (NICE Guidelines) with typically three sessions per week (duration of 45–60 min) for a duration of 10 to 12 weeks (National collaborating centre for mental health, 2010). It should be critically noted that a more recent review (Krogh et al., 2017)—similar to the most recent Cochrane meta-analysis (Cooney et al., 2013)—assumes that with increasing control of potentially outcome-relevant variables, the informative value of data on direct effects of exercise programs on depressive disorders tends to decline. Nevertheless, based on the available literature, it can be summarized that exercise as a supplement to cognitive-behavioral treatment approaches shows positive effects.

Effects of Exercise in Persons with Depressive Disorders

Exercise can have an antidepressant effect on people with depressive disorders. Exercise programs lasting several weeks show medium- to large-sized positive effects on depressive symptoms. The effects of exercise programs were comparable to the effects of pharmacological or psychotherapeutic approaches. There is less evidence of acute effects of exercise bouts; however, initial results indicate that single exercise bouts have a positive effect on the patient's affective state—a strategy that might be used to augment other empirically supported treatments, particularly until the patient responds to those treatments.

28.2.1.2 Anxiety Disorders

Phobic anxiety disorders and **other phobic anxiety disorders** belong to the group of neurotic, stress-related, and somatoform disorders (F40–F48). In patients with anxiety disorders, for the majority harmless situations cause anxiety, which leads to avoidance of the situation or to experiencing the situation with fear. Anxiety co-occurs often with a depressive disorder. Common forms of anxiety disorders include agoraphobia or generalized anxiety disorder.

A basic distinction is made between **trait anxiety** and **state anxiety** in the psychological approach to the construct of anxiety. Trait anxiety can be described as a general disposition to perceive stimuli as threatening, while state anxiety is described as the acute psychological and physiological reaction to a perceived threat (Spielberger et al., 1970). In the context of exercise psychology, state anxiety is assessed when focusing on acute effects of single bouts of exercise. When focusing on chronic exercise interventions, changes in trait anxiety, or general anxiety symptoms, are assessed.

In 2010, 274 million cases of anxiety disorders were registered worldwide. Anxiety disorders globally accounted for 390 disability-adjusted life years per 100,000 persons, making them the sixth leading cause of disability worldwide (Baxter et al., 2014; Whiteford et al., 2013) (◘ Fig. 28.3).

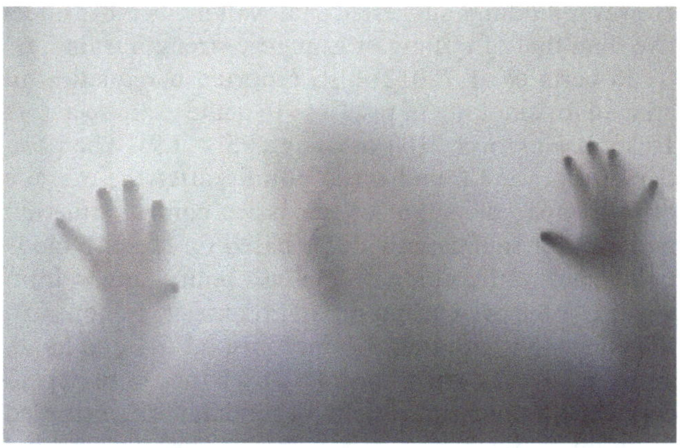

◘ **Fig. 28.3** Anxiety disorders are relatively common mental disorders and lead to severe impairment of quality of life

▪ Acute Effects of Single Bouts of Exercise

In the 1960s and 1970s, exercise was assumed to be associated with anxiety symptoms and panic attacks due to increased **lactate concentration** (Pitts Jr. & McClure Jr., 1967). This assumption was refuted (Grosz & Farmer, 1972; Morgan, 1979). However, compared to the healthy population, there are currently only a few studies on the direct effects of exercise and exercise in people with clinical anxiety disorders. Ensari et al. (2015) examined, in their meta-analysis of 36 RCTs, the acute effects of exercise bouts on symptoms of anxiety in healthy and diseased populations and reported small but significant anxiety-reducing effects (ES = 0.2). The authors noted that it is difficult to draw any meaningful conclusions about the acute effects of exercise among people with clinically relevant anxiety given only three randomized controlled trials (151 patients in total). However, the results were promising, as the observed effect strength was higher in clinical populations than that in healthy populations; large positive effects were reported in two of the three randomized controlled trials (ES $\geq$ 0.8).

More recent evidence has highlighted the anxiolytic effects of acute exercise among young adults with elevated worry symptoms indicative of subclinical or analogue generalized anxiety disorder (GAD), who are more likely to develop future clinically significant psychopathologies (Wolitzky-Taylor et al., 2014). In the first study, compared to 30 min of quiet rest, 17 young adult women with analogue GAD showed moderate to large (ES = 0.44 to 1.69) improvements in state anxiety and feelings of energy following 30 min of vigorous-intensity (~70% heart rate reserve) treadmill running (Herring et al., 2017b). A second study replicated the positive effects of 30 min of vigorous acute aerobic exercise among young adult women with analogue GAD, including clinically meaningful improvement in feelings of energy (ES = 1.35) and a potentially clinically meaningful improvement in worry (ES = 0.53); additionally, this study extended the previous study to support positive effects among young adult men with analogue GAD, including a clinically meaningful improvement in feelings of energy (ES = 0.92) (Herring et al., 2019).

With regard to the type, intensity, and duration of the exercise bouts, the following recommendations were given for acute reduction of anxiety symptoms: Walking on a treadmill seems to be more effective compared to that of cycling, weight training, or rowing. The effects of aerobic exercise bouts among those with clinically relevant symptoms seems to be similar to that of healthy populations (Petruzzello et al., 1991). It is possible that high-intensity exercise has larger benefits compared to that of low or moderate exercise, although there are also conflicting observations from healthy populations (Bartholomew & Linder, 1998). Regarding duration, no difference was observed between short (20 min or shorter) or longer exercise bouts (longer than 20 min) after controlling for potential confounding variables. Moreover, exercise seems to be most effective in people who are not regularly physically active, as well as in women and those over 25 years of age (Petruzzello et al., 1991).

▪ **Chronic Effects of Exercise Programs Lasting for Several Weeks**

Compared to the available evidence for exercise effects among depressed patients, few studies have been conducted on the chronic effects of exercise in people with anxiety disorders. However, four of five recently published reviews concluded that the available evidence supports that exercise training may be an effective adjuvant or adjunct therapy for clinically relevant anxiety (Asmundson et al., 2013; Herring et al., 2010; Jayakody et al., 2014; Stubbs et al., 2017), and the effects appear to be similar to those in healthy populations (▶ Chap. 26). Although a meta-analysis of seven RCTs of aerobic exercise among anxiety disorder patients suggested that exercise is not an effective treatment for anxiety disorders (Bartley et al., 2013), the most recent meta-analysis conducted by Stubbs et al. (2017), which included more than 250 persons with anxiety disorders and—due to the high level of comorbidity—persons with posttraumatic stress disorder, reported a moderate positive effect of exercise programs on anxiety symptoms compared to that of control interventions (ES = 0.6).

Due to the small number of studies, at the present stage of research, no recommendations can be made for clinical populations regarding the influence of frequency, intensity, and duration. However, the highest effects for healthy and clinical populations were observed in programs lasting 4 to 9 weeks, with three to four interventions per week (each bout between 1 and 1.5 h). There were no significant differences between moderate- and vigorous-intensity exercise. Regarding the mode of exercise, the majority of studies among patients with anxiety disorders have focused on aerobic exercise modes. However, in a small RCT that Stubbs et al. (2017) classified as a high-quality trial, demonstrating a low risk of bias, 6 weeks of either lower body resistance exercise training or cycling significantly improved clinical severity (Herring et al., 2012), associated signs and symptoms (Herring et al., 2011), quality of life (Herring et al., 2016), and dimensions of sleep quality and efficiency (Herring et al., 2015); larger-magnitude improvements were shown for resistance exercise training, supporting that both aerobic and resistance exercise modes improve outcomes among people with clinically relevant anxiety.

Effects of Exercise on Persons with Anxiety Disorders

Exercise programs lasting several weeks show medium positive effects on symptoms of anxiety in people with anxiety disorders. Contrary to earlier assumptions that exercise could have an acute anxiety-increasing effect, current findings show that even single exercise bouts (especially aerobic exercise activities) can reduce anxiety symptoms.

28.2.1.3 Mental and Behavioral Disorders Due to Psychoactive Substance Use

Substance use disorders such as **dependence syndrome** or **withdrawal state** belong to the group of mental and behavioral disorders caused by psychotropic substances (F10–F19) and develop after repeated substance use. Addiction disorders include behavioral, cognitive, emotional, and physical phenomena. It is mainly characterized by a strong desire to take one or more substances (craving) and problems in controlling consumption. Typical substances are tobacco, alcohol, or illegal drugs.

A study on the prevalence of substance use disorders showed that 147 million people worldwide were affected by substance use disorders in 2010. When substance use disorders related to illegal drugs and alcohol are combined, substance use disorders are responsible for more than 20% of DALYs lost due to mental and behavioral disorders worldwide (Whiteford et al., 2013).

▪ **Acute Effects of Single Bouts of Exercise**

Acute effects of single exercise bouts have primarily been studied in smokers. Haasova et al. (2013) found a reduction in the desire to smoke immediately after exercise. The large effect size of ES = 2.0 was based on more than 800 observations. Little information was provided about the type, intensity, and duration of the exercise. However, findings suggested that walking is more effective than that of cycling or isometric strength training.

Roberts et al. (2012) also reported a reduction in craving for smoking in response to acute exercise across 15 studies of over 2100 persons. (ES = 1.9). The positive effects were found up to 30 min after the exercise bout compared to that of a passive control situation and did not significantly differ based on exercise mode or intensity—the mode of exercise bouts ranged from yoga to intensive cycling on an ergometer. In contrast, the effects on withdrawal symptoms, on the one hand, and the affective state, on the other hand, were dependent on the intensity: Slight to moderate intensity led to an immediate decrease in withdrawal symptoms and positive effects on the affective state, while high intensity had a negative effect on withdrawal symptoms and affective state. For this reason and for reasons of compliance and better tolerance of exercise, the authors recommended exercise bouts with light intensity, although there is a need to clarify the ideal intensity of exercise. Intensity preference may also influence exercise response among smokers. Monroe et al. (2020) recently showed that 20 min of cycling at the preferred intensity reduced mood disturbances which occurred shortly after smoking a cigarette and blunted dorsolateral prefrontal cortex hemodynamic response to emotionally arousing scenes among 15 cigarette smokers. Similar effects are reported in other review articles (Ledochowski et al., 2013; Taylor et al., 2007).

Research has less focused on the acute effects of exercise in persons with alcohol or illegal drug use disorders. Zschucke et al. (2012) described in their review article only one study on acute effects in alcohol-dependent persons and could not identify any studies in drug-dependent populations. Although alcohol-dependent persons showed a reduction in the desire for alcohol during moderately intensive 10-min cycling, the effect did not last until after the exercise bout and a tendency to higher craving after exercise compared to that before the exercise bout was observed (Study Box: Cycling Against Craving).

Study Box

Cycling Against Craving

A strong desire (craving) is a precursor—and a characteristic of dependence—of the harmful behavior of alcohol dependence (alcohol consumption). Ussher et al. (2004) investigated in a rehabilitation clinic shortly after physical detoxification whether a short exercise bout of medium intensity can reduce the desire for alcohol (alcohol urges) and affective state in patients with substance use disorders. The patients bicycled for 10 min at medium intensity (experimental condition) and at very low intensity (control condition). Craving for alcohol was measured with the questionnaire "Alcohol Urge Questionnaire" (MacKillop, 2006) using items such as "I want a drink so bad I can almost taste it" and "Nothing would be better than a drink right now" before and after exercise. The results showed that a short cycling session of 10 min at medium intensity was able to reduce craving for alcohol for a short time.

Chronic Effects of Exercise Programs Lasting for Several Weeks

Ussher et al. (2014) described in their Cochrane review the effectiveness of exercise programs in the context of tobacco cessation. A meta-analytical consideration of the effects was dispensed due to the large heterogeneity of the included studies. The primary outcome variable was the abstinence rate, but secondary psychological variables such as symptoms of anxiety or depression were also reported. However, the combined results of 11 randomized controlled trials do not suggest a clear influence of exercise programs on psychological variables (e.g., symptoms of anxiety or depression) in persons with tobacco use disorder. The authors concluded that the data available are not yet sufficient to make solid statements about the effects of exercise programs for people with tobacco addiction and recommend large-scale randomized controlled trials for further research.

Wang et al. (2014) came to different conclusions, including not only studies in persons with tobacco use disorder but also studies in persons with alcohol and drug use disorder in their meta-analysis. On the basis of 22 randomized controlled trials, the authors reported a reduction in anxiety symptoms (ES = 0.3) and depression symptoms (ES = 0.5) after exercise intervention. The effects were larger in persons with alcohol and drug use disorder compared to that of persons with tobacco use disorder.

There were no differences regarding the type and intensity of the exercise programs, which led to the conclusion that low-, moderate-, or high-intensity exercise programs should be similarly effective. It should be noted here that in most low-intensity studies, so-called mind-body exercise such as Qigong, TaiChi, or Yoga were used. In addition to the exercise component, these modes of exercise also include meditative elements and breathing techniques, which might have a beneficial effect on symptoms of anxiety and depression. No conclusion was presented on the ideal duration of the exercise programs. The exercise programs ranged from 10 days to 6 months, with the majority of studies involving interventions of between 8 and 12 weeks (Wang et al., 2014).

With regard to tobacco cessation, the chronic effects of exercise in most forms appear questionable (Klinsophon et al., 2017). Based on 19 randomized controlled trials, the authors could only find a positive influence of yoga exercise programs combined with cognitive behavioral therapy on smoking cessation.

In a narrative review, Zschucke et al. (2012) included studies in persons with alcohol and drug use disorder and provided information on the design of exercise programs. For persons with tobacco use disorder, it seems more effective to intervene at least three times a week. Due to the data available, it is difficult to give concrete advice on the design of exercise for persons with alcohol and drug use disorder. The authors concluded that in persons with alcohol use disorder, a period of 4 weeks might be too short to have positive effects on symptoms of anxiety or depression.

Hallgren et al. (2017) reported a positive effect (ES = 0.9) on depressive symptoms in persons with alcohol use disorder, but not on the amount of alcohol consumed after the intervention. Although more than 20 randomized controlled trials were included in this meta-analytical study, only the results of four studies were included in the calculation of the effect sizes since depressive (concomitant) symptoms were not included in the other studies. However, only two (alcohol consumption per day) and three (alcohol consumption per week) studies were included in the analysis of alcohol consumption. The authors also noted that future research should focus on the dropout rate, as this was more than 40% in the studies examined.

Exercise and Substance Use

Individual bouts of exercise were highly effective in reducing the acute craving for substance. The reduction lasts up to 30 min after individual exercise bouts. The effect of exercise on the craving for substances in the long term is questionable due to the heterogeneous current findings. However, people with mental and behavioral disorders caused by psychotropic substances can benefit from the positive effects of exercise programs on symptoms of depression or anxiety. Exercise programs should pay particular attention to the dropout rate and countermeasures should be taken at an early stage.

28.2.1.4 Potential Mechanisms

In the previous sections of the chapter, it was summarized whether and to which amount exercise and exercise can contribute to the treatment of mental health disorders. So far, however, there are only few reliable research results on potential **mechanisms** of exercise. Although there are various hypotheses, some of which are supported by results in animal experiments, the hypotheses have rarely been tested in humans. Potential mechanisms are mostly derived from healthy populations. For people with health disorders, these are considered collectively for different disorders, since the mechanisms in the different disorders overlap. The hypotheses can be differentiated into biological and psychosocial explanatory approaches. However, it seems to be accepted that not a single hypothesis, but rather a multifactorial approach may explain the manifold effects of exercise on affective state. A synopsis of hypotheses relevant to clinical populations will be presented here. An overview table of potential mechanisms in healthy persons can be found in ► Chap. 26 (► Table 26.2).

- **Biological Explanations**

Several previous reviews have discussed plausible biological mechanisms for the effects of exercise (Dishman et al., 2006; Schuch et al., 2016; Sciolino & Holmes, 2012). Some of the biological explanations assume that lower quantities in certain neurobiological substrates, including neurotransmitters and neurotrophic factors, are present in people with mental disorders. For example, patients with depressive disorders show lower concentrations of metabolites of the monoamine metabolism such as norepinephrine and serotonin. Exercise can have a positive influence on the release of these neurobiological messengers, which can have an acute effect in terms of regulating the affective state and, in the longer term, plausibly reduce symptoms of depression or anxiety. This regulatory influence may also have a positive effect on craving for substances, the strength of craving for substances, and withdrawal symptoms in patients with substance use disorders (Zschucke et al., 2012).

Important messenger substances include norepinephrine, dopamine, adrenaline, and serotonin (**"monoamine depletion hypothesis,"** **"catecholamine hypothesis,"** **"serotonin hypothesis"**), endogenous cannabinoids (**"endocannabinoid hypothesis"**) or interleukins, and tumor necrosis factors (**"immune system modulation hypothesis"**). The "immune system modulation hypothesis" also includes hormonal chronic changes in the hypothalamic-pituitary-adrenal cortex axis, which have a positive effect on stress reactions. These changes are particularly relevant in patients with substance use, anxiety, and depressive disorders (Buckworth et al., 2013; Roberts et al., 2012). Exercise may also promote the formation of new nerve cells by activating the brain-derived neurotrophic factor, which is a partial target of drug therapies, especially in patients with depressive disorders (Pedersen & Saltin, 2015).

The **"endorphin hypothesis,"** which is known beyond research, assumes that pain-inhibiting endorphins are released through (intense) exercise. This hypothesis has now only been accepted sporadically, as empirical studies have not been able to show a connection between endorphin levels and changes in the affective state (Goldfarb et al., 1987). Although elevated endorphin levels have been detected in blood plasma after intense physical exercise (Boecker et al., 2010), there is evidence that these levels are not able to cross the blood-brain barrier, particularly at temperatures characteristic of intense exercise, and studies have shown that opioid antagonists do not block mood improvements following exercise (Buckworth et al., 2013). Since a moderate intensity is often recommended and chosen for exercise in health disorders, the "endorphin hypothesis" additionally appears less relevant in patients.

Furthermore, the **"thermoregulation hypothesis"** postulates that exercise leads to an increased blood supply to the brain, a rise in body temperature, and increased metabolic activity. These factors have a particularly positive effect on the affective state and, in the longer term, on anxiety symptoms.

The "**transient hypofrontality hypothesis**" assumes that during exercise, areas of the brain that do not immediately contribute to the execution of exercise are less supplied with blood (Dietrich, 2003). This may limit the neuronal resources that are necessary for emotional and cognitive processes such as anxiety or depression symptoms. However, current findings do not confirm the "transient hypofrontality hypothesis"(Rooks et al., 2010).

- **Psychosocial Explanations**

The "**distraction hypothesis**" can be seen as a psychological consequence of the "transient hypofrontality hypothesis." However, the hypothesis does not consider the physiological background, but focuses on the individual momentary assessment of stressors during exercise. Exercise distracts people from stressors and worries and results in a fading of the negative affective state. The hypothesis is particularly relevant for acute changes in the affective state due to exercise.

Reflection

Distraction to Alleviate Discomfort?

Usually, being distracted is not considered desirable. For example, being distracted by a thought of the upcoming nice evening with friends concentrating is less helpful when concentrating on a train of thought in this chapter. However, a distraction can be positive when the issue being distracted from is something negative and burdensome (so certainly not this chapter), such as a painful stimulus, long-lasting thoughts on failure, or the suffering of social rejection. Think specifically about an event where you were distracted by exercise in a positive sense. Was that (and why) positive for your health and affective state in the short, medium, or long term?

For chronic changes, the "**self-efficacy hypothesis**" offers a psychological explanation. It is assumed that repeated mastering of tasks and the achievement of athletic goals have a positive effect on self-efficacy, and thus, symptoms of anxiety and depression are reduced in the long term (Muris, 2002).

So-called nonspecific concomitant effects are also plausible. Accordingly, the positive effect of exercise is not attributed to the intervention itself, but to other variables, e.g., the group setting or cognitive aspects.

28.2.2 Exercise for Persons with Physical Health Disorders

In the following, effects of exercise on psychological parameters in physical health disorders are reported. Physical health disorders, such as cardiovascular or respiratory diseases, are responsible for most deaths, disabilities, and the resulting burden of disease. In the European Region, the leading causes of premature death (before age 65 years) are cardiovascular diseases (50%) followed by oncological diseases (about 20%).

Cardiovascular Diseases

Cardiovascular diseases include all diseases of the heart, vessels, and blood circulation. Typical heart diseases are heart failure or coronary heart disease. Vascular diseases such as arteriosclerosis or thrombosis also fall into this category.

Research on physical disorders is mainly interested in "hard data," i.e., easily objectifiable data for the evaluation of therapies (e.g., 5-year mortality, end of sick leave, physiological parameters, physical performance). The positive effects of exercise seem to be sufficiently corroborated in various patient populations in regularly updated meta-analyses, for example, in patients after stroke (Saunders et al., 2016), with cardiovascular diseases (Anderson et al., 2016), with oncological diseases (Fong et al., 2012; Furmaniak et al., 2016), and with respiratory diseases (Lahham et al., 2016; Paneroni et al., 2017).

For people with physical health disorders, primarily chronic effects of exercise programs on the (health-related) quality of life are intensively studied. Additionally, symptoms of anxiety and depression are reported in meta-analyses since it is known that patients with chronic diseases have an increased incidence of such symptoms (Kessler et al., 2005). The mechanism between chronic disease and depression seems to be bidirectional: chronic (physical) health disorders increase the risk for the development of depressive disorders, but depression also increases the risk for the development of chronic diseases most likely through behavioral patterns. Research is currently broadly based and both metabolic and lifestyle-relevant factors are discussed. In the following, the evidence for chronic effects of exercise on quality of life and symptoms of depression and anxiety is summarized. Fatigue syndrome also plays a major role, especially in oncological diseases, as between 60% and 100% of oncological patients report symptoms of fatigue (Scott & Posmontier, 2017).

Similar to mental disorders, a brief definition of the health disorders is given firstly, based on the International Statistical Classification of Diseases and Related Health Problems (ICD-10).

28.2.2.1 Cardiovascular Diseases

Cardiovascular diseases are listed in the ICD-10 under **diseases of the circulatory system** (I00–I99) and include diseases of the arteries, arterioles, and capillaries (atherosclerosis), cerebrovascular diseases (e.g., cerebral infarction), ischemic heart diseases (e.g., acute myocardial infarction), and hypertension (high blood pressure).

Herring and colleagues conducted meta-analyses of studies of exercise training effects on anxiety (Herring et al., 2010) and depressive symptoms in persons with chronic diseases. For anxiety, compared with those with no treatment conditions, exercise training significantly reduced anxiety symptoms among 2914 patients with a diverse range of diseases by a small mean effect (ES = 0.29). Exercise programs lasting no more than 12 weeks and session durations of 30 min or more resulted in the largest anxiety reductions. Similarly, for depression, exercise programs significantly reduced depressive symptoms by a small mean effect (ES = 0.30), independent of the type of disease. Depressive symptom reductions were largest among patients with elevated depressive symptoms at the beginning of the intervention and for whom exercise resulted in functional improvements, supporting that it seems to be important whether the exercise program leads to a functional physical improvement among chronically ill adults. Although the majority of evidence has focused on aerobic exercise training, recent meta-analytic evidence supported the anxiolytic and antidepressant effects of resistance exercise training. Gordon and colleagues reported a significant small (ES = 0.31) reduction in anxiety symptoms among 922 healthy and chronically ill adults across 31 effects derived from 16 RCTs, regardless of health status, age, sex, or features of the resistance exercise training (Gordon et al., 2017). Similarly, a meta-analysis of 33 RCTs of 1877 healthy and chronically ill adults showed that resistance exercise training significantly reduced depressive symptoms by a moderate-sized mean effect (ES = 0.66), regardless of health status, total prescribed volume of resistance exercise training, or significant strength improvements (Gordon et al., 2018).

Anderson et al. (2016) reported a reduced cardiovascular mortality rate and a reduced risk of hospital admissions after exercise-based rehabilitation programs in the aforementioned Cochrane meta-analysis. Effects on quality of life were also reported. However, due to the heterogeneity of the reported assessments, no effect sizes for quality of life were reported. However, the researchers concluded that exercise programs have a positive effect on the quality of life of patients with cardiovascular disease since significant improvements in quality of life were reported in 5 of the 20 studies examined.

The results in patients after stroke seem less clear. The group of authors around van de Port et al. (2007) included 21 randomized controlled trials with a total of more than 500 patients and could not detect a significant effect on quality of life despite functional improvement in walking speed and endurance. Saunders et al. (2016) reported in a meta-analysis including more than 50 randomized controlled trials and almost 3000 patients that the available data are not sufficient to reliably determine the effects of exercise on quality of life.

In contrast, Chen and Rimmer (2011) reported a small positive effect on quality of life (ES = 0.3) immediately after exercise programs in a meta-analysis including more than 400 stroke patients. However, this effect disappeared in the follow-up (3 to 4 months after the exercise intervention). The authors explain the discrepancy to the other meta-analyses by the fact that three additional randomized controlled trials were included that showed positive effects. Moreover, according to their statement, the group of authors was the only one to examine the mental dimension of quality of life separately. So far evidence is limited regarding the relation of quality of life to various characteristics of exercise programs (e.g., intensity, frequency, duration) in persons after stroke.

Controlled studies on acute effects on the affective state are rare among people with cardiovascular diseases. In current reviews, the acute effects refer to the results found in nonclinical populations, where anxiety-reducing effects of single exercise bouts were found. The intensity seems to have an important influence: A reduction in state anxiety was observed after exercise bouts with low or moderate intensity, whereas high-intensity bouts appear to be less effective in this population (Strickland & Smith, 2014).

Niedermeier et al. (2017) examined the effects of a single therapy bout with exercise components in a sample of mainly patients after stroke and reported positive effects on affective state for robot-supported gait training.

Effects of Exercise on Cardiovascular Diseases

The findings on the positive effect of exercise programs on the quality of life or symptoms of depression and anxiety must be considered as inconsistent. One reason might be found in the heterogeneity of the cardiovascular diseases studied. Possible improvements in mental health seem to be closely linked to functional improvements in motor skills. However, exercise-based rehabilitation programs are recommended for per-

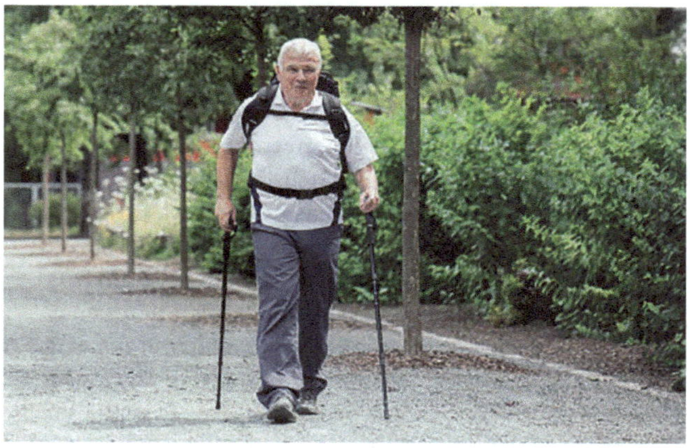

Fig. 28.4 Exercise against cardiovascular diseases

sons with cardiovascular disease due to the positive cardiovascular effects and the reduction of hospital admissions regardless of the effect on quality of life (Anderson et al., 2016) (Fig. 28.4).

28.2.2.2 Oncological Diseases

Oncological diseases are listed in the ICD-10 in the disease group **neoplasms** (C00-D48) and include benign and malignant neoplasms. Neoplasms are caused by a change in cells and result in an uncontrolled proliferation (tumor). The tumors can affect surrounding tissue and spread to other parts of the body (metastases). The subdivision of oncological diseases is based on the localization of the new formations, e.g., digestive organs, mammary glands, or respiratory organs. "Cancer" is an umbrella term for all the subdivisions mentioned and includes carcinomas, sarcomas, lymphomas, leukemia, other specified and localized types, and unspecified cancers.

With a prevalence of 3.7 million diseases and 1.9 million deaths per year, the group of oncological diseases can be described as the second most frequent cause of death and disease in Europe (World Health Organization, 2012). In addition to tobacco and alcohol consumption, unhealthy diet, overweight, and lack of exercise are seen as risk factors for oncological diseases (Ezzati et al., 2002). The risk of a person developing cancer during their lifetime is about 30% in more developed countries (Torre et al., 2015).

Data regarding the effect of exercise programs on the quality of life of people with oncological diseases can be described as positive. Ferrer et al. (2011) report in their meta-analysis based on more than 3500 persons and 78 studies a small positive effect (ES = 0.3) of exercise programs on the (self-reported) quality of life approximately 1 week after an exercise intervention. This effect increased when quality of life was recorded 18 weeks after the intervention (ES = 0.4). The effects were larger when exercise intensity was moderate (about six times the basal metabolic rate) compared to that of low-intensity exercise (about four times the basal metabolic rate). The authors noted that it was not possible to determine the influence of group effects (e.g., social support) of exercise.

Speck et al. (2010) studied more than 60 target variables in their extensive analysis (more than 6800 patients, 82 studies) and reported similar positive effects on quality of life (ES = 0.3) and fatigue (ES = 0.5) after an exercise program. During the intervention, the authors found small positive effects on anxiety symptoms (ES = 0.4). In terms of intensity, the researchers recommend to avoid high-intensity exercise with regard to a possible negative influence on the immune system.

Further confirmation is reported in the Cochrane articles by Mishra et al. (2012), Larun et al. (2016), and Cramp and Byron-Daniel (2012). Fatigue symptoms were significantly reduced immediately after several weeks of exercise intervention (ES = 0.3, low effect). Aerobic exercise seems to be most effective here. At the follow-up after 12 weeks and 6 months, the fatigue symptoms were still reduced. In addition, positive effects were reported on symptoms of anxiety (ES = 0.3) and sleep quality (ES = 0.5).

Chiu et al. (2015) described a medium positive effect of exercise (ES = 0.5) on sleep quality based on nine randomized controlled trials and almost 600 patients. Moderate walking as an exercise intervention seems to be particularly effective. It should be noted that positive effects on sleep quality were not reported in all studies. Mercier et al. (2016) found no significant effects. The authors mentioned possible floor effects as an explanation since the examined patient group already reported a good sleep quality at the beginning of the study. The authors expect positive effects especially for outdoor exercise interventions.

When comparing different interventions to reduce fatigue, Mustian et al. (2017) concluded that psychological (ES = 0.3) or exercise interventions (ES = 0.3) are more effective compared to pharmaceutical interventions (ES = 0.1, not significant), which is based on 113 controlled studies with more than 11,000 patients with cancer. Professionally guided exercise interventions seem to be important, as Sweegers et al. (2018) reported significant differences between instructed (ES = 0.2) and uninstructed exercise programs (ES = 0.04).

Exercise training effects on cancer-related fatigue may differ in patients during and following treatment. In a meta-analysis of 70 studies of 4881 cancer patients, Puetz and Herring et al. (2012) reported that exercise significantly reduced cancer-related fatigue by a small mean effect (ES = 0.32 and 0.38) during and following cancer treatment, respectively. The effects, however, were moderated differentially over the time course of treatment and recovery, such that during treatment patients with lower baseline fatigue scores and higher exercise adherence realized larger improvements. Following treatment, fatigue reductions were largest for trials with longer durations between treatment completion and exercise initiation, trials with shorter exercise program lengths, and trials using wait-list comparisons. These findings highlighted that exercise has a palliative effect in patients during treatment and a recuperative effect posttreatment (Puetz & Herring, 2012).

Effects of Exercise in Persons with Oncological Diseases

The evidence for the analysis of exercise effects in persons with oncological diseases can be described as well established. Several meta-analyses confirm low to medium positive effects of exercise programs lasting several weeks on quality of life and fatigue, effects which may differ during treatment and following treatment. In addition, the importance of supervised exercise programs to increase compliance and intensity of exercise and to promote helpful social interactions is emphasized.

28.2.2.3 Chronic Respiratory Diseases

Chronic diseases such as chronic obstructive pulmonary disease (COPD) and asthma are particularly relevant in the group of **diseases of the respiratory system** (J00–J99). COPD is characterized by coughing, increased sputum, and shortness of breath on exertion and difficulty in breathing out.

In 2010, the estimated prevalence of COPD was almost 14% in Europe (Adeloye et al., 2015). COPD is believed to be the fourth most common cause of death (Mannino & Kiri, 2006).

Coventry and Hind (2007) investigated the effect of exercise programs on symptoms of anxiety and depression and on quality of life in people with COPD. The authors reported a stronger reduction in symptoms of anxiety (ES = 0.3) and depression (ES = 0.6) compared to that of standard treatment in their review of six randomized controlled trials with a total of more than 500 COPD patients. Both the psychological (ES = 0.7) and physical components (ES = 0.4) of quality of life were positively influenced.

Exercise-induced improvements in quality of life are supported by Paneroni et al. (2017), who found large effects (ES = 1.2) in 10 randomized controlled trials of severely affected patients. Lacasse et al. (2007) reported almost identical results regarding quality of life in their meta-analysis of 31 randomized controlled trials. Spruit et al. (2013) provided details on potential exercise programs for patients with COPD, which are discussed below.

Exercise in Practice

Exercise for Persons with Diseases of the Respiratory System

The following training recommendations are given by Spruit et al. (2013) to effectively improve quality of life (as well as disease symptoms and exercise tolerance) in persons with respiratory diseases:

Aerobic training (cycling or walking) is primarily used in rehabilitation. Recommended is a frequency of three to five bouts per week and a bout duration of 20 to 60 min at an intensity of about 60% of the maximum exertion, which corresponds to a perceived exertion of 12–14 according to Borg (1982). The optimal duration of the exercise program is still controversially discussed, but the authors recommend about 12 weeks. Muscle-strengthening exercises of the respiratory muscles, general strength training, training of the upper extremities, and electrical stimulation are used in addition to aerobic training.

Furthermore, the following basic principles apply:

- Before starting the exercise program, a thorough medical examination of the physical condition to ensure safety and training control is indicated.
- Reduced performance capacity of patients due to increased energy consumption for breathing activity, restrictions on gas exchange and the cardiovascular system, and muscular dysfunctions of the lower extremities should be considered.
- Home-based exercise programs should be considered for ambulatory patients.

Effects of Exercise in Persons with Chronic Respiratory Diseases

Consistently low- to medium-sized positive effects of exercise interventions on quality of life and symptoms of anxiety and depression were reported in persons with chronic respiratory diseases. Data, however, are somewhat less consistent compared to that of persons with oncological diseases.

28.2.2.4 Other Physical Health Disorders

In the following, effects of exercise on psychological variables in other physical health disorders are presented.

- **Multiple Sclerosis**

Pilutti et al. (2013) conducted a meta-analysis including 17 randomized controlled trials with a total of more than 500 patients with multiple sclerosis (G35.-). Symptoms of fatigue were positively influenced by exercise programs compared to control interventions (ES = 0.5). The ideal mode, frequency, intensity, or duration of the exercise programs is still unclear; however, larger effect sizes were observed in strength training compared to that of aerobic exercise training. The average frequency was three bouts per week with a duration of approximately 45 min. The exercise programs were carried out over a period of 3 to 26 weeks. More recently, Herring et al. (2017a) showed that exercise training significantly reduced depressive symptoms by a moderate mean effect (ES = 0.55) across 14 RCTs that included 624 patients with MS; improvements were significantly larger when exercise also significantly improved fatigue symptoms.

▪ Parkinson's Disease

There is currently little evidence of the effects of exercise programs on mental health and quality of life in patients with Parkinson's disease (G20.-). Goodwin et al. (2008) stated that available studies indicate a positive effect on quality of life, but included only four randomized controlled trials. Sumec et al. (2015) similarly reported positive effects on quality of life and depressive symptoms, but also highlighted mixed methodological quality. Although Wu et al. (2017) did not conduct a meta-analysis of the 11 included studies with approximately 350 patients; they recommended aerobic activities to reduce depressive symptoms and to improve quality of life among patients with Parkinson's disease.

▪ Diabetes Mellitus

Chronic effects of exercise programs on psychological parameters are unclear in patients with diabetes (E11.-). Heterogeneous effects were reported in the meta-analysis by van der Heijden et al. (2013), with 20 randomized controlled trials with more than 1700 patients. Aerobic exercise training did not show any significant effects on quality of life and no conclusions could be drawn for strength training. Positive effects on symptoms of depression or anxiety were reported sporadically in studies. No significant effects on quality of life were found in the Cochrane analysis by Thomas et al. (2006).

To the best of our knowledge, no meta-analyses are yet available for the acute effects. Kopp et al. (2012) reported positive effects of a single 20-min bout of brisk walking. After the bout, patients reported an increase in the basic dimensions of activation and valence compared to that of a sedentary control condition.

▪ Chronic Pain

It is difficult to classify chronic pain conditions in the ICD-10 classification system because pain syndromes are described from both a stronger physical health perspective (e.g., low back pain, M54.5) and a psychological perspective (e.g., persistent somatoform pain disorder, F45.4). In the multidisciplinary treatment of chronic pain, a biopsychosocial model was established that uses an appropriate weighting of these factors in the etiology and course of the pain disorder (Engel, 1977). Here, we focus on the effect of exercise on chronic pain exclusively.

It should be mentioned that exercise may also cause painful conditions, especially if the intensity is too high (see ▶ Sect. 28.3.2). However, exercise is used to reduce chronic pain. In a Cochrane article by Geneen et al. (2017), 21 reviews based on more than 37,000 patients with various pain conditions were summarized. Despite the large amount of data, the authors were unable to report effect sizes or draw a definitive conclusion. However, it was noted that exercise is an intervention with few harmful side effects and possibly pain-reducing and may also have a positive effect on quality of life.

Searle et al. (2015) reported a small pain-reducing effect (ES = 0.3) in patients with chronic back pain based on 45 randomized controlled trials. The authors recommend mainly strengthening exercises and interventions with coordinative elements for the whole body or the trunk. Aerobic interventions did not show positive effects. However, this does not seem to apply generally to patients with musculoskeletal pain disorders, as positive pain-reducing effects have been reported as a result of longer aerobic interventions (moderate walking for 6 to 12 months). O'Connor et al. (2015) summarized data from 26 studies with more than 2300 patients in a meta-analysis. The authors recommend that exercise programs should be designed for long-term application and include strategies to increase participation.

Summary

The following is a rough summary to classify the findings. However, it has to be considered as somewhat imprecise since it is a complex and differentiated picture.

- **Multiple sclerosis**: It is relatively certain that exercise programs result in reduced fatigue; however, the ideal design of exercise (also in terms of frequency, intensity, or duration) needs further study.
- **Parkinson's disease**: Initial findings show a positive effect of exercise programs on quality of life and depressive symptoms.
- **Diabetes mellitus**: So far, there is no evidence that the quality of life can be positively influenced by exercise programs. Positive effects on depression or anxiety symptoms have been reported.
- **Chronic pain**: Although exercise programs are used to reduce chronic pain, data are conflicting. It should be noted that symptoms might increase by exercise (especially at a high exercise intensity), but repeated exposure to exercise bouts seems to reduce chronic pain.

28

28.3 Exercise: Risks and Side Effects

Up to now, the present chapter has primarily focused on the positive aspects of exercise in patients with various health disorders. However, the positive effects of exercise may turn negative, e.g., when exercise is conducted excessively and injuries are ignored, when substances are (ab)used to enhance performance, and goals stimulate the development of eating disorders among athletes. In the following, an attempt will be made to separate mental from physical risks. However, the presence of mental risks (e.g., exercise dependence) may also cause negative physical effects (e.g., injuries) and vice versa.

28.3.1 Exercise and Mental Risks

28.3.1.1 Eating Disorders

Empirical data suggest that the prevalence of mental disorders such as depression is comparable between athletes and nonathletes (Reardon & Factor, 2010). However, both female and male competitive athletes seem to be at higher risk of developing eating disorders than nonathletes (Reardon & Factor, 2010). Eating disorders (F.50-), with anorexia nervosa and bulimia nervosa as the most important representatives, belong to the group of mental and behavioral disorders. Anorexic persons define a very low weight threshold for themselves and induce weight loss in order to achieve this, e.g., by restrictive eating or excessive exercise. Persons with bulimia show repeated bouts of overeating and subsequent vomiting. The prevalence of anorexia nervosa and bulimia nervosa in athletes varies between sports and is comparatively high in sports where a competitive advantage is achieved by a lower weight (Joy et al., 2016). Prevalence rates range from 2% in ball sports to over 40% in aesthetic sports, such as gymnastics (Joy et al., 2016) (◘ Fig. 28.5). Even though prevalence rate is higher among female compared to that of male athletes, eating disorders in exercise clearly cannot be classified as a purely female phenomenon (Werner et al., 2013).

The first step recommended to prevent and identify eating disorders as a systematic screening of athletes in suspected cases since early detection of eating disorders increases the chances of treatment. In addition, the supporting team should be trained on the warning signs of eating disorders and the importance of weight should be less emphasized, especially in sports where weight is a key factor (Joy et al., 2016). With regard to the treatment of eating disorders in athletes, Petrie & Greenleaf, 2014 point out that stigmatization of those affected should be avoided and suggest a proactive approach to eating disorders within the whole team. The primary criterion should be the health of the athletes, when deciding whether athletes with eating disorder should continue training or participate in competitions. However, the authors explicitly point out that this does not necessarily mean that athletes are prohibited from participating in training and/or competitions (Petrie and Greenleaf (2014).

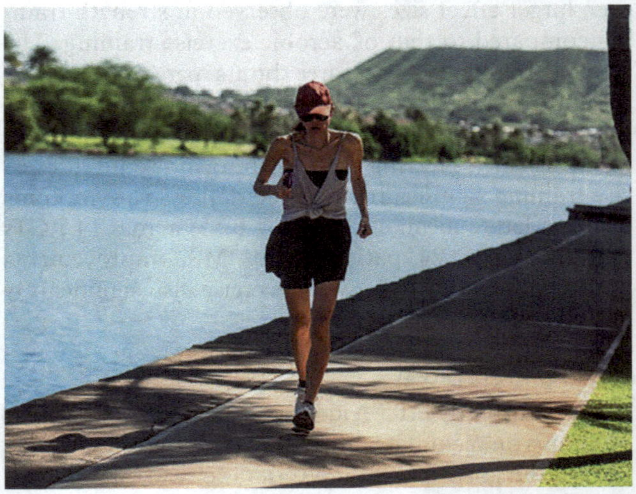

◘ **Fig. 28.5** Exercising with the intention to reduce weight in eating disorders

Eating disorders may be accompanied by (secondary) exercise dependence, which is discussed below. Some authors refer to anorexia athletica as a subclinical eating disorder with changes in eating behavior that do not (yet) meet the criteria for anorexia nervosa (Pugliese et al., 1983). However, these eating disorders are not considered here, since these are not mentioned in the ICD-10 classification system.

28.3.1.2 Exercise Dependence

Negative effects of exercise primarily occur at a very high training volume. In addition to the overtraining syndrome (a decrease in performance despite continued training), chronic fatigue, sleep disorders, and negative affective state (Kreher & Schwartz, 2012; Morgan et al., 1987), **exercise dependence** should be mentioned here. Exercise dependence is referred to a depressive state where it is impossible to not exercise, continuous mental occupation with exercise, engaging in exercise despite negative health consequences or against medical advice, and neglect of social contacts in order to be able to practice more exercise (Breuer & Kleinert, 2009; Grüsser & Thaleman, 2006; Zeeck et al., 2013).

Prevalence rates show a large variety in different populations and sports, ranging from 3% to 50% (Magee et al., 2016). However, the prevalence rate in the general population is assumed to be low since only a small percentage of the population exercises at all. Breuer and Kleinert (2009) reported that only one in 1000 athletes manifest the disorder characteristics and that about one in 10,000 athletes is in need of treatment.

So far, exercise dependence is not mentioned in the ICD-10 classification system, which might be an illustration of the problematic research situation in this area. On the one hand, there are very different definitions of the construct of exercise dependence; on the other hand, there are hardly any studies, longitudinal studies or meta-analyses, on the underlying psychological risk factors (Hausenblas & Symons Downs, 2002). In addition, a classification in the ICD-10 classification system seems difficult at present since dependencies that are not bound to substances are partly included in the group of obsessive-compulsive disorders (F42.-) and partly in the category of abnormal habits and impulse disorders (F63.-), where pathological gambling is mentioned.

A differentiation into primary and secondary exercise dependence was already made in the 1980s despite this classification-related uncertainty. In the case of primary exercise dependence, exercising as a behavioral pattern is considered the "addictive object," and in the case of secondary exercise dependence, exercising is regarded as a means of weight regulation in the context of eating disorders (Davis et al., 1995). Research efforts are also existent in the field of psychological diagnostics with the aim of psychometrically assessing exercise dependence, e.g., the "Exercise Dependence Scale" (EDS-R) by Downs et al. (2004) and a short scale "Exercise Addiction Inventory" by Griffiths et al. (2005). The authors point out that exercise dependence should only be "diagnosed" with the inclusion of an additional clinical assessment (Methods: Measurement of Exercise Dependence).

Methods: Measurement of Exercise Dependence

The "Exercise Addiction Inventory" by Griffiths et al. (2005) is based on the components of substance addiction modified to exercise (in the order of the items: salience, conflict, mood modification, tolerance, withdrawal, and relapse). The items are rated on a 1–5 scale, and the sum of the six items is considered an indicator of exercise dependence, whereby the team of authors describes a sum score of more than 24 as "at risk" for exercise dependence. The scale can be found in Griffiths et al. (2005).

Vallerand et al. (2014) proposed another approach via the term "passion" and distinguished between a harmonic and an obsessive form of this passion. On the one hand, the authors offer in their underlying construct an access via the well-established "self-determination theory" (▶ Chap. 8); on the other hand, the theoretical approach of a dualistic model on the passion for exercise could avoid a potential pathologization of intensive exercise. From a methodological point of view, it is difficult to distinguish between commitment for a behavior and dependence. Exercise has less potential for harm and represents a priori a health-promoting pattern of behavior from the point of view of both the individual and society in contrast to other problematic behavior such as intensive gambling or unnecessary shopping.

28.3.1.3 Substance Use

Usually, use of illegal and/or performance-enhancing substances (doping) is associated with substance use in exercise. However, alcohol and drug use for the purpose of relaxation and distraction needs consideration, even if the public interest is mainly focused on doping.

There is a controversial debate in literature whether there is a general positive correlation between alcohol consumption behavior and exercise (Lisha et al., 2011). However, sociodemographic characteristics and different sports must be taken into account in this relationship from the perspective of the authors of this chapter. Particularly, younger men excessively exercising are likely to show higher alcohol consumption behavior compared to that of the general population, as Kopp et al. (2015) reported in their study. The extent to which athletes are more susceptible to intensive alcohol consumption cannot be clearly answered on the basis of current research. However, it should be mentioned that competitive sport should not be considered a protective factor (Diehl et al., 2012; Martens & Martin, 2014). There seems to be a difference in the use of illegal substances such as marijuana, cocaine, or psychedelics where athletes use fewer of these substances compared to that of their age cohort (Diehl et al., 2012; Lisha & Sussman, 2010).

Probably the most important association that readers may have in this context is the illegal use of performance-enhancing substances with the aim of achieving better results in competitions. Doping is classified as an undesirable behavior because it undermines the spirit of fair competition; in addition, it poses a health risk to athletes that should not be underestimated. Nevertheless, this behavior is reported to be relatively common in some sports (including weight training), with prevalence rates of 10–78% in various studies (Blouin & Goldfield, 1995; Dunn et al., 2009). Furthermore, there seems to be a willingness to take illegal substances to improve performance in recreational sports, which should not be underestimated. For example, the use of painkillers is reported to realize a high training workload despite pain (Blank et al., 2016a).

? Which Factors Are Associated with the Use of Illegal Substances?

Ntoumanis et al. (2014) revealed in a meta-analysis the following psychological factors to be associated with an increased likelihood of taking performance-enhancing illegal substances:

- Use of legal supplements
- Perceived social norms
- Positive attitudes towards doping

28

Identifying the underlying mechanisms for doping behavior remains a major challenge in research despite the great diversity of psychological approaches since information on actual behavior is often biased by social desirability. Alternative assessment strategies (e.g., implicit associations, covert survey approaches) are not undisputed in psychodiagnostics, and it remains questionable whether breakthroughs might be expected here. It was suggested previously to conduct a restart and to examine doping behavior in an integrative, qualitative, and interdisciplinary (psychology and sociology) research model (Blank et al., 2016b).

28.3.2 Exercise and Physical Risks

Exercise involves physical risks in addition to mental risks. Possible negative physical consequences of incorrect exercise with high intensity include injuries, an increased probability of sudden cardiac death, impaired immune functions, and the female athlete triad.

28.3.2.1 Injuries

So far, exercise science has focused most intensively on injuries. Injuries can be divided into two categories: injuries caused by overstrain, such as postural or muscular imbalances, or injuries caused by trauma. The incidence of fatal injuries in exercise can be described as very low. For the European Union, Kisser and Bauer (2012) and Bauer et al. (2014) reported between 0.2 and 1.4 fatal injuries per 100,000 persons per year. The range in fatal injuries results from the inclusion of death by drowning, which the authors see as an overestimated figure, since not every death by drowning must have occurred during exercise. Activities with the highest rate of fatal injuries are swimming, mountain climbing, and cycling. The authors summarize mountaineering and climbing activities under mountain exercise. Alpine skiing and aviation sports (e.g., paragliding) are listed separately (Kisser & Bauer, 2012).

In the European Union, 6.1 million nonfatal injuries treated in hospital annually are attributable to sports and exercise corresponding to an incidence of nonfatal injuries of about 1200 injuries per 100,000 people annually. Exercise injuries account for about 15% of injuries compared to that of road traffic (11%), home and leisure (58%), or work (10%) (Bauer et al., 2014). Almost half of the accidents (40%) occur in ball sports with the lower extremities most frequently affected (Fig. 28.6).

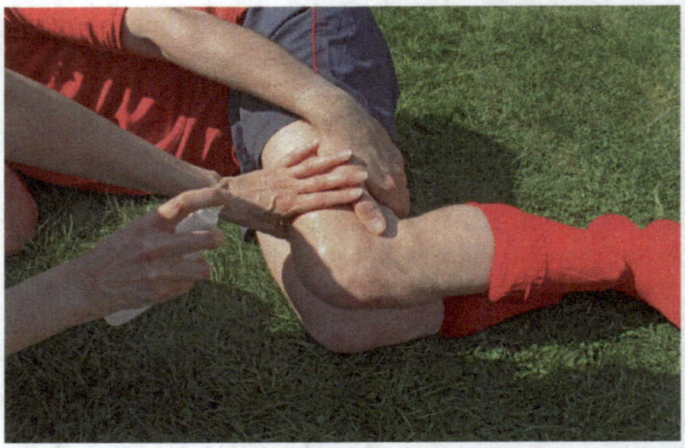

Fig. 28.6 Injuries often occur in ball sports

Two approaches in exercise psychology are particularly important when focusing on injuries. On the one hand, focus is put on the questions whether and to what extent psychological factors may lead to an increased risk of injuries and whether there are possibilities for intervention in this respect. On the other hand, research is conducted on the psychological prerequisites for return to sports after injury.

Previously, intensive research was conducted on personality traits in various so-called high-risk sports on a potential link between psychological factors and the risk of injuries. In the meantime, this spectrum changed in a way that now also prophylactic behavior is considered including the wearing of protective clothing, the choice of route, or consideration of weather conditions. **High-risk sports** in literature usually contains sports, where an increased potential of a serious or fatal injury is present. It is gratifying to note that a consensus in this research area seems to present that people who engage in high-risk sports should not be labelled "adrenaline junkies" or "sensation-seekers." Present research approaches instead focus on underlying motives with interesting approaches in the areas of identity, emotion regulation, and alexithymia (deficits in the identification and description of emotional states).

There is also evidence from a review article that there is a higher probability of injuries in athletes who are considered "more prone to stress" in the sense of neurocognitive or attention-related capacity loss and increased distractibility and who were confronted with a higher density of negative life events (Ivarsson et al., 2017). The authors assumed that these two factors can contribute to an increased likelihood of injury and suggest that injury research should focus more on behavioral variables. Furthermore, the authors conclude that psychological interventions for injury prophylaxis are effective in general and especially in athletes with an increased risk of injury, which might be explained by optimized conditions due to a change in stress-relevant variables (Ivarsson et al., 2017).

The second approach in the field of injuries is a consideration of the psychological requirements for return to sports after injury. In this respect, Ardern et al. (2013) reported that a higher probability of return to sports is related to positive psychological responses to the course of the rehabilitation process such that motivation and trust are linked to (thus accompanying) reduced expression of negative emotions such as fear, depression, and anger. The systematic overview of Ardern et al. (2013) is based on the "self-determination theory" (▶ Chap. 8). However, it is important to point out that the role of psychological factors in injuries has to be cautiously assessed (and thus not be overestimated) due to the low effect sizes in the available meta-analyses.

28.3.2.2 Sudden Cardiac Death

Regular exercise is primarily associated with the prevention of cardiovascular disease (Varghese et al., 2016). However, intensive physical exertion is considered a potential cause of sudden cardiac death. Determining the prevalence of sudden cardiac death during exercise is difficult, because it is a very rare event and strongly influenced by characteristics of the population under study (e.g., age, previous diseases). Albert et al. (2000) studied more than 20,000 men between 40 and 84 years of age for 12 years and found an extremely low risk of sudden cardiac (one death in 1.5 million intensive exercise bouts). The authors reported the highest prevalence in physically inactive persons and recommended regular exercise as the best prevention of sudden cardiac death. Moreover, postmortem analyses showed that previous cardiac disease is the reason for sudden cardiac death in about 70% of the cases (Semsarian et al., 2015). Therefore, a medical examination before starting exercise programs is recommended in the presence of cardiovascular or metabolic risk factors (American College of Sports Medicine, 2018).

28.3.2.3 Impaired Immune Function

Regular exercise can improve immune function of the body—similar to the prevention of cardiovascular diseases. However, the immune function of the body is impaired, at least in the short term, after longer exercise bouts to complete exhaustion (e.g., marathon runs). Nieman et al. (1990) reported that 13% of marathoners suffered from a respiratory infection within the week after the marathon. In contrast, only 2.2% of the people, who had been prepared to run the marathon but ultimately did not participate, suffered a respiratory infection. It is currently assumed that the immune function is impaired between 3 and up to 72 h after high-intensity training sessions.

28.3.2.4 Female Athlete Triad

The female athlete triad is a combination of the three factors amenorrhea (absence of menstruation), osteoporosis, and listlessness (with or without eating disorder; ▶ Sect. 28.3.1.1). The prevalence in the female population is between 2% and 5% (Nazem & Ackerman, 2012). However, the prevalence of secondary amenorrhea is up to over 60% among female ballet or running athletes (Nazem & Ackerman, 2012). The female athlete triad can be associated with an increased risk of injury and reduced fertility. Therefore, vigilance on the supporting team is recommended in concerning sports.

28.4 Conclusion

In summary, it can be stated that exercise almost always results in an increase in the outcome variables affective state and quality of life in persons with both mental and physical health disorders. Importantly, exercise training results in medium-sized effects on symptoms of anxiety and depression and low-sized effects on quality of life. While chronic effects are already well documented in some disorders (e.g., depressive disorders), acute effects of exercise on psychological parameters are less well represented in the existing literature in clinical populations. For the chronic effects, various authors conclude that a differentiated view of different types, intensities, frequencies, and durations of exercise is necessary to optimize exercise recommendations and implementation in medical settings.

Furthermore, ongoing research is needed focusing on potential mechanisms of exercise in various disorders. In this context, interdisciplinary approaches taking into account both biological and psychosocial aspects might help given the number of theories discussed.

From a health-economic perspective weighting of the advantages and disadvantages of exercise, the undesirable side effects of exercise are considered less prominent compared to that of the gains of exercise in the treatment of mental and physical disorders according to the positive research results shown.

This does not mean that the undesirable side effects and effects of exercise should not receive attention in research, teaching, and practice. However, the clearly predominant overall benefit should lead to even greater efforts in the field of research on exercise, disorders, and injuries. A promising field for research and practice seems to be the investigation of acute as well as chronic effects of exercise that can contribute to a significant symptom improvement in a variety of mental disorders. This is also where exercise psychology as a scientific discipline still has some catching up to do since there seems to be a certain restraint when studying clinical populations. Consequently, researchers sometimes prefer, for example, exercise interventions on students with mildly depressive impairments instead of severely affected psychiatric in-patients. These are the challenges that should be positively addressed in the field of exercise psychology, when the current social situation with rising prevalence and incidence rates of mental disorders is considered. An expansion of the field of clinical exercise psychology should be pushed at all levels.

28

Learning Control Questions

Basic:

1. List mental disorders for which the effects of exercise have been tested. How strong are the effects?
2. Which psychological variables are linked to doping behavior?
3. Name and explain possible risks and side effects of exercise.

Advanced:

4. Why is it important to differentiate into effects of acute (single bouts) and chronic exercise?
5. Which characteristics of exercise potentially moderate the influence of exercise in persons with depressive disorders?
6. What are the primary psychological outcome variables in studies to assess the chronic effects of exercise in chronic physical health disorders?
7. Describe the acute effects of single exercise bouts in persons with the following mental disorders: depressive disorders, anxiety disorders, and mental and behavioral disorders due to psychoactive substance use.
8. Describe the chronic effects of exercise programs in persons with the following mental disorders: depressive disorders, anxiety disorders, and mental and behavioral disorders due to psychoactive substance use.
9. Describe the chronic effects of exercise programs in persons with the following physical health disorders: cardiovascular diseases, oncological diseases, and chronic respiratory diseases.

Experts:

10. What effect sizes can be expected and what exactly does the effect size mean? What can it describe and what questions cannot be answered by knowing the size of an effect?
11. Which guidelines for exercise programs for people with depressive disorders do you know? Provide the most important contents.
12. As a coach, are you responsible for the mental and physical health of your athletes? Do you have the expertise to assess mental health? Where would experts be found?
13. Is it justified to recommend exercise as a method to improve mental health? What are advantages and possible disadvantages of such a recommendation?
14. What are the hypothesized mechanisms of exercise in persons with disorders?

References

Adeloye, D., Chua, S., Lee, C., Basquill, C., Papana, A., Theodoratou, E., Nair, H., Gasevic, D., Sridhar, D., Campbell, H., Chan, K. Y., Sheikh, A., Rudan, I., & Global Health Epidemiology Reference Group. (2015). Global and regional estimates of COPD prevalence: Systematic review and meta-analysis. *Journal of Global Health, 5*(2), 020415.

Albert, C. M., Mittleman, M. A., Chae, C. U., Lee, I. M., Hennekens, C. H., & Manson, J. E. (2000). Triggering of sudden death from cardiac causes by vigorous exertion. *The New England Journal of Medicine, 343*(19), 1355–1361.

American College of Sports Medicine. (2018). *ACSM's guidelines for exercise testing and prescription*. Lippincott, Williams, & Wilkins.

Anderson, L., Thompson, D. R., Oldridge, N., Zwisler, A.-D., Rees, K., Martin, N., & Taylor, R. S. (2016). Exercise-based cardiac rehabilitation for coronary heart disease. *Cochrane Database of Systematic Reviews, 2016*(1), CD001800.

Ardern, C. L., Taylor, N. F., Feller, J. A., & Webster, K. E. (2013). A systematic review of the psychological factors associated with returning to sport following injury. *British Journal of Sports Medicine, 47*(17), 1120–1126.

Asmundson, G. J., Fetzner, M. G., Deboer, L. B., Powers, M. B., Otto, M. W., & Smits, J. A. (2013). Let's get physical: A contemporary review of the anxiolytic effects of exercise for anxiety and its disorders. *Depression and Anxiety, 30*(4), 362–373.

Bailey, A. P., Hetrick, S. E., Rosenbaum, S., Purcell, R., & Parker, A. G. (2018). Treating depression with physical activity in adolescents and young adults: a systematic review and meta-analysis of randomised controlled trials. *Psychological medicine*, 48(7), 1068–1083.

Bartholomew, J. B., & Linder, D. E. (1998). State anxiety following resistance exercise: The role of gender and exercise intensity. *Journal of Behavioral Medicine, 21*(2), 205–219.

Bartholomew, J. B., Morrison, D., & Ciccolo, J. T. (2005). Effects of acute exercise on mood and well-being in patients with major depressive disorder. *Medicine and Science in Sports and Exercise, 37*(12), 2032.

Bartley, C. A., Hay, M., & Bloch, M. H. (2013). Meta-analysis: Aerobic exercise for the treatment of anxiety disorders. *Progress in Neuro-Psychopharmacology & Biological Psychiatry, 45*, 34–39.

Bauer, R., Steiner, M., Kisser, R., Macey, S. M., & Thayer, D. (2014). Unfälle in der EU. *Bundesgesundheitsblatt - Gesundheitsforschung - Gesundheitsschutz, 57*(6), 673–680.

Baxter, A. J., Vos, T., Scott, K. M., Ferrari, A. J., & Whiteford, H. A. (2014). The global burden of anxiety disorders in 2010. *Psychological Medicine, 44*(11), 2363–2374.

Beck, A. T., Steer, R. A., & Brown, G. K. (1996). *Beck depression inventory-II*. Psychological Corporation.

Blank, C., Brunner, J., Kreische, B., Lazzeri, M., Schobersberger, W., & Kopp, M. (2016a). Performance-enhancing substance use in university students: Motives, attitudes, and differences in normative beliefs. *Journal of Substance Use, 22*(3), 324–330.

Blank, C., Kopp, M., Niedermeier, M., Schnitzer, M., & Schobersberger, W. (2016b). Predictors of doping intentions, susceptibility, and behaviour of elite athletes: A meta-analytic review. *Springerplus, 5*(1), 1–14.

Blouin, A. G., & Goldfield, G. S. (1995). Body image and steroid use in male bodybuilders. *The International Journal of Eating Disorders, 18*(2), 159–165.

Boecker, H., Othman, A., Mueckter, S., Scheef, L., Pensel, M., Daamen, M., Jankowski, J., Schild, H., Tölle, T., & Schreckenberger, M. (2010). Advocating neuroimaging studies of transmitter release in human physical exercise challenges studies. *Open access Journal of Sports Medicine, 1*, 167–175.

Borg, G. (1982). Psychophysical bases of perceived exertion. *Medicine and Science in Sports and Exercise, 14*, 377–381.

Breuer, S., & Kleinert, J. (2009). Primäre Sportsucht und bewegungsbezogene Abhängigkeit—Beschreibung, Erklärung und Diagnostik. In D. Batthyany & A. Pritz (Eds.), *Rausch ohne Drogen* (pp. 191–218). Springer.

Buckworth, J., Dishman, R. K., O'Connor, P. J., & Tomporowski, P. D. (2013). *Exercise psychology*. Champaign, IL.

Caspersen, C. J., Powell, K. E., & Christenson, G. M. (1985). Physical activity, exercise, and physical fitness: Definitions and distinctions for health-related research. *Public Health Reports, 100*(2), 126–131.

Chen, M. D., & Rimmer, J. H. (2011). Effects of exercise on quality of life in stroke survivors: A meta-analysis. *Stroke, 42*(3), 832–837.

Chiu, H.Y., Huang, H.C., Chen, P.Y., Hou, W.H., & Tsai, P.S. (2015). Walking improves sleep in individuals with cancer: a meta-analysis of randomized, controlled trials. *Oncology Nursing Forum* 42(2): E54–62.

Cohen, J. (1988). *Statistical power analysis for the behavioral sciences*. Lawrence Erlbaum Associates.

Cooney, G. M., Dwan, K., Greig, C. A., Lawlor, D. A., Rimer, J., Waugh, F. R., McMurdo, M., & Mead, G. E. (2013). Exercise for depression. *Cochrane Database of Systematic Reviews, 9*, CD004366.

Coventry, P. A., & Hind, D. (2007). Comprehensive pulmonary rehabilitation for anxiety and depression in adults with chronic obstructive pulmonary disease: Systematic review and meta-analysis. *Journal of Psychosomatic Research, 63*(5), 551–565.

Cramp, F., & Byron-Daniel, J. (2012). Exercise for the management of cancer-related fatigue in adults. *Cochrane Database of Systematic Reviews, 11*, CD006145.

Davis, C., Kennedy, S. H., Ralevski, E., Dionne, M., Brewer, H., Neitzert, C., & Ratusny, D. (1995). Obsessive compulsiveness and physical activity in anorexia nervosa and high-level exercising. *Journal of Psychosomatic Research, 39*(8), 967–976.

Davis, H., Sullivan, J. P., Carr, C., Coppel, D. B., Shunk, A., Carter, J., Goldman, S., Hammond, T., & Baillie, P. H. F. (2014). Issues in the diagnosis of psychopathological disorders. In A. G. Papaioannou & D. Hackfort (Eds.), *Routledge companion to sport and exercise psychology: Global perspectives and fundamental concepts* (pp. 936–952). Routledge.

Diehl, K., Thiel, A., Zipfel, S., Mayer, J., Litaker, D. G., & Schneider, S. (2012). How healthy is the behavior of young athletes? A systematic literature review and meta-analyses. *Journal of Sports Science and Medicine, 11*(2), 201–220.

Dietrich, A. (2003). Functional neuroanatomy of altered states of consciousness: The transient hypofrontality hypothesis. *Consciousness and Cognition, 12*(2), 231–256.

Ding, D., Lawson, K. D., Kolbe-Alexander, T. L., Finkelstein, E. A., Katzmarzyk, P. T., van Mechelen, W., & Pratt, M. (2016). The economic burden of physical inactivity: A global analysis of major non-communicable diseases. *The Lancet, 388*(10051), 1311–1324.

Dishman, R. K., Berthoud, H. R., Booth, F. W., Cotman, C. W., Edgerton, V. R., Fleshner, M. R., Gandevia, S. C., Gomez-Pinilla, F., Greenwood, B. N., Hillman, C. H., Kramer, A. F., Levin, B. E., Moran, T. H., Russo-Neustadt, A. A., Salamone, J. D., Van Hoomissen, J. D., Wade, C. E., York, D. A., & Zigmond, M. J. (2006). Neurobiology of exercise. *Obesity (Silver Spring), 14*(3), 345–356.

Dittner, A. J., Wessely, S. C., & Brown, R. G. (2004). The assessment of fatigue: A practical guide for clinicians and researchers. *Journal of Psychosomatic Research, 56*(2), 157–170.

Downs, D. S., Hausenblas, H. A., & Nigg, C. R. (2004). Factorial validity and psychometric examination of the exercise dependence scale-revised. *Measurement in Physical Education and Exercise Science, 8*(4), 183–201.

Dunn, A. L., Trivedi, M. H., Kampert, J. B., Clark, C. G., & Chambliss, H. O. (2005). Exercise treatment for depression: Efficacy and dose response. *American Journal of Preventive Medicine, 28*(1), 1–8.

Dunn, M., Mazanov, J., & Sitharthan, G. (2009). Predicting future anabolic-androgenic steroid use intentions with current substance use: Findings from an internet-based survey. *Clinical Journal of Sport Medicine, 19*(3), 222–227.

Ekkekakis, P. (2015). Honey, I shrunk the pooled SMD! Guide to critical appraisal of systematic reviews and meta-analyses using the Cochrane review on exercise for depression as example. *Mental Health and Physical Activity, 8*, 21–36.

Ekkekakis, P., Hall, E. E., & Petruzzello, S. J. (2004). Practical markers of the transition from aerobic to anaerobic metabolism during exercise: Rationale and a case for affect-based exercise prescription. *Preventive Medicine, 38*(2), 149–159.

Ekkekakis, P., Lind, E., & Vazou, S. (2010). Affective responses to increasing levels of exercise intensity in normal-weight, overweight, and obese middle-aged women. *Obesity, 18*(1), 79–85.

Ekkekakis, P., Parfitt, G., & Petruzzello, S. J. (2011). The pleasure and displeasure people feel when they exercise at different intensities: Decennial update and progress towards a tripartite rationale for exercise intensity prescription. *Sports Medicine, 41*(8), 641–671.

Engel, G. (1977). The need for a new medical model: A challenge for biomedicine. *Science, 196*(4286), 129–136.

Ensari, I., Greenlee, T. A., Motl, R. W., & Petruzzello, S. J. (2015). Meta-analysis of acute exercise effects on state anxiety: An update of randomized controlled trials over the past 25 years. *Depression and Anxiety, 32*(8), 624–634.

Ezzati, M., Lopez, A. D., Rodgers, A., Vander Hoorn, S., & Murray, C. J. L. (2002). Selected major risk factors and global and regional burden of disease. *The Lancet*, 360(9343), 1347–1360.

Fayers, P. M., & Machin, D. (2013). *Quality of life: The assessment, analysis and interpretation of patient-reported outcomes*. John Wiley & Sons.

Ferrer, R. A., Huedo-Medina, T. B., Johnson, B. T., Ryan, S., & Pescatello, L. S. (2011). Exercise interventions for cancer survivors: A meta-analysis of quality of life outcomes. *Annals of Behavioral Medicine, 41*(1), 32–47.

Fong, D. Y. T., Ho, J. W. C., Hui, B. P. H., Lee, A. M., Macfarlane, D. J., Leung, S. S. K., Cerin, E., Chan, W. Y. Y., Leung, I. P. F., Lam, S. H. S., Taylor, A. J., & Cheng, K.-K. (2012). Physical activity for cancer survivors: Meta-analysis of randomised controlled trials. *BMJ, 344*, e70.

Fox, K. R. (2000). The effects of exercise on self-perceptions and self-esteem. In H. Biddle, K. R. Fox, & S. H. Boutcher (Eds.), *Physical activity and psychological well-being* (pp. 88–117). Routledge.

Frühauf, A., Niedermeier, M., Elliott, L. R., Ledochowski, L., Marksteiner, J., & Kopp, M. (2016). Acute effects of outdoor physical activity on affect and psychological well-being in depressed patients—A preliminary study. *Mental Health and Physical Activity, 10*, 4–9.

Furmaniak, A. C., Menig, M., & Markes, M. H. (2016). Exercise for women receiving adjuvant therapy for breast cancer. *Cochrane Database of Systematic Reviews, 9*(9), CD005001.

GBD 2015 Mortality and Causes of Death Collaborators. (2016). Global, regional, and national life expectancy, all-cause mortality, and cause-specific mortality for 249 causes of death, 1980–2015: A systematic analysis for the Global Burden of Disease Study 2015. *Lancet, 388*(10053), 1459–1544.

Geneen, L. J., Moore, R. A., Clarke, C., Martin, D., Colvin, L. A., & Smith, B. H. (2017). Physical activity and exercise for chronic pain in adults: An overview of Cochrane Reviews. *Cochrane Database of Systematic Reviews, 1*, CD011279.

Goldfarb, A. H., Hatfield, B. D., Sforzo, G. A., & Flynn, M. G. (1987). Serum beta-endorphin levels during a graded exercise test to exhaustion. *Medicine and Science in Sports and Exercise, 19*(2), 78–82.

Goodwin, V. A., Richards, S. H., Taylor, R. S., Taylor, A. H., & Campbell, J. L. (2008). The effectiveness of exercise interventions for people with Parkinson's disease: A systematic review and meta-analysis. *Movement Disorders, 23*(5), 631–640.

Gordon, B. R., McDowell, C. P., Hallgren, M., Meyer, J. D., Lyons, M., & Herring, M. P. (2018). Association of Efficacy of resistance exercise training with depressive symptoms: Meta-analysis and meta-regression analysis of randomized clinical trials. *JAMA Psychiatry, 75*(6), 566–576.

Gordon, B. R., McDowell, C. P., Lyons, M., & Herring, M. P. (2017). The effects of resistance exercise training on anxiety: A meta-analysis and meta-regression analysis of randomized controlled trials. *Sports Medicine, 47*(12), 2521–2532.

Griffiths, M. D., Szabo, A., & Terry, A. (2005). The exercise addiction inventory: A quick and easy screening tool for health practitioners. *British Journal of Sports Medicine, 39*(6), e30.

Grosz, H. J., & Farmer, B. B. (1972). Pitts' and McClure's lactate-anxiety study revisited. *British Journal of Psychiatry, 120*(557), 415–418.

Grüsser, S., & Thaleman, C. (2006). *Verhaltenssucht—Diagnostik, Therapie, Forschung*. Huber.

Haasova, M., Warren, F. C., Ussher, M., Janse Van Rensburg, K., Faulkner, G., Cropley, M., Byron-Daniel, J., Everson-Hock, E. S., Oh, H., & Taylor, A. H. (2013). The acute effects of physical activity on cigarette cravings: Systematic review and meta-analysis with individual participant data. *Addiction, 108*(1), 26–37.

Hallgren, M., Vancampfort, D., Giesen, E. S., Lundin, A., & Stubbs, B. (2017). Exercise as treatment for alcohol use disorders: Systematic review and meta-analysis. *British Journal of Sports Medicine, 51*(14), 1058–1064.

Hamilton, M. (1967). Development of a rating scale for primary depressive illness. *The British Journal of Social and Clinical Psychology, 6*(4), 278–296.

Hausenblas, H. A., & Symons Downs, D. (2002). Exercise dependence: A systematic review. *Psychology of Sport and Exercise, 3*(2), 89–123.

Hedges, L. V. (1981). Distribution theory for Glass's estimator of effect size and related estimators. *Journal of Educational Statistics, 6*(2), 107–128.

Heggelund, J., Kleppe, K. D., Morken, G., & Vedul-Kjelsas, E. (2014). High aerobic intensity training and psychological states in patients with depression or schizophrenia. *Frontiers in Psychiatry, 5*, 148.

Herring, M. P., Fleming, K. M., Hayes, S. P., Motl, R. W., & Coote, S. B. (2017a). Moderators of exercise effects on depressive symptoms in multiple sclerosis: A meta-regression. *American Journal of Preventive Medicine, 53*(4), 508–518.

Herring, M. P., Hallgren, M., & Campbell, M. J. (2017b). Acute exercise effects on worry, state anxiety, and feelings of energy and fatigue among young women with probable generalized anxiety disorder: A pilot study. *Psychology of Sport and Exercise, 33*, 31–36.

Herring, M. P., Jacob, M. L., Suveg, C., Dishman, R. K., & O'Connor, P. J. (2012). Feasibility of exercise training for the short-term treatment of generalized anxiety disorder: A randomized controlled trial. *Psychotherapy and Psychosomatics, 81*(1), 21–28.

Herring, M. P., Jacob, M. L., Suveg, C., & O'Connor, P. J. (2011). Effects of short-term exercise training on signs and symptoms of generalized anxiety disorder. *Mental Health and Physical Activity, 4*(2), 71–77.

Herring, M. P., Johnson, K. E., & O'Connor, P. J. (2016). Exercise training and health-related quality of life in generalized anxiety disorder. *Psychology of Sport and Exercise, 27*, 138–141.

Herring, M. P., Kline, C. E., & O'Connor, P. J. (2015). Effects of exercise on sleep among young women with generalized anxiety disorder. *Mental Health and Physical Activity, 9*, 59–66.

Herring, M. P., Monroe, D. C., Gordon, B. R., Hallgren, M., & Campbell, M. J. (2019). Acute exercise effects among young adults with analogue generalized anxiety disorder. *Medicine and Science in Sports and Exercise, 51*(5), 962–969.

Herring, M. P., & O'Connor, P. J. (2009). The effect of acute resistance exercise on feelings of energy and fatigue. *Journal of Sports Sciences, 27*(7), 701–709.

Herring, M. P., O'Connor, P. J., & Dishman, R. K. (2010). The effect of exercise training on anxiety symptoms among patients: A systematic review. *Archives of Internal Medicine, 170*(4), 321–331.

Ivarsson, A., Johnson, U., Andersen, M. B., Tranaeus, U., Stenling, A., & Lindwall, M. (2017). Psychosocial factors and sport injuries: Meta-analyses for prediction and prevention. *Sports Medicine, 47*(2), 353–365.

Jayakody, K., Gunadasa, S., & Hosker, C. (2014). Exercise for anxiety disorders: Systematic review. *British Journal of Sports Medicine, 48*(3), 187–196.

Joormann, J., Siemer, M., & Gotlib, I. H. (2007). Mood regulation in depression: Differential effects of distraction and recall of happy memories on sad mood. *Journal of Abnormal Psychology, 116*(3), 484–490.

Joy, E., Kussman, A., & Nattiv, A. (2016). 2016 update on eating disorders in athletes: A comprehensive narrative review with a focus on clinical assessment and management. *British Journal of Sports Medicine, 50*(3), 154–162.

Kahneman, D. (1999). Objective happiness. In D. Kahneman, E. Diener, & N. Schwarz (Eds.), *Well-being: Foundations of hedonic psychology* (pp. 3–25). Russell-Sage.

Kessler, R. C., Berglund, P., Demler, O., Jin, R., Merikangas, K. R., & Walters, E. E. (2005). Lifetime prevalence and age-of-onset distributions of DSM-IV disorders in the National Comorbidity Survey Replication. *Archives of General Psychiatry, 62*(6), 593–602.

Kisser, R., & Bauer, R. (2012). *The burden of sports injuries in the European Union*. Austrian Road Safety Board.

Klinsophon, T., Thaveeratitham, P., Sitthipornvorakul, E., & Janwantanakul, P. (2017). Effect of exercise type on smoking cessation: A meta-analysis of randomized controlled trials. *BMC Research Notes, 10*(1), 442.

Kopp, M., Burtscher, M., Kopp-Wilfling, P., Ruedl, G., Kumnig, M., Ledochowski, L., & Rumpold, G. (2015). Is there a link between physical activity and alcohol use? *Substance Use & Misuse, 50*(5), 546–551.

Kopp, M., Steinlechner, M., Ruedl, G., Ledochowski, L., Rumpold, G., & Taylor, A. H. (2012). Acute effects of brisk walking on affect and psychological well-being in individuals with type 2 diabetes. *Diabetes Research and Clinical Practice, 95*(1), 25–29.

Kreher, J. B., & Schwartz, J. B. (2012). Overtraining syndrome: A practical guide. *Sports Health, 4*(2), 128–138.

Krogh, J., Hjorthoj, C., Speyer, H., Gluud, C., & Nordentoft, M. (2017). Exercise for patients with major depression: A systematic review with meta-analysis and trial sequential analysis. *BMJ Open, 7*(9), e014820.

Lacasse, Y., Martin, S., Lasserson, T. J., & Goldstein, R. S. (2007). Meta-analysis of respiratory rehabilitation in chronic obstructive pulmonary disease. A Cochrane systematic review. *Europa Medicophysica, 43*(4), 475–485.

Lahham, A., McDonald, C. F., & Holland, A. E. (2016). Exercise training alone or with the addition of activity counseling improves physical activity levels in COPD: A systematic review and meta-analysis of randomized controlled trials. *International Journal of Chronic Obstructive Pulmonary Disease, 11*, 3121–3136.

Larun, L., Brurberg, K. G., Odgaard-Jensen, J., & Price, J. R. (2016). Exercise therapy for chronic fatigue syndrome. *Cochrane Database of Systematic Reviews, 12*, CD003200.

Ledochowski, L., Taylor, A. H., Haasova, M., Faulkner, G. E., Ussher, M. H., & Kopp, M. (2013). Unmittelbare Auswirkungen einzelner Bewegungseinheiten auf das Bedürfnis zu rauchen. *Zeitschrift für Gesundheitspsychologie, 21*(3), 122–137.

Legrand, F. D., Race, M., & Herring, M. P. (2018). Acute effects of outdoor and indoor exercise on feelings of energy and fatigue in people with depressive symptoms. *Journal of Environmental Psychology, 56*, 91–96.

Lisha, N. E., Martens, M., & Leventhal, A. M. (2011). Age and gender as moderators of the relationship between physical activity and alcohol use. *Addictive Behaviors, 36*(9), 933–936.

Lisha, N. E., & Sussman, S. (2010). Relationship of high school and college sports participation with alcohol, tobacco, and illicit drug use: A review. *Addictive Behaviors, 35*(5), 399–407.

Liu, N. H., Daumit, G. L., Dua, T., Aquila, R., Charlson, F., Cuijpers, P., Druss, B., Dudek, K., Freeman, M., Fujii, C., Gaebel, W., Hegerl, U., Levav, I., Munk Laursen, T., Ma, H., Maj, M., Elena Medina-Mora, M., Nordentoft, M., Prabhakaran, D., Pratt, K., Prince, M., Rangaswamy, T., Shiers, D., Susser, E., Thornicroft, G., Wahlbeck, K., Fekadu Wassie, A., Whiteford, H., & Saxena, S. (2017). Excess mortality in persons with severe mental disorders: A multilevel intervention framework and priorities for clinical practice, policy and research agendas. *World Psychiatry, 16*(1), 30–40.

Loy, B. D., O'Connor, P. J., & Dishman, R. K. (2013). The effect of a single bout of exercise on energy and fatigue states: A systematic review and meta-analysis. *Fatigue: Biomedicine, Health & Behavior, 1*(4), 223–242.

MacKillop, J. (2006). Factor structure of the alcohol urge questionnaire under neutral conditions and during a cue-elicited urge state. *Alcoholism, Clinical and Experimental Research, 30*(8), 1315–1321.

Magee, C. A., Buchanan, I., & Barrie, L. (2016). Profiles of exercise dependence symptoms in ironman participants. *Psychology of Sport and Exercise, 24*, 48–55.

Mannino, D. M., & Kiri, V. A. (2006). Changing the burden of COPD mortality. *International Journal of Chronic Obstructive Pulmonary Disease, 1*(3), 219–233.

Martens, M. P., & Martin, J. L. (2014). Substance abuse. In A. G. Papaioannou & D. Hackfort (Eds.), *Routledge companion to sport and exercise psychology*. Routledge.

Mercier, J., Savard, J., & Bernard, P. (2016). Exercise interventions to improve sleep in cancer patients: A systematic review and meta-analysis. *Sleep Medicine Reviews, 36*, 43–56.

Meyer, J., McDowell, C., Lansing, J., Brower, C., Smith, L., Tully, M., & Herring, M. (2020). Changes in physical activity and sedentary behavior in response to COVID-19 and their associations with mental health in 3052 US adults. *International Journal of Environmental Research and Public Health*, 17(18), 6469.

Meyer, J. D., Ellingson, L. D., Koltyn, K. F., Stegner, A. J., Kim, J. S., & Cook, D. B. (2016a). Psychobiological responses to preferred and prescribed intensity exercise in major depressive disorder. *Medicine and Science in Sports and Exercise, 48*(11), 2207–2215.

Meyer, J. D., Koltyn, K. F., Stegner, A. J., Kim, J. S., & Cook, D. B. (2016b). Influence of exercise intensity for improving depressed mood in depression: A dose-response study. *Behavior Therapy, 47*(4), 527–537.

Meyer, T. J., Miller, M. L., Metzger, R. L., & Borkovec, T. D. (1990). Development and validation of the Penn State Worry Questionnaire. *Behaviour Research and Therapy, 28*(6), 487–495.

Mishra, S. I., Scherer, R. W., Geigle, P. M., Berlanstein, D. R., Topaloglu, O., Gotay, C. C., & Snyder, C. (2012). Exercise interventions on health-related quality of life for cancer survivors. *Cochrane Database of Systematic Reviews, 2012*(8), CD007566.

Monroe, D. C., Patel, N. R., McCully, K. K., & Dishman, R. K. (2020). The effects of exercise on mood and prefrontal brain responses to emotional scenes in smokers. *Physiology & Behavior, 213*, 112721.

Morgan, W., Brown, D., Raglin, J., O'connor, P., & Ellickson, K. (1987). Psychological monitoring of overtraining and staleness. *British Journal of Sports Medicine, 21*(3), 107–114.

Morgan, W. P. (1979). Anxiety reduction following acute physical activity. *Psychiatric Annals, 9*(3), 36–45.

Muris, P. (2002). Relationships between self-efficacy and symptoms of anxiety disorders and depression in a normal adolescent sample. *Personality and Individual Differences, 32*(2), 337–348.

Murray, C. J., Vos, T., Lozano, R., Naghavi, M., Flaxman, A. D., Michaud, C., Ezzati, M., Shibuya, K., Salomon, J. A., Abdalla, S., Aboyans, V., Abraham, J., Ackerman, I., Aggarwal, R., Ahn, S. Y., Ali, M. K., Alvarado, M., Anderson, H. R., Anderson, L. M., Andrews, K. G., Atkinson, C., Baddour, L. M., Bahalim, A. N., Barker-Collo, S., Barrero, L. H., Bartels, D. H., Basanez, M. G., Baxter, A., Bell, M. L., Benjamin, E. J., Bennett, D., Bernabe, E., Bhalla, K., Bhandari, B., Bikbov, B., Abdulhak, A. B., Birbeck, G., Black, J. A., Blencowe, H., Blore, J. D., Blyth, F., Bolliger, I., Bonaventure, A., Boufous, S., Bourne, R., Boussinesq, M., Braithwaite, T., Brayne, C., Bridgett, L., Brooker, S., Brooks, P., Brugha, T. S., Bryan-Hancock, C., Bucello, C., Buchbinder, R., Buckle, G., Budke, C. M., Burch, M., Burney, P., Burstein, R., Calabria, B., Campbell, B., Canter, C. E., Carabin, H., Carapetis, J., Carmona, L., Cella, C., Charlson, F., Chen, H., Cheng, A. T., Chou, D., Chugh, S. S., Coffeng, L. E., Colan, S. D., Colquhoun, S., Colson, K. E., Condon, J., Connor, M. D., Cooper, L. T., Corriere, M., Cortinovis, M., de Vaccaro, K. C., Couser, W., Cowie, B. C., Criqui, M. H., Cross, M., Dabhadkar, K. C., Dahiya, M., Dahodwala, N., Damsere-Derry, J., Danaei, G., Davis, A., De Leo, D., Degenhardt, L., Dellavalle, R., Delossantos, A., Denenberg, J., Derrett, S., Jarlais, D. C. D., Dharmaratne, S. D., Dherani, M., Diaz-Torne, C., Dolk, H., Dorsey, E. R., Driscoll, T., Duber, H., Ebel, B., Edmond, K., Elbaz, A., Ali, S. E., Erskine, H., Erwin, P. J., Espindola, P., Ewoigbokhan, S. E., Farzadfar, F., Feigin, V., Felson, D. T., Ferrari, A., Ferri, C. P., Fevre, E. M., Finucane, M. M., Flaxman, S., Flood, L., Foreman, K., Forouzanfar, M. H., Fowkes, F. G., Fransen, M., Freeman, M. K., Gabbe, B. J., Gabriel, S. E., Gakidou, E., Ganatra, H. A., Garcia, B., Gaspari, F., Gillum, R. F., Gmel, G., Gonzalez-Medina, D., Gosselin, R., Grainger, R., Grant, B., Groeger, J., Guillemin, F., Gunnell, D., Gupta, R., Haagsma, J., Hagan, H., Halasa, Y. A.,

28

Hall, W., Haring, D., Haro, J. M., Harrison, J. E., Havmoeller, R., Hay, R. J., Higashi, H., Hill, C., Hoen, B., Hoffman, H., Hotez, P. J., Hoy, D., Huang, J. J., Ibeanusi, S. E., Jacobsen, K. H., James, S. L., Jarvis, D., Jasrasaria, R., Jayaraman, S., Johns, N., Jonas, J. B., Karthikeyan, G., Kassebaum, N., Kawakami, N., Keren, A., Khoo, J. P., King, C. H., Knowlton, L. M., Kobusingye, O., Koranteng, A., Krishnamurthi, R., Laden, F., Lalloo, R., Laslett, L. L., Lathlean, T., Leasher, J. L., Lee, Y. Y., Leigh, J., Levinson, D., Lim, S. S., Limb, E., Lin, J. K., Lipnick, M., Lipshultz, S. E., Liu, W., Loane, M., Ohno, S. L., Lyons, R., Mabweijano, J., MacIntyre, M. F., Malekzadeh, R., Mallinger, L., Manivannan, S., Marcenes, W., March, L., Margolis, D. J., Marks, G. B., Marks, R., Matsumori, A., Matzopoulos, R., Mayosi, B. M., McAnulty, J. H., McDermott, M. M., McGill, N., McGrath, J., Medina-Mora, M. E., Meltzer, M., Mensah, G. A., Merriman, T. R., Meyer, A. C., Miglioli, V., Miller, M., Miller, T. R., Mitchell, P. B., Mock, C., Mocumbi, A. O., Moffitt, T. E., Mokdad, A. A., Monasta, L., Montico, M., Moradi-Lakeh, M., Moran, A., Morawska, L., Mori, R., Murdoch, M. E., Mwaniki, M. K., Naidoo, K., Nair, M. N., Naldi, L., Narayan, K. M., Nelson, P. K., Nelson, R. G., Nevitt, M. C., Newton, C. R., Nolte, S., Norman, P., Norman, R., O'Donnell, M., O'Hanlon, S., Olives, C., Omer, S. B., Ortblad, K., Osborne, R., Ozgediz, D., Page, A., Pahari, B., Pandian, J. D., Rivero, A. P., Patten, S. B., Pearce, N., Padilla, R. P., Perez-Ruiz, F., Perico, N., Pesudovs, K., Phillips, D., Phillips, M. R., Pierce, K., Pion, S., Polanczyk, G. V., Polinder, S., Pope, C. A., 3rd, Popova, S., Porrini, E., Pourmalek, F., Prince, M., Pullan, R. L., Ramaiah, K. D., Ranganathan, D., Razavi, H., Regan, M., Rehm, J. T., Rein, D. B., Remuzzi, G., Richardson, K., Rivara, F. P., Roberts, T., Robinson, C., De Leon, F. R., Ronfani, L., Room, R., Rosenfeld, L. C., Rushton, L., Sacco, R. L., Saha, S., Sampson, U., Sanchez-Riera, L., Sanman, E., Schwebel, D. C., Scott, J. G., Segui-Gomez, M., Shahraz, S., Shepard, D. S., Shin, H., Shivakoti, R., Singh, D., Singh, G. M., Singh, J. A., Singleton, J., Sleet, D. A., Sliwa, K., Smith, E., Smith, J. L., Stapelberg, N. J., Steer, A., Steiner, T., Stolk, W. A., Stovner, L. J., Sudfeld, C., Syed, S., Tamburlini, G., Tavakkoli, M., Taylor, H. R., Taylor, J. A., Taylor, W. J., Thomas, B., Thomson, W. M., Thurston, G. D., Tleyjeh, I. M., Tonelli, M., Towbin, J. A., Truelsen, T., Tsilimbaris, M. K., Ubeda, C., Undurraga, E. A., van der Werf, M. J., van Os, J., Vavilala, M. S., Venketasubramanian, N., Wang, M., Wang, W., Watt, K., Weatherall, D. J., Weinstock, M. A., Weintraub, R., Weisskopf, M. G., Weissman, M. M., White, R. A., Whiteford, H., Wiebe, N., Wiersma, S. T., Wilkinson, J. D., Williams, H. C., Williams, S. R., Witt, E., Wolfe, F., Woolf, A. D., Wulf, S., Yeh, P. H., Zaidi, A. K., Zheng, Z. J., Zonies, D., Lopez, A. D., AlMazroa, M. A., & Memish, Z. A. (2012). Disability-adjusted life years (DALYs) for 291 diseases and injuries in 21 regions, 1990–2010: A systematic analysis for the Global Burden of Disease Study 2010. *Lancet, 380*(9859), 2197–2223.

Mustian, K. M., Alfano, C. M., Heckler, C., Kleckner, A. S., Kleckner, I. R., Leach, C. R., Mohr, D., Palesh, O. G., Peppone, L. J., & Piper, B. F. (2017). Comparison of pharmaceutical, psychological, and exercise treatments for cancer-related fatigue: A meta-analysis. *JAMA Oncology, 3*(7), 961–968.

National Collaborating Centre for Mental Health. (2010). *Depression: The Treatment and Management of Depression in Adults* (Updated ed.). The British Psychological Society & The Royal College of Psychiatrists.

Nazem, T. G., & Ackerman, K. E. (2012). The female athlete triad. *Sports Health, 4*(4), 302–311.

Niedermeier, M., Ledochowski, L., Mayr, A., Saltuari, L., & Kopp, M. (2017). Immediate affective responses of gait training in neurological rehabilitation—A randomized crossover trial. *Journal of Rehabilitation Medicine, 49*(4), 341–346.

Nieman, D. C., Johanssen, L. M., Lee, J. W., & Arabatzis, K. (1990). Infectious episodes in runners before and after the los Angeles Marathon. *The Journal of Sports Medicine and Physical Fitness, 30*(3), 316–328.

Ntoumanis, N., Ng, J. Y., & Barkoukis, V. (2014). Personal and psychosocial predictors of doping use in physical activity settings: a meta-analysis. *Sports Medicine*, 44.

O'Connor, S. R., Tully, M. A., Ryan, B., Bleakley, C. M., Baxter, G. D., Bradley, J. M., & McDonough, S. M. (2015). Walking exercise for chronic musculoskeletal pain: Systematic review and meta-analysis. *Archives of Physical Medicine and Rehabilitation, 96*(4), 724–734.e723.

OCEBM Levels of Evidence Working Group. (2009). *The oxford levels of evidence*. http://www.cebm.net/oxford-centre-evidence-based-medicine-levels-evidence-march-2009/.

Paneroni, M., Simonelli, C., Vitacca, M., & Ambrosino, N. (2017). Aerobic exercise training in very severe chronic obstructive pulmonary disease: A systematic review and meta-analysis. *American Journal of Physical Medicine & Rehabilitation, 96*(8), 541–548.

Pedersen, B. K., & Saltin, B. (2015). Exercise as medicine—Evidence for prescribing exercise as therapy in 26 different chronic diseases. *Scandinavian Journal of Medicine & Science in Sports, 25*(Suppl 3), 1–72.

Petrie, T. A., & Greenleaf, C. (2014). Eating disorders. In A. Papaioannou, & D. Hackfort (Eds.). Routledge Companion to Sport and Exercise Psychology: *Global perspectives and fundamental concepts* (pp. 837–851). Routledge.

Petruzzello, S., Landers, D., Hatfield, B., Kubitz, K., & Salazar, W. (1991). A meta-analysis on the anxiety-reducing effects of acute and chronic exercise. *Sports Medicine, 11*(3), 143–182.

Physical Activity Guidelines Advisory Committee. (2018). *2018 physical activity guidelines advisory committee scientific report*. U.S. Department of Health and Human Services.

Pilutti, L. A., Greenlee, T. A., Motl, R. W., Nickrent, M. S., & Petruzzello, S. J. (2013). Effects of exercise training on fatigue in multiple sclerosis: A meta-analysis. *Psychosomatic Medicine, 75*(6), 575–580.

Pitts, F. N., Jr., & McClure, J. N., Jr. (1967). Lactate metabolism in anxiety neurosis. *The New England Journal of Medicine, 277*(25), 1329–1336.

Puetz, T. W., & Herring, M. P. (2012). Differential effects of exercise on cancer-related fatigue during and following treatment: A meta-analysis. *American Journal of Preventive Medicine, 43*(2), e1–e24.

Pugliese, M. T., Lifshitz, F., Grad, G., Fort, P., & Marks-Katz, M. (1983). Fear of obesity. A cause of short stature and delayed puberty. *The New England Journal of Medicine, 309*(9), 513–518.

Radloff, L. S. (1977). The CES-D scale: A self-report depression scale for research in the general population. *Applied Psychological Measurement, 1*(3), 385–401.

Reardon, C. L., & Factor, R. M. (2010). Sport psychiatry: A systematic review of diagnosis and medical treatment of mental illness in athletes. *Sports Medicine, 40*(11), 961–980.

Rhodes, R. E., & Kates, A. (2015). Can the affective response to exercise predict future motives and physical activity behavior? A systematic review of published evidence. *Annals of Behavioral Medicine, 49*(5), 715–731.

Roberts, V., Maddison, R., Simpson, C., Bullen, C., & Prapavessis, H. (2012). The acute effects of exercise on cigarette cravings, withdrawal symptoms, affect, and smoking behaviour: Systematic review update and meta-analysis. *Psychopharmacology, 222*(1), 1–15.

Rooks, C. R., Thom, N. J., McCully, K. K., & Dishman, R. K. (2010). Effects of incremental exercise on cerebral oxygenation measured by near-infrared spectroscopy: A systematic review. *Progress in Neurobiology, 92*(2), 134–150.

Rosenbaum, S., Tiedemann, A., Sherrington, C., Curtis, J., & Ward, P. B. (2014). Physical activity interventions for people with mental illness: a systematic review and meta-analysis. *The Journal of clinical psychiatry*, 75(9), 964–974.

Saunders, D. H., Sanderson, M., Hayes, S., Kilrane, M., Greig, C. A., Brazzelli, M., & Mead, G. E. (2016). Physical fitness training for stroke patients. *Cochrane Database of Systematic Reviews, 3*(3), CD003316.

Sayette, M. A., Shiffman, S., Tiffany, S. T., Niaura, R. S., Martin, C. S., & Shadel, W. G. (2000). The measurement of drug craving. *Addiction, 95*(Suppl 2), S189–S210.

Schuch, F. B., Deslandes, A. C., Stubbs, B., Gosmann, N. P., Silva, C. T., & Fleck, M. P. (2016). Neurobiological effects of exercise on major depressive disorder: A systematic review. *Neuroscience and Biobehavioral Reviews, 61*, 1–11.

Schuch, F. B., Morres, I. D., Ekkekakis, P., Rosenbaum, S., & Stubbs, B. (2017). A critical review of exercise as a treatment for clinically depressed adults: Time to get pragmatic. *Acta Neuropsychiatrica, 29*(2), 65–71.

Sciolino, N. R., & Holmes, P. V. (2012). Exercise offers anxiolytic potential: A role for stress and brain noradrenergic-galaninergic mechanisms. *Neuroscience and Biobehavioral Reviews, 36*(9), 1965–1984.

Scott, K., & Posmontier, B. (2017). Exercise interventions to reduce cancer-related fatigue and improve health-related quality of life in cancer patients. *Holistic Nursing Practice, 31*(2), 66–79.

Searle, A., Spink, M., Ho, A., & Chuter, V. (2015). Exercise interventions for the treatment of chronic low back pain: A systematic review and meta-analysis of randomised controlled trials. *Clinical Rehabilitation, 29*(12), 1155–1167.

Semsarian, C., Ingles, J., & Wilde, A. A. M. (2015). Sudden cardiac death in the young: The molecular autopsy and a practical approach to surviving relatives. *European Heart Journal, 36*(21), 1290–1296.

Speck, R. M., Courneya, K. S., Mâsse, L. C., Duval, S., & Schmitz, K. H. (2010). An update of controlled physical activity trials in cancer survivors: A systematic review and meta-analysis. *Journal of Cancer Survivorship, 4*(2), 87–100.

Spielberger, C. D., Gorsuch, R. L., & Lushene, R. E. (1970). *Manual for the state-trait anxiety inventory*. Consulting Psychologists Press.

Spruit, M. A., Singh, S. J., Garvey, C., ZuWallack, R., Nici, L., Rochester, C., Hill, K., Holland, A. E., Lareau, S. C., Man, W. D., Pitta, F., Sewell, L., Raskin, J., Bourbeau, J., Crouch, R., Franssen, F. M., Casaburi, R., Vercoulen, J. H., Vogiatzis, I., Gosselink, R., Clini, E. M., Effing, T. W., Maltais, F., van der Palen, J., Troosters, T., Janssen, D. J., Collins, E., Garcia-Aymerich, J., Brooks, D., Fahy, B. F., Puhan, M. A., Hoogendoorn, M., Garrod, R., Schols, A. M., Carlin, B., Benzo, R., Meek, P., Morgan, M., Rutten-van Molken, M. P., Ries, A. L., Make, B., Goldstein, R. S., Dowson, C. A., Brozek, J. L., Donner, C. F., & Wouters, E. F. (2013). An official American Thoracic Society/European Respiratory Society statement: Key concepts and advances in pulmonary rehabilitation. *American Journal of Respiratory and Critical Care Medicine, 188*(8), e13–e64.

Stark, R., Schöny, W., & Kopp, M. (2012). Auswirkungen einer moderaten Bewegungseinheit auf die psychische Befindlichkeit bei PatientInnen mit affektiven Störungen in stationär psychiatrischer Behandlung. [Acute effects of a single bout of moderate exercise on psychological well-being in patients with affective disorder during hospital treatment]. *Neuropsychiatrie, 26*(4), 166–170.

Strickland, J. C., & Smith, M. A. (2014). The anxiolytic effects of resistance exercise. *Frontiers in Psychology, 5*, 753.

Stubbs, B., Vancampfort, D., Rosenbaum, S., Firth, J., Cosco, T., Veronese, N., Salum, G. A., & Schuch, F. B. (2017). An examination of the anxiolytic effects of exercise for people with anxiety and stress-related disorders: A meta-analysis. *Psychiatry Research, 249*, 102–108.

Sumec, R., Filip, P., Sheardova, K., & Bares, M. (2015). Psychological benefits of nonpharmacological methods aimed for improving balance in Parkinson's disease: A systematic review. *Behavioural Neurology, 2015*, 620674.

Sweegers, M. G., Altenburg, T. M., Chinapaw, M. J., Kalter, J., Verdonck-de Leeuw, I. M., Courneya, K. S., Newton, R. U., Aaronson, N. K., Jacobsen, P. B., Brug, J., & Buffart, L. M. (2018). Which exercise prescriptions improve quality of life and physical function in patients with cancer during and following treatment? A systematic review and meta-analysis of randomised controlled trials. *British Journal of Sports Medicine, 52*(8), 505–513.

Taylor, A. H., & Faulkner, G. (2008). Inaugural editorial. *Mental Health and Physical Activity, 1*(1), 1–8.

Taylor, A. H., Ussher, M. H., & Faulkner, G. (2007). The acute effects of exercise on cigarette cravings, withdrawal symptoms, affect and smoking behaviour: A systematic review. *Addiction, 102*(4), 534–543.

Thomas, D., Elliott, E. J., & Naughton, G. A. (2006). Exercise for type 2 diabetes mellitus. *Cochrane Database of Systematic Reviews, 2006*(3), CD002968.

Trivedi, M. H., Fava, M., Wisniewski, S. R., Thase, M. E., Quitkin, F., Warden, D., Ritz, L., Nierenberg, A. A., Lebowitz, B. D., Biggs, M. M., Luther, J. F., Shores-Wilson, K., & Rush, A. J. (2006). Medication augmentation after the failure of SSRIs for depression. *The New England Journal of Medicine, 354*(12), 1243–1252.

Trivedi, M. H., Greer, T. L., Church, T. S., Carmody, T. J., Grannemann, B. D., Galper, D. I., Dunn, A. L., Earnest, C. P., Sunderajan, P., Henley, S. S., & Blair, S. N. (2011). Exercise as an augmentation treatment for nonremitted major depressive disorder: A randomized, parallel dose comparison. *The Journal of Clinical Psychiatry, 72*(5), 677–684.

Torre, L. A., Bray, F., Siegel, R. L., Ferlay, J., Lortet-Tieulent, J., & Jemal, A. (2015). Global cancer statistics, 2012. CA: *A Cancer Journal for Clinicians*, 65(2), 87–108.

Ussher, M., Sampuran, A. K., Doshi, R., West, R., & Drummond, D. C. (2004). Acute effect of a brief bout of exercise on alcohol urges. *Addiction, 99*(12), 1542–1547.

Ussher, M. H., Taylor, A. H., & Faulkner, G. E. (2014). Exercise interventions for smoking cessation. *Cochrane Database of Systematic Reviews, 2014*(8), CD002295.

Vallerand, R. J., Verner-Filion, J., & Paquet, Y. (2014). Passion for sport and exercise. In A. G. Papaioannou & D. Hackfort (Eds.), *Routledge companion to sport and exercise psychology: Global perspectives and fundamental concepts*. Routledge.

van de Port, I. G., Wood-Dauphinee, S., Lindeman, E., & Kwakkel, G. (2007). Effects of exercise training programs on walking competency after stroke: A systematic review. *American Journal of Physical Medicine & Rehabilitation, 86*(11), 935–951.

van der Heijden, M. M. P., van Dooren, F. E. P., Pop, V. J. M., & Pouwer, F. (2013). Effects of exercise training on quality of life, symptoms of depression, symptoms of anxiety and emotional well-being in type 2 diabetes mellitus: A systematic review. *Diabetologia, 56*(6), 1210–1225.

Varghese, T., Schultz, W. M., McCue, A. A., Lambert, C. T., Sandesara, P. B., Eapen, D. J., Gordon, N. F., Franklin, B. A., & Sperling, L. S. (2016). Physical activity in the prevention of coronary heart disease: Implications for the clinician. *Heart, 102*(12), 904–909.

Wang, D., Wang, Y., Wang, Y., Li, R., & Zhou, C. (2014). Impact of Physical Exercise on Substance Use Disorders: *A Meta-Analysis. PloS One*, 9(10), e110728.

Ware, J. E., & Sherbourne, C. D. (1992). The MOS 36-item short-form health survey (SF-36): I. Conceptual framework and item selection. *Medical Care, 30*(6), 473–483.

Werner, A., Thiel, A., Schneider, S., Mayer, J., Giel, K. E., & Zipfel, S. (2013). Weight-control behaviour and weight-concerns in young elite athletes—A systematic review. *Journal of Eating Disorders, 1*, 18–18.

Whiteford, H. A., Degenhardt, L., Rehm, J., Baxter, A. J., Ferrari, A. J., Erskine, H. E., Charlson, F. J., Norman, R. E., Flaxman, A. D., Johns, N., Burstein, R., Murray, C. J. L., & Vos, T. (2013). Global burden of disease attributable to mental and substance use disorders: Findings from the Global Burden of Disease Study 2010. *The Lancet, 382*(9904), 1575–1586.

Williams, D. M., Dunsiger, S., Ciccolo, J. T., Lewis, B. A., Albrecht, A. E., & Marcus, B. H. (2008). Acute affective response to a moderate-intensity exercise stimulus predicts physical activity participation 6 and 12 months later. *Psychology of Sport and Exercise, 9*(3), 231–245.

Wolitzky-Taylor, K., Dour, H., Zinbarg, R., Mineka, S., Vrshek-Schallhorn, S., Epstein, A., Bobova, L., Griffith, J., Waters, A., Nazarian, M., Rose, R., & Craske, M. G. (2014). Experiencing core symptoms of anxiety and unipolar mood disorders in late adolescence predicts disorder onset in early adulthood. *Depression and Anxiety, 31*(3), 207–213.

World Health Organization. (1998a). Development of the World Health Organization WHOQOL-BREF quality of life assessment. *Psychological Medicine, 28*(03), 551–558.

World Health Organization. (1998b). The World Health Organization quality of life assessment (WHOQOL): Development and general psychometric properties. *Social Science & Medicine, 46*(12), 1569–1585.

World Health Organization. (2012). *Noncommunicable diseases*. http://www.euro.who.int/en/health-topics/noncommunicable-diseases.

World Health Organization. (2015). *The ICD-10 classification of mental and behavioural disorders: Clinical descriptions and diagnostic guidelines*. World Health Organization.

World Health Organization. (2017). *Depression and other common mental disorders: Global Health estimates*. World Health Organization.

Wu, P. L., Lee, M., & Huang, T. T. (2017). Effectiveness of physical activity on patients with depression and Parkinson's disease: A systematic review. *PLoS One, 12*(7), e0181515.

Zeeck, A., Leonhart, R., Mosebach, N., Schlegel, S., Linster, H. W., & Hartmann, A. (2013). Psychopathologische Aspekte von Sport. *Zeitschrift für Sportpsychologie, 20*(3), 94–106.

Zigmond, A. S., & Snaith, R. P. (1983). The hospital anxiety and depression scale. *Acta Psychiatrica Scandinavica, 67*(6), 361–370.

Zschucke, E., Heinz, A., & Ströhle, A. (2012). Exercise and physical activity in the therapy of substance use disorders. *The Scientific World Journal, 2012*, 901741.

Supplementary Information

J. Schüler et al. (eds.), *Sport and Exercise Psychology*, https://doi.org/10.1007/978-3-031-03921-8

Index

A

B

C

D

E

F

G

J

K

L

M

N

O

P

Q

R

S

T

U

V

W

Y

Z